12/6/01

Atlas of Neuroradiologic Embryology, Anatomy, and Variants

Atlas of Neuroradiologic Embryology, Anatomy, and Variants

J. Randy Jinkins, M.D., F.A.C.R.
Director of Neuroimaging Research
Department of Radiology
University of Nebraska Medical Center
Omaha, Nebraska

LIPPINCOTT WILLIAMS & WILKINS
A **Wolters Kluwer** Company
Philadelphia • Baltimore • New York • London
Buenos Aires • Hong Kong • Sydney • Tokyo

Acquisitions Editor: Joyce-Rachel John
Developmental Editors: Brian Brown and Sonya Seigafuse
Production Editor: Rosemary Palumbo
Manufacturing Manager: Tim Reynolds
Cover Designer: David Levy
Compositor: Maryland Composition Company, Inc.
Printer: Maple Press

530 Walnut Street
Philadelphia, PA 19106-3780 USA
LWW.com

Printed in the USA

Library of Congress Cataloging-in-Publication Data

Atlas of neuroradiologic embryology, anatomy, and variants/[edited
by] J. Randy Jinkins.
p. cm.
Includes bibliographical references and index.
ISBN 0-7817-1652-7
1. Neuroanatomy Atlases. 2. Nervous system—Radiography Atlases.
3. Skull—Anatomy Atlases. 4. Skull—Radiography Atlases.
5. Spine—Anatomy Atlases. 6. Spine—Radiography Atlases.
I. Jinkins, J. Randy.
[DNLM: 1. Brain—anatomy & histology Atlases. 2. Neck—anatomy &
histology Atlases. 3. Skull—anatomy & histology Atlases.
4. Spine—anatomy & histology Atlases. WL 17 A8838 2000]
QM451A85 2000
611′.8′0222—dc21
DNLM/DLC
for Library of Congress 99-40671
CIP

Care has been taken to confirm the accuracy of the information presented and to describe generally accepted practices. However, the author and publisher are not responsible for errors or omissions or for any consequences from application of the information in this book and make no warranty, expressed or implied, with respect to the currency, completeness, or accuracy of the contents of the publication. Application of this information in a particular situation remains the professional responsibility of the practitioner.

The author and publisher have exerted every effort to ensure that drug selection and dosage set forth in this text are in accordance with current recommendations and practice at the time of publication. However, in view of ongoing research, changes in government regulations, and the constant flow of information relating to drug therapy and drug reactions, the reader is urged to check the package insert for each drug for any change in indications and dosage and for added warnings and precautions. This is particularly important when the recommended agent is a new or infrequently employed drug.

Some drugs and medical devices presented in this publication have Food and Drug Administration (FDA) clearance for limited use in restricted research settings. It is the responsibility of the health care provider to ascertain the FDA status of each drug or device planned for use in their clinical practice.

10 9 8 7 6 5 4 3 2 1

To you. . .

The patients who intrigue, the students who challenge, the colleagues who encourage, the mentors who inspire, and the technical support staff who together and in their own unique ways have made it possible to present this body of radioanatomic information.

And especially,

To Carol

Contents

Contributors

Author
J. Randy Jinkins, M.D., F.A.C.R.
Director of Neuroimaging Research, Department of Radiology, 981045 Nebraska Medical Center, Omaha, Nebraska 68198-1045

Senior Contributors
Shakeeb Chinoy, M.D.
Neuroradiology Research Fellow, Department of Radiology, University of Texas Health Science Center at San Antonio, Mail Code 7800, 7703 Floyd Curl Drive, San Antonio, Texas 78229-3900

Claudia da Costa Leite, M.D.
Neuroradiology Research Fellow, Department of Radiology, University of Texas Health Science Center at San Antonio, Mail Code 7800, 7703 Floyd Curl Drive, San Antonio, Texas 78229-3900; Presently, Department of Radiology, University of Sao Paulo, School of Medicine, Sao Paulo, Brazil

Contributors
Canan Abusoglu, M.D.
Neuroradiology Research Fellow, Department of Radiology, University of Texas Health Science Center at San Antonio, Mail Code 7800, 7703 Floyd Curl Drive, San Antonio, Texas 78229-3900

Manohar Aribandi, M.D.
Neuroradiology Fellow, Department of Radiology, University of Texas Health Science Center at San Antonio, Mail Code 7800, 7703 Floyd Curl Drive, San Antonio, Texas 78229-3900

Ronald Cervantes, M.D.
Neuroradiology Fellow, Department of Radiology, University of Texas Health Science Center at San Antonio, Mail Code 7800, 7703 Floyd Curl Drive, San Antonio, Texas 78229-3900

Lap-Kin Chan, M.B.Ch.B., F.R.C.R.
Neuroradiology Research Fellow, Department of Radiology, University of Texas Health Science Center at San Antonio, Mail Code 7800, 7703 Floyd Curl Drive, San Antonio, Texas 78229-3900; Presently, Senior Medical Officer, Diagnostic Radiology Department, Kwong Wah Hospital, 25 Waterloo Road, Kowloon, Hong Kong

Ki Yau Chow, M.B.Ch.B., F.R.C.R.
Neuroradiology Research Fellow, Department of Radiology, University of Texas Health Science Center at San Antonio, Mail Code 7800, 7703 Floyd Curl Drive, San Antonio, Texas 78229-3900; Presently, Senior Medical Officer, Department of Diagnostic Radiology, Tuen Mun Hospital, Tsing Chong Koon Road, Tuen Mun, New Territories, Hong Kong

Chi Sing Cheng, M.B.B.S., F.R.C.R.
Neuroradiology Research Fellow, Department of Radiology, University of Texas Health Science Center at San Antonio, Mail Code 7800, 7703 Floyd Curl Drive, San Antonio, Texas 78229-3900; Presently, Chairman, Department of Diagnostic Radiology, Ruttonjee Hospital, Wanchai, Hong Kong

Zuhair U. El Zimmili, M.B., B.Ch.
Neuroradiology Research Fellow, Department of Radiology, University of Texas Health Science Center at San Antonio, Mail Code 7800, 7703 Floyd Curl Drive, San Antonio, Texas 78229-3900

Beatriz E. Escobar, M.D.
Neuroradiology Research Fellow, Department of Radiology, University of Texas Health Science Center at San Antonio, Mail Code 7800, 7703 Floyd Curl Drive, San Antonio, Texas 78229-3900

Se-Jong Kim, M.D.
Neuroradiology Research Fellow, Department of Radiology, University of Texas Health Science Center at San Antonio, Mail Code 7800, 7703 Floyd Curl Drive, San Antonio, Texas 78229-3900; Presently, Director, Section of Neuroradiology, Department of Radiology, Kwangju Christian Hospital, 264 Yangrim-Dong, Nam-Ku, Kwangju 503-040, Korea

Yeong-Man Lai, M.B.Ch.B., F.R.C.R.
Neuroradiology Research Fellow, Department of Radiology, University of Texas Health Science Center at San Antonio, Mail Code 7800, 7703 Floyd Curl Drive, San Antonio, Texas 78229-3900; Presently, Senior Medical Officer, Department of Radiology, Princess Margaret Hospital, Lai King Hill Road, Kowloon, Hong Kong

Jin Foo Liu, M.B.B.S., F.R.C.R.
Neuroradiology Research Fellow, Department of Radiology, University of Texas Health Science Center at San Antonio, Mail Code 7800, 7703 Floyd Curl Drive, San Antonio, Texas 78229-3900; Presently, Senior Medical Officer, Diagnostic Radiology Department, Kwong Wah Hospital, 25 Waterloo Road, Kowloon, Hong Kong

Mehmet Teksam, M.D.
Neuroradiology Research Fellow, Department of Radiology, University of Texas Health Science Center at San Antonio, Mail Code 7800, 7703 Floyd Curl Drive, San Antonio, Texas 78229-3900

Illustrators

David Baker
Medical Illustrator, Graphic Services, University of Texas Health Science Center at San Antonio, 7703 Floyd Curl Drive, San Antonio, Texas 78229-3900

Nick Lang
Medical Illustrator, Graphic Services, University of Texas Health Science Center at San Antonio, 7703 Floyd Curl Drive, San Antonio, Texas 78229-3900

Nancy Place
Medical Illustration Supervisor, Graphic Services, University of Texas Health Science Center at San Antonio, 7703 Floyd Curl Drive, San Antonio, Texas 78229-3900

Preface

A sincere attempt was made in the anatomic renderings throughout this book to create a schematic, idealized depiction of the anatomy under discussion. Because of variations between individual patients and patient groups, this approach is intended to assist the reader in conceptualizing the general anatomic principles that lie behind the medical images.

The generalized anatomical configuration of the artwork has important implications for understanding basic normal anatomy presenting at medical imaging: Certain anatomic relationships are only clearly understandable by means of a summary anatomic diagram, because the anatomy is only poorly, if ever, reliably or reproducibly visualized via imaging.

Normal anatomy is the foundation of the study of medicine in general and medical imaging in particular; the many variations of normal anatomy must be recognized so that they are not confused with disease. An effort was made to include as many of the common variations as possible, knowing that the possibilities are infinite.

The primary goal of this book is to make those of us in the neurosciences better at what we do, and to achieve this improvement more quickly and at a more fundamental level than was practically possible in the past using single or multiple reference source(s). The intention is to accelerate the process of individual creativity and future discovery by more clearly and concisely defining the contents and presently known limits of the domain of neuroscience as it applies to neuroanatomy, and in turn, how neuroanatomy applies to neurodiagnostic imaging.

J. Randy Jinkins

Note to the Reader

If any reader feels that a significant reference source has been inadvertently omitted, or has a relevant anatomical drawing, or a medical image of a normal or variant structure that should be included, please forward the information/case to the author at the address below.

The goal of this process is to improve the fundamental, universally applicable data contained herein in the next edition. Contributor credit will be clearly detailed in future editions.

This undertaking of neuroradiologic anatomy revealed many points of anatomy for which no recorded term could be found. For this reason, new terminology is notated the first time it is used in each chapter by following the italicized term with the author's name. An effort has been made to choose logical nomenclature when such new terminology was required. Alternative terms will be included in later editions if the suggested nomenclature is supplied in writing with a clear explanation and documentation, if available.

Address correspondence to:

J. Randy Jinkins, M.D., F.A.C.R.
Director of Neuroimaging Research
Department of Radiology
981045 Nebraska Medical Center
Omaha, Nebraska 68198-1045

Acknowledgments

A great deal of thanks goes to those who made the production of this book possible. These individuals include: Cheryl Portenier Howard for administrative assistance, Joanne Murray for transcription work, and Cono Farias for photographic reproduction. I also thank Brian Brown, Joyce-Rachel John, Rosemary Palumbo, and James D. Ryan at Lippincott Williams & Wilkins. I salute their talent and professionalism.

J. Randy Jinkins

Introduction

This book outlines normal embryologic development, normal anatomy, and variants of the cranium, spine, face, and neck. The general definitions of categories of nonpathological anatomy include:

Embryologic Anatomy The progressive morphologic ontologic anatomic development of tissues and organ systems.

Normal Anatomy The morphologic end result of the normal embryologic development of tissues and organ systems that continues to evolve variably from birth to early adulthood.

Variant Anatomy The morphologic end result of embryologic development of tissues and organ systems that differs to a minor degree from the majority of otherwise normal subjects, but nevertheless is not invariably associated with dysfunction.

Aging Anatomy The progressive morphologic evolution of tissues and organ systems from early adulthood onward that does not always entail cell loss and is not necessarily associated with dysfunction.

Any departure from these types of normal anatomy are considered abnormal and include *pathologic anatomy* (e.g., trauma, infection, neoplasia, degenerative alteration, etc. that is associated with dysfunction). With certain exceptions, pathologic anatomy will not be included in this textbook.

It should also be noted that since all anatomy is congenital, the distinction between *variant anatomy* and congenital anomalies is not a clear one. For this reason, some commonly encountered "congenital anomalies" will be included in the variant sections of various chapters.

Atlas of Neuroradiologic Embryology, Anatomy, and Variants

CHAPTER 1

Embryology

EMBRYOLOGY OF THE BRAIN AND CALVARIA

Embryology of the Brain

Development of the Notochord and Neural Tube

1. The formation of the human central nervous system (CNS) is a progressive, complex process. The basic events of CNS development include dorsal induction; ventral induction; neuronal proliferation, differentiation and histogenesis; neuronal migration; and, finally, axonal myelination.
2. *Dorsal induction* is a very early stage that includes the formation of the neural plate, notochord, neural groove, neural folds, and neural tube. Dorsal induction includes two different steps: primary and secondary neurulation. Primary neurulation refers to the formation of the neural tube from its cranial end to the end of the notochord at the L-1 and L-2 levels. This process occurs during the third and fourth weeks of gestation. Secondary neurulation refers to the formation of the lower lumbar, sacral, and coccygeal vertebral segments from the caudal cell mass. This process occurs between the fourth and seventh weeks of gestation.
3. *Ventral induction* includes the formation and development of the brain vesicles and the formation of the telencephalon, diencephalon, mesencephalon, metencephalon, myelencephalon. This occurs between the fifth and tenth weeks of gestation.
4. *Neuronal proliferation, differentiation, and histogenesis* commence between the second and fifth months of gestation and continue into the postnatal period. These events include germinal matrix formation, cellular proliferation and differentiation, choroid plexus, formation, and initiation of cerebrospinal fluid production.
5. *Neuronal migration* of the neurons that are generated in the ventricular and subventricular layers of the brain surrounding the primitive cerebral vesicles toward the superficial cortex and deep nuclei of the cerebrum and cerebellum occurs in the third, fourth, and fifth months of gestation. The formation of the corpus callosum and other commissures is associated with interhemispheric cerebral axonal migrational events, which take place between 10 and 20 weeks of gestation.
6. *Axonal myelination* begins in the 3-week embryo. In the third semester of gestation, myelin appears in the brain stem and in the central parts of the cerebellum. Later, it appears in the thalamus and posterior limb of the internal capsule. After birth, myelination progresses in the remainder of the cerebellar hemispheres, the optic radiations, and in both centra semiovale. During the first and second years of life, the myelination process spreads throughout the remaining brain. Although the majority of CNS axons are myelinated by 2 years of age, a minor degree of myelination continues into later adolescence.
7. Overview of CNS development
   a. The notochord serves as the developmental precursor for the induction of the neuroectoderm to form the neural tube (the origin of the CNS) and the neural crest (the origin of the peripheral nervous system). The notochord also actuates the induction of the mesodermal germ layer, to give rise to the mesenchymal elements forming the spinal column and paraspinal tissues, including bone, muscle, ligaments, intervertebral disc, connective tissue, blood vessels, and meninges.
   b. The CNS appears at the beginning of the third week as a slipper-shaped plate (viewed from above) of thickened endoderm and overlying neural plate. The neural plate is located in the middorsal region in front of the primitive pit. Its lateral edge soon becomes elevated to form the neural folds.
   c. With further development, the neural folds become more elevated, approach each other in the midline, and finally fuse, thus forming the closed neural tube. This fusion begins in the cervical region and proceeds in a somewhat irregular fashion in the cephalic and caudal directions.
   d. The proximal two-thirds of the neural tube thickens to form the future brain, while the caudal one-third forms most of the future spinal cord.

e. The neural tube lumen will become the cerebral ventricular system and the central canal of the spinal cord.
f. Some neuroectodermal cells are not included in the neural tube but remain situated between it and the cutaneous ectoderm as the neural crest. The neural crest cells will later differentiate into the sensory neurons of the dorsal root and cranial nerve ganglia and into the sympathetic and parasympathetic motor neurons of the autonomic ganglia.
g. The mesenchyme around the neural tube forms bilaterally symmetrical longitudinal columns of solid mesoderm that begin to segment into paired blocks called somites. The dorsolateral portion (dermatomyotome) of each somite will form the skeletal muscles and the dermis. The ventromedial portion (sclerotome) will form the cartilage, bone, and ligaments of the vertebral column.

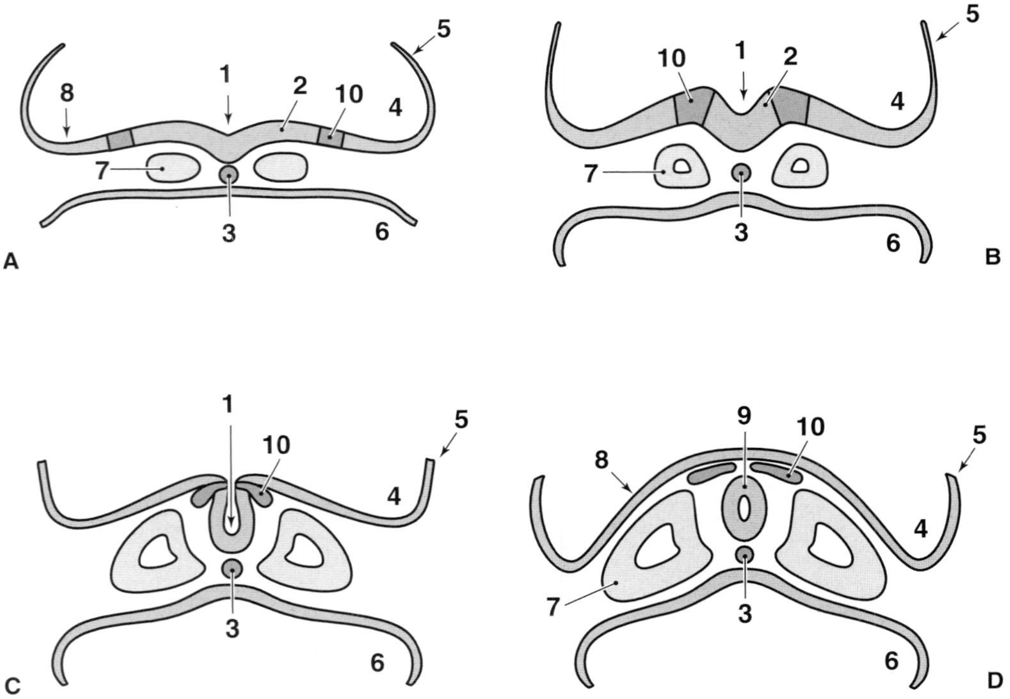

Figure 1-1: Transverse schematics of the development of the notochord and neural tube from 18 to 22 days' gestation. **A:** Transverse schematic of an embryo at day 18 of gestation. **B:** Transverse schematic of an embryo between 18 and 22 days' gestation. **C:** Transverse schematic of an embryo between 18 and 22 days' gestation. **D:** Transverse schematic of embryo at day 22 of gestation.

1 Neural groove
2 Neural ectoderm
3 Notochord
4 Amniotic cavity
5 Amnion
6 Yolk sac
7 Embryonic mesoderm
8 Surface ectoderm
9 Neural tube
10 Neural crest

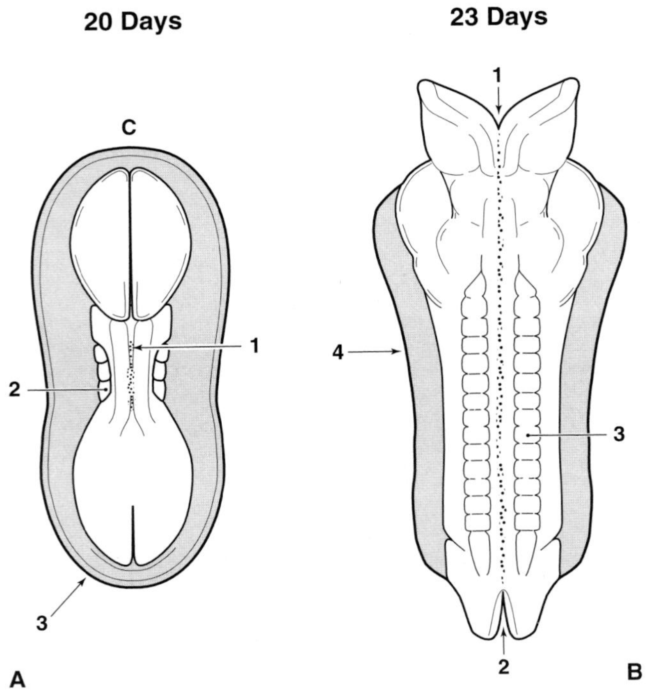

Figure 1-2A: Dorsal view of embryo at 20 days' gestation. The amnion has been removed. *C*, cranial end of embryo.

1 Neural groove
2 Somite
3 Cut edge of amnion

Figure 1-2B: Dorsal view of embryo at 23 days' gestation. The nervous system is connected to the amniotic cavity through the cranial and caudal neuropores.

1 Cranial neuropore
2 Caudal neuropore
3 Somite
4 Cut edge of amnion

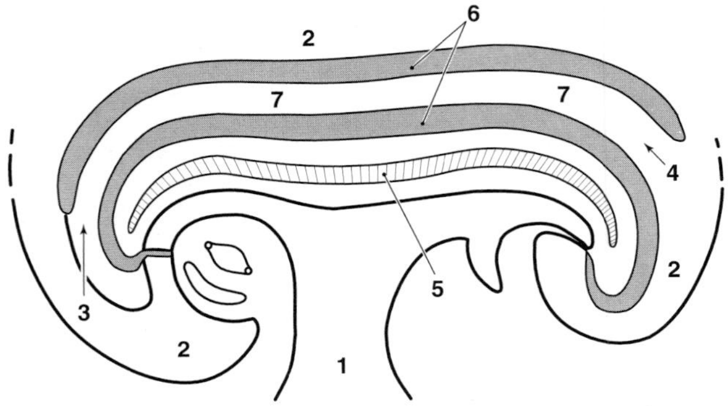

Figure 1-3: Sagittal schematic of an embryo at day 24 of gestation.

1 Yolk sac
2 Amniotic cavity
3 Cranial neuropore
4 Caudal neuropore
5 Notochord
6 Neural tube
7 Neural canal

Formation of the Neurenteric Canal

1. By the seventeenth day of gestation, ectodermal cells that entered the primitive pit have advanced cephalically in the midline to the protochordal plate to create the notochordal process.
2. The primitive pit deepens and invaginates into the previously solid notochordal process, forming a hollow notochord canal. This quickly fuses with the endoderm.
3. At the points of fusion, breakdown of cells opens the notochordal canal to the yolk sac. As a result, there is transient communication from the amnion through the notochordal canal to the yolk sac. This is the canal of Kovalevsky, or the neurenteric canal.
4. Subsequently, the notochordal canal undergoes complex changes that close the communication with the yolk sac, reestablishing complete layers of endoderm and ectoderm, and reform a solid core of tissue—the true notochord.
5. The endoderm ultimately forms the gut.

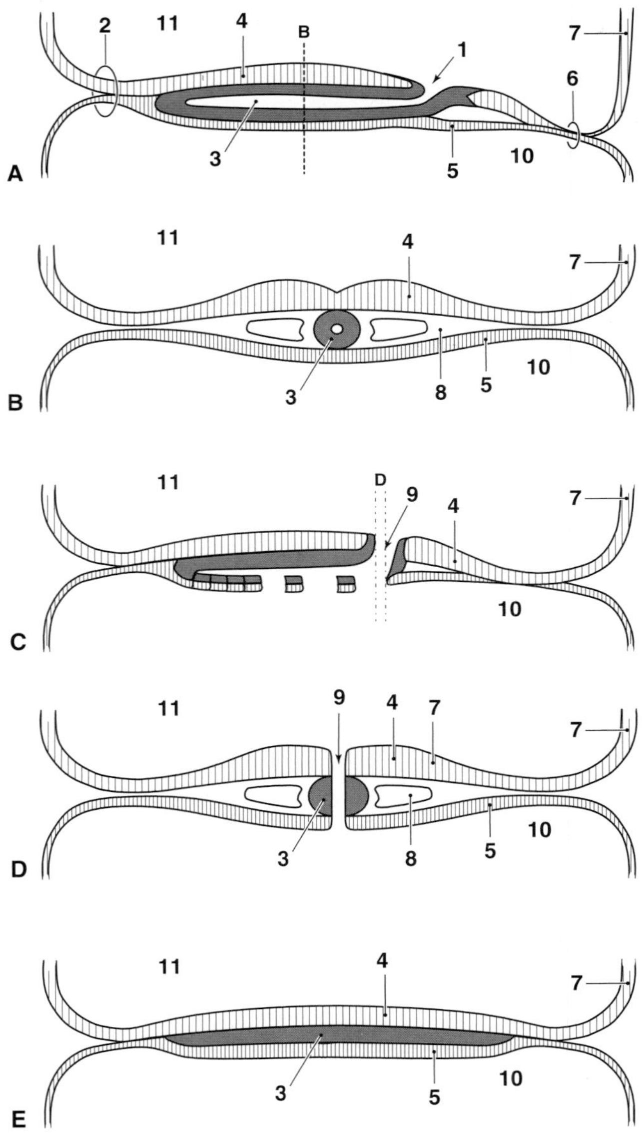

Figure 1-4: Formation of the neurenteric canal. **A:** Midline sagittal schematic of an embryo at day 16 of gestation. *B*, the level of cross section shown in Fig. 1-4B. **B:** Cross section of Fig. 1-4A. **C:** Midline sagittal schematic of an embryo at day 17 of gestation showing the neurenteric canal. D, the level of cross-section shown in Fig. 1-4D. **D:** Cross section of Fig. 1-4C at the level of the neurenteric canal. **E:** Midline sagittal schematic of an embryo following reestablishment of the continuity of the notochord, ectoderm, and endoderm.

1 Primitive pit
2 Protochordal plate
3 Notochord process and canal
4 Neural plate
5 Endoderm
6 Cloacal membrane
7 Ectoderm
8 Intra-embryonic mesoderm
9 Neurenteric canal
10 Yolk sac
11 Amniotic cavity

Embryologic Development of the Brain

1. The cervical flexure demarcates the hindbrain from the developing spinal cord.
2. The pontine flexure divides the hindbrain into the metencephalon (rostral) and the myelencephalon (caudal).
3. The metencephalon is separated from the mesencephalon by the rhombencephalic isthmus.
4. At 6 weeks' gestation, two optic vesicles develop in the embryo on each side of the forebrain. These optic vesicles are the primordia of the retina and optic nerves (see also section on Embryology of the Visual Apparatus).
5. The metencephalon develops into the pons and the cerebellum.
6. Three swellings develop in the lateral walls of the third ventricles of the diencephalon: the epithalamus, thalamus, and hypothalamus.
7. The diencephalon also gives rise to the infundibulum, which will form the neurohypophysis.
8. Meanwhile, the cerebral hemispheres are expanding, and the optic chiasm is being formed.
9. At about 10 weeks' gestation, cerebral commissures begin their development.
10. The cerebral hemispheres subsequently expand anteriorly, posteriorly, superiorly, and inferiorly to form the frontal, occipital, parietal, and temporal lobes.

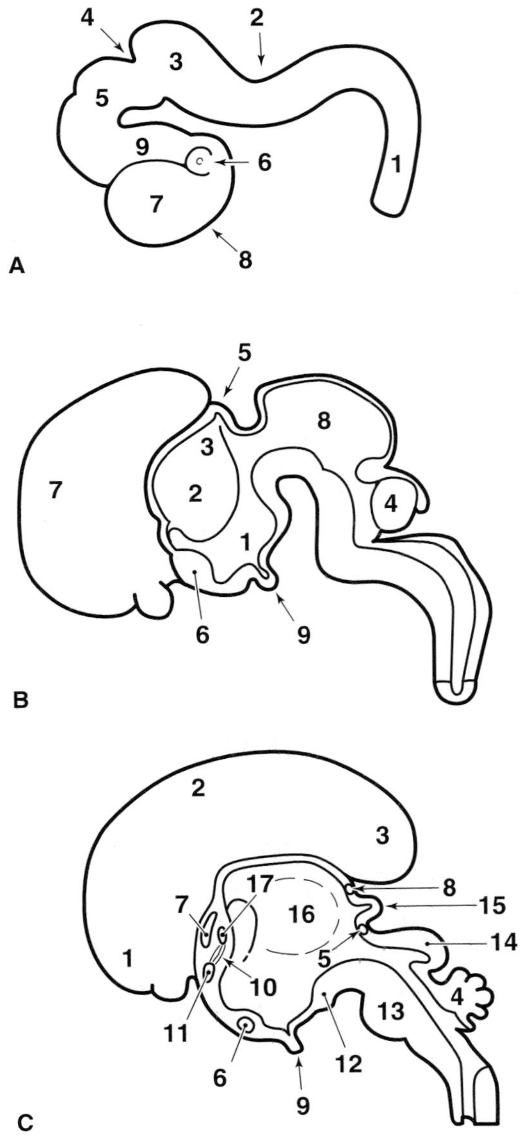

Figure 1-5: Embryologic development of the brain.

A: Lateral schematic of the brain at approximately 6 weeks' gestation.
1 Myelencephalon
2 Pontine flexure
3 Metencephalon
4 Rhombencephalic isthmus
5 Mesencephalon
6 Optic cup
7 Primitive cerebral hemisphere
8 Telencephalon
9 Diencephalon

B: Lateral schematic of an 8-week embryo.
1 Hypothalamus
2 Thalamus
3 Epithalamus
4 Cerebellum
5 Pineal body
6 Optic chiasm
7 Cerebral hemispheres
8 Mesencephalon
9 Infundibulum

C: Lateral schematic of a 10-week embryo. The cerebral commissures begin their development. The cerebral hemispheres expand anteriorly, posteriorly, superiorly, and inferiorly to form the frontal, occipital, parietal, and temporal lobes.
1 Frontal lobe
2 Parietal lobe
3 Occipital lobe
4 Cerebellum
5 Posterior commissure
6 Optic chiasm
7 Corpus callosum
8 Habenular commissure
9 Infundibulum
10 Lamina terminalis
11 Anterior commissure
12 Mamillary bodies
13 Pons
14 Colliculi
15 Epiphysis
16 Third ventricle
17 Hippocampal commissure

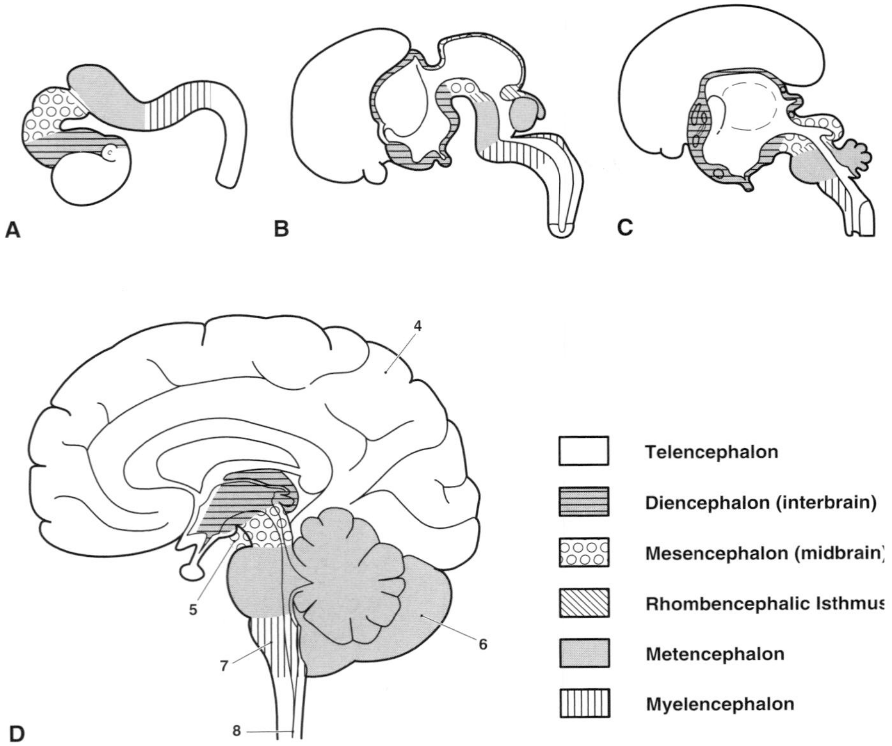

Figure 1-6: Sagittal schematics depicting the developing brain segmented according to region. **A:** Five-week embryo. **B:** Seven-week embryo. **C:** Eight-week embryo. **D:** Sagittal schematic of an adult depicting the structures and corresponding brain regions.

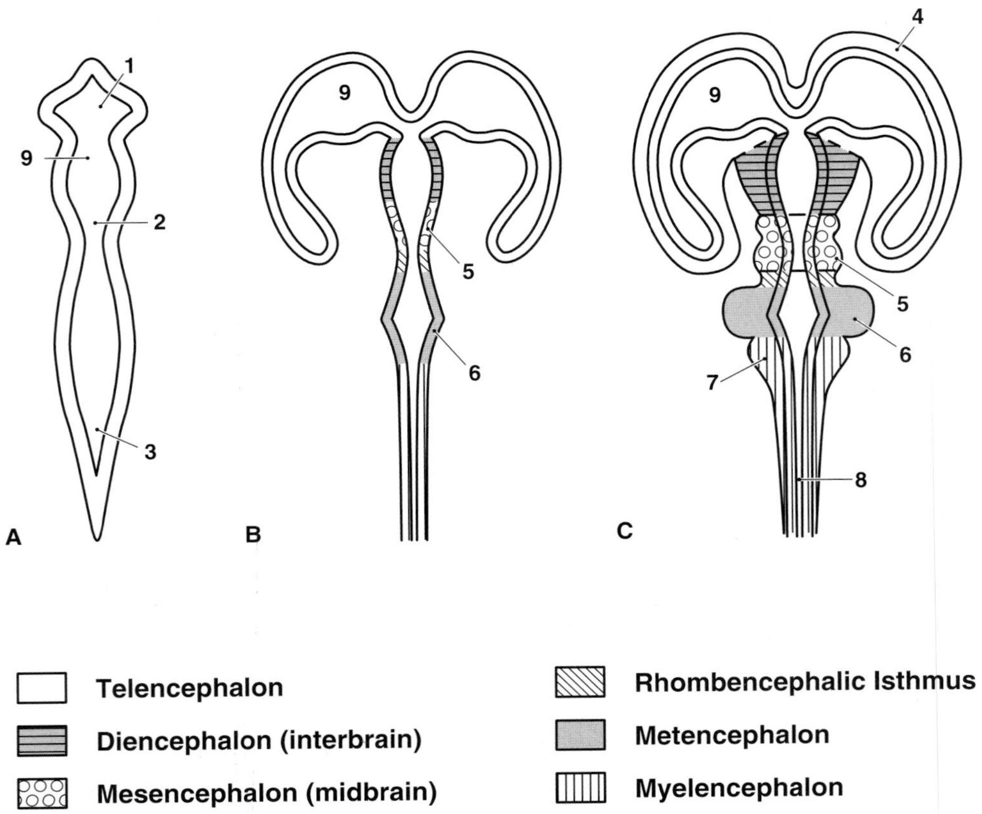

Figure 1-7: Coronal schematics corresponding to Fig. 1-5. **A:** Corresponds to Fig. 1-5A. **B:** Corresponds to Fig. 1-5B. **C:** Corresponds to Fig. 1-5C.
1 Forebrain or prosencephalon
2 Midbrain or mesencephalon
3 Rhombencephalon or hindbrain
4 Cerebral hemispheres
5 Tectum and midbrain
6 Pons and cerebellum
7 Medulla oblongata
8 Spinal cord
9 Developing cerebral vesicles

Embryologic Development of the Cerebral Ventricular System

Formation of the Brain Vesicles and Regional Adult Derivatives

1. The ciliated epithelial cells lining the developing neural tube begin to secrete a watery liquid that distends the cavity of the tube, while the cephalic end (rostral neuropore) constricts to form the three primary brain vesicles.
2. In the fourth week of gestation, during formation of the rostral aspect of the neural tube and after closure of the rostral neuropore, three dilations evolve and surround the primary brain vesicles. The uppermost cephalic vesicle is surrounded by the forebrain, or prosencephalon, the middle vesicle is surrounded by the midbrain, or mesencephalon, and the lower vesicle is surrounded by the hindbrain, or rhombencephalon.
3. Unequal cell growth rate and migration result in flexures, constrictions, invagination, and evaginations of the rostral neural tube. This leads to the appearance in the fifth week of gestation of five secondary brain vesicles within (rostrally to ventrally): the telencephalon, diencephalon, mesencephalon, metencephalon, and myelencephalon.
4. The adult derivatives of these secondary vesicles/regions include
   a. telencephalon: cerebral hemispheres, lateral ventricles
   b. diencephalon: epithalamus, thalami, hypothalamus, subthalamus, third ventricle
   c. mesencephalon: midbrain, cerebral aqueduct
   d. metencephalon: pons, cerebellum, upper aspect of fourth ventricle
   e. myelencephalon: lower aspect of fourth ventricle, medulla oblongata

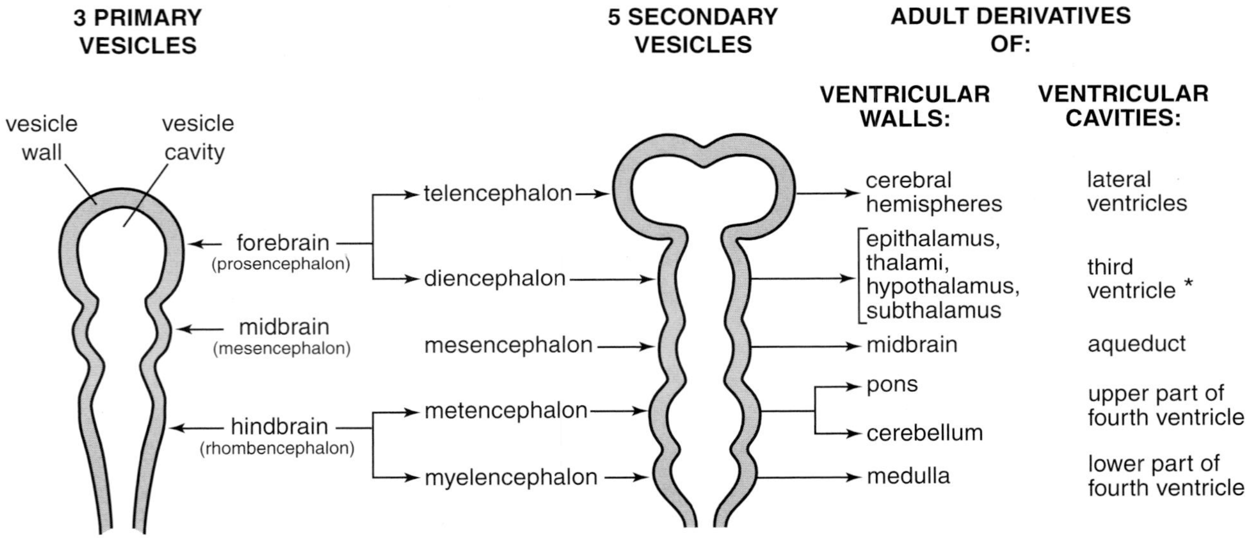

Figure 1-8: Schematics of the embryonic brain vesicles and the mature derivatives. *The rostral one-third of the third ventricle is formed from the lumen of the telencephalon; the caudal two-thirds of the third ventricle is formed from the lumen of the diencephalon.

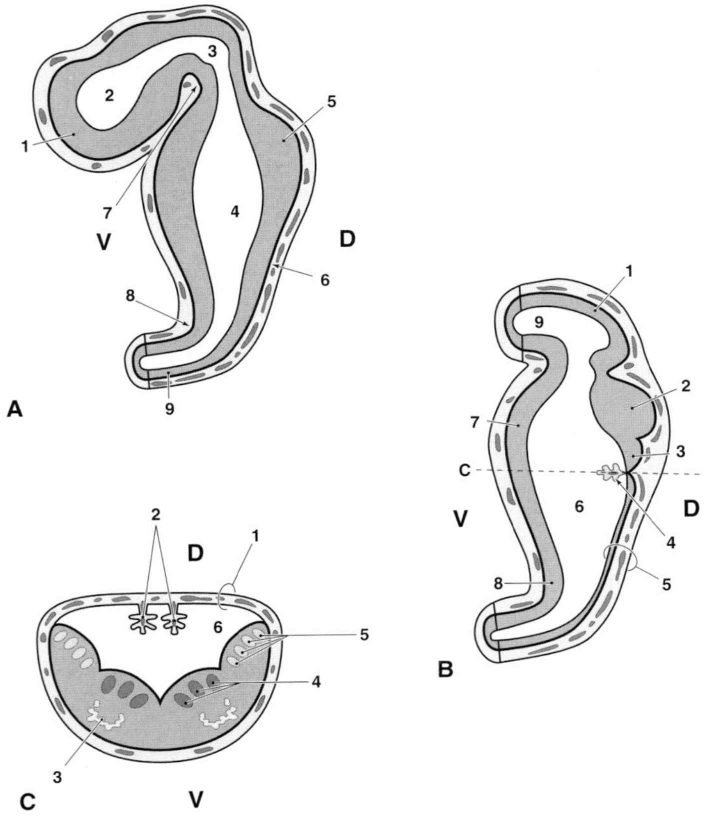

Figure 1-9: Schematics of the developing cerebral ventricular system and choroid plexi.

A: Midline sagittal schematic of developing brain at 5 weeks' gestation. *V*, ventral; *D*, dorsal.

1 Forebrain (prosencephalon)
2 Primary forebrain (prosencephalon) vesicle
3 Primary midbrain (mesencephalon) vesicle
4 Primary hindbrain (rhombencephalon) vesicle
5 Cerebellum
6 Pontine flexure
7 Midbrain flexure
8 Cervical flexure
9 Spinal cord

B: Midline sagittal schematic of developing brain at 6 weeks' gestation. *C*, level of axial section in Fig. 1-9C; *V*, ventral; *D*, dorsal.

1 Midbrain
2 Anterior lobe of cerebellum
3 Nodule
4 Fourth ventricle choroid plexus
5 Tela choroidea of fourth ventricle
6 Fourth ventricle
7 Pons
8 Medulla oblongata
9 Aqueduct of Sylvius

C: Axial schematic through the fourth ventricle at the level of the choroid plexus. *V*, ventral; *D*, dorsal.

1 Tela choroidea of fourth ventricle
2 Fourth ventricle choroid plexus
3 Olivary nucleus
4 Somatic and visceral efferent fibers
5 Somatic and visceral afferent fibers
6 Fourth ventricle

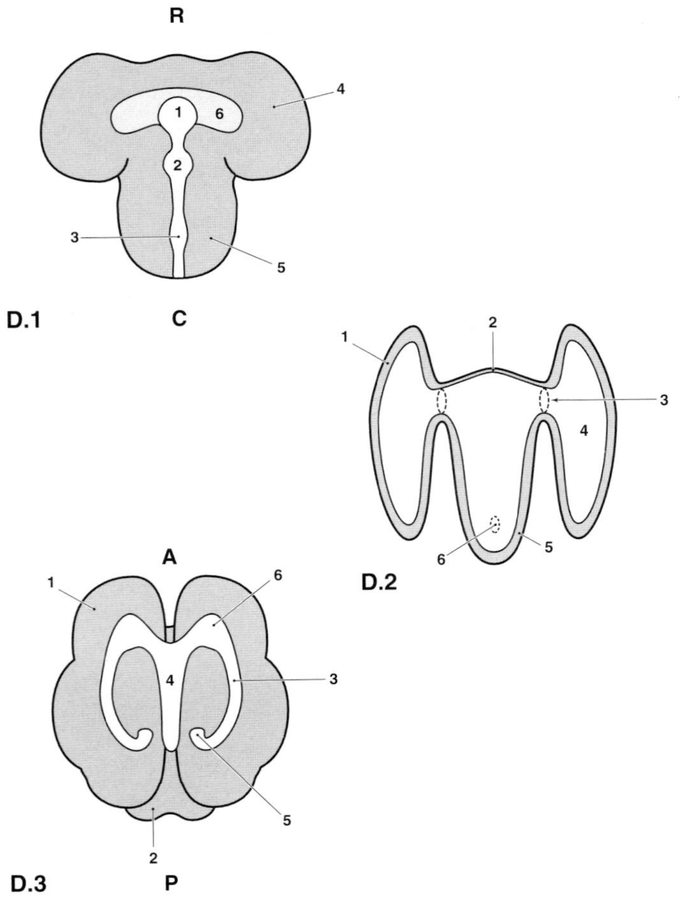

Figure 1-9D: Schematic of developing cerebral ventricular system from the superior dorsal aspect (schematics not to size).

(*1*) First month of gestation
1 Primary forebrain vesicle
2 Primary midbrain vesicle
3 Primary hindbrain vesicle
4 Cerebral hemisphere
5 Cerebellum/brain stem
6 Developing ependyma
R, rostral; *C*, caudal.

(*2*) Thirteen weeks' gestation
1 Cerebral hemisphere
2 Lamina terminalis
3 Foramen of Monro
4 Lateral ventricle
5 Diencephalon
6 Aqueduct of Sylvius

(*3*) Twenty-one weeks' gestation
1 Cerebral hemisphere
2 Cerebellum
3 Body of lateral ventricle
4 Third ventricle
5 Temporal horn of lateral ventricle
6 Anterior horn of lateral ventricle
A, anterior; *P*, posterior.

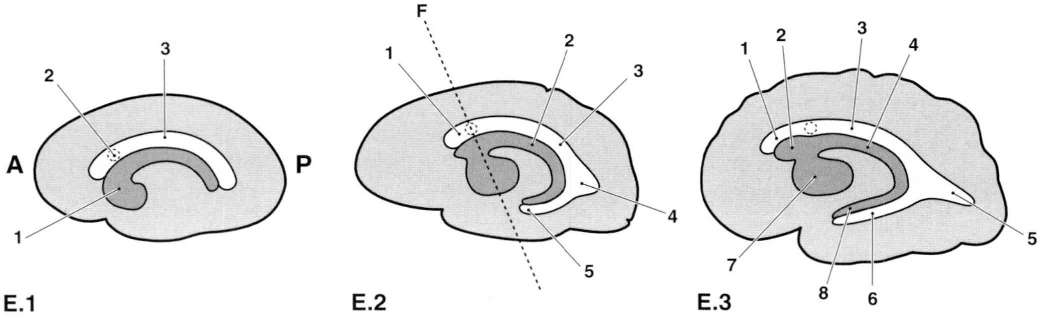

Figure 1-9E: Schematic of developing lateral cerebral ventricular system on one side, from the lateral aspect.
(*1*) Thirteen weeks' gestation
1 Corpus striatum
2 Foramen of Monro
3 Lateral ventricle
A, anterior; *P*, posterior.
(*2*) Twenty-one weeks' gestation
1 Frontal horn of lateral ventricle
2 Corpus striatum
3 Body of lateral ventricle
4 Atrium of lateral ventricle
5 Temporal horn of lateral ventricle
F, level of coronal section in Fig. 1-9F.
(*3*) Thirty-two weeks' gestation
1 Frontal horn of lateral ventricle
2 Head of caudate nucleus
3 Body of lateral ventricle
4 Body of caudate nucleus
5 Occipital horn of lateral ventricle
6 Temporal horn of lateral ventricle
7 Lentiform nucleus
8 Tail of caudate nucleus

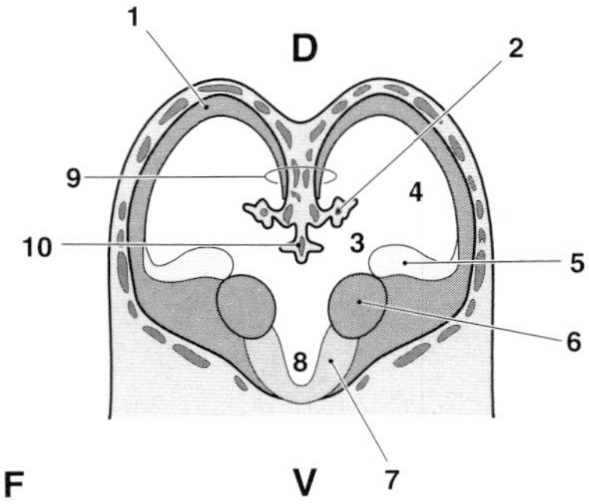

Figure 1-9F: Axial (coronal) schematic of the developing ventricular system at the level of the foramina of Monro at 11 weeks' gestation. *D*, dorsal; *V*, ventral.
1 Cerebral hemisphere
2 Lateral ventricle choroid plexus on left side
3 Foramen of Monro on left side
4 Lateral ventricle
5 Corpus striatum
6 Thalamus
7 Hypothalamus
8 Third ventricle
9 Tela choroidea of the lateral and third ventricles
10 Third ventricle choroid plexus

The Mature Ventricular System

1. The mature telencephalon has two cavities: the right and the left lateral ventricles. Each lateral ventricle consists of a body, an atrium, a frontal horn, an occipital horn, and a temporal horn.
2. The cavity of the telencephalon–diencephalon junction is termed the third ventricle. Each lateral ventricle communicates with the third ventricle through a foramen of Monro (interventricular foramen).
3. The cavity of the mesencephalon is narrow and appears as a canal, termed the aqueduct of Sylvius; this aqueduct is the communication between the third and the fourth ventricles.
4. The cavity of the rhombencephalon is the fourth ventricle. It has two lateral recesses (right and left lateral recesses), at the termination of which are openings into the basal subarachnoid cisterns, termed the foramina of Luschka. In the midline posteriorly there is a third opening of the fourth ventricle into the basal subarachnoid cisterns termed the foramen of Magendie.

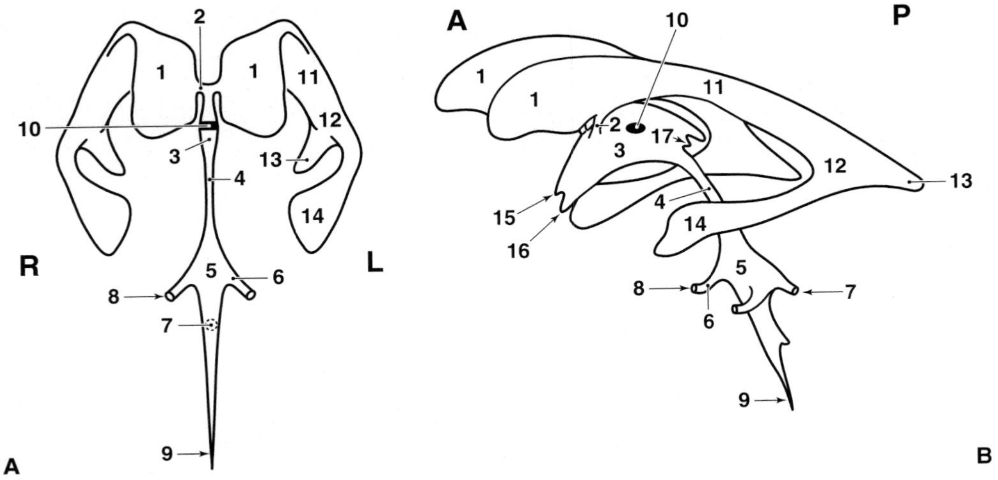

Figure 1-10: Three-dimensional configuration of the mature lumina of the cerebral ventricular system. **A:** Frontal schematic of the ventricular system. **B:** Lateral schematic of the ventricular system. *A*, anterior; *P*, posterior; *R*, right; *L*, left.

1 Frontal horn of lateral ventricle
2 Foramen of Monro
3 Third ventricle
4 Aqueduct of Sylvius
5 Fourth ventricle
6 Lateral recess of fourth ventricle
7 Foramen of Magendie
8 Foramen of Luschka
9 Obex
10 Massa intermedia
11 Body of lateral ventricle
12 Atrium of lateral ventricle
13 Occipital horn of lateral ventricle
14 Temporal horn of lateral ventricle
15 Chiasmatic recess of third ventricle
16 Infundibular recess of the third ventricle
17 Pineal recess of third ventricle

Formation of the Lobes, Gyri and Sulci/Fissures of the Cerebral Hemispheres

1. The cerebral hemispheres arise at the beginning of the fifth week of gestation as bilateral evaginations of the lateral wall of the forebrain. As the hemispheres expand, they gradually cover the lateral aspect of the diencephalon, mesencephalon, and cephalic portion of the metencephalon. Growth of the hemispheres in the anterior, posterior, and inferior directions results in the formation of the frontal, occipital, and temporal lobes.
2. Differential growth between the frontal and temporal lobes results in a depression called the insula.
3. The smooth, primordial cerebral hemispheres are initially lissencephalic. During the development of the cerebral hemispheres, the superficial cortex grows more rapidly than the underlying white matter, so that many convolutions or gyri, separated by sulci and fissures, are formed in its surface. In general, basic gyral formation and sulcation takes place between 8 and 29 weeks of gestation. After this age, brain maturation is characterized by increasing complexity of the sulci and gyri.
4. In the newborn, the entire surface of the brain is gyrated, but the gyri are less numerous and less complex in morphologic features than in the adult.

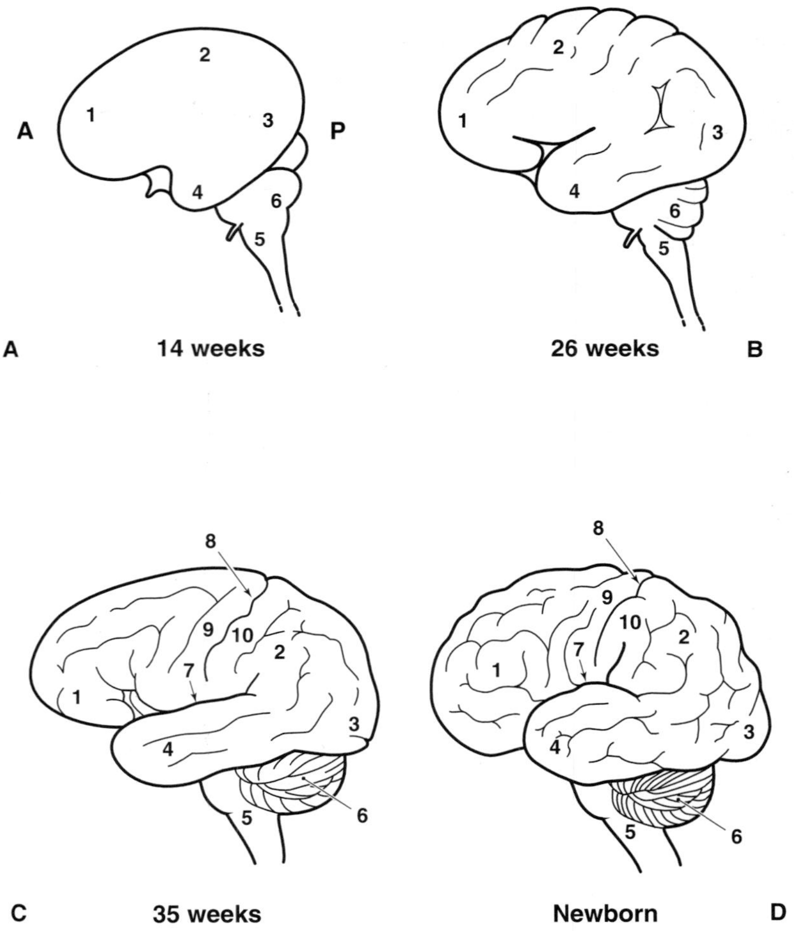

Figure 1-11: Lateral schematic showing the progressive formation of gyri, sulci, and fissures of the brain. **A:** Fourteen weeks' gestation. *A,* anterior; *P,* posterior. **B:** Twenty-six weeks' gestation. **C:** Thirty weeks' gestation. **D:** Thirty-eight weeks' gestation.

1 Frontal lobe
2 Parietal lobe
3 Occipital lobe
4 Temporal lobe
5 Brain stem
6 Cerebellum
7 Lateral (Sylvian) fissure
8 Central sulcus
9 Precentral gyrus
10 Postcentral gyrus

Embryologic Development of the Cerebral Commissures

1. The cerebral commissures are groups of axonal fibers that connect generally corresponding areas of the cerebral hemispheres with one another.
2. The largest of these commissures is the corpus callosum.
3. The first commissure to appear is the anterior commissure, which arises by the third week of gestation. The second commissure to appear is the forniceal, or hippocampal, commissure. It regresses as the corpus callosum grows.
4. The corpus callosum begins at the lamina terminalis at 10 weeks of gestation; as the cerebral cortex enlarges, more fibers are added to the corpus callosum, and it expands posteriorly, arching over the thin roof of the diencephalon.
5. The lamina terminalis becomes progressively stretched to form the thin septa pellucida.
6. The posterior and habenular commissures will form posterior to the lamina terminalis.
7. The optic chiasm, which develops in the ventral part of the lamina terminalis, also is considered by some researchers to be a cerebral commissure (see Embryology of the Visual Apparatus). Others consider the optic chiasm to be more properly a decussation.

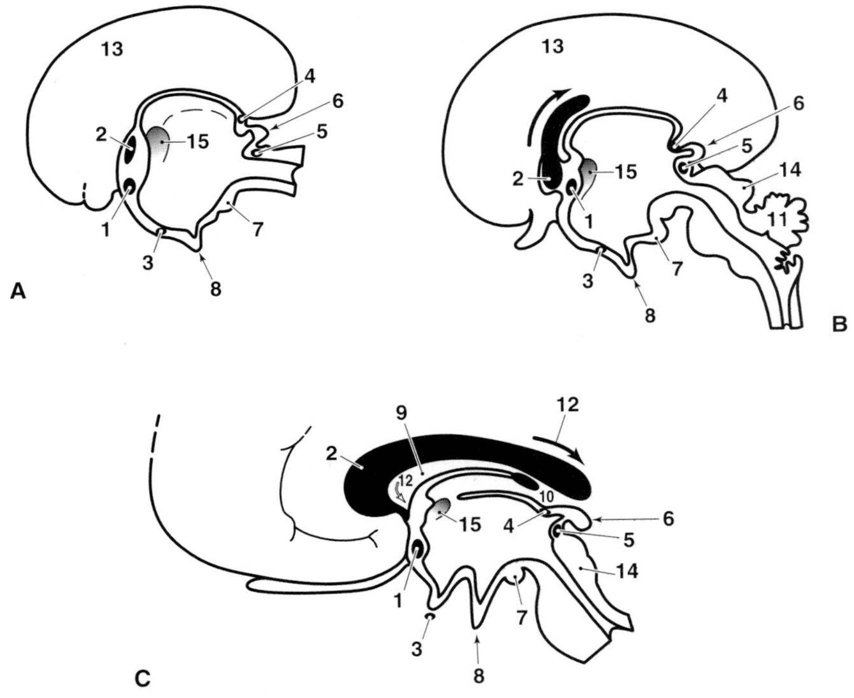

Figure 1-12: Development of the cerebral commissures. **A:** Lateral schematic of the development of the cerebral commissures in a 10-week embryo. **B:** Lateral schematic of the development of the cerebral commissures in a 4-month embryo. **C:** Lateral schematic of the development of the cerebral commissures in a newborn infant.

1 Anterior commissure
2 Corpus callosum
3 Optic chiasm
4 Habenular commissure
5 Posterior commissure
6 Epiphysis (pineal)
7 Mamillary body
8 Pituitary infundibulum
9 Septum pellucidum
10 Hippocampal commissure
11 Cerebellum
12 Direction of the expansion of the corpus callosum
13 Cerebral hemispheres
14 Quadrigeminal plate
15 Foramen of Monro

TABLE 1-1: Timetable of Normal Developmental Cerebral Myelination as Determined by Comparison with Mature (Normal Adult) Signal on MR Imaging

	T1-weighted images	T2-weighted images
Infratentorial tissue		
Brain stem	Birth	Birth
Cerebellar peduncles		
Superior/inferior	Birth	Birth to 6 months
Middle	Birth	2–3 months
Cerebellum, deep white matter (deep to superficial)	1–3 months	3–18 months
Supratentorial tissue		
Thalamus	Birth	Birth
Internal capsule		
Posterior limb	Birth	Birth
Anterior limb	3 months	3–6 months
Corpus callosum		
Splenium	3 months	4 months
Genu	6 months	8 months
Postcentral gyrus	Birth	Birth
Precentral gyrus	Birth	2–3 weeks
Centrum semiovale	Birth to 1 month	Birth to 2 months
Optic nerves and tracts	Birth	1–2 months
Occipital lobes	6 months	6.5–15 months
Posterior frontal, posterior temporal, and posterior parietal lobes	6 months	6.5–15 months
Anterior frontal, anterior parietal, and midtemporal lobes	8 months	6.5–15 months
Frontal and temporal poles	12 months	24 months

Embryology of the Calvaria

Embryologic Development of the Calvaria (Skull)

1. The paraxial mesoderm forms a segmented series of tissue blocks on each side of the neural tube. These are known as somatomeres in the cranial region and as somites from the occipital region of the skull extending caudally.
2. The skull can be divided into two parts: the *neurocranium*, which is derived from the mesoderm of the somatomeres and occipital somites, and the *viscerocranium*, which is derived from the neural crest. The neurocranium will form the cranial vault and skull base, while the viscerocranium will form the skeleton of the face.
3. The neurocranium is divided into two portions: the *membranous part*, consisting of the flat bones that will form the cranial vault, and the *cartilaginous part* that will form the skull base (*chondrocranium*).
4. The mesenchyme in the roof and sides of the skull will form flat bones. During fetal life these membranous bones will enlarge by an apposition of new layers of membranous bone and by osteoclastic resorption.
5. In the newborn these flat bones are separated from each other by the connective tissue in the sutures. At points where more than two calvarial bones meet, the sutures are relatively wider and are known as fontanelles. The anterior fontanelle, located at the intersection of the sagittal and coronal sutures, will usually close by the end of the second year. The posterior fontanelle, located between the sagittal and lambdoid sutures, will usually close by about 2 months of age.
6. Additional, smaller, paired fontanelles include the anterolateral, or sphenoidal, fontanelles at the junction of the frontal, parietal, temporal, and sphenoid bones and the posterolateral, or mastoid, fontanelles at the junction of the occipital, parietal, and temporal bones.
7. The cartilaginous neurocranium is formed initially by several separate cartilages (i.e., ossification centers) that will fuse and ossify to form the skull base.

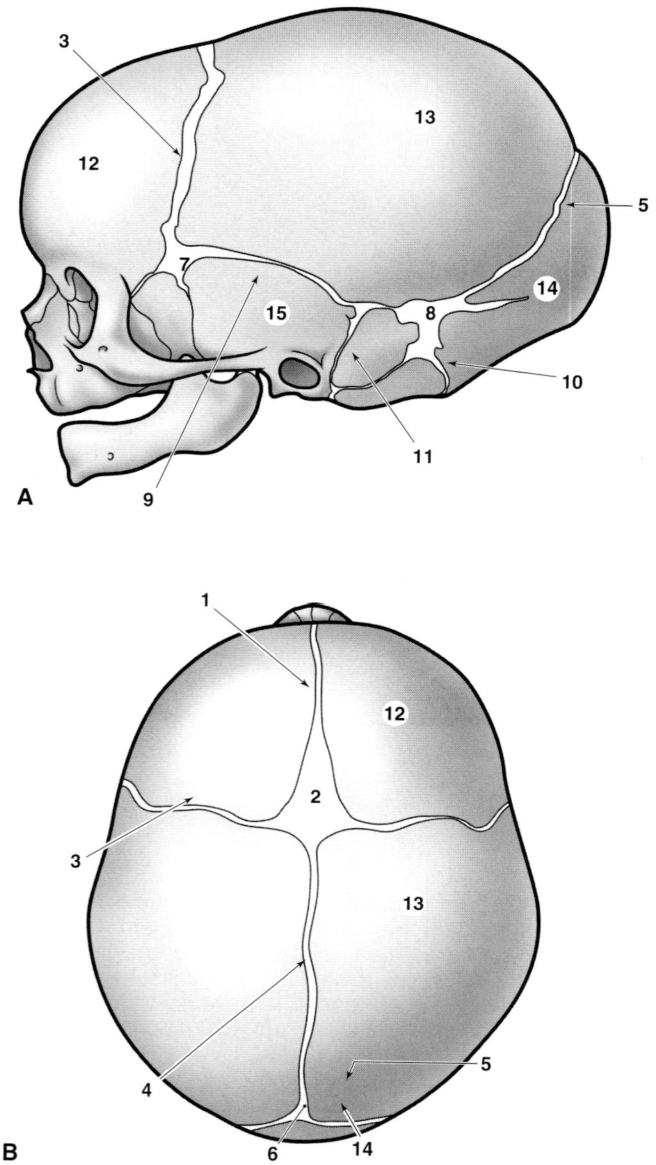

Figure 1-13: Schematic of the skull of a newborn. **A:** Lateral schematic of the skull of a newborn. **B:** Schematic of the skull of a newborn viewed from above.

1 Frontal or metopic suture
2 Anterior fontanelle
3 Coronal suture
4 Sagittal suture
5 Lambdoid suture
6 Posterior fontanelle
7 Anterolateral or sphenoidal fontanelle
8 Posterolateral or mastoid fontanelle
9 Squamous suture
10 Mendosal suture (posterior intraoccipital suture)
11 Petrosquamosal suture
12 Frontal bone
13 Parietal bone
14 Occipital bone
15 Temporal bone

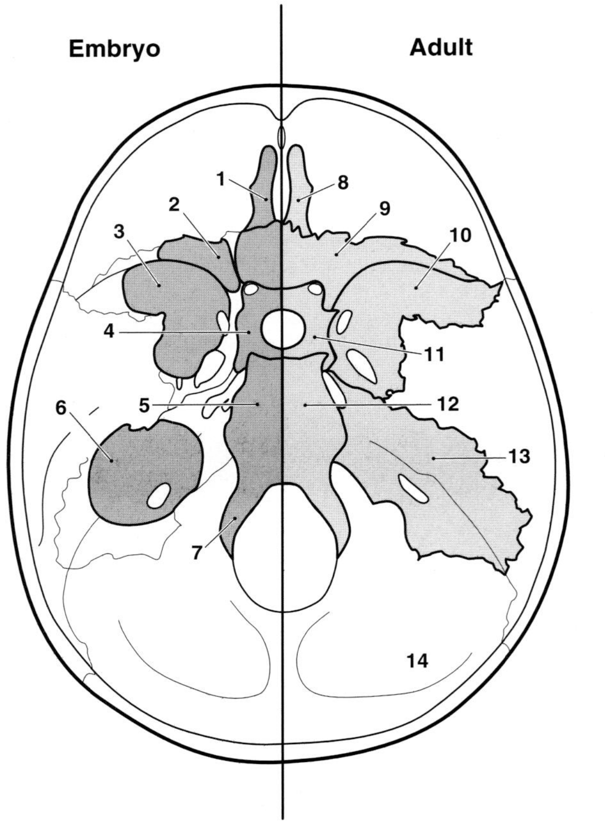

Figure 1-14: Development of the skull base. Schematic showing the embryonic components of condrocranium (cartilaginous neurocranium) that will form the skull base in an embryo and the corresponding skull base in an adult.
1 Trabeculae cranii
2 Ala orbitalis
3 Ala temporalis
4 Hypophyseal cartilage
5 Parachordal cartilage
6 Periotic capsule
7 Occipital sclerotomes
8 Ethmoid bone
9 Lesser wing of sphenoid bone
10 Greater wing of sphenoid bone
11 Body of sphenoid bone
12 Base of occipital bone
13 Petrous bone
14 Occipital bone

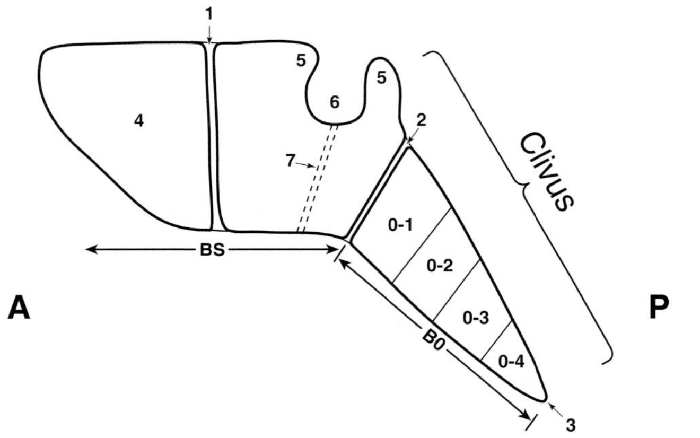

Figure 1-15: Lateral midline schematic showing the components of the clivus and central skull base with their embryologic precursors. The basisphenoid and basiocciput are separated before fusion by the sphenooccipital synchondrosis. The presphenoid and basisphenoid are the central precursors of the sphenoid bone. The basiocciput is formed from the four primary occipital sclerotomes or "vertebrae" (OI-O-4). Fusion of the sphenooccipital synchondrosis generally occurs after age 12 years. *A*, anterior; *P*, posterior; *O-1/O-4*, occipital sclerotomes or "vertebrae"; *BS*, basisphenoid; *BO*, basiocciput; *BS* + posterior part of BO: clivus.
1 Anterior intrasphenoid synchondrosis
2 Sphenooccipital synchondrosis
3 Basion
4 Presphenoid ossification center (n = 1)
5 Sphenoid ossification centers
6 Sella turcica
7 Region of pharangohypophyseal (craniopharyngeal) canal

Embryology of the Brachiocephalic and Cerebral Vasculature

Embryologic Development of the Left-sided Aortic Arch

1. The atrium, ventricle, and bulbous cordis of the developing embryonic heart tube continues in the craniad direction into the aortic sac (root). Two vessels emerge from the aortic sac on each side and represent the two primitive ventral aortas. These vessels then grow dorsally and form a transverse connecting segment known as the first aortic arch. Further caudal growth from this arch forms the primitive dorsal aorta.
2. Five additional pairs of aortic arches form in succession, connecting the ipsilateral primitive ventral and dorsal aortas.
3. The eventual fate of the six aortic arches is mixed. The first aortic arch involutes completely. The second aortic arch gives rise to the hyoid and stapedial arteries. The third aortic arch forms the proximal common carotid arteries. The fourth aortic arch on the left side forms the main adult left aortic arch; the right side forms the right subclavian artery. The fifth aortic arch is transient. The sixth aortic arch on the right becomes the right pulmonary artery, while on the left it persists during the fetal period as the ductus arteriosus.

Early Embryologic Development of the Cerebral Arterial and Venous Systems

1. The developing neural tube is invested in a superficial arterial network. Initially, three primitive arteries penetrate the ventral aspect of the neural tube.
2. All stages of development of the cerebral venous system lag considerably behind the development of the cerebral arterial system.
3. The early venous system consists of a network of primitive collecting veins that drain into a superficial venous network on the surface of the neural tube.
4. The primitive venous network is superficial to the primitive arterial network.
5. Early arterial flow is predominately from the periphery to the center, with venous flow the reverse of this pattern. In other words, the basic early arterial flow is centripetal and the venous flow is centrifugal.
6. Subsequent growth of the cerebral hemispheres results in a shift of this pattern of blood flow. Deep medullary veins develop along the lines of the peripheral migration of neurons, from the primitive vesicles outward toward the superficial cerebral cortex.
7. Therefore, while the developing cerebral arterial flow remains centripetal, the later venous drainage is mixed: superficial cerebral tissues have centrifugal venous drainage, and deep cerebral tissues have centripetal venous drainage.

Embryologic Development of the Internal Carotid Artery

1. The roots of the internal carotid arteries develop at the origin of the third primitive aortic arch from the primitive aorta.
2. The proximal cervical internal carotid artery consists of the third primitive aortic arch.
3. The distal cervical internal carotid artery originates from the junction of the distal third primitive aortic arch and the primitive dorsal aorta.
4. The distal cervical internal carotid artery consists of a persistent segment of the craniad extent of the primitive dorsal aorta.

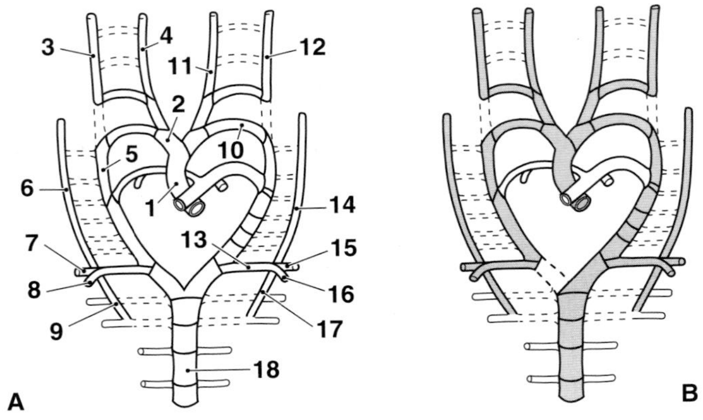

Figure 1-16: Embryologic anatomy of common (typical) aortic arch and cephalic artery anomalies. Origins of normal left aortic arch and the brachiocephalic vessels. **A:** Template from which the various aortic arches and brachiocephalic vessels are derived. **B:** Origins of normal left aortic arch and brachiocephalic vessels.

1 Ascending aorta
2 Innominate artery
3 Right internal carotid artery
4 Right external carotid artery
5 Right subclavian artery
6 Right vertebral artery
7 Right thyrocervical trunk
8 Right subclavian artery
9 Right internal mammary artery
10 Aortic arch
11 Left external carotid artery
12 Left internal carotid artery
13 Left subclavian artery
14 Vertebral artery
15 Left thyrocervical trunk
16 Left subclavian artery
17 Left internal mammary artery
18 Descending aorta

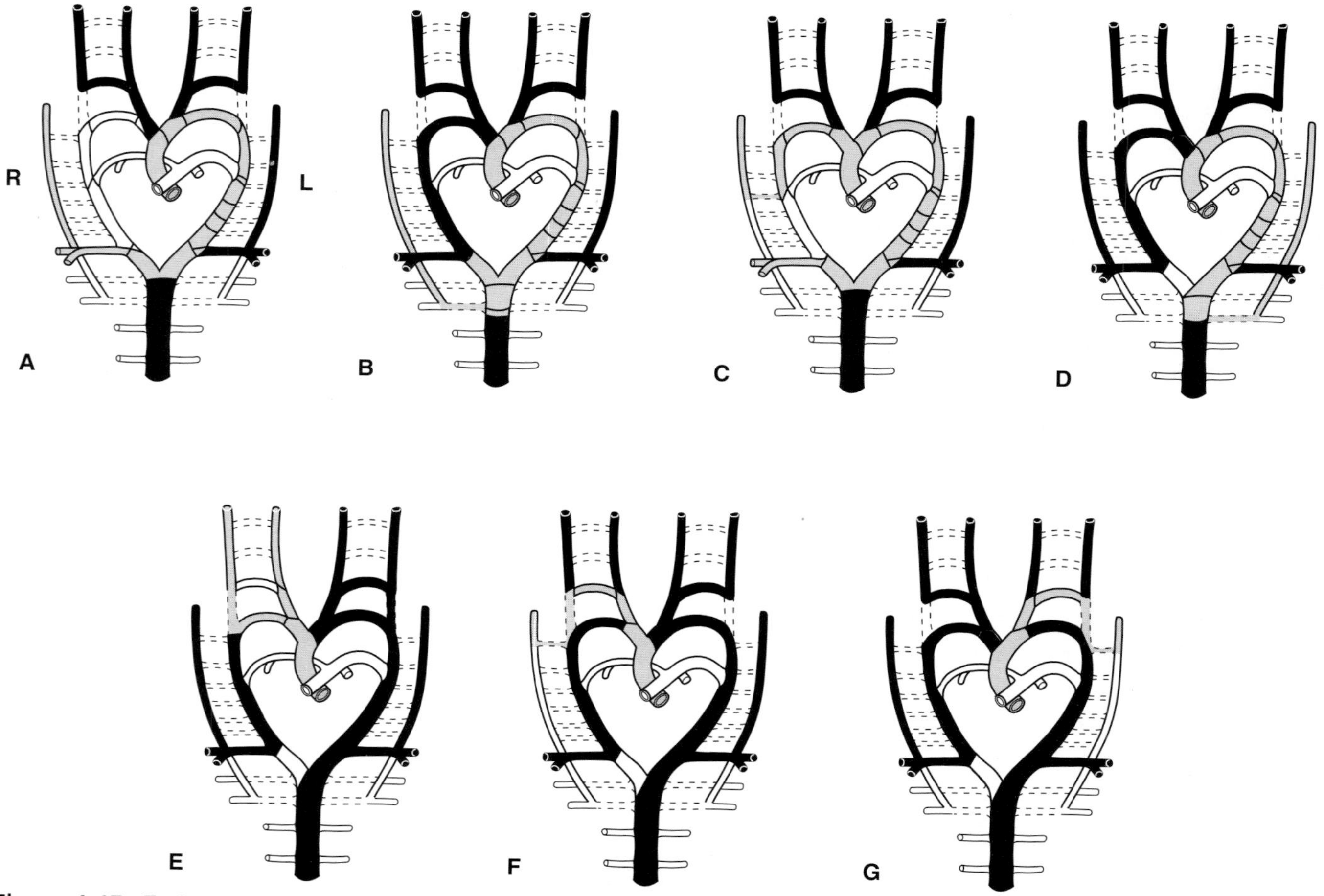

Figure 1-17: Embryologic anatomy of common (typical) aortic arch and cephalic artery anomalies. Common left aortic arch anomalies. **A:** Aberrant right subclavian artery with left aortic arch. **B:** Right vertebral artery arising from distal left aortic arch. **C:** Right vertebral artery arising from the right common carotid artery in the presence of an aberrant right subclavian artery in the left aortic arch. **D:** Left vertebral artery arising from the left aortic arch distal to the left subclavian artery. **E:** Separate origins of internal and external carotid arteries from the innominate artery in a left aortic arch. **F:** Right proatlantal artery arising from right internal carotid artery in a left aortic arch. **G:** Left proatlantal artery arising from left internal carotid artery in a left aortic arch. *R*, right; *L*, left; *gray shading*, basic left-sided aortic arch and specific variation; *black shading*, otherwise normal branching from left-sided aortic arch; *unshaded vessels*, involutionally atretic connections.

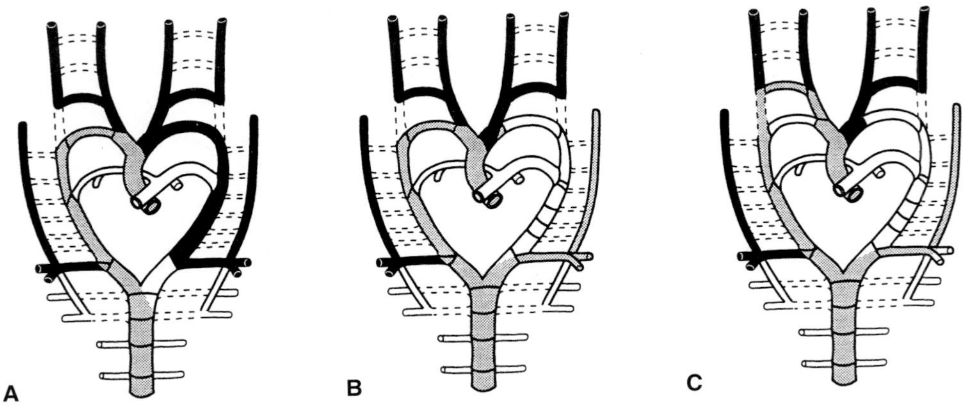

A B C

Figure 1-18: Embryologic anatomy of common (typical) aortic arch and cephalic artery anomalies. Common right aortic arch anomalies. **A:** Mirror-image right aortic arch. **B:** Right aortic arch with aberrant left subclavian artery. **C:** Right cervical aortic arch with aberrant left subclavian artery.

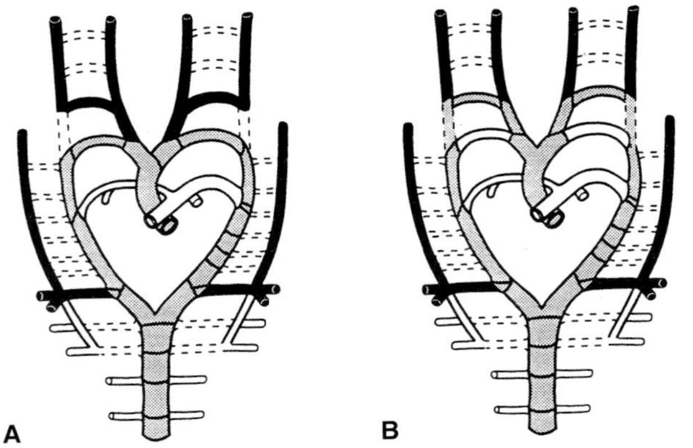

A B

Figure 1-19: Embryologic anatomy of common (typical) aortic arch and cephalic artery anomalies. Common double aortic arch anomalies. **A:** Complete double aortic arch at normal level. **B:** Double cervical aortic arch.

Figure 1-20: Schematics showing normal theoretical development of the cerebral vascular system and anastomoses.

A: Primitive vascular supply to cerebral hemispheres before neuronal migration.

1 Primitive hemispheric capillary network
2 Primitive hemispheric venous network
3 Primitive cerebral hemisphere
4 Primitive cerebral vesicle
5 Primitive hemispheric arterial network

B: Developing vascular supply to cerebral hemispheres after neuronal migration.

1 Arterial inflow (centripetal)
2 Hemispheric cerebral cortex
3 Cerebral ventricle
4 Deep venous drainage (centripetal)
5 Subcortical cerebral hemisphere
6 Superficial (centrifugal) venous drainage

C: Developing cerebral capillary hemisphere arterial vascular watershed (*asterisk*).

D: Developing cerebral hemispheric venous vascular watershed (*asterisk*).

E: Mature systems of combined (Figs. 1-20C and 1-20D) cerebral hemispheric parenchymal arterial vascular watersheds.

1 Capillary arterial watershed
2 Venous watershed

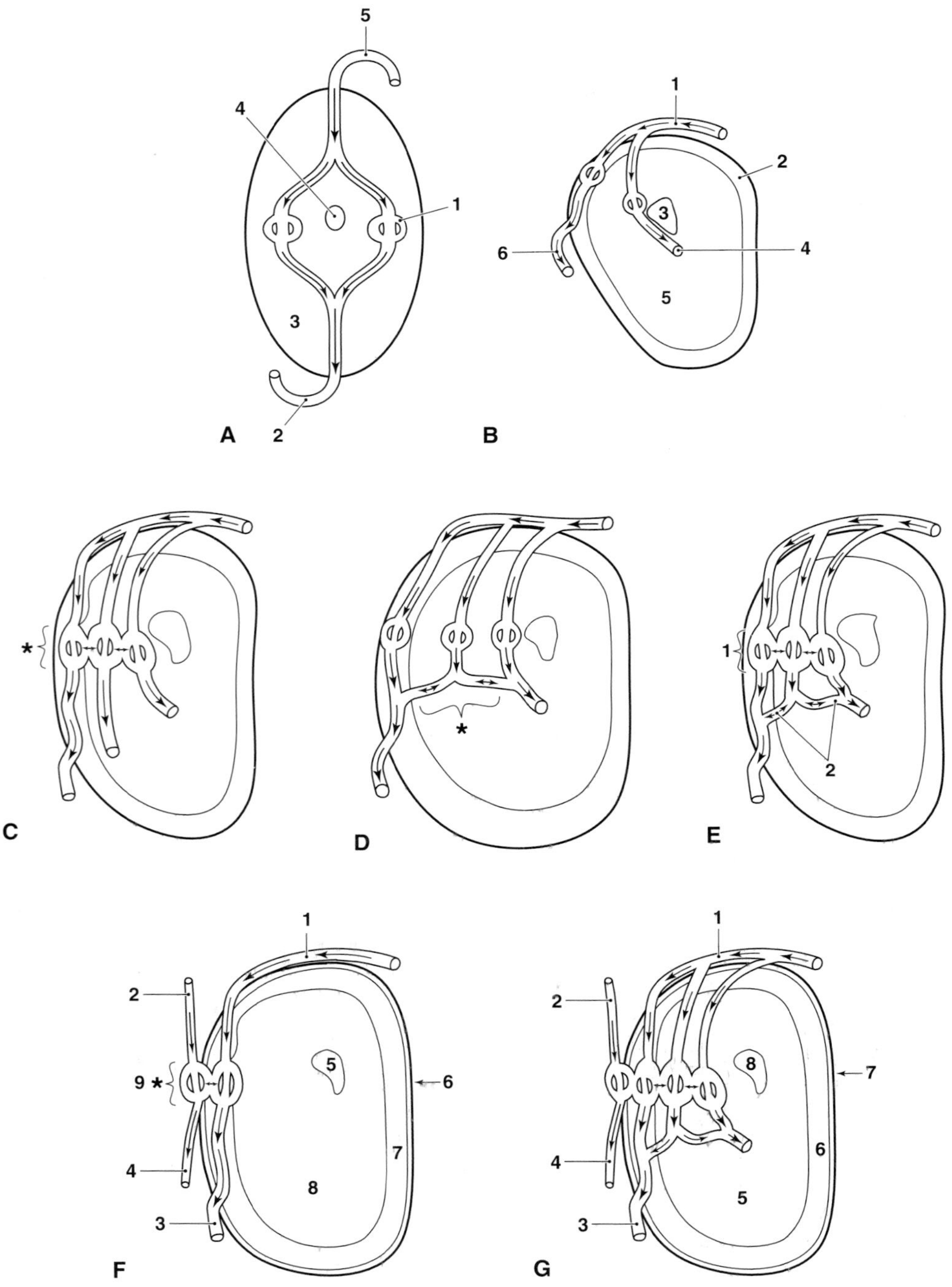

F: Mature cerebral hemispheric leptomeningeal–cortical watershed (*asterisk*).
1 Branch artery to cerebral cortex from internal circulation
2 Branch artery to leptomeninges from external circulation
3 Vein draining cerebral cortex
4 Vein draining leptomeninges
5 Cerebral ventricle
6 Leptomeninges
7 Cerebral cortex
8 Cerebral hemisphere
9 Leptomeningeal capillary watershed

G: Mature adult system of combined leptomeningeal, superficial, and deep hemispheric arterial and venous watersheds (refer to Fig. 1-20C, D, and F).
1 Branch artery to cerebral cortex
2 Branch artery to leptomeninges from external circulation
3 Vein draining cerebral cortex
4 Vein draining leptomeninges
5 Cerebral hemisphere
6 Cerebral cortex
7 Leptomeninges
8 Cerebral ventricle

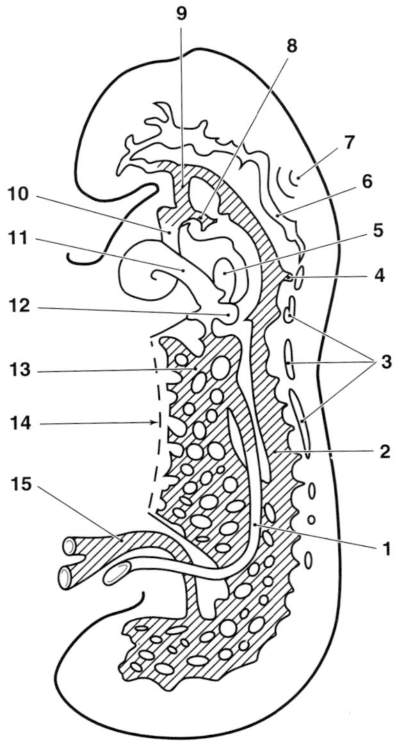

A

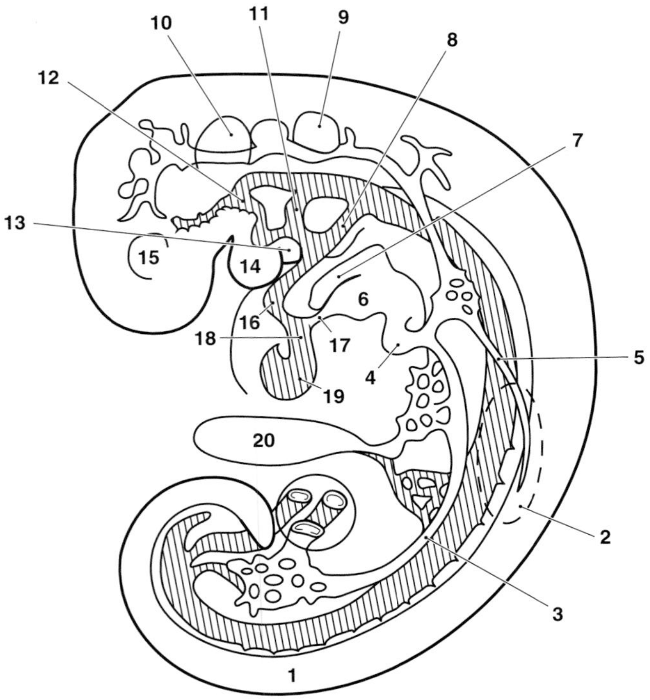

B

Figure 1-21A: Sagittal schematic of the vascular system of a human embryo with 14 paired somites.

1 Left umbilical vein
2 Dorsal aorta
3 Rudiments of postcardinal vein
4 Rudiment of common cardinal vein
5 Right atrium
6 Primitive head vein
7 Otocyst
8 Rudiment of second aortic arch
9 First aortic arch
10 Aortic sac
11 Ventricle
12 Left atrium
13 Vitelline plexus
14 Yolk sac
15 Umbilical arteries

Figure 1-21B: Sagittal schematic of the vascular system of a human embryo with 28 somites (age 26 days).

1 Spinal cord
2 Upper limb bud
3 Left umbilical vein
4 Left horn of sinus venoses
5 Left postcardinal vein
6 Left atrium
7 Right atrium
8 Third aortic arch
9 Otocyst
10 Trigeminal ganglion
11 Second aortic arch
12 First aortic arch
13 Hyoid arch
14 Mandibular arch
15 Optic rudiment
16 Aortic sac
17 Atrioventricular canal
18 Bulbous cordis
19 Left ventricle
20 Yolk sac

Embryologic Development of the Anterior Cerebral Artery

1. Initially, the terminal end of the cranial (distal) segment of the developing internal carotid artery ends in branches to the nasal fossa and the olfactory nerve; this primitive olfactory artery will become the anterior cerebral artery.
2. The primitive olfactory artery is a paired structure. The two parts join in the midline in a plexiform manner to give rise to the anterior communicating artery.
3. The anterior cerebral artery, as a continuation of the primitive olfactory artery, extends upward and backward between the developing cerebral hemispheres.
4. The primitive olfactory artery eventually regresses to supply a small arterial branch to the nasal cavity and to the anterior perforated substance.

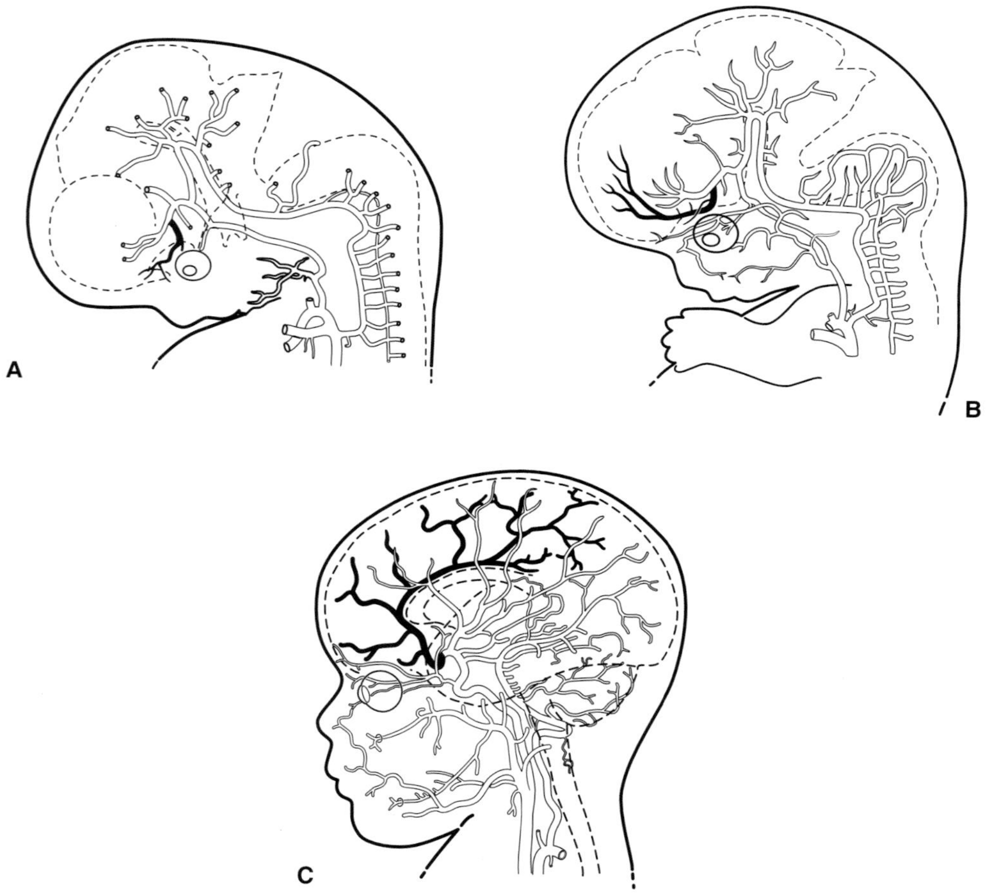

Figure 1-22: Embryologic development of the anterior cerebral artery (*shaded*). **A:** Early. **B:** Intermediate. **C:** Late.

Embryologic Development of the Middle Cerebral Artery

1. The middle cerebral artery arises directly from the internal carotid artery just distal to the anterior choroidal artery.
2. The branches of the middle cerebral artery extend outward over the surface of the developing cerebral hemispheres in a curvilinear, outwardly convex course.
3. In the second month of fetal life, a depression appears over the lateral aspect of the cerebral hemispheres. The depression gradually deepens, eventually forming a fossa with a broad floor, the insula.
4. Folds then form along the edge of this fossa, which cover over the enclosed developing insula. The folds, or opercula, carry with them the branches of the middle cerebral artery lying on their surface.

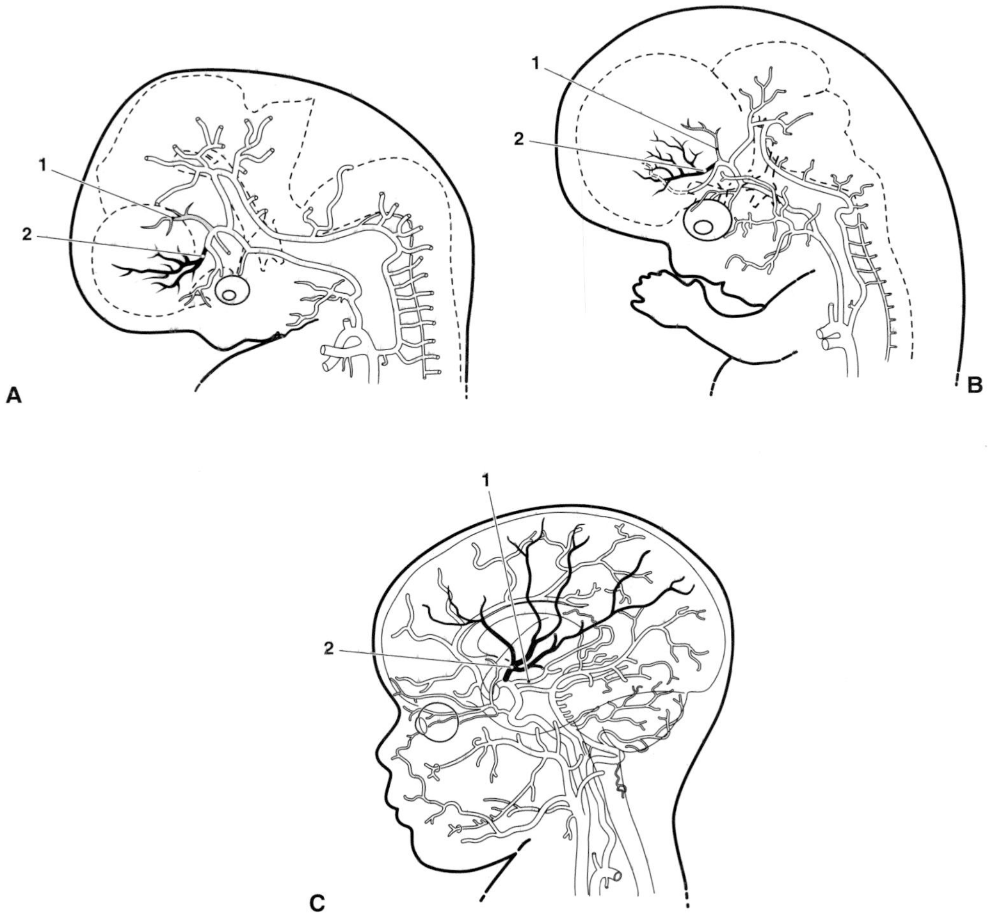

Figure 1-23: Embryologic development of the middle cerebral artery. **A:** Early. **B:** Intermediate. **C:** Late.
1 Anterior choroidal artery
2 Middle cerebral artery

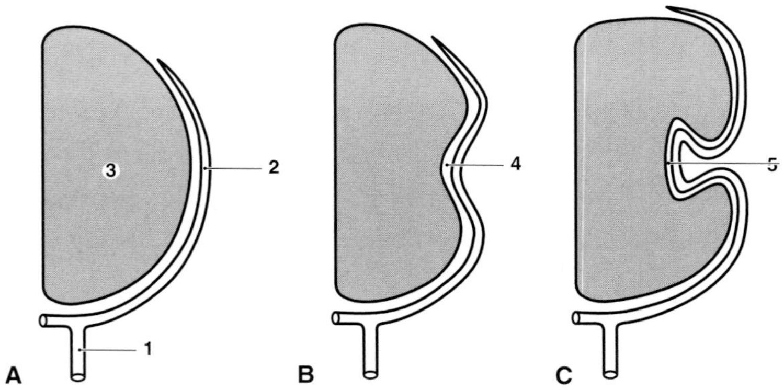

Figure 1-24: Frontal schematic of embryologic Sylvian region development of intermediate and distal middle cerebral artery branches. **A:** Early. **B:** Intermediate. **C:** Late.

1 Internal carotid artery
2 Middle cerebral artery
3 Cerebral hemisphere
4 Depression over lateral aspect of the cerebral hemisphere
5 Developing insula

Embryologic Development of the Posterior Cerebral Artery

1. The proximal posterior cerebral artery originates as a fusion of several developing vessels supplying the mesencephalon, diencephalon, and choroid plexus.
2. These primitive mesencephalic, diencephalic, posterior choroidal, and posterior cerebral arteries arise from a common stem at the caudal end of the embryonic posterior communicating artery.
3. The posterior cerebral artery then grows backward and upward over the surface of the posterior temporal lobe and occipital lobes as an extension of the internal carotid artery and posterior communicating artery.
4. In the majority of cases, the posterior cerebral artery then shifts its dominant connection to the basilar artery, with subsequent partial regression of the posterior communicating artery.

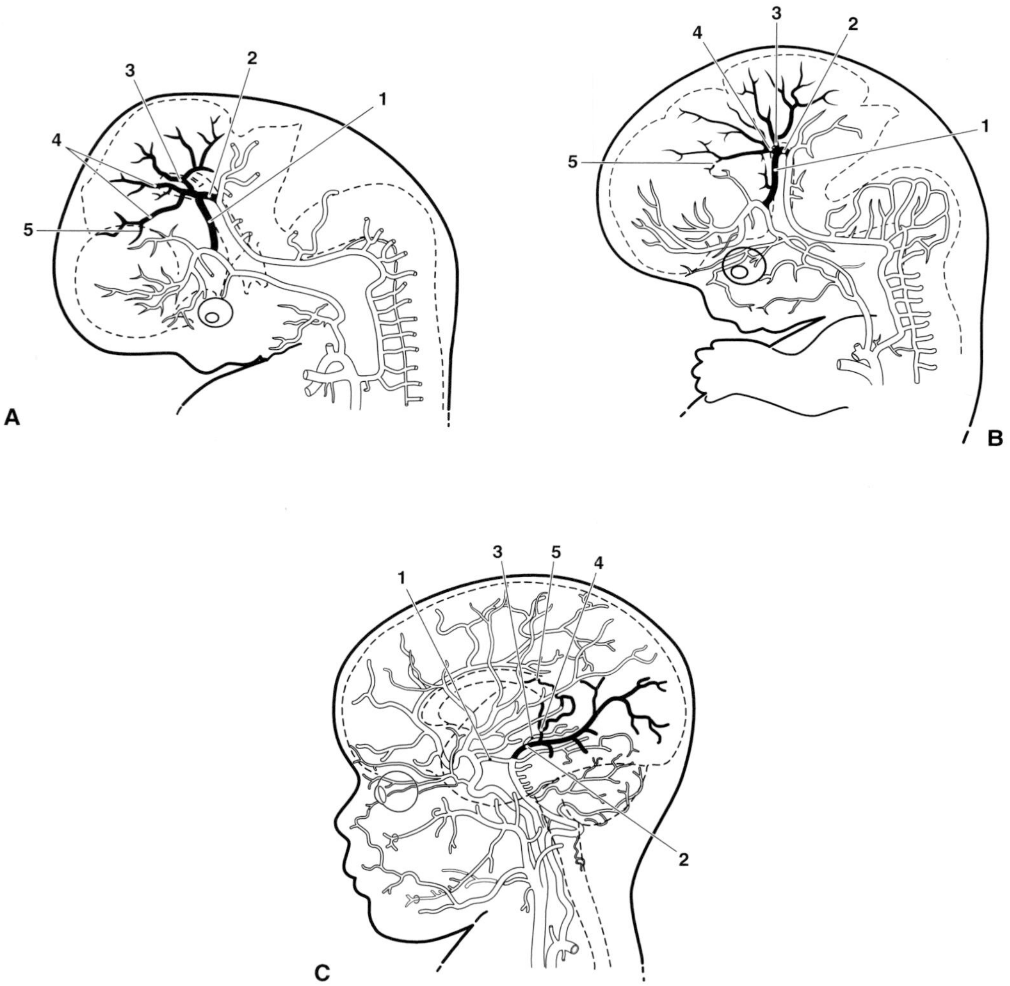

Figure 1-25: Embryologic development of posterior cerebral artery (*shaded areas*). **A:** Early. **B:** Intermediate. **C:** Late.
1 Posterior communicating artery
2 Stem of postcerebral artery
3 Mesencephalic artery
4 Diencephalic artery
5 Posterior choroidal artery

Embryologic Development of the External Carotid Artery

1. The external carotid trunk is formed as an outgrowth of the ventral aspect of the third primitive aortic arch.
2. At the same time, the stapedial artery forms from the dorsal portion of the second aortic arch, which, in turn, originates from the internal carotid artery.
3. An anastomosis occurs between the internal maxillary branch of the cranially developing external carotid trunk and the caudally growing maxillomandibular branch of the stapedial artery.
4. The connection of the stapedial artery with the internal carotid artery involutes by the third fetal month. The external carotid artery trunk then takes over the vascular supply of the stapedial artery. Among other branch arteries, this vascular territory includes that of the middle meningeal artery and the inferior alveolar artery.

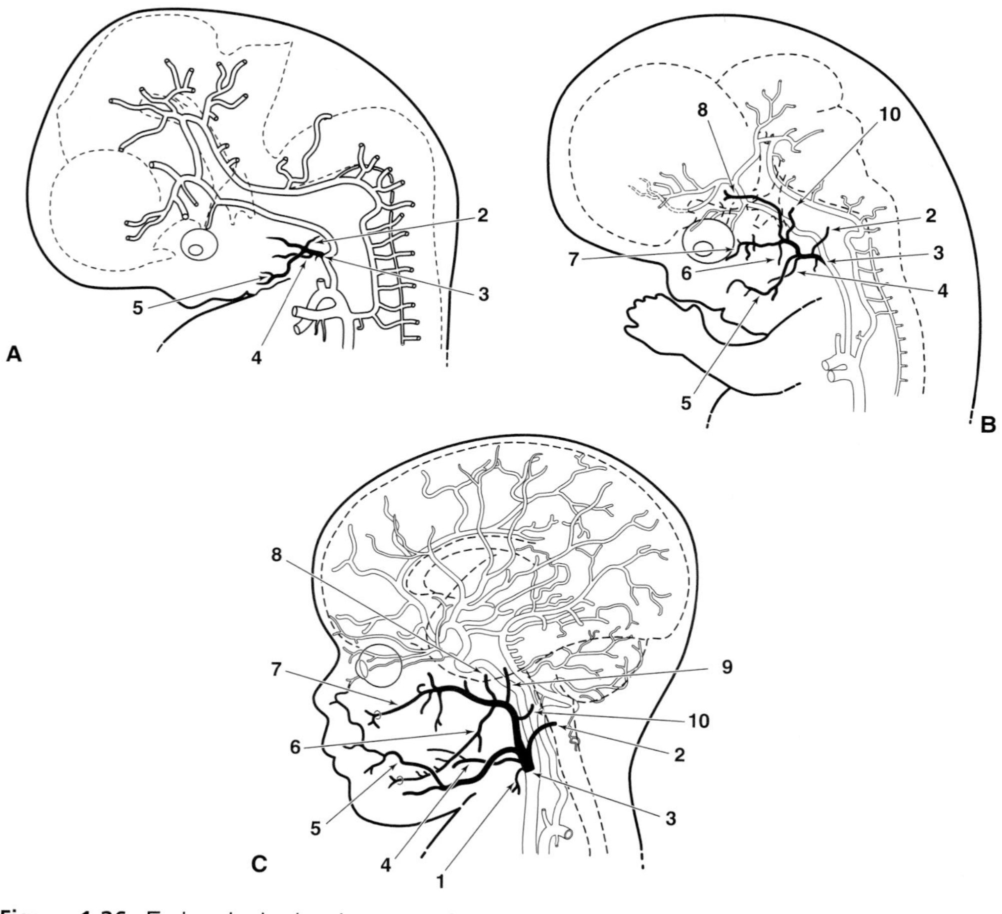

Figure 1-26: Embryologic development of the external carotid artery (*shaded*). **A:** Early. **B:** Intermediate. **C:** Late.

1 Superior thyroidal artery
2 Occipital artery
3 External carotid artery
4 Lingual artery
5 Facial artery
6 Inferior alveolar artery
7 Internal maxillary artery
8 Middle meningeal artery
9 Superficial temporal artery
10 Posterior auricular artery

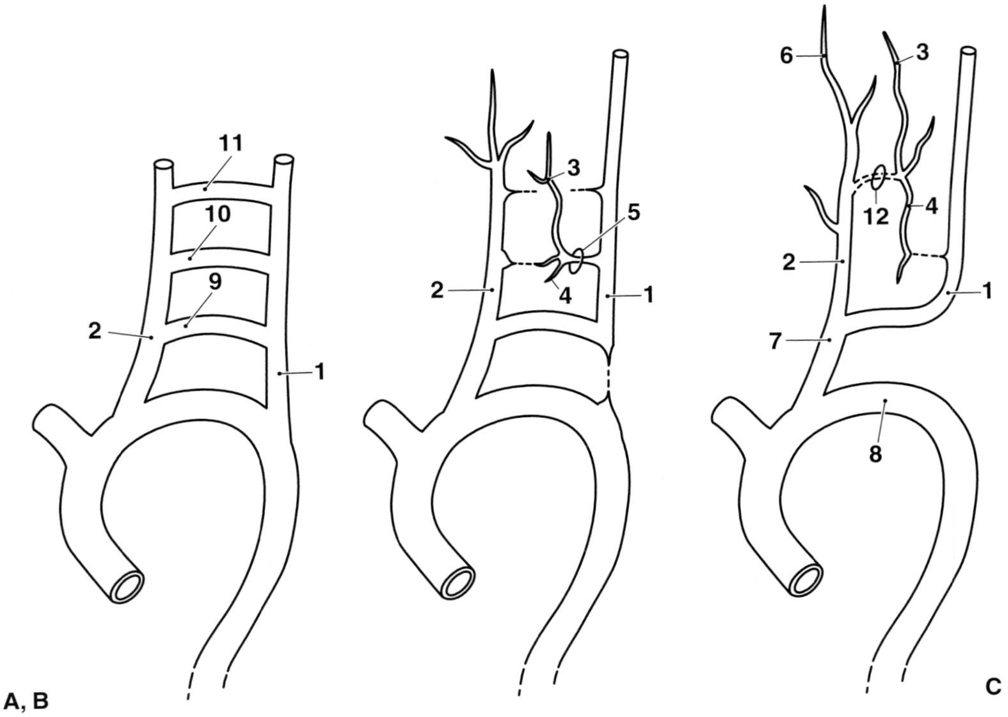

Figure 1-27: Embryologic development of the external carotid artery from the aortic arch. **A:** Early. **B:** Intermediate. **C:** Late. *Dashed line*, vascular regression; *dashed lumen*, reestablished vascular connection.

1 Internal carotid artery
2 External carotid artery
3 Middle meningeal artery
4 Internal maxillary artery
5 Stapedial artery
6 Superficial temporal artery
7 Common carotid artery
8 Left aortic arch
9 First primitive aortic arch
10 Second primitive aortic arch
11 Third primitive aortic arch
12 Maxillomandibular branch of the stapedial artery

Embryologic Development of the Cranial Vertebrobasilar Arterial Vascular System

1. The basilar artery forms initially as a paired structure that is closely applied to the ventral surface of the hindbrain.
2. The rostral vascular connections of these paired primitive basilar arteries are with the posterior divisions of the developing primitive internal carotid arteries. The caudal vascular connections of these paired primitive basilar arteries are with the craniad extensions of the developing vertebral arteries.
3. In the intermediate developmental stages, the paired primitive basilar arteries fuse to form a single, though plexiform, midline basilar artery.
4. In most cases, the basilar artery fenestrations eventually disappear to constitute an adult-form single basilar artery trunk.

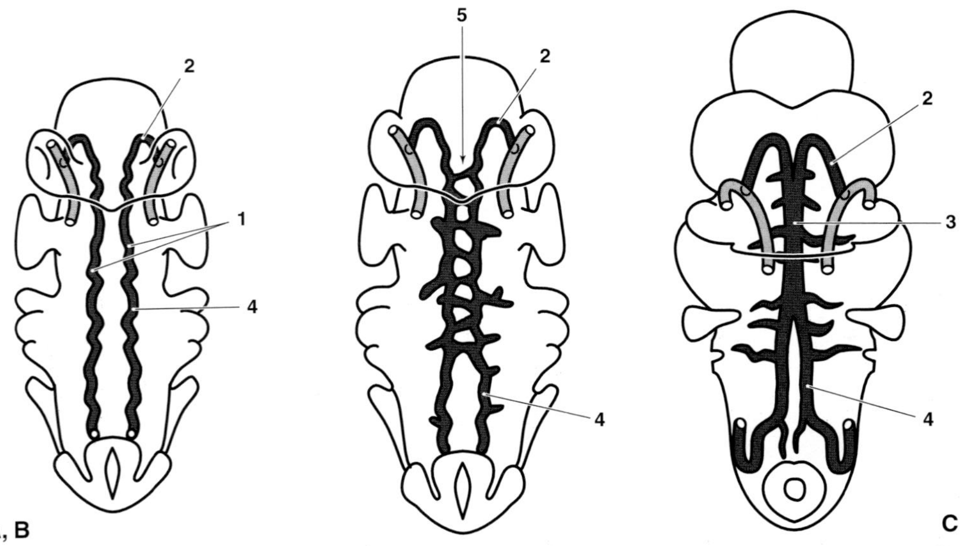

Figure 1-28: Embryologic development of the cranial vertebrobasilar arterial system. **A:** Early development of vertebrobasilar vascular system with paired primitive basilar arteries. **B:** Intermediate development of vertebrobasilar vascular system with interbasilar fenestra. **C:** Late development of vertebrobasilar vascular system with primitive basilar arteries fully fused into single trunk.

1 Paired primitive basilar arteries
2 Posterior cerebral artery
3 Mature basilar artery
4 Vertebral artery
5 Primitive plexiform basilar artery connections

Intermediate and Late Cerebral Venous Development

1. The development of the deep cerebral veins occurs during embryogenesis and maturation of the cerebral hemispheres.
2. The development of the cerebral veins lags behind that of the developing cerebral arteries.
3. The earliest cerebral venous drainage is to the superficial pial venous plexus.
4. The deep venous system develops later, with the maturation of the deep cerebral structures.
5. The deep medullary cerebral veins follow the pathway of the peripheral embryonic migration of the gray cells during development of the cerebral hemispheres, extending from the subependymal region of the cerebral ventricles to the superficial cerebral cortex.
6. Generally speaking, the normal mature venous flow is from the center of the brain outward toward the brain surfaces (i.e., the cerebral ventricles and outer cerebral cortex). This will result in both superficial and deep venous drainage.
7. The final development of the dural venous sinuses takes place following birth.

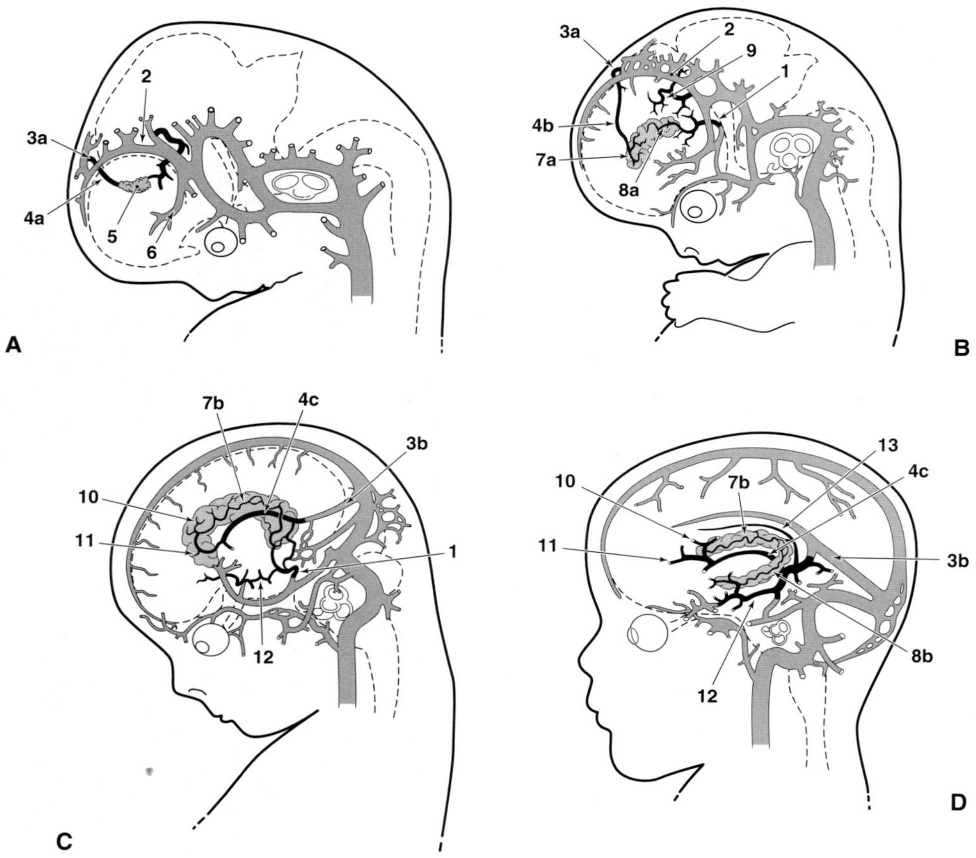

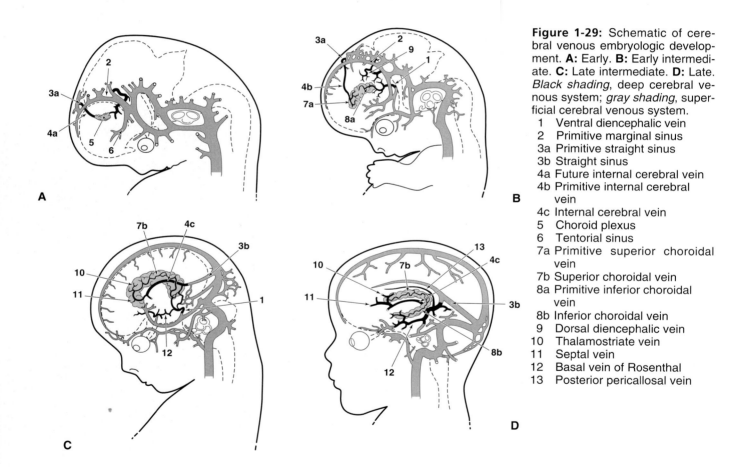

Figure 1-29: Schematic of cerebral venous embryologic development. **A:** Early. **B:** Early intermediate. **C:** Late intermediate. **D:** Late. *Black shading*, deep cerebral venous system; *gray shading*, superficial cerebral venous system.

1 Ventral diencephalic vein
2 Primitive marginal sinus
3a Primitive straight sinus
3b Straight sinus
4a Future internal cerebral vein
4b Primitive internal cerebral vein
4c Internal cerebral vein
5 Choroid plexus
6 Tentorial sinus
7a Primitive superior choroidal vein
7b Superior choroidal vein
8a Primitive inferior choroidal vein
8b Inferior choroidal vein
9 Dorsal diencephalic vein
10 Thalamostriate vein
11 Septal vein
12 Basal vein of Rosenthal
13 Posterior pericallosal vein

EMBRYOLOGY OF THE SPINE

Embryologic Development of the Spinal Column

1. The formation of the vertebral column follows a series of steps categorized as membrane development, chondrification, and ossification. Each vertebra goes through these steps sequentially.
2. The process starts in the future occipital region and sweeps along the length of the spine, so that different parts of the spine exhibit different stages at any moment in time during development.
3. By day 17 of gestation, mesodermal cells at the cephalic end of the embryo form a thick mass of paraxial mesenchyme situated lateral to the notochord and ventrolateral to the neural plate. This paraxial mesoderm forms bilaterally symmetrical, longitudinal columns of solid mesoderm that begin to segment into paired blocks called somites by day 20.
4. The dorsolateral portion of each somite differentiates into the dermatomyotome, which will form the skeletal muscle and dermis.
5. The ventromedial portion of each somite differentiates into the sclerotome, which will form the cartilage, bone, and ligaments of the vertebral column. Cells from the sclerotome portion migrate medially to form the perichordal tube after the notochord separates from the neural tube and the endoderm. This process takes place first in the cervical segments and then proceeds cranially and caudally.
6. The vertebral bodies formed from the perichordal tube of mesoderm and other sclerotomic cells migrate dorsally to eventually surround the neural tube, giving rise to the posterior bony elements of the spinal column.
7. Starting at about day 24 of gestation, a major resegmentation takes place in the membranous vertebral bodies. The caudal and cephalic halves of each segment differentiate from each other. Fissures form in the midportion of each segment, between the two halves, and the two halves cleave from each other. These halves then unite with adjacent half-segments, such that the lower half of one older primitive segment joins with the upper half of the older primitive segment below, forming a new structure designated the precartilaginous primitive vertebra.
8. The arteries situated between the two older primitive segments become trapped within the middle of the new precartilaginous primitive vertebrae. The lower halves of the older primitive segments now abut the newly formed gaps between two newly formed adjacent precartilaginous primitive vertebrae and contribute the cells that form the anulus fibrosus of the intervertebral disc and the cartilaginous end plates.
9. The dermatomyotomes attach to adjacent vertebrae across the disc. The portion of the notochord within the gaps between adjacent primitive vertebrae expands and undergoes mucoid degeneration to form the nucleus pulposus.
10. Starting at 4 weeks of gestation, each vertebral unit develops from three separate mesenchymal centers: the single mesenchymal center of the centrum that will give rise to the vertebral body surrounding the notochord, the paired mesenchymal centers of the two neural processes that will give rise to the posterior bony neural arches, and the dorsal aspect of the vertebral body. Between 6 and 8 weeks, each mesenchymal vertebra becomes cartilaginous. Around the ninth week, these chondrification centers begin the ossification process.
11. After birth, there are three separate primary centers of ossification for each vertebral segment. These three centers, the two posterior neural processes and the centrum, are joined by the preossified cartilaginous neurocentral synchondrosis. At approximately 16 years of age, secondary centers of ossification form at the upper and lower surfaces of the vertebral bodies as well as the tips of the spinous process and two transverse processes. These secondary ossification centers generally fuse with the adjacent bone of the vertebrae by 25 years of age.

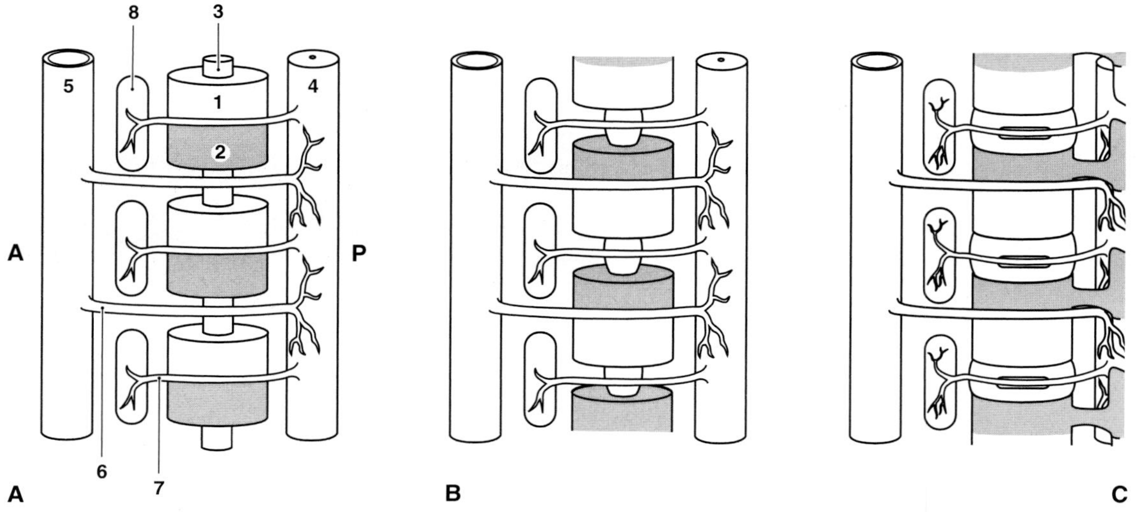

Figure 1-30: Lateral schematic of the progressive resegmentation of the spinal sclerotomes. **A:** Early. **B:** Intermediate. **C:** Final arrangement of the sclerotomes after resegmentation. *A*, anterior; *P*, posterior.

1 Cranial sclerotome
2 Caudal sclerotome
3 Notochord
4 Spinal cord
5 Aorta
6 Raduculomedullary artery
7 Spinal nerve
8 Perispinal muscle

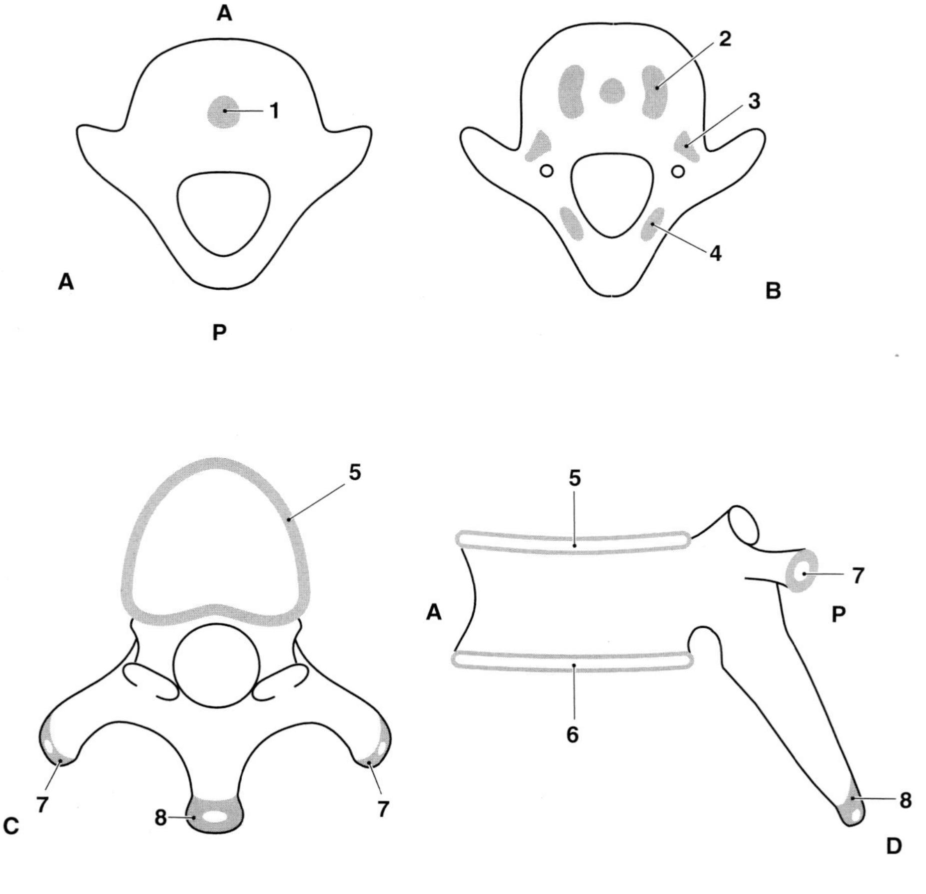

Figure 1-31: Schematics of the embryologic development of the vertebrae. **A:** Four-week-old embryo. **B:** Embryo at 6–8 weeks. **C, D:** A 16-year-old. **A–C:** Axial view. **D:** Sagittal view. *A*, anterior; *P*, posterior.

1 Early mesenchymal center of the centrum (primary ossification center)
2 Cartilaginous mesen-chymal center of the centrum (primary ossification center)
3 Neurocentral synchondrosis
4 Cartilaginous mesen-chymal center of the posterior neural processes (primary ossification center)
5 Secondary ossification center of the upper end plate of the vertebral body
6 Secondary ossification center of the lower end plate of the vertebral body
7 Secondary ossification center(s) of transverse processes
8 Secondary ossification center of spinous process

Embryologic Development of the Spinal Cord and Nerves

1. The cephalic portion of the spinal cord forms by the mechanism of *neurulation*. This process establishes the cervical and thoracic segments of the spinal cord and the upper portion of the lumbar cord up to the midlumbar segment. The more distal portions of the spinal cord and the filum terminalis are formed in a process called *canalization* and *retrogressive differentiation* of the caudal cell mass.
2. The undifferentiated caudal cell mass of the primitive streak is found caudal to the posterior neuropore and extends to the tail fold under an intact covering of cutaneous ectoderm. The caudal cell mass develops vacuoles around which the cells assume a neural appearance. Subsequently, these vacuoles coalesce to form the distal part of the neural tube, which then fuses with the rostral neural tube that is simultaneously undergoing formation by neurulation. The transient ventriculus terminalis, which marks the level of the future conus medullaris, becomes identifiable by day 43 to 48 of gestation. This process of canalization of the caudal cell mass is less precise than that of neurulation.
3. The walls of the neural tube consist of neuroepithelial cells. These cells extend through the entire thickness of the wall. Collectively, these cells are referred to as the neuroepithelial layer or neuroepithelium.
4. After neural tube closure, the neuroepithelial cells give rise to neuroblasts. These neuroblasts form a zone around the neuroepithelial layer known as the mantle layer. The mantle layer will eventually form the gray matter of spinal cord. The mantle layer has ventral and dorsal areas of thickening (horns)—the basal plates and alar plates—that will form the motor and sensory areas, respectively. Between these two areas in the thoracic and upper lumbar levels there is also a small intermediate horn that contains a part of the sympathetic portion of the autonomic nervous system.
5. The outermost layer of the spinal cord contains the nerve fibers emerging from the neuroblasts in the mantle layer. It is known as the marginal layer. The marginal layer will form the white matter of the spinal cord.
6. The neural crest forms the sensory ganglia (dorsal root ganglia) on each side of the neural tube. During further development, the neuroblasts (eventual dorsal root neurons) from the sensory ganglia form two processes—proximal and distal. These two processes are known as the dorsal sensory root of the spinal nerve. The proximal process penetrates the dorsal portion of the neural tube and will either connect with the dorsal horn or ascend through the marginal layer to one of the higher brain centers. The distal process will join the fibers of the ventral motor root and thus participate in the formation of the trunk of the spinal nerve. Eventually, these distal processes terminate in the sensory receptor organs.
7. Around the third month of gestation, the spinal cord extends the entire length of the developing spinal column. However, during further development, the vertebral column and the dura lengthen more rapidly than the spinal cord, with the result that the terminal end of the cord gradually shifts to a higher spinal segment level. At birth, this end is located at the level of the third lumbar vertebra. Because of this disproportionate growth, the lower spinal nerves descend obliquely from their segment of origin in the spinal cord to the corresponding level of the vertebral column. The terminal dura remains attached to the vertebral column at the coccygeal level.
8. In the adult, the spinal cord terminates at the L-1 level. Below this point the CNS is represented only by the filum terminate, which marks the tract of regression of the terminal spinal cord.

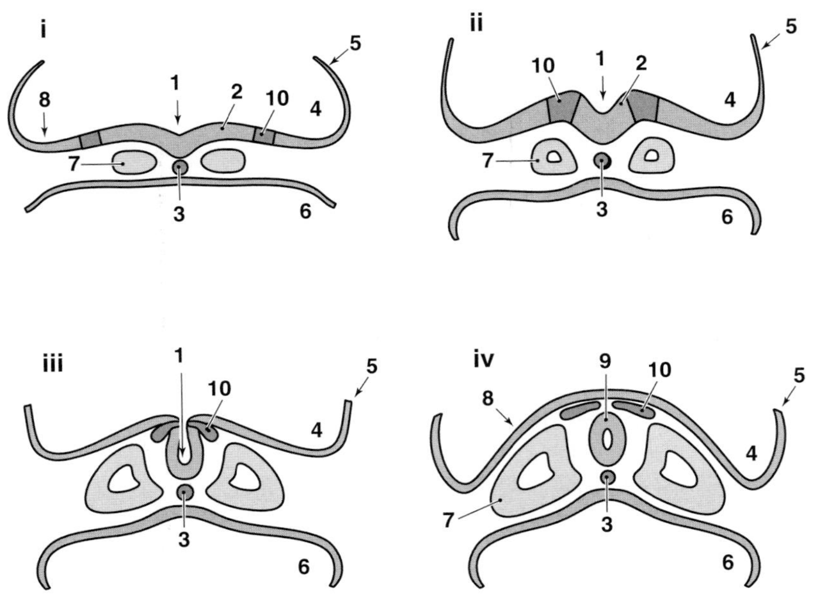

A

Figure 1-32A: Axial cross-sectional schematic of the embryologic development of the neural tube.
i Transverse schematic of an embryo at day 18 of gestation
ii Transverse schematic of an embryo between 18 and 22 days' gestation
iii Transverse schematic of an embryo between 18 and 22 days' gestation
iv Transverse schematic of an embryo at day 28 of gestation
1 Neural groove
2 Neural ectoderm
3 Notochord
4 Amniotic cavity
5 Amnion
6 Yolk sac
7 Embryonic mesoderm
8 Surface ectoderm
9 Neural tube
10 Neural crest

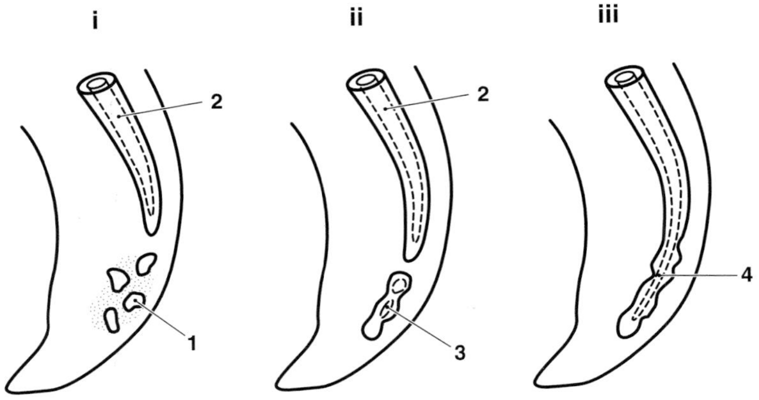

B

Figure 1-32B: Sagittal schematic of the embryologic development of the caudal cell mass (28–48 days' gestation).
1 Primitive caudal cell mass
2 Neural tube
3 Coalition and vacuolation of the caudal cell mass
4 Fusion between the neural tube and the vacuolated caudal cell mass

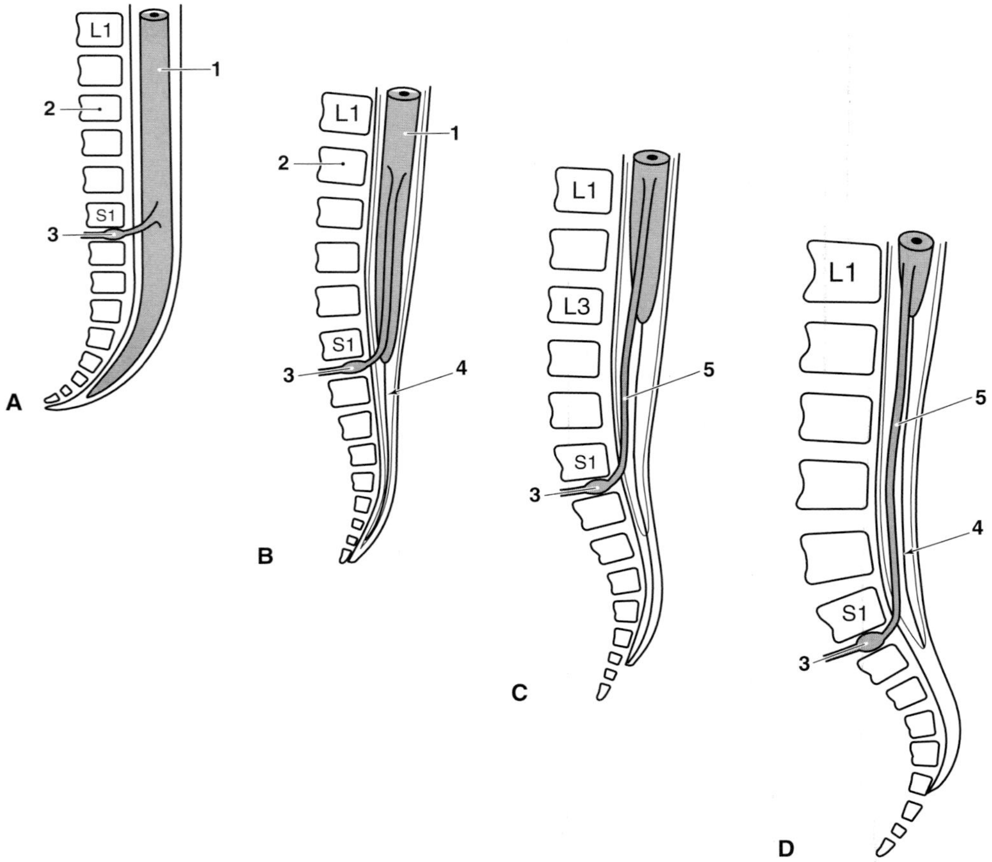

Figure 1-33: Sagittal schematic of the development and spatial relationship of the spinal cord and spinal column. **A:** The spinal column and cord of a 3-month embryo. Note neural segmental level of the spinal cord and the spinal column segmental level are approximately the same. **B:** The spinal column and cord of a 5-month embryo. Note the spinal cord termination at the S-1 spinal column segmental level and the elongation of the S-1 nerve root. **C:** The spinal column and cord of a newborn infant. Note the spinal cord termination at the L3 spinal column segmental level and the progressive elongation of the S-1 nerve root. **D:** The spinal column and cord level of termination (approximately L-1) from age 2 years onward.

1 Spinal cord
2 Vertebral body
3 S-1 nerve root
4 Filum terminate
5 Cauda equina

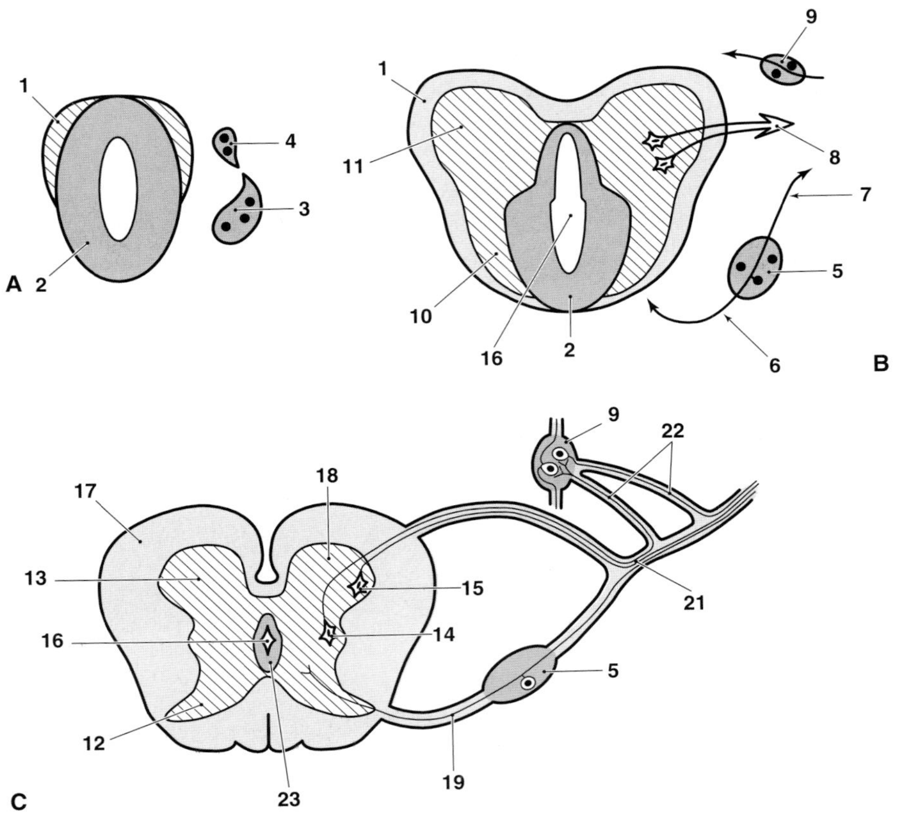

Figure 1-34: Axial schematic of the embryologic development of gray and white matter of the spinal cord and spinal nerves. **A:** Migration of neuroblast from matrix layer to mantle layer. **B:** Formation of marginal layer. **C:** Formation of mixed (sensory and motor) spinal nerve.

1 Marginal layer
2 Mantle layer
3 Dorsal root ganglion primordium
4 Sympathetic ganglion primordium
5 Dorsal root ganglion
6 Central axonal process of dorsal spinal nerve root
7 Distal axonal process of dorsal spinal nerve root
8 Ventral spinal nerve root
9 Paravertebral sympathetic ganglion
10 Alar plate of mantle layer
11 Basal plate of mantle layer
12 Sensory area (dorsal horn)
13 Motor area (ventral horn)
14 Intermediolateral cell
15 Motor neuron
16 Central canal of spinal cord
17 White matter
18 Gray matter
19 Dorsal nerve root
20 Ventral nerve root
21 Spinal nerve
22 Gray and white rami communicantes
23 Ependymal cells

EMBRYOLOGY OF THE PITUITARY GLAND

1. The hypophysis develops from two completely different origins—one from an ectodermal outpocketing of the stomodeum in front of the buccopharyngeal membrane known as Rathke's pouch and the other from a downward extension of the diencephalon, the infundibulum.
2. At 3 weeks of gestation, Rathke's pouch is seen as an invagination of the stomodeum and grows dorsally as the budding diencephalic infundibulum grows ventrally.
3. In approximately the second month, Rathke's pouch loses its connection with the oral cavity. The anterior wall of Rathke's pouch will form the anterior lobe of the hypophysis (*adenohypophysis*). The posterior wall will develop the *pars intermedia*.
4. Occasionally, a small ectopic part of Rathke's pouch called the "ectopic pharyngeal hypophysis" persists in the pharyngeal wall; persistence of an ectopic osseous part of Rathke's pouch (i.e., sphenoid bone) results in intraosseous accessory anterior pituitary lobe tissue. Ectopic pituitary tissue can also be displaced into the developing sphenoid sinus (i.e., "ectopic intrasphenoid hypophysis").
5. The infundibulum will form the median eminence, the pituitary stalk, and the posterior lobe of the hypophysis (*neurohypophysis*).

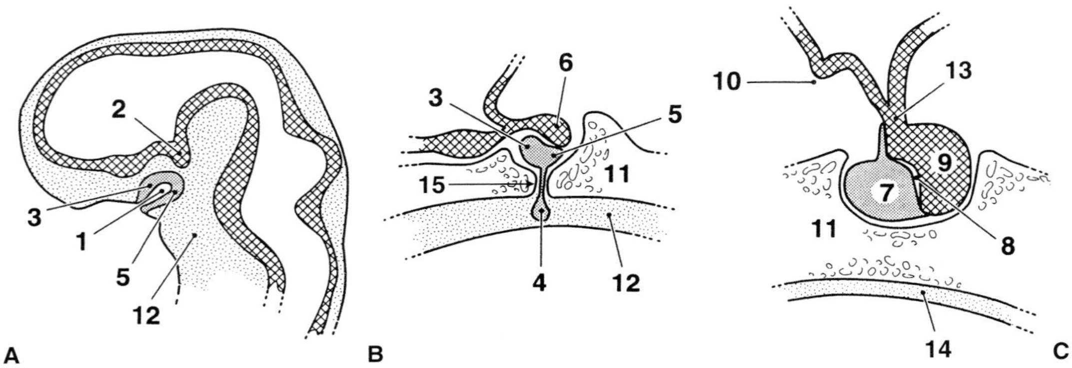

Figure 1-35: Embryologic development of the pituitary gland. **A:** Sagittal schematic of a 6-week embryo. **B:** Sagittal schematic of an 11-week embryo. **C:** Sagittal schematic of a 16-week embryo.

1 Rathke's (hypophyseal) pouch
2 Budding pituitary infundibulum
3 Anterior wall of Rathke's pouch
4 Pharyngeal hypophysis (temporary)
5 Posterior wall of Rathke's pouch
6 Expanding pituitary infundibulum
7 Anterior lobe of the hypophysis (adenohypophysis)
8 Pars intermedia
9 Posterior lobe of hypophysis (neurohypophysis)
10 Optic chiasm
11 Sphenoid bone
12 Endoderm
13 Mature pituitary infundibulum
14 Pharyngeal mucosa
15 Pathway of regressed Rathke's pouch (craniopharyngeal canal)

EMBRYOLOGIC DEVELOPMENT OF THE AUDITORY APPARATUS

1. The ear consists of three parts of different origin: the internal ear, the middle ear, and the external ear.
2. The internal ear originates from the otic vesicle, which in the fourth week of gestation splits off from the surface ectoderm.
3. The otic vesicle divides into a ventral component, which gives rise to the saccule and the cochlear duct, and a dorsal component, which gives rise to the utricle, semicircular canal, and endolymphatic duct. These epithelial structures are known collectively as the membranous labyrinth.
4. The middle ear, consisting of the tympanic cavity and auditory tube, is lined with epithelium of endodermal origin, as is derived from the first pharyngeal pouch.
5. The ossicles are derived from the first (malleus and incus) and second (stapes) pharyngeal arches. As the tympanic cavity expands, it gradually envelops the ossicles.
6. The mastoid antrum is also derived from an expansion of the tympanic cavity. Pneumatization occurs after birth.
7. The external auditory canal develops from the first pharyngeal cleft and is separated from the tympanic cavity by the tympanic membrane. The ectodermal cells in the bottom of this funnel-shaped tube proliferate and form a meatal plug, which later degenerates to produce a cavity.
8. The external tympanic membrane has an external covering derived from ectoderm, an internal covering derived from endoderm, and an intermediate layer of mesenchyme.
9. The auricle develops from mesenchymal enlargements.

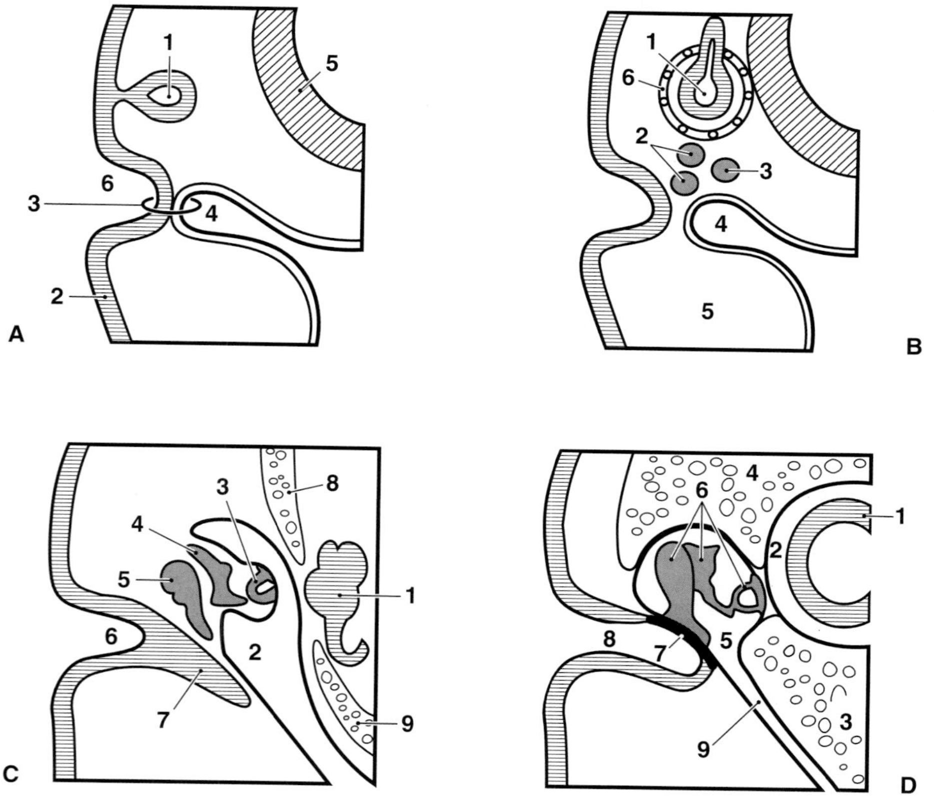

Figure 1-36: Frontal schematic representation of the embryologic development of the middle and internal ear on the right.

A: Frontal schematic of a 4-week embryo.
1 Otic vesicle
2 Ectoderm
3 First branchial membrane
4 First pharyngeal pouch
5 Wall of hindbrain
6 First branchial groove

B: Frontal schematic of a 5-week embryo.
1 Otic vesicle
2 Derives from the first pharyngeal arch cartilage (precursors of malleus and incus)
3 Derives from the second pharyngeal arch cartilage (precursor of stapes)
4 Tubotympanic recess
5 Second branchial arch
6 Condensing mesenchyme

C: Frontal schematic depicting the tubotympanic recess enveloping the ossicles.
1 Otic vesicle
2 Tympanic cavity
3 Stapes
4 Incus
5 Malleus
6 Primitive external acoustic meatus
7 Meatal plug
8 Squamous temporal bone
9 Petrous temporal bone

D: Frontal schematic depicting the final stages of the development of the ear.
1 Membranous labyrinth
2 Perilymphatic space
3 Petrous temporal bone
4 Squamous temporal bone
5 Tympanic cavity
6 Ossicles
7 Tympanic membrane
8 External acoustic canal
9 Endolymphatic duct

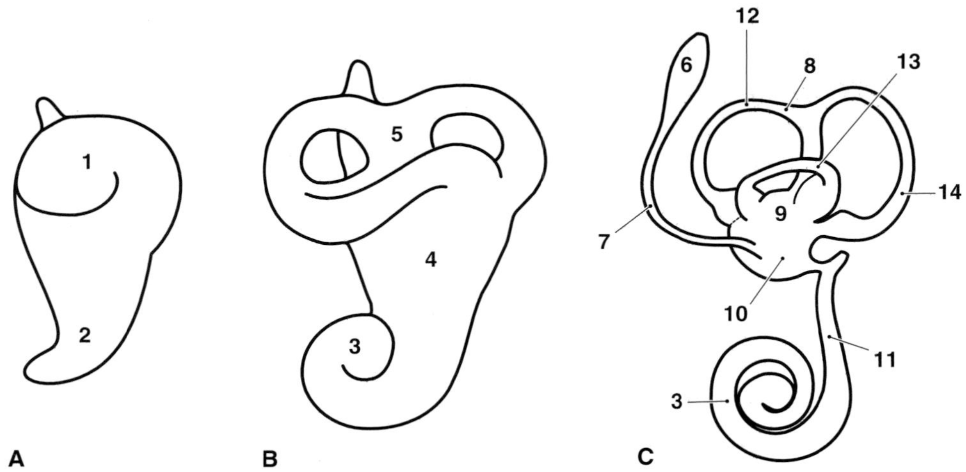

Figure 1-37: Schematic depicting the embryologic development of the otocyst at 6 weeks **(A)**, 7 weeks **(B)**, 8 weeks **(C)** of gestation, forming the internal ear.

1 Utricular portion of otic vesicle
2 Saccular portion of otic vesicle
3 Cochlea
4 Saccule
5 Developing semicircular canals
6 Endolymphatic sac
7 Endolymphatic duct
8 Semicircular duct
9 Utricule
10 Saccule
11 Cochlear duct
12 Lateral semicircular canal
13 Superior semicircular canal
14 Posterior semicircular canal

EMBRYOLOGIC DEVELOPMENT OF THE VISUAL APPARATUS

1. The neural ectoderm of the forebrain will form the retina, iris, and optic nerve.
2. The surface ectoderm of the head will form the lens, and the surrounding mesoderm will create the vascular and fibrous coats of the globes.
3. At the fourth week of gestation, the optic sulci appear in the neural fold at the cranial end of the embryo. When the forebrain vesicle is formed, the optic sulci evaginate to shape the optic vesicle on each side of the forebrain.
4. The surface ectoderm adjacent to the optic vesicle thickens to form the lens placode.
5. As the optic vesicles grow laterally, their distal ends expand. Their connections with the forebrain are hollow and are termed the optic stalks.
6. Concomitantly, the distal portion of the optic vesicle invaginates and becomes a double-walled structure called the optic cup.
7. The wall of the optic cup will develop into the retina and the anterior part of the optic cup will form the iris.
8. The central region of each lens placode soon invaginates and sinks deep to the surface to form the lens pit.
9. The edges of the lens pit gradually approach each other and fuse to form the lens vesicle, which soon detaches from the surface (cutaneous) ectoderm. The lens vesicle develops into the lens.
10. Linear grooves called choroid fissures evolve on the ventral surface of the optic cups and along the optic stalk.
11. The optic fissure contains the hyaloid artery and the hyaloid vein.
12. The surface layer of the retina has axons that connect directly with the brain in the wall of the optic stalk.
13. The cavity (lumen) within the optic stalk subsequently involutes. Many of the axons within the optic stalk eventually form the mature optic nerve.

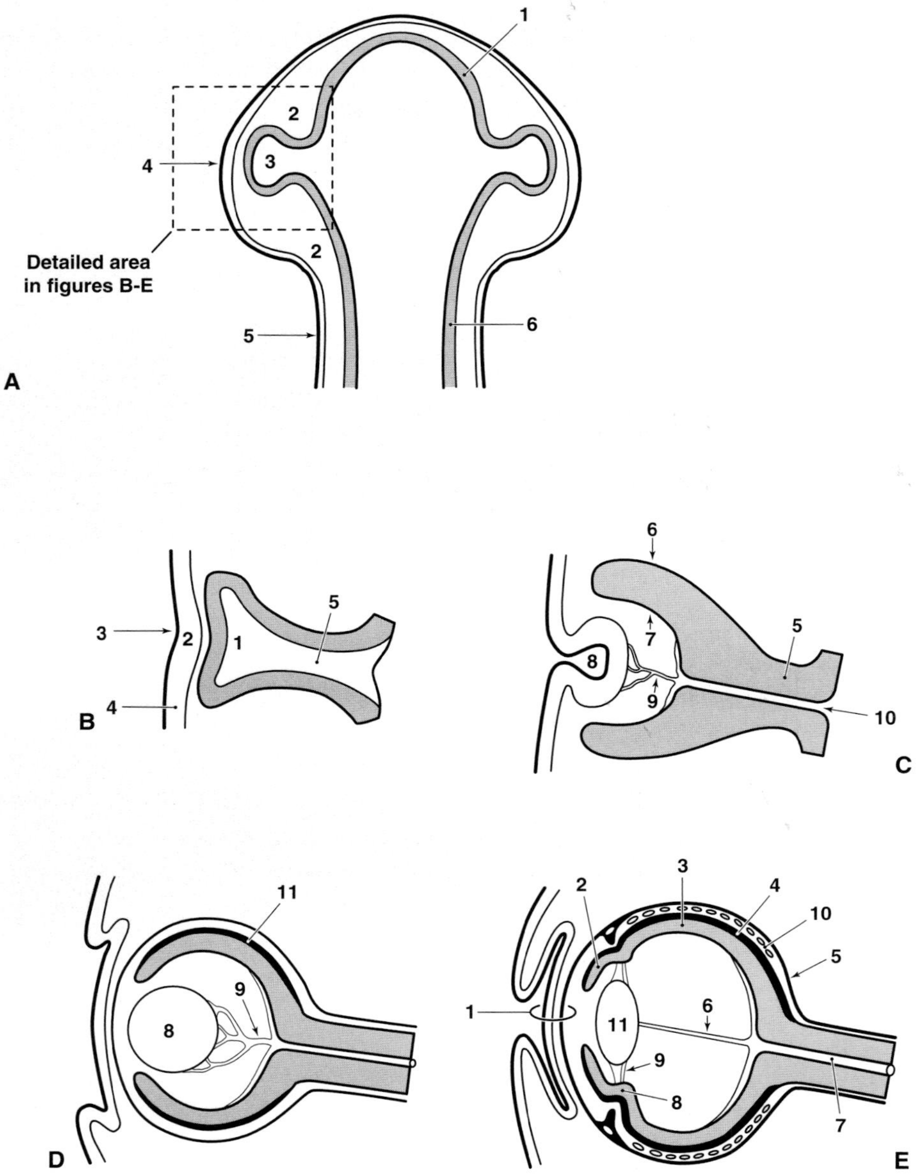

Figure 1-38: Embryologic development of the eye.

A: Coronal schematic of the forebrain at 28 days' gestation.
1 Forebrain
2 Mesenchyme
3 Optic vesicle
4 Placode
5 Surface ectoderm
6 Midbrain

B–D: Sagittal schematics depicting successive development of the optic vesicle and lens placode.
1 Optic cup
2 Lens placode
3 Lens pit
4 Surface ectoderm
5 Optic stalk
6 Outer layer of optic cup
7 Inner layer of the optic cup
8 Lens vesicle
9 Hyaloid artery
10 Lumen of optic stalk
11 Intraretinal space

E: Sagittal schematic of the newborn (mature) eye.
1 Cornea
2 Iris
3 Neural layer of retina
4 Pigmented layer of retina
5 Sclera
6 Hyaloid canal
7 Central artery of retina
8 Ciliary body
9 Suspensory ligament
10 Choroid
11 Lens

TABLE 1-2: Embryonic Sources of Adult Ocular Structures

Embryonic sources	Adult structures
Neural ectoderm of forebrain	Retina, iris, optic nerve
Mesoderm	Vascular and fibrous coats of the globe
Surface ectoderm of the anterior cranium	Lens

EMBRYOLOGIC DEVELOPMENT OF THE PARANASAL SINUSES

1. The paranasal sinuses are derived from ectoderm and originate as outpouchings or diverticula from the walls of the nasal cavities.
2. These sinuses become air-filled extensions into the craniofacial bones for which they are named, including the frontal, ethmoid, maxillary, and sphenoid sinuses.

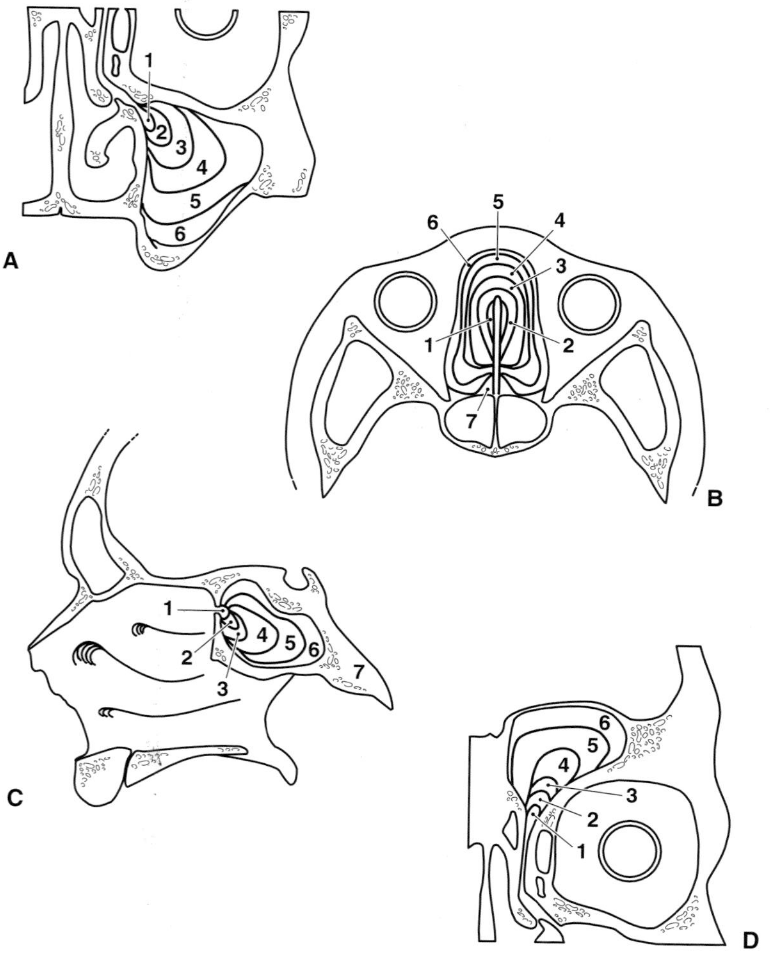

Figure 1-39: Embryologic development of the paranasal sinuses.
A: Coronal schematic showing the temporal and morphologic changes that occur from birth to maturity in the aeration of the paranasal sinuses.
1 Newborn
2 One year
3 Four years
4 Seven years
5 Twelve years
6 Adult
B: Axial schematic showing the morphologic changes from birth to maturity in the aeration of the ethmoid sinuses.
1 Newborn
2 Three years
3 Five years
4 Seven years
5 Twelve years
6 Adult
7 Spheno-ethmoidal recess
C: Sagittal schematic showing the morphologic changes that occur in the aeration of the sphenoidal sinus from birth to maturity.
1 Newborn
2 Three years
3 Five years
4 Seven years
5 Twelve years
6 Adult
7 Sphenoid bone
D: Coronal schematic showing the morphologic changes that occur from birth to maturity in the aeration of the frontal sinuses.
1 Newborn
2 One year
3 Four years
4 Seven years
5 Twelve years
6 Adult

TABLE 1-3: Developmental Aeration of the Paranasal Sinuses

Paranasal sinus	Onset of development	Adult configuration
Maxillary	Third month of gestation	12 years of age
Sphenoid	Fourth month of gestation	Puberty
Ethmoid	Fifth month of gestation	Puberty
Frontal	After birth	Adulthood

EMBRYOLOGY OF THE NECK AND FACE

Overview

1. Mesenchyme forming the tissues of the neck is derived from three main sources: the lateral plate mesoderm, the neural crest, and the ectodermal placodes.
   a. The lateral plate mesoderm forms the laryngeal cartilages and regional connective tissue.
   b. Neural crest cells from the forebrain, midbrain, and hindbrain migrate ventrally and rostrally to shape the midface and pharyngeal arch skeletal structures and the remaining regional tissues, including bone, cartilage, teeth, tendons, skin, meninges, glandular stroma, and some neuronal tissue.
   c. Ectodermal placodes give rise to the neurons of the fifth, seventh, ninth, and tenth cranial nerve ganglia.
2. The pharyngeal pouches are a number of outpocketings that arise from the pharyngeal gut, the most cranial portion of the foregut. These pouches partially penetrate the overlying mesenchymal tissue but do not open externally.
3. The pharyngeal (branchial) arches consist of bars of mesenchymal tissue that are separated by deep clefts known as branchial (pharyngeal) clefts.
4. The pharyngeal arches then give rise to five mesenchymal prominences: the mandibular prominences (branchial arches 1 and 2), the maxillary prominences (branchial arches 3 and 4), the frontonasal prominence (branchial arch number 5).
5. The face is subsequently further formed by the appearance of the nasal prominences.
6. The center of the face is formed by the stomodeum.

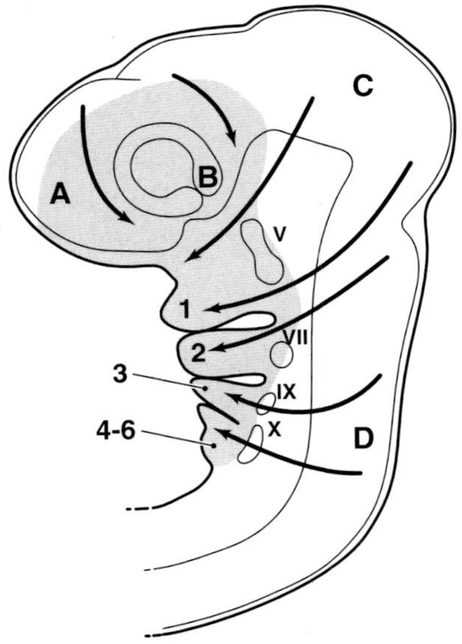

Figure 1-40: Sagittal schematic of the migration pathways (*arrows*) of neural crest cells from fore-, mid-, and hindbrain regions into their final location (*shaded areas*) in the areas of the pharyngeal arches (*1–6*) and face. Note also the regions of ectodermal thickening (placodes) that assist in the formation of the lens of the globe and the fifth (V), seventh (VII), ninth (IX), and tenth (X) cranial sensory ganglia (ovals). *A*, forebrain; *B*, lens placode; *C*, midbrain; *D*, hindbrain.

Specifics of the Embryologic Development of the Neck

The Pharyngeal Arches

1. The early human embryo has five pharyngeal arches: I, II, III, IV, and VI. The fourth and sixth arches partially fuse during development to form a combined fourth pharyngeal arch (IV).
2. Each pharyngeal arch is made up of an inner epithelium of endodermal origin, a central core of mesenchymal tissue, and an outer epithelium of ectoderm.
3. Each pharyngeal arch also has a component of neural crest cells that migrate into the core of the arch.
4. Each pharyngeal arch is alternately characterized by its own skeletal, muscular, neural, and vascular components and derivatives.

TABLE 1-4: Derivatives of the Pharyngeal Arches (I–IV)

Pharyngeal arch	Cranial nerve	Muscles	Skeletal structures
I. Mandibular	V. Trigeminal nerve: mandibular division	Muscles of mastication (temporal, masseter, medial and lateral pterygoid muscles); mylohyoid, anterior belly of digastric muscles, tensor palatine and tensor tympani muscles	Incus, malleus, anterior ligament of the malleus, sphenomandibular ligament, parts of the mandible and temporal and zygomatic bones, maxilla
II. Hyoid	VII. Facial nerve	Muscles of facial expression (buccinator, auricularis, frontalis, platysma, orbicularis oris and oculi muscles), posterior belly of digastric, stylohyoid, stapedius muscles	Stapes, styloid process, stylohyoid ligament, lesser horn and upper portion of the body of the hyoid bone
III.	IX. Glossopharyngeal nerve	Stylopharyngeus muscle, possibly the upper pharyngeal constrictors	Greater horn and lower portion of the body of the hyoid bone
IV.	X. Vagus nerve: superior laryngeal branch	Cricothyroid, levator palatini muscles, constrictors of the pharynx	Most of the laryngeal cartilages (thyroid, arytenoid, corniculate, and cuneiform)
	X. Vagus nerve: recurrent laryngeal branch	Intrinsic muscles of the larynx	Remaining laryngeal cartilage (cricoid)

Modified from Sadler TW. *Langman's Medical Embryology*. Baltimore: Williams & Wilkins, 1990.

The Pharyngeal Pouches

1. The human embryo has five paired pharyngeal pouches (I–V). The fifth pharyngeal pouch is usually considered part of the fourth in discussions of this topic.
2. The endodermal lining of the pharyngeal pouches gives rise to several structures and organs, including the middle ear cavity, the eustachian tube, part of the tympanic membrane, the palatine tonsil, the parathyroid glands, the thymus, and the ultimobranchial body—the latter being part of the thyroid gland, which contains the parafollicular or "C" cells that secrete calcitonin.

TABLE 1-5: The Pharyngeal Pouches and their Derivatives

Pharyngeal pouch	Structures derived
I	Middle ear cavity, eustachian tube, tympanic membrane
II	Palatine tonsil, tonsillar fossa
III	Inferior parathyroid glands, thymus
IV	Superior parathyroid glands
V	Ultimobranchial body (part of thyroid gland giving rise to parafollicular or C cells)

The Pharyngeal Clefts

1. The human embryo has four paired pharyngeal clefts.
2. The first cleft gives rise to the external auditory meatus and, with the first pharyngeal pouch, contributes to the formation of the tympanic membrane.
3. Proliferation of mesenchymal cells in the second pharyngeal arch results in an overgrowth of tissue covering over the third and fourth pharyngeal arches, which subsequently fuse with the epicardial ridge. This causes the second, third, and fourth pharyngeal clefts to lose external contact. These clefts form a temporary cavity, the cervical sinus, that normally disappears with further development of this region.

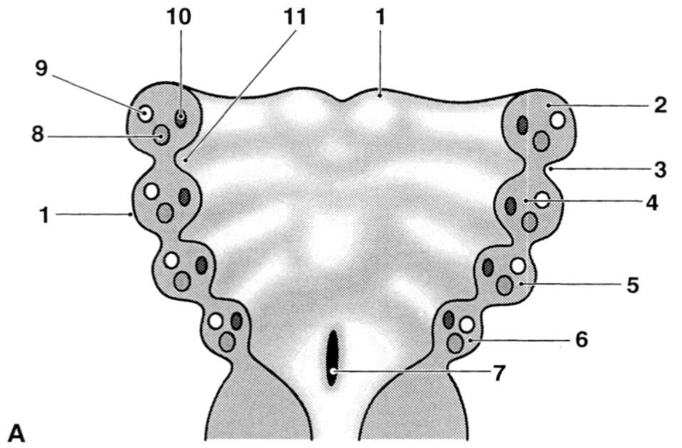

Figure 1-41A: Coronal schematic of the embryonic pharyngeal arches at a very early stage of development. Each arch contains a cartilaginous component, a nerve, an artery, and a muscular component.

1 Endodermal epithelium
2 First pharyngeal arch
3 Pharyngeal cleft
4 Second pharyngeal arch
5 Third pharyngeal arch
6 Fourth pharyngeal arch
7 Laryngeal orifice
8 Cartilage
9 Nerve
10 Artery
11 Pharyngeal pouch

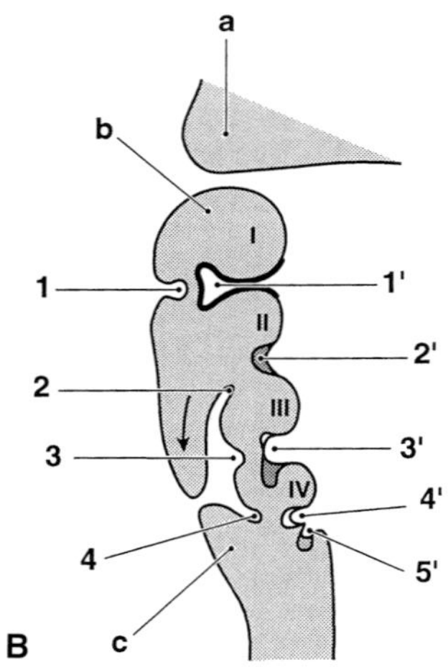

Figure 1-41B: Coronal schematic of the development of the embryonic pharyngeal clefts and pouches on the right at a later stage than that of Fig. 1-41A. Note that the second arch has grown over the third and fourth arches (*arrow*), covering over the second, third, and fourth pharyngeal clefts.

a. Maxillary process
b. Mandibular process
c. Epicardial ridge
1–4: Pharyngeal clefts
I–IV: Pharyngeal arches
1′–5′: Pharyngeal pouches

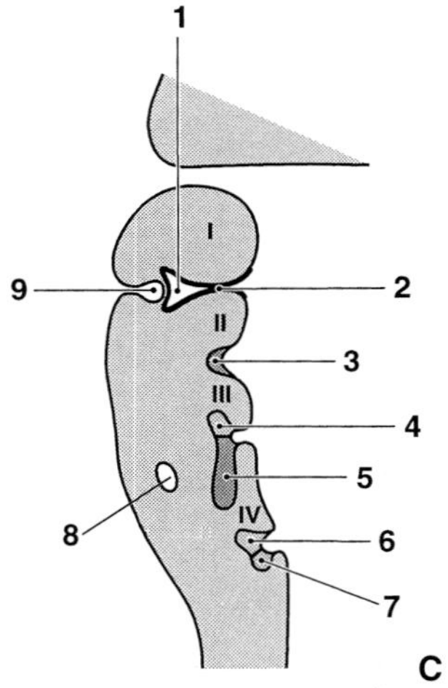

Figure 1-41C: Coronal schematic still later in development than shown in Fig. 1-41B. The remnants of the second, third, and fourth pharyngeal clefts form the transient cervical sinus. Note the neck structures eventually formed by the various pharyngeal pouches.

1 Primary tympanic cavity
2 Auditory (eustachian) tube
3 Palatine tonsil
4 Parathyroid gland (inferior)
5 Thymus
6 Parathyroid gland (superior)
7 Ultimobranchial body
8 Cervical sinus
9 External auditory meatus

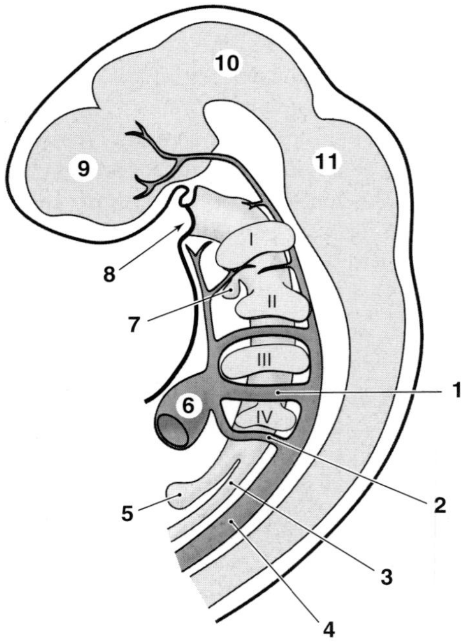

Figure 1-42: Sagittal schematic of the embryonic pharyngeal pouches (I–IV) as outpocketings of the foregut. Note also the primordium of the thyroid gland and the developing aortic arches.
I–IV: Pharyngeal pouches
1 Fourth aortic arch
2 Sixth aortic arch
3 Esophagus
4 Dorsal aorta
5 Trachea and lung bud
6 Aortic sac
7 Thyroid primordium
8 Stomodeum
9 Forebrain
10 Midbrain
11 Hindbrain

Embryologic Development of the Tongue

1. The tongue develops from the pharyngeal arches in the form of several swellings.
   a. There are two lateral lingual swellings and a first medial swelling, the tuberculum impar, originating from the first pharyngeal arch.
   b. A second median swelling, the copula or hypobranchial eminence, originates from the second, third, and fourth pharyngeal arches.
   c. A third median swelling gives rise to the epiglottis evolving from the fourth pharyngeal arch.
2. The anterior two-thirds, or body, of the tongue arises from the first pharyngeal arch, while the root of the tongue originates from the second, third, and fourth pharyngeal arches.

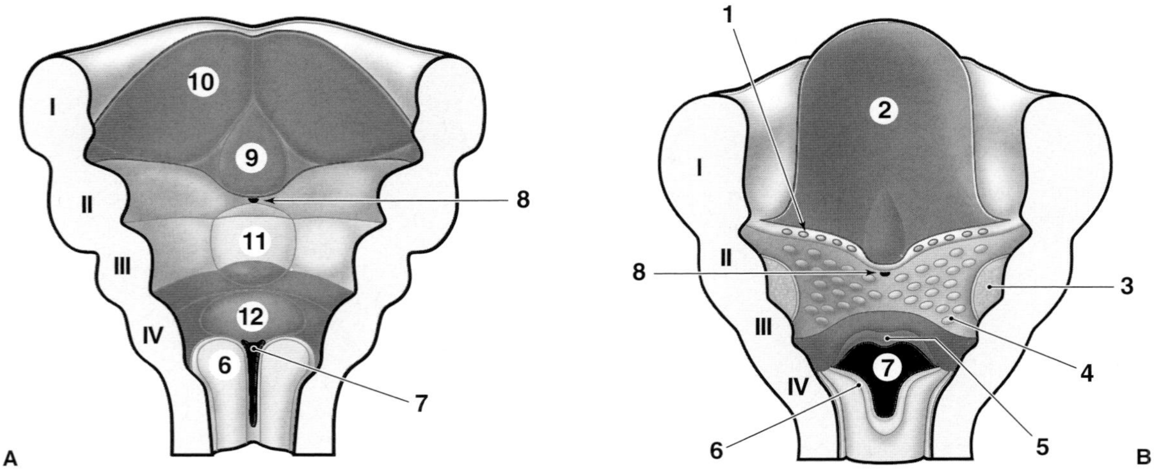

Figure 1-43: Coronal schematic of the ventral portions of the embryonic pharyngeal arches as seen from above, to show development of the tongue. The cut surfaces of the pharyngeal arches are indicated by numbers I to IV. **A:** Five-week embryo. **B:** Five-month embryo.

1 Terminal sulcus
2 Body of tongue
3 Palatine tonsil
4 Root of tongue
5 Epiglottis
6 Arytenoid swellings
7 Laryngeal orifice
8 Foramen cecum
9 Tuberculum impar
10 Lateral lingual swelling
11 Copula (hypobranchial eminence)
12 Epiglottal swelling

Development of the Thyroid Gland

1. The thyroid gland develops from an epithelial proliferation in the floor of the primitive pharynx between the developing tuberculum impar and copula (see Development of the Tongue). This point of origin will later become the foramen cecum.
2. The thyroid tissue then begins a descent in the neck anterior to the pharynx. During migration, the thyroid tissue maintains its connection to the tongue (foramen cecum) via the transient thyroglossal duct.
3. The thyroid tissue eventually descends to its final position anterior to the upper trachea. It assumes its definitive configuration as the mature thyroid gland with two lateral lobes connected by a narrow median isthmus.

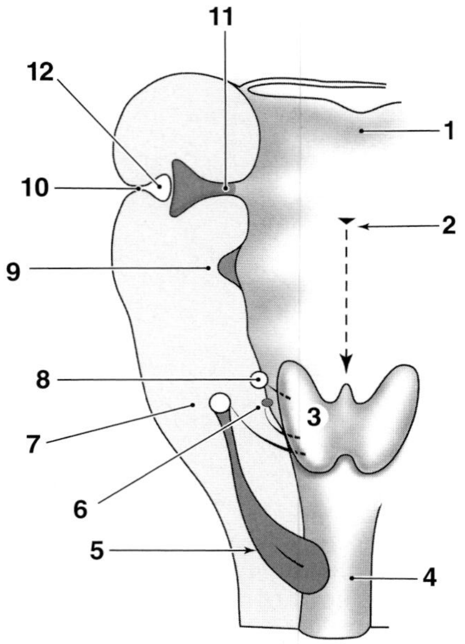

Figure 1-44: Coronal schematic showing embryonic migration of the thyroid gland, thymus, and parathyroid glands (*dashed arrow*). The thyroid gland originates at the level of the foramen cecum in the tongue and descends to the level of the first tracheal rings.

1 Ventral aspect of pharynx
2 Foramen cecum
3 Thyroid gland
4 Foregut
5 Thymus
6 Ultimobranchial body
7 Inferior parathyroid gland (from third pouch)
8 Superior parathyroid gland (from fourth pouch)
9 Palatine tonsil
10 External auditory canal
11 Auditory (eustachian) tube
12 Primary (early) tympanic cavity

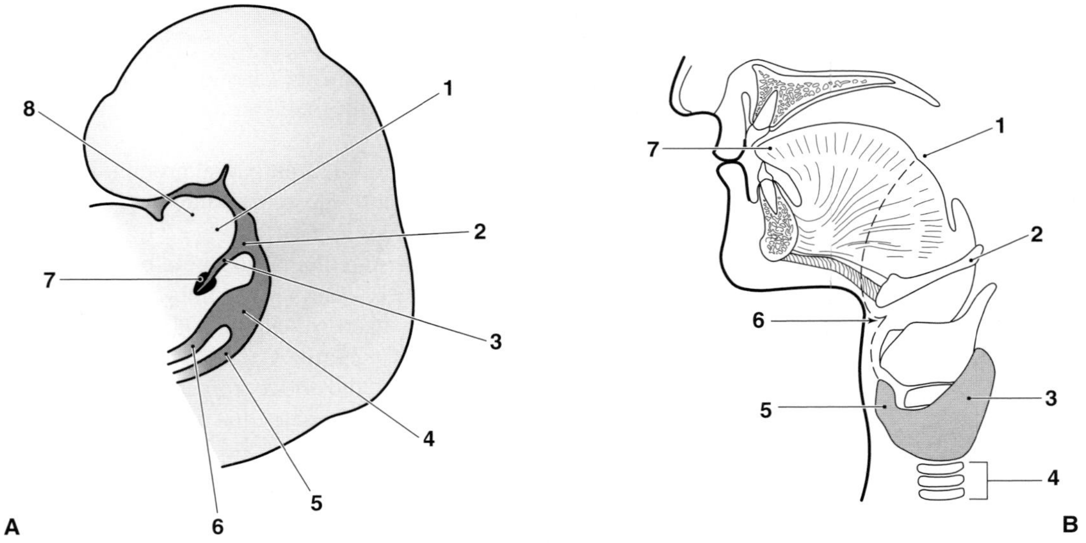

Figure 1-45: The normal development of the thyroid gland.
A: Sagittal schematic of early thyroid gland development. The thyroid primordium arises as an epithelial diverticulum in the middle of the pharynx immediately caudal to the tuberculum impar.
1 Tuberculum impar
2 Foramen cecum
3 Thyroglossal duct
4 Pharyngeal gut
5 Esophagus
6 Trachea
7 Thyroid gland primordium
8 Primitive tongue
B: Sagittal schematic of the position of the thyroid gland in the adult as related to regional structures of the neck. The *dashed line* indicates the downward path of migration of thyroid tissue.
1 Foramen cecum
2 Hyoid bone
3 Thyroid gland
4 Upper tracheal rings
5 Pyramidal lobe of thyroid gland (inconstant)
6 Migratory path of thyroid gland (*dashed line*)
7 Tongue

Embryologic Development of the Face

1. The face is formed initially from pairs of facial prominences arising from the pharyngeal arches that surround the primitive stomodeum: the facial prominences, the maxillary prominences, and the frontonasal prominence.
2. The nasal (olfactory) placodes form on either side of the frontonasal prominence from surface ectoderm. These nasal placodes subsequently invaginate into nasal pits. The lateral and medial nasal prominences border the nasal pits.
3. The nasolacrimal groove initially separates the maxillary and lateral nasal prominences. A solid epithelial cord is formed from the ectoderm in the floor of this groove, which eventually canalizes to give rise to the nasolacrimal duct and lacrimal sac.
4. The maxillary prominences give rise to the cheeks and maxillae.
5. The nose develops from five facial prominences: (a) the bridge from the frontal prominences, (b) the crest and tip of the nose from the two fused medial nasal prominences, and (c) the alae (sides) from the paired lateral nasal prominences.
6. The intermaxillary segment emerges from the fusion of the maxillary and medial nasal prominences. The intermaxillary segment consists of the following.
   a. A labial component forms the philtrum of the upper lip.
   b. An upper jaw component gives rise to the four incisor teeth.
   c. A palatal component forms the primary palate.
7. The secondary palate arises from two extensions of the maxillary prominences, the palatine shelves. These two shelves ascend and fuse to form the secondary palate. The palatine shelves further fuse with the primary palate; the incisive foramen and transient incisive suture are the midline landmarks between the primary and secondary palates.
8. The nasal cavities form initially from a deepening of the nasal pits. A rupture of the oronasal membrane, temporarily separating the exterior from the oral cavity, results in the formation of the paired primitive choanae. With further development of the nasal chambers, the definitive choanae form at the junction of the nasal cavity and pharynx.
9. The paranasal sinuses arise as diverticula from the lateral nasal wall. These sinuses are named for the maxillary, ethmoid, frontal, and sphenoid bones in which they form.

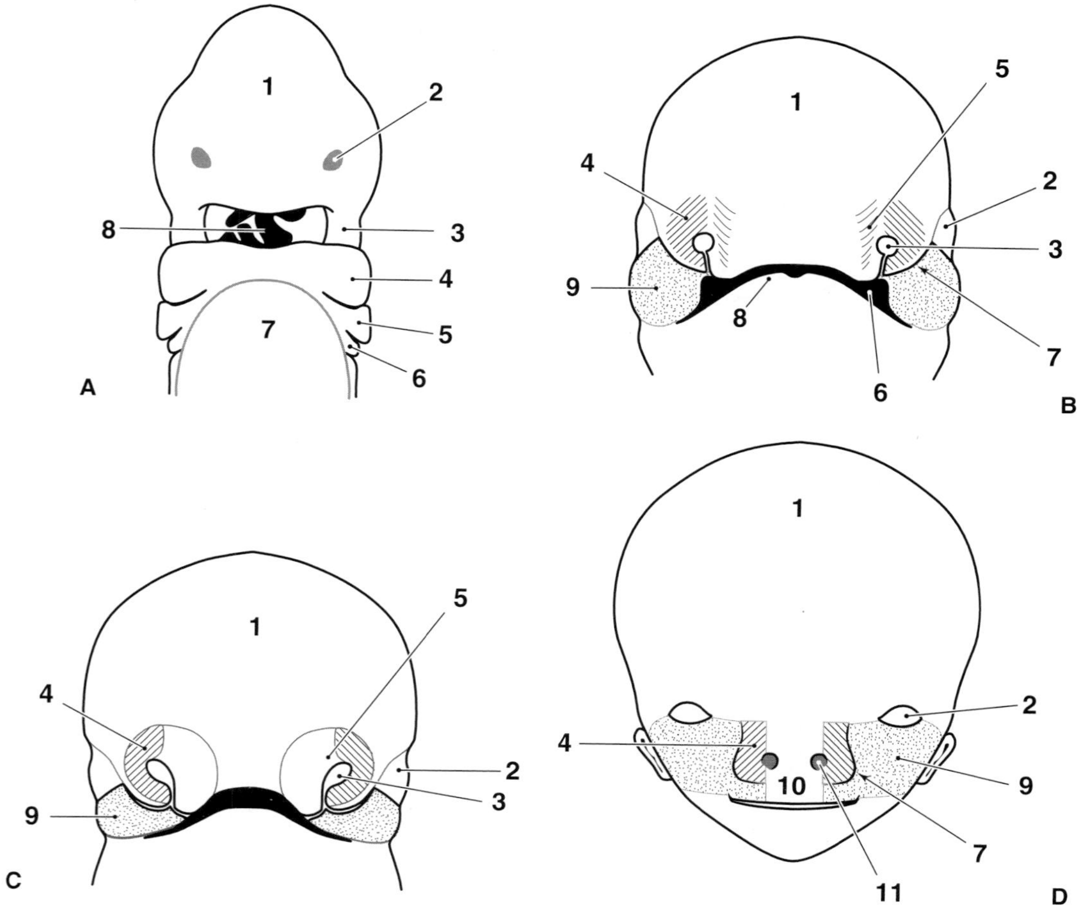

Figure 1-46: Frontal schematics showing the embryologic development of the face.
A: Embryo at 4½ weeks.
1 Frontonasal prominence
2 Nasal placode
3 Maxillary prominence
4 Mandibular prominence
5 Second pharyngeal arches
6 Third pharyngeal arches
7 Cardiac bulge
8 Stomodeum
B: Five-week embryo.
C: Six-week embryo.
D: Ten-week embryo.
1 Frontonasal prominence
2 Eye
3 Nasal pit
4 Lateral nasal prominence
5 Medial nasal prominence
6 Stomodeum
7 Nasolacrimal groove
8 Mandibular prominence
9 Maxillary prominence
10 Philtrum
11 Nose

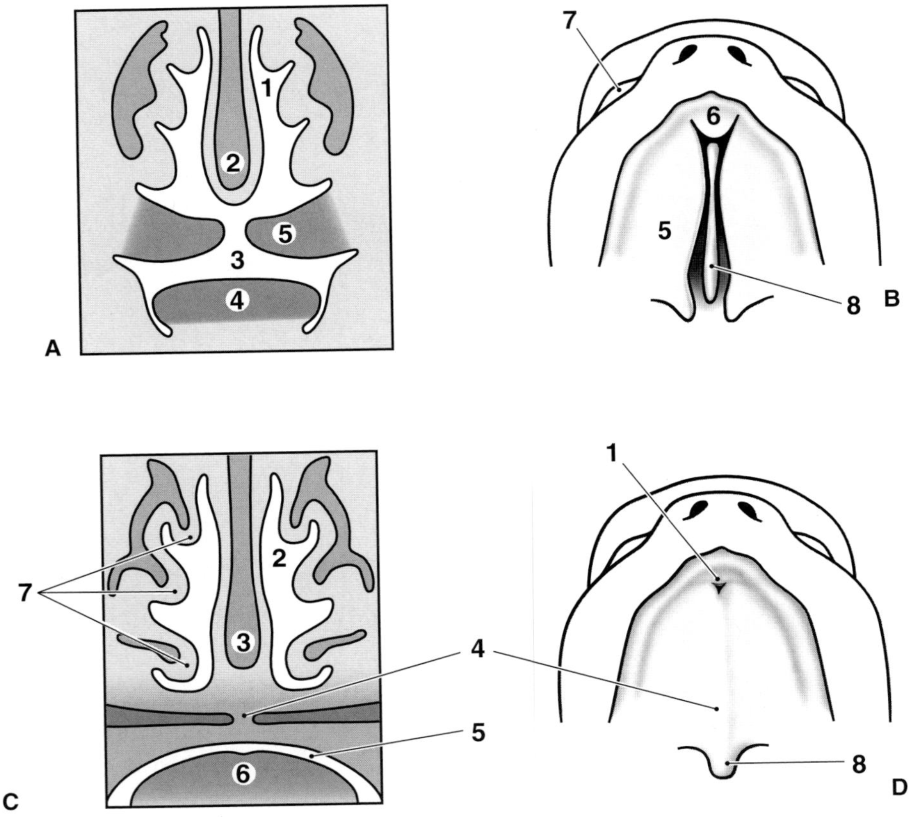

Figure 1-47: Schematics showing the embryologic development of the palate.
A: Embryo at 7½ weeks gestation. Coronal schematic through the face.
B: Embryo at 7½ weeks gestation. Ventral view of the palatine shelves after removal of the lower jaw and tongue. The shelves are approximating in the midline.
1 Nasal chamber
2 Nasal septum
3 Oral cavity
4 Tongue
5 Palatine shelf (paired, unfused)
6 Primary palate
7 Eye
8 Nasal septum
C: Embryo at 10 weeks gestation. Coronal schematic through the face. The two palatine shelves have fused with each other and with the nasal septum.
D: Embryo at 10 weeks gestation. Ventral view of the palate showing fusion of the palatal shelves in the midline. The incisive foramen forms the midline landmark between the primary and secondary palate.
1 Incisive foramen
2 Nasal chamber
3 Nasal septum
4 Fused palatal shelves
5 Oral cavity
6 Tongue
7 Nasal conchae
8 Uvula

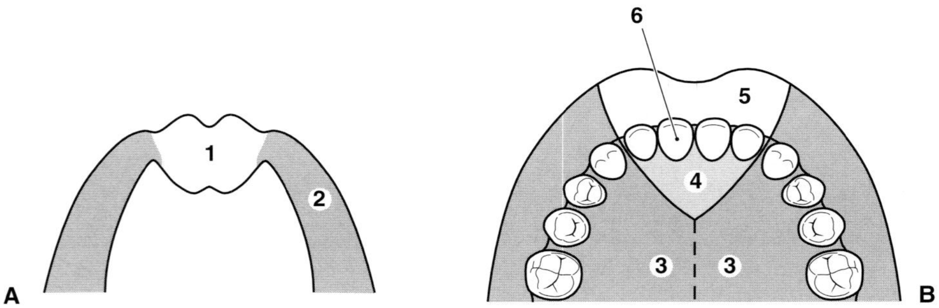

Figure 1-48: Schematic from below showing the embryologic development of the palate.
A: The developing intermaxillary segment and maxillary process.
B: The intermaxillary segment gives rise to the philtrum of the upper lip, the median part of the maxillary bone and its four incisor teeth, and the triangular primary palate.
1 Intermaxillary segment
2 Maxillary process
3 Fused palatal plates
4 Primary palate
5 Philtrum of lip
6 Maxilla with four incisor teeth

TABLE 1-6: Embryonic Structures Contributing to the Formation of the Face

Facial prominence	Structures formed
Frontonasal [a]	Forehead, bridge of nose, medial and lateral nasal prominences
Maxillary	Cheeks, lateral portion of upper lip
Medial nasal	Philtrum of upper lip, crest and tip of nose
Lateral nasal	Alae of nose
Mandibular	Lower lip

[a] The frontonasal prominence represents a single unpaired structure, whereas the other prominences are paired.
Modified from Sadler TW. Head and neck. In: *Langman's medical embryology*. Baltimore: Williams & Wilkins, 1990.

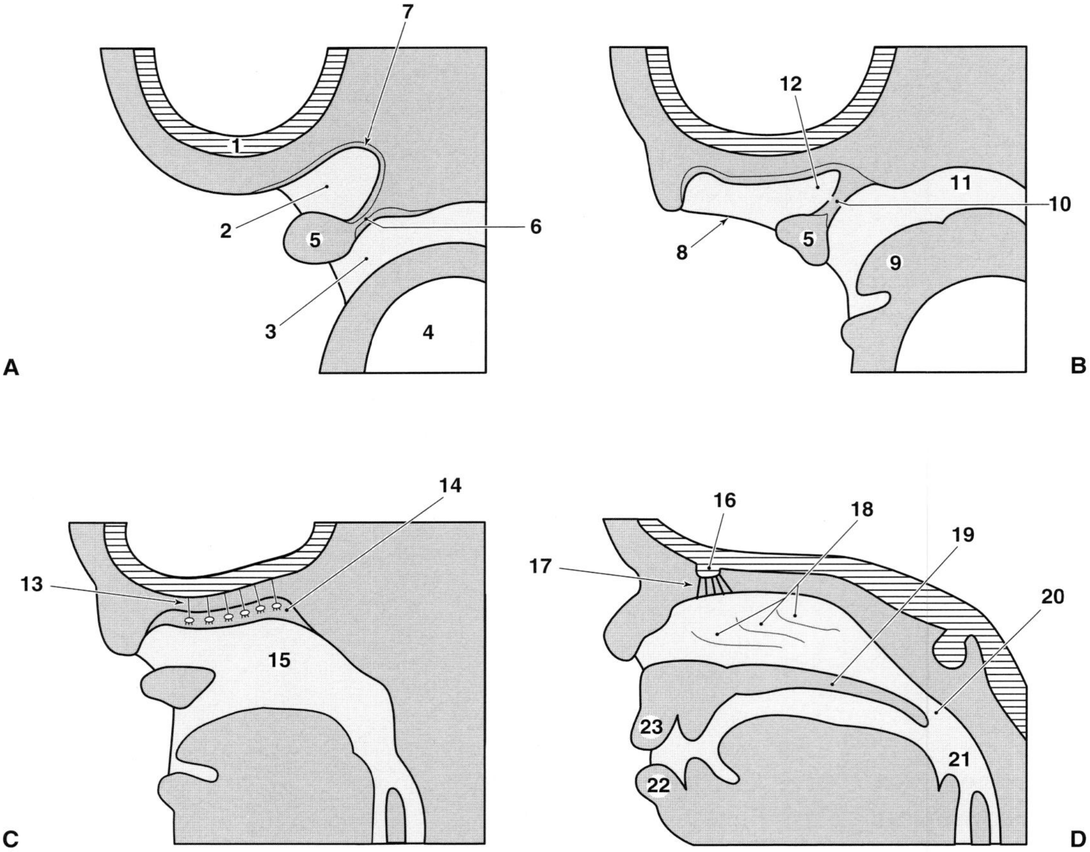

Figure 1-49: Embryologic development of the nasal passageways. **A**: Sagittal schematic at 5 weeks' gestation. **B:** Sagittal schematic at 6 weeks' gestation. **C:** Sagittal schematic at 7 weeks' gestation. **D:** Sagittal schematic at 12 weeks' gestation.

1 Wall of developing brain
2 Nasal sac
3 Oral cavity
4 Heart
5 Primary palate
6 Oronasal membrane
7 Surface ectoderm
8 Nostril
9 Tongue
10 Rupturing oronasal membrane
11 Pharynx
12 Nasal cavity
13 Olfactory nerve fibers
14 Olfactory epithelium
15 Primitive choana
16 Olfactory bulb
17 Olfactory nerves
18 Nasal conchae
19 Secondary palate
20 Definitive choana
21 Oropharynx
22 Lower lip
23 Upper lip

Embryologic Development of the Teeth

1. The teeth evolve initially from the dental lamina, part of the basal layer of the epithelial lining of the oral cavity extending along the length of the upper and lower jaws. Outbuddings of the dental lamina form the primordia of the ectodermal component of the teeth. The bud subsequently invaginates, and the resulting cap shape consists of several layers—the outer dental epithelium, the inner dental epithelium, and an intervening core of tissue, the stellate reticulum.
2. Within the indentation of the cap-shaped invagination, mesenchyme of neural crest origin forms the dental papilla. The outermost of these mesenchymal cells of the dental papilla differentiate into odontoblasts that provide predentin, which form dentine. The other cells of the dental papilla constitute the tooth pulp. The epithelial cells of the outer dental epithelium differentiate into ameloblasts, which give rise to tooth enamel. Mesenchymal cells on the outer surface of the developing tooth differentiate into cementoblasts, which produce cementum, a thin layer of specialized bone. Finally, the mesenchyme outside the cementum forms the periodontal ligament, which serves to hold the tooth in position. This forms the deciduous teeth.
3. The buds for the permanent teeth are located in the lingual aspect of the deciduous teeth. These buds grow in the third month of embryonic development and are dormant until the sixth year of life. As the permanent tooth begins to grow, it assists in shedding the deciduous tooth by displacement. The root of the deciduous tooth is eventually resorbed by osteoclasts.

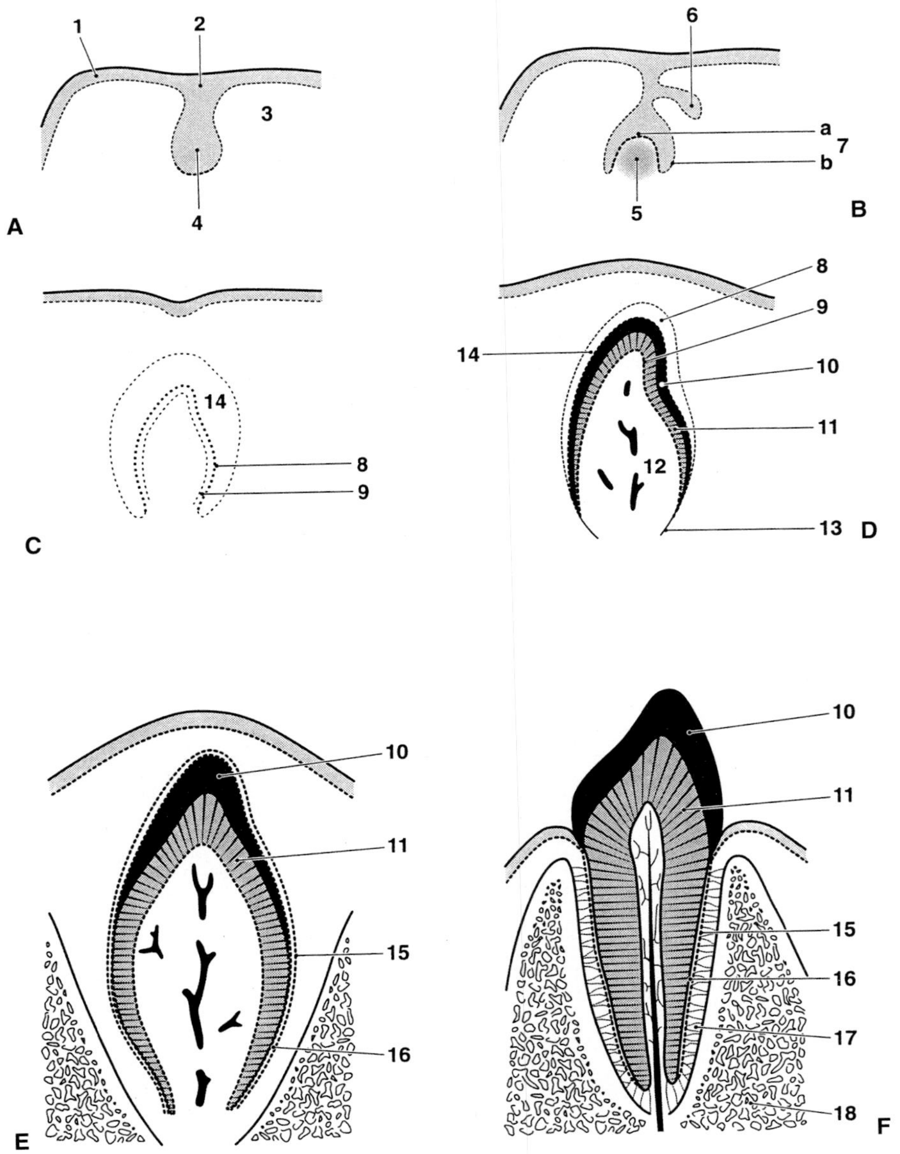

Figure 1-50: Schematics showing the embryologic development of the tooth at successive stages. **A:** 8 weeks. **B:** 10 weeks. **C:** 3 months. **D:** 6 months. **E:** At birth. **F:** After tooth eruption.

1 Oral epithelium
2 Dental lamina
3 Mesenchyme of jaw
4 Dental bud
5 Dental papilla
6 Permanent tooth bud
7 Dental epithelium
   a. Inner
   b. Outer
8 Ameloblasts
9 Odontoblasts
10 Enamel
11 Dentine
12 Dental pulp
13 Root sheath
14 Stellate reticulum
15 Cementoblasts
16 Cementum
17 Periodontal ligament
18 Bone of tooth socket

CHAPTER 2

Cranium

2A. THE SKULL

OVERVIEW

1. The skull is the most modified part of the axial skeleton. It harbors the brain and serves to protect the rostral central nervous system.
2. The skull is made up of separate bones joined in adulthood by partially or completely fused sutures and synchondroses.
3. The bones of the skull in the normal adult either are in symmetrical pairs or are single and situated midline. The paired bones include the parietal and temporal bones. The single midline bones include the frontal, occipital, ethmoid, and sphenoid bones.
4. There are also inconsistent accessory calvarial bones that lie between the sutures and in the fontanelles, termed sutural (wormian) bones.
5. The calvaria is the domelike superior portion of the skull. It consists of the superior portions of the frontal, parietal, and occipital bones. "Calvarium" is an incorrect term that is often improperly used to mean calvaria.
6. The bones of the skull are either of ossified membranous bone (e.g., cranial vault) or of ossified cartilaginous elements (e.g., base of skull).
7. The calvarial foramina provide entry and exit of nerves and blood vessels (e.g., arteries, veins). The foramen magnum is the largest foramen, where the brain stem is continuous with the spinal cord.
8. The major external landmarks of the cranial vault include the nasion, representing the junction between the internasal and frontonasal sutures; the glabella, a median frontal elevation immediately above the frontonasal junction; the bregma, or the point at which the coronal and sagittal sutures meet the vertex or apex of the cranial vault; the lambda at the junction of the sagittal and lambdoid sutures; the inion, demarcating the summit of the external occipital protuberance; the pterion, marking the H-shaped junction of the frontal, sphenoid, parietal, and temporal squama; and the asterion at the junction of the occipital, temporal, and parietal bones.

SKULL ANATOMY

The Frontal Bone

1. The frontal bone forms the forehead and roofs of the orbits on either side of the skull.
2. The frontal bone articulates with the parietal bones at the coronal suture, the nasal bones at the frontonasal suture, the ethmoid bone at the fronto-ethmoidal sutures, the zygoma at the zygomaticofrontal suture, the maxilla at the frontomaxillary suture, and the lacrimal and sphenoid bones.
3. The frontal bone is the main component of the floor of the anterior fossa, together with the lesser wing of the sphenoid bone and the cribriform plate of the ethmoid bone.
4. The frontal bone has two primary ossification centers that are separated embryologically by the metopic suture at the midline. This suture may persist into adulthood in up to 10% of cases.
5. The external bony elevation superiomedial to the orbits in the midline is termed the glabella.
6. The frontal bones commonly undergo a form of benign internal hyperostosis, hyperostosis frontalis interna, in middle-aged women.

The Parietal Bones

1. The parietal bones are a pair of convex plates with a quadrangular shape situated on either side of the skull.
2. The two parietal bones meet at the midline at the sagittal suture.

3. They articulate with the frontal bone anteriorly at the coronal suture and at the occipital bone posteriorly at the lambdoid suture.
4. The lateral inferior borders of the parietal bones articulate with the greater wing of sphenoid bone anteriorly and the squamous portion of the temporal bone in its mid and posterior parts.
5. Each parietal bone ossifies from two separate centers on each side that unite early during fetal life.
6. The parietal bones rarely undergo a form of benign internal hyperostosis, hyperostosis parietalis interna, in middle-aged women.

The Occipital Bone

1. The occipital bone is situated at the lower posterior part of the skull in the midline. It consists of four parts surrounding the foramen magnum: the basilar, squamous, and two condylar parts.
2. Basilar part of the occipital bone (basiocciput)
   a. The basilar part of the occipital bone is called the basiocciput, which is formed from the fusion of four primary (cranial) vertebrae.
   b. It fuses with the basisphenoid at the sphenooccipital synchondrosis to become the clivus. The clivus represents the central anterior wall of the posterior cranial fossa and the central skull base.
3. Squamous part of the occipital bone
   a. The squamous part of the occipital bone forms the posterior border of the foramen magnum.
   b. Its concave interior surface forms the lateral and posterior wall of the posterior cranial fossa.
   c. Superolaterally, the squamous part of the occipital bone articulates with the parietal bones on either side at the lambdoid suture and the mastoid part of the temporal bone at the occipital mastoid suture.
   d. Superoposteriorly, the occipital bone has two protuberances: the internal and external occipital protuberances.
   e. Especially in the region surrounding the torcular Herophili, the occipital bone may have excavations or impressions of the inner table extending into the diploic space occupied in part by arachnoid granulations.
4. Condylar (exoccipital) parts of the occipital bone
   a. The paired exoccipital or condylar parts of the occipital bone form the lateral borders of the foramen magnum.
   b. The condylar part of the occipital bone lies between the basiocciput and the squamous part of the occiput and fuses with them by a synchondrosis in early life.

The Temporal Bones

1. The paired temporal bones are located on either side of the skull and form a part of the skull base as well as the lateral cranial vault.
2. The individual temporal bones consist of four parts, including the squamous, tympanic, petromastoid, and styloid parts.
3. The squamous part of the temporal bone
   a. The squamous part of the temporal bone is placed vertically and is approximately oval in shape.
   b. It articulates with the parietal bone superiorly and the greater wing of sphenoid bone anteriorly.
   c. The zygomatic process extends forward to articulate with the zygomaticotemporal suture.
   d. The glenoid or mandibular fossa lies inferiorly and forms the temporomandibular articulation.

4. The tympanic part of the temporal bone
   a. The tympanic part of the temporal bone is a ringlike structure placed near the root of the zygomatic process in front of the mastoid process.
   b. It encircles the external auditory meatus and fuses with the petromastoid part medially and the squamous part posteriorly.
   c. Inferiorly, the sheath of the styloid process gives rise to the styloid part of the temporal bone.
5. The petromastoid part of the temporal bone
   a. The petromastoid part of the temporal bone consists of the developmentally fused petrous and mastoid bones.
   b. The petrous bone is a wedge-shaped piece of bone that lies between the greater wing of sphenoid bone and the occipital bone.
      i. It forms the petrous ridges on the floor of the skull bilaterally and separates the middle and posterior cranial fossae.
      ii. The tentorium cerebelli arises from the superior margin of the petrous bone.
      iii. The anterior—-superior surface of the petrous bone forms part of the middle cranial fossa.
      iv. The posterior surface of the petrous bone becomes a part of the anterior wall of the posterior cranial fossa, with the internal auditory meatus piercing its medial aspect.
      v. The paired carotid canals pass through the medial aspects of petrous bones and enter the middle cranial fossae.
      vi. The paired jugular foramina open into the posterior fossa between the lateral edges of the occipital bones and the inferomedial aspects of the petrous bones.
      vii. The petrous bone provides housing for the auditory complex and the facial nerve canal.
   c. The mastoid part of the temporal bone lies posterior to the petrous part. It forms part of the anterolateral wall of the posterior cranial fossa and harbors the mastoid air cells.
6. The styloid part of the temporal bone
   a. The styloid process is a rod-shaped, pointed structure projecting from the inferior aspect of the temporal bone.
   b. The stylohyoid ligament on each side arises from the apex of the styloid process and inserts into the lesser cornu of the hyoid bone.
7. All four parts of the temporal bone ossify individually and fuse with one another early in life.

The Ethmoid Bone

1. The ethmoid bone is a small, irregular bone in the floor of the anterior cranial fossa; it lies between the part of the frontal bone forming the orbital roof at the midline and the front of the body of sphenoid bone.
2. The upper surface of the ethmoid bone forms the perforated cribriform plate through which the terminal branches of the olfactory nerves pass.
3. The crista galli is an upward bony projection from the floor of the anterior cranial fossa in the midline anteriorly.
4. Below the cribriform plate, the perpendicular plate of the ethmoid bone forms part of the midline nasal septum. The ethmoid air cells are found on either side of the midline.
5. The ethmoid bone gives rise to the superior and middle nasal conchae on each side.

The Sphenoid Bone

1. The sphenoid bone is the central osseous structure of the skull base.
2. It has a complex composition consisting of a body (basisphenoid), a pair of greater wings, a pair of lesser wings, and two pterygoid processes.
3. The body of the sphenoid bone (basisphenoid)
   a. The body of the sphenoid bone is a cuboid structure located at the center of the skull base.
   b. The dorsum of the body has a small depression on its superior surface that eventually forms the pituitary fossa (bony sella turcica).
   c. The basisphenoid fuses in early life with the basiocciput (basilar part of the occipital bone), across the cartilaginous sphenooccipital synchondrosis, to form the clivus.
   d. The body harbors the sphenoid air cells.
4. Greater wings of the sphenoid bone
   a. The greater wings of the sphenoid bone lie postero-inferiorly on either side of the body and form the anterior wall and floor of the middle cranial fossa.
   b. The foramina rotundum (CN-V2) are situated in the medial part of the anterior walls bilaterally; the pterygoid (Vidian) canals (Vidian nerve or nerve of the pterygoid canal) are located immediately supramedial to the foramina rotundum.
   c. The foramina ovale (CN-V3) and spinosum (middle meningeal artery) are located in the posterior part of the sphenoid wings bilaterally.
   d. The greater wings articulate with the temporal bone posteriorly and the frontal and parietal bones anteriorly on either side.
   e. The medial and lateral alae (wings) of the pterygoid plates are thin plates of vertically placed bone that extend downward from the inferior surface of the greater wing, to which attach the medial and lateral pterygoid muscles bilaterally, respectively.
5. Lesser wings of the sphenoid bone
   a. The lesser wings of the sphenoid bone extend anterolaterally from the body; the optic foramina (CN-II) are found at their base.
   b. The anterior clinoid processes project medially and attach to the anterior medial free end of the tentorium cerebelli.

The Clivus

1. The clivus forms from the developmental fusion of the basiocciput and the basisphenoid across the sphenooccipital synchondrosis.
2. The clivus forms a part of the central skull base.
3. Postero-inferiorly the clivus terminates in the basion, the anterior margin of the foramen magnum.

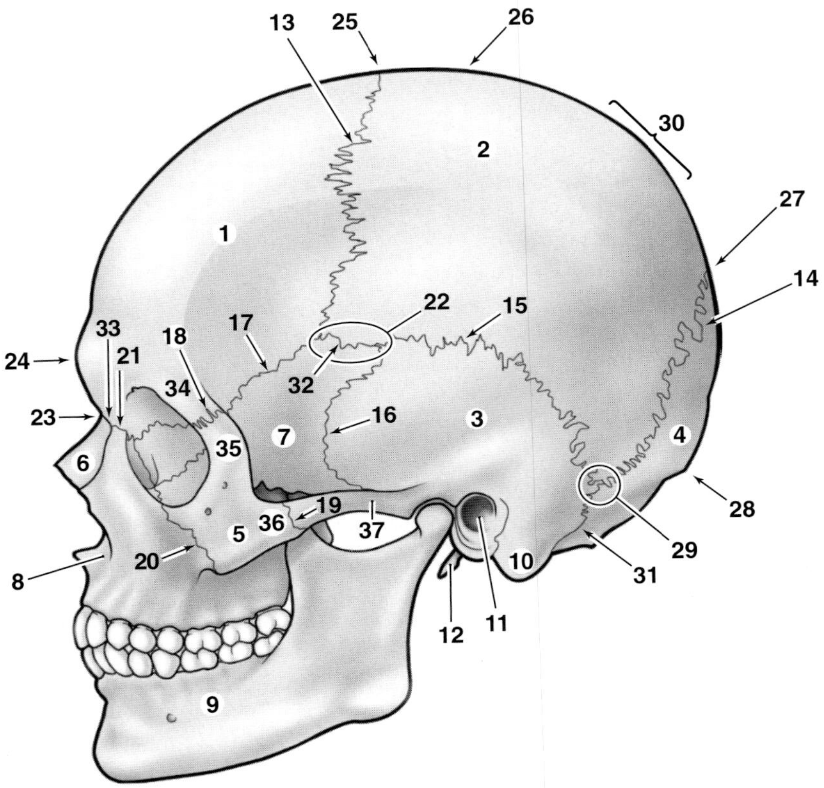

Figure 2A-1: Lateral schematic of the skull, showing the normal anatomic features.

1 Frontal bone
2 Parietal bone
3 Temporal bone (squamous part)
4 Occipital bone
5 Zygomatic bone
6 Nasal bone
7 Sphenoid bone (greater wing)
8 Maxilla
9 Mandible
10 Mastoid process
11 External acoustic meatus
12 Styloid process
13 Coronal suture
14 Lambdoid suture
15 Temporoparietal (squamosal) suture
16 Sphenosquamosal suture
17 Sphenofrontal suture
18 Zygomaticofrontal suture
19 Zygomaticotemporal suture
20 Zygomaticomaxillary suture
21 Frontomaxillary suture
22 Pterion
23 Nasion
24 Glabella
25 Bregma
26 Vertex
27 Lambda
28 External occipital protuberance (inion)
29 Asterion
30 Sagittal suture (not seen: extends from bregma to lambda in midline)
31 Temporooccipital suture
32 Sphenoparietal suture
33 Frontonasal suture
34 Zygomatic process of the frontal bone
35 Frontal process of the zygomatic bone
36 Zygomatic process of the zygoma
37 Zygomatic process of the temporal bone

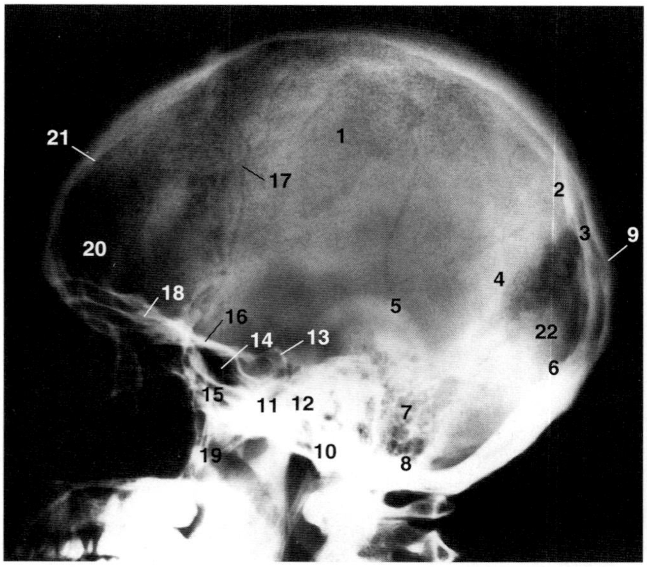

Figure 2A-2: Skull radiograph in the lateral projection, showing many of the normal anatomic features.

1 Parietal bone
2 Inner table of skull
3 Diploë
4 Lambdoid suture
5 Auricle
6 Internal occipital protuberance
7 Posterior cranial fossa
8 Mastoid air cells
9 External table of skull
10 Basilar portion of occipital bone
11 Floor of sella turcica
12 Pituitary fossa
13 Dorsum sella
14 Anterior clinoid processes
15 Sphenoid sinus
16 Planum sphenoidale
17 Groove for middle meningeal artery
18 Roof of orbit
19 Pterygoid processes
20 Anterior cranial fossa
21 Frontal bone
22 Occipital bone

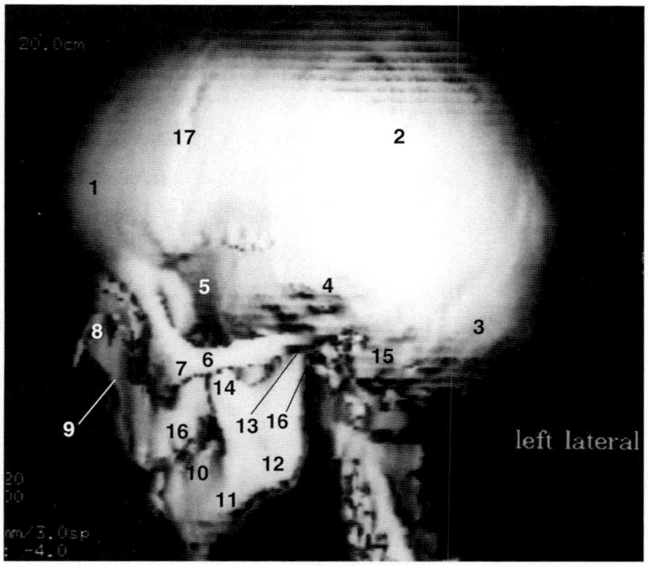

Figure 2A-3: Three-dimensional CT reconstruction of the skull in the lateral projection, showing many of the normal anatomic surface features.

1 Frontal bone
2 Parietal bone
3 Occipital bone
4 Temporal bone squamosa
5 Deep temporal fossa
6 Zygomatic arch
7 Zygomatic bone
8 Nasal bone(s)
9 Alveolar process of maxilla
10 Alveolar process of mandible
11 Body of mandible
12 Angle of mandible
13 Ramus of mandible
14 Coronoid process of mandible
15 Mastoid process of temporal bone
16 Condylar process of mandible
17 Coronal suture

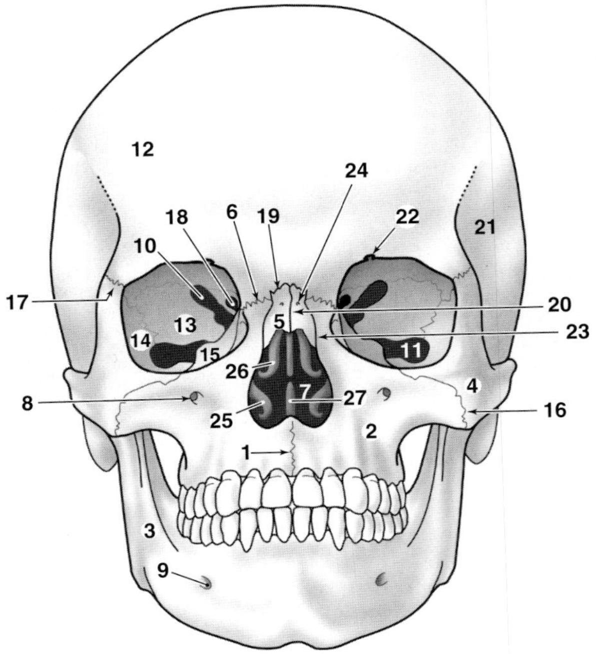

Figure 2A-4: Frontal schematic of the skull, showing the normal anatomic features.

1 Intermaxillary suture
2 Maxilla
3 Mandible
4 Zygomatic bone
5 Nasal bone
6 Frontomaxillary suture
7 Piriform aperture (anterior nasal aperture)
8 Infraorbital foramen
9 Mental foramen
10 Superior orbital fissure
11 Inferior orbital fissure
12 Frontal bone
13 Greater wing of sphenoid bone
14 Orbital process of zygomatic bone
15 Maxillary process of orbit
16 Zygomaticomaxillary suture
17 Zygomaticofrontal suture
18 Optic foramen
19 Frontonasal suture
20 Internasal suture
21 Temporal squamosa
22 Supraorbital notch
23 Nasomaxillary suture
24 Nasal vascular foramen
25 Inferior nasal concha
26 Middle nasal concha
27 Nasal septum

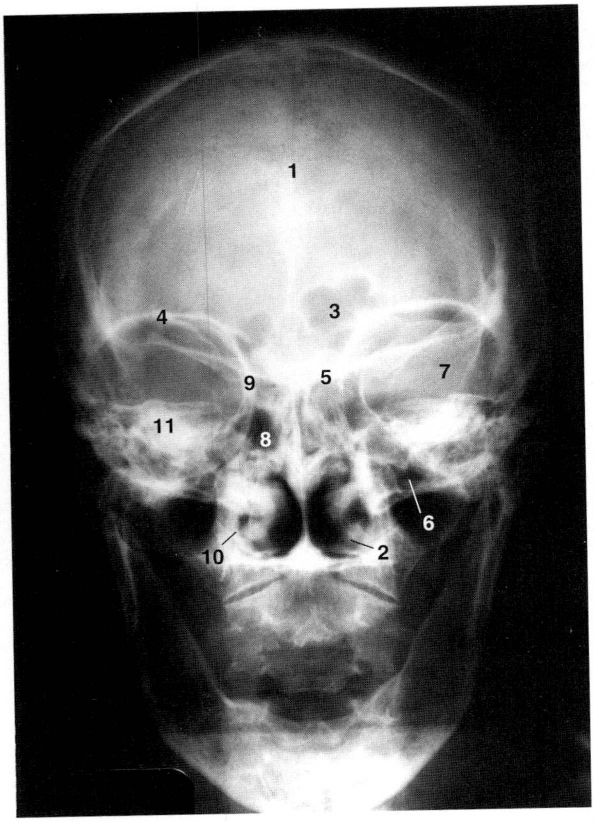

Figure 2A-5: Skull radiograph in the frontal projection, showing many of the normal anatomic features.

1 Sagittal suture
2 Nasal cavity
3 Frontal sinus
4 Roof of orbit
5 Cribriform plate
6 Maxillary sinus
7 Greater wing of sphenoid bone
8 Ethmoid sinus air cells
9 Medial orbital wall (lamina papyracea)
10 Lateral wall of nasal cavity
11 Upper border of petrous part of temporal bone

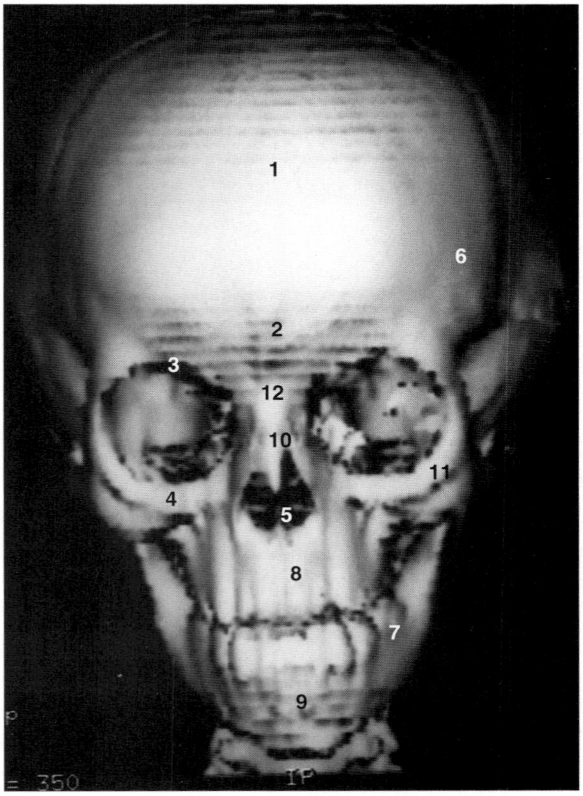

Figure 2A-6: Three-dimensional CT reconstruction of the skull in the frontal projection, showing many of the normal anatomic surface features.

1 Frontal bone
2 Glabella
3 Supraorbital margin
4 Infraorbital margin
5 Nasal passageway
6 Temporal bone squamosa
7 Ramus of mandible
8 Alveolar process of maxilla
9 Alveolar process of mandible
10 Nasal bone
11 Zygomatic bone
12 Nasion

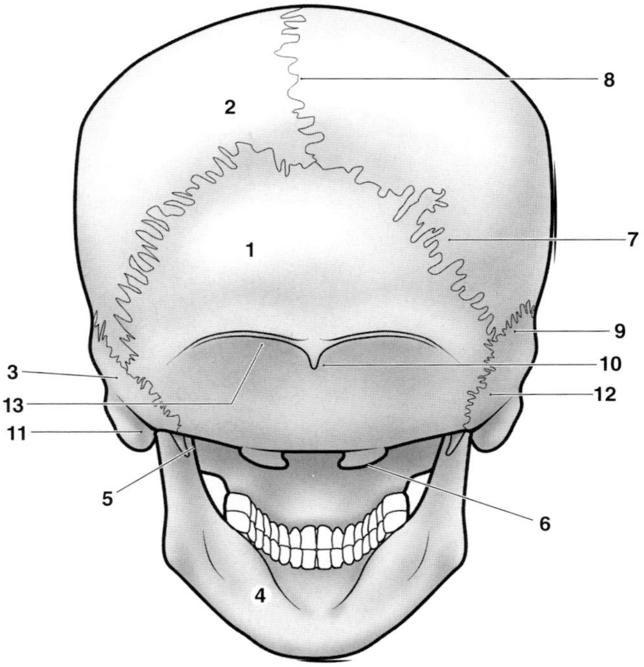

Figure 2A-7: Posterior schematic of the skull, showing the normal anatomic features.

1 Occipital bone
2 Parietal bone
3 Temporal bone
4 Mandible
5 Styloid process
6 Occipital condoyle
7 Lambdoid suture
8 Sagittal suture
9 Parietotemporal suture
10 External occipital protuberance (inion)
11 Mastoid process
12 Occipital temporal suture
13 Superior nuchal line

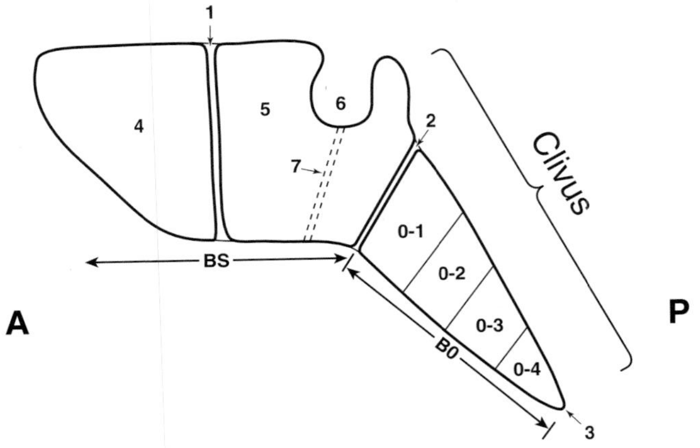

Figure 2A-8: Lateral midline schematic, showing the components of the clivus and central skull base with their embryologic precursors. The basisphenoid and basiocciput are separated before fusion by the sphenooccipital synchondrosis. The presphenoid and basisphenoid are the central precursors of the sphenoid bone. The basiocciput is formed from the four primary occipital sclerotomes or primitive "vertebrae" (O1-O-4). Fusion of the sphenooccipital synchondrosis generally occurs after the age of 12 years. *A*, anterior; *P*, posterior; *O-1/O-4*, occipital sclerotomes or primitive "vertebrae"; *BS*, basisphenoid; *BO*, basiocciput.

1 Anterior intrasphenoid synchondrosis (temporary)
2 Sphenooccipital synchondrosis (temporary)
3 Basion
4 Presphenoid ossification center
5 Central (primary) sphenoid ossification centers
6 Sella turcica (pituitary fossa)
7 Embryonic region of pharyngohypophyseal (craniopharyngeal) canal

The Sutures, Synchondroses, and Fontanelles

1. The cranial sutures separate the bones of the cranium and are composed of fibrous connective tissue. They are continuous with the pericranium on their external aspect and the outer (periosteal) layer of the dura mater on the inside of the skull. Clinical closure of the sutures does not always indicate that bony fusion has occurred. Persistent suture lines can sometimes be observed on radiography after the sutures are functionally "closed."
2. The cranial synchondroses are narrow regions of residual cartilaginous tissue that persist for limited periods between two enchondral centers of ossification in the cranial bones at the base of the skull after calvarial ossification has occurred.
3. The cranial fontanelles are temporary irregular, nonossified areas of connective tissue lying between two or more bones of the cranial vault during development.

TABLE 2A-1: The Sutures of the Skull

Suture	Location
Coronal suture	Paired sutures between the frontal and parietal bones on both sides of the skull anteriorly; continuous through the anterior fontanelle in the midline at the bregma
Lambdoid suture	Paired sutures between the parietal bones on both sides of the skull and the occipital bone posteriorly; continuous through the posterior fontanelle in the midline at the lambda; terminates laterally at the asterion
Sagittal suture	Single suture between the pair of parietal bones at the midline superiorly running anterioposteriorly; continuous at the bregma anteriorly with the coronal sutures; continuous posteriorly at the lambda with the lambdoid sutures
Metopic (frontal) suture	Single suture between the pair of frontal bones at midline anteriorly
Temporoparietal (squamosal) suture	Paired sutures between the parietal and temporal bones on both sides of the skull
Sphenofrontal suture	Paired sutures continuous from the coronal suture, between the frontal and sphenoidal bones on both sides of the skull, and extending to the base of the anterior cranial fossa
Temporooccipital suture	Paired sutures between the petrous part of the temporal bone and the occipital bone (basioccipital part of the temporal bone) continuous with the lambdoid suture from above
Occipital-petrosal suture	Paired sutures between the greater wing of sphenoid bone and the anterior margin of petrous bone in the floor of middle cranial fossa
Sphenopetrosal suture	Paired sutures between the greater wing of the sphenoid bone and the anterior margin of petrous bone in the floor of middle cranial fossa
Sphenosquamosal suture	Paired sutures between the greater wing of sphenoid bone and the temporal bone, extending from the pterion downward to the floor of the middle cranial fossa on both sides
Sphenoparietal suture	Paired short sutures between the greater wing of the sphenoid bone and the parietal bone on the two sides of skull; located at the pterion
Superior-median intraoccipital suture	An incomplete single sagittal suture in the midline of the interparietal part of the occipital bone, extending from its superior margin and continuous above with the junction of the two lambdoid sutures and the sagittal suture
Mendosal suture	See posterior intraoccipital synchondrosis.

TABLE 2A-2: The Synchondroses of the Skull

Synchondrosis	Location
Sphenooccipital synchondrosis	Between the basisphenoid (part of sphenoid bone) and basioccipital (part of occipital bone) bones
Anterior intrasphenoidal synchondrosis	Between the presphenoid part and the sphenoid (central) part of the sphenoid bone during formation
Median longitudinal intrasphenoidal synchrondosis (Jinkins)	In the midline between the halves of the developing basisphenoid
Superior median longitudinal intraoccipital synchondrosis (Jinkins)	In the midline between the two halves of the central basisphenoid ossification center
Inferior-median longitudinal intraoccipital synchondrosis (Jinkins)	In the midline occipital squama inferiorly communicating with the foramen magnum
Anterior intraoccipital synchondrosis	Between the basioccipital and condylar (exoccipital) parts of the occipital bones
Posterior intraoccipital (mendosal, innominate) synchondrosis	Between the squamous and condylar (exoccipital) parts of the occipital bone
Temporooccipital (petrooccipital) synchrondrosis	Between the petrous part of the temporal bone and the basioccipital part of the bone
Sphenopetrosal synchondrosis	Between the basisphenoid bone and petrous part of the temporal bone
Spheno-ethmoidal synchondrosis	Between the basisphenoid and ethmoid bones

TABLE 2A-3: The Fontanelles of the Skull

Fontanelle	Location
Anterior fontanelle	Diamond-shaped single fontanelle lying in the midline between the frontal and paired parietal bones
Posterior fontanelle	Triangle-shaped single fontanelle lying in the midline between the paired parietal bones and the squamous part of the occipital bone
Anterolateral sphenoidal fontanelles	Paired fontanelles at the lateral extremes of the coronal suture (pterion) bilaterally
Posterolateral fontanelles	Paired fontanelles lying at the junction of the parietal, occipital, and temporal bones (asterion) bilaterally
Glabellar fontanelle	Single fontanelle lying at the midline between the frontal bone and the nasal bones in the region of the future glabella
Metopic fontanelle	Single fontanelle lying in the midline within the metopic suture over the forehead
Parietal fontanelle	Single fontanelle lying in the midline within the sagittal suture over the vertex

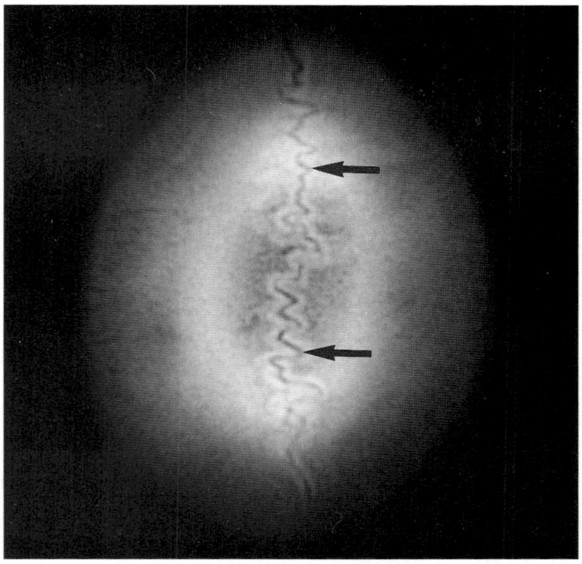

Figure 2A-9A: Cranial sutures and fontanelles. Axial CT image showing the interdigitating sagittal suture (*arrows*).

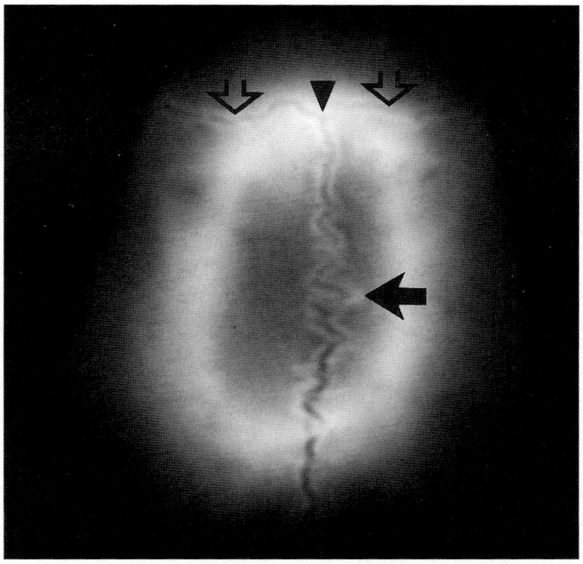

Figure 2A-9B: Axial CT image showing the coronal (*open arrows*) and sagittal (*closed arrow*) sutures at their junction (bregma: *arrowhead*).

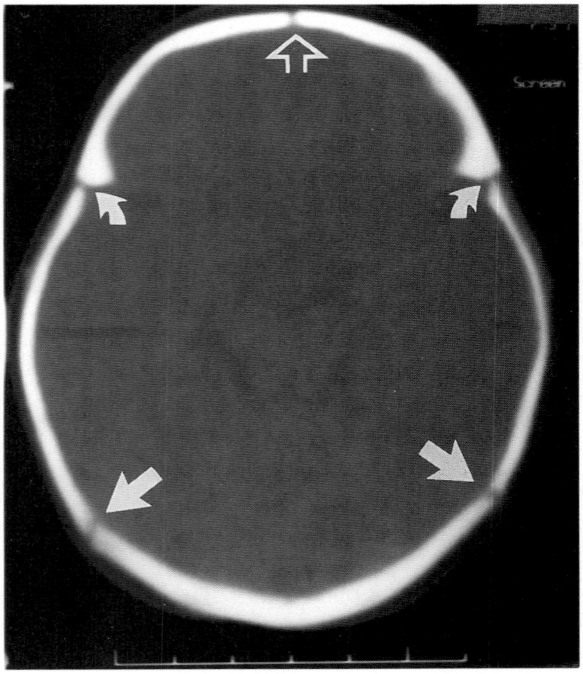

Figure 2A-9C: Axial CT image of a neonate, showing several unfused sutures, including the metopic suture (*open arrow*), the coronal sutures (*curved arrows*), and the lambdoid sutures (*straight arrows*).

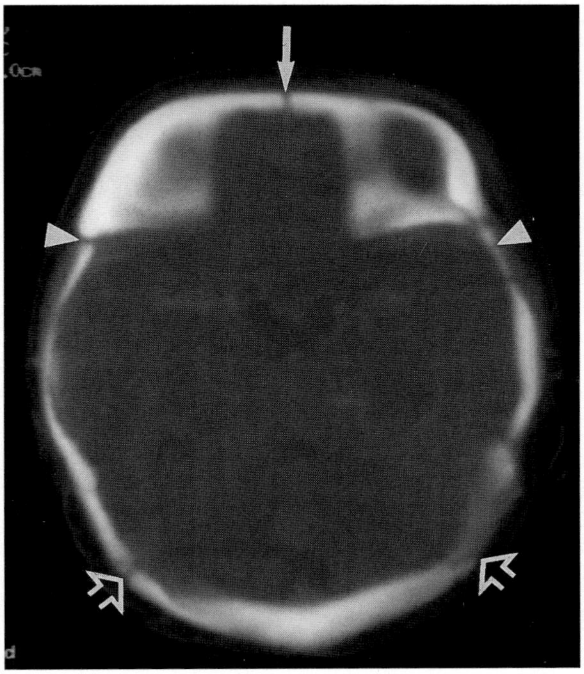

Figure 2A-9D: Axial CT image of a neonate, showing several unfused cranial sutures, including the metopic suture (*closed arrow*), the coronal sutures at the level of the anterolateral (sphenoidal) fontanelles (*arrowheads*), and the lambdoid sutures (*open arrows*).

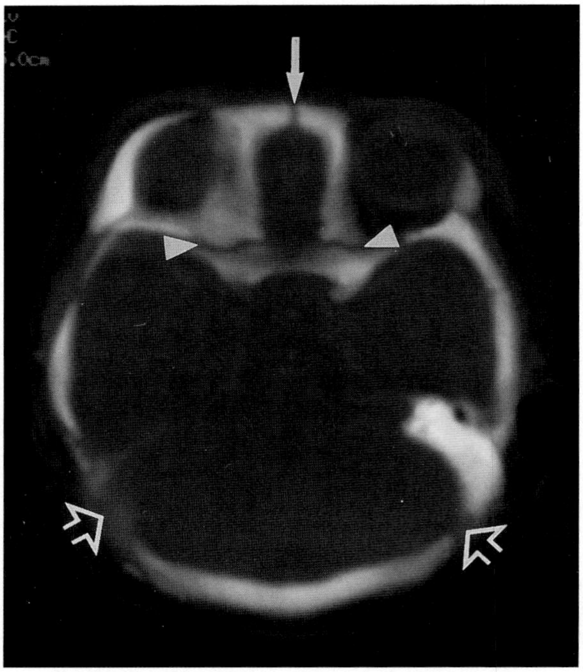

Figure 2A-9E: Axial CT image of a newborn, showing several of the unfused sutures and fontanelles, including the metopic suture (*solid arrow*), the frontosphenoid suture (*arrowheads*), and the posterolateral fontanelles (*open arrows*).

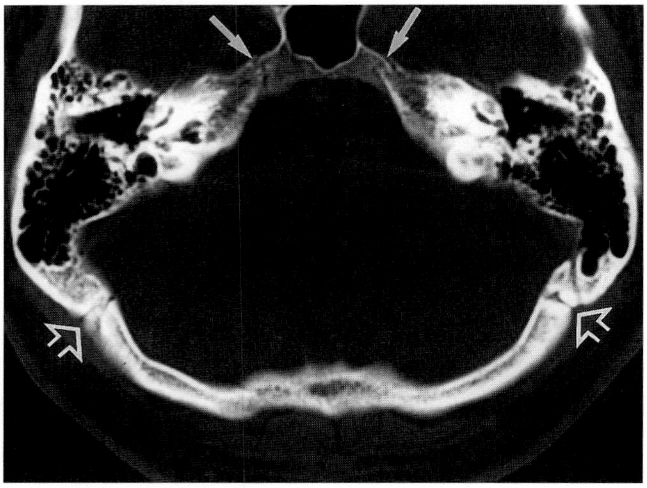

Figure 2A-9F: Magnified axial CT image of an adult, showing the sphenopetrosal sutures (*solid arrows*) and the inferior aspect of the lambdoid sutures (*open arrows*).

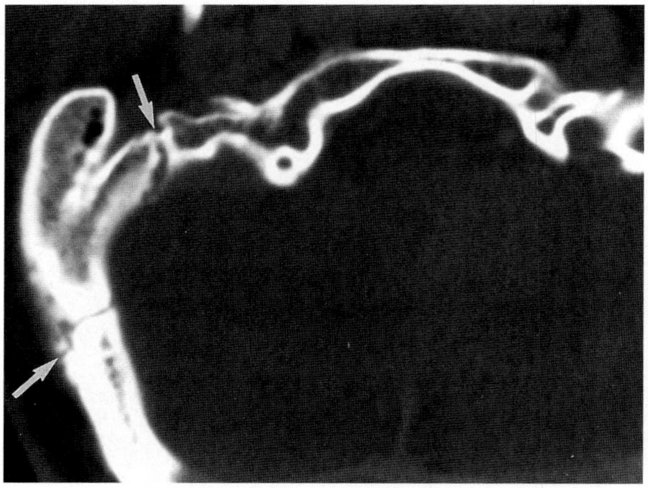

Figure 2A-9G: Temporooccipital suture. Axial CT image showing the temporooccipital suture (*arrows*).

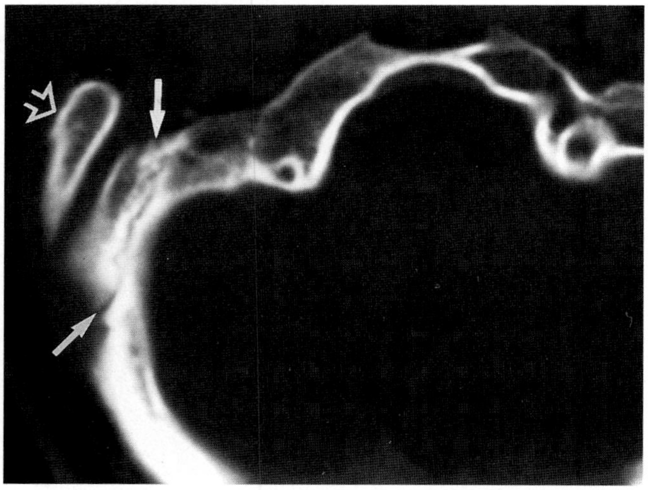

Figure 2A-9H: Axial CT showing the inferior extent of the temporooccipital suture (*solid arrows*). Also note the tip of the mastoid process (*open arrow*).

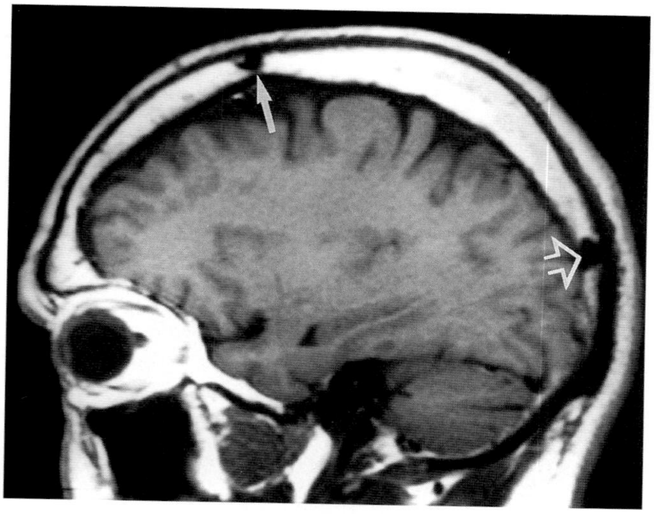

Figure 2A-9I: Parasagittal T1-weighted MR image showing the coronal (*solid arrow*) and lambdoid sutures (*open arrow*).

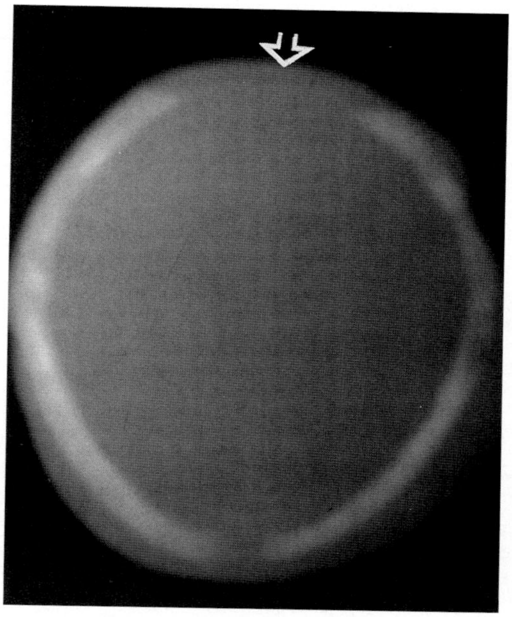

Figure 2A-9J: Axial CT image of a neonate, showing the anterior (*arrow*) fontanelle.

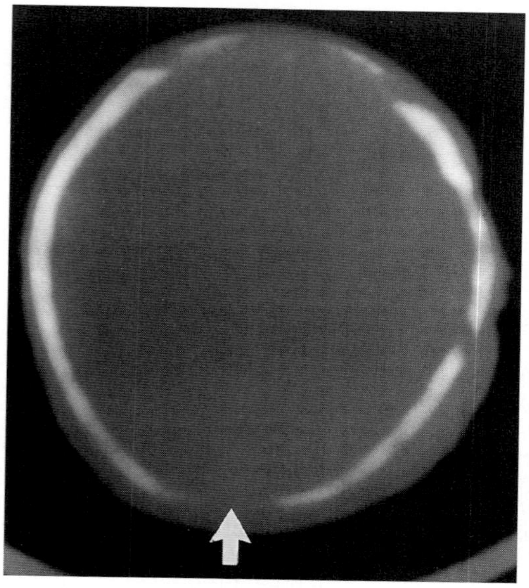

Figure 2A-9K: Axial CT image of a neonate, showing the posterior fontanelle (*arrow*).

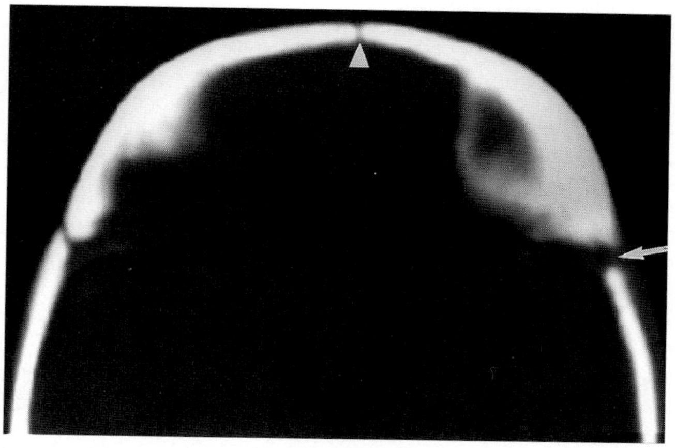

Figure 2A-9L: Magnified axial CT image showing the anterolateral (sphenoidal) fontanelle on the left side (*arrow*) and the metopic suture (*arrowhead*).

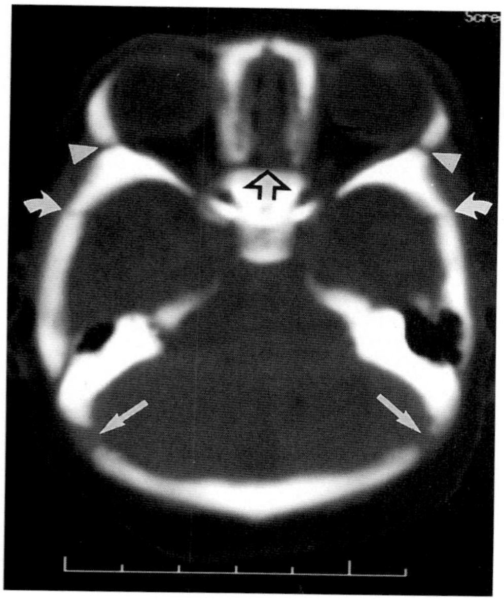

Figure 2A-9M: Axial CT image of a newborn, showing the posterolateral fontanelles (*solid arrows*) between the temporal and occipital bones, the spheno-ethmoidal suture (*open arrow*) between the ossified sphenoid bone and the unossified ethmoid bones, the frontosphenoidal sutures (*arrowheads*), and the sphenosquamosal sutures (*curved arrows*).

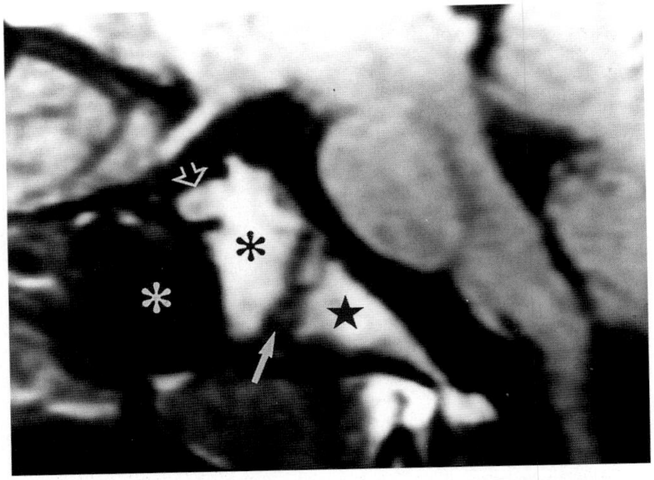

Figure 2A-10A: Skull base sutures and synchondroses. Sagittal T1-weighted MR image in a child shows the relatively hypointense sphenooccipital synchondrosis (*arrow*) between the basisphenoid (*black asterisk*) and the basiocciput (*star*) of the clivus. Also note the pituitary gland (*open arrow*) and the air within the sphenoid sinus (*white asterisk*).

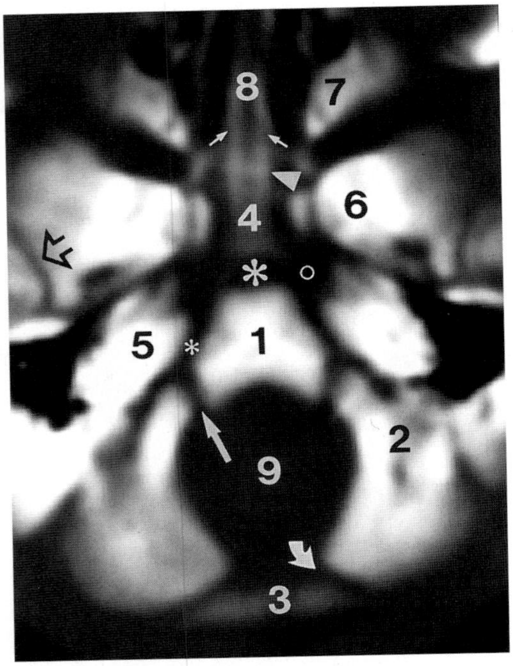

Figure 2A-10B: Axial CT image of a newborn skull base shows the anterior intraoccipital synchondrosis(es) (*large, straight, solid arrow*) between the basioccipital (1) and condylar (2) (exoccipital) parts of the occipital bone, the posterior intraoccipital (mendosal or innominate) synchondrosis(es) (*curved arrow*) between exoccipital and squamous part (3) of the occipital bones, the sphenooccipital synchondrosis (*large asterisk*) between the sphenoid (4, basisphenoid) and occipital (1, basioccipital) bones, the temporooccipital (petrooccipital) synchondrosis(es) (*small asterisk*) between the temporal (5) and the basioccipital (1) bones, the sphenopetrosal synchondrosis(es) (*small circle*) between the basisphenoid bone (4) and the petrous part (5) of the temporal bone (5), the fused remnant of the intrasphenoid synchondrosis (*arrowhead*) and the faintly seen spheno-ethmoidal synchondrosis between the basisphenoid bone (4) and the ethmoid bones (8) (*double small, solid arrows*). Also note the greater (6) and lesser (7) wings of the sphenoid bone, the sphenosquamosal suture(s) (*open arrow*), and the foramen magnum (9).

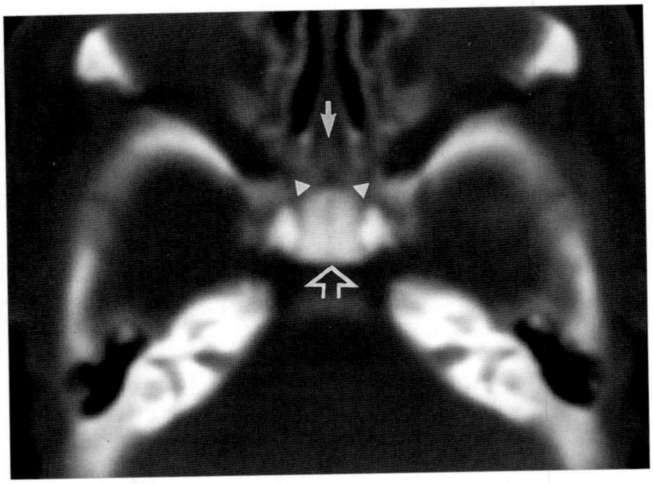

Figure 2A-10C: Axial CT image showing the presphenoid ossification center (*solid arrow*), the anterior intrasphenoidal synchondrosis (*arrowheads*) and the median longitudinal intrasphenoidal synchondrosis (*open arrow*).

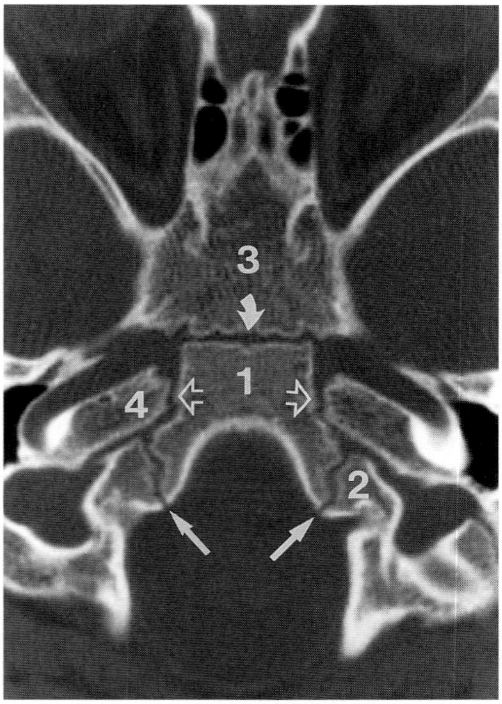

Figure 2A-10D: Axial CT image in an older infant shows the anterior intraoccipital synchondrosis (*straight arrows*) between the basioccipital (1) and exoccipital (2) bones, the sphenooccipital synchondrosis (*curved arrow*) between the basisphenoid (3) and basioccipital (1) bones, and the temporooccipital (petrooccipital) synchondrosis (*open arrows*) between the basiocciput (1) and the petrous part of the temporal bone (4).

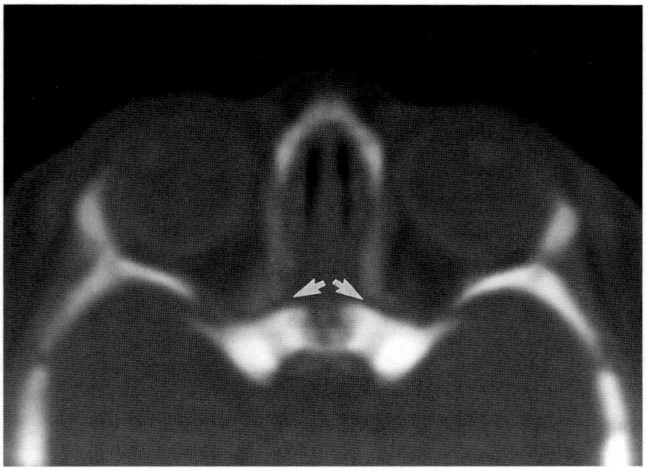

Figure 2A-10E: The frontosphenoid sutures. Axial CT showing the frontosphenoid sutures (*arrows*) bilaterally.

SKULL VARIANTS

Accessory Bones/Ossification Centers of the Skull

- Sutural bones (wormian bones) are most often seen at fontanelles and at the junction of two or more sutures, especially in the region of the lambdoid suture.
- A prominent sutural bone at the lambda (junction of the lambdoid and sagittal sutures) is sometimes referred to as the Inca bone or Garthe's ossicle.
- The epipteric bone(s) (pterion ossicle[s]) is a sutural bone that sometimes can be found at the pterion of the skull; unnamed accessory ossicles may occasionally be found at the asterion, the site of the posterolateral fontanelle.
- Kerckring's bone (ossification center) is a bone or ossification center that undergoes cartilaginous ossification at the posterior margin of the foramen magnum before it fuses early in life with the occipital bone.
- Other unnamed accessory bones or ossification centers are occasionally observed (e.g., skull base accessory ossification centers).

Vascular Variants of the Skull

- Venous lakes
- Emissary venous channels
- Diploic venous channels
- Arterial impressions (e.g., middle meningeal artery groove)
- Venous impressions (e.g., superior sagittal and transverse venous sinus groove)

Arachnoid Granulation Impressions (Excavations) of the Skull

- Occipital arachnoid granulation impressions (excavations)
- Parietal arachnoid granulation impressions (excavations)

Protuberances of the Skull

- Internal occipital protuberance
- External occipital protuberance

Hyperostosis Interna of the Skull

- Hyperostosis frontalis interna
- Hyperostosis parietalis interna

Sutural/Synchondrosal Variants of the Calvaria

- Metopic suture
- Superior median intraoccipital suture
- Sutural (wormian) bones
- Secondary sutural ossification centers
- Secondary synchondrosal ossification centers
- Sclerotic synchondrosal ossification centers

Calvarial Thinning and Anomalous Foramina

- Parietal thinning
- Parietal foramina

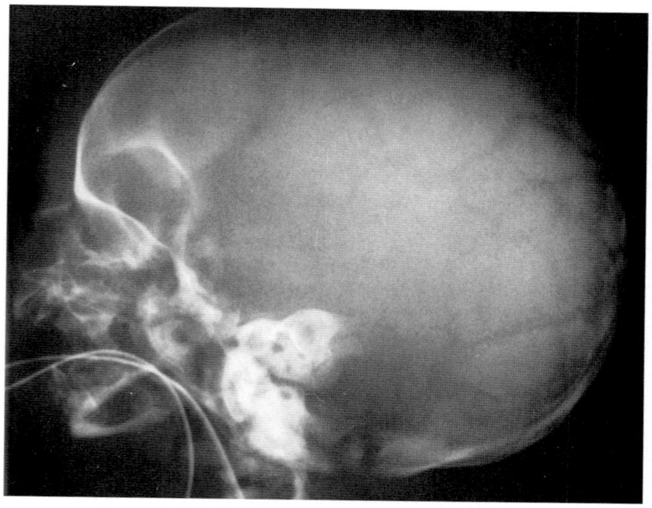

Figure 2A-11A: Sutural (wormian) bones. Skull radiograph in a child in the lateral projection showing multiple parietooccipital sutural (wormian) bones in a newborn.

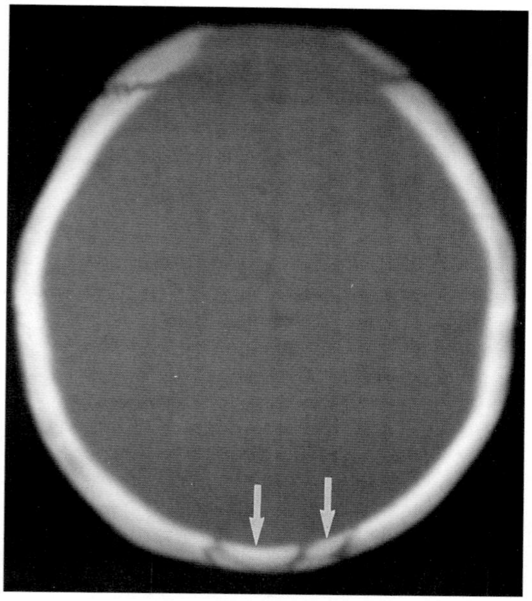

Figure 2A-11B: Sutural (wormian) bones. Axial CT image in a different child showing multiple wormian bones (*arrows*).

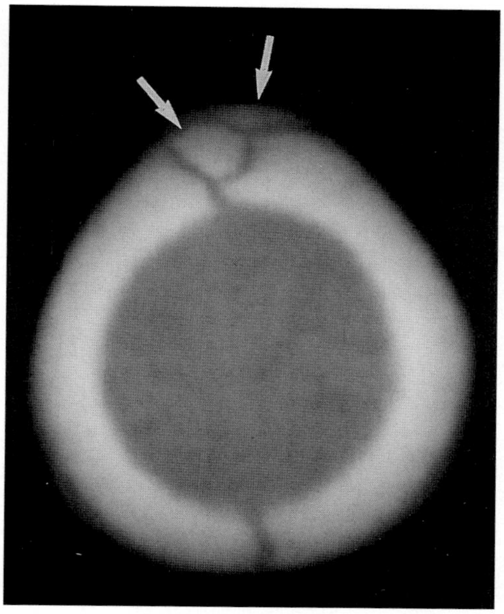

Figure 2A-11C: Sutural (wormian) bone in the anterior calvarial fontanelle (bregma). Axial CT of a third child, showing two sutural bones (*arrows*) at the level of the bregma.

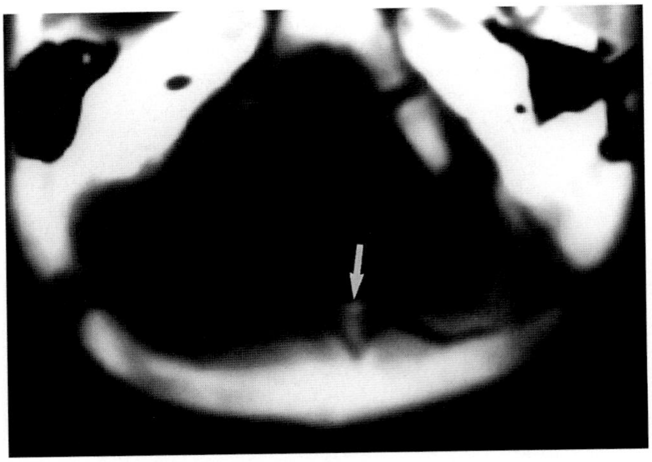

Figure 2A-12: Kerckring's bone (ossicle). Magnified axial CT image showing Kerckring's bone (*arrow*).

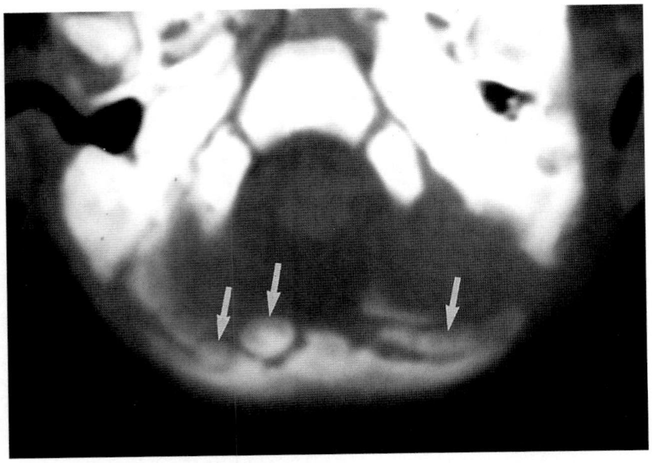

Figure 2A-13: Intraoccipital sutural (wormian) bones. Axial CT scan showing multiple intraoccipital sutural bones (*arrows*).

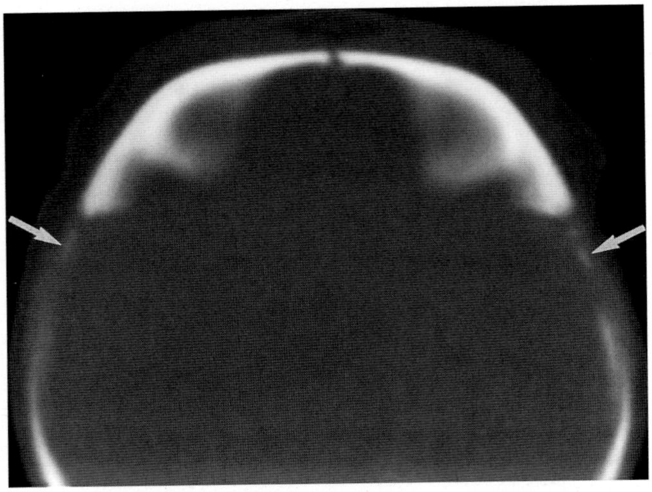

Figure 2A-14: Epiteric sutural (wormian) bones. Axial CT image showing bilateral epipteric sutural bones (*arrows*) in the region of the anterolateral (pterion) fontanelle bilaterally.

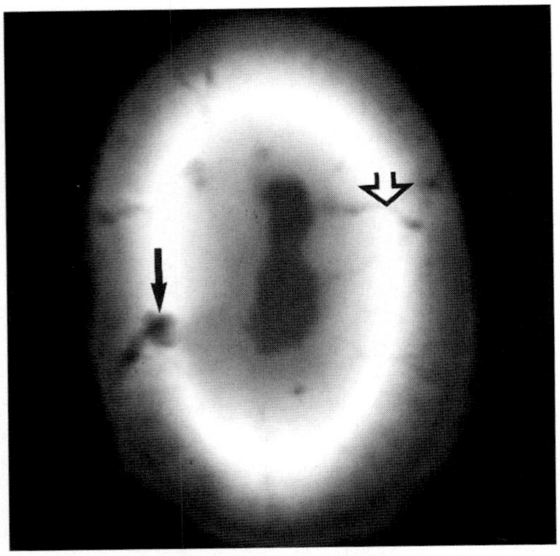

Figure 2A-15: Calvarial venous lake and emissary venous channel. Axial CT image showing a venous lake (*solid arrow*) with a communicating vein and a calvarial emissary venous channel (*open arrow*).

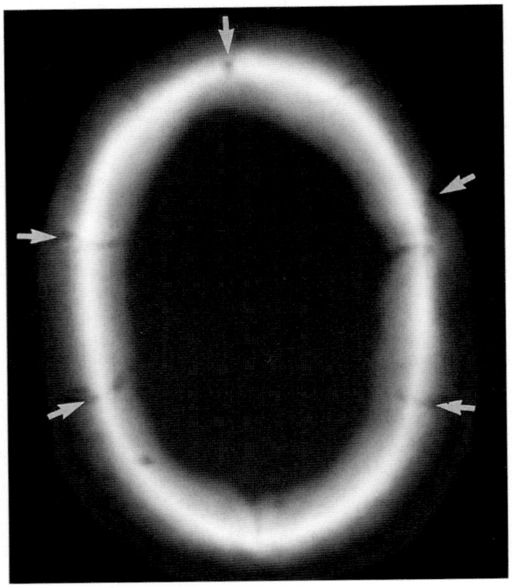

Figure 2A-16: Calvarial diploic and emissary veins. Axial CT image showing multiple diploic and emissary veins (*arrows*).

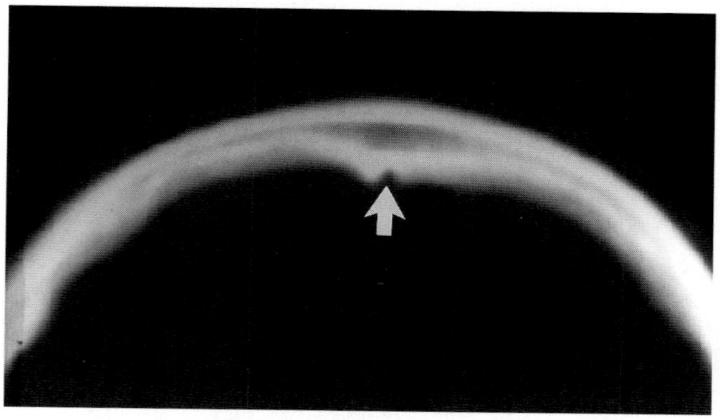

Figure 2A-17A: Venous sinus calvarial groove. Axial CT image shows the anterior aspect of the superior sagittal venous sinus groove (*arrow*) in the internal crest of the frontal bone.

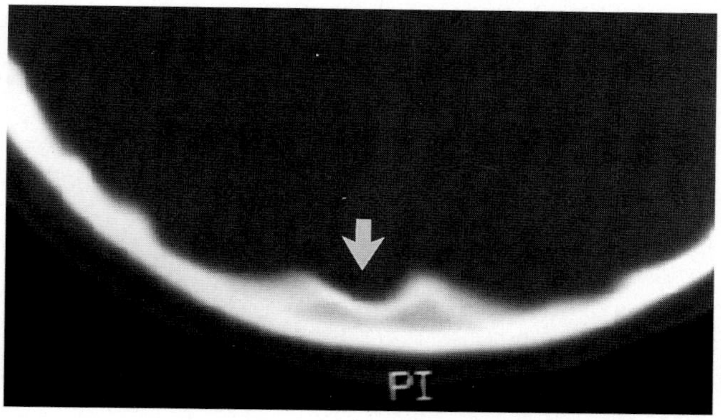

Figure 2A-17B: Venous sinus calvarial groove. Axial CT image shows the posterior aspect of the sagittal venous sinus groove (*arrow*) in the occipital bone.

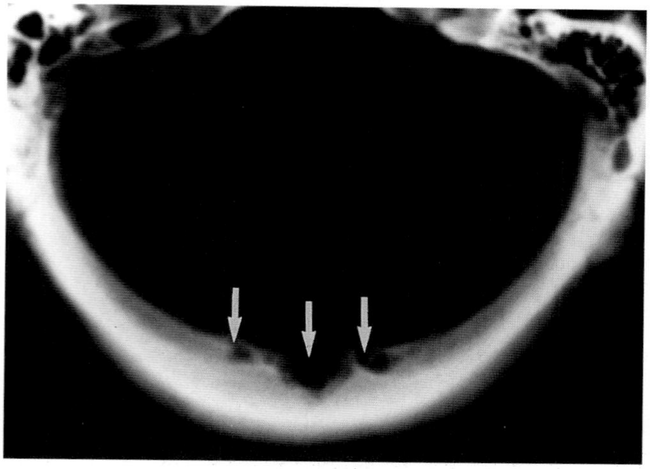

Figure 2A-18: Calvarial arachnoid granulation excavations. Axial CT image showing multiple large arachnoid granulation impressions (excavations) in the occipital bone (*arrows*).

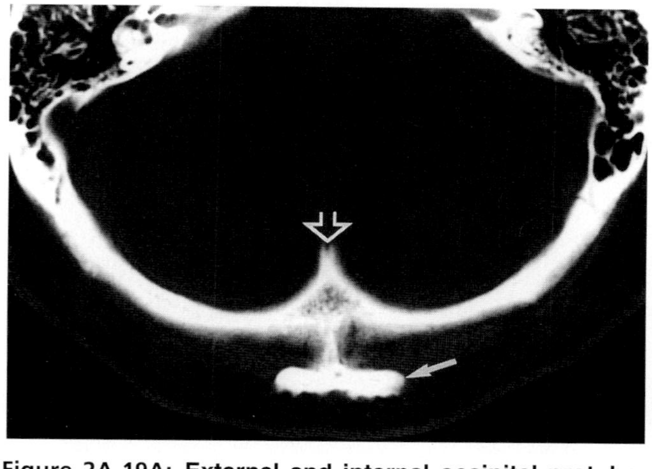

Figure 2A-19A: External and internal occipital protuberance. Axial CT image showing large external (*solid arrow*) and internal (*open arrow*) occipital protuberances.

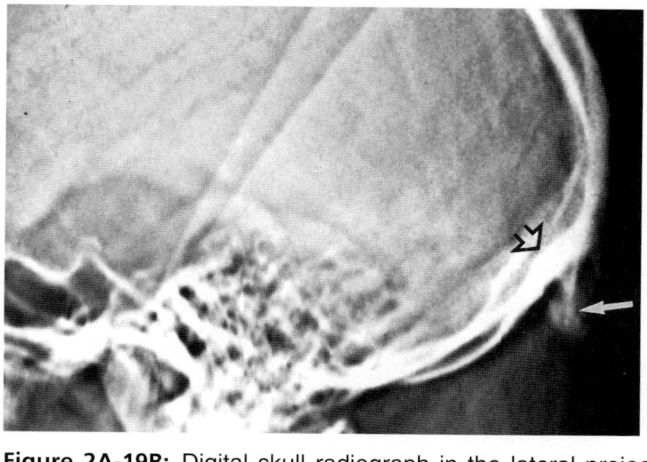

Figure 2A-19B: Digital skull radiograph in the lateral projection, showing the large external (*solid arrow*) and internal (*open arrow*) occipital protuberances.

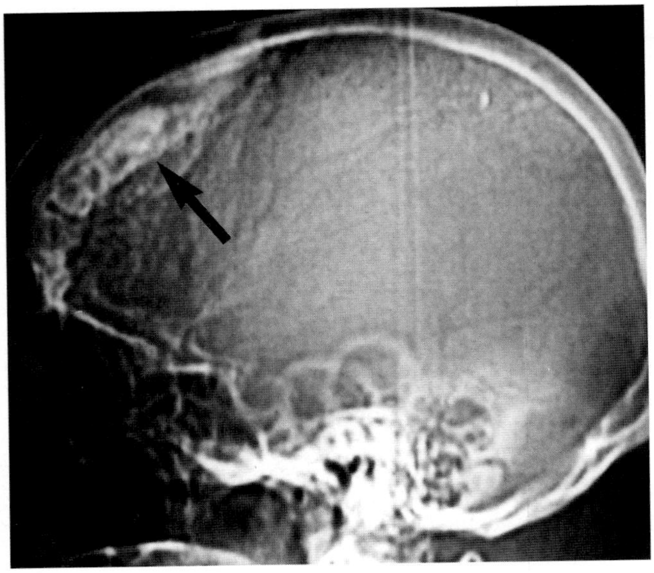

Figure 2A-20A: Hyperostosis frontalis interna. Digital skull radiograph in the lateral projection showing hyperostosis frontalis interna (*arrow*).

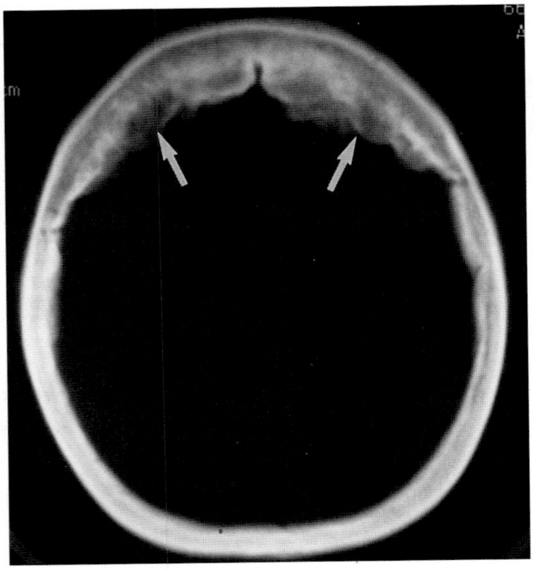

Figure 2A-20B: Axial CT image showing the hyperostosis frontalis interna (*arrows*).

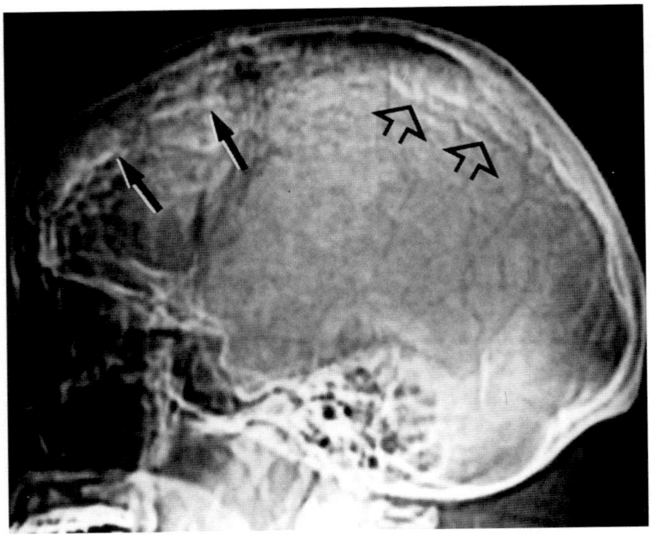

Figure 2A-21A: Hyperostosis frontalis and parietalis interna. Digital skull radiograph in the lateral projection showing hyperostosis frontalis (*closed arrows*) and parietalis (*open arrows*) interna.

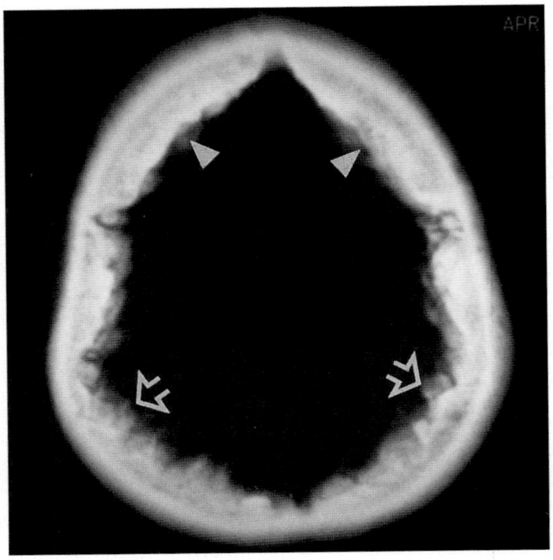

Figure 2A-21B: Axial CT image showing hyperostosis frontalis (*arrowheads*) and parietalis (*open arrows*) interna.

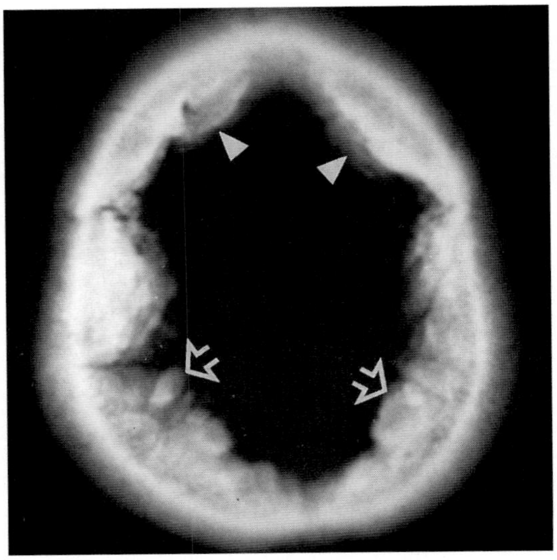

Figure 2A-21C: Axial CT image at a level higher than that of Fig. 2A-21B shows the hyperostosis frontalis (*arrowheads*) and parietalis (*open arrows*) interna.

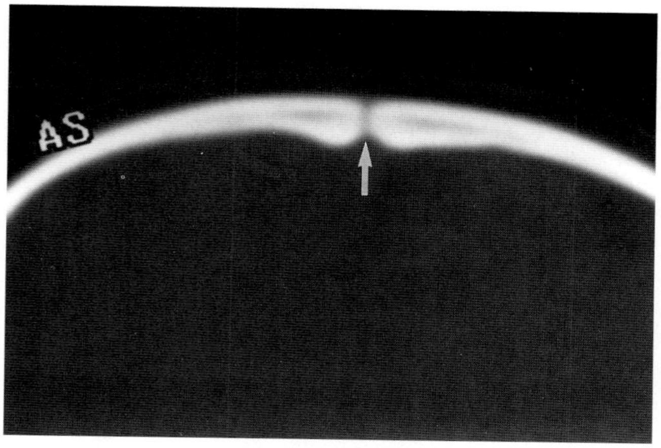

Figure 2A-22A: Metopic suture. Axial CT image in bone window showing metopic suture (*arrow*).

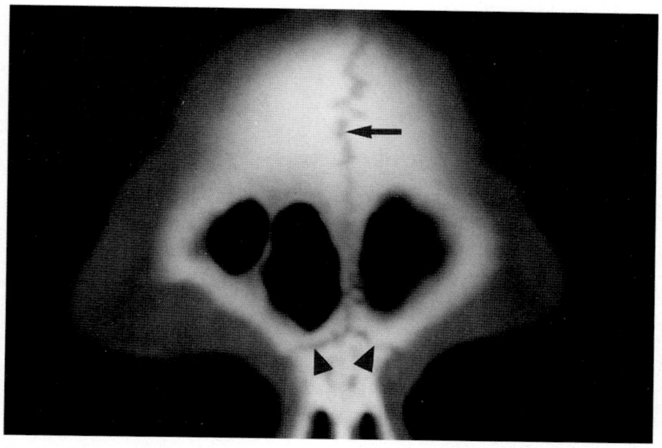

Figure 2A-22B: Coronal CT image showing the metopic sutures (*arrow*) communicating with the frontonasal suture (*arrowheads*).

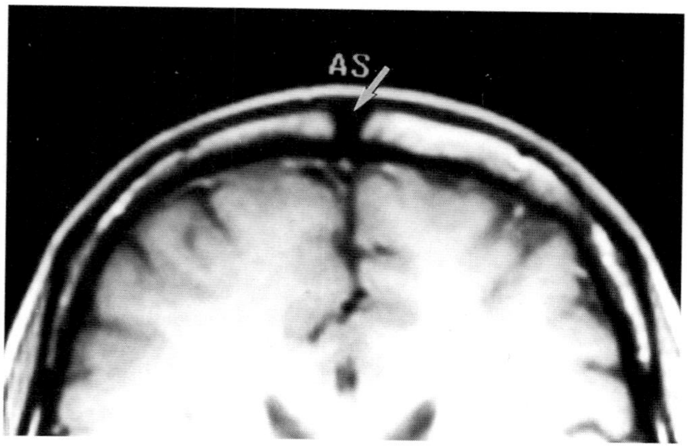

Figure 2A-22C: T1-weighted MR image showing the metopic suture (*arrow*).

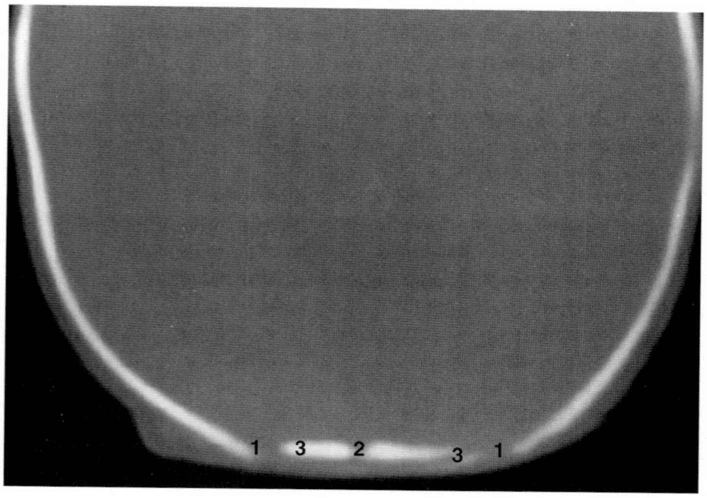

Figure 2A-23A: Superior-median longitudinal intraoccipital suture. Axial CT image in a neonate showing the superior-median intraoccipital suture.
1 Lambdoid sutures
2 Superior-median longitudinal intraoccipital suture
3 Occipital bone

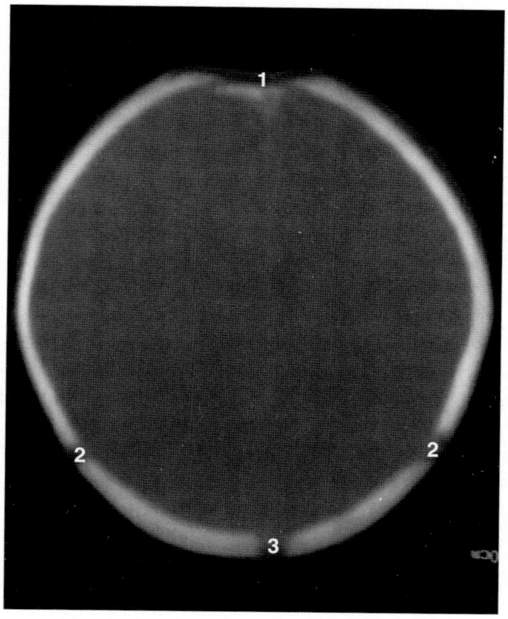

Figure 2A-23B: Axial CT image in a different neonate from the one represented in Fig. 2A-23A, showing the superior median intraoccipital suture.
1 Anterior fontanelle
2 Lambdoid sutures
3 Superior-median longitudinal intraoccipital suture

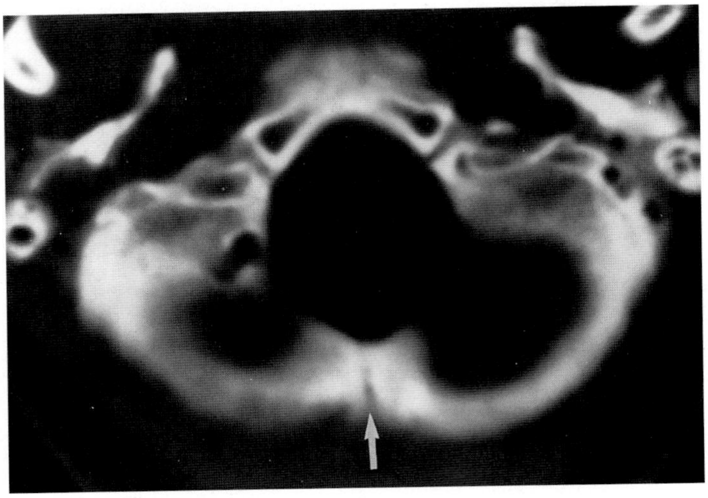

Figure 2A-23C: Inferior-median longitudinal intraoccipital suture/synchondrosis (midline cranium bifidum of the occipital squama). Axial CT image in a child, showing the inferior-median longitudinal intraoccipital suture/synchondrosis (*arrow*), representing an unfused split (cranium bifidum) in the occipital squama in the midline.

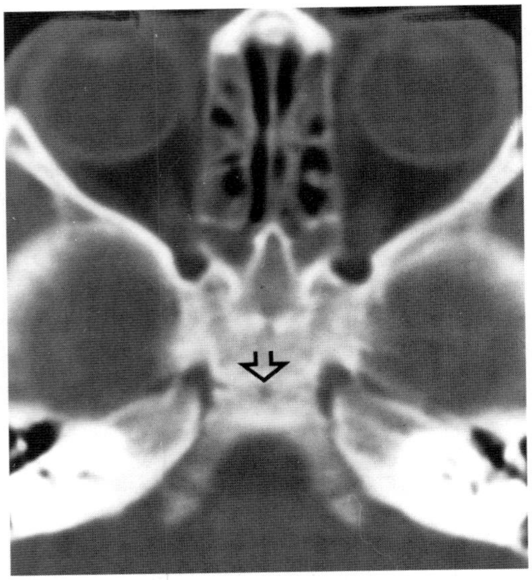

Figure 2A-24: Variation in fusion of the sphenooccipital synchondrosis. Axial CT image in an infant, showing a transient radiolucency in the midline sphenooccipital synchondrosis (*open arrow*).

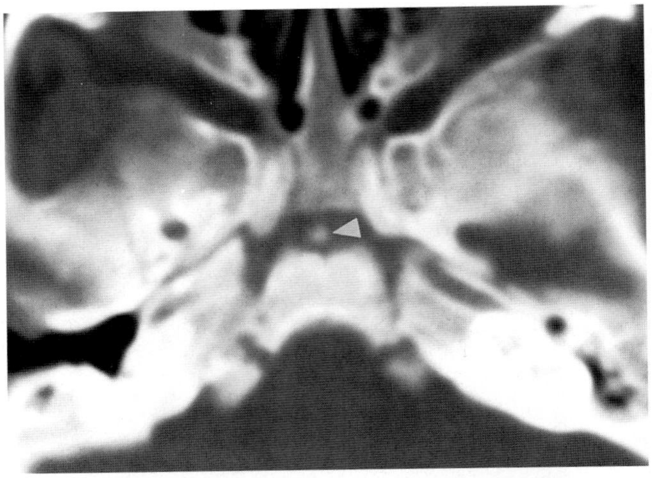

Figure 2A-25A: Accessory ossification center within the sphenooccipital synchondrosis. Axial CT in a child showing an accessory ossification center (*arrowhead*) within the sphenooccipital synchondrosis.

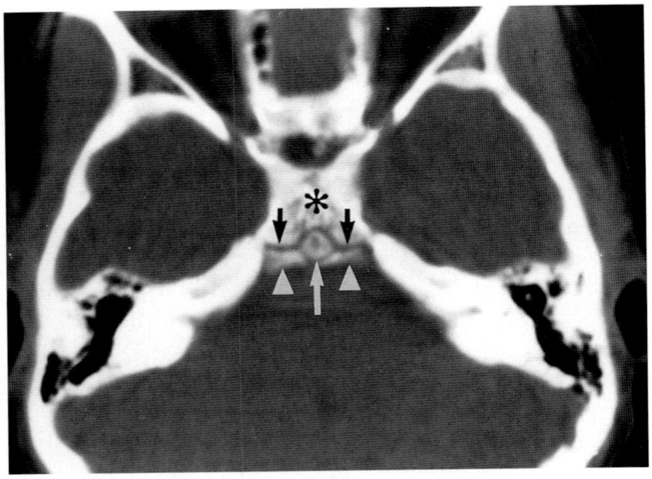

Figure 2A-25B: Accessory calvarial synchondrosis ossification center. Axial CT image in a child, showing the unfused sphenooccipital synchondrosis (*black arrows*) and a rounded accessory sphenooccipital ossification center (*white arrow*) interposed between the basisphenoid (*asterisk*) and the basiocciput (*arrowheads*).

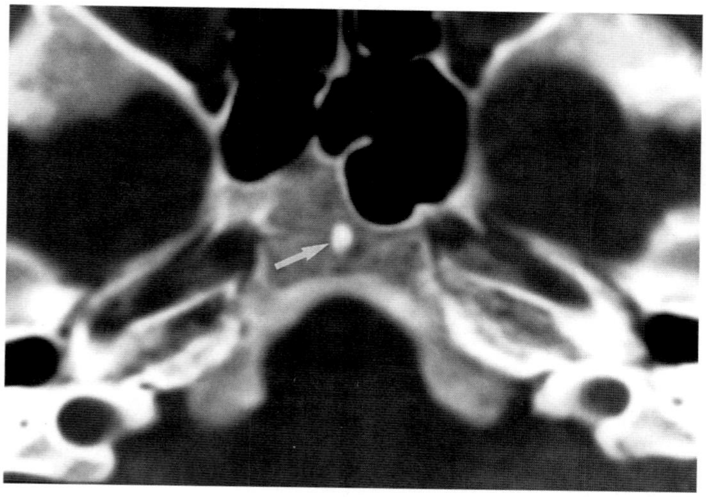

Figure 2A-26A: Sclerotic remnant of sphenooccipital synchondrosis. Axial CT image showing sclerotic remnant (*arrow*) of the sphenooccipital synchondrosis.

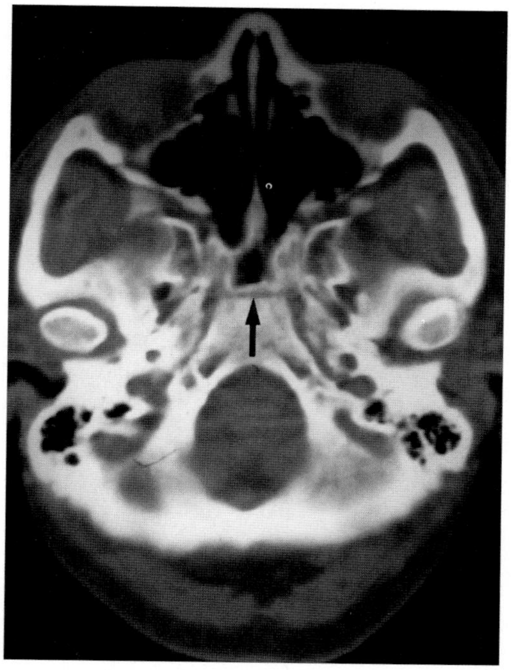

Figure 2A-26B: Persistent sphenooccipital synchondrosis. Axial CT image in a 33-year-old adult, showing persistence of the sphenooccipital synchondrosis (*arrow*).

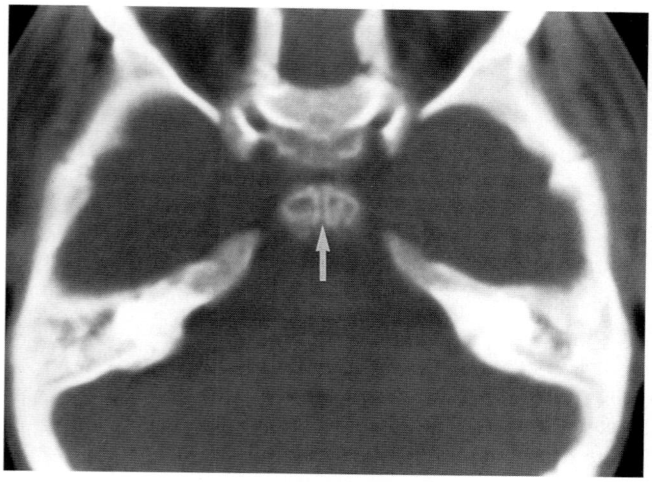

Figure 2A-27: Split ossification center (median longitudinal intrasphenoidal synchrondrosis) involving the basisphenoid (spina bifida occulta of the first embryonic occipital sclerotome/vertebra [O-1]). Axial CT image in a young adult showing a split (*arrow*) in the dorsum sella representing spina bifida occulta of the first embryonic occipital sclerotome/vertebra (O-1). This may result from a persistent median longitudinal intrasphenoidal synchondrosis. The petrous air cells are opacified, and the petrous bones are sclerotic, suggesting chronic petromastoiditis.

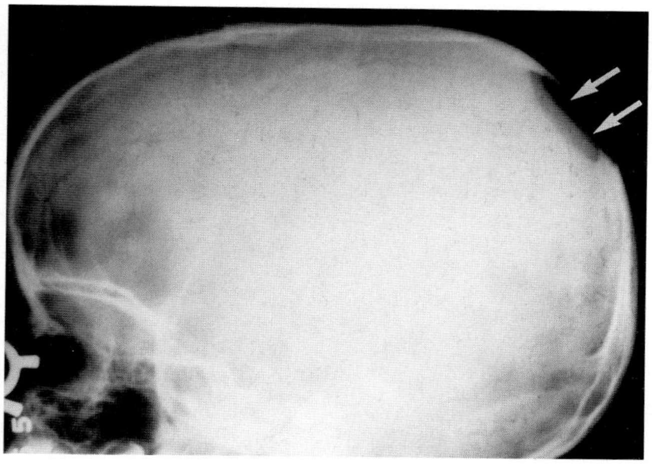

Figure 2A-28: Parietal foramina. Radiograph of the skull in the lateral projection shows the typical appearance of parietal foramina (*arrows*).

2B. Skull Base

OVERVIEW

Interior of the Skull Base

The interior of the skull base is composed of the floors of the anterior, middle, and posterior cranial fossae.

Floor of the Anterior Cranial Fossa

1. The floor of the anterior cranial fossa is formed anteriorly by the frontal bone orbital plates on both sides, the cribriform plate of the ethmoid bone in the midline, and the lesser wings and anterior part of the sphenoid body posteriorly.
2. The terminal branches of the olfactory nerves pass through the foramina in the cribriform plate into the nasal cavity.
3. The chiasmatic sulcus is posterior to the planum sphenoidale. Within it rests the optic chiasm.
4. The lesser wings of the sphenoid bones mark the posterior edge of the anterior cranial fossa and taper to form the anterior clinoid process at its medial extent, on each side of the body of the sphenoid. The free anteromedial border of the tentorium cerebelli attaches to the apex of the anterior clinoid process bilaterally. The anterior clinoid process on each side is grooved medially by the internal carotid artery. Occasionally, an osseous bar surrounds the carotid artery at this point, forming a caroticoclinoid foramen.
5. Optic canals penetrate the sphenoid bone medial and inferior to the anterior clinoid processes and transmit the optic nerves (second cranial nerve: CN-II).
6. The crista galli is an intracranial bony projection of the ethmoid bone in the midline, anterior to which the anterior extent of the falx cerebri is attached.
7. The foramen caecum is located anterior to the crista galli in the midline. Normally it is blind ending, but occasionally it transmits a vein from the nasal mucosa draining into the anterior aspect of the superior sagittal venous sinus.
8. The anterior ethmoidal canal penetrates at the cribrifrontal suture just behind the crista galli; it transmits the anterior ethmoidal vessels and nerve. The posterior ethmoidal canal is found at the posterolateral corner of the cribriform plate and transmits the posterior ethmoidal vessels. The ethmoidal arteries are branches of the ophthalmic artery.

Floor of the Middle Cranial Fossa

1. The floor of the middle cranial fossa is formed by the greater wing of the sphenoid bone anteriorly and the temporal bone posteriorly.
2. Anteriorly it is bordered by the posterior edge of the lesser wing of the sphenoid bone and posteriorly by the ridge of the petrous portion of the temporal bone.
3. Medially it is bordered by the body of sphenoid bones including the sella turcica.
4. Laterally it is bordered by the squamous part of the temporal bone and the greater wing of the sphenoid bone. The superior orbital fissure is an oblique opening between the greater and lesser wings of the sphenoid bone and the body of the sphenoid bone anteriorly. The superior orbital fissure transmits the terminal branches of the ophthalmic nerve (ophthalmic [first] division of the fifth cranial nerve: CN-V1), the ophthalmic veins, and the oculomotor (CN-III), trochlear (CN-IV), and abducens (CN-VI) nerves.
5. The foramen rotundum pierces the greater wing of the sphenoid bone below and posterior to the superior orbital fissure. The maxillary nerve (maxillary [second] division of the fifth cranial nerve: CN-V2) branch of the trigeminal (CN-V) nerve passes into the pterygopalatine fossa via the foramen rotundum and canal.
6. The foramen ovale is posterolateral to the foramen rotundum in the greater wing of the sphenoid bone. The mandibular (mandibular [third] division of the fifth cranial nerve: CN-V3) passes into the infratemporal fossa via the foramen rotundum.
7. Meckel's cave is on the lateral surface of the tip of the petrous bone just posterior to the foramen ovale. The trigeminal nerve (CN-V) ganglion rests in an impression within

Meckel's cave. Meckel's cave is otherwise filled with cerebrospinal fluid and freely communicates with the subarachnoid space.

8. The foramen spinosum is a small opening in the greater wing of the sphenoid bone lateral and posterior to the foramen ovale. The foramen spinosum transmits the middle meningeal artery and the meningeal branch of the mandibular nerve (mandibular [third] division of the fifth cranial nerve: CN-V3).
9. The foramen lacerum is an irregular opening formed between the tip of the petrous bone and the body and greater wing of the sphenoid bone. Throughout its course it transmits the meningeal branches of the ascending pharyngeal artery and small unnamed veins. The internal carotid artery pierces the foramen lacerum in its posterior wall superior to its origin and exits through its upper end. It does not traverse its entire course.
10. The carotid canal proper is an oblique tunnel containing the internal carotid artery. This canal enters into the inferior surface of the petrous part of the temporal bone and opens into the middle cranial fossa at the tip of the petrous bone just behind the foramen lacerum. The internal carotid artery sympathetic plexus accompanies the artery.
11. The vidian (pterygoid) canal traverses the greater wing of the sphenoid bone. It transmits the vidian (pterygoid) nerve and artery and runs from the anterior border of the foramen lacerum anteriorly, to end in the pterygopalatine fossa. The vidian nerve (nerve of the pterygoid canal) transmits parasympathetic fibers of the greater petrosal nerve, itself a branch of the facial nerve (CN-VII), to the pterygopalatine ganglion. Sympathetic fibers from the internal carotid sympathetic plexus, initially transmitted within the deep petrosal nerve, and the vidian artery (artery of the pterygoid canal), a branch of the distal internal carotid artery, also traverse the vidian canal. The parasympathetic fibers will subsequently join the palatine, nasopalatine, and pharyngeal nerves, branches of the maxillary nerve (second division of the fifth cranial nerve: CN-V2), as secretomotor fibers to the mucosa of the nasal passageways, palate, and pharynx and the lacrimal gland. The sympathetic fibers supply the same mucosal areas as well as the lacrimal gland.
12. The paired pterygopalatine fossae lie beneath the orbital apexes on each side. The pterygopalatine fossa is bordered anteriorly by maxilla, posteriorly by the sphenoid bone (pterygoid process and greater wing), superiorly by the inferior orbital fissure (communicating with the orbit inferiorly), laterally by the pterygomaxillary fissure (communicating with the infratemporal fossa) communicating with the middle cranial fossa, inferomedially by the palatovaginal canal, and medially by the sphenopalatine foramen (communicating with the nasal cavity) and the orbital/sphenoidal processes of the palatine bone. The foramen rotundum and vidian (pterygoid) canal open into the posterior aspect of the pterygopalatine fossa (communicating with the middle cranial fossa). The pterygopalatine fossa contains the pterygopalatine ganglion, (in which synapse parasympathetic nerves from the greater petrosal nerve/vidian [pterygoid] nerve), the maxillary nerve (CN-V2), and the vidian/petrosal nerve and artery.
13. The pterygomaxillary fissure transmits the lesser and greater palatine nerves (branches of the maxillary [second] division of the fifth cranial nerve: CN-V2) and branches of the internal maxillary artery.
14. The foramen rotundum (and canal) transmits the maxillary nerve (maxillary [second] division of the fifth cranial nerve: CN-V2) to the pterygopalatine fossa, en route to the infraorbital fissure. Parasympathetic fibers from the pterygopalatine ganglion temporarily join the maxillary nerve on their way to the lacrimal gland. The direct communication of the sphenopalatine fossa with the infraorbital fissure allows the transmission of parasympathetic fibers to the lacrimal gland.
15. The sphenopalatine foramen communicates with the posterior aspect of the superior nasal meatus and transmits the sphenopalatine vessels and the posterior–superior nasal nerves.
16. The palatovaginal canal transmits the pharyngeal nerve from the pterygopalatine ganglion to the pharyngeal roof.

The Floor of The Posterior Cranial Fossa

1. The floor of the posterior cranial fossa is formed by the clivus anteriorly, the petrous and mastoid parts of the temporal bone anterolaterally, and the occipital bone inferiorly, posteriorly, and posterolaterally.
2. The foramen magnum is the largest opening in the base of posterior fossa, where the brain stem continues into the spinal cord. The vertebral arteries enter the skull via the foramen magnum on two sides of the medulla oblongata.
3. Posterior to the foramen magnum, the internal occipital crest runs sagittally in the midline upward, to end in the internal occipital protuberance. The transverse occipital sulci run laterally on either side of the internal occipital protuberance to accommodate the transverse venous sinuses.
4. The internal auditory meatus perforates the medial third of the posterior surface of the petrous part of the temporal bones bilaterally. The internal auditory meatus transmits the facial (CN-VII) and vestibulocochlear/auditory (CN-VIII) cranial nerves to the internal auditory canal of the temporal bone on each side; it also transmits the nervus intermedius and the labyrinthine vessels.
5. The paired jugular foramina are local widenings at the petrooccipital suture. They consist of two parts: (a) the pars nervosa, which transmits the glossopharyngeal (CN-IX) cranial nerve, and (b) the pars venosa, which transmits the jugular vein and the vagus (CN-X) and spinal accessory (CN-XI) cranial nerves.
6. The hypoglossal canal is located at the base of the occipital condyle on either side of the foramen magnum. The paired hypoglossal canals transmit the hypoglossal nerve (CN-XII) on each side. The hypoglossal emissary vein also commonly exits via the hypoglossal canal.

TABLE 2B-1: The Foramina/Fissures of the Skull and the Structures Transmitted

Foramina	Structure(s) transmitted
Arnold's foramen (inconstant)	Superficial and deep minor petrosal nerves and emissary vein
Carotid canal	Internal carotid artery, sympathetic neural plexus
Foramen lacerum	Meningeal branch of mandibular nerve (CN-V3), artery and emissary vein
Foramen magnum	Spinal cord, spinal accessory nerve (CN-XI), vertebral arteries, anterior and posterior spinal arteries
Foramen ovale	Mandibular nerve (CN-V3)
Foramen rotundum	Maxillary nerve (CN-V2), emissary veins and artery of the foramen rotundum
Foramen spinosum	Middle meningeal artery and meningeal branch of the mandibular nerve (CN-V3)
Foramina innominata	Unnamed venous emissary veins in skull base
Hypoglossal canal	Hypoglossal nerve (CN-XII), hypoglossal emissary vein connecting sigmoid venous sinus with internal jugular vein or pterygoid venous plexus
Inferior orbital fissure	Infraorbital nerve (CN-V2) Infraorbital artery and inferior ophthalmic vein, sympathetic/parasympathetic nerves
Infraorbital foramen/canal	Infraorbital nerve (branch of CN-V2), inferior ophthalmic vein
Internal acoustic meatus	Facial nerve (CN-VII) and vestibulocochlear (acoustic) nerve (CN-VIII), nervus intermedius, labyrinthine vessels
Jugular foramen	Pars venosa: vagus nerve (CN-X) and spinal accessory nerve (CN-XI), internal jugular vein; pars nervosa: glossopharyngeal nerve (CN-IX)
Mastoid foramen	Emissary vein connecting the sigmoid venous sinus with the extracranial veins (e.g., vertebral venous plexus)
Olfactory foramina	Olfactory nerve (CN-1) branches
Optic foramen	Optic nerve (CN-II), ophthalmic artery
Parietal foramen(-ina)	Venous emissary vein(s); alternatively, large (several cm) functionless foramina in the parietal bones on either side of the midline
Pharyngohypophyseal (craniopharyngeal) canal (inconstant)	Capsular arterial branch (sinusal)
Posterior condylar canal	Emissary vein connecting the suboccipital venous plexus with the sigmoid venous sinus
Sphenoid emissary foramen (foramen of Vesalius) (inconstant)	Cavernous venous sinus emissary vein to the pterygoid venous plexus, cavernous venous sinus branch of the accessory meningeal artery
Stylomastoid foramen	Facial (CN-VII) nerve
Superior orbital fissure	Oculomotor nerve (CN-III), trochlear nerve (CN-IV), ophthalmic nerve (CN-V1), abducens nerve (CN-VI), autonomic nervous system branches (sympathetic and parasympathetic nerves), deep recurrent ophthalmic artery, superior, lacrimal/meningeal artery branch(es), ophthalmic vein
Supraorbital notch (foramen)	Supraorbital nerve (branch of CN-V1), supraorbital artery and vein
Vidian (pterygoid) canal	Vidian nerve (nerve of the pterygoid canal), vidian artery (artery of the pterygoid canal)

CN, cranial nerve.

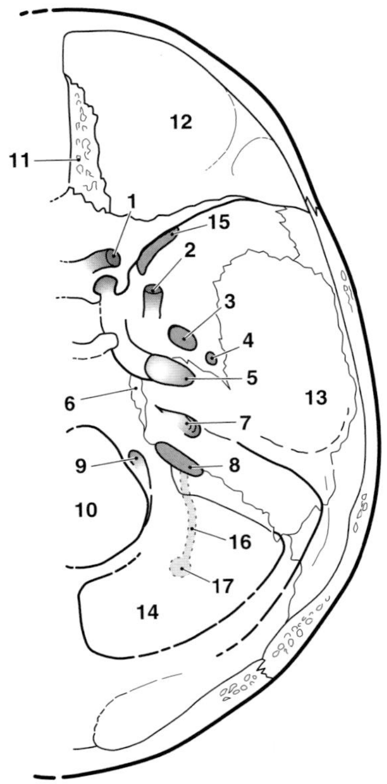

Figure 2B-1: Schematic of the interior of the skull base on the left, showing the foramina and canals.
1 Optic foramen
2 Foramen rotundum
3 Foramen ovale
4 Foramen spinosum
5 Carotid canal
6 Foramen lacerum
7 Internal auditory meatus
8 Jugular foramen
9 Hypoglossal canal
10 Foramen magnum
11 Cribriform plate and foramina
12 Anterior cranial fossa
13 Middle cranial fossa
14 Posterior cranial fossa
15 Superior orbital fissure
16 Posterior condylar emissary vein canal
17 Posterior condylar foramen

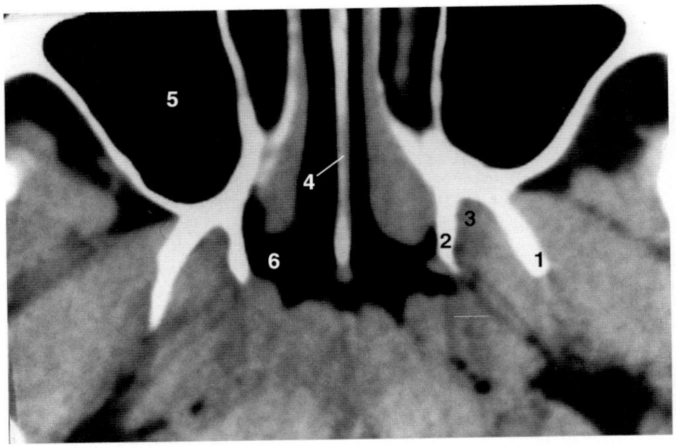

Figure 2B-2A: Normal anatomy of the skull base. A series of axial and coronal CT images showing the normal anatomy of the skull base. **A:** Axial CT image showing the pterygoid plate and fossa.
1 Lateral pterygoid plate
2 Medial pterygoid plate
3 Pterygoid fossa
4 Vomer of the nasal septum
5 Maxillary sinus
6 Nasopharynx

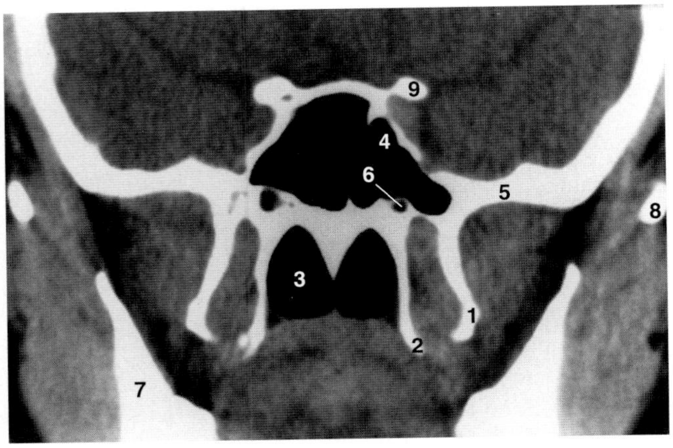

Figure 2B-2B: Coronal CT image showing the pterygoid plates.
1 Lateral pterygoid plate
2 Medial pterygoid plate
3 Nasopharynx
4 Sphenoid sinus
5 Floor of middle cranial fossa
6 Pterygoid (vidian) canal
7 Mandible
8 Zygomatic arch
9 Anterior clinoid process

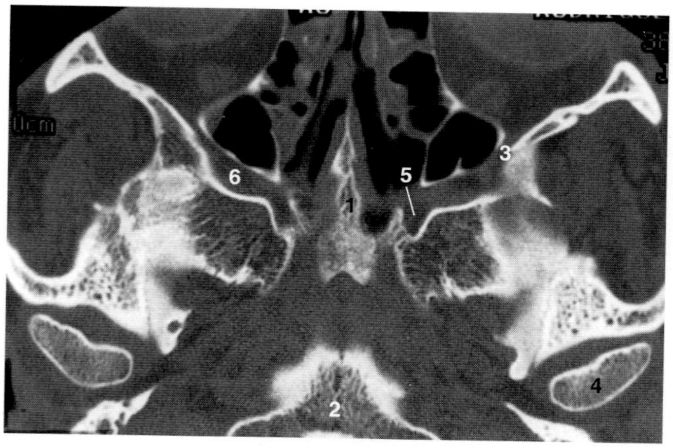

Figure 2B-2C: Axial section at the level of the pterygopalatine fossa.

1 Rostrum of sphenoid bone
2 Clivus
3 Inferior orbital fissure
4 Mandibular condyle
5 Sphenopalatine foramen
6 Pterygopalatine fossa

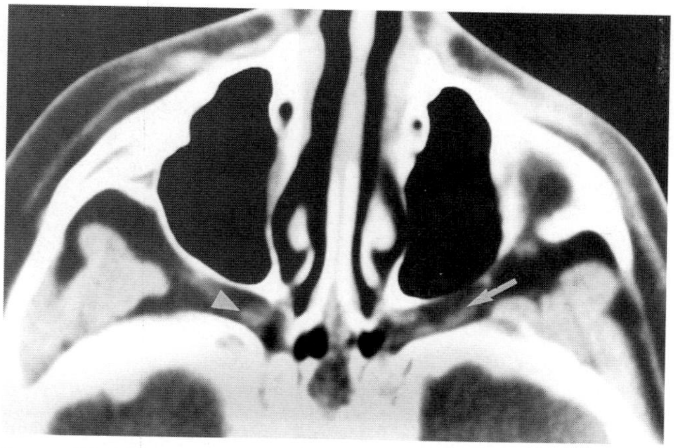

Figure 2B-2D: Axial CT image showing pterygopalatine fossa (*arrow*) and ganglion (*arrowhead*).

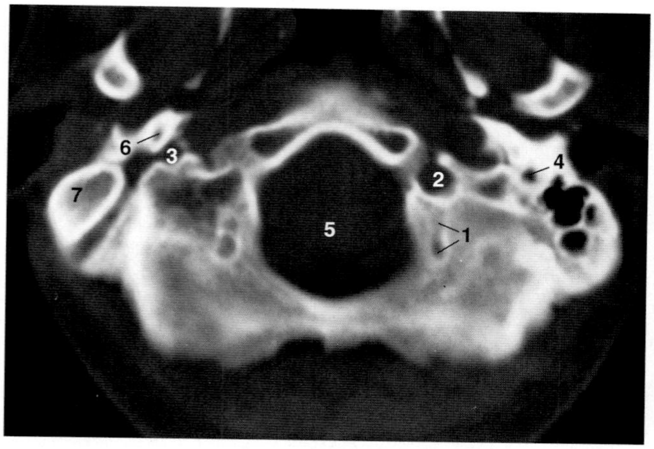

Figure 2B-2E: Axial CT image at the level of the foramen magnum.

1 Posterior condylar venous canal and foramen
2 Jugular vein fossa
3 Stylomastoid foramen
4 Lower facial nerve canal (continuation of 3)
5 Foramen magnum
6 Upper end (base) of styloid process
7 Mastoid process

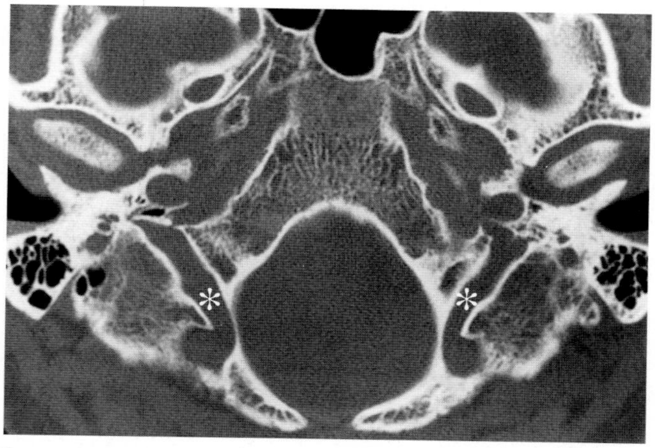

Figure 2B-2F: Axial CT image showing the posterior condylar canals bilaterally (*asterisks*).

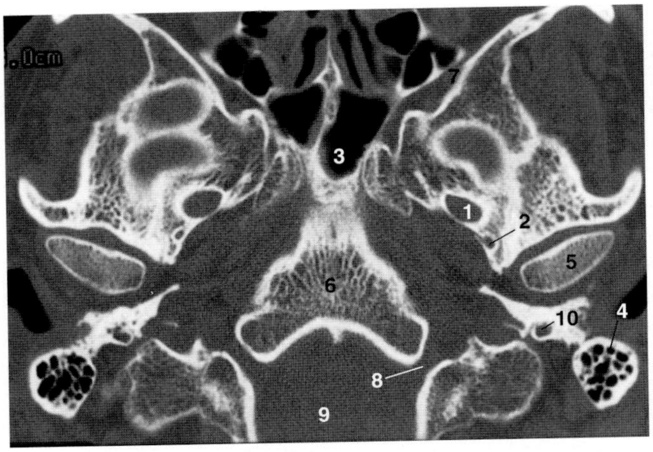

Figure 2B-2G: Axial CT image at the level of the hypoglossal canals.

1 Foramen ovale
2 Foramen spinosum
3 Sphenoid sinus
4 Mastoid air cells
5 Mandibular condyle
6 Clivus
7 Inferior orbital fissure
8 Hypoglossal canal
9 Foramen magnum
10 Facial nerve canal

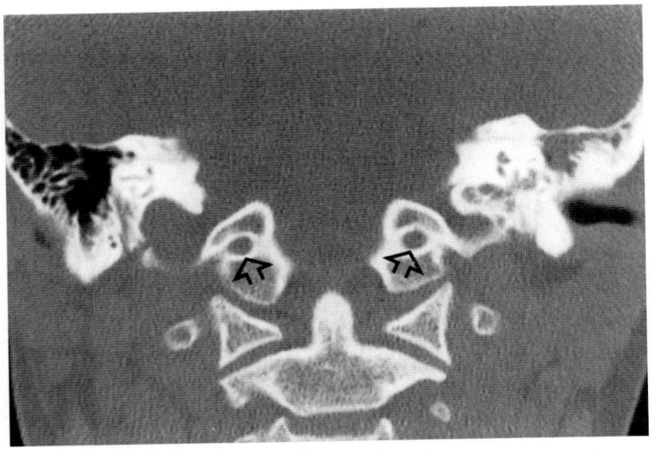

Figure 2B-2H: Coronal CT image showing the hypoglossal canals bilaterally (*arrows*).

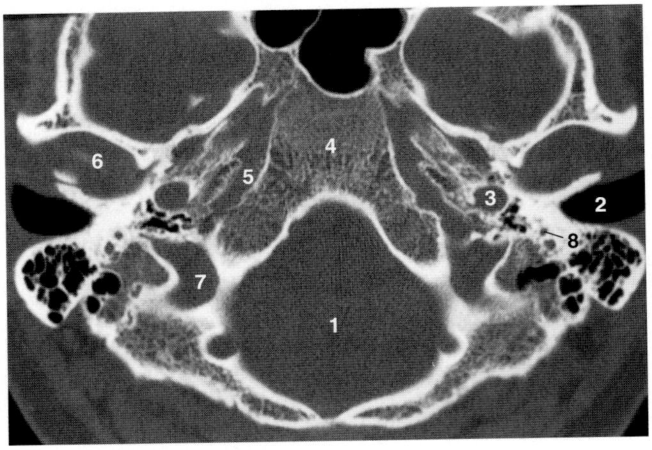

Figure 2B-2I: Axial CT image at the level of the clivus.

1 Foramen magnum
2 Lateral extent of the external auditory canal
3 Carotid canal
4 Clivus
5 Foramen lacerum
6 Glenoid fossa
7 Jugular vein fossa
8 Lower facial nerve canal

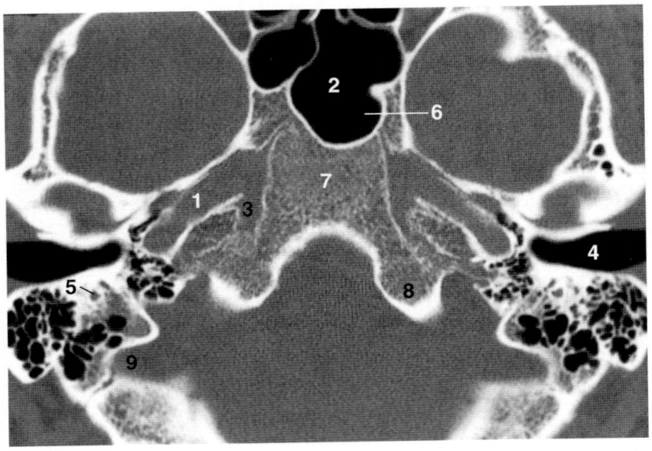

Figure 2B-2J: Axial CT image at the level of the carotid canals.

1 Carotid canal
2 Sphenoid sinus
3 Foramen lacerum
4 External auditory canal
5 Facial nerve canal
6 Sphenoid sinus
7 Clivus
8 Jugular tubercle
9 Jugular siphon sulcus

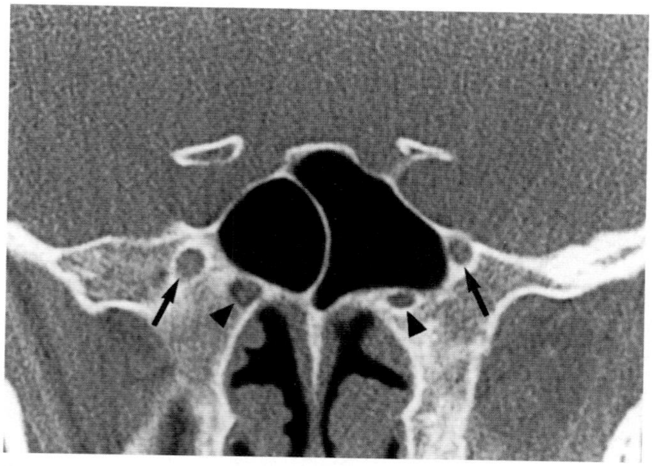

Figure 2B-2K: Foramina rotunda and vidian canals. Coronal CT image showing foramina rotunda (*arrows*) and vidian (pterygoid) canals (*arrowheads*) bilaterally.

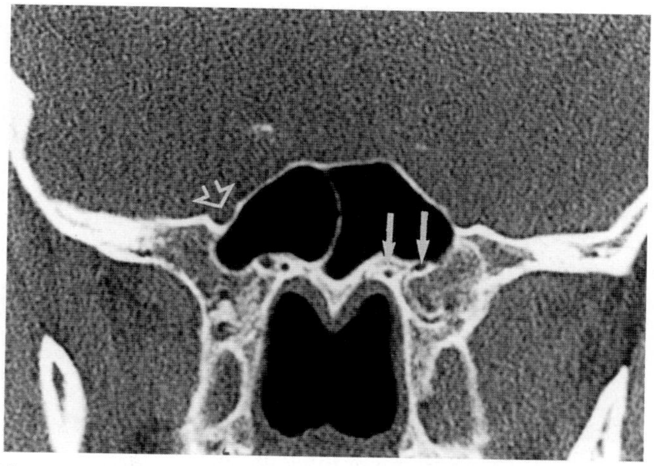

Figure 2B-2L: Duplication of the vidian canals. Coronal CT image posterior to that of Fig. 2B-2K, showing duplication of the pterygoid (vidian) canals bilaterally (*arrows*), perhaps one component carrying neural structures and the other vascular structures. The incomplete bony foramen rotundum [*sulcus rotundum* (Jinkins)] is also seen (*open arrow*), a typical feature observed posteriorly.

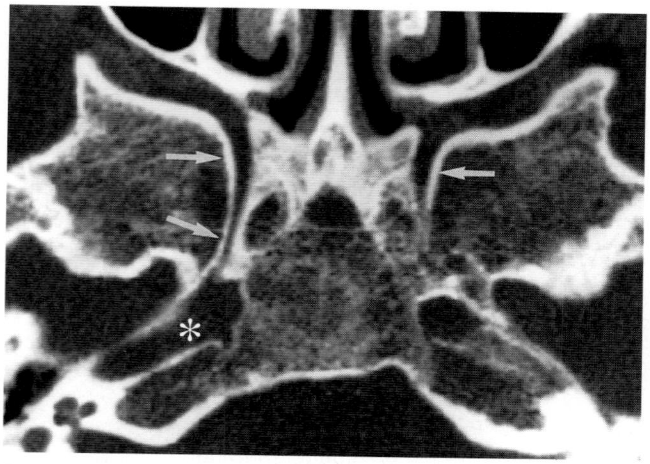

Figure 2B-2M: Vidian canals. Magnified axial CT image showing the vidian (pterygoid) (*arrows*) bilaterally. The communication with the carotid canal (*asterisks*) is noted on the right side.

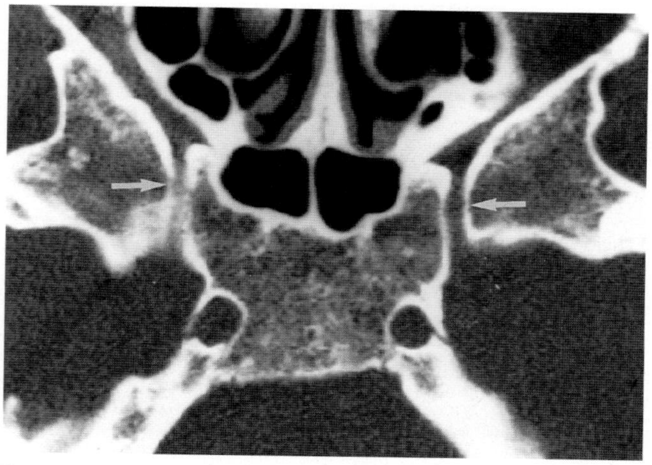

Figure 2B-2N: Foramina rotunda. Magnified axial CT image at a higher level than that of Fig. 2B-2M, showing the foramina rotunda (*arrows*).

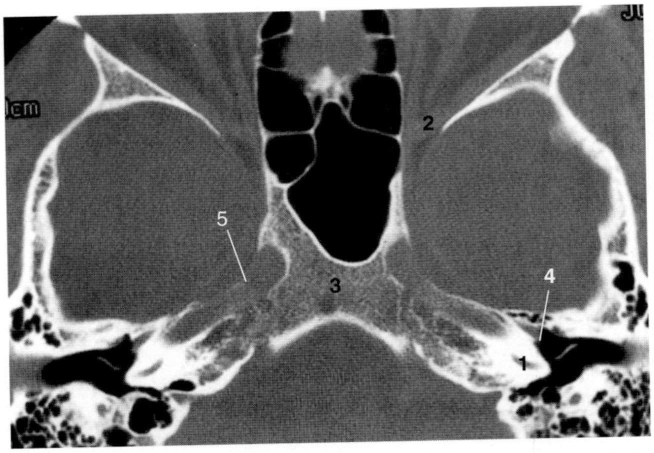

Figure 2B-2O: Anatomy at the level of the superior orbital fissure. Axial CT image at the level of the superior orbital fissure.

1 Basal turn of the cochlea
2 Superior orbital fissure
3 Clivus
4 Termination of eustachian tube
5 Carotid canal

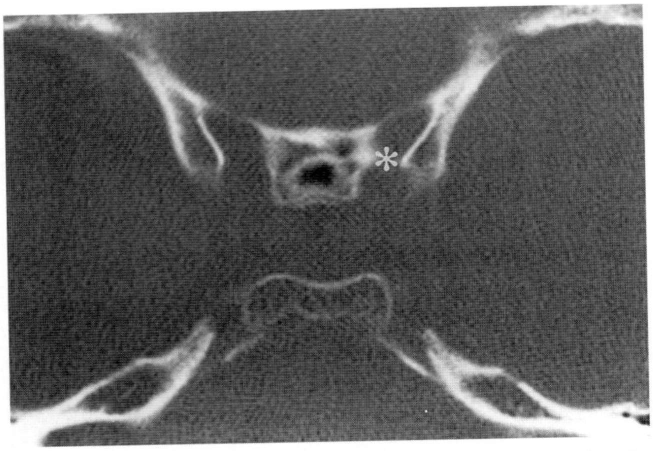

Figure 2B-2P: The optic canals. Axial CT scan showing the proximal extent of the optic canals (*asterisk*).

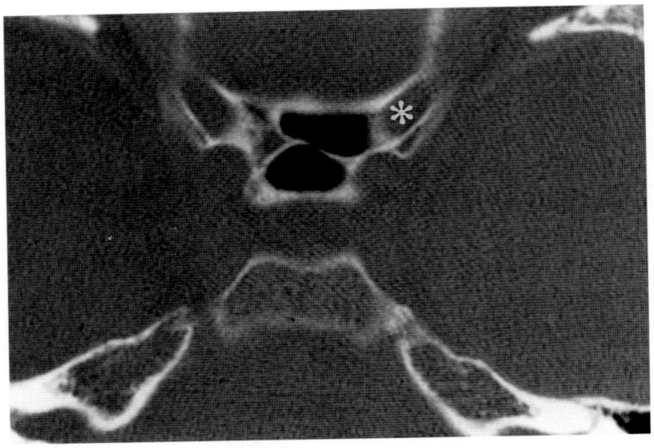

Figure 2B-2Q: Axial CT image at a level just inferior to Fig. 2B-2P, showing the middle extent of the optic canals (*asterisk*).

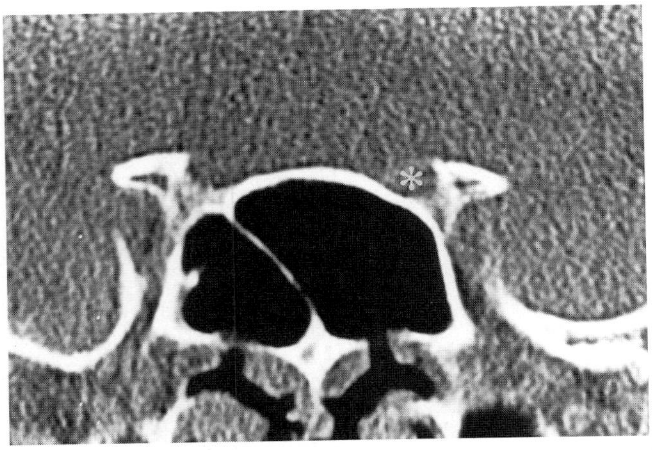

Figure 2B-2R: Coronal CT image showing the most proximal extent of the optic canals (*asterisk*), the junctions of the optic canals, and the suprasellar cistern.

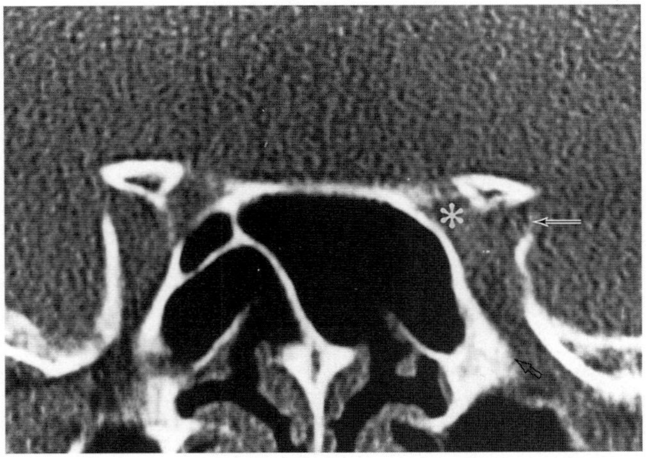

Figure 2B-2S: Coronal CT image acquired immediately anterior to that of Fig. 2B-2R shows the junction (*asterisk*) of the optic canals with the orbital apex. Also note the superior (*solid arrow*) and inferior (*open arrow*) orbital fissures.

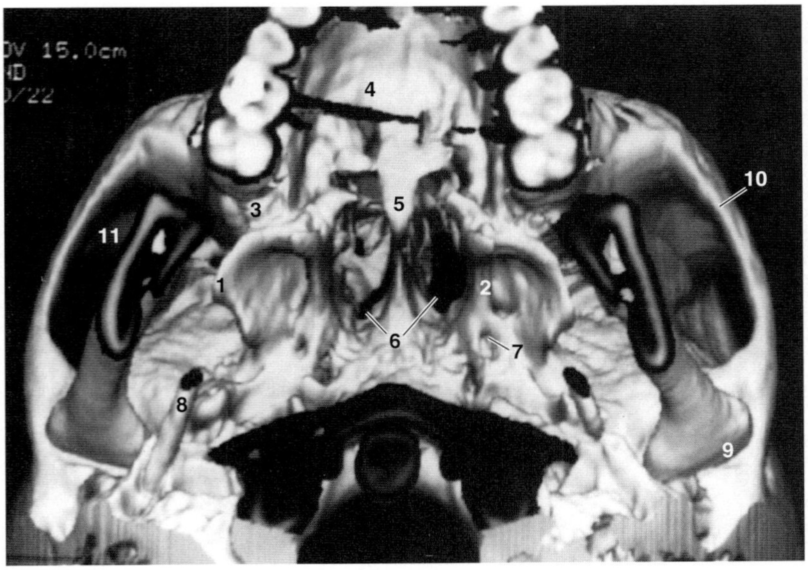

Figure 2B-2T: Skull base from below. Three-dimensional CT image showing the surface features of the skull base from below.

1 Lateral pterygoid plate
2 Medial pterygoid plate
3 Pterygopalatine fossa
4 Hard palate
5 Posterior nasal spine
6 Nasal choanae
7 Foramen ovale
8 Styloid process
9 Temporomandibular joint
10 Zygomatic arch
11 Deep temporal fossa

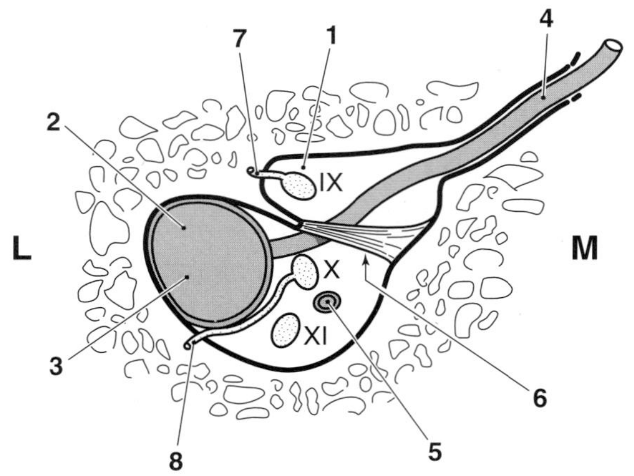

Figure 2B-3: Axial schematic of the jugular vein foramen and its contents on the right side. *IX*, glossopharyngeal nerve; *X*, vagus nerve; *XI*, spinal accessory nerve; *A*, anterior; *P*, posterior; *M*, medial; *L*, lateral.

1 Pars nervosa
2 Pars vascularis (jugular vein)
3 Proximal internal jugular vein/terminal end of sigmoid venous sinus
4 Inferior petrosal venous sinus
5 Posterior meningeal artery
6 Septum
7 Jacobson's nerve (CN-IX)
8 Arnold's nerve (CN-X)

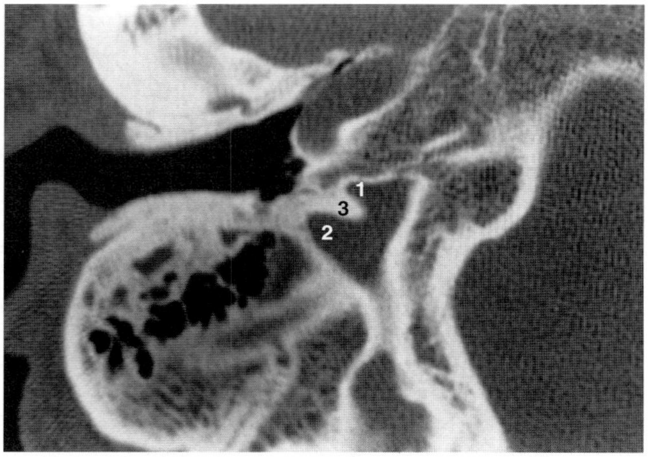

Figure 2B-4: Jugular foramen. Axial CT image showing the components of the jugular foramen on the right side.

1 Pars nervosa
2 Pars vascularis
3 Bony septum

CALVARIAL FORAMINA VARIANTS

- Asymmetric jugular venous foramina
- Sphenoid emissary venous foramen (foramen of Vesalius)
- Persistent pharyngohypophyseal (craniopharyngeal) canal, partial or complete (Jinkins)
- Arnold's foramen
- Foramina innominata (unnamed venous emissary foramina)
- Other asymmetric neurovascular foramina (e.g., foramen ovale)

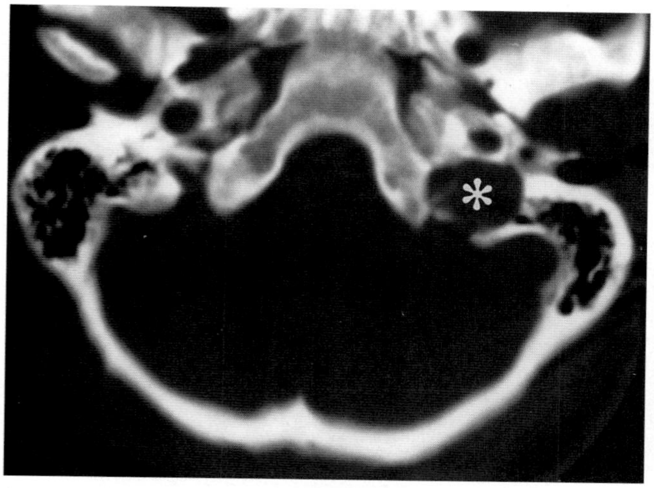

Figure 2B-5A: Dominant internal jugular vein foramen. Axial CT image showing a dominant internal jugular vein canal (*asterisk*) on the left side.

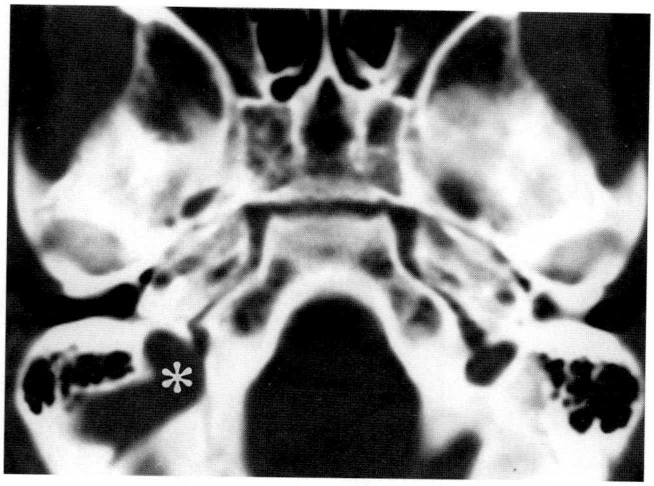

Figure 2B-5B: Asymmetric jugular foramina. Axial CT image of a different patient, showing a dominant internal jugular vein canal (*asterisk*) on the right side.

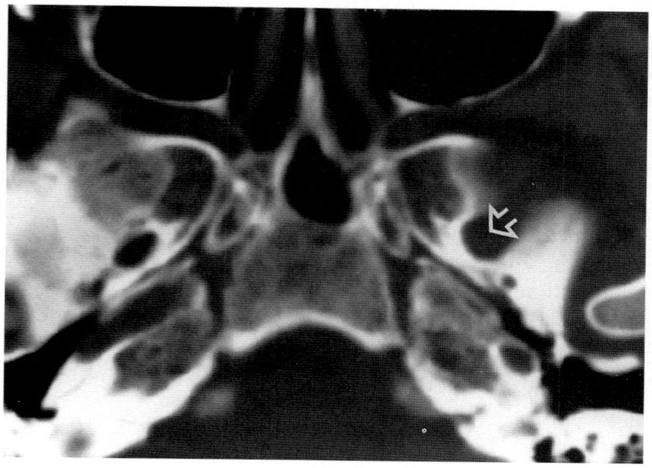

Figure 2B-5C: Asymmetric foramina ovale. Axial CT image showing a larger foramen ovale (*arrow*) on the left side.

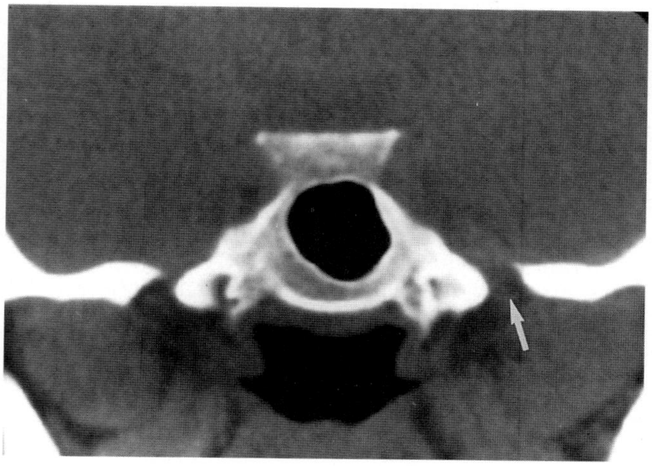

Figure 2B-5D: Asymmetric foramina ovale. Coronal CT image in the same case as Fig. 2B-5C showing the larger foramen ovale (*arrows*) on the left side.

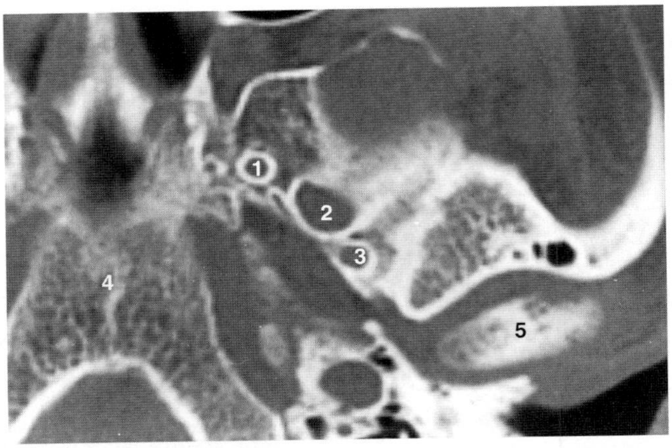

Figure 2B-6: Sphenoid emissary foramen (foramen of Vesalius). Axial CT showing the foramen of Vesalius anteromedial to the foramen ovale.

1 Sphenoid emissary foramen (foramen of Vesalius: inconstant opening that contains an emissary vein that connects the cavernous venous sinus to the pterygoid venous plexus)
2 Foramen ovale
3 Foramen spinosum
4 Clivus
5 Left mandibular condyle

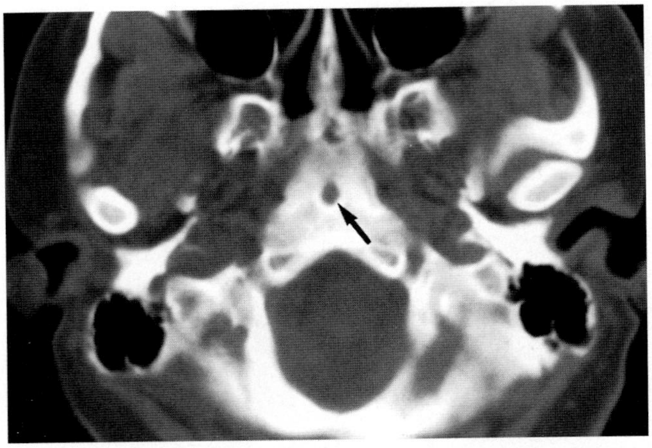

Figure 2B-7A: Persistent remnant of pharyngohypophyseal (craniopharyngeal) canal. Axial CT image in an adult shows a probable persistent remnant of the pharyngohypophyseal (craniopharyngeal) canal (*arrow*).

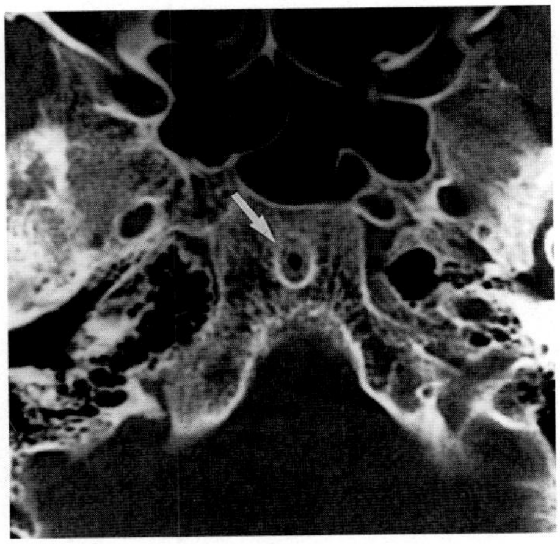

Figure 2B-7B: Axial CT showing a foramen in the basisphenoid (*arrow*) of the clivus containing air within its lumen, indicating communication with the nasopharynx. This pharyngohypophyseal canal was incomplete and ended blindly without communicating with the sella turcica.

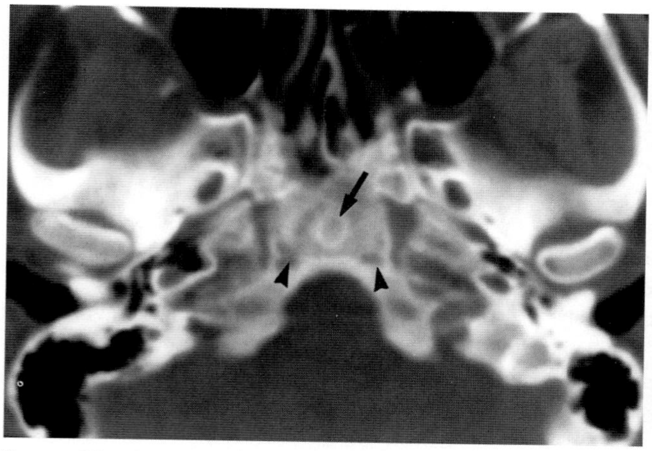

Figure 2B-7C: Axial CT image showing a sclerotic remnant (*arrow*) of the pharyngohypophyseal (craniopharyngeal) canal. Note that this remnant is anterior to the residual lucency of the sphenooccipital synchondrosis (*arrowheads*).

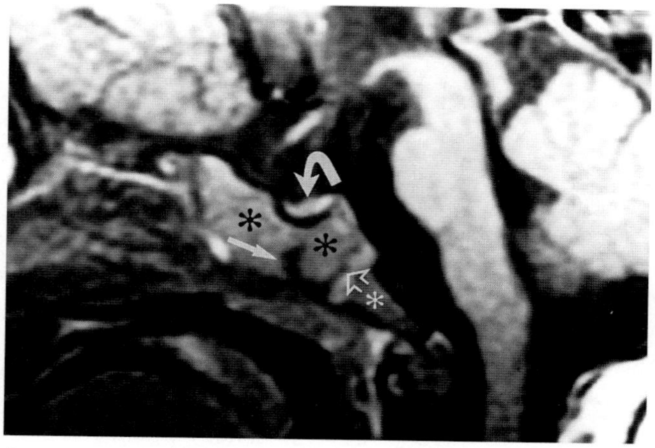

Figure 2B-7D: Sagittal T1-weighted MR image showing a remnant of the pharyngohypophyseal (craniopharyngeal) canal (*closed straight arrow*) inferior to the sella turcica/pituitary gland (*curved arrow*). Also note the basiocciput (*white asterisk*), the basisphenoid (*black asterisks*), and the sphenoccipital synchondrosis (*open straight arrow*).

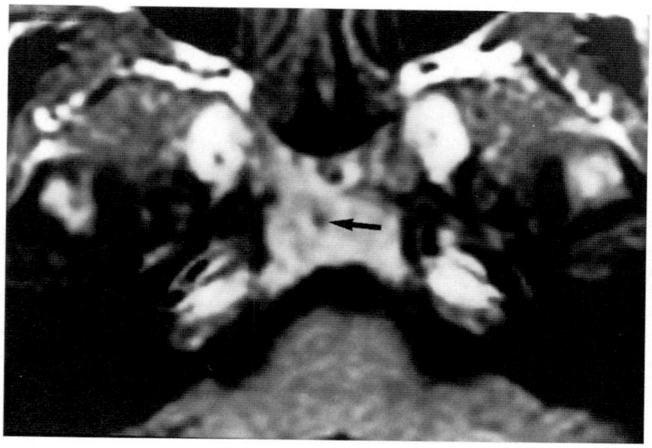

Figure 2B-7E: Axial T1-weighted MR image showing a small remnant of the pharyngohypophyseal (craniopharyngeal) canal (*arrow*) traversing the fatty marrow of the clivus.

THE CLIVUS

1. The term clivus literally means a "downward sloping surface."
2. The clivus refers to that part of the skull base just anterior to the foramen magnum in the midline.
3. The clivus is a wedge-shaped bone formed by a combination of the basal part of the occipital bone (basiocciput) and the body of the sphenoid bone (basisphenoid) at the sphenooccipital synchondrosis. After an average age of approximately 20 years, the sphenooccipital synchondrosis is replaced by bony fusion.
4. The lower part of the pons and the medulla oblongata of the brain stem lie against the posterior surface of the clivus, which is normally concave posterosuperiorly. The pons and the medulla are separated from the clivus by the prepontine and perimedullary cisterns.
5. The boundaries of the clivus
   a. Anteriorly the boundary of the clivus is not well defined; it joins with the bony structure of the sphenoid bone surrounding the sphenoid sinus.
   b. Posteriorly the boundary of the clivus is the anterior margin of the foramen magnum (the basion).
   c. Laterally the boundary of the clivus is the petrooccipital fissure superiorly and the synchondrosis between the basioccipital and exoccipital parts of the occipital bone inferiorly.
   d. Inferiorly the boundary of the clivus is the nasopharyngeal surface overlying the lower portion of the basisphenoid and basiocciput.
   e. Superiorly the clivus borders upon the basal subarachnoid spaces anterior to the brain stem.
6. The free surfaces of the clivus
   a. The inferior (exocranial) surface has attachments with the fibrous raphe of the pharynx, the muscles of the nasopharynx, and the anterior ligaments of the spinal column.
   b. The posterior (endocranial) surface is usually smooth and is covered by dura mater.
7. The clivus has cortical bone on its surfaces and cancellous bone in its central portion, which may be variably pneumatized from the sphenoid sinus.
8. Two small bony protuberances, jugular tubercles, project posteriorly from the lateral inferior margin of the clivus. These jugular tubercles are bony elevations of the occipital bone projecting from the medial side of the two jugular foramina.

CLIVUS VARIANTS

- Superiorly displaced or congenitally flat clivus (i.e., platybasia, basilar impression/invagination)
- Shortened clivus (e.g., achondroplasia, idiopathic)

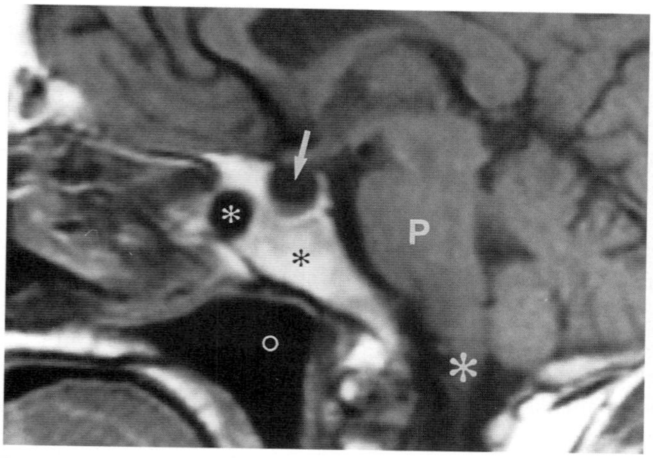

Figure 2B-8A: The clivus. Sagittal T1-weighted MR image showing the typical hyperintensity of the marrow of the clivus (*black asterisk*) in an adult. Note the air within the sphenoid sinus (*small white asterisk*). *P*, pons; *large white asterisk*, foramen magnum; *arrow*, sella turcica (partially empty); *circle*, nasopharynx.

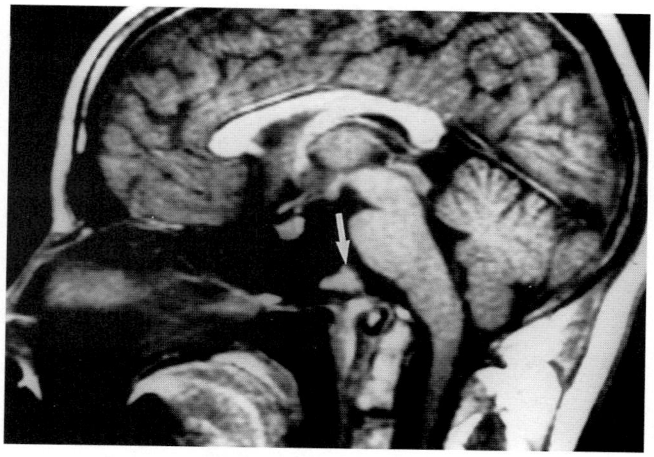

Figure 2B-8B: Hypoplastic clivus. Sagittal T1-weighted MR image showing a short (hypoplastic) clivus (*arrow*), platybasia, a large anteroposterior foramen diameter, and posterosuperior displacement of the odontoid process and anterior arch of C-1. Note the sharp posterior deflection of the cervicomedullary junction.

THE PETROUS PORTION OF THE TEMPORAL BONE

The External Auditory Canal

1. The external auditory canal (EAC) is directed anteromedially from the external auditory meatus at the concha of the auricle, or pinna, to the tympanic membrane.
2. The total length of the EAC is about 2.5 cm in the adult; the outer third is cartilaginous, and the inner two-thirds is composed of bone.
3. The tympanic membrane at its medial end separates the EAC from the tympanic cavity.

The Tympanic Membrane

1. The tympanic membrane (TM) is an oval-shaped, thin membrane measuring approximately 9 × 10 mm in the adult; it is continuous with the skin of the EAC, but it contains no dermal papillae.
2. It is tightly adherent to the medial end of the osseous EAC at the tympanic sulcus by means of a circumferential ring of thickened fibrocartilage. The TM makes an angle of approximately 55 degrees with the floor of the medial end of the EAC.
3. The TM is slightly drawn inward at its center, the umbo, where the handle of the malleus is firmly attached.
4. The anterior and posterioı malleolar folds are formed in the superior part of the TM; the lateral process of the malleus is attached to the middle parts of the folds.
5. The pars flaccida is the part of the relatively lax membrane between the malleolar folds; the pars tensa, which is relatively taut, forms the remaining portion of the membrane.

The Tympanic Cavity (Tympanum, Middle Ear)

1. The tympanic cavity is an irregular airspace in the temporal bone measuring approximately 15 × 15 × 6 mm in the adult.
2. The tympanic cavity proper includes the mesotympanum and the hypotympanum. It contains the upper half of the malleus and most of the incus.
3. The epitympanum is the attic above the level of the tympanic membrane. The tympanic cavity communicates with the nasopharynx via the eustachian (pharyngotympanic, auditory) tubes. The eustachian tube runs anteromedially and slopes downward from the anteromedial end of the tympanic cavity. It consists of bony and cartilaginous sections. The bony part (~12 mm) begins at the anterior tympanic wall and ends at the outer skull base; the cartilaginous part (~24 mm) extends to and opens into the nasopharynx via the fibrous terminal. A lymphoid mass, the tubal tonsil is found submucosally at the pharyngeal orifice. The mucosa of the eustachian tube is continuous between the tympanic and pharyngeal mucosal surfaces.
4. The tegmen tympani is the bony roof of the tympanic cavity that separates it from the middle cranial fossa.
5. The tensor tympani is a muscle that occupies its canal in the anterior wall of the cavity. It originates from the cartilaginous part of the eustachian tube, the adjacent greater wing of the sphenoid bone, and its own canal, and it is attached to the handle of the malleus. It is innervated by a branch of the mandibular nerve (CN-V3). The tensor tympani muscle tenses the tympanic membrane and seats the stapes more firmly in the oval window.
6. The stapedius muscle originates from the pyramidal eminence in the posterior wall of the tympanic cavity and is attached to the neck of the stapes. It is innervated by a branch of the facial nerve (CN-VII). The stapedius muscle opposes the tensor tympani;

together these two muscles dampen auditory vibrations (especially those of high intensity).

7. The facial nerve canal
   a. The facial nerve canal is S-shaped and arises at the lateral end of the internal auditory canal.
   b. The genu of the canal is in the anteromedial wall of the tympanic cavity; the genu turns posterolaterally and harbors the geniculate nucleus of the facial nerve.
   c. The facial nerve canal subsequently courses posteriorly in the medial wall of the tympanic cavity, producing a bony prominence on the upper part of the wall.
   d. The second turn of the facial nerve canal is in the posteromedial wall of the tympanic cavity, where it descends inferiorly.
   e. The chorda tympani nerve arises from the facial nerve in the descending part of the canal.
   f. The facial nerve canal ends at the stylomastoid foramen in the base of the skull.
8. The chorda tympani is a branch nerve that arises from the descending part of the facial nerve (CN-VII) in the facial canal.
   a. The chorda tympani enters the tympanic cavity through a canaliculus in the posterior wall.
   b. The nerve passes upward and anteriorly and traverses the tympanic cavity at the level of the upper end of the malleolus.
   c. The chorda tympani leaves the tympanic cavity and the petrous part of the temporal bone through another canaliculus in the anterior wall of the tympanic cavity.
9. The promontory is a prominence on the anterior part of the medial wall of the tympanic cavity overlying the basal turn of the cochlea.
10. The oval window (vestibular window) is an opening situated posterosuperior to the promontory. It connects the tympanic cavity to the vestibule. The oval window is covered by the end plate (base) of the stapes.
11. The round window is an opening posterosuperior to the promontory that connects the tympanic cavity to the scala tympani of the cochlea. It is covered by the so-called secondary tympanic membrane.
12. The carotid canal ascends into the petrous part of the temporal bone in front of and medial to the tympanic cavity and cochlea. The carotid canal turns 90 degrees anteromedially, lying medial to the eustachian tube, and enters the cranium near the petrous tip.
13. The epitympanic recess of the tympanic cavity is continuous with the mastoid air cells posteriorly via the aditus of the mastoid antrum.
14. The vascular supply of the tympanic cavity includes the anterior tympanic branch of the internal maxillary artery, the stylomastoid branch of the occipital or posterior auricular arteries, a petrosal branch of the middle meningeal artery, the superior tympanic branch of the middle meningeal artery, a branch of the ascending pharyngeal artery and a branch of the vidian (pterygoid) artery, and a tympanic branch from the internal carotid artery.
15. The innervations of the tympanic cavity, the tympanic neural plexus, ramifies within the mucosa of the tympanic cavity, the eustachian tube, and mastoid air cells; this sympathetic plexus includes input from the tympanic branch of the glossopharyngeal nerve (CN-IX) and caroticotympanic nerves of sympathetic origin. The tympanic plexus continues as the lesser petrosal nerve; this nerve eventually joins the otic ganglion and subsequently supplies the parotid gland.

The Auditory Ossicles

1. The malleus consists of a head, neck, handle, anterior process, and lateral process.
   a. The head articulates with the body of the incus.
   b. The neck is a narrow part joining with the head and the two processes.
   c. The anterior process is attached to the wall of the tympanic cavity via the tendon of the aditus and directly to the center of the tympanic membrane at the umbo.

   d. The anterior process is attached to the petrotympanic fissure by ligamentous fibers.
   e. The lateral process is attached to the upper part of the tympanic membrane and the anterior and posterior malleolar folds.
2. The incus consists of a body, a lenticular process, and a short and a long process.
   a. The body articulates with head of the malleus.
   b. The short process is attached by ligamentous fibers to the posterior wall of the epitympanic recess of the tympanic cavity.
   c. The long process ends in the lenticular process, which articulates with the stapes.
   d. The lenticular process articulates with the head of the stapes via a cartilaginous facet.
3. The stapes consist of a head, a neck, two limbs, and a base.
   a. The head articulates with the lenticular process of the incus via a cartilaginous facet.
   b. The neck is attached to the tendon of the stapedius muscle.
   c. Anterior and posterior limbs (crura) join the head with the end plate (base).
   d. The end plate (base) covers the oval window and is fixed to it by the annular ligament.
4. Otic ossicular joints
   a. The articulations between the auditory ossicles are synovial joints.

The Inner Ear

1. The inner ear consists of an osseous labyrinth, a membranous labyrinth, endolymph, and perilymph.
   a. The osseous labyrinth is made up of cavities within the petrous part of the temporal bone.
   b. The membranous labyrinth is a membranous sac within the osseous labyrinth.
   c. Endolymph is fluid within the membranous labyrinth.
   d. Perilymph is fluid outside the membranous labyrinth but within the osseous labyrinth.
2. The vestibular endolymphatic aqueduct is an extension of the vestibular membranous labyrinth through the osseous vestibular aqueduct. It ends in the blind endolymphatic sac over the posterior surface of the petrous bone. The endolymphatic sac lies partially between the two layers of dura of the cranial cavity.
3. The three parts of the inner ear are the vestibule, the three semicircular canals, and the cochlea.
   a. The vestibule
      i. The vestibule lies medial to the tympanic cavity, posterior to the cochlea, and antero-inferior to the semicircular canals.
      ii. The membranous vestibule consists of the utricle (from which the cochlea originates); the two are joined by the utriculosacular duct.
      iii. The oval window is on the lateral wall of the vestibule.
   b. The semicircular canals
      i. There are three semicircular canals arising from the vestibule: lateral, posterior, and superior.
      ii. The posterior and superior semicircular canals share an entry into the vestibule; consequently, the semicircular canals have five ostia communicating with the vestibule.
      iii. Each semicircular canal communicates with the utricle of the vestibule.
      iv. Each semicircular canal has a dilated ampulla in one of its arms joining the vestibule.
   c. The cochlea
      i. The cochlea has a conical, snail shape and one and a half to two and three-fourths turns.
      ii. The apex points anterosuperiorly toward the medial wall of the tympanic cavity.

iii. The base faces the internal auditory canal and is perforated by the cochlear nerve (branch of CN-VIII).
iv. The cochlear duct communicates with the saccule of the vestibule via the ductus reuniens.
v. The modiolus is the central conical axis of the cochlea.
vi. There are three longitudinal channels within the cochlea: the blind-ending cochlear duct in the center, containing endolymph, and two flanking channels intercommunicating at the apex of the modiolus, the scala vestibuli and the scala tympani, containing perilymph.
vii. The perilymphatic space surrounding the semicircular canals communicates with the scala vestibuli, which subsequently communicates with the scala tympani via the helicotrema. The scala tympani is separated from the tympanic cavity by the secondary tympanic membrane at the round window; the scala tympani is continuous with the cranial subarachnoid space via the cochlear aqueduct.

The Internal Auditory Canal

1. The internal auditory canal is directed posteromedially from the base of the cochlea toward the posterior fossa of the cranium; it opens onto the medial part of the posterior surface of the petrous part of the temporal bone.
2. It transmits the facial (CN-VII) and vestibulocochlear/auditory (CN-VIII) cranial nerves.
3. The thinner facial (CN-VII) cranial nerve is located in the superoanterior quadrant of the internal auditory canal, whereas the thicker vestibulocochlear (CN-VIII) cranial nerve occupies the remainder.

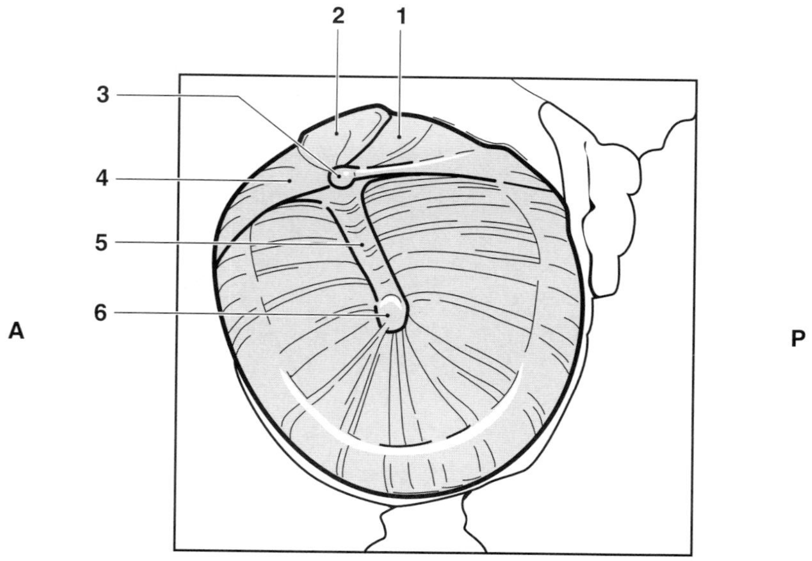

Figure 2B-9: Lateral schematic of external aspect of the tympanic membrane on the right side. *A*, anterior; *P*, posterior.
1 Posterior malleolar fold
2 Pars flaccida
3 Lateral process of malleus
4 Anterior malleolar fold
5 Handle of malleus
6 Umbo

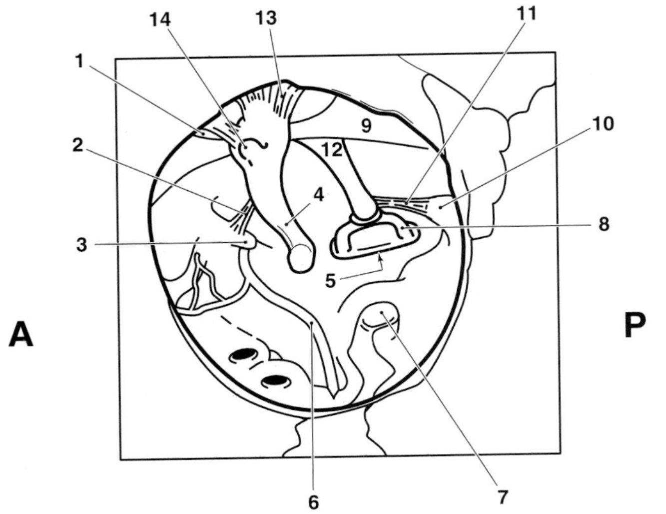

Figure 2B-10: Lateral schematic of the tympanic cavity on the right side after removal of tympanic membrane (inferolateral view). *A*, anterior; *P*, posterior.

1 Anterior malleolar fold
2 Tensor tympani
3 Processus cochleariformis
4 Handle of malleus
5 Oval window
6 Tympanic nerve on promontory
7 Round window (fossa fenestrae cochlea)
8 Posterior crus of stapes
9 Posterior mallear fold
10 Pyramid
11 Stapedius
12 Long process of incus
13 Lateral ligament of malleus
14 Lateral process of malleus

Figure 2B-11: Schematic of the auditory ossicles. **A:** Articulated auditory ossicles on the right side, viewed from the front. M, medial; L, lateral. **B:** Medial and posterior aspect of the malleus. **C:** Anterior and medial aspect of the left incus. **D:** Superior and anteromedial aspect of the stapes.

1 Head (caput)
2 Facet for incus
3 Neck
4 Handle (manubrium)
5 Anterior process
6 Lateral process
7 Facet for malleus
8 Long limb (crus longum)
9 Lenticular process
10 Short limb (crus breve)
11 Body (corpus)
12 Head (caput)
13 Anterior limb (crus anterius)
14 Neck
15 Posterior limb (crus posterius)
16 Base (for oval window)
17 Facet for stapes
18 Facet for incus
19 Incudomalleolar joint
20 Incudostapedial joint

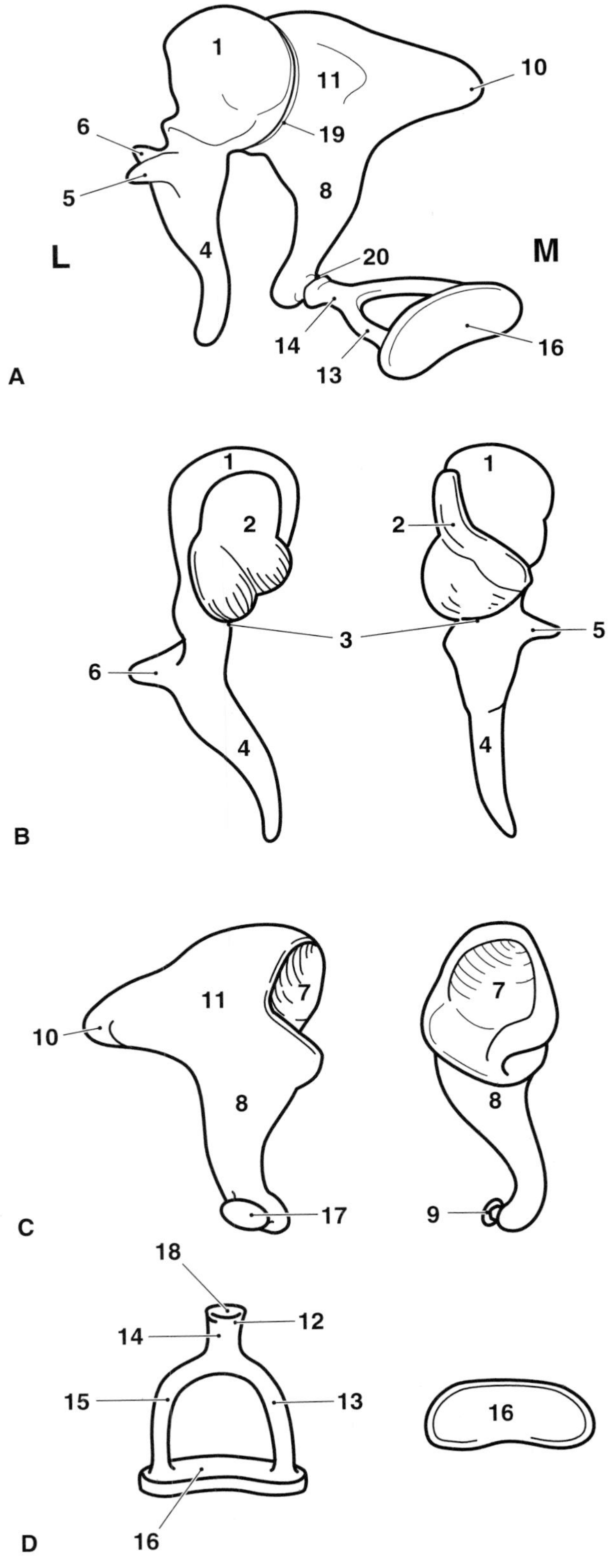

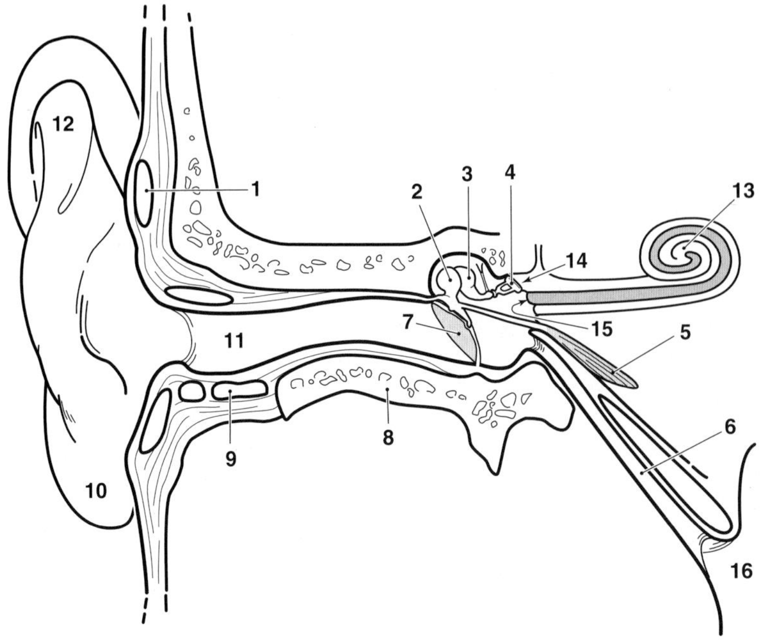

Figure 2B-12: Schematic of the external and middle portions of the right ear opened in its anterior aspect to show the structures of the ear.

1 Cartilage of auricle
2 Head of malleus
3 Incus
4 Stapes
5 Tensor tympani muscle
6 Eustachian (auditory) tube
7 Tympanic membrane
8 Osseous part of meatus
9 Cartilaginous part of external auditory canal
10 Lobule of auricle
11 External auditory meatus
12 Auricle
13 Cochlea (not to scale or orientation)
14 Oval window
15 Round window
16 Nasopharynx

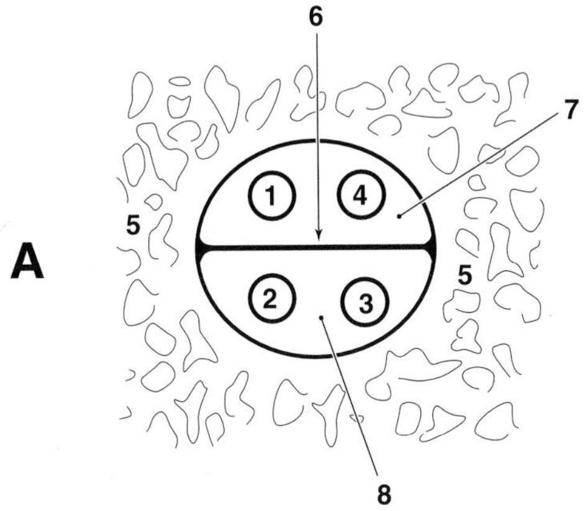

Figure 2B-13: Cross-sectional schematic of the primary contents of the apex (fundus) of the internal auditory canal on the right side, as viewed medially. *A*, anterior; *P*, posterior.

1 Facial nerve (CN-VII)
2 Cochlear nerve (branch of CN-VIII)
3 Inferior vestibular nerve (branch of CN-VIII)
4 Superior vestibular nerve (branch of CN-VIII)
5 Petrous part of temporal bone
6 Crista falciformis (transverse crest)
7 Superior fossa of the internal auditory canal (filled primarily with cerebrospinal fluid)
8 Inferior fossa of the internal auditory canal (filled primarily with cerebrospinal fluid)

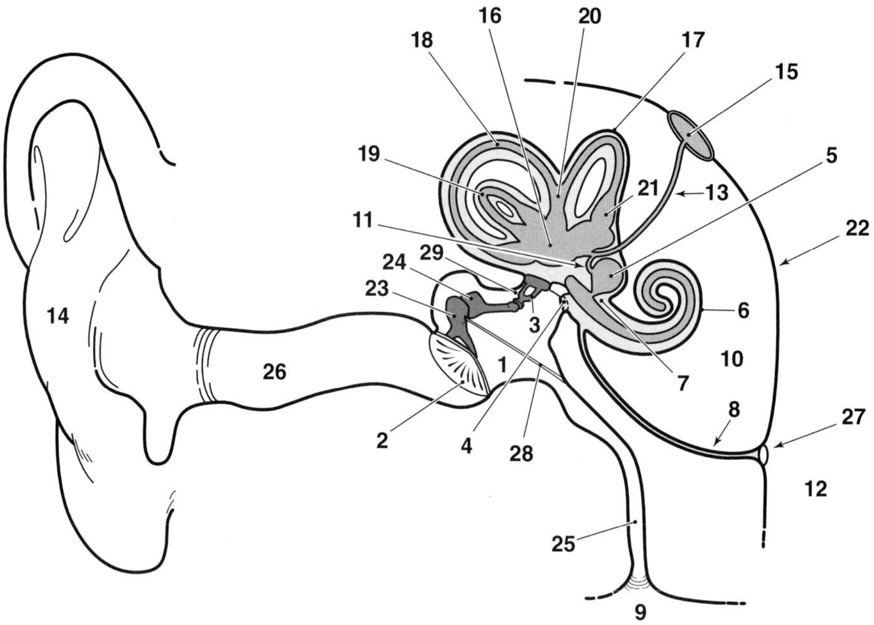

Figure 2B-14: Schematic of the auditory apparatus on the right side (not to scale or to three-dimentional anatomic configuration).

1 Middle ear
2 Tympanic membrane
3 Stapes in oval window
4 Round window
5 Saccule
6 Cochlea
7 Ductus reuniens
8 Cochlear aqueduct
9 Nasopharynx
10 Petrous part of temporal bone
11 Utriculosaccular duct
12 Subarachnoid space
13 Vestibular (endolymphatic) aqueduct
14 Pinna of external ear
15 Endolymphatic sac located between inner and outer (periosteal) layers of cranial dura mater
16 Utricle
17 Superior semicircular canal
18 Posterior semicircular canal
19 Lateral semicircular canal
20 Crus commune
21 Ampulla
22 Dura mater
23 Malleus
24 Incus
25 Eustachian tube
26 External auditory canal
27 Orifice of cochlear aqueduct into subarachnoid space
28 Tensor tympani muscle
29 Stapedius muscle

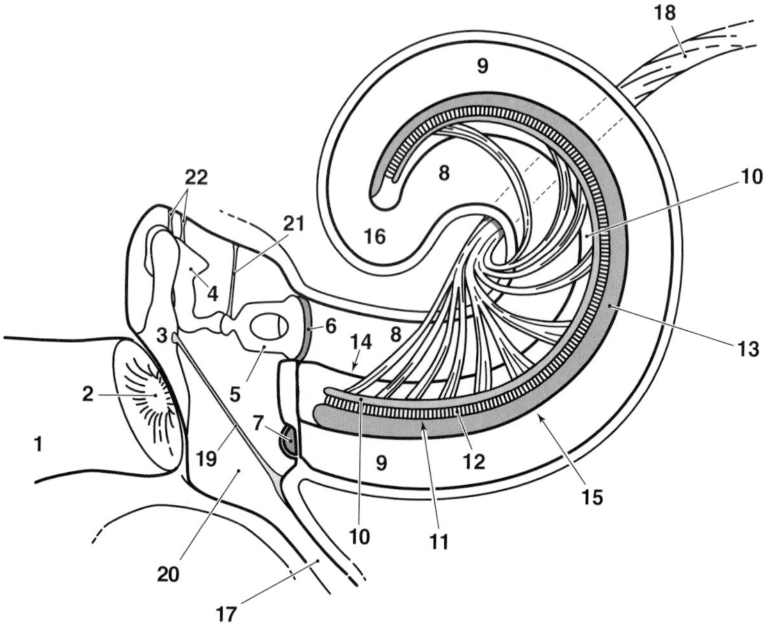

Figure 2B-15: Schematic of the middle ear and cochlea on the right side (not to scale).

1 External auditory canal
2 Tympanic membrane
3 Malleus
4 Incus
5 Stapes
6 Oval window
7 Round window
8 Scala vestibuli (filled with perilymph)
9 Scala tympani (filled with perilymph)
10 Cochlear duct (scala media) (filled with endolymph)
11 Tectorial membrane
12 Hair cells (neuro-epithelial sensory end organs)
13 Spiral organ (organ of Corti) (*shaded*)
14 Vestibular membrane
15 Basilar membrane
16 Helicotrema
17 Eustachian (auditory) tube
18 Cochlear branch of vestibulocochlear (auditory, CN-VIII) nerve
19 Tensor tympani muscle
20 Middle ear
21 Stapedius muscle
22 Suspensory ligaments

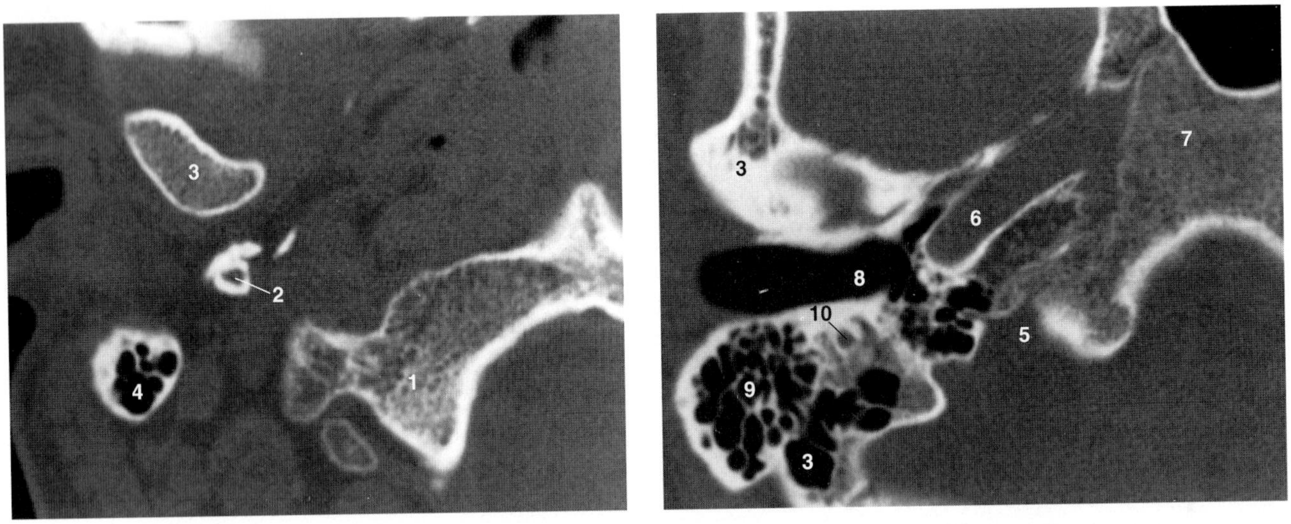

A B

Figure 2B-16A–L: The temporal bone. Axial CT images showing the normal anatomy of the right temporal bone.

1 Occipital condyle
2 Styloid process
3 Mandibular condyle
4 Mastoid tip
5 Jugular fossa
6 Carotid canal
7 Clivus
8 External auditory canal
9 Mastoid air cells
10 Descending portion of facial canal
11 Proximal end of eustachian tube
12 Basal turn of cochlea
13 Second turn of cochlea
14 Petrous tip
15 Round window
16 Manubrium malleus
17 Head of malleus
18 Incus
19 Vestibule
20 Posterior semicircular canal
21 Horizontal portion of facial nerve canal
22 Internal auditory canal
23 Genu of facial nerve canal
24 Mastoid antrum
25 Lateral semicircular canal
26 Superior semicircular canal
27 Incudomalleolar joint
28 Distal segment of vestibular aqueduct
29 Proximal segment of vestibular aqueduct

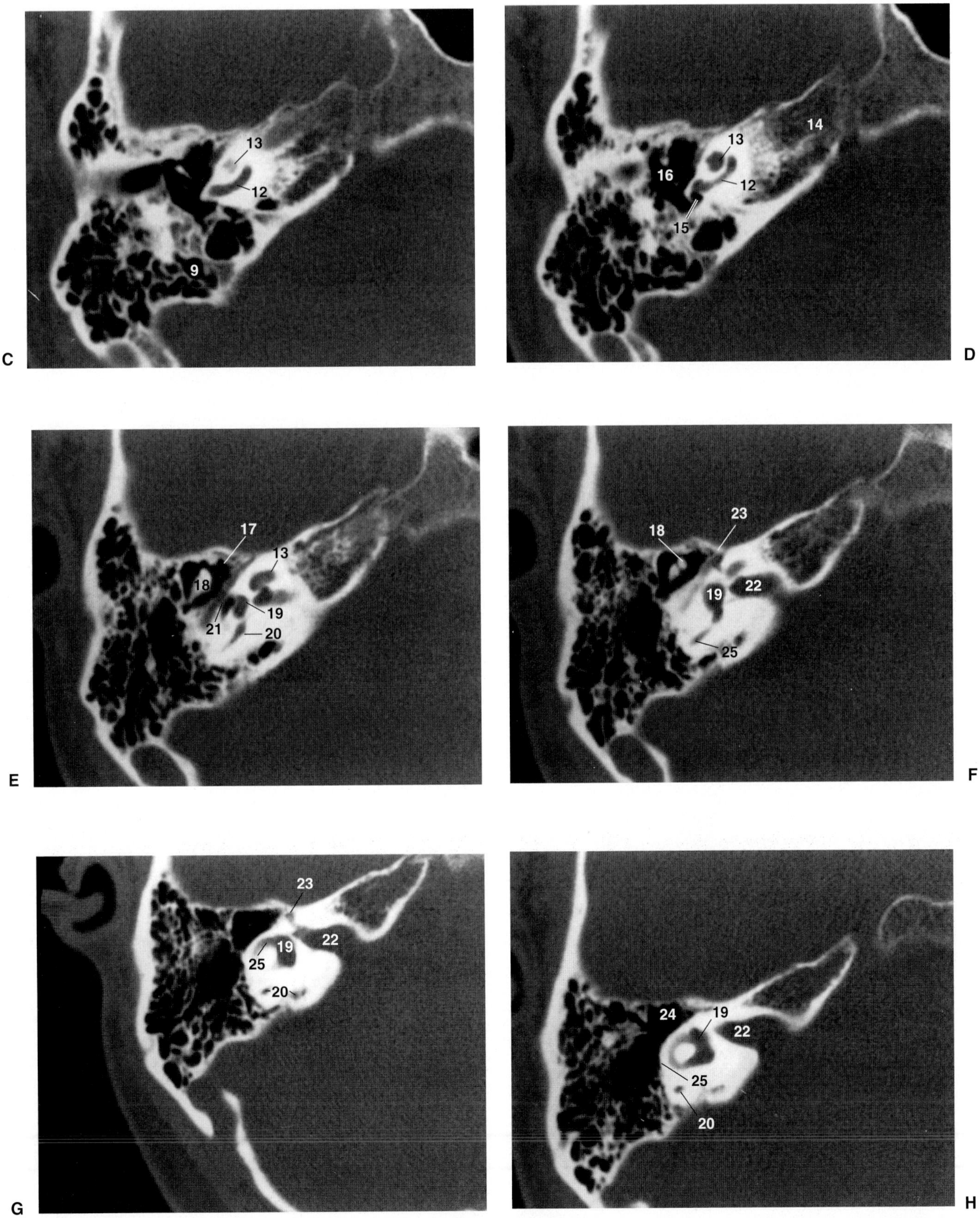

Figure 2B-16: Continued.

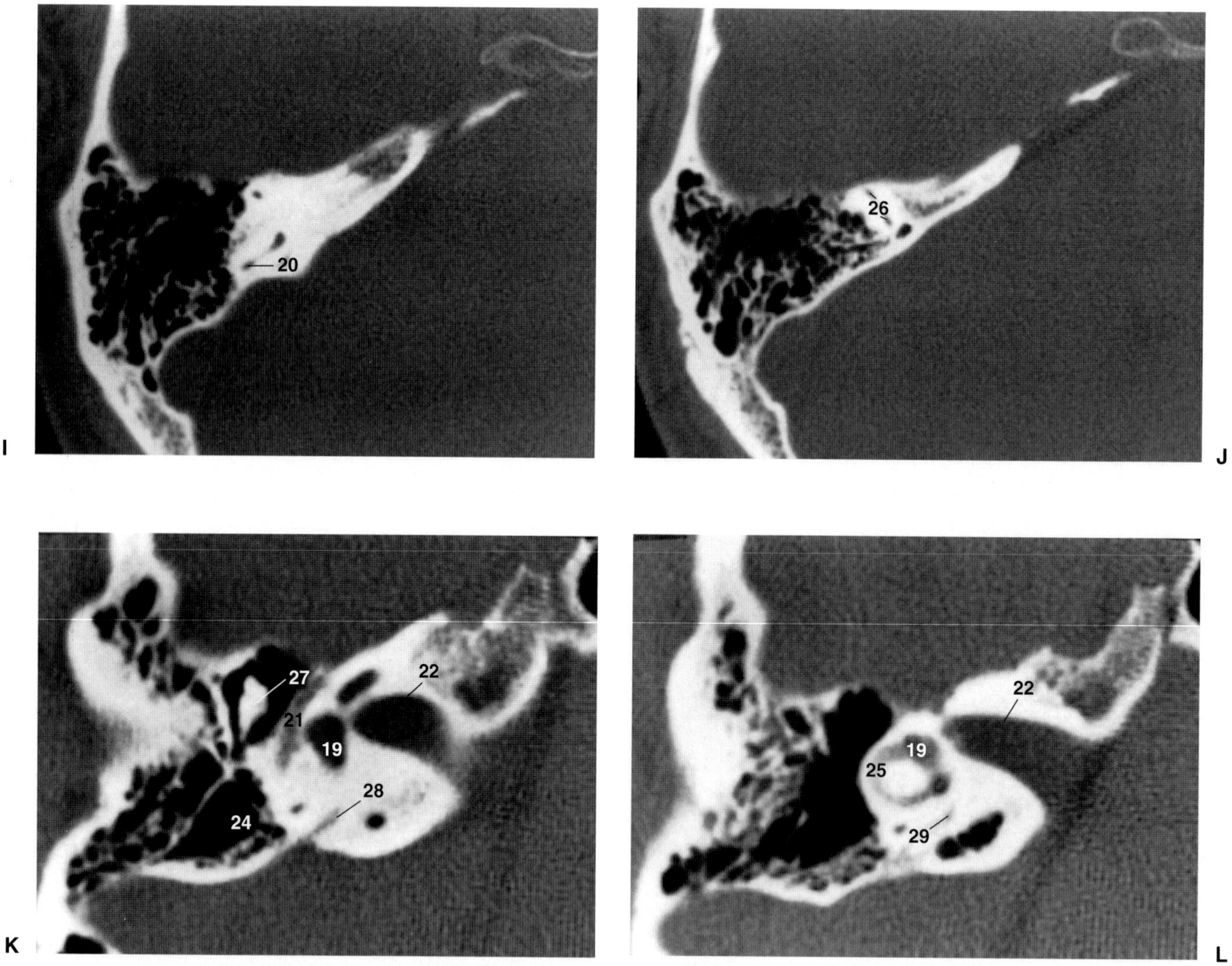

Figure 2B-16: Continued.

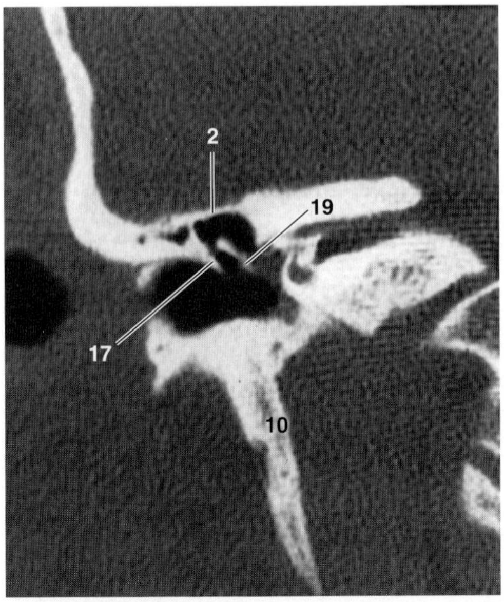

A

Figure 2B-17A–E: The temporal bone. Coronal CT images showing the normal anatomy of the right temporal bone.

1 Mastoid air cells
2 Tegmen tympani
3 Epitympanum
4 Stapes
5 Oval window
6 Hypotympanum
7 Basal turn of cochlea
8 Head of malleus
9 External auditory canal
10 Styloid process
11 Cochlea
12 Vestibule
13 Internal auditory canal
14 Crista falciformis
15 Lateral semicircular canal
16 Round window
17 Scutum
18 Superior semicircular canal
19 Incudostapedial joint
20 Incus

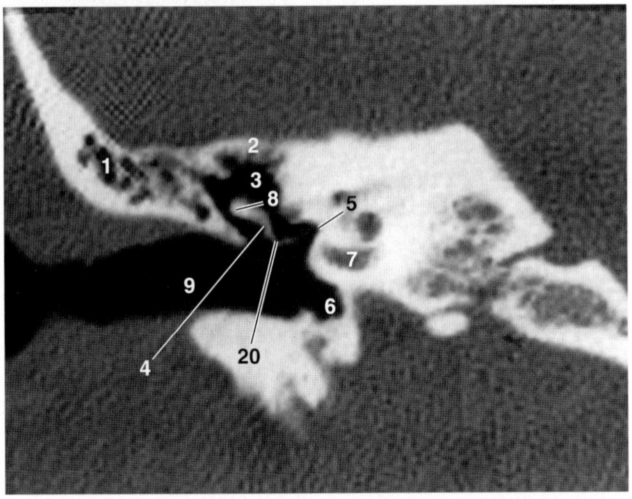

B

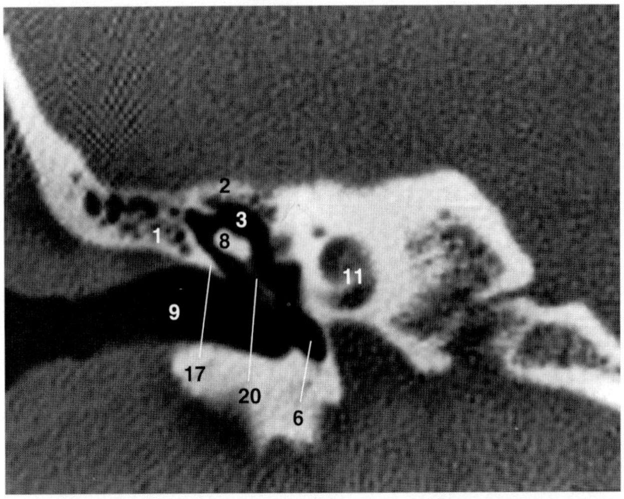

C

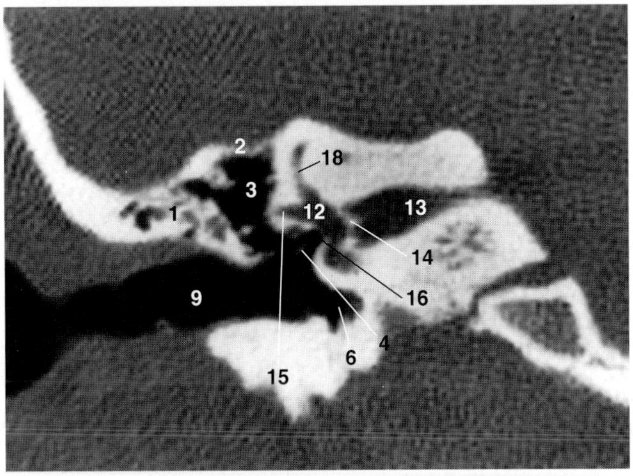

D

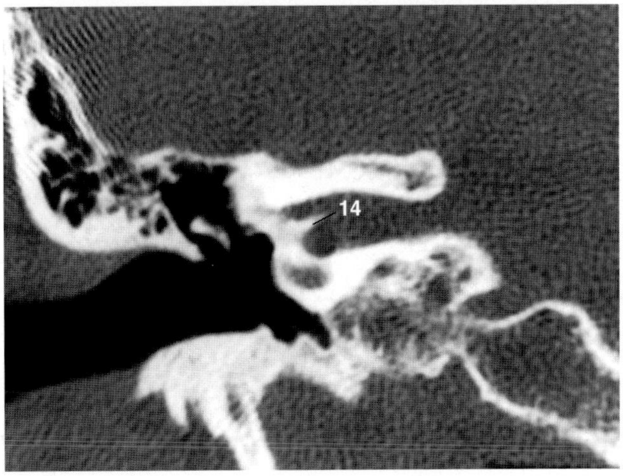

E

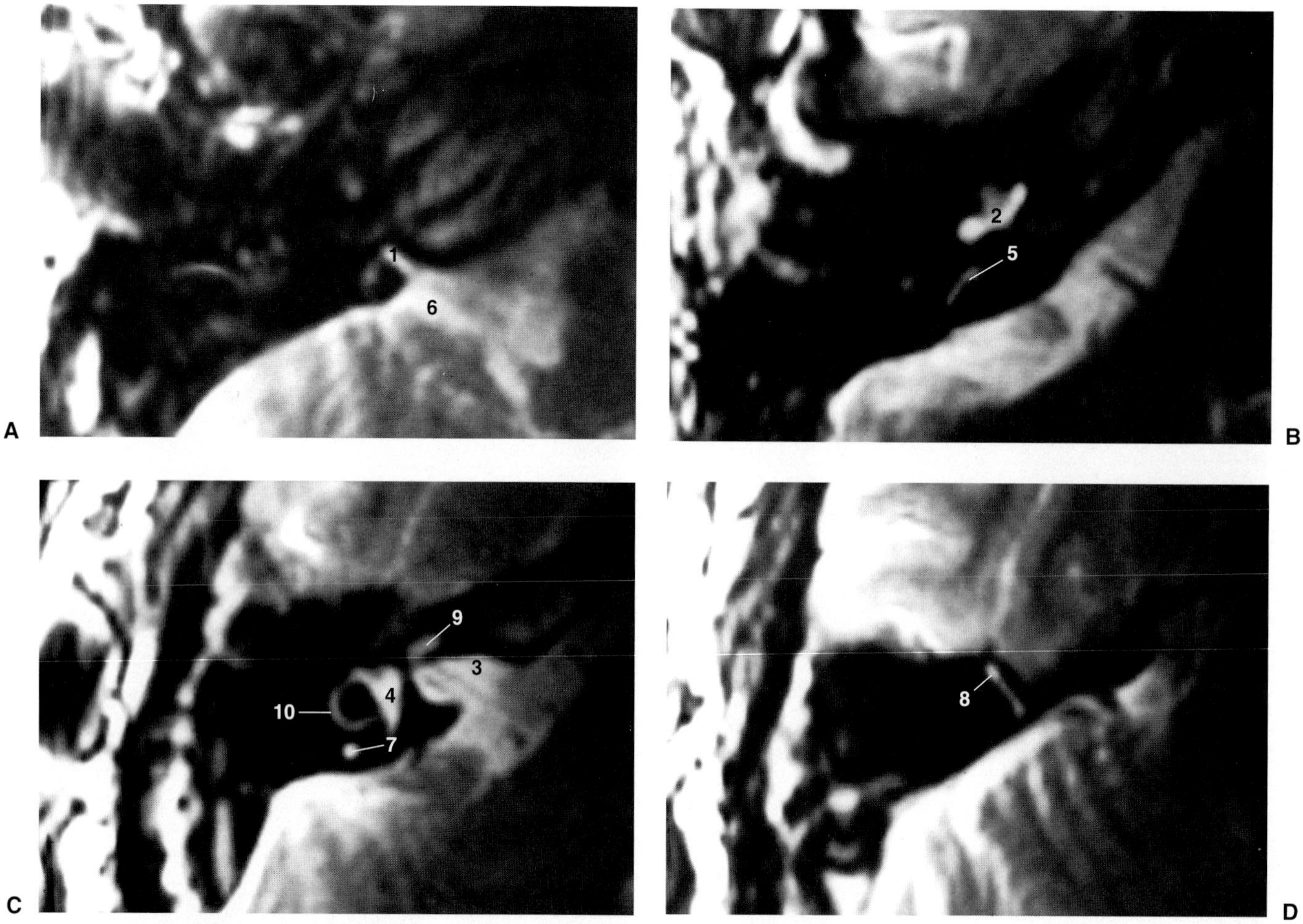

Figure 2B-18A–D: The temporal bone. Axial T2-weighted MR images (from inferior to superior) on the right side.

1 Cochlear aqueduct
2 Basal turn of cochlea
3 Internal auditory canal with cranial nerves VII (facial: anterior) and VIII (vestibulocochlear: posterior).
4 Vestibule
5 Vestibular aqueduct
6 Subarachnoid space
7 Posterior semicircular canal
8 Superior semicircular canal
9 Proximal facial nerve canal
10 Lateral semicircular canal

THE CRANIOCERVICAL JUNCTION

1. *Chamberlain's line* is drawn from the posterior edge of the hard palate to the posterior border of the foramen magnum (opisthion). Normally, Chamberlain's line lies above the odontoid process (dens). Projection of 2.5 mm or up to one-third of the odontoid process above this line is considered normal. If the tip of the odontoid projects 6 mm or more above this line, basilar invagination/impression is considered to be present; if the odontoid tip projects above the line between 2.5 and 6 mm, platybasia/basilar invagination/basilar impression should only be suspected.
2. *McGregor's line* is a modification of Chamberlain's line; it is drawn from the hard palate to the undersurface of the occipital bone. The dens should normally lie no more than 4.5 mm above McGregor's line; if it lies more than this, platybasia/basilar invagination or basilar impression should be suspected.
3. *Welcher's basal angle* is the angle formed between a line drawn between the nasion and the tuberculum sellae and a line drawn between the tuberculum sellae and the basion (anterior margin of foramen magnum). A normal angulation is less than 140 degrees. An angle greater than 140 degrees suggests basilar invagination/platybasia or basilar impression.

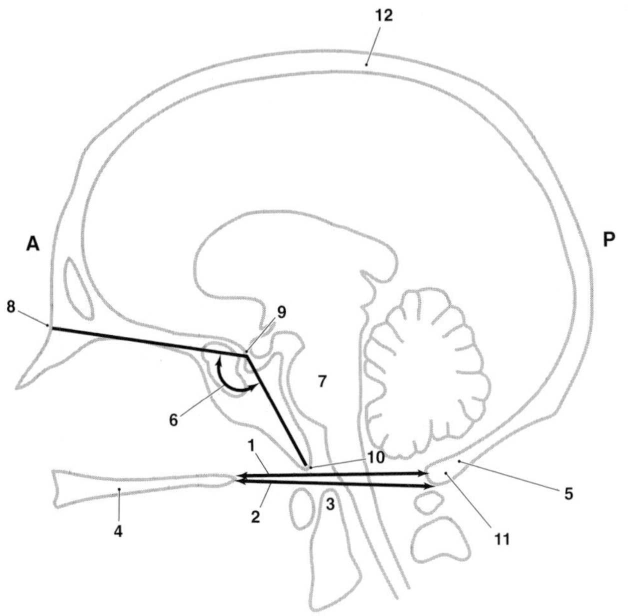

Figure 2B-19: Lateral schematic showing the normal linear, angular measurements of the skull base and at the craniocervical junction. *A*, anterior; *P*, posterior.
1 Chamberlain's line
2 McGregor's line
3 Dens
4 Hard palate
5 Occipital bone
6 Welcher's basal angle
7 Pons
8 Nasion
9 Tuberculum sellae
10 Basion
11 Opisthion
12 Cranial vertex

SKULL BASE VARIANTS

- Variations in marrow fat/aeration of crista galli
- Fat in cavernous venous sinus
- Skull base dural insertion calcification (e.g., petroclinoid ligament)
- Variations in aeration of the petromastoid air cells
  - Hypo-hyperaeration of the petromastoid air cells
  - Symmetric/asymmetric aeration of the tips of the petrous portion of the temporal bone
  - Aeration of the skull base emanating from the paranasal sinuses or petromastoid air cells
- Abnormalities in the formation and segmentation of the primary occipital vertebrae/sclerotomes (0-1/0-4).
  - Abnormality in the formation of one or more of the primary occipital vertebrae/sclerotomes (e.g., aplasia, spinal bifida)
  - Partial/complete segmentation anomaly of one or more primary occipital vertebrae/sclerotomes
  - Clival hypoplasia (short clivus)
  - Flat skull base(platybasia, basilar impression, basilar invagination)

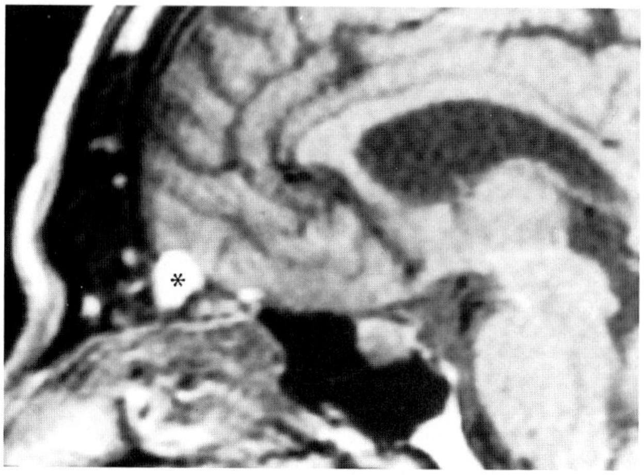

Figure 2B-20A: Marrow fat in crista galli. Sagittal T1-weighted MR image showing hyperintense marrow fat within the crista galli (*asterisk*) anteriorly in the floor of the anterior cranial fossa.

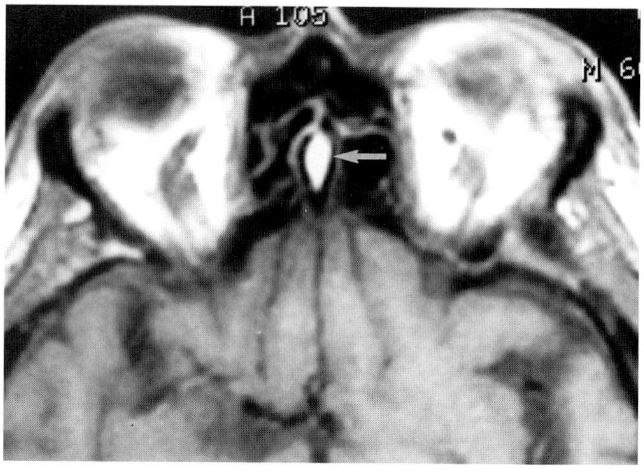

Figure 2B-20B: Marrow fat in crista galli. Axial T1-weighted MR image showing the hyperintense fat in the crista galli (*arrow*).

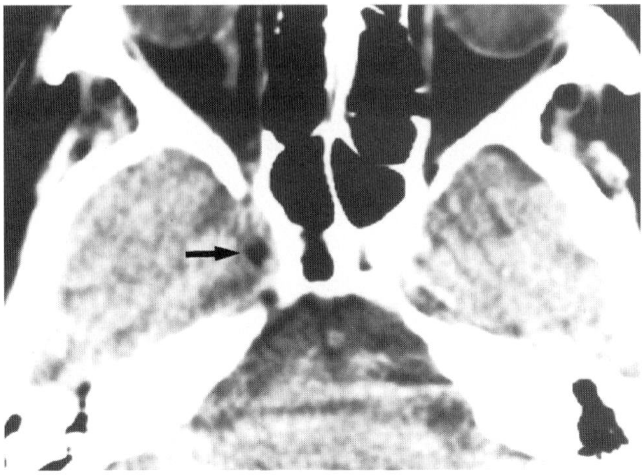

Figure 2B-21: Fat in the cavernous venous sinus. Coronal CT image showing hypodense fat in the cavernous venous sinus (*arrow*).

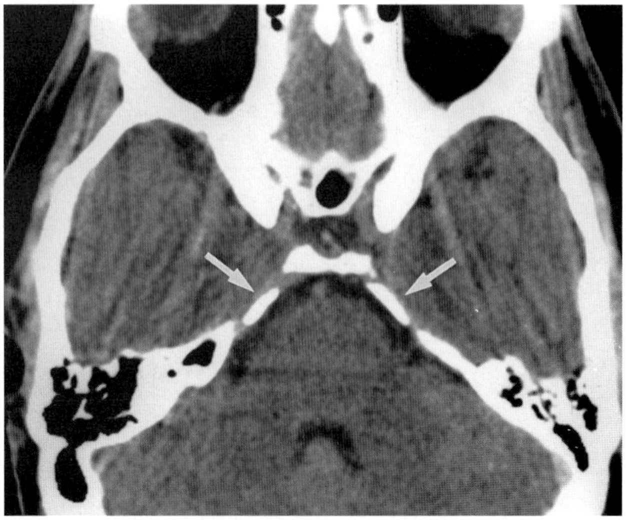

Figure 2B-22: Petroclinoid ligament calcification. Unenhanced axial CT image showing petroclinoid ligament calcification (*arrows*).

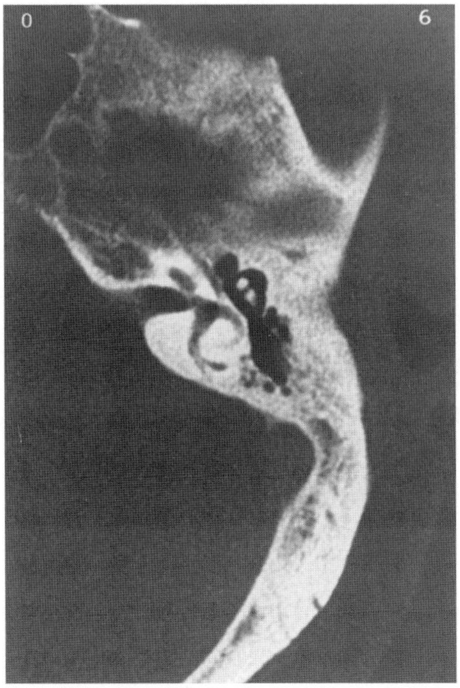

Figure 2B-23A: Hypo-aeration of the petromastoid air cells. Axial CT image showing marked hypo-aeration of the petromastoid air cells on the left side. There were similar findings on the right side (not shown).

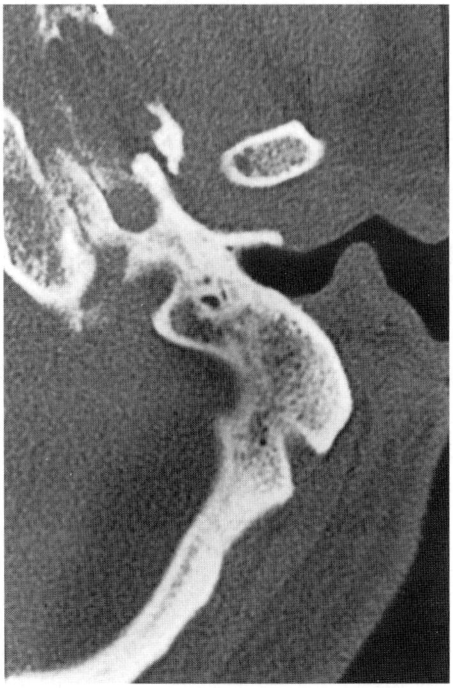

Figure 2B-23B: Axial CT image at a lower level than that of Fig. 2B-23A, showing hypo-aeration of the mastoid process of the temporal bone.

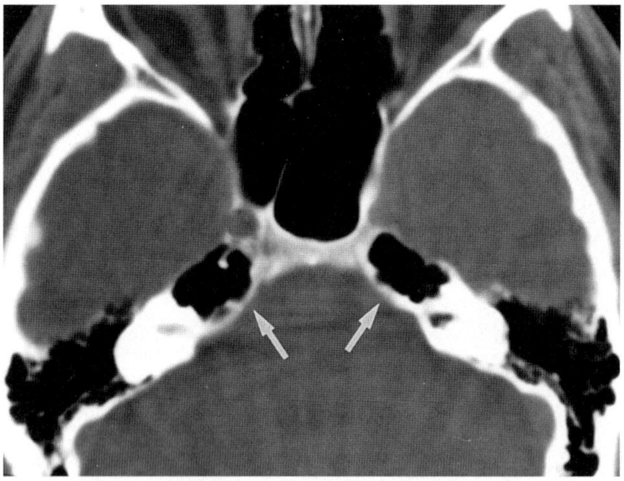

Figure 2B-24A: Hyperaeration of the petromastoid air cells. Axial CT image showing aeration of the medial tips (apexes) of the petrous part of the temporal bones bilaterally (*arrows*).

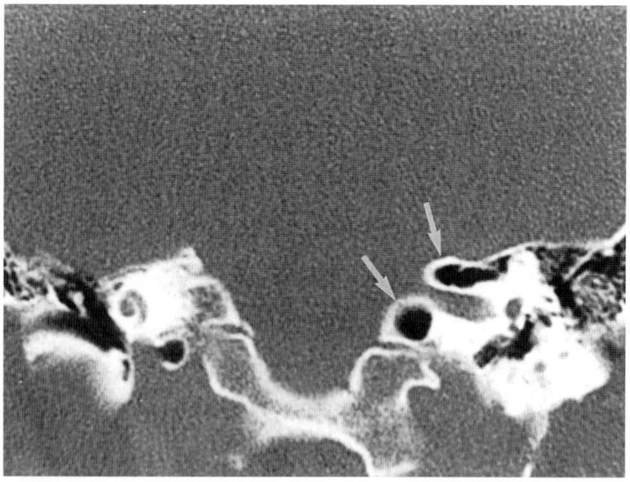

Figure 2B-24B: Coronal CT image showing unilateral aeration of petrous tip and occipital condyle (*arrows*) on the left side.

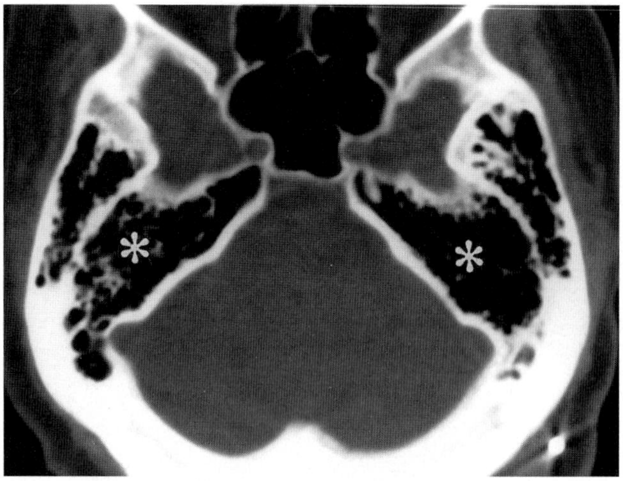

Figure 2B-24C: Axial CT image showing bilateral hyperplastic petromastoid air cells (*asterisks*).

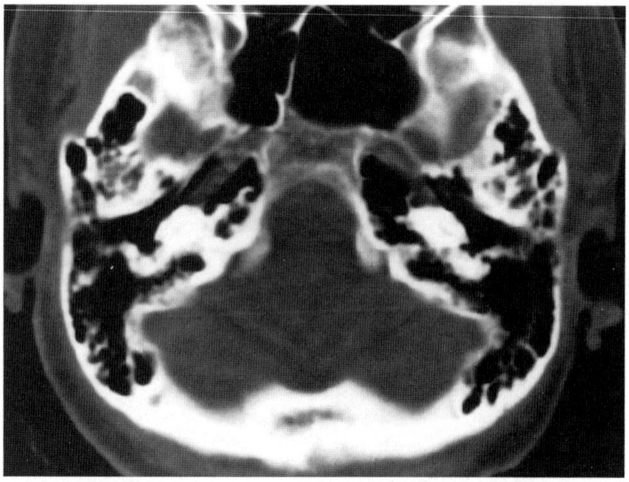

Figure 2B-24D: Axial CT image inferior to Fig. 2B-24C showing enlarged petromastoid air cells.

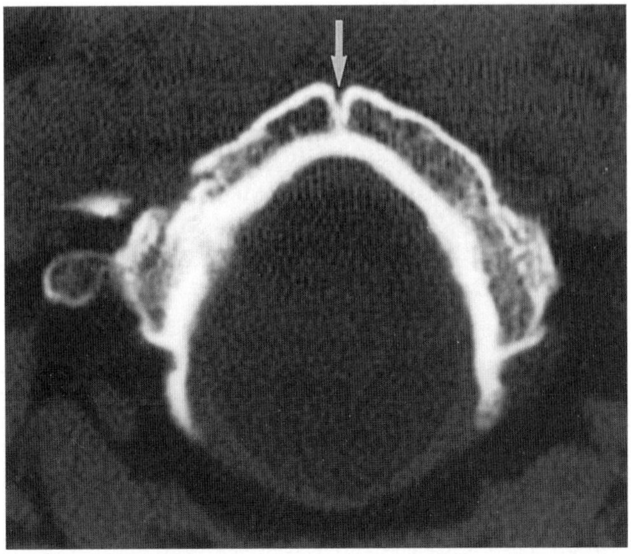

Figure 2B-25: Basioccipital cranium bifidum (spina bifida occulta of the fourth embryonic occiptal vertebra—0-4). Axial CT image showing a split in the anterior margin of the foramen magnum (basion), representing a basioccipital cranium bifidum occulta (*arrow*). This results from a persistent split in the primitive stages of development of the fourth occipital vertebrae or sclerotome (0-4).

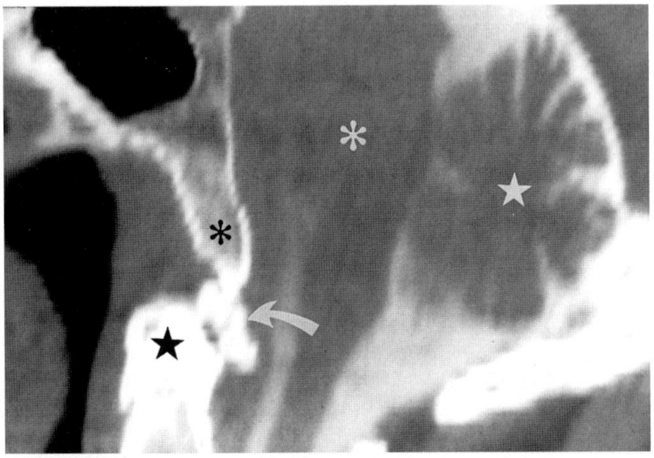

Figure 2B-26A: Abnormality in segmentation of the basiocciput: occipital vertebra sclerotomes. Reformatted sagittal CT myelogram showing a remnant (O-4 ossicle) of the fourth occipital vertebra/sclerotome (O-4) (*arrow*) interposed between the clivus (*black asterisk*) and the odontoid process of C-2 (*black star*). The brain stem (*white asterisk*) and cerebellum (*white star*) are also noted.

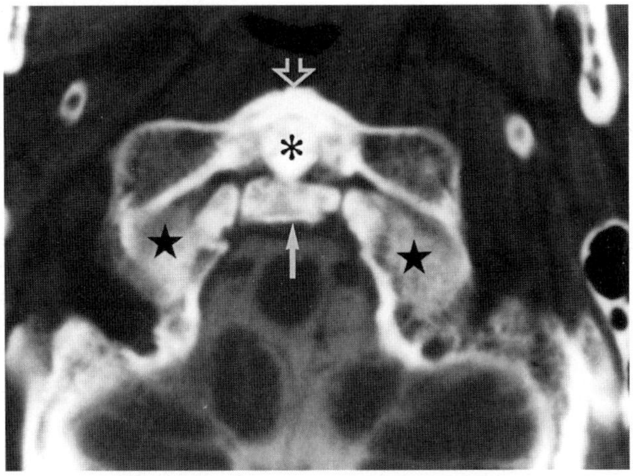

Figure 2B-26B: Axial CT image showing the fourth occipital vertebra (O-4 ossicle) (*arrow*). The surrounding odontoid process of C-2 (*asterisk*), the anterior arch of C-1 (*open arrow*), and the occipital condyles (*stars*) are also noted.

2c. Cerebral Hemispheres

OVERVIEW

1. On gross examination, the two cerebral hemispheres are lateral mirror images of each other, partially separated by the longitudinal interhemispheric fissure in the midline.
2. On a smaller scale, there are asymmetries between the hemispheres that may be represented by differences in size, cytoarchitecture, neuron number, neuron size, and dendritic arborization.
3. The outer surface of each hemisphere is marked by outwardly rounded gyri and inwardly invaginating fissures and sulci.

THE LOBES OF THE CEREBRAL HEMISPHERES

Each cerebral hemisphere is subdivided into six major regions or lobes: frontal, parietal, occipital, temporal, insular, and limbic.

The Frontal Lobe

Lateral Aspect

1. The frontal lobe extends forward from the central sulcus.
2. The precentral gyrus forms the posterior margin of the frontal lobe. It is the primary motor cortex, where the corticospinal and corticobulbar tracts originate. The precentral gyrus has a spatial functional anatomic (somatotopic) organization that can be represented by a motor homunculus.
3. The precentral sulcus is the anterior border of the precentral gyrus and is parallel to the central sulcus.
4. The superior and inferior frontal sulci extend forward and separate the anterolateral surface of the frontal lobe into the superior, middle, and inferior frontal gyri.

Medial Aspect

1. The medial frontal gyrus is located anterior to and above the cingulate sulcus.
2. The paracentral lobule is located posterior to and above the cingulate sulcus. It is continuous with the precentral gyrus anteriorly and is invaded by the central sulcus posteriorly.

Inferior Aspect

1. Medially and running longitudinally, the gyrus rectus is separated from the medial orbital gyrus by the olfactory sulcus.
2. The H-shaped orbital sulci divide the remainder of the inferior surface of the frontal lobe into the medial, anterior, posterior, and lateral orbital gyri.

The Parietal Lobe

Lateral Aspect

1. The parietal lobe is situated posterior to the central sulcus and anterior to the parietooccipital sulcus.
2. The postcentral gyrus is parallel to the precentral gyrus and is bordered posteriorly by the postcentral sulcus. It is the primary sensory cortex for the contralateral side of the body. The postcentral gyrus has a spatial functional anatomic (somatotopic) configuration that can be represented by a sensory homunculus.
3. The area posterior to the postcentral sulcus is subdivided into the superior and inferior parietal lobules by the intraparietal sulcus.
4. The inferior parietal lobule is divided into three parts: the supramarginal gyrus (anteriorly), the angulaı gyrus (intermediate), and the arcus temporooccipitalis (posteriorly).

Medial Aspect

1. The part of the paracentral lobule posterior to the central sulcus is an element of the parietal lobe.
2. The remaining medial surface part of the parietal lobe is formed by the precuneus located posterior to the paracentral lobule.

The Occipital Lobe

Lateral Aspect

1. The occipital lobe is posterior to the parietooccipital sulcus.
2. The transverse occipital sulcus descends from the parietooccipital sulcus and intersects the interparietal sulcus.
3. The lateral occipital sulcus divides the occipital lobe into superior and inferior occipital gyri.
4. The vertically oriented lunate sulcus is located anterior to the occipital pole. Superior and inferior polar occipital sulci may radiate away from the lunate sulcus.

Medial Aspect

1. Posterior to the parietooccipital sulcus is the cuneus; it is bordered inferiorly by the calcarine sulcus.
2. Inferior to the calcarine sulcus is the lingual gyrus.

Inferior Aspect

1. Lateral to the lingual gyrus is the collateral sulcus running longitudinally.
2. The occipitotemporal sulcus runs parallel to the collateral sulcus and is located laterally. It separates the medial and lateral occipitotemporal gyri. These gyri connect the occipital and temporal lobes inferiorly.

The Temporal Lobe

Lateral Aspect

1. The temporal lobe is separated from the frontal and parietal lobes by the Sylvian (lateral) fissure.
2. The superior, middle, and inferior temporal gyri are separated by the superior and middle temporal sulci.

Superior Aspect

One or two (anterior and posterior) transverse temporal gyri extend medially from the superior temporal gyrus.

Medial Aspect

1. The parahippocampal gyrus is on the medial surface of the temporal lobe.
2. The parahippocampal gyrus continues into the uncus, its anterior end.

Inferior Aspect

1. The occipitotemporal sulcus extends from the occipital lobe anteriorly.
2. The occipitotemporal sulcus separates the medial and lateral occipitotemporal gyri extending from the occipital to the temporal poles.

The Insula

1. The insula is buried deep in the Sylvian (lateral) fissure.
2. The insula is covered by three lids, or opercula: frontal, frontoparietal, and temporal.
3. The surface of the insula appears triangular in shape and is divided into anterior and

posterior parts by the sulcus centralis insula. It consists of a cortical area that is almost completely surrounded by a circular sulcus.

4. The anterior part is divided into three to four gyri breves; the posterior part consists of one longer gyrus that may be divided superiorly.

The Limbic Lobe

1. The limbic lobe is an arbitrary cortical area on the medial surface of the hemisphere surrounding the brain stem and the corpus callosum. It includes the subcallosal gyrus, the cingulate gyrus, the parahippocampal gyrus, the hippocampal formation, and the dentate gyrus.
2. The limbic lobe proper is often functionally linked (e.g., emotion) to the hippocampus and its subcortical connections (amygdala, septal region, hypothalamus, habenula, mesencephalic tectum, anterior thalamic nuclei, mammillary body, and fornix), and in this context these combined regions are referred to as the "limbic system."

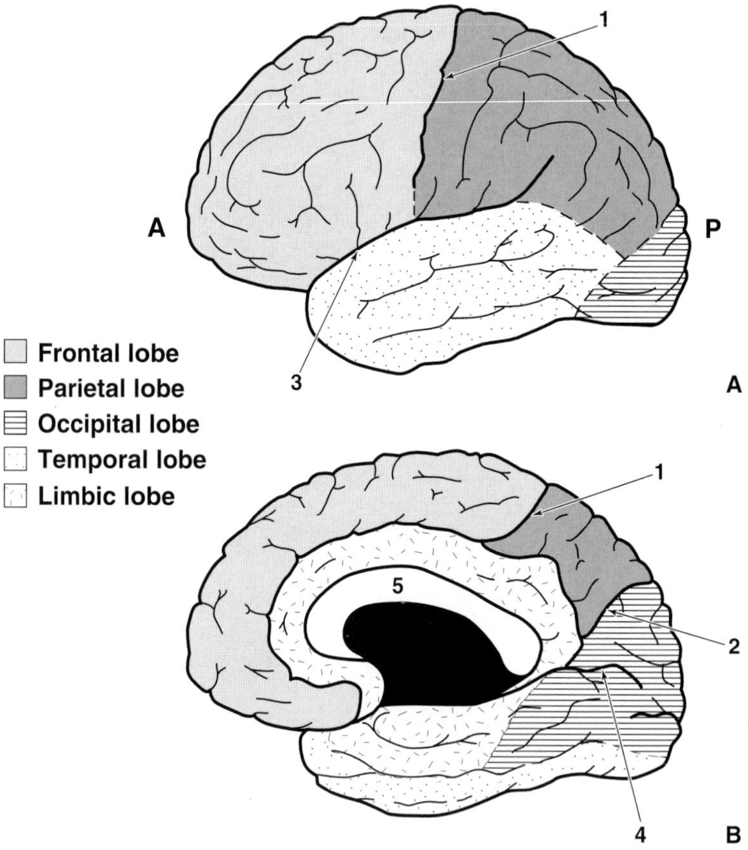

Figure 2C-1: Schematics of the lobes and major sulci/fissures of the cerebral hemispheres. **A:** Lateral aspect. **B:** Medial aspect. *A*, anterior; *P*, posterior.
1 Central sulcus
2 Parietooccipital sulcus
3 Sylvian fissure
4 Calcarine fissure
5 Corpus callosum

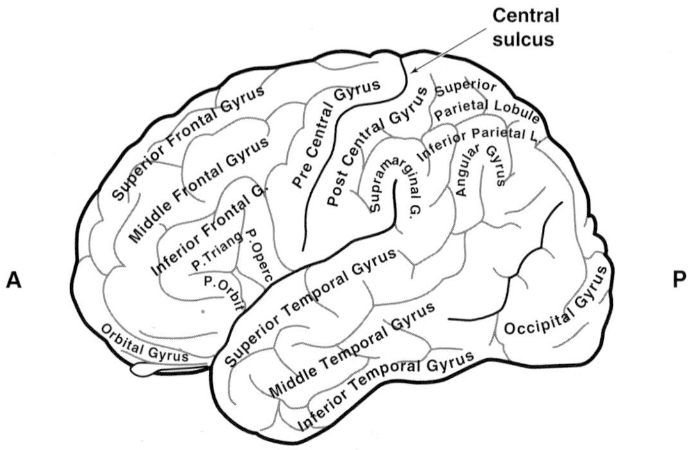

Figure 2C-2A: Schematic of the superficial sulci and gyri of the lateral aspect of the left hemisphere. *A*, anterior; *P*, posterior.

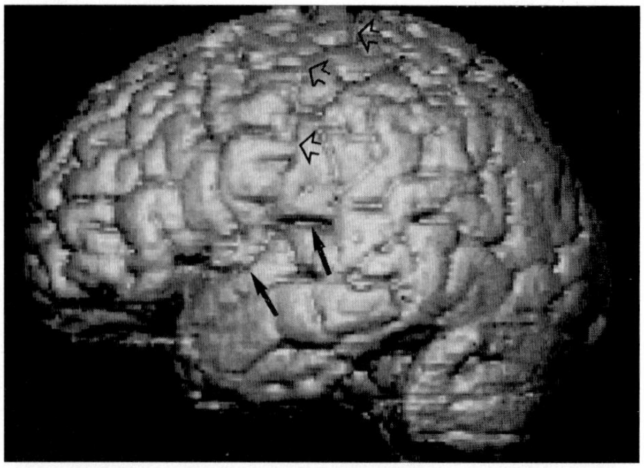

Figure 2C-2B: Lateral aspect of a three-dimensional MR image of the brain. Note, among other features, the central sulcus (*open arrows*) and the Sylvian fissure (*solid arrows*) (compare with Fig. 2C-2A) (courtesy of J. Lancaster).

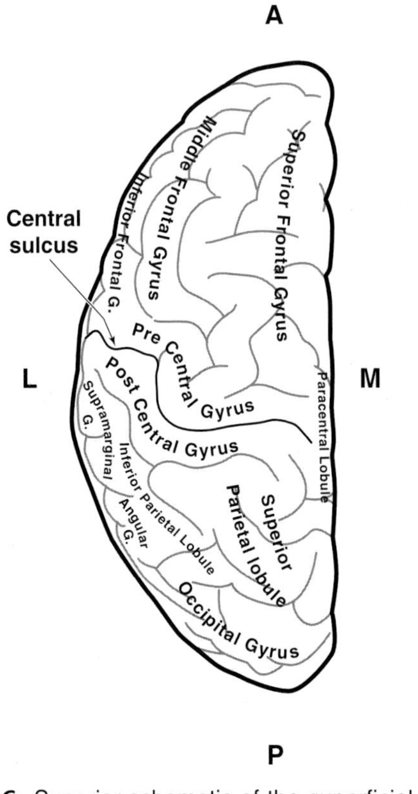

Figure 2C-2C: Superior schematic of the superficial sulci and gyri of the left hemisphere. *A*, anterior; *P*, posterior; *M*, medial; *L*, lateral.

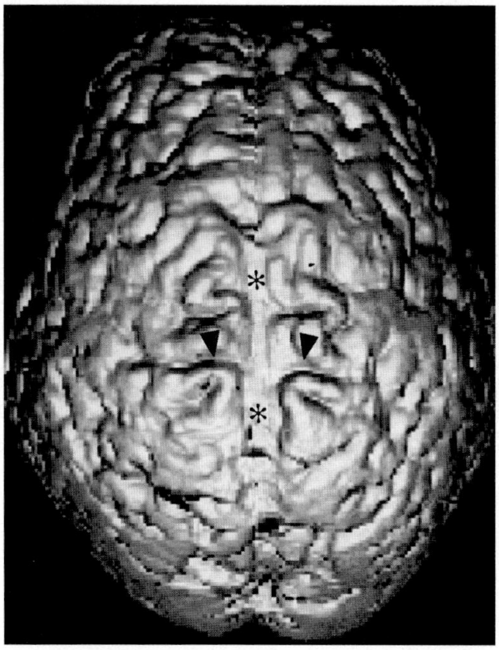

Figure 2C-2D: Superior aspect of a three-dimensional MR image of the brain. Note the interhemispheric fissure (*asterisks*) and the central sulci (*arrowheads*) (compare with Fig. 2C-2C). (Courtesy of J. Lancaster.)

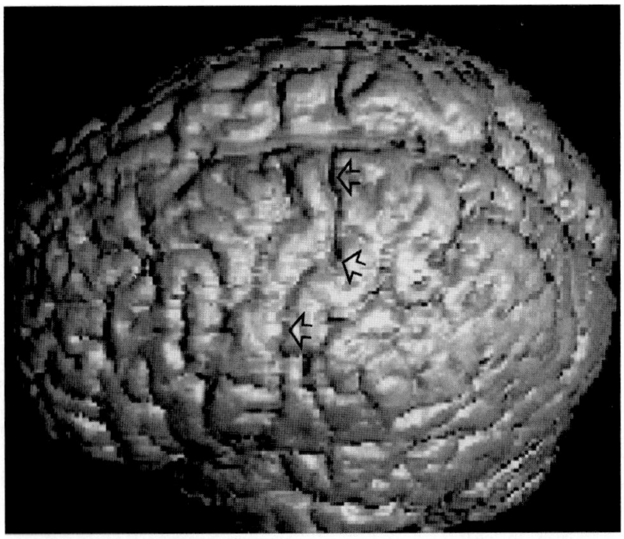

Figure 2C-2E: Oblique lateral aspect of a three-dimensional MR image of the brain (refer to Fig. 2C-2C). Note the central sulcus (*arrows*) (courtesy of J. Lancaster).

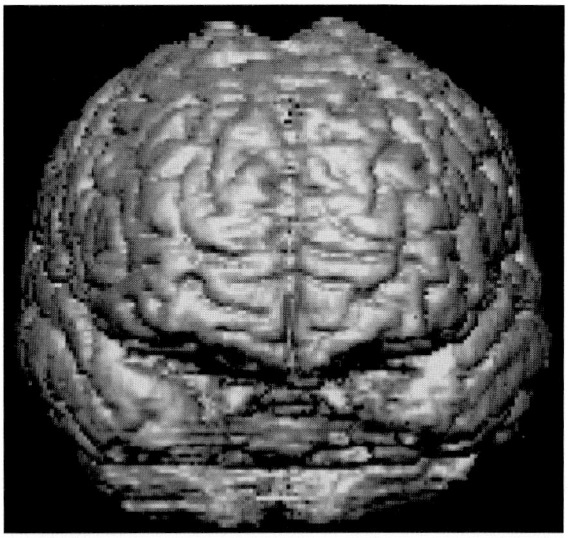

Figure 2C-2F: Frontal aspect of a three-dimensional MR image of the brain. (Courtesy of J. Lancaster.)

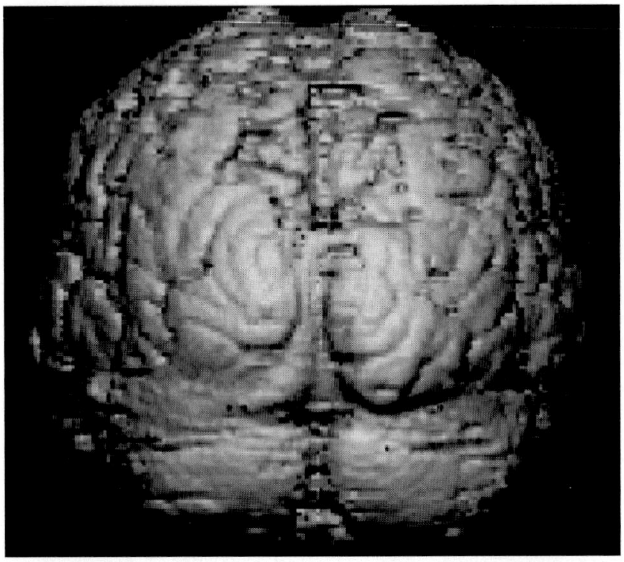

Figure 2C-2G: Posterior aspect of a three-dimensional MR image of the brain. (Courtesy of J. Lancaster.)

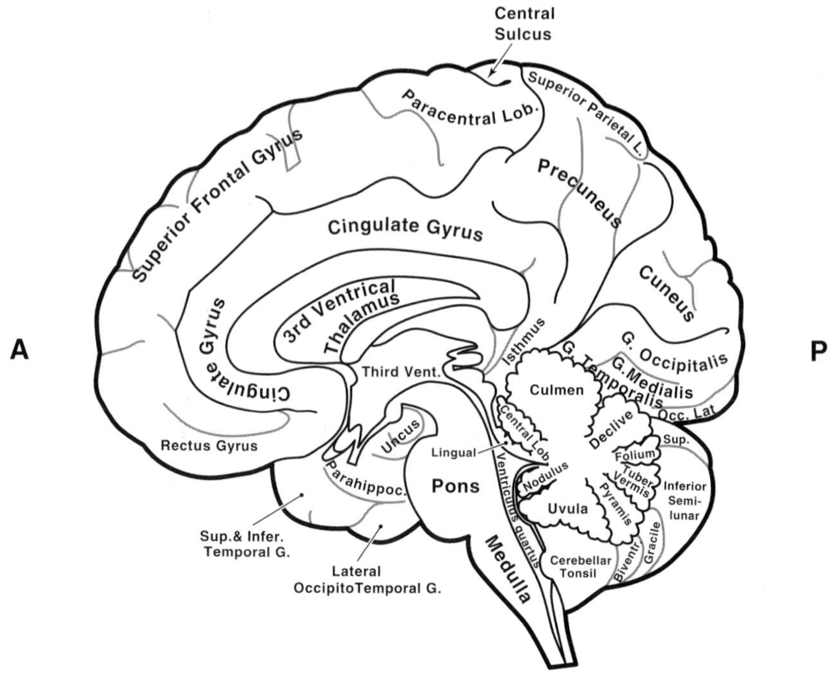

Figure 2C-2H: Schematic of the superficial sulci and gyri of the medial aspect of the right hemisphere. The left hemisphere has been removed. *A*, anterior; *P*, posterior.

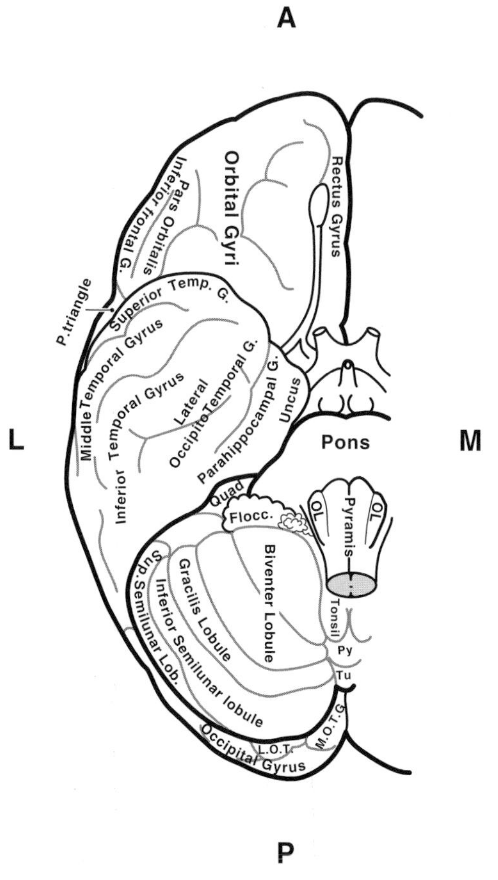

Figure 2C-2I: Schematic of the superficial sulci and gyri of the inferior aspect of the right hemisphere and cerebellum. *A*, anterior; *P*, posterior; *M*, medial; *L*, lateral.

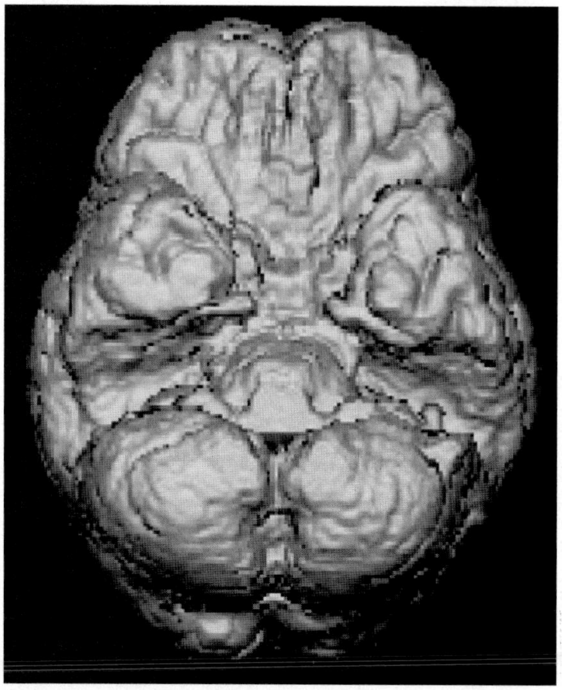

Figure 2C-2J: Inferior aspect of a three-dimensional MR image of the brain (compare with Fig 2C-2I).

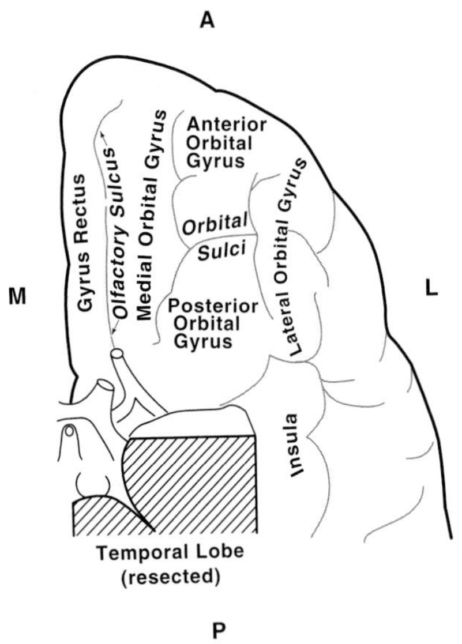

Figure 2C-3A: Schematic of the orbital surface of the left frontal lobe. *A*, anterior; *P*, posterior; *M*, medial; *L*, lateral.

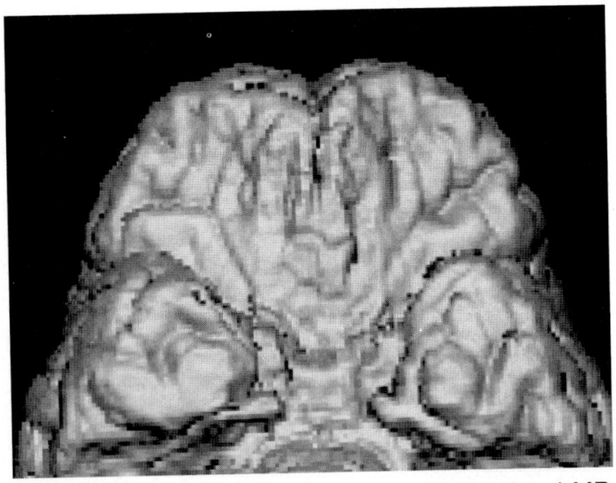

Figure 2C-3B: Inferior aspect of a three-dimensional MR image of the frontal lobes (refer to Fig. 2C-3A) (Courtesy of J. Lancaster).

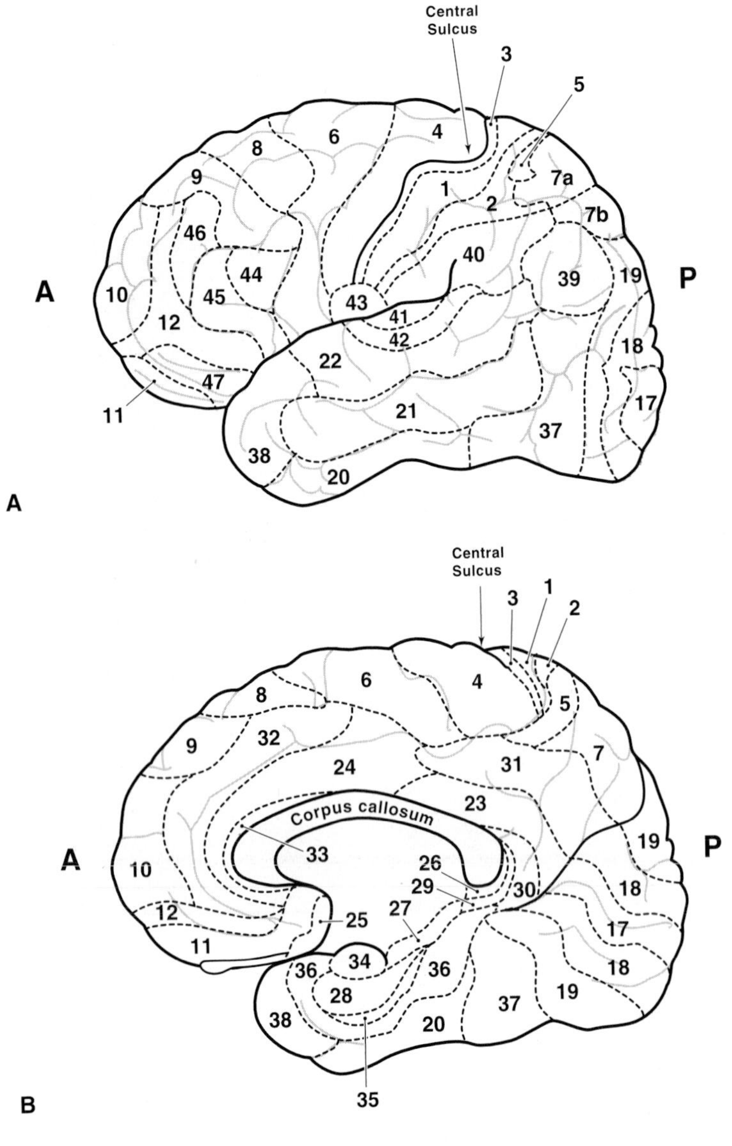

Figure 2C-4: Schematic of Brodman's cytoarchitectonic areas of the cerebrum by number. **A:** Lateral aspect of left hemisphere. **B:** Medial aspect of right hemisphere (left hemisphere removed). *A*, anterior; *P*, posterior. Numbers refer to Brodman's cytoarchitectonic areas.

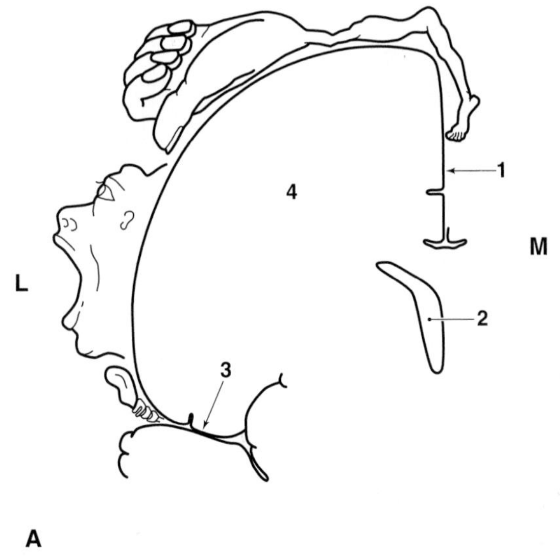

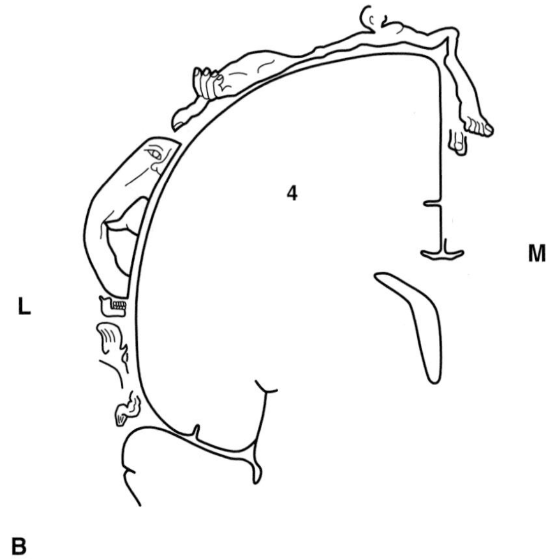

Figure 2C-5A: Coronal schematic of the precentral gyrus on the right side, with an overlay of the motor homunculus, or somatotopic motor organization of the gyrus. *M*, medial; *L*, lateral.
Figure 2C-5B: Coronal schematic of the postcentral gyrus on the right side with an overlay of the sensory homunculus, or somatotopic sensory organization of the gyrus. *M*, medial; *L*, lateral.

1 Interhemispheric fissure
2 Body of lateral ventricle
3 Sylvian fissure
4 Right cerebral hemisphere

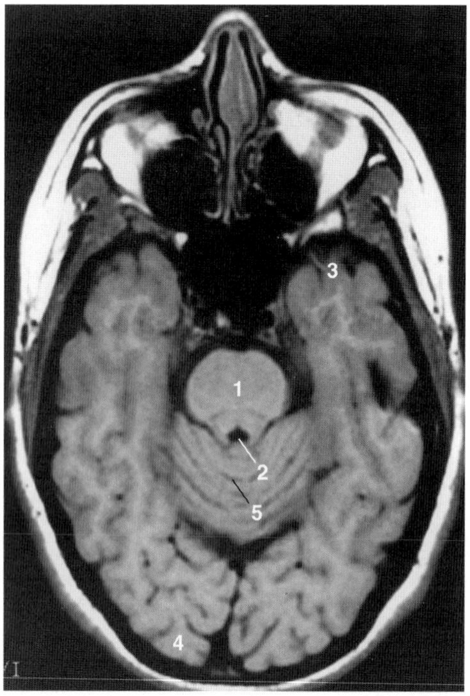

Figure 2C-6A: **Axial cross-sectional anatomy of the cerebral hemispheres.** Axial T1-weighted MR image at the level of the temporal and occipital lobes.

1 Upper pons
2 Upper aspect of fourth ventricle
3 Pole of temporal lobe
4 Pole of occipital lobe
5 Superior cerebellar vermis

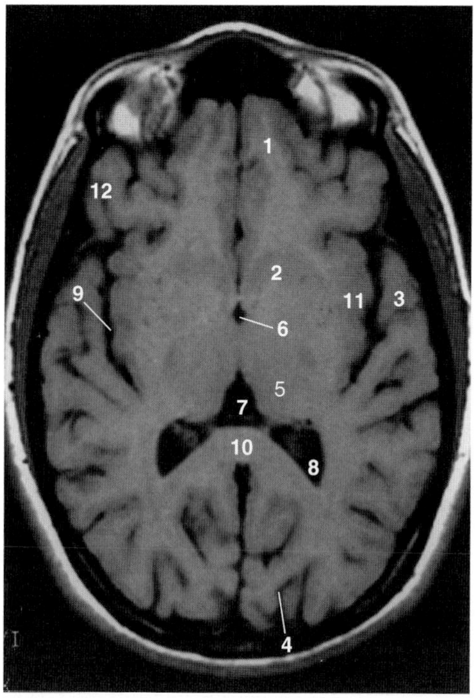

Figure 2C-6B: **Axial and sagittal cross-sectional anatomy of the cerebral hemispheres.** Axial T1-weighted MR image at the level of the insula and occipital lobes.

1 Basal aspect of the frontal lobe
2 Anterior commissure
3 Temporal operculum
4 Occipital lobe
5 Thalamus
6 Third ventricle
7 Cistern of the velum interpositum
8 Atrium (trigone) of lateral ventricle
9 Sylvian fissure
10 Splenium of corpus callosum
11 Insula
12 Frontal operculum

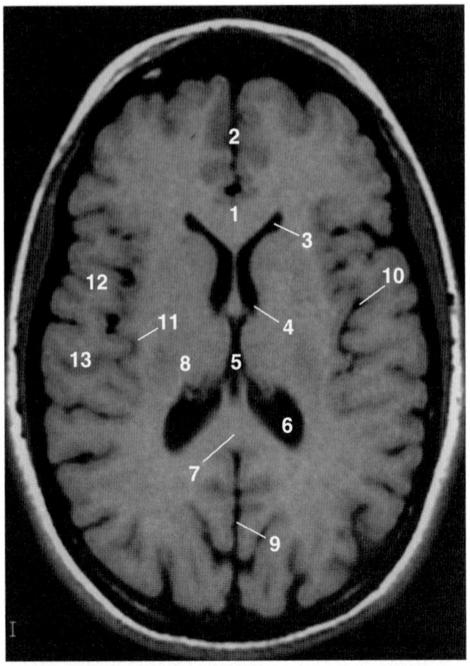

Figure 2C-6C: Axial cross-sectional anatomy of the cerebral hemispheres. Axial T1-weighted MR image at the level of the upper and Sylvian fissures.

1 Genu of corpus callosum
2 Anterior aspect of interhemispheric fissure
3 Anterior horn of lateral ventricle
4 Foramen of Monro
5 Third ventricle
6 Atrium of lateral ventricle
7 Splenium of corpus callosum
8 Thalamus
9 Posterior aspect of interhemispheric fissure
10 Upper Sylvian fissure
11 Insula
12 Frontal operculum
13 Parietal operculum

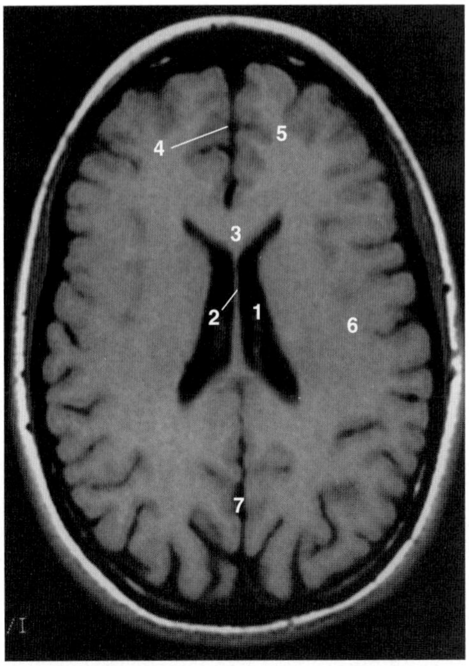

Figure 2C-6D: Axial and sagittal cross-sectional anatomy of the cerebral hemispheres. Axial T1-weighted MR image at the level of the frontal and parietal lobes.

1 Body of lateral ventricle
2 Septum pellucidum (septi pellucidi)
3 Genu of corpus callosum
4 Anterior aspect of interhemispheric fissure
5 Frontal lobe
6 Parietal lobe
7 Posterior aspect of interhemispheric fissure

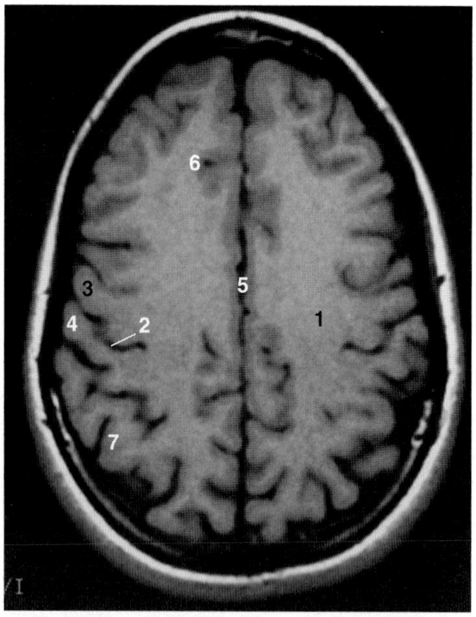

Figure 2C-6E: Axial cross-sectional anatomy of the cerebral hemispheres. Axial T1-weighted MR image at the level of the centrum semiovale.
1 Centrum semiovale
2 Central sulcus
3 Precentral gyrus
4 Postcentral gyrus
5 Central aspect of interhemispheric fissure
6 Frontal lobe
7 Parietal lobe

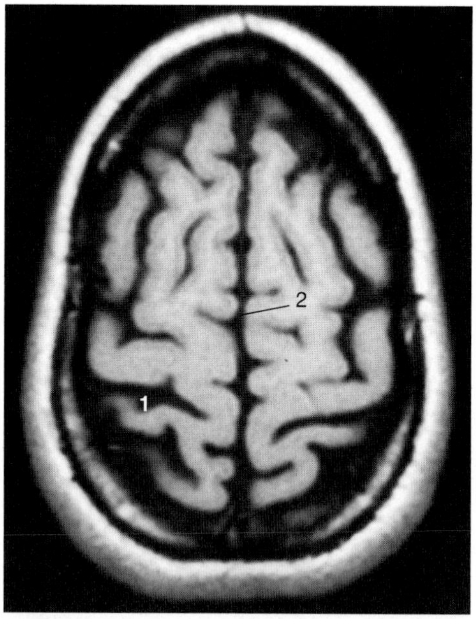

Figure 2C-6F: Axial cross-sectional anatomy of the cerebral hemispheres. Axial T1-weighted MR image at the level of the vertex.
1 Upper aspect of the central sulcus
2 Central upper aspect of interhemispheric fissure

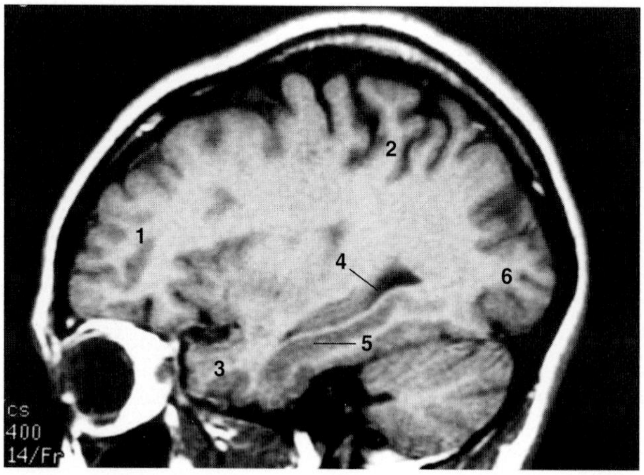

Figure 2C-6G: Sagittal cross-sectional anatomy of the cerebral hemispheres. Parasagittal T1-weighted MR image at the level of the temporal lobe.
1 Frontal lobe
2 Parietal lobe
3 Pole of temporal lobe
4 Temporal horn of lateral ventricle
5 Parahippocampal gyrus
6 Occipital lobe

CEREBRAL HEMISPHERE VARIANTS

- Gross lateral differences between sizes of the lobes of the cerebral hemispheres
- Gross lateral difference between the gyri, sulci, and fissures

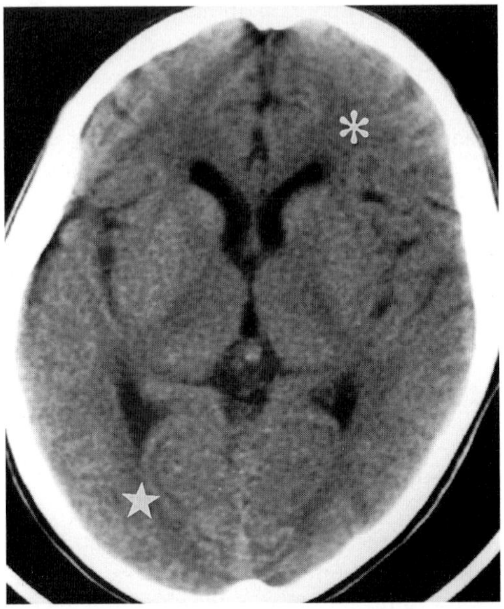

Figure 2C-7A: Normal gross brain asymmetry. Axial CT image showing that the left frontal (*asterisk*) and right occipital (*star*) lobes are perceptibly grossly larger than their contralateral counterparts.

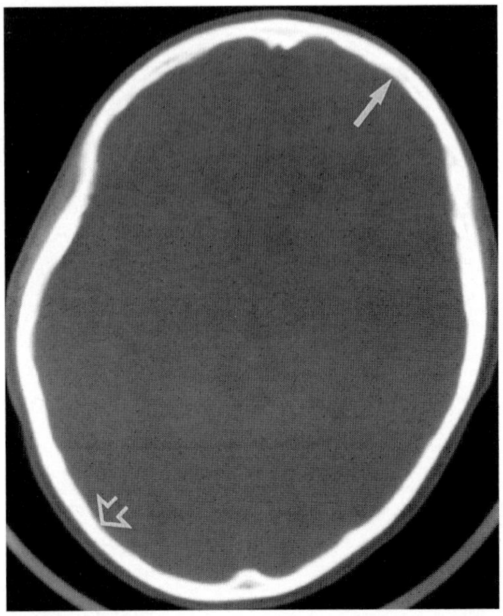

Figure 2C-7B: Normal gross brain asymmetry. Axial CT image showing consonant asymmetry in the overlying calvarium. The left side of the frontal bone (*solid arrow*) and the right side of the occipital bone (*open arrow*) are larger and protrude outward more than their contralateral counterparts.

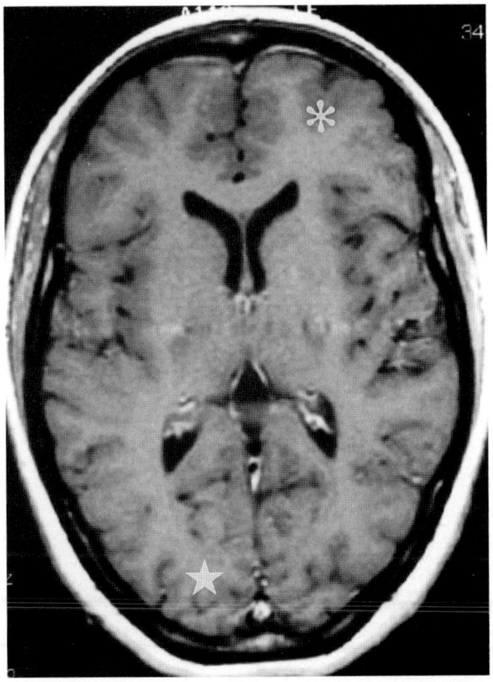

Figure 2C-7C: Normal gross brain asymmetry. Enhanced axial Tl-weighted MR image showing the typical asymmetry between the cerebral hemispheres. Note that the left frontal lobe (*asterisk*) and right occipital lobes (*star*) are grossly larger than their contralateral counterparts.

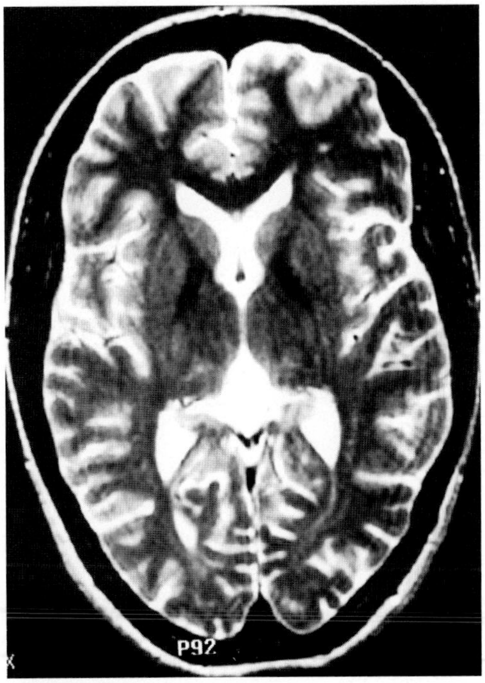

Figure 2C-7D: Normal gross brain asymmetry. Axial T2-weighted MR image showing the typical asymmetry of the cerebral hemispheres.

2D. DIENCEPHALON

OVERVIEW

1. The diencephalon is the medial ventral part of the forebrain.
2. It is a paired structure that lies craniad to the midbrain of the brain stem.
3. The diencephalon is continuous anteriorly and laterally with the cerebral hemispheres.
4. The diencephalon has two major and two minor subregions that are bilaterally represented.
   a. The major subregions are the thalamus (dorsal thalamus) and the hypothalamus.
   b. The minor subregions are the epithalamus and the subthalamus (ventral thalamus).
5. The boundaries of the diencephalon include:
   a. Rostrally, it joins the lamina terminalis.
   b. Caudally, it joins the midbrain.
   c. Ventrally, it forms part of the ventral surface of the brain.
   d. Dorsally, it forms part of the floor of the bodies of the lateral ventricles.
   e. Medially, it forms part of the walls of the third ventricle.
   f. Laterally, it borders on the posterior portion of the internal capsule.

THE THALAMUS (DORSAL THALAMUS)

1. The thalami are paired ovoid masses of diencephalic neurons arranged into nuclei.
2. The thalami lie medial to the posterior limbs of the internal capsules.
3. The two thalami form the lateral walls of the third ventricle superior to the hypothalamic sulcus.
4. A nuclear/axonal mass called the massa intermedia (interthalamic adhesion) is inconsistent in size, sometimes multiple, and sometimes absent altogether. It may connect up to 80% of the medial surfaces of the two thalami across the lumen of the third ventricle. Although it contains neurons whose axonal processes may cross the midline, many of these axons recurve back across the median plane.
5. Each thalamus has rostral and caudal poles in addition to dorsal, ventral, medial, and lateral surfaces.
   a. The rostral pole commences just behind the plane of the foramen of Monro and the genu of the internal capsule.
   b. The caudal pole, or the pulvinar, overhangs the geniculate bodies and superior colliculi of the quadrigeminal plate.
   c. Dorsolaterally, the thalamus borders on the body and tail of the caudate nucleus and on the thalamostriate vein and stria terminalis.
   d. Dorsomedially, the thalamus forms the floor of the body of the lateral ventricle. The tela choroidea covers the dorsomedial aspect of the thalamus and bridges the lumen of the third ventricle as its roof. The tela choroidea consists of an inner lining of pia mater and an outer layer of ependyma; it invests the blood vessels and matrix of the choroid plexus.
   e. Medially, the thalamus borders on the lumen of the third ventricle.
   f. Ventrally, the thalamic fasciculus separates the thalamus from the zona incerta of the subthalamus (ventral thalamus).
   g. Laterally, the external medullary lamina, a thin sheet of white matter, separates the thalamus from the nucleus reticularis thalami. The reticular nucleus(i) in turn separates the thalamus proper from the posterior limb of the internal capsule.
6. The capsules and laminae of the myelinated axons of thalamus include the myelinated capsule and the internal medullary lamina.
   a. The myelinated capsule
      i. The myelinated capsule begins dorsal to the myelin-free area on the medial aspect of the thalamus.
      ii. It commences at the stria terminalis and extends laterally, ventrally, and medially.

iii. It consists of thin sheets of white matter, the stratum zonale (superiorly), and the external medullary lamina (laterally).

b. The internal medullary lamina
   i. The internal medullary lamina cleaves the thalamus sagittally into two roughly equal medial and lateral nuclear groups and then splits dorsally around the anterior nucleus of the thalamus.
   ii. The internal medullary lamina thereby separates the thalamic nuclei into medial, lateral, and dorsal nuclear groups.

7. The thalamus is a major source of afferent fibers to the cerebral cortex.
8. The thalamus modulates almost all of the neural activity into and out of the cerebral cortex through the thalamocortical and corticothalamic circuits.
9. The major thalamic nuclei
   a. The anterior thalamic nuclear group consists of the anterodorsal nuclei, anteroventral nuclei, and anteronuclei.
   b. The medial thalamic nuclear group consists of a single component, the mediodorsal nucleus.
   c. The ventral thalamic nuclear group consists of the ventral anterior nucleus, the ventral lateral nuclear complex, and the ventral posterior complex.
   d. The dorsal thalamic nuclear group consists of the lateral dorsal nucleus, the lateral posterior nucleus, and the pulvinar.
   e. The intralaminar thalamic nuclear group are collections of neurons within the internal medullary lamina. This group consists of the anterior (central medial, paracentral, and central lateral nuclei) and posterior (centromedian and parafascicular nuclei) intralaminar nuclei.
   f. The midline thalamic nuclear group consists of the rhomboidalis, reuniens, and parataenialis nuclei. The paraventricular nuclei (paraventricularis) and the central medial nucleus are also sometimes included in this group.
   g. The medial (medial, ventral, dorsal nuclei) and lateral (dorsal, lateral, geniculate nucleus) geniculate bodies (metathalamus).
10. The major connections of the thalamic nuclei
   a. The anterior thalamic nuclear group are primarily recipients of the mammillothalamic tract. They project to cortical targets in the anterior limbic area, the cingulate gyrus, and the parahippocampal gyrus.
   b. The ventral thalamic nuclei are mainly general and special somatomotor nuclei.
      i. The ventral anterior nucleus receives neural input primarily from the cerebellum and projects to the cerebral motor area.
      ii. The ventral posterior nucleus receives input primarily from the general somatic afferent axons and projects to the somatosensory cerebral cortex of the postcentral gyrus.
      iii. The ventral lateral nucleus is made up of several divisions: the anterior division, with input from the globus pallidus and projection to the premotor and supplementary motor areas; the medial division, with input from the pars reticulata of the substantia nigra and projection to the dorsolateral and medial frontal lobe; and the posterior division, with input from the deep cerebellar nuclei, spinothalamic tract, vestibular nuclei, and primary motor cortex and projection to the primary motor cortex.
   c. The metathalamus includes the medial and lateral geniculate bodies.
      i. The medial geniculate bodies receive auditory input and project to the transverse temporal gyri.
      ii. The lateral geniculate bodies receive visual input and project to the calcarine cortex.
   d. The dorsal thalamic nuclei
      i. The lateral dorsal nucleus (nucleus lateralis dorsalis)
         - The lateral dorsal nucleus is located behind the anterior nucleus.
         - The lateral dorsal nucleus receives afferent neural input from the amygdala and fornix.
         - The lateral dorsal nucleus projects to the cingulate gyrus.

ii. The lateral posterior nucleus (nucleus lateralis posterior)
- The lateral posterior nucleus covers the ventral thalamic nuclei.
- The lateral posterior nucleus forms reciprocal connections with the parietal lobe behind the somatosensory receptive cortex.

iii. The pulvinar (nucleus pulvinaris)
- The pulvinar forms reciprocal connections with the cortex of the parietal lobe and with the occipital and temporal lobes.

e. The medial thalamic nuclear group

i. The mediodorsal nucleus
- The mediodorsal nucleus receives subcortical afferent neural input from the basal olfactory structures, the hypothalamus, the periventricular fiber system, the striatum, and the cerebellum.
- The mediodorsal nucleus projects to the frontal lobe anterior to the motor strip of the precentral gyrus.

f. The anterior intralaminar nuclei

i. The anterior intralaminar nuclei have reciprocal connections with widespread hemispheric cortical areas; the posterior intralaminar nuclei have more restricted connections (motor, premotor, supplementary motor areas). Both anterior and posterior groups also project to the striatum.

g. The midline thalamic nuclei

i. The midline nuclei receive afferent fibers from the hypothalamus, the periaqueductal gray matter, the spinothalamic tract, and the medullary and pontine reticular formation.

ii. Efferent fibers project to the hippocampal formation, the amygdala, the nucleus accumbens, the cingulate gyrus, and the orbitofrontal cortex.

THE HYPOTHALAMUS

1. The hypothalamus is the most ventral part of the diencephalon and extends from the optic chiasm to the caudal border of the mammillary bodies.
2. The hypothalamus comprises the floor and the inferior and lateral walls of the third ventricle ventral to the hypothalamic sulcus.
3. The hypothalamus exerts control over the viscera, somatic tissues, endocrine system, homeostasis, and some behaviors.
4. The hypothalamic boundaries

a. The ventral boundary of the hypothalamus

i. The ventral aspect of the hypothalamus is bordered upon by the optic chiasm and tracts and the posterior lobe of the hypophysis (pituitary gland).

ii. The postmammillary sulcus separates the hypothalamus from the midbrain basis.

b. The rostral boundary of the hypothalamus

i. The rostral border of the hypothalamus medially is formed by the junction of the lamina terminalis with the anterior commissure of the telencephalon.

ii. The rostral border of the hypothalamus laterally is formed by the ventromedial edge of the internal capsule, the medial tip of the globus pallidus and the ansa lenticularis, the substantia innominata of the anterior perforated substance, and the diagonal band.

c. The caudal boundary of the hypothalamus

i. The caudal border of the hypothalamus medially is formed by a line drawn from the posterior margin of the mammillary bodies to the posterior commissure.

ii. The caudal border of the hypothalamus laterally is formed by the continuation of the ventromedial edge of the internal capsule as it descends into the midbrain basis.

d. The dorsal boundary of the hypothalamus

i. The dorsal border of the hypothalamus is formed by the hypothalamic sulcus, running longitudinally in the wall of the third ventricle.

5. The divisions and nuclei of the hypothalamus
   a. The hypothalamus may be divided anteroposteriorly and mediolaterally.
      i. Anteroposteriorly, the hypothalamus consists of chiasmatic (supraoptic), tuberal (infundibulotuberal), and posterior (mammillary) areas.
      ii. Mediolaterally, the hypothalamus consists of periventricular, intermediate (medial), and lateral zones.
   b. Periventricular zone
      i. The periventricular zone borders on the third ventricle.
      ii. Periventricular zone nuclei include preoptic, suprachiasmatic, and arcuate nuclei.
   c. Intermediate (medial) zone nuclei include paraventricular and supraoptic nuclei, intermediate nuclear groups, ventromedial and dorsomedial nuclei, mammillary body nuclei, and tuberomammillary nuclei.
   d. The lateral zone forms a continuum of cells that extends through the lateral hypothalamic area.
6. The connections of the hypothalamic nuclei
   a. The hypothalamus exerts effects by three means: direct neural connection, the bloodstream, and the cerebrospinal fluid. The latter two are hormonally effected.
   b. The afferent connections to the hypothalamus include the ascending somatic and visceral sensory systems, various brain stem tracts, the olfactory and visual systems, the thalamus, the limbic system, and the neocortex.
   c. The efferent connections of the hypothalamus include reciprocal connections with the afferent projections. Prominent are the effects of the hypothalamus upon the central origins of autonomic nerve fibers.

THE EPITHALAMUS

1. The epithalamus is the most dorsal part of all the nuclear zones of the diencephalon.
2. The epithalamus consists of the following.
   a. Pineal body
   b. Habenular commissure
   c. Stria medullaris thalami
   d. Posterior commissure
   e. Medial and lateral habenular nuclei
   f. Anterior and posterior paraventricular nuclei
3. The connections of the epithalamus
   a. The paraventricular nuclei
      i. Afferent connections: the hypothalamus, the septal nuclei, the stria terminalis, the hippocampal formation, and the brain stem
      ii. Efferent connections: the nucleus accumbens, the amygdaloid nuclear complex, and the hippocampal formation
   b. The habenular commissure and nuclei
      i. The habenular commissure connects the habenular nuclei of the two sides, the amygdaloid nuclear complexes, and the hippocampal cortices. Crossed tectohabenular fibers also travel in this commissure.
      ii. Afferent connections: the piriformis cortex, the basal nucleus of Maynert, the hypothalamus, the globus pallidus, the pars compacta of the substantia nigra, the midbrain raphe nuclei, the lateral dorsal tegmental nucleus, and the septofimbrial nucleus
      iii. Efferent connections: the interpeduncular midbrain nucleus, the raphe nuclei, the reticular formation of the midbrain, the pars compacta of the substantia nigra, the ventral tegmental area, the hypothalamus, and the basal forebrain
   c. The stria medullaris thalami
      i. The stria medullaris thalami sends fibers to the ipsilateral habenular nucleus and through the habenular commissure to the contralateral habenular nucleus.

d. The pineal body
   i. Connections are to the habenular nuclei via the habenulopineal tract and the dorsal ascending tegmental nonadrenergic bundle and to the superior cervical ganglia via sympathetic fibers.

e. The posterior commissure
   i. The posterior commissure is associated with the interstitial nuclei of the posterior commissure, the dorsal nuclei of the posterior commissure nucleus, and the interstitial nucleus of Cajal. Fibers from these nuclei and the medial longitudinal fasciculus cross the midline in this commissure. Other axonal components include contributions from the dorsal thalamic nuclei, pretectal nuclei, superior colliculi, and tectal and habenular nuclei.

THE SUBTHALAMUS (VENTRAL THALAMUS)

1. The subthalamus is a transitional zone ventral to the thalamus and lateral to the hypothalamus.
2. The subthalamus is bounded by the thalamus dorsally, the hypothalamus medially, and the internal capsule laterally.
3. The main nuclear groups of the subthalamus include the reticular nucleus, the zona incerta, the fields of Forel, the pregeniculate nucleus, the upper poles of the red nucleus and substantia nigra, and the endopeduncular nucleus.
4. The connections of the subthalamic nuclei
   a. The reticular nucleus
      i. Afferent connections: corticothalamic, thalamocortical, thalamostriatal, and palidothalamic fibers and the nucleus cuneiformis
      ii. Efferent connections: the dorsal thalamus
   b. The pregeniculate nucleus
      i. Afferent connections: the retina, the visual cortex, the pretectum, the superior colliculus, the cerebellum, the vestibular nuclei, the subthalamic nucleus, and the locus ceruleus
      ii. Efferent connections: superior colliculus, pretectal nuclei, pontine nuclei, hypothalamus, and dorsal thalamus
   c. The zona incerta
      i. Afferent connections: the sensory motor cortex, the pregeniculate nucleus, the deep cerebellar nuclei, the trigeminal nuclear complex, and the spinal cord
      ii. Efferent connections: the pretectal region of the midbrain and the spinal cord
   d. The fields of Forel
      i. Afferent connections: the globus pallidus, the spinal cord, and the reticular formation of the brain stem
      ii. Efferent connection: the spinal cord

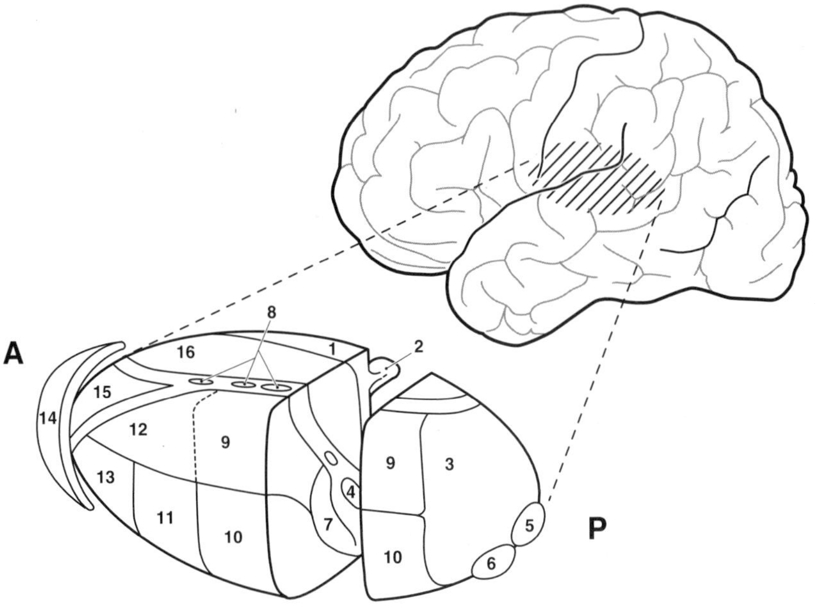

Figure 2D-1: Lateral oblique schematic of the main nuclear masses of the thalamus (dorsal thalamus). *A*, anterior; *P*, posterior.

1 Midline nuclei
2 Massa intermedia (interthalamic adhesion)
3 Pulvinar
4 Centromedian nucleus
5 Medial geniculate body
6 Lateral geniculate body
7 Ventral posterior medial nucleus
8 Intralaminar nuclei
9 Lateral posterior nucleus
10 Ventral posterior lateral nucleus
11 Ventral lateral nucleus
12 Dorsal lateral nucleus
13 Ventral anterior nucleus
14 Reticular nucleus
15 Anterior nuclear group
16 Mediodorsal nucleus

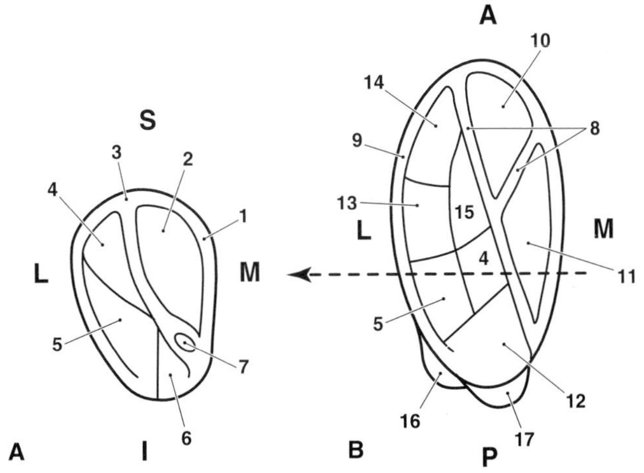

Figure 2D-2: Schematic cross sections of the nuclei of the thalamus (dorsal thalamus). **A:** Coronal section. **B:** Axial section. *A*, anterior; *P*, posterior; *S*, superior; *I*, inferior; *M*, medial; *L*, lateral; *dashed arrow*, plane of section of Fig. 2D-2A.

1 Midline nuclei
2 Mediodorsal nucleus
3 Reticularis nucleus
4 Lateral posterior nucleus
5 Ventral posterior lateral nucleus
6 Ventral posterior medial nucleus
7 Intralaminar nucleus
8 Internal medullary lamina
9 External medullary lamina
10 Anterior nuclear division
11 Medial nuclear division
12 Pulvinar
13 Ventral lateral nucleus
14 Ventral anterior nucleus
15 Lateral dorsal nucleus
16 Lateral geniculate body
17 Medial geniculate body

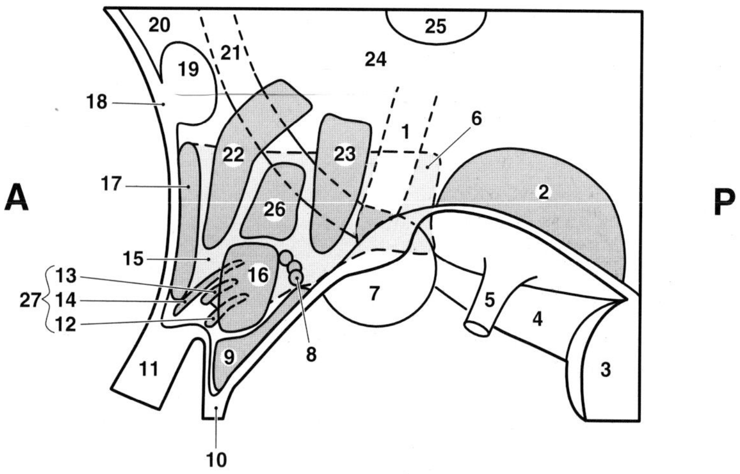

Figure 2D-3: Lateral schematic of the hypothalamic region of the right cerebral hemisphere from the medial aspect, showing the major underlying hypothalamic nuclei. The left hemisphere has been removed. *A*, anterior; *P*, posterior.

1 Mammillothalamic tract
2 Red nucleus
3 Pons
4 Basis pedunculi
5 Oculomotor nerve (cut edge)
6 Lateral hypothalamic area
7 Mammillary body
8 Nuclei tuberis lateralis
9 Nucleus infundibularis (arcuate nucleus)
10 Infundibular stalk (cut edge)
11 Optic chiasm (cut edge)
12 Pars ventromedialis
13 Pars dorsomedialis
14 Pars dorsolateralis
15 Intermediate nucleus
16 Ventromedial nucleus
17 Preoptic nucleus
18 Lamina terminalis
19 Anterior commissure
20 Septum pellucidum
21 Fornix
22 Paraventricular nucleus
23 Posterior nucleus
24 Third ventricle surface overlying the right thalamus
25 Massa intermedia (interthalamic adhesion)
26 Dorsal medial nucleus
27 Supraoptic nucleus

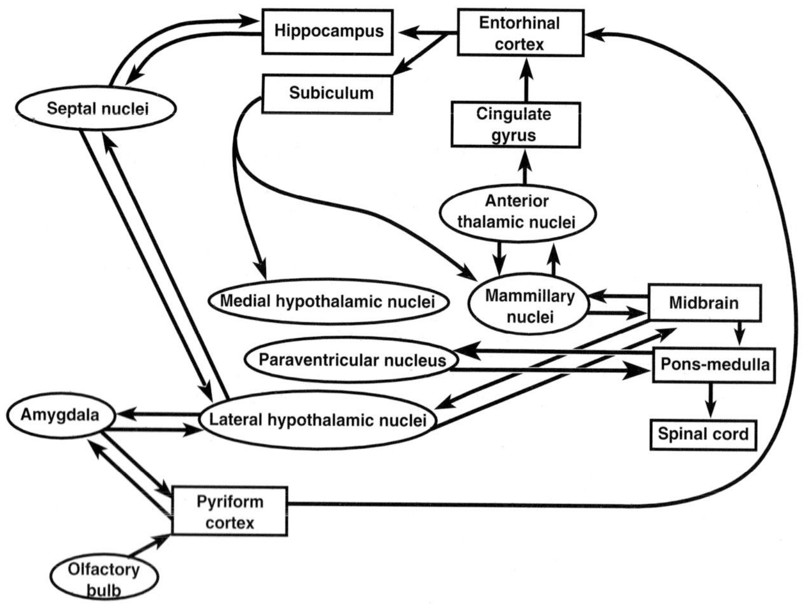

Figure 2D-4: Schematic diagram of the principal fiber connections of the hypothalamus.

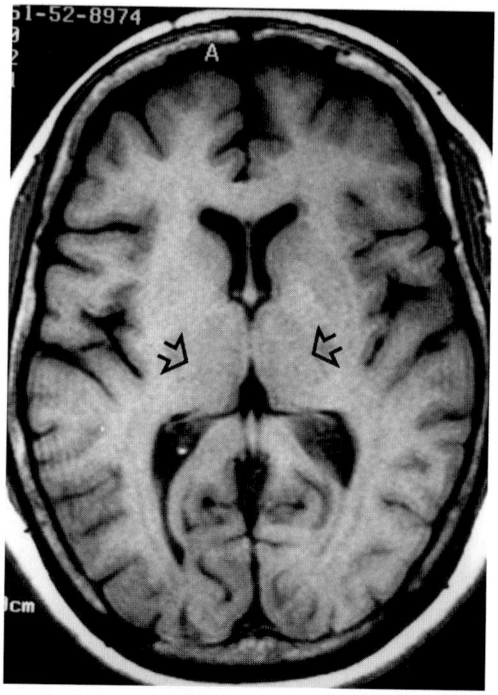

Figure 2D-5A: The thalami. Axial T1-weighted MR image showing the thalami (*arrows*) bilaterally.

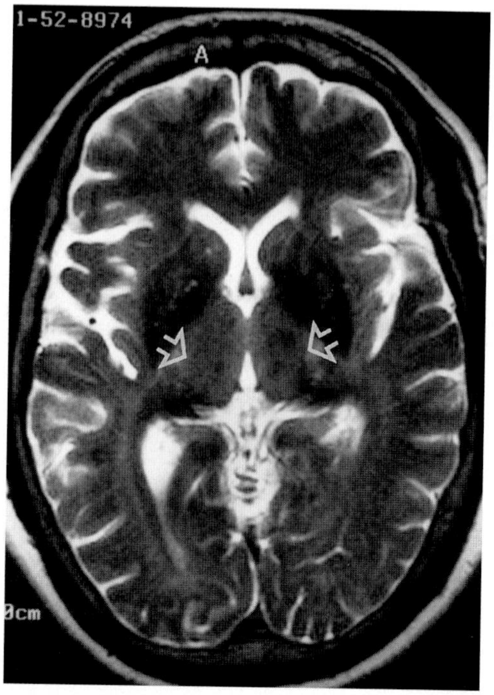

Figure 2D-5B: The thalami. Axial T2-weighted MR image showing the thalami (*arrows*) bilaterally.

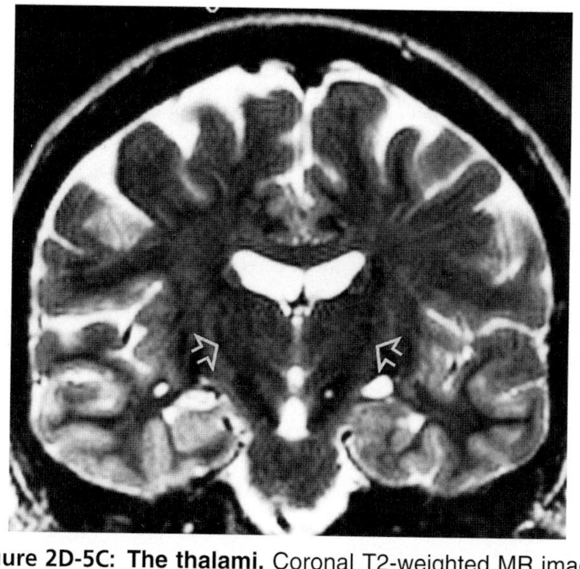

Figure 2D-5C: The thalami. Coronal T2-weighted MR image showing the thalami (*arrows*).

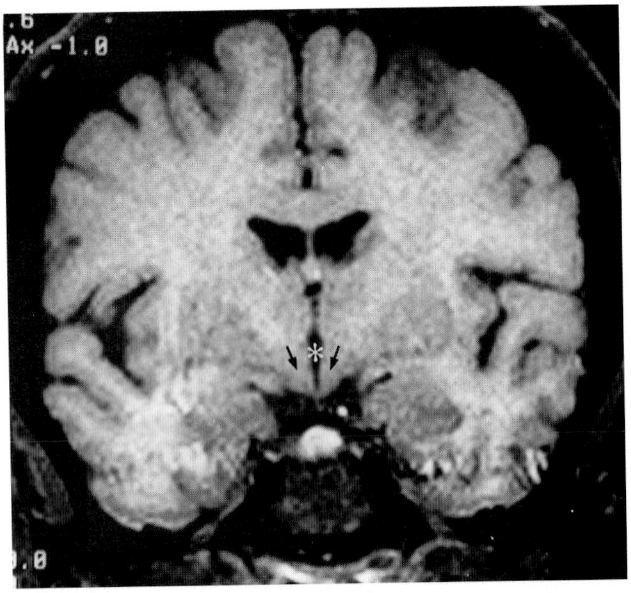

Figure 2D-6A: **The hypothalamus.** Coronal T1-weighted MR image showing the hypothalamus (*arrows*) on either side of the third ventricle (*asterisk*).

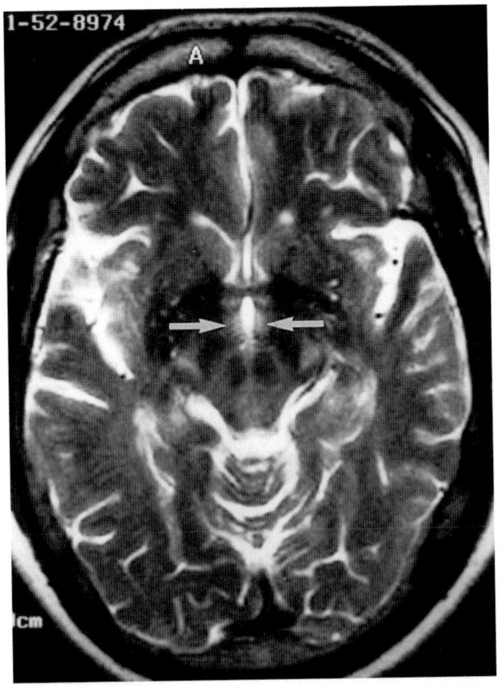

Figure 2D-6B: **The hypothalamus.** Axial T2-weighted MR image showing the region of the hypothalamic nuclei (*arrows*) lateral to the third ventricle.

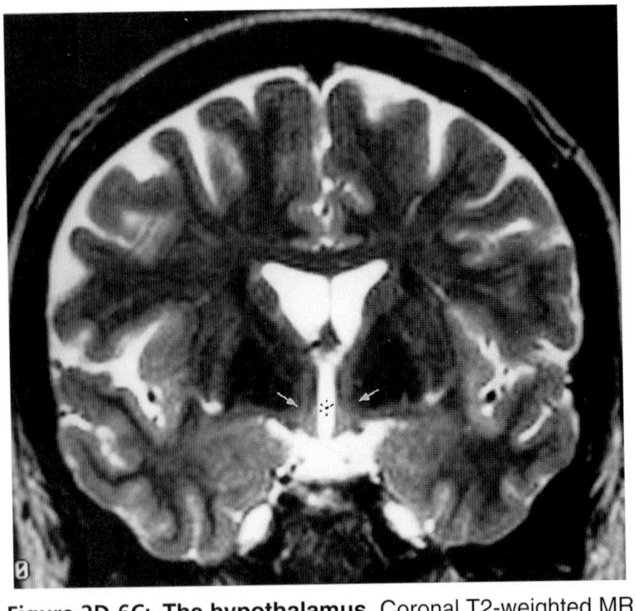

Figure 2D-6C: **The hypothalamus.** Coronal T2-weighted MR image showing some of the thalamic nuclei (*arrows*) on either side of the third ventricle (*asterisk*).

TABLE 2D-1: Components of the Diencephalon

Thalamus (dorsal thalamus)
Hypothalamus
Epithalamus
Pineal body
Habenular commissure
Striae medullaris thalami
Posterior commissure
Medial and lateral habenular nuclei
Anterior and posterior paraventricular nuclei
Subthalamus (ventral thalamus)
Reticular nucleus
Zona incerta
Fields of Forel
Pregeniculate nucleus
Upper pole of the red nucleus
Upper aspect of substantia nigra
Endopeduncular nucleus

TABLE 2D-2: Thalamic (Dorsal Thalamic) Nuclei: Classification and Main Connections

Name	Sources of subcortical input	Destination of output	Nucleus type	Functional classification
Specific nuclei				
Anterior group	Mammillary body	Cingulate gyrus	R	Limbic
Anterior ventralis				
Anterior dorsalis				
Anterior medialis				
Medial group	Amygdala	Prefrontal cortex	A	Association and limbic
Medialis dorsalis	Olfactory areas	Medial temporal cortex	R	
Lateral group: ventral tier	Thalamus			
Ventralis anterior	Globus pallidus	Premotor cortex (6)	R	Motor and nonspecific
	Substantia nigra	Prefrontal cortex	NS	
	Cerebellum	Thalamus		
	Thalamus			
Ventralis lateralis	Intracerebellar nuclei	Motor cortex (4)	R	Motor
	Substantia nigra			
	Globus pallidus			
Ventralis posterior lateralis	Dorsal column nuclei	Sensorimotor cortex	R	Somatosensory (body)
	Spinal cord			
	Vestibular nuclei			
Ventralis posterior medialis	Trigeminal nuclei	Sensorimotor cortex	R	Somatosensory (head)
	Solitary nucleus			Taste
Ventralis posterior inferior	Vestibular nuclei	Sensorimotor cortex	R	Somatosensory
				Vestibular
Lateral group: dorsal tier				
Lateralis dorsalis	Thalamus	Parietal association cortex	A	Association
		Cingulate gyrus		Limbic
Lateralis posterior	Thalamus	Parietal association	A	Association (somatosensory/ visual)
Pulvinar	Superior colliculus	Occipital, parietal, and temporal association cortex	A	Association
	Pretectal area	Frontal eye field	R	Visual, speech
	Thalamus			
Posterior group				
Suprageniculatus	Reticular formation	Insular cortex	NS	Nonspecific?
Limitans	Midbrain tectum			
Posterior	Spinal cord	Retro-insular cortex	R	Somatosensory
	Trigeminal nuclei	Postauditory cortex	NS	Nociceptive
Metathalamus				
Lateral geniculate body	Retina	Primary visual cortex	R	Visual

continued

TABLE 2D-2 *(continued)*

Name	Sources of subcortical input	Destination of output	Nucleus type	Functional classification
Medial geniculate body	Inferior colliculus	Primary auditory cortex	R	Auditory
	Spinal cord Superior colliculus	Insular and opercular cortex		Association (nociceptive?)
Nonspecific nuclei				
Midline group				
Parataenialis Paraventricularis Reuniens Rhomboidalis	Hypothalamus Thalamus Reticular formation	Hippocampal region Cingulate gyrus Amygdala	NS	Limbic
Intralaminar nuclei				
Centrum medianum Parafascicularis Paracentralis	Reticular formation Thalamus Sensory and motor systems	Caudate nucleus Putamen Cortex	NS	Reticular
Centralis lateralis Centralis medialis	Thalamus Reticular formation			
Reticular nucleus Reticularis	Thalamus Cortex	Thalamus Reticular formation Superior colliculus	NS	Reticular (Attention?)

A, association nucleus: NS, nonspecific nucleus; R, relay nucleus;
Modified from Berkovitz BKB, Moxham BJ. In: *A textbook of head and neck anatomy*, Chicago: Year Book Medical Publishers, 1988:530–531.

2E. Basal Ganglia

OVERVIEW

1. The basal ganglia represent the central gray matter of the telencephalon.
2. The basal ganglia lie between the thalamus and the centrum semiovale.
3. The basal ganglia consist of the caudate nucleus, the putamen, the globus pallidus, the amygdaloid nuclear complex (amygdala), and the claustrum.
4. The corpus striatum refers to a combination of the caudate nucleus, the putamen, the globus pallidus, the ventral striatum, and the ventral pallidum (see later discussion).
5. The striatum proper includes the caudate nucleus, the putamen, and the ventral striatum (see later discussion).
   a. At present, the definition of the corpus striatum has been expanded to include a dorsal division and a ventral division.
      i. The dorsal division of the corpus striatum includes the caudate nucleus, the globus pallidus, and the putamen.
      ii. The ventral division of the corpus striatum includes the ventral striatum (the nucleus accumbens and the olfactory tubercle) and the ventral pallidus in the posterior aspect of the anterior perforated substance.
6. The lentiform nucleus consists of the putamen and the globus pallidus (pallidus). The lateral medullary lamina divides the putamen and the globus pallidus. The medial medullary lamina divides the globus pallidus into medial and lateral parts.
7. The neostriatum consists of the caudate nucleus and the putamen and is a synonym for the striatum.
8. The paleostriatum is a synonym for the globus pallidus.
9. The archistriatum is a synonym for the amygdaloid nuclear complex (amygdala).

THE CORPUS STRIATUM

1. The caudate nucleus
   a. The caudate nucleus is an elongated, arched gray matter structure closely related throughout its extent to the lateral ventricle.
   b. The caudate nucleus consists of a head, body, and tail.
   c. The head of the caudate nucleus is the enlarged rostral part, which forms the lateral wall of the anterior horn of the lateral ventricle.
   d. The body of the caudate nucleus lies along the dorsolateral border of the thalamus near the lateral wall of the lateral ventricle.
   e. The tail of the caudate nucleus follows the curvature of the temporal horn of the lateral ventricle and sweeps into the temporal lobe. It terminates in the region of the amygdaloid nuclear complex.
2. The putamen
   a. The putamen is the largest and most lateral component of the lentiform nucleus.
   b. The putamen is separated from the caudate nucleus by the anterior limb of the internal capsule except in the rostral part of the putamen, where it is continuous with the head of the caudate.
   c. The putamen lies between the lateral medullary lamina of the globus pallidus and the external capsule.
3. The globus pallidus
   a. The globus pallidus is the most medial part of the lentiform nucleus.
   b. The globus pallidus is divided into medial and lateral parts by the medial medullary lamina.
   c. The globus pallidus is separated from the putamen by the lateral medullary lamina and from the thalamus by the posterior limb of the internal capsule.
4. Blood supply of the basal ganglia
   a. The major blood supply to the basal ganglia is via the lenticulostriate arteries,

branches of the proximal anterior and middle cerebral arteries. These arteries enter the brain through the anterior perforated substance.

b. The caudate nucleus receives additional blood supply from the anterior and posterior choroidal arteries.

c. The postero-inferior aspect of the lentiform nucleus (putamen and globus pallidus) receives its blood supply from the thalamostriate (thalamoperforating) arteries, branches of the proximal posterior cerebral artery.

5. The interconnections of the corpus striatum include the following projections. The cerebral cortex projects to the striatum (caudate, putamen, ventral striatum). In turn, the corpus striatum projects to the globus pallidus and substantia nigra (pars reticulata). Finally, these latter structures project back to the cerebral cortex and to the superior colliculus in the quadrigeminal plate of the midbrain.

THE AMYGDALA (AMYGDALOID NUCLEAR COMPLEX)

1. The amygdala is an ovoid mass of gray matter situated in the dorsomedial part of the temporal lobe internal to the uncus of the hippocampus and near the terminal tail of the caudate nucleus.
2. The amygdala is also in contact with the putamen, the globus pallidus, and the claustrum.
3. The amygdala forms the ventral, superior, and medial walls of the tip of the temporal horn of the lateral ventricle on each side.
4. Its principal extrinsic interconnections are with the limbic and olfactory systems; these connections include the stria terminalis and amygdalofugal pathways to the hypothalamus and brain stem, respectively. Other external connections include the forebrain, thalamus, and corpus striatum.
5. Extensive intrinsic interconnections are present between the many nuclei of the amygdaloid nuclear complex.

THE CLAUSTRUM

1. The claustrum is a thin layer of gray matter lying between the putamen and the insular cortex.
2. The claustrum is separated from the putamen by the external capsule.
3. The claustrum is separated from the cortex of the insula by the extreme capsule.
4. The claustrum is continuous anteriorly and inferiorly with the anterior perforated substance, the amygdala, and the prepiriform cortex.
5. The claustrum is believed to have interconnections with the insula.

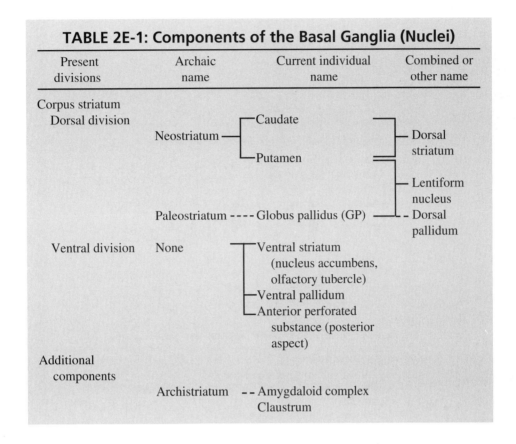

TABLE 2E-1: Components of the Basal Ganglia (Nuclei)

Present divisions	Archaic name	Current individual name	Combined or other name
Corpus striatum			
Dorsal division	Neostriatum	Caudate	Dorsal striatum
		Putamen	Lentiform nucleus
	Paleostriatum	Globus pallidus (GP)	Dorsal pallidum
Ventral division	None	Ventral striatum (nucleus accumbens, olfactory tubercle)	
		Ventral pallidum	
		Anterior perforated substance (posterior aspect)	
Additional components	Archistriatum	Amygdaloid complex	
		Claustrum	

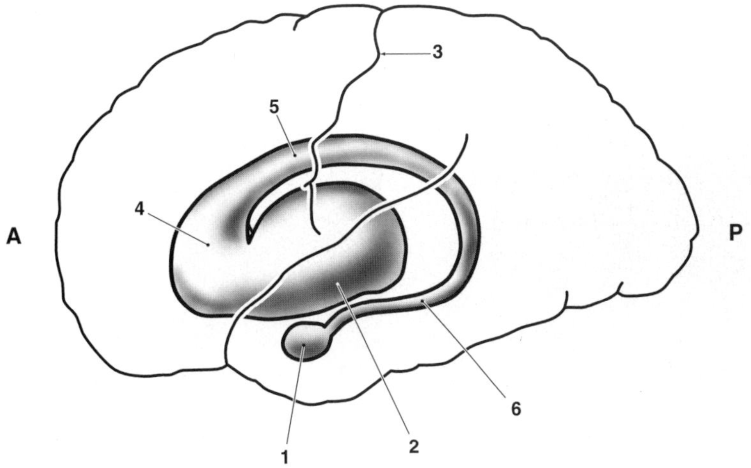

Figure 2E-1: Schematic showing the relationship between the regions of the basal ganglia. *A*, anterior; *P*, posterior.

1 Amygdaloid nuclear complex
2 Lentiform nucleus (putamen and globus pallidus)
3 Central sulcus
4 Head of caudate nucleus
5 Body of caudate nucleus
6 Tail of caudate nucleus

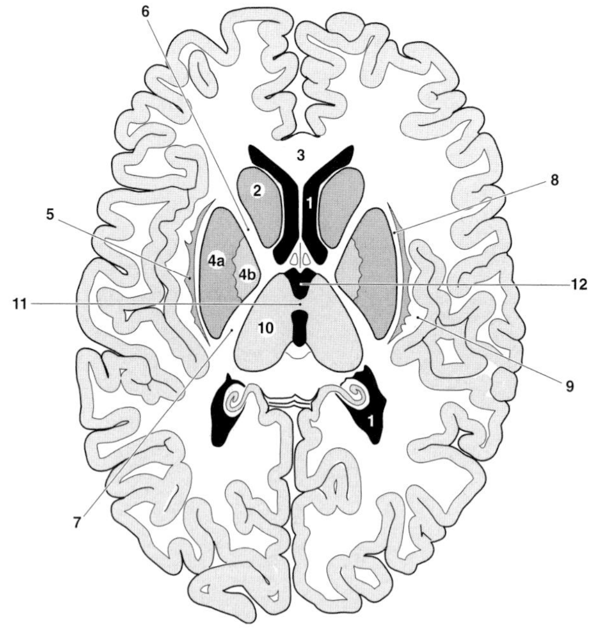

Figure 2E-2: Axial schematic of the basal ganglia.
1 Lateral ventricle
2 Head of caudate nucleus
3 Anterior aspect of corpus callosum
4 Lentiform nucleus (*a*, putamen; *b*, globus pallidus)
5 Claustrum
6 Anterior limb of internal capsule
7 Posterior limb of internal capsule
8 External capsule
9 Extreme capsule
10 Thalamus
11 Massa intermedia (interthalamic adhesion)
12 Third ventricle

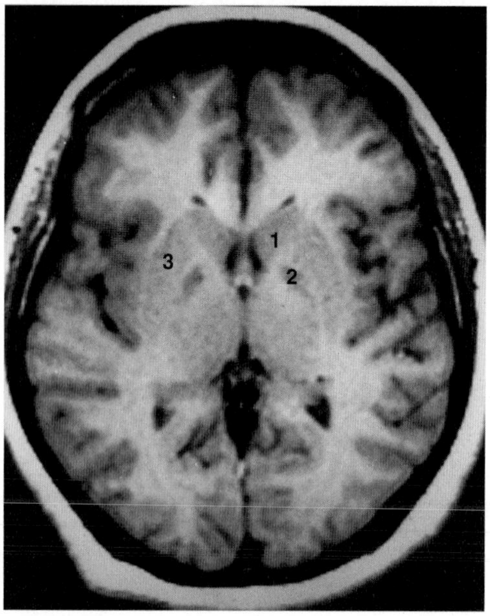

Figure 2E-3A: The basal ganglia.
1 Head of caudate nucleus
2 Globus pallidus
3 Putamen

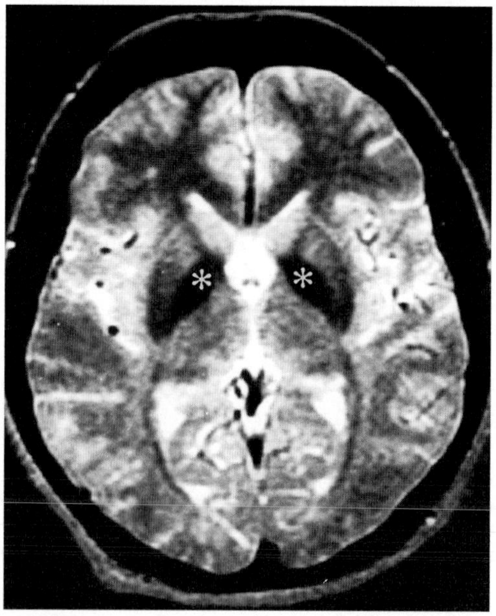

Figure 2E-3B: Axial T2-weighted MR image shows relatively marked hypointensity of globus pallidus bilaterally (*asterisks*) due to iron content.

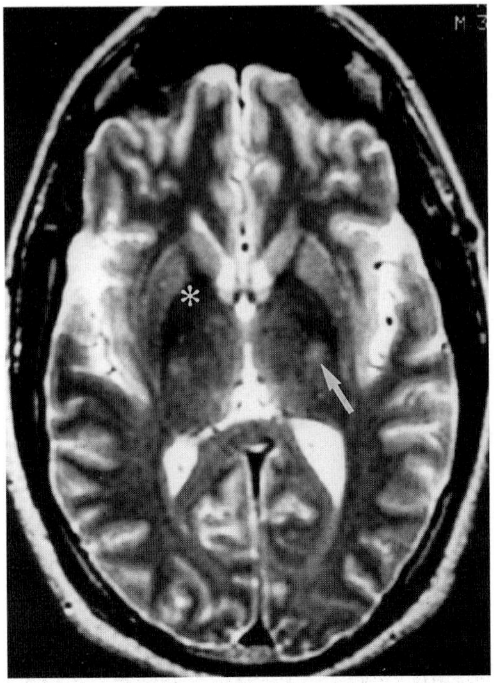

Figure 2E-3C: Axial T2-weighted MR image showing the normally hypointense globus pallidus (*asterisk*) due to iron content. Also note the normal hyperintense area (*arrow*) within the posterior limb of the internal capsule bilaterally.

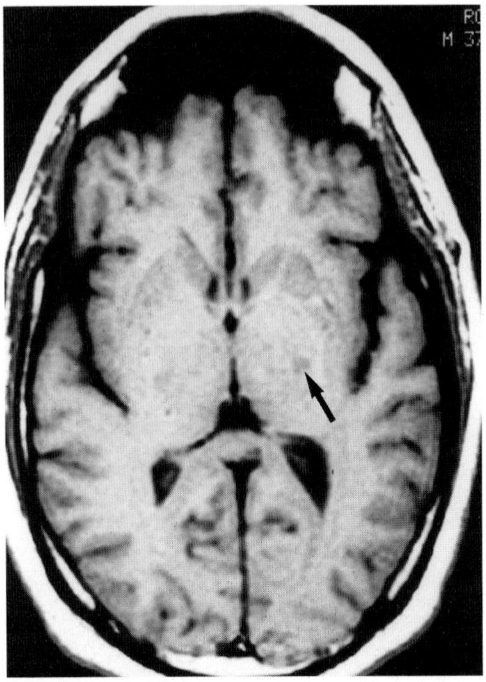

Figure 2E-3D: Axial T1-weighted MR image showing that the area in the posterior limb of the internal capsule (*arrow*) observed in Fig. 2E-3C is relatively hypointense on this acquisition.

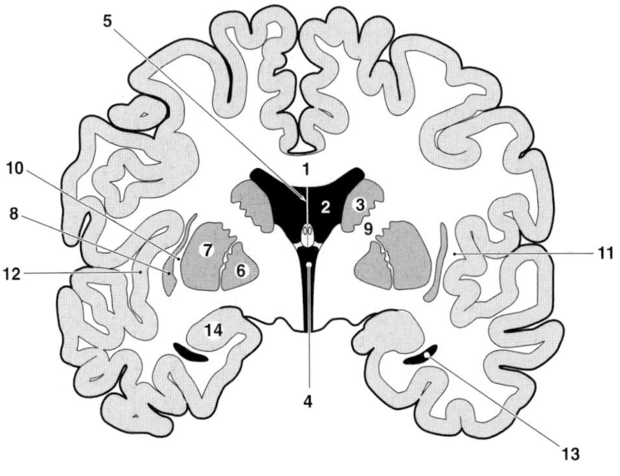

Figure 2E-4A: Coronal schematic of the basal ganglia.

1 Corpus callosum
2 Body of lateral ventricle
3 Caudate nucleus
4 Third ventricle
5 Septum pellucidum
6 Globus pallidus
7 Putamen
8 Claustrum
9 Internal capsule
10 External capsule
11 Extreme capsule
12 Insula
13 Temporal horn of lateral ventricle
14 Amygdala

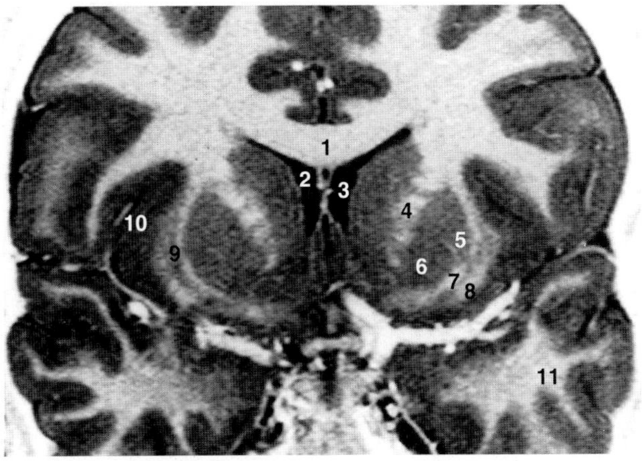

Figure 2E-4B: The basal ganglia. Reversed filming of a T2-weighted fast spin echo MR image shows the basal ganglia. (Case courtesy of C. L. Truwitt, M.D.)

1 Corpus callosum
2 Lateral ventricle
3 Caudate nucleus
4 Internal capsule
5 Putamen
6 Globus pallidus
7 External capsule
8 Extreme capsule
9 Claustrum
10 Insula
11 Temporal lobe

BASAL GANGLIA VARIANTS

- Non-calcified globus pallidus
- Calcified globus pallidus
- Varying degree of iron deposition

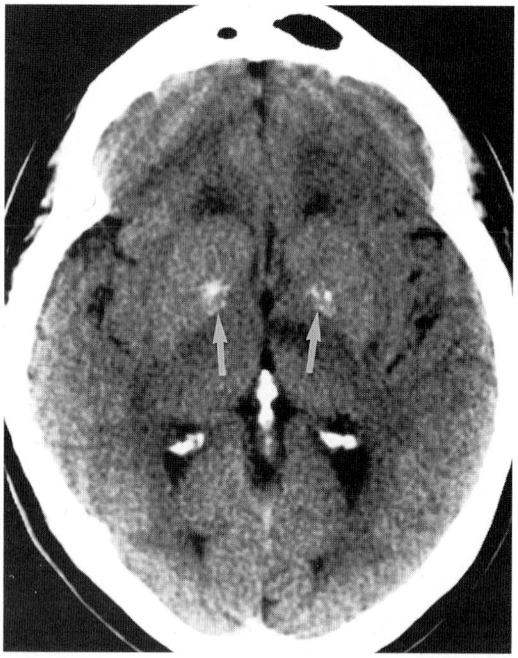

Figure 2E-5A: Basal ganglia calcifications. Unenhanced axial CT image in an asymptomatic middle-aged woman, showing bilateral calcifications in the globus pallidus (*arrows*). Also note the normal pineal and choroid plexus calcifications.

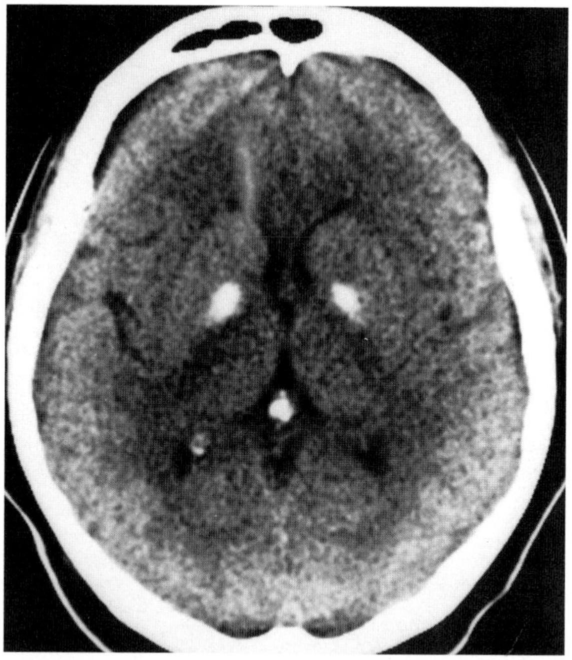

Figure 2E-5B: Basal ganglia calcifications. Unenhanced axial CT image in a different adult patient, showing more dense globus pallidus calcifications bilaterally. Note also pineal and choroid plexus calcifications on the right.

2F. Limbic System and Hippocampus

THE LIMBIC LOBE AND SYSTEM

1. Historically, the *limbic lobe* proper consists of the subcallosal, cingulate, and parahippocampal gyri, the hippocampal formation, and the dentate gyrus.
2. The *limbic system*, on the other hand, is a collection of cortical and subcortical structures whose connections are located on the medial side of the cerebral hemispheres surrounding the brain stem and corpus callosum. The limbic system includes the limbic lobe as well as many associated regions.
3. The cortical structures of the limbic system include the hippocampus proper (Ammon's horn), dentate gyrus, subicular complex (subiculum, presubiculum, parasubiculum), entorhinal cortex, and subcallosal, supracallosal (indusium grisium and medial/lateral longitudinal stria of Lancisii), cingulate, parahippocampal, and paraterminal gyri.
4. The subcortical structures of the limbic system include the amygdala (amygdaloid nuclear complex), habenular nuclei, septal nuclei, hypothalamus, epithalamus, anterior nuclei of the thalamus, mesencephalic tegmentum (medial tegmental region of the midbrain), mammillary bodies, and fornices.
5. The limbic system exerts control over important bodily functions by influencing the endocrine and autonomic nervous systems (visceral activities). It also appears to regulate motivation and emotional status and is believed to be important for memory functions (behavioral activities).

TABLE 2F-1: Components of the Limbic System

Cortical Limbic System Structures
- Parahippocampal gyrus
- Cingulate gyrus
- Isthmus of the cingulate gyrus
- Subcallosal gyrus
- Hippocampus proper
- Subicular complex (subiculum, presubiculum, and parasubiculum)
- Dentate gyrus
- Supracallosal gyrus (indusium grisium and medial/lateral longitudinal stria of Lancisii)
- Paraterminal gyrus
- Entorhinal cortex

Associated Subcortical Limbic System Structures
- Amygdala (amygdaloid nuclear complex)
- Habenular nuclei
- Mammillary bodies
- Septal nuclei
- Epithalamus
- Portions of the hypothalamus
- Anterior thalamic nuclei
- Mesencephalic tegmentum
- Fornices

THE HIPPOCAMPUS

1. The hippocampus is a longitudinal, comma-shaped structure running anteroposteriorly, medial to the temporal horn of the lateral ventricle within each cerebral hemisphere.
2. The hippocampal formation includes the dentate gyrus, the hippocampus proper (Ammon's horn: "cornu ammonis"), the subicular complex (subiculum, presubiculum, and parasubiculum), and the entorhinal cortex. Some anatomists also include hippocampal rudiments (e.g., diagonal band, supracallosal and subsplenial gyri, or the indusium grisium).
3. Grossly, the hippocampus is divided into three parts: the head, the body, and the tail.
4. The hippocampus proper (cornu ammonis) has a primitive configuration with superficial rather than deep white matter and a deeply situated, three-layered cortex. The ventricular surface of the hippocampus is covered by a layer of white matter, the alveus, which converges to form the fimbria on its medial surface and from which the fornix arises. The subiculum is the transition zone between the three-layered cortex of the hippocampus and the six-layered cortex of the temporal lobe.
5. In the coronal plane, the hippocampus is seen to be a bilaminar U-shaped structure of gray matter with one lamina rolled up and interlocked inside the other—the outer lamina, or cornu ammonis (Ammon's horn, hippocampus proper), and the inner lamina, or dentate gyrus.
6. The hippocampus proper is continuous with the subiculum on the surface of the parahippocampal gyrus.
7. The closed circuit linking the hippocampus proper, mammillary body, thalamic nuclei, cingulate gyrus, and entorhinal area of the temporal lobe (Broca area 28: anterior part of parahippocampal gyrus) is called the "circuit of Papez." The fiber tracts linking the circuit include the cingulum, the temporoammonic tract, the fornix, the mammillothalamic tract, and the superior thalamic peduncle. The circuit is believed to perform regulatory functions within the limbic system, especially those involved with emotion.
8. The two hippocampi are joined across the midline by the hippocampal commissure (psalterium), transmitted via the posterior aspect of the bodies of the fornices.

CONNECTIONS OF THE LIMBIC SYSTEM

Limbic system connections include extensive, complex groups of afferent, intrinsic, and efferent fibers (see schematics).

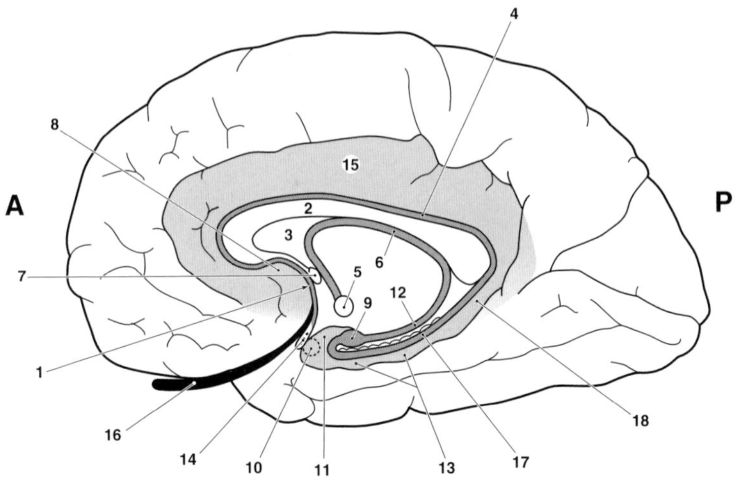

Figure 2F-1A: Medial schematic of the combined limbic system on the right side. The left hemisphere has been removed. *A*, anterior; *P*, posterior.

1 Paraolfactory area
2 Corpus callosum (cut surface)
3 Septum pellucidum
4 Supracallosal gyrus (indusium grisium and medial/lateral longitudinal stria)
5 Mammillary body
6 Fornix
7 Anterior commissure (cut surface)
8 Subcallosal gyrus
9 Hippocampus proper
10 Amygdaloid (amygdaloid nuclear complex)
11 Uncus of hippocampus
12 Fimbria
13 Parahippocampal gyrus
14 Septal region/anterior perforated substance
15 Cingulate gyrus
16 Olfactory bulb and tract (first cranial nerve)
17 Facia dentata of dentate gyrus
18 Isthmus of cingulate gyrus

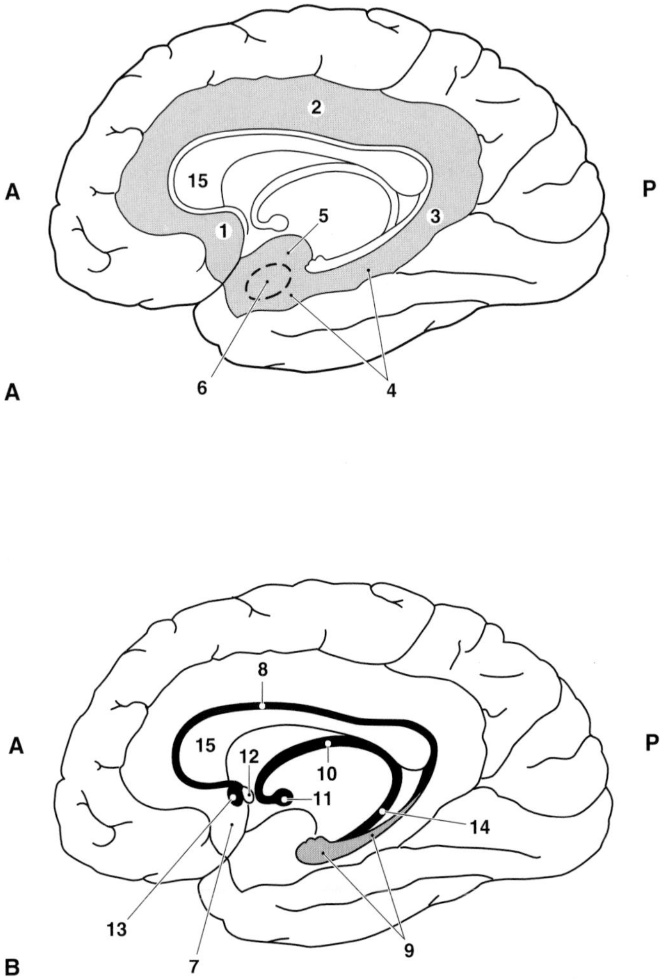

Figure 2F-1B: Medial schematics of the limbic system separated into outer and inner "gyri" on the right side. The left hemisphere has been removed. *A*, anterior; *P*, posterior.

A: *Outer gyrus.*

1 Subcallosal gyrus
2 Cingulate gyrus
3 Isthmus of cingulate gyrus
4 Parahippocampal gyrus
5 Uncus
6 Amygdala (amygdaloid nuclear complex)

B: *Inner gyrus.*

7 Paraterminal gyrus
8 Supracallosal gyrus (indusium grisium, longitudinal stria)
9 Hippocampus proper (cornu ammonis)
10 Fornix
11 Mammillary body
12 Anterior commissure (cut surface)
13 Septal region/anterior perforated substance
14 Fimbria
15 Corpus callosum (cut surface)

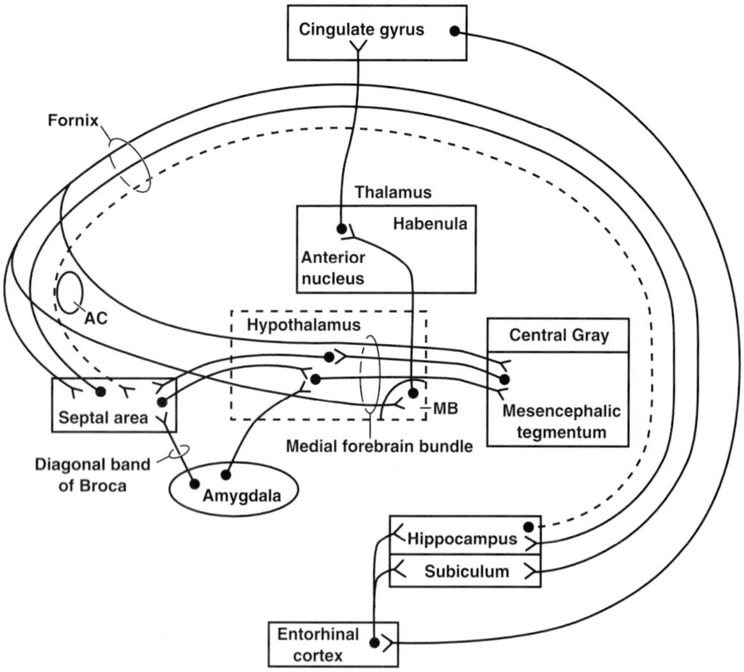

Figure 2F-2: Schematic of the major interconnections between the structures making up the "limbic system." *AC*, anterior commissure; *MB*, mammillary body.

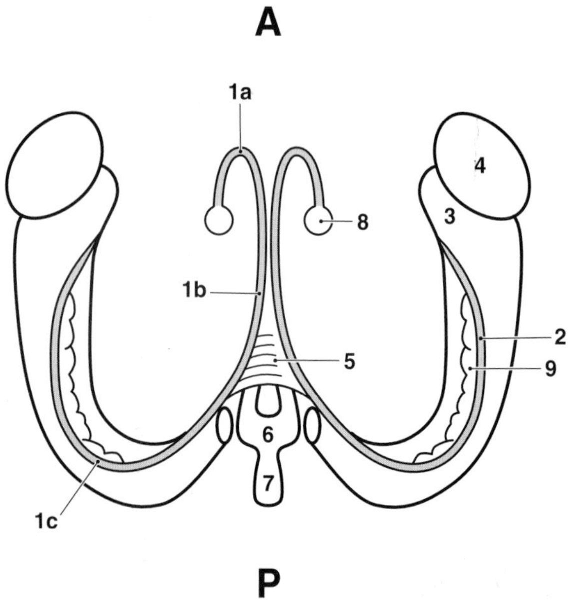

Figure 2F-3: Superior schematic of the fornices and related structures. *A*, anterior; *P*, posterior.

1 Fornix
   a. Anterior column (pillar)
   b. Body
   c. Posterior column (pillar)
2 Fimbria
3 Hippocampus proper
4 Amygdaloid nuclear complex (amygdala)
5 Hippocampal commissure (psalterium)
6 Habenular commissure
7 Pineal gland
8 Mammillary body
9 Dentate gyrus

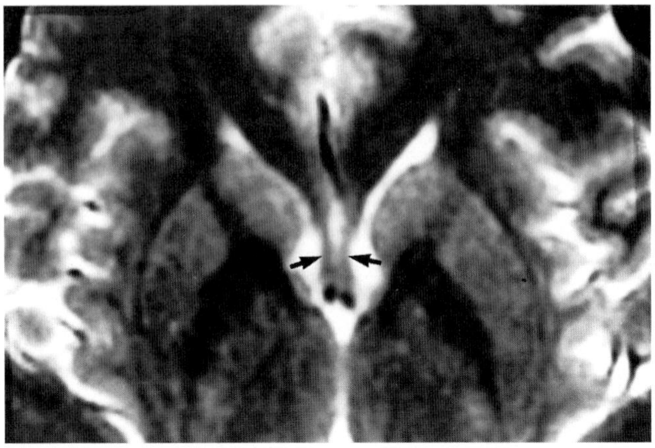

Figure 2F-4A: The fornices. Coronal T2-weighted MR image showing the anterior columns (pillars) of the fornices (*arrows*).

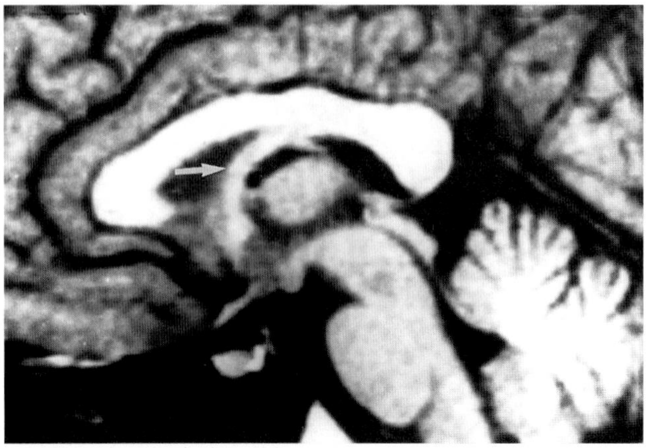

Figure 2F-4B: The fornices. Sagittal T1-weighted MR image showing the anterior aspect of the body(ies) of the fornix(ices) (*arrow*).

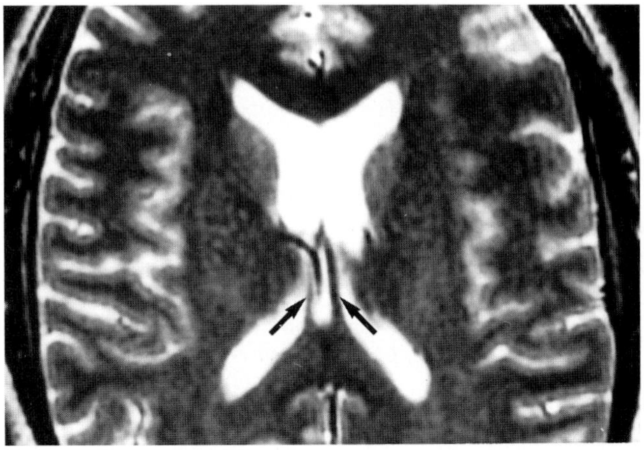

Figure 2F-4C: The fornices. Magnified axial T2-weighted MR image showing the posterior aspect of the bodies of the fornices (*arrows*).

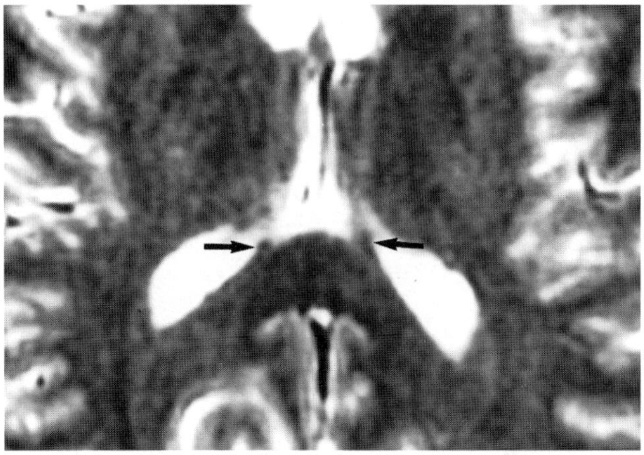

Figure 2F-4D: The fornices. Coronal T2-weighted MR image showing the posterior columns (pillars) of the fornices (*arrows*).

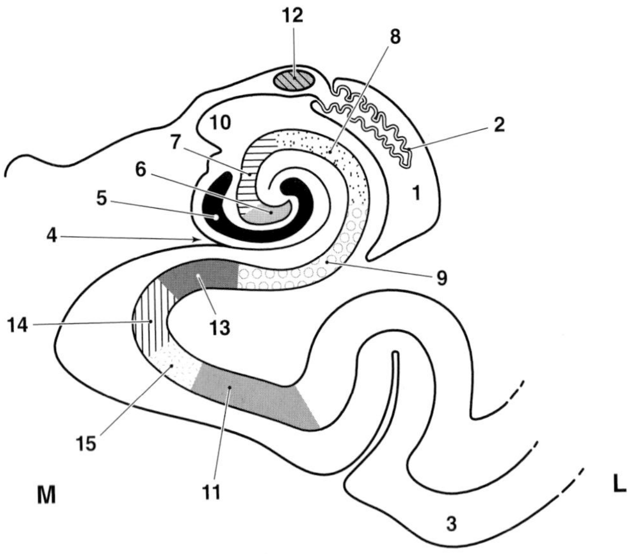

Figure 2F-5: Coronal section schematic of the substructure of the hippocampus on the left side. *M*, medial; *L*, lateral; *CA*, Cornu ammonis (Ammon's horn, hippocampus proper); *CA 1-4*, subregion designation of central hippocampus.

1 Temporal horn of the lateral ventricle
2 Choroid plexus of the temporal horn of the lateral ventricle
3 Occipitotemporal gyrus
4 Hippocampal sulcus (uncal fissure)
5 Dentate gyrus
6 CA4
7 CA3
8 CA2
9 CA1
10 Fimbria
11 Parahippocampal gyrus
12 Optic tract
13 Subiculum
14 Presubiculum
15 Parasubiculum

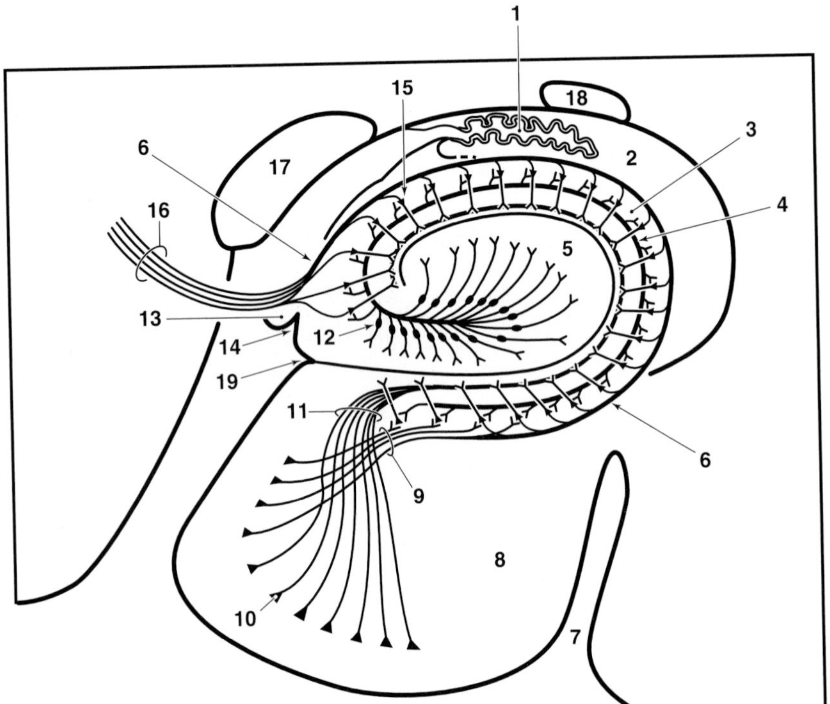

Figure 2F-6: Coronal section schematic of the hippocampal formation showing the major axonal connections on the left side.

1 Choroid plexus of temporal horn of lateral ventricle.
2 Temporal horn of the lateral ventricle
3 Hippocampal gyrus
4 Dentato-hippocampal tract
5 Dentate gyrus
6 Alveus
7 Rhinal sulcus
8 Parahippocampal gyrus
9 Temporoalveolar tract
10 Pyramidal neurons of the parahippocampal gyrus (entorhinal area)
11 Temporoammonic (perforant) tract
12 Granular neurons of the dentate gyrus
13 Fimbria
14 Fimbria-dentate sulcus
15 Pyramidal neurons of the hippocampus
16 Fornix
17 Optic tract
18 Tail of caudate nucleus
19 Hippocampal sulcus (uncal fissure)

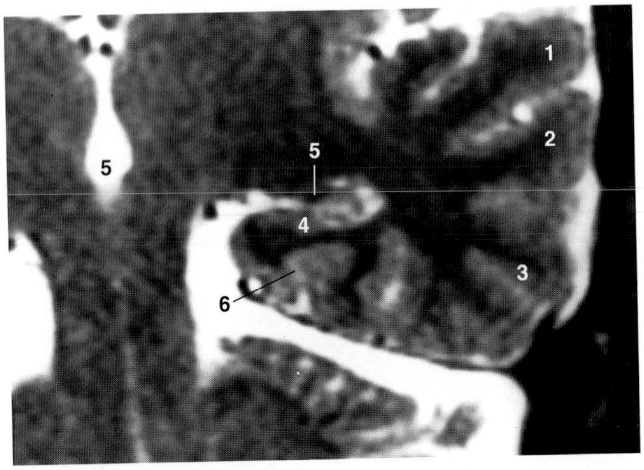

Figure 2F-7: T2-weighted MR image in the coronal plane showing the temporal lobe anatomy.

1 Superior temporal gyrus
2 Middle temporal gyrus
3 Inferior temporal gyrus
4 Subiculum
5 Hippocampus proper
6 Parahippocampal gyrus

2G. Cerebellum

OVERVIEW

1. The cerebellum consists of a midline vermis and two lateral hemispheres.
2. The cerebellum borders on the fourth ventricle posteriorly, leaving three apertures: two foramina of Luschka laterally and a single foramen of Magendie in the midline.
3. The cerebellum is attached to the dorsum of the brain stem through three pairs of cerebellar peduncles, which contain the nerve fibers entering and exiting the cerebellum
   a. Superior cerebellar peduncles join to the midbrain.
   b. Middle cerebellar peduncles join to the pons.
   c. Inferior cerebellar peduncles join to the medulla oblongata.
4. The interval between the two superior cerebellar peduncles is bridged by a membrane formed of pia mater and ependyma, termed the superior medullary velum.
5. The membrane between the caudal cerebellum and the medulla oblongata is termed the inferior medullary velum.
6. Structurally, the two hemispheres of the cerebellum consist of a gray cortical mantle representing the cerebellar cortex, a medullary core of white matter, and four pairs of gray matter nuclei embedded in the hemispheric central white matter: the dentate, emboliform, globose, and fastigial nuclei. The emboliform and globose nuclei are sometimes referred to as the interposed nuclei (i.e., interposed between the dentate and fastigial nuclei).
7. The surface of the cerebellum is thrown into many thin folds called the cerebellar folia, separated by shallow cerebellar sulci.
8. Transverse clefts or fissures, which are much deeper than the sulci, separate groups of folia into lobes and lobules.
9. There are three cerebellar lobes that are phylogenetically and functionally distinct: the anterior, posterior, and flocculonodular lobes.

THE LOBES OF THE CEREBELLUM

The Anterior Lobe

1. The anterior lobe of the cerebellum lies anterior to the primary cerebellar fissure.
2. The hemispheric lobules of the anterior lobe are the alar lobule, central lobule, and the anterior quadrangular lobule.
3. The vermian lobules of the anterior lobe include the lingula, centralis (central lobule), and culmen.
4. The anterior lobe receives neural input through the spinocerebellar tract.
5. The anterior lobe plays a major role in the regulation of muscle tone.

The Posterior Lobe

1. The posterior lobe lies between the primary fissure and the posterolateral cerebellar fissure.
2. The horizontal fissure passes midway through the posterior lobe.
3. The lateral hemispheric lobules of the posterior lobe include the posterior quadrangular lobule, superior semilunar lobule, inferior semilunar lobule, gracile lobule, biventral lobule (medial and lateral belly), and tonsil.
4. The vermian lobules of the posterior lobe include the declive, folium, tuber, pyramis, and uvula.
5. The posterior lobe receives neural input through the corticopontocerebellar fibers.
6. The posterior lobe primarily serves in the coordination of voluntary motor activity.

The Flocculonodular Lobe

1. The flocculonodular lobe lies anterior to the posterolateral fissure, along the inferior aspect of the cerebellum.

2. The hemispheric lobules of the flocculonodular lobe include the floccular lobule and the accessory paraflocculus of Henle.
3. The vermian lobule of the flocculonodular lobe is the nodule (nodulus).
4. The flocculonodular lobe receives neural input from the vestibular system.
5. The flocculonodular lobe primarily serves to maintain posture and balance.

FUNCTIONAL DIVISIONS OF THE CEREBELLUM AND MAJOR CEREBELLAR PATHWAYS

1. The spinocerebellum consists of the vermis and the paravermian cortex.
   a. The vermis consists of the vermian cortex. Its connections are via the vermian spinocerebellar pathway.
      i. Neural input is from the spinal cord (spinocerebellar tracts) and the labyrinth of the inner ear.
      ii. Neural output is to the fastigial nucleus.
      iii. The fastigial nucleus in turn projects the vestibular nuclei and the ventral lateral nucleus of the thalamus.
      iv. The vestibular nucleus in turn projects to the spinal cord; the ventral lateral nucleus projects to the trunk (body) area of the precentral gyrus.
      v. Neural function is to maintain muscle tone and postural control over truncal and proximal limb muscles.
   b. The paravermian cortex consists of the cerebellar hemispheric cortex in the paravermian area. Its connections are via the paravermian spinocerebellar pathway.
      i. Neural input is from the spinal cord (spinocerebellar tracts) from distal muscles.
      ii. Neural output is to the interposed (emboliform and globose) nuclei.
      iii. The interposed nuclei in turn project to the ventral lateral nucleus of the thalamus and the red nucleus.
      iv. The ventral lateral nucleus subsequently projects to the precentral gyrus, which in turn gives rise to the lateral corticospinal tract. The red nucleus gives rise to the rubrospinal tract.
2. The cerebrocerebellum consists of the cerebellar hemispheres, excluding the paravermian cortex. Its connections are via the lateral hemispheric cerebellar (pontocerebellar) pathway.
   a. Neural input is from the contralateral motor and sensory cerebral cortex (corticopontocerebellar tract).
   b. Neural output is to the dentate nucleus, which in turn projects to the following:
      i. The red nucleus, which in turn projects to the inferior olivary nucleus; the inferior olivary nucleus subsequently projects to the cerebellum.
      ii. The ventral lateral nucleus of the thalamus, which in turn projects to the motor and premotor cerebral cortex; the cerebral cortex subsequently gives rise to the corticobulbar, lateral corticospinal, and corticopontocerebellar tracts.
      iii. The inferior olivary nucleus, which in turn projects to the contralateral dentate nucleus.
   c. The neural function of the cerebrocerebellum is to regulate initiation, planning, and timing of voluntary motor activity.
3. The vestibulocerebellum consists of the flocculonodular lobe. Its connections are via the vestibulocerebellar pathway.
   a. Neural input is from the vestibular apparatus (semicircular canals and otolith organs).
   b. Neural output is to the vestibular nuclei.
   c. The vestibular nuclei in turn project via the medial longitudinal fasciculi to the ocular motor nuclei (cranial nerves III, IV, and VI) and via the medial and lateral vestibulospinal tracts to the spinal cord.
   d. The neural function of the vestibulocerebellum is to maintain posture, balance, and eye movement coordination.

THE CEREBELLAR PEDUNCLES

1. There are three paired cerebellar peduncles: the superior, middle, and inferior peduncles.
2. The superior cerebellar peduncle contains both afferent and efferent fibers. It decussates in the caudal mesencephalon (midbrain).
3. The middle cerebral peduncle is entirely afferent and primarily consists of pontocerebellar fibers.
4. The inferior cerebellar peduncle consists of two subparts: the restiform body and the juxtarestiform body. This peduncle contains both afferent and efferent fibers.
5. The major tracts of the cerebellar peduncles are detailed in Table 1.

CEREBELLAR WHITE MATTER AND CEREBELLAR COMMISSURE

1. Beneath the cerebellar cortex lies the white matter core of the cerebellum. The medullary laminae of the white matter take a branching pattern in the sagittal phase, known as the arbor vitae. This white matter primarily consists of the efferent and afferent axons projecting from or traversing toward the cerebellar gray matter. Intrinsic fibers projecting between areas within one cerebellar hemisphere or between the two hemispheres are also present.
2. Axons crossing the midline in the deep core of the cerebellum and in the anterior medullary velum make up the cerebellar commissure.
3. The cerebellar commissure
   a. The cerebellar commissure has two components.
      i. A rostral afferent portion contains fibers from the restiform body and the middle cerebellar peduncle.
      ii. A caudal efferent portion contains fibers of the fastigial nucleus (uncinate tract).
   b. The cerebellar commissure is essentially a decussation of afferent and efferent fibers traversing to heterotopic points in the two cerebellar hemispheres. The cerebellar commissural fibers do not cross to homotopic sites in the cerebellar hemispheres, as is the case with some cerebral commissures.
4. The central mass of white matter within each cerebellar hemisphere contains the four paired cerebellar nuclei: dentate, emboliform, globose, and fastigial nuclei.

THE NEURAL INPUT AND GENERAL SOMATOTOPIC ORGANIZATION OF THE CEREBELLUM

1. Mossy fiber system and somatotopic localization in the cerebellum: The mossy fiber projections account for all of the input to the cerebellum, with the exception of the climbing fibers that link the inferior olivary nucleus with the Purkinje cells of the cerebellum, the olivocerebellar fibers.
2. Mossy fibers from different sources project to different regions of the cerebellum: spinal afferents project to the spinocerebellum, vestibular afferents project to the vestibulocerebellum and fastigial nucleus, and pontocerebellar afferents project to the cerebrocerebellum and dentate nuclei.
3. The spinocerebellum has regions that have a somatotopic representation of the somatosensory information coming in from the ipsilateral half of the body. In the anterior lobe this somatotopic representation spans the vermian paravermian regions, and in the posterior lobe it is found in the paravermian area.
4. Auditory and visual afferents generally terminate in the dorsal aspect of the midline vermis.
5. The cerebropontocerebellar afferents primarily project to the contralateral cerebrocerebellum with a small ipsilateral projection.

THE CEREBELLAR BLOOD SUPPLY

1. The superior cerebellar artery (SCA)
   a. Penetrating branches of the SCA supply the superior and middle cerebellar peduncles, the deep cerebellar nuclei, the cerebellar white matter, and the dorsolateral quadrant of the caudal midbrain.
   b. Cortical branches of the SCA supply the anterior vermis, the anterior aspect of the cerebellar hemispheres, and the lateral margins of the cerebellum.
2. The anterior–inferior cerebellar artery (AICA)
   a. Penetrating branches of the AICA supply the dorsolateral quadrant of the rostral medulla oblongata and caudal pons, the inferior portion of the middle cerebellar peduncle, and the inferior cerebellar peduncle.
   b. Cortical branches of the AICA supply the flocculus, part of the vermis, and the inferior portion of the cerebellar hemisphere anteriorly.
3. The posterior–inferior cerebellar artery (PICA)
   a. Penetrating branches of the PICA supply part of the dentate nucleus.
   b. Cortical branches of the PICA supply the dorsolateral quadrant of the medulla oblongata, the inferior and posterior vermis, the cerebellar tonsils, and the inferolateral surface of the cerebellar hemisphere.

TABLE 2G-1: Major Tracts Within the Cerebellar Peduncles

Peduncle	Tracts	Afferent/efferent fibers
Superior	Ventral spinocerebellar tract	Afferent
	Trigeminocerebellar tract	Afferent
	Tectocerebellar tract	Afferent
	Ceruleocerebellar tract	Afferent
	Dentatorubrothalamic tract	Efferent
	Interpositorubrothalamic tract	Efferent
	Fastigiothalamic tract	Efferent
	Fastigiovestibular tract	Efferent
Middle	Pontocerebellar tracts	Afferent
Inferior		
Restiform body subdivision	Dorsal spinocerebellar tract	Afferent
	Olivocerebellar tract	Afferent
	Reticulocerebellar tract	Afferent
Juxtarestiform body subdivision	Cuneocerebellar tract	Afferent
	Direct and secondary: Vestibulocerebellar tracts	Afferent
	Cerebellovestibular tracts	Efferent

TABLE 2G-2: Corresponding Subdivisions of the Cerebellum with Intervening Fissures[a]

	Lobule		
Lobe	Vermian	Hemispheric	Fissure
Anterior	Lingula (I)		Precentral
	Centralis (II, III)	Alar central	Postcentral (preculminate)
	Culmen (IV)	Anterior quadrangular	
			Primary
Posterior	Declive (V)	Posterior quadrangular	
			Posterior–superior (postlunate)
	Folium (VI)	Superior semilunar	Horizontal
	Tuber (VII)	Inferior semilunar	Anterior–inferior
		Gracile	Prepyramidal
			Posterior–inferior
	Pyramis (VIII)	Biventral (lateral and medial belly)	Secondary (postpyramidal or retrotonsillar)
	Uvula (IX)	Tonsil and paraflocculus	Posterolateral
Flocculonodular	Nodule (X)	Flocculus	

[a]Note alternative names (numbers) in parentheses.

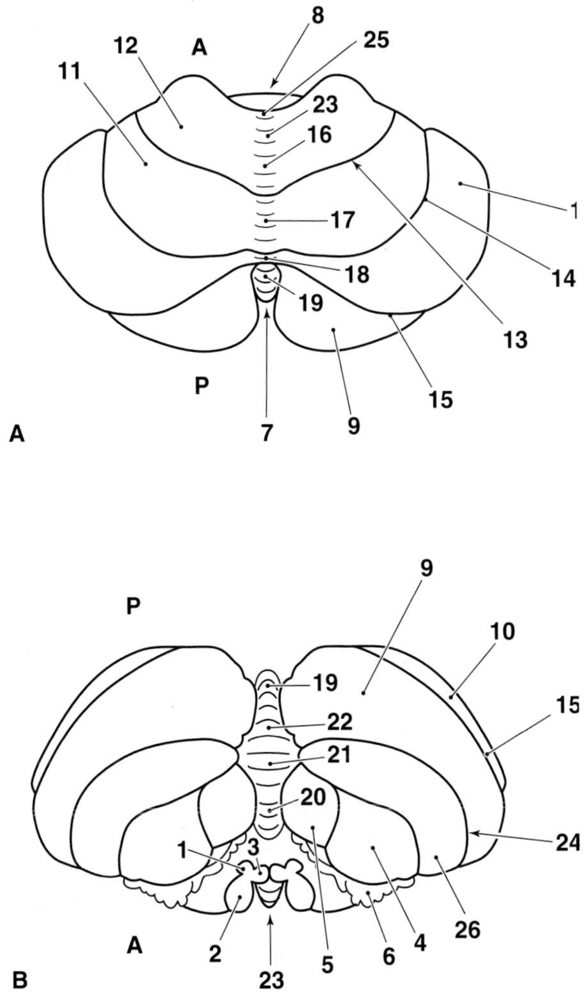

Figure 2G-1: Schematics of the cerebellar lobules. **A:** Superior–posterior aspect. **B:** Inferior aspect. *A*, anterior; *P*, posterior.

1 Inferior cerebellar peduncle (cut surface)
2 Middle cerebellar peduncle (cut surface)
3 Superior cerebellar peduncle (cut surface)
4 Biventral lobule
5 Cerebellar tonsil
6 Flocculus
7 Posterior incisure
8 Anterior incisure
9 Inferior semilunar lobule
10 Superior semilunar lobule
11 Posterior quadrangular lobule
12 Anterior quadrangular lobule
13 Primary fissure
14 Posterior–superior fissure
15 Horizontal fissure
16 Culmen
17 Declive
18 Folium
19 Tuber
20 Nodulus
21 Uvula
22 Pyramis
23 Centralis (central lobule)
24 Anterior inferior fissure
25 Lingula
26 Gracile lobule

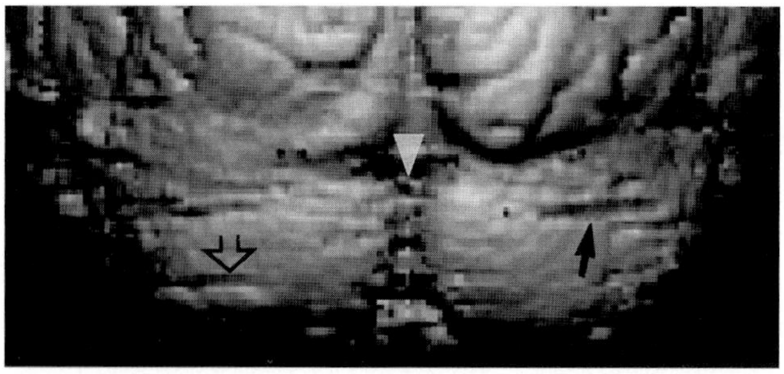

Figure 2G-2A: Posterior aspect of a three-dimensional MR image of the cerebellum. Note the primary fissure (*solid arrow*), the posterosuperior fissure (*open arrow*), and the vermis (*arrowhead*) (**A–D** courtesy of J. Lancaster).

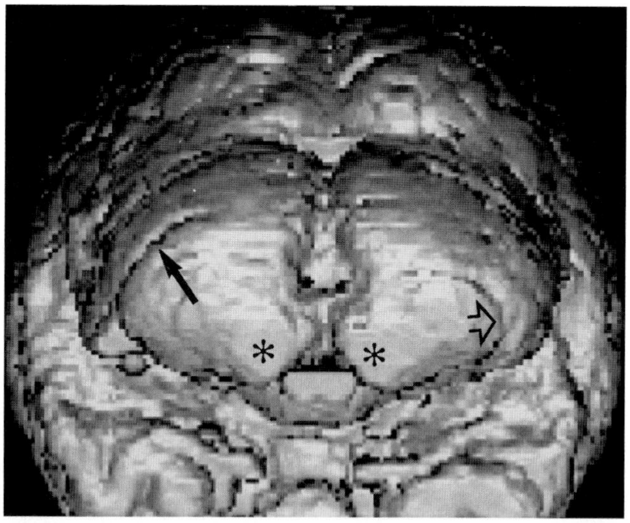

Figure 2G-2B: Postero-inferior aspect of a three-dimensional MR image of the cerebellum. Note the horizontal fissure (*solid arrow*), the antero-inferior fissure (*open arrow*), and the cerebellar tonsils (*asterisks*).

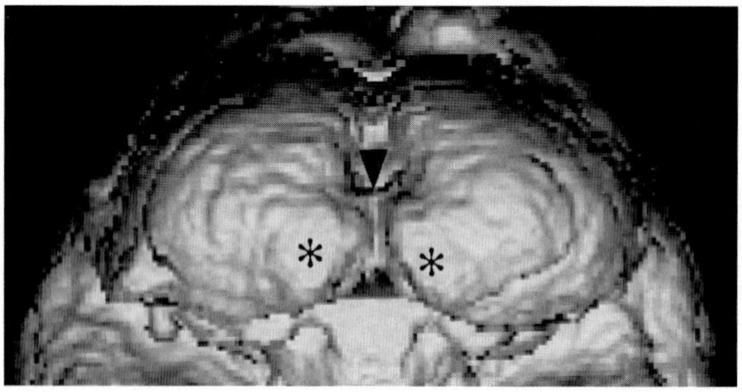

Figure 2G-2C: Inferior aspect of a three-dimensional MR image of the cerebellum (posterior at top). Note the cerebellar tonsils (*asterisks*) and inferior vermis (*arrowhead*). The inferior aspect of the fourth ventricle and part of the medulla oblongata have been resected.

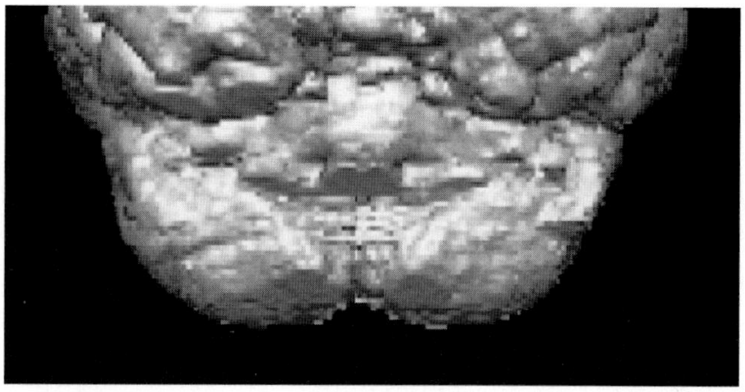

Figure 2G-2D: Antero-inferior aspect of a three-dimensional MR image of the cerebellum. The inferior aspect of the medulla oblongata and inferior medullary vellum has been resected.

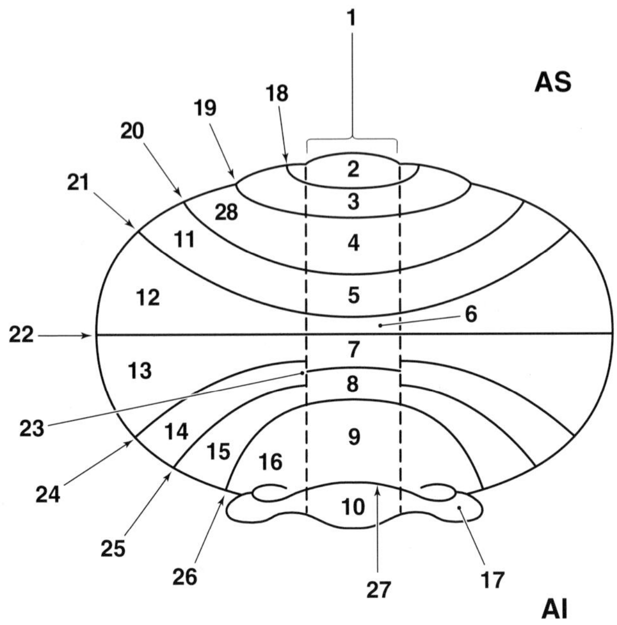

Figure 2G-3: Schematic of the "flattened" surface of the cerebellum. *AS*, anterior–superior; *AI*, anterior–inferior.

1 Vermis
2 Lingula
3 Centralis (central lobule) and ala
4 Culmen
5 Declive
6 Folium
7 Tuber
8 Pyramis
9 Uvula
10 Nodulus
11 Posterior portion of the quadrangular lobule
12 Superior portion of the semilunar lobule
13 Inferior portion of the semilunar lobule
14 Gracile lobule
15 Biventral lobule
16 Tonsil
17 Flocculus
18 Precentral fissure
19 Postcentral (preculminate) fissure
20 Primary fissure
21 Posterior–superior fissure
22 Horizontal fissure
23 Prepyramidal fissure
24 Anterior–inferior fissure
25 Posterior–inferior fissure
26 Secondary fissure
27 Posterolateral fissure
28 Anterior portion of quadrangular lobule

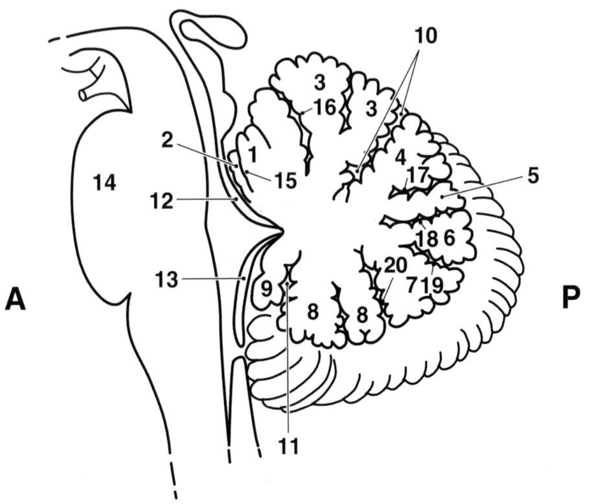

Figure 2G-4: Sagittal schematic of the cerebellar lobules. *A*, anterior; *P*, posterior.

1 Centralis (central lobule)
2 Lingula
3 Culmen
4 Declive
5 Folium
6 Tuber
7 Pyramis
8 Uvula
9 Nodulus
10 Primary fissure
11 Posterolateral fissure
12 Anterior (superior) medullary velum
13 Posterior (inferior) medullary velum
14 Pons
15 Precentral fissure
16 Postcentral (preculminate) fissure
17 Posterior-superior fissure
18 Horizontal fissure
19 Prepyramidal fissure
20 Secondary fissure

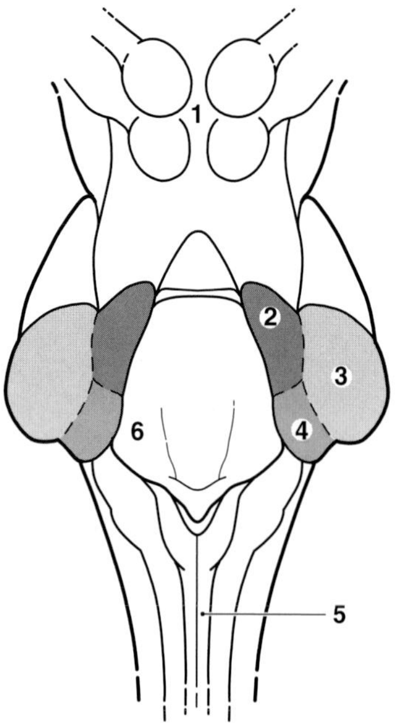

Figure 2G-5: Posterior schematic of the cerebellar peduncles. The cerebellum has been removed.
1 Quadrigeminal plate
2 Superior cerebellar peduncle (cut surface)
3 Middle cerebellar peduncle (cut surface)
4 Inferior cerebellar peduncle (cut surface)
5 Medulla oblongata
6 Fourth ventricle (open, with superior and inferior medullary velum removed)

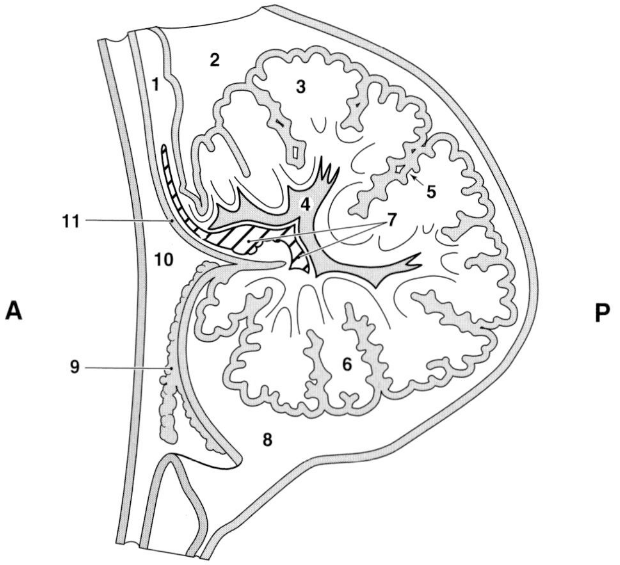

Figure 2G-6: Sagittal schematic of the cerebellar commissure. *A*, anterior; *P*, posterior.
1 Quadrigeminal plate
2 Quadrigeminal cistern
3 Anterior lobe
4 Rostral (afferent) portion of the cerebellar commissure (*gray shading*)
5 Primary fissure
6 Posterior lobe
7 Caudal (efferent) portion of the cerebellar commissure (decussation of the uncinate tract) (*cross-hatched area*)
8 Cisterna magna
9 Choroid plexus
10 Fourth ventricle
11 Anterior medullary velum

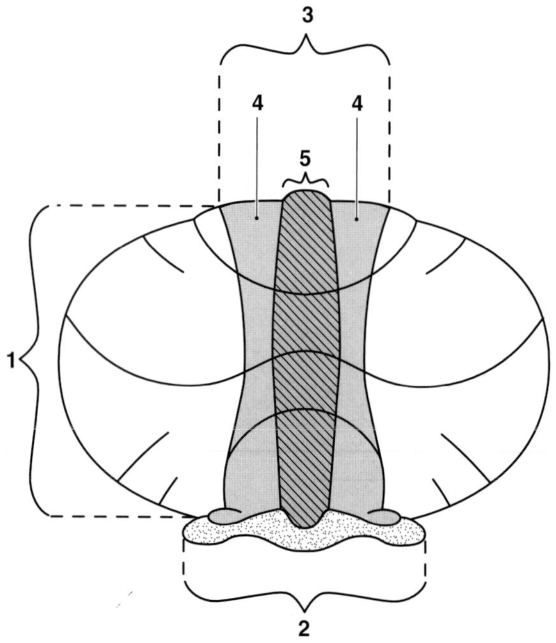

Figure 2G-7: Schematic representation of the cerebellar cortex in a single plane.
1 Cerebrocerebellum
2 Vestibulocerebellum
3 Spinocerebellum
4 Paravermian areas
5 Vermis

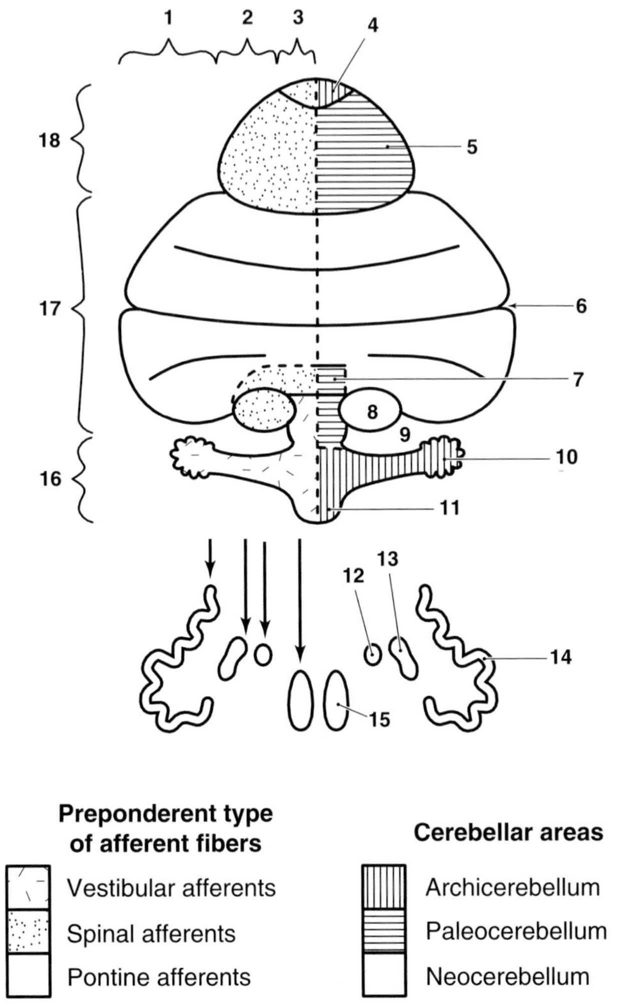

Figure 2G-8: Schematic of the afferent topographical regions of the cerebellum.
1 Lateral region
2 Paravermian region
3 Vermian region
4 Lingula
5 Primary fissure
6 Horizontal fissure
7 Uvula
8 Tonsil
9 Dorsolateral (posterolateral) fissure
10 Flocculus
11 Nodule
12 Globose nucleus
13 Emboliform nucleus
14 Dentate nucleus
15 Fastigial nucleus
16 Flocculonodular lobe
17 Middle lobe
18 Anterior lobe

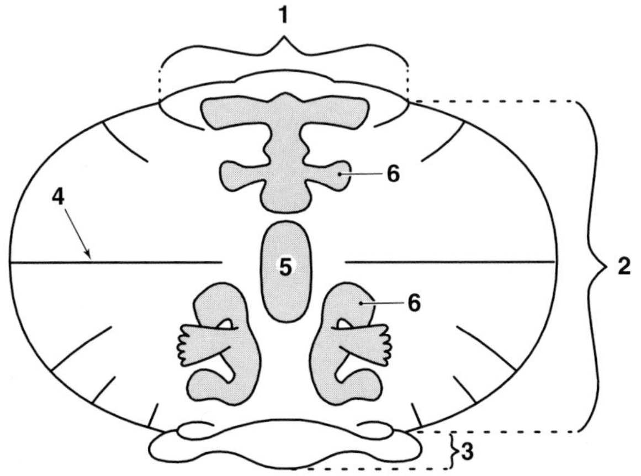

Figure 2G-9: Schematic of the somatotopic sensory representations of the cerebellar cortex.
1 Anterior lobe
2 Posterior lobe
3 Flocculonodular lobe
4 Horizontal fissure
5 Auditory and visual area
6 Sensory homunculus for the body

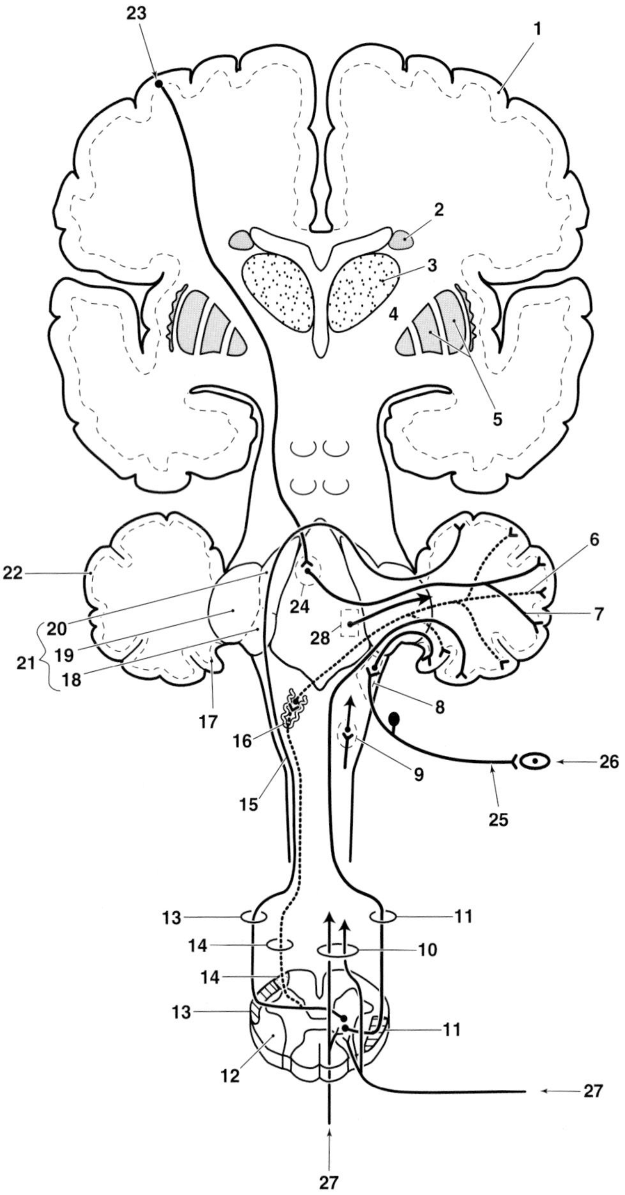

Figure 2G-10: Coronal schematic of the major afferent connections of the cerebellum.
1 Cerebral cortex
2 Caudate nucleus
3 Thalamus
4 Internal capsule
5 Lentiform nucleus
6 Climbing fiber
7 Mossy fiber
8 Vestibular nuclei
9 Accessory (lateral) cuneate nucleus
10 Ascending sensory tracts
11 Dorsal spinocerebellar tract
12 Spinal cord
13 Ventral spinocerebellar tract
14 Spinoolivary tract
15 Medulla oblongata
16 Inferior olivary nucleus
17 Flocculonodular lobe of cerebellum
18 Inferior cerebellar peduncle
19 Middle cerebellar peduncle
20 Superior cerebellar peduncle
21 Cerebellar peduncles
22 Cerebellar hemisphere
23 Corticopontine neuron
24 Pontine nuclei (pontocerebellar neuron)
25 Vestibulocochlear nerve (cranial nerve VIII)
26 Vestibular hair cell
27 Sensory afferent nerves
28 Reticular formation

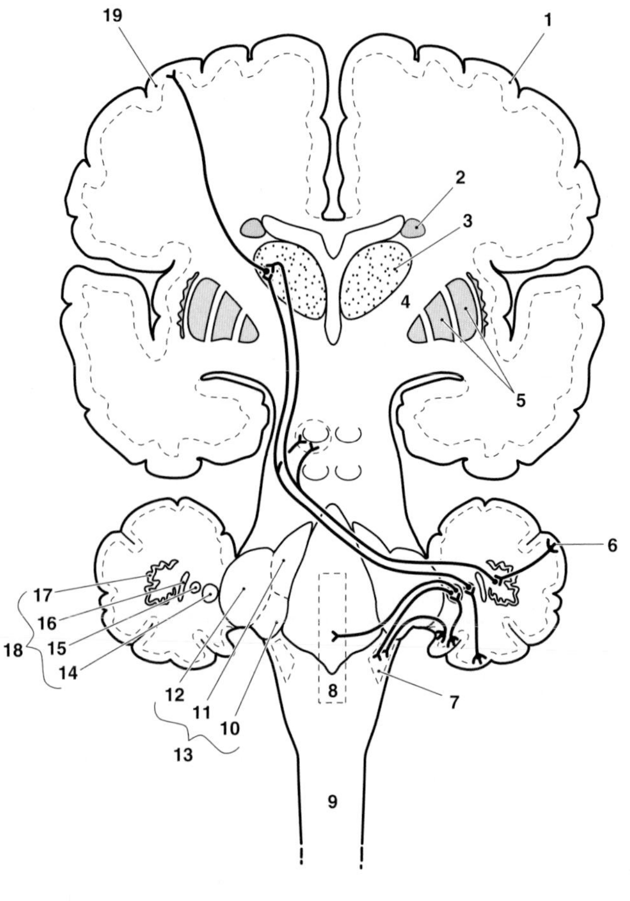

Figure 2G-11: Coronal schematic of the major efferent connections of the cerebellum.
1 Cerebral cortex
2 Caudate nucleus
3 Ventral lateral nucleus of the thalamus
4 Internal capsule
5 Lentiform nucleus
6 Purkinje cell
7 Vestibular nuclei
8 Reticular formation
9 Spinal cord
10 Inferior peduncle
11 Superior peduncle
12 Middle peduncle
13 Cerebellar peduncles
14 Fastigial nucleus
15 Globose nucleus
16 Emboliform nucleus
17 Dentate nucleus
18 Intracerebellar nuclei
19 Precentral gyrus (motor)

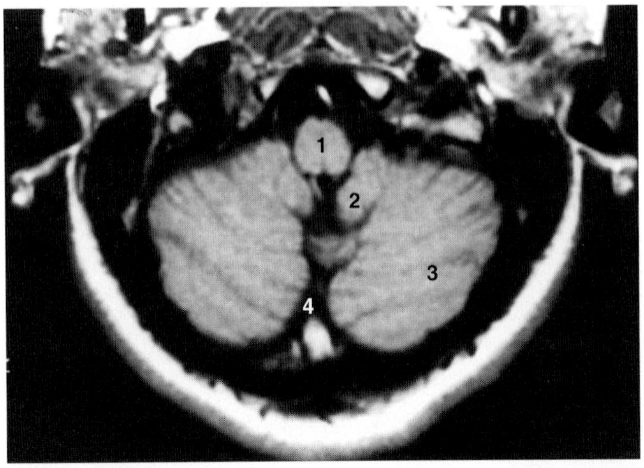

Figure 2G-12A: Cerebellar anatomy. Axial T1-weighted MR image showing:
1 Medulla oblongata
2 Cerebellar tonsil
3 Cerebellar hemisphere
4 Cisterna magna

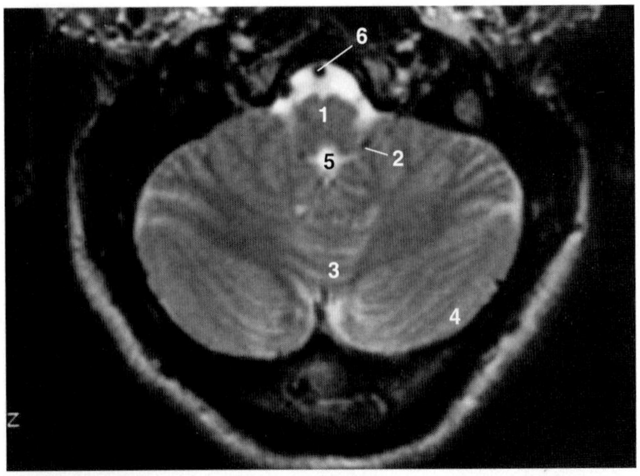

Figure 2G-12B: Cerebellar anatomy. Axial T1-weighted MR image showing:
1 Medulla oblongata
2 Inferior cerebellar peduncle
3 Cerebellar vermis
4 Cerebellar hemisphere
5 Fourth ventricle
6 Basilar artery

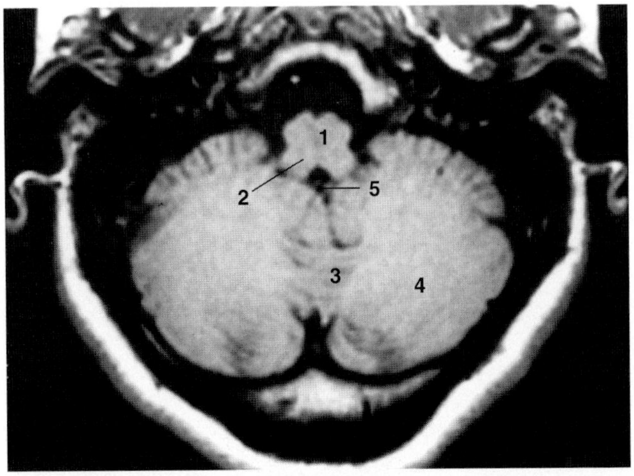

Figure 2G-12C: Cerebellar anatomy. Axial T2-weighted fast spin echo MR image showing:
1 Medulla oblongata
2 Inferior cerebellar peduncles
3 Cerebellar vermis
4 Cerebellar hemisphere
5 Fourth ventricle

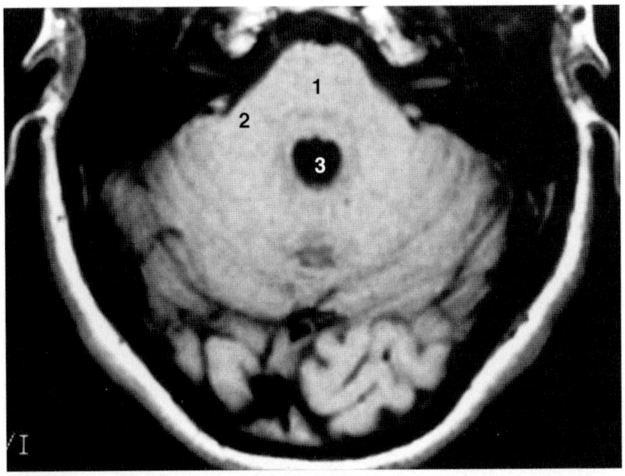

Figure 2G-12D: Cerebellar anatomy. Axial T1-weighted MR image showing:
1 Pons
2 Middle cerebellar peduncle
3 Fourth ventricle

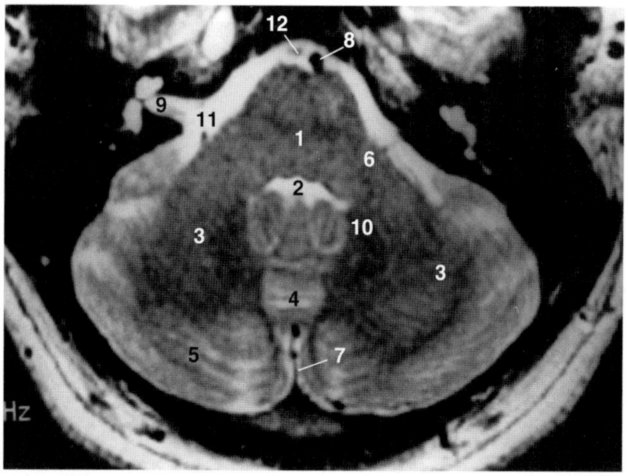

Figure 2G-12E: Cerebellar anatomy. Axial T2-weighted MR image showing:
1 Pons
2 Fourth ventricle
3 Cerebellar hemispheres
4 Posterior–inferior cerebellar vermis
5 Cerebellar folia and sulci/fissures
6 Middle cerebellar peduncle
7 Falx cerebelli
8 Basilar artery flow void
9 Internal auditory canal
10 Dentate nucleus
11 Cerebello-pontine angle cistern
12 Prepontine cistern

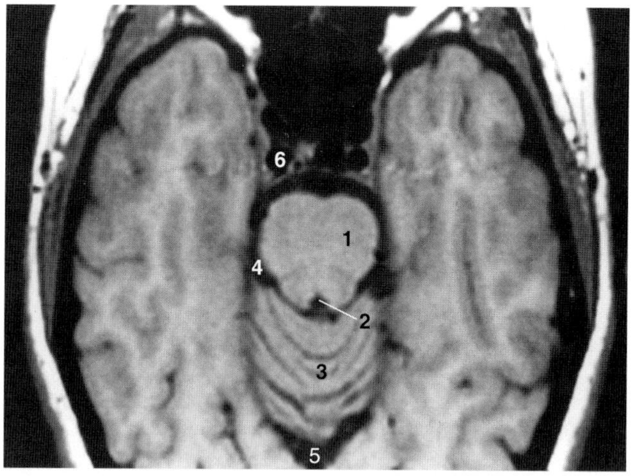

Figure 2G-12F: Cerebellar anatomy. Axial T1-weighted MR image showing:
1 Upper pons
2 Fourth ventricle
3 Superior vermis
4 Ambient cistern
5 Superior cerebellar cistern
6 Cavernous portion of internal carotid artery

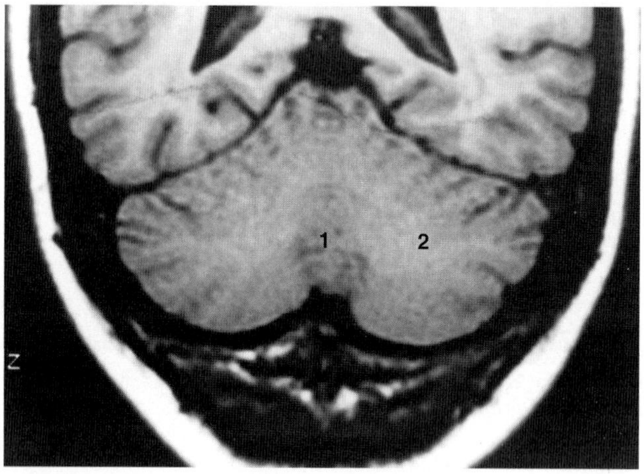

Figure 2G-12G: Cerebellar anatomy. Coronal T1-weighted MR image showing:
1 Cerebellar vermis
2 Cerebellar hemisphere

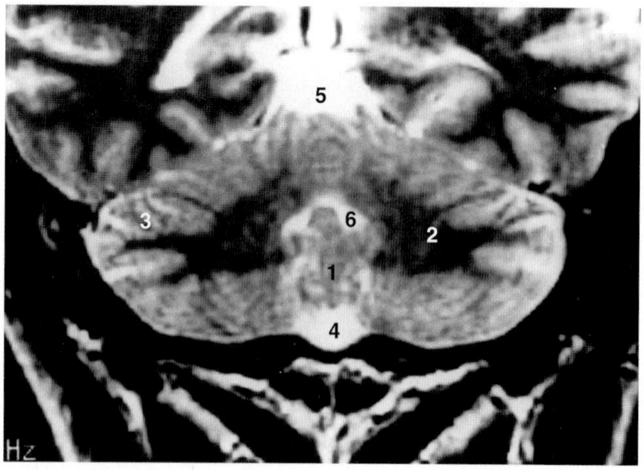

Figure 2G-12H: Cerebellar anatomy. Coronal T2-weighted MR image showing:
1 Inferior cerebellar vermis
2 Deep cerebellar white matter
3 Cerebellar folia and sulci/fissures
4 Cisterna magna
5 Superior cerebellar/vermian cistern
6 Fourth ventricle

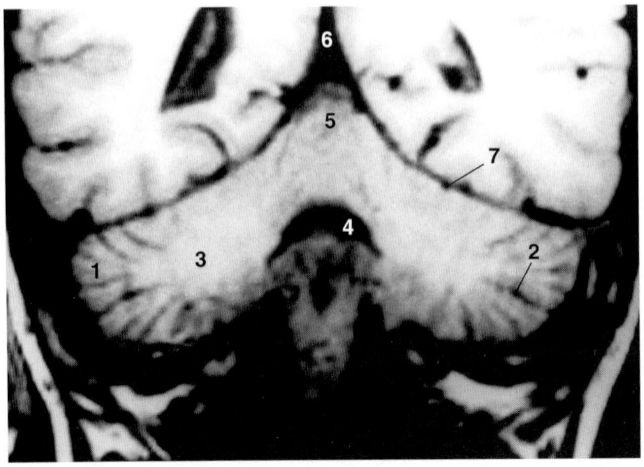

Figure 2G-12I: Cerebellar anatomy. Coronal T1-weighted MR image showing:
1 Cerebellar folia
2 Cerebellar fissure
3 Cerebellar hemisphere deep white matter
4 Fourth ventricle
5 Superior vermis
6 Superior vermian cistern
7 Tentorium cerebelli

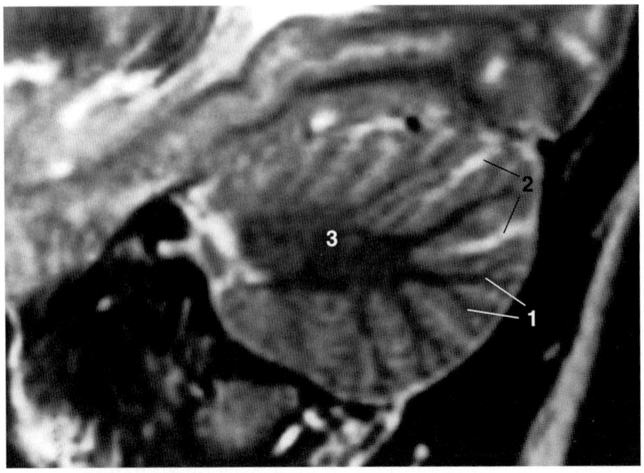

Figure 2G-12J: Cerebellar anatomy. Sagittal T2-weighted MR image showing:
1 Cerebellar folia
2 Cerebellar sulci and fissures
3 Cerebellar hemisphere deep white matter

2H. Brain Stem

ANATOMY

1. In rostrocaudal order, the three transverse subdivisions of the brain stem include the midbrain, the pons, and the medulla oblongata.
2. In dorsoventral order, the longitudinal laminae of the brain stem include the tectum, the tegmentum, and the basis.

The Brain Stem Tectum

1. The midbrain tectum (i.e., roof) consists of the quadrigeminal plate that roofs the cerebral aqueduct.
2. The pontine tectum consists of the anterior medullary velum that roofs the rostral fourth ventricle.
3. The medullary tectum consists of the posterior medullary velum that roofs the caudal fourth ventricle.
4. The anterior and posterior medullary vela meet dorsally at the peak of the roof of the fourth ventricle, or the fastigium.
5. The tectum contains no longitudinal motor or sensory tracts, no cranial nerve nuclei, and no portion of the reticular formation.

The Brain Stem Basis

1. The brain stem basis consists of nuclei in the basis pontis and the descending motor tracts, including the following.
   a. The pyramidal tracts, including the corticobulbar and corticospinal tracts
   b. The corticopontine tracts, part of the corticopontocerebellar pathway
2. The midbrain basis conveys the pyramidal and corticopontine motor tracts. It contains no nuclei.
3. The pontine basis contains the above-mentioned motor tracts in transit to the medulla oblongata as well as the pontine nuclei, part of the corticopontocerebellar pathway.
4. The medullary basis primarily contains the corticospinal tracts, most of the corticobulbar tract (i.e., corticopontine fibers) having already terminated in the pontine basis, with some exceptions.

The Brain Stem Tegmentum

1. The tegmentum (i.e., covering) is the plate of tracts and brain stem neurons lying between the tectum and basis. It is the most complex subdivision of the brain stem.
2. The gray matter of the tegmentum consists of the motor and sensory nuclei of cranial nerves III to X and XII, the reticular formation, and the supplementary motor and sensory nuclei.
3. The white matter of the tegmentum consists of all ascending long sensory tracts from the spinal cord or cranial nerve nuclei to the cerebellum, brain stem, and thalamus; afferent and efferent cerebellar pathways; the medial longitudinal fasciculus; the central tegmental tract; and the unnamed reticular formation pathways.

The Substantia Nigra

1. The substantia nigra is a paired nuclear complex in each cerebral peduncle.

2. The substantia nigra consists of a cell-rich area, the pars compacta; a less cellular area, the pars reticulata; and the pars lateralis, a smaller cellular area lateral to the pars compacta.
3. Together, the pars compacta and pars lateralis make up the majority of the dopaminergic neuron population of the midbrain.
4. The pars compacta (A9 as designated by Dahlström and Fuxe) is continuous across the midline through the paranigral nucleus, the ventral dopamine group (A10).
5. Serotoninergic cell groups include B7 and B8 (of Dahlström and Fuxe) in the raphe.
6. The substantia nigra forms important connections with the dorsal striatum (the caudate nucleus and putamen) and the ventral striatum (nucleus accumbens and olfactory tubercle). Briefly, the cerebral cortex projects to the dorsal/ventral striatum, which in turn projects to the pallidus (globus pallidus) and pars reticulata of the substantia nigra, which subsequently projects to the cerebral cortex, either in the supplementary motor area or in the prefrontal and cingulate region.

The Reticular Formation

1. The reticular formation consists of loosely arranged nuclear groups separated by large dendritic trees the nuclear groups are connected by large numbers of collateral afferent and efferent axons.
2. The reticular formation extends throughout the brain stem tegmentum.
3. The four reticular formation nuclei (nuclear regions) are the raphe and the medial (central) gigantocellular nucleus, lateral paraventricular (small-celled nucleus), and cerebellar reticular formation nucleus.
4. The reticular formation receives the most heterogeneous brain and spinal cord input of any grouping of neurons in the entire nervous system. Reticular efferents influence most regions of the central nervous system, including the cerebral cortex and spinal cord.
5. The reticular formation mediates the following:
   a. Mental activity: consciousness, attention span, alerting responses, and the sleep–wake cycle
   b. Homeostasis: visceral and glandular activity
   c. Reflexes: somatomotor and sensorimotor reflexes

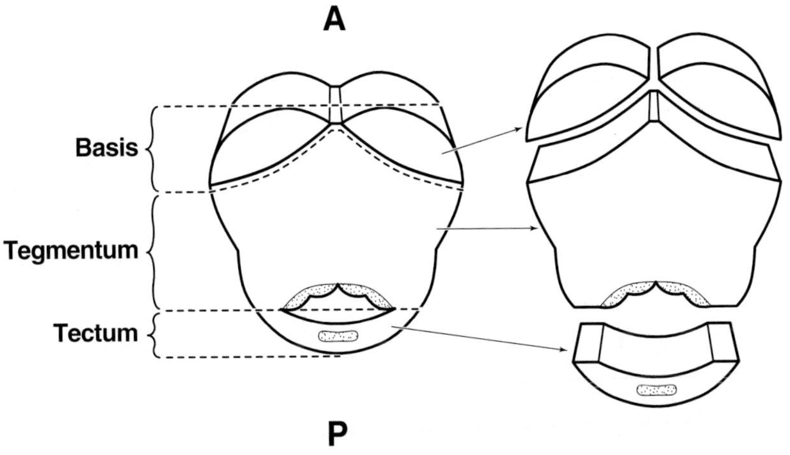

Figure 2H-1: Intact and exploded schematics of a composite axial cross section of the brain stem to show the three longitudinal subdivisions (laminae) of the tectum, tegmentum, and basis. *A*, anterior; *P*, posterior.

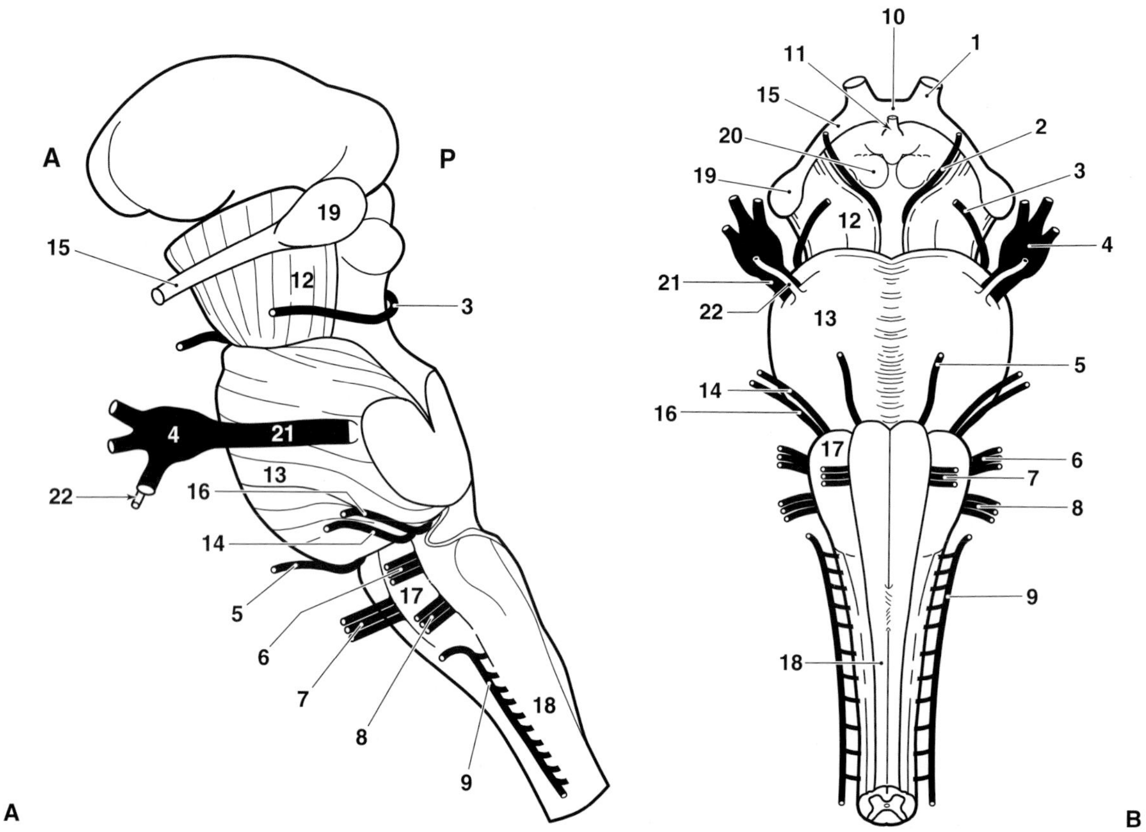

Figure 2H-2: Lateral **(A)** and inferofrontal **(B)** schematics of the brain stem and exiting cranial nerves after removal of the cerebellum. *A*, anterior; *P*, posterior.

1 Optic (II) nerve
2 Oculomotor (III) nerve
3 Trochlear (IV) nerve
4 Trigeminal (V) ganglion
5 Abducens (IV) nerve
6 Glossopharyngeal (IX) nerve
7 Hypoglossal (XII) nerve
8 Vagus (X) nerve
9 Spinal accessory (XI) nerve
10 Optic chiasm (II)
11 Transected pituitary infundibulum
12 Midbrain
13 Pons
14 Facial (VII) nerve
15 Optic (CN-II) tract
16 Vestibulocochlear (auditory: VIII) nerve
17 Medulla oblongata
18 Spinal cord
19 Lateral geniculate body
20 Mammillary body
21 Trigeminal (V) sensory root
22 Trigeminal (V) motor root

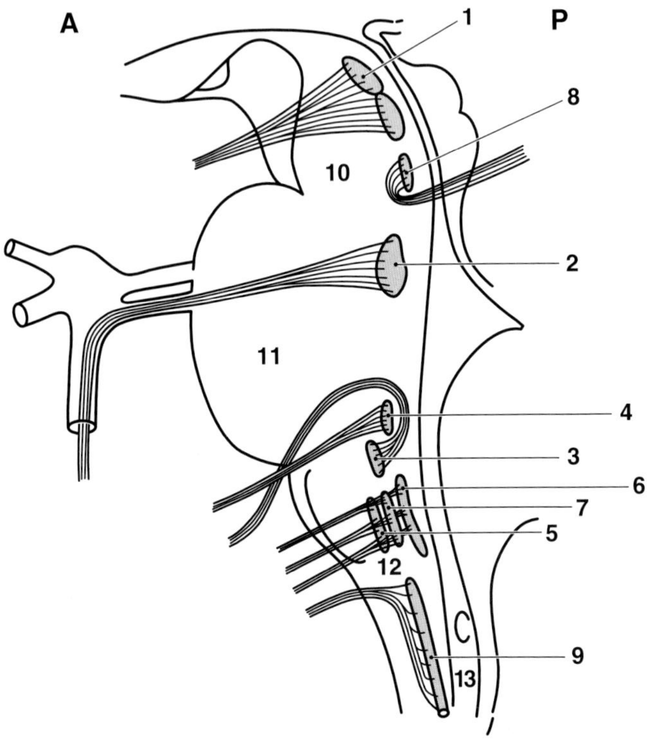

Figure 2H-3A: Lateral schematic of the cranial nerve motor nuclei. *A*, anterior; *P*, posterior.

1 Oculomotor (III) nerve nucleus (Edinger-Westphal)
2 Motor nucleus of trigeminal (V) nerve
3 Facial (VII) nerve nucleus
4 Abducens (VI) nerve
5 Nucleus ambiguus (IX, X)
6 Vagus (X) nerve nucleus
7 Hypoglossal (VII) nerve nucleus
8 Trochlear (IV) nerve
9 Spinal accessory (IX) nerve
10 Midbrain
11 Pons
12 Medulla oblongata
13 Spinal cord

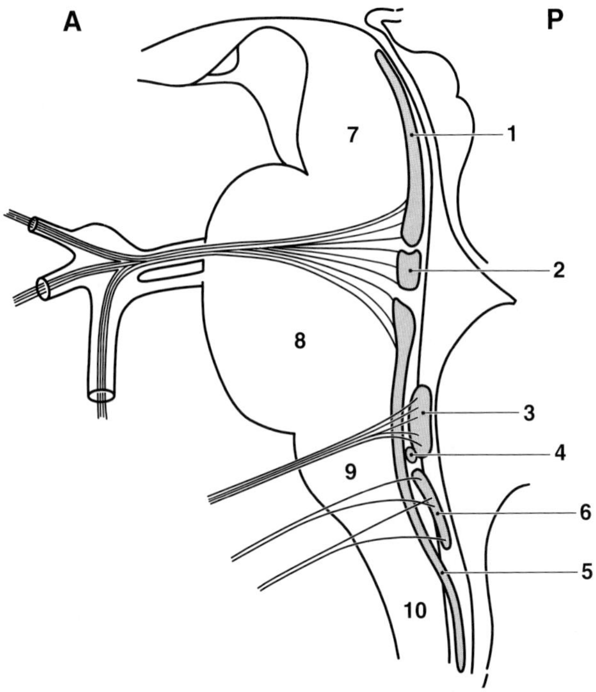

Figure 2H-3B: Lateral schematic of the cranial nerve sensory nuclei. *A*, anterior; *P*, posterior.

1 Trigeminal (V) mesencephalic nucleus
2 Trigeminal (V) pontine nucleus
3 Vestibular (VIII) nucleus
4 Cochlear (VIII) nucleus
5 Spinal trigeminal (V) nerve
6 Nucleus solitarius (IX, X)
7 Midbrain
8 Pons
9 Medulla oblongata
10 Spinal cord

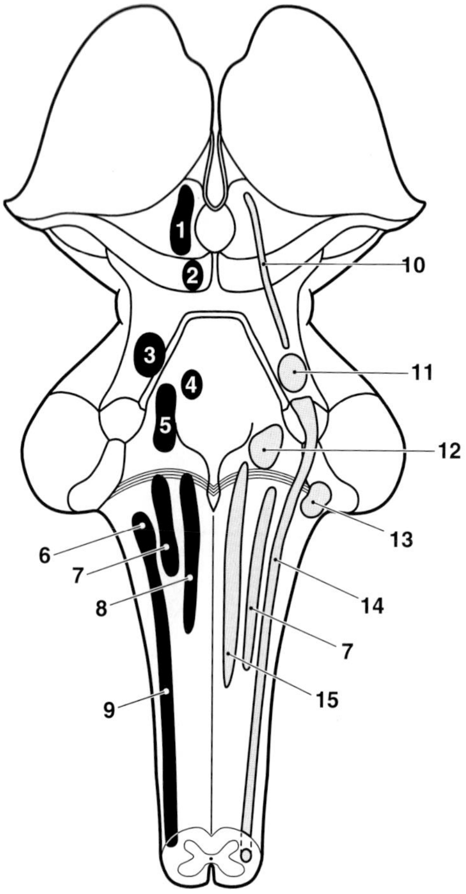

Figure 2H-3C: Posterior schematic of the cranial nerve nuclei of the brain stem. *Black area*, motor nuclei; *stippled area*, sensory nuclei.

1 Oculomotor (III) nucleus
2 Trochlear (IV) nucleus
3 Trigeminal motor (V) nucleus
4 Abducens (VI) nucleus
5 Facial nucleus (VII)
6 Nucleus ambiguus (IX, X)
7 Dorsal nucleus of vagus (X)
8 Hypoglossal (XII) nucleus
9 Spinal (XI) accessory
10 Trigeminal (V) mesencephalic nucleus
11 Trigeminal (V) pontine nucleus
12 Vestibular (VIII) nucleus
13 Cochlear (VIII) nucleus
14 Trigeminal (V) spinal nucleus
15 Nucleus solitarius (VII, IX, X)

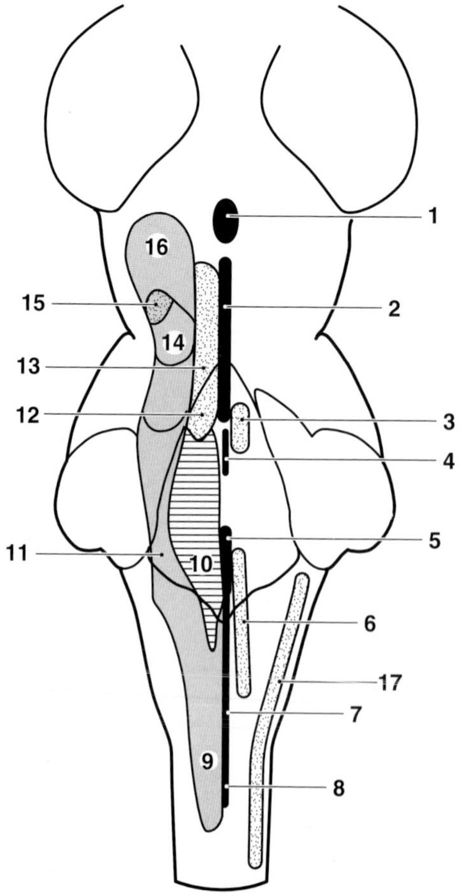

Figure 2H-4: Posterior schematic of the brain stem showing the location of the four groups of reticular formation nuclei.

1 Dorsal and ventral raphe nuclei
2 Superior central sulcus nuclei
3 Pontine reticulotegmental nuclei
4 Nucleus raphe pontis
5 Nucleus raphe magnus
6 Paramedian reticular nucleus
7 Nucleus raphe pallidus
8 Nucleus raphe obscurus
9 Ventral (central) reticular nucleus
10 Gigantocellular reticular nucleus
11 Parvicellular reticular nucleus
12 Caudal pontine reticular nucleus
13 Oral pontine reticular nucleus
14 Parabrachial nuclei
15 Pediculopontine nucleus
16 Cuneiform and subcuneiform nuclei
17 Lateral reticular nucleus

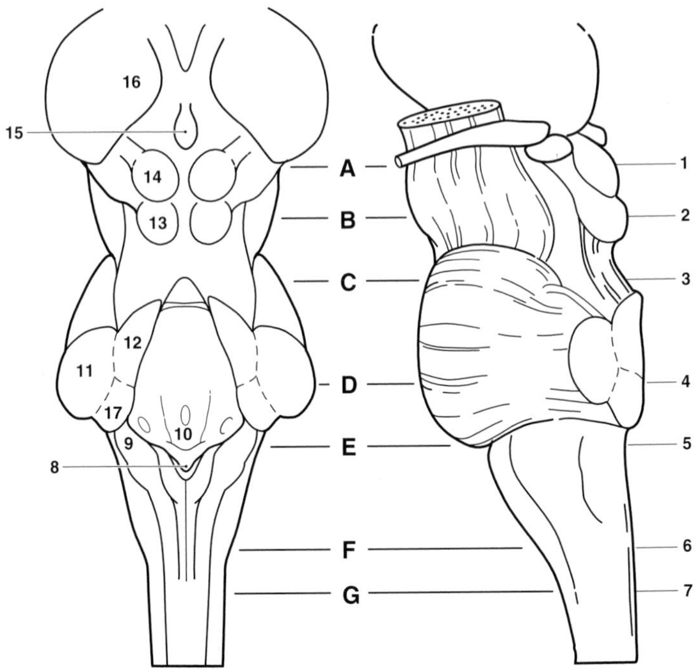

Figure 2H-5: Schematics of the brain stem showing the levels of transverse sections in Fig. 2H-6. The levels of the transverse sections (A–G) are shown after removal of the cerebellum.

1 Rostral midbrain
2 Caudal midbrain
3 Rostral pons
4 Caudal pons
5 Rostral medulla oblongata
6 Caudal medulla oblongata
7 Junction of medulla oblongata and spinal cord
8 Obex
9 Inferior cerebellar peduncle
10 Rhomboid fossa (floor of fourth ventricle)
11 Middle cerebellar peduncle
12 Superior cerebellar peduncle
13 Inferior colliculus
14 Superior colliculus
15 Pineal body (gland)
16 Thalamus
17 Inferior cerebellar peduncle

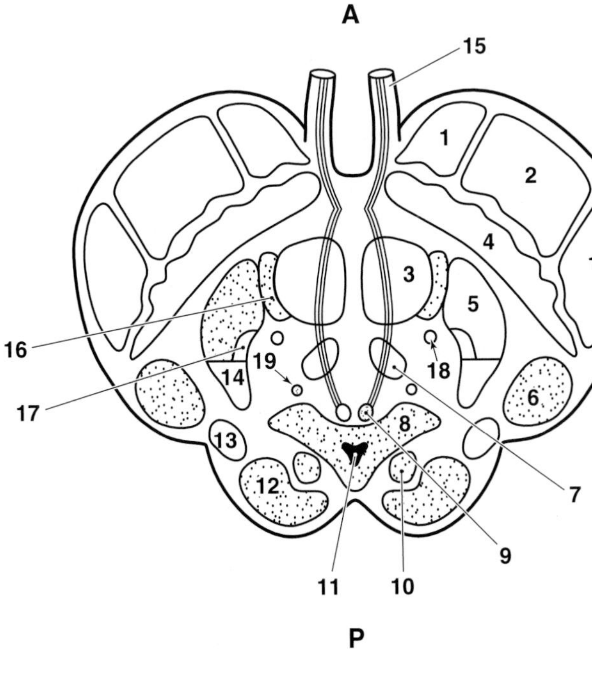

Figure 2H-6A: Axial schematic of the rostral midbrain at the level of the superior colliculus. *A*, anterior; *P*, posterior.

1 Corticopontine tracts
2 Pyramidal (corticospinal) tracts and corticobulbar tracts
3 Red nucleus
4 Substantia nigra
5 Medial lemniscus
6 Medial geniculate body
7 Medial longitudinal fasciculus
8 Periaqueductal gray matter
9 Oculomotor (III) nerve nucleus
10 Trigeminal (V) nerve (mesencephalic) nucleus
11 Cerebral aqueduct of Sylvius
12 Superior colliculus
13 Spinothalamic lateral tract
14 Ventral spinothalamic tract (trigeminal lemniscus)
15 Oculomotor (III) nerve
16 Dentothalamic tract
17 Spinal lemniscus
18 Dorsal trigeminothalamic tract
19 Interstitial nucleus of Cajal

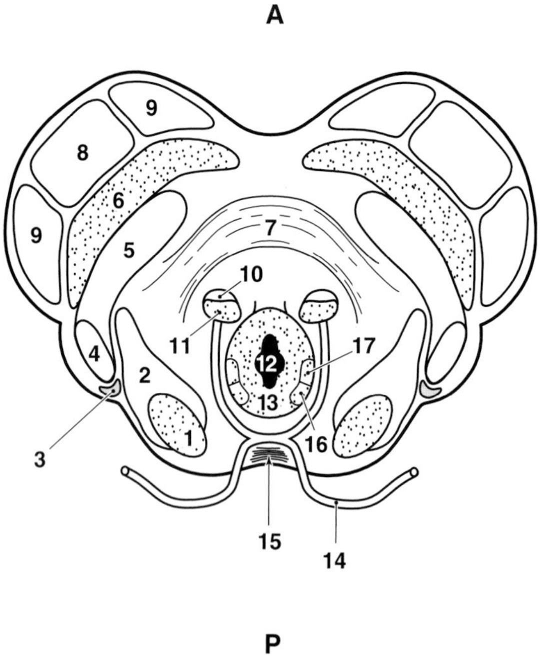

Figure 2H-6B: Axial schematic of the caudal midbrain at the level of the inferior colliculus. *A*, anterior; *P*, posterior.

1 Inferior colliculus nucleus
2 Lateral lemniscus
3 Spinothalamic anterolateral tract (spinal lemniscus)
4 Ventral spinothalamic tract (trigeminal lemniscus)
5 Medial lemniscus
6 Substantia nigra (nucleus)
7 Decussation of superior cerebellar peduncles
8 Pyramidal (corticospinal) tract and corticobulbar tract
9 Corticopontine tract
10 Medial longitudinal fasciculus
11 Trochlear (IV) nerve nucleus
12 Cerebral aqueduct of Sylvius
13 Periaqueductal gray matter
14 Trochlear (IV) nerve
15 Commissure of inferior colliculus
16 Mesencephalic nucleus of the trigeminal (V) nerves
17 Mesencephalic tract of the trigeminal (V) nerves

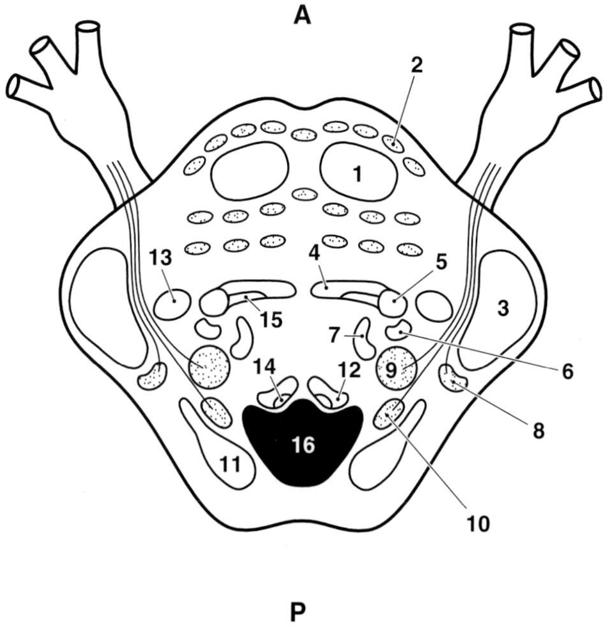

Figure 2H-6C: Axial schematic of the rostral pons. *A*, anterior; *P*, posterior.

1 Pyramidal (corticospinal) tract and corticobulbar tract
2 Pontine nuclei
3 Middle cerebellar peduncle
4 Medial lemniscus
5 Spinal lemniscus (anterolateral tract)
6 Lateral spinothalamic tract
7 Dorsal trigeminothalamic tract
8 Trigeminal (V) nerve nucleus (sensory)
9 Trigeminal (V) nerve nucleus (motor)
10 Trigeminal (V) nerve nucleus (mesencephalic)
11 Superior cerebellar peduncle
12 Medial longitudinal fasciculus
13 Lateral lemniscus
14 Tectospinal tract
15 Ventral trigeminothalamic tract (trigeminal lemniscus)
16 Fourth ventricle

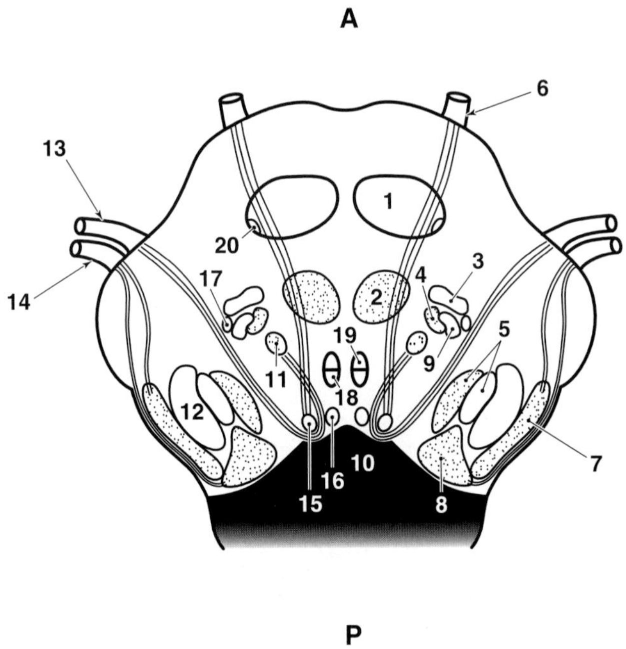

Figure 2H-6D: Axial schematic of the brain stem at the level of the caudal pons. *A*, anterior; *P*, posterior.

1 Pyramidal (corticospinal) tract and corticobulbar tract
2 Medial lemniscus
3 Anterolateral tract (spinal lemniscus)
4 Superior olivary nucleus
5 Trigeminal (V) nerve nucleus (*stippled*) and trigeminal tract
6 Abducens (VI) nerve
7 Vestibulocochlear (VIII) nerve nucleus (cochlear)
8 Vestibulocochlear (VIII) nerve nucleus (vestibular)
9 Lateral lemniscus
10 Fourth ventricle
11 Facial (VII) nerve nucleus
12 Inferior cerebellar peduncle
13 Facial (VII) nerve
14 Vestibulocochlear (auditory: VIII) nerve
15 Abducens nerve nucleus
16 Medial longitudinal fasciculus
17 Lateral lemniscus
18 Medial longitudinal fasciculus
19 Tectospinal tract
20 Ventral trigeminothalamic tract

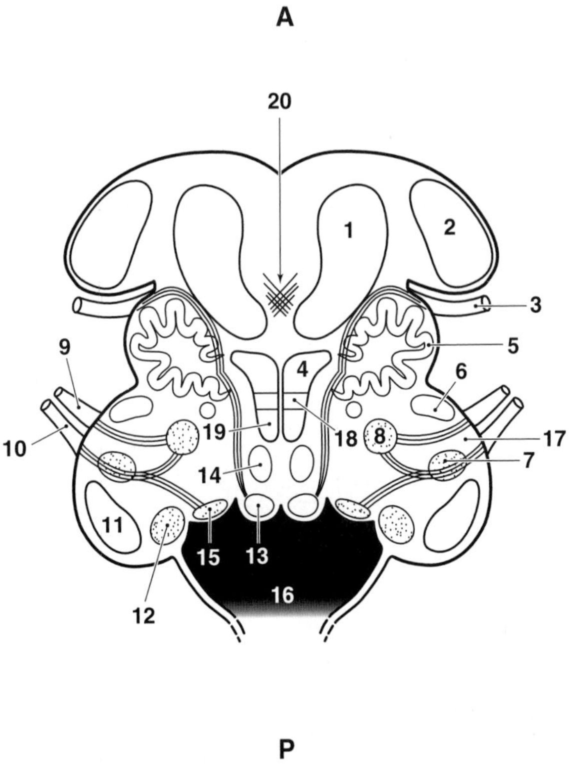

Figure 2H-6E: Schematic of the brain stem at the level of the rostral medulla oblongata. *A*, anterior; *P*, posterior.

1 Pyramidal (corticospinal) tract and corticobulbar tract
2 Middle cerebellar peduncle
3 Hypoglossal (XII) nerve
4 Medial lemniscus
5 Inferior olivary nucleus
6 Spinothalamic tracts (ventral, anterolateral, rubrospinal)
7 Trigeminal (V) nerve nucleus and tract
8 Nucleus ambiguus (IX, X)
9 Accessory (XI) nerve
10 Vagus (X) nerve
11 Inferior cerebellar peduncle
12 Vestibulocochlear (VIII) nerve nuclei
13 Hypoglossal (XII) nerve nucleus
14 Vestibulospinal tract
15 Solitary nucleus
16 Fourth ventricle
17 Ventral spinothalamic tract
18 Tectospinal tract
19 Medial longitudinal fasciculus
20 Olivocerebellar tract decussation

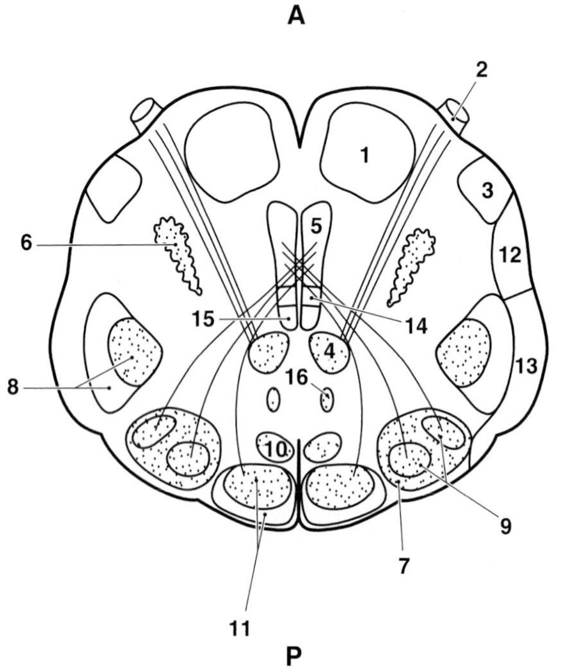

Figure 2H-6F: Axial schematic of the brain stem at the level of the caudal medulla oblongata. *A*, anterior; *P*, posterior.

1 Pyramidal (corticospinal) tract and corticobulbar tract
2 Hypoglossal (XII) nerve
3 Anterolateral tract
4 Hypoglossal (XII) nerve nucleus
5 Medial lemniscus
6 Accessory olivary nucleus
7 Cuneate nucleus
8 Trigeminal (V) nerve nucleus (*stippled*) and tract
9 Cuneate fasciculus
10 Solitary nucleus (IX, X)
11 Gracile nucleus (*stippled*) and fasciculus
12 Ventral spinocerebellar tract
13 Dorsal spinocerebellar tract
14 Tectospinal tract
15 Medial longitudinal fasciculus
16 Dorsal motor nucleus of vagus

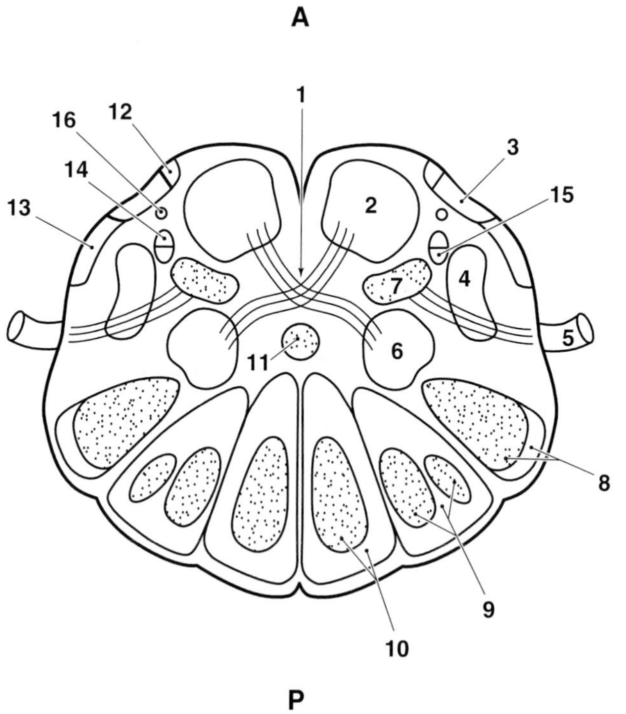

Figure 2H-6G: Axial schematic of the brain stem at the level of the lowermost caudal medulla near the cervicomedullary junction. *A*, anterior; *P*, posterior.

1 Pyramidal decussation
2 Pyramidal (corticospinal) tract and corticobulbar tract
3 Ventral spinothalamic tract
4 Anterolateral spinothalamic tract
5 Accessory (XI) nerve
6 Lateral corticospinal tract
7 Accessory (XI) nerve nucleus
8 Trigeminal (V) nerve nucleus (*stippled*) and tract
9 Cuneate nucleus (*stippled*) and fasciculus
10 Gracile nucleus (*stippled*) and fasciculus
11 Central gray matter
12 Spinoolivary tract
13 Dorsal spinocerebellar tract
14 Tectospinal tract
15 Medial longitudinal fasciculus
16 Lateral vestibulospinal tract

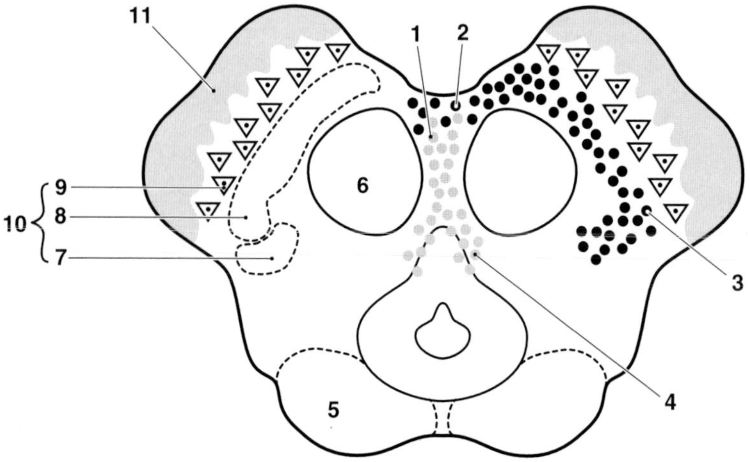

Figure 2H-6H: Axial schematic of the midbrain to show the substantia nigra and the position of dopaminergic cell groups (A9, A10) and the serotoninergic cell groups (B7, B8) in the raphe.

1 Ventral raphe seritonergic group (group B8)
2 Dopamine cell group (group A10: paranigral nucleus)
3 Dopamine cell group (group A9)
4 Dorsal raphe seritonergic (group B7)
5 Superior colliculus
6 Red nucleus
7 Pars lateralis
8 Pars compacta
9 Pars reticulata
10 Substantia nigra
11 Crus cerebri junction with cerebral peduncle

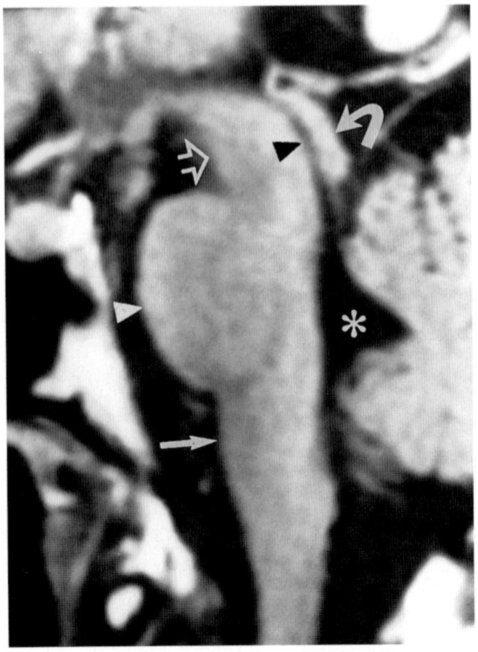

Figure 2H-7A: The brain stem. Sagittal T1-weighted MR image of the brain stem showing the midbrain (*open arrow*), the pons (*white arrowhead*), the medulla oblongata (*solid straight arrow*), the quadrigeminal plate (*curved arrow*), the cerebral aqueduct (*black arrowhead*), and the fourth ventricle (*asterisk*).

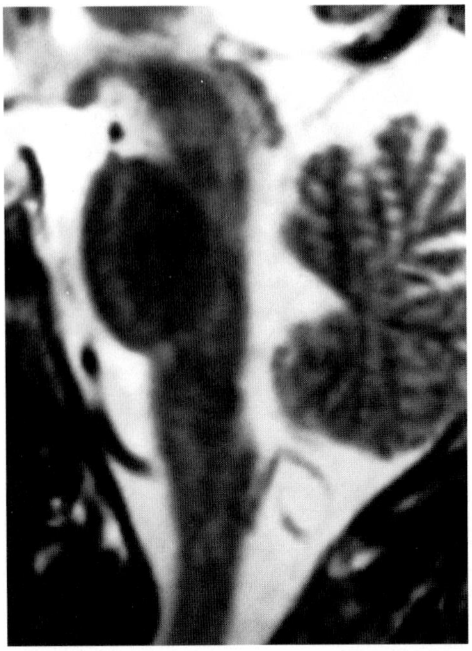

Figure 2H-7B: The brain stem. Sagittal T2-weighted MR image showing the gross brain stem anatomy.

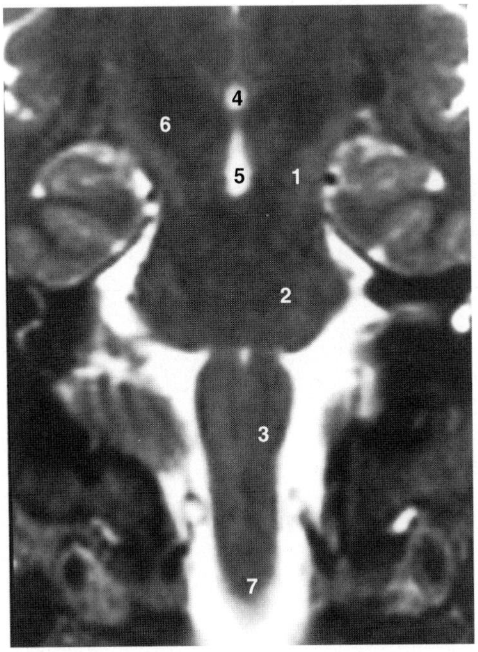

Figure 2H-7C: The brain stem. Coronal T2-weighted MR image of the brain stem.

1 Cerebral peduncle of midbrain
2 Pons
3 Medulla oblongata
4 Third ventricle
5 Interpeduncular cistern
6 Crus cerebri
7 Upper cervical spinal cord

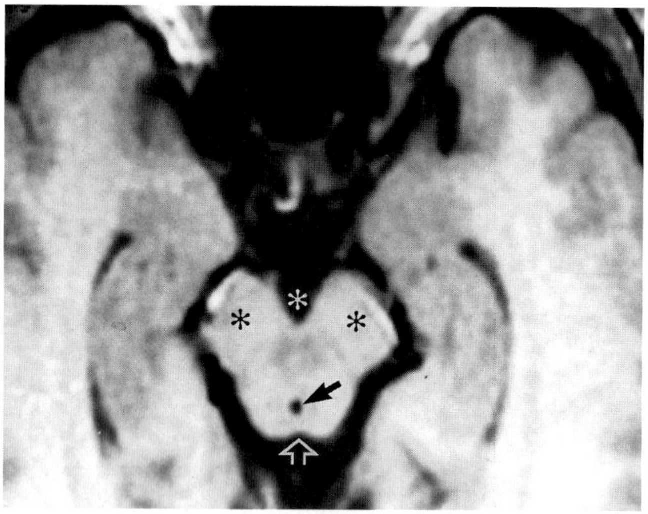

Figure 2H-8A: Midbrain anatomy. Axial T1-weighted MR image showing the midbrain with the cerebral peduncles (*black asterisks*), the quadrigeminal plate (*open arrow*), the cerebral aqueduct of Sylvius (*solid arrow*), and the interpeduncular cistern (*white asterisk*).

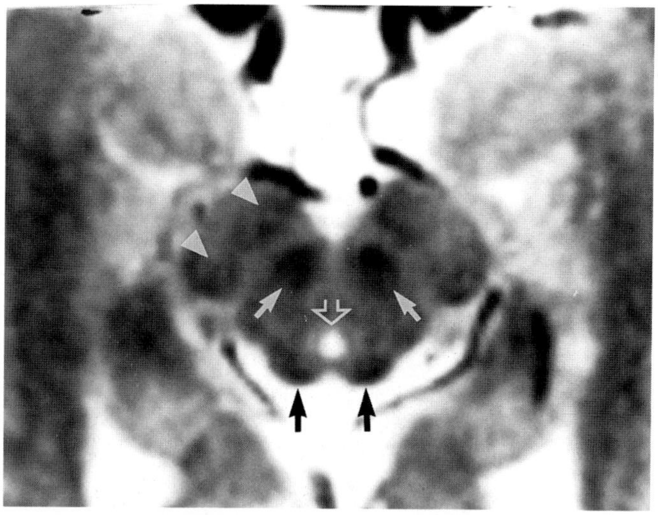

Figure 2H-8B: Midbrain anatomy. Axial T2-weighted MR image showing the normal hypointensity of the substantia nigra (*arrowheads*) and the red nuclei (*solid white arrows*). The distal aqueduct of Sylvius (*open arrow*) is also identified, as are the inferior colliculi (*small solid black arrows*).

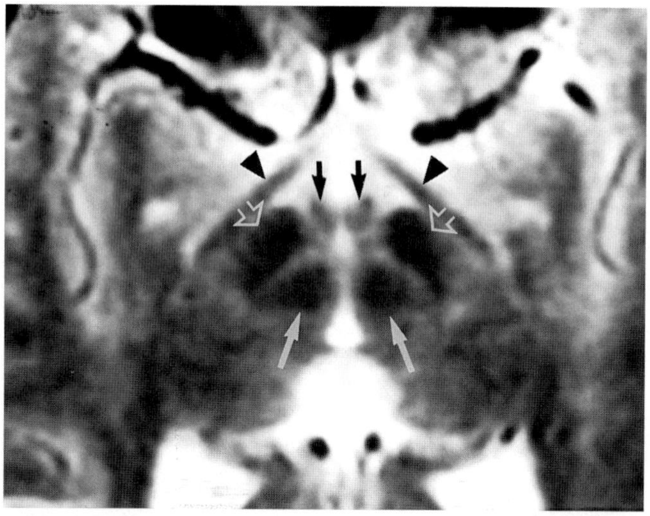

Figure 2H-8C: Midbrain anatomy. Axial T2-weighted MR image at a level just superior to that of Fig. 2H-8B, showing the red nuclei (*white solid arrows*), the substantia nigra (*open arrows*) bilaterally, the mammillary bodies (*black arrows*), and the optic tracts (*arrowheads*).

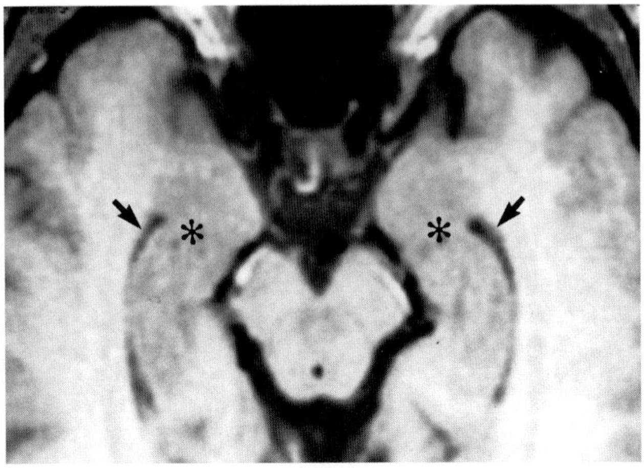

Figure 2H-9A: Amygdaloid nuclear complex. Axial T1-weighted MR image showing the amygdaloid nuclear complexes (*asterisks*) medial to the temporal horns (*arrows*) of the lateral ventricles.

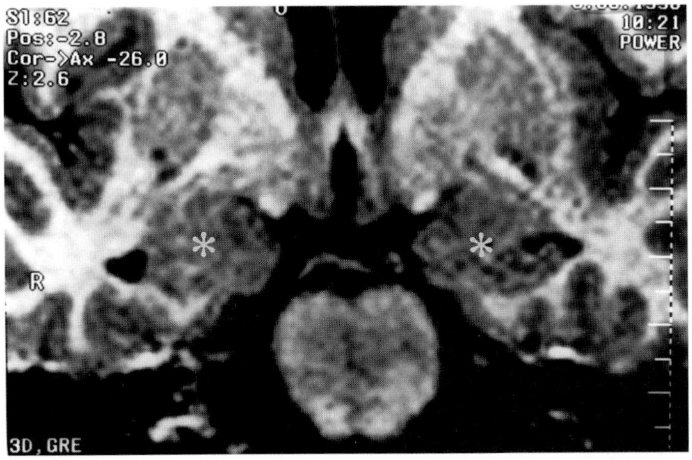

Figure 2H-9B: Amygdaloid nuclear complex. Coronal T1-weighted MR image showing the amygdaloid nuclear complexes bilaterally (*asterisks*).

2I. Peripheral Segments of the Cranial Nerves

THE OLFACTORY NERVE COMPLEX (CN-I)

1. Olfactory stimuli are sensed by the peripheral processes of bipolar olfactory neurons, located in the olfactory mucosa in the superoposterior aspect of the nasal cavity. Their central processes are grouped together to form approximately 20 olfactory nerves on each side.
2. These nerves pass through the perforated cribriform plate of the ethmoid bone and terminate in the olfactory bulbs. Here they form synapses with mitral and tufted cells at the glomerulus. Efferent fibers from these cells pass into the olfactory tract.
3. In the anterior part of the olfactory tract, there is a small grouping of neurons called the anterior olfactory nucleus. Their cells form synapses with mitral cells via interneurons and also with fibers from the contralateral anterior olfactory nucleus. Efferent fibers from the anterior olfactory nucleus also enter the olfactory tract.
4. The olfactory tract terminates by forming three striae: the lateral, intermediate, and medial olfactory striae.
5. The lateral olfactory stria contains most of the fibers from the mitral and tufted cells. It terminates in the primary olfactory area located at the anteromedial part of the temporal pole. The primary olfactory area includes the uncus, the amygdaloid nuclear complex, and the anterior part of the parahippocampal gyrus.
6. The intermediate olfactory stria ends in an ill-defined area in the anterior perforated substance. Its exact role is unclear.
7. Fibers of the medial olfactory stria mainly originate from the anterior olfactory nucleus. They cross in the anterior commissure to terminate in the contralateral anterior olfactory nucleus. They serve to interconnect the two olfactory centers (nuclei).

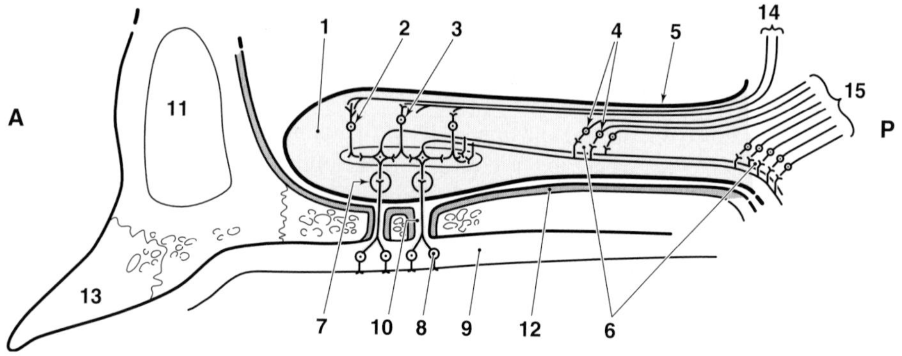

Figure 2I-1: Lateral schematic of the olfactory neurons, bulb, and tract (CN-I) (not to scale, enlarged to illustrate detail). *A*, anterior; *P*, posterior.

1 Olfactory bulb
2 Tufted cell
3 Mitral cell
4 Interneurons
5 Olfactory tract
6 Anterior olfactory nucleus
7 Olfactory glomerulus
8 Bipolar olfactory neuron
9 Nasal olfactory mucosa
10 Foramen in cribriform plate of ethmoid bone lined by meninges
11 Frontal air cells
12 Meninges of anterior cranial fossa
13 Nasal bones
14 Fibers from contralateral anterior olfactory nucleus
15 Centrally projecting fibers from the anterior olfactory nucleus

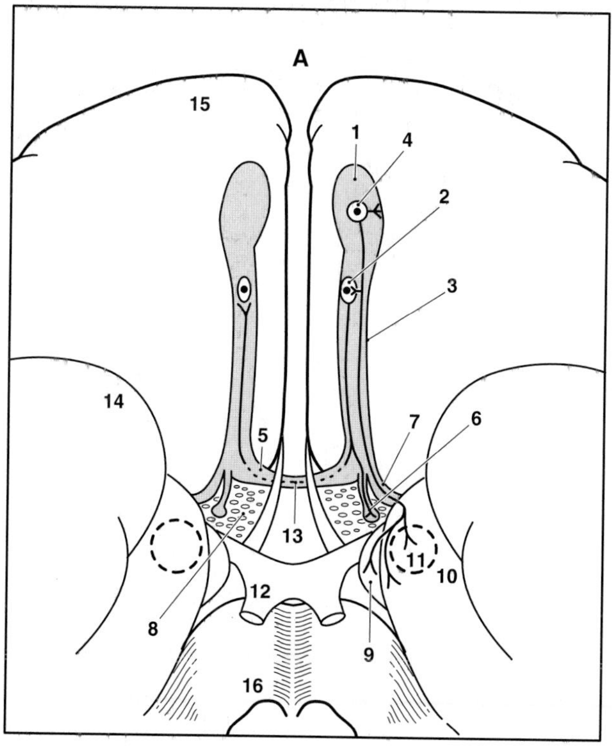

Figure 2I-2: Schematic of the olfactory nerve pathway (CN-I) viewed from below. *A*, anterior.

1 Olfactory bulb
2 Anterior olfactory nucleus
3 Olfactory tract
4 Mitral and tufted cells
5 Medial olfactory stria
6 Intermediate olfactory stria
7 Lateral olfactory stria
8 Anterior perforated substance (Primary olfactory area)
9 Uncus
10 Anterior part of the parahippocampal gyrus
11 Amygdaloid nuclear complex
12 Optic chiasm and cut edges of optic nerves
13 Anterior commissure
14 Temporal lobe
15 Frontal lobe
16 Brain stem

THE OPTIC NERVE COMPLEX (CN-II)

1. The photoreceptors of the visual system—the rod and cone cells—are located in the retina.
2. Optical signals from the rod and cone cells of the retina are transmitted to large multipolar ganglion cells, whose axons converge at the optic disc (optic papilla, optic nerve head) to form the optic nerve.
3. The optic nerve extends to the optic chiasm.
4. Optic fibers from the nasal half of the retina (temporal visual field) cross to the opposite side in the optic chiasm, whereas fibers from the temporal half of the retina (nasal visual field) remain on the same side.
5. Most of the optic fibers terminate in the paired lateral geniculate bodies (thalamic nuclei).
6. Axons from the lateral geniculate bodies form the optic radiation (geniculocalcarine tracts) on each side, which end in the calcarine areas (calcarine or visual cortex) in the medial occipital lobes bilaterally.

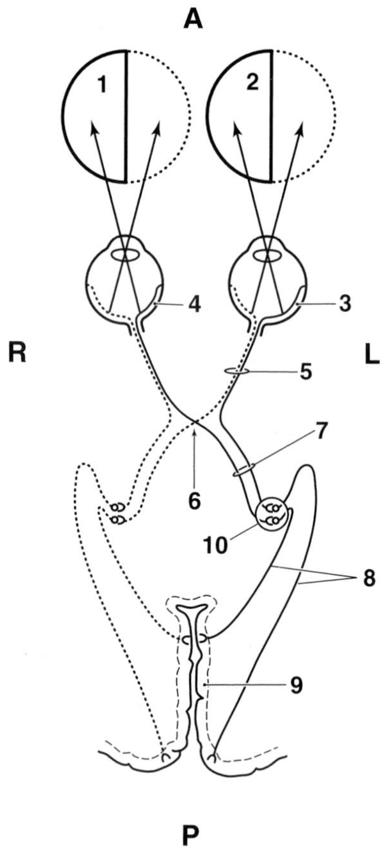

Figure 21-3: Schematic of the visual pathway (CN-II) viewed from above. *L*, left; *R*, right; *A*, anterior; *P*, posterior.

1 Temporal visual field of the left hemispheric visual (calcarine) cortex
2 Nasal visual field of the left hemispheric visual (calcarine) cortex
3 Temporal retina
4 Nasal retina
5 Optic nerve
6 Optic chiasm
7 Optic tract
8 Optic radiation
9 Visual (calcarine) cortex of the left hemisphere
10 Lateral geniculate body on the left side

THE OCULOMOTOR NERVE (CN-III)

1. The oculomotor nerve nucleus is situated in the midbrain at the level of the superior colliculus.
2. The nerve exits from the anterior surface of the midbrain. It then travels through the interpeduncular fossa to enter the lateral wall of the cavernous venous sinus. From there it enters the orbit via the superior orbital fissure.
3. Within the orbit, the oculomotor nerve innervates five of the total of seven extraocular muscles, including the levator palpebrae superioris, superior rectus, inferior rectus, medial rectus, and inferior oblique muscles.
4. The oculomotor nerve also carries parasympathetic fibers from the Edinger-Westphal nucleus. This nucleus is situated in the midbrain, medial and dorsal to the oculomotor nerve nucleus.
5. At the orbit, the parasympathetic fibers leave the main nerve to form synapses within the ciliary ganglion. The postganglionic parasympathetic fibers then exit the ciliary ganglion and are carried by the ciliary nerve (branch of the ophthalmic [first] division of the fifth cranial nerve: CN-V1) to supply the sphincter papillae muscle (muscle of pupillary constriction) and the ciliary muscle (muscle of lens accommodation) of the eye (see also The Parasympathetic Neural Supply to the Head and Neck, pp. 212–213).

THE TROCHLEAR NERVE (CN-IV)

1. The trochlear nerve nucleus is situated in the midbrain at the level of the inferior colliculus.
2. The trochlear nerve passes posteriorly around the cerebral aqueduct of Sylvius and crosses the midline to exit the posterior surface of the brain stem.
3. The trochlear nerve then travels forward around the cerebral peduncle to enter the lateral wall of the cavernous venous sinus. Here it is situated between the oculomotor nerve (CN-III) above and the first and second divisions of the trigeminal nerve (CN-V1 and CN-V2 divisions) below.
4. The trochlear nerve then passes through the superior orbital fissure to enter the orbit, where it innervates the superior oblique muscle.

THE ABDUCENS NERVE (CN-VI)

1. The abducens nerve nucleus is situated at the lower border of the pons.
2. The abducens nerve exits the anterior surface of the brain stem at the pontomedullary junction.
3. The abducens nerve then travels anteriorly to course within the cavernous venous sinus.
4. The abducens subsequently passes through the superior orbital fissure to enter the orbit, where it innervates the lateral rectus muscle.

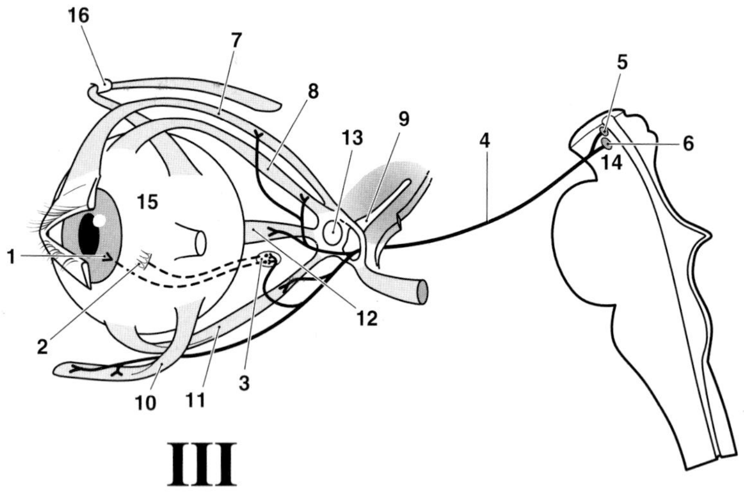

Figure 21-4: Lateral schematic of the oculomotor nerve pathway (CN-III) on the left. (The lateral rectus has been cut, and the lateral aspect of the lids has been removed.)

1 Sphincter papillae muscle (muscle of papillary constriction)
2 Ciliary muscle (muscle of lens accommodation)
3 Ciliary ganglion
4 Oculomotor nerve
5 Edinger-Westphal nucleus
6 Oculomotor nerve nucleus
7 Levator palpebrae superioris
8 Superior rectus muscle
9 Superior orbital fissure
10 Inferior oblique muscle
11 Inferior rectus muscle
12 Medial rectus muscle
13 Aperture for the optic nerve/sheath complex
14 Midbrain
15 Left globe
16 Fibrocartilaginous trochlea

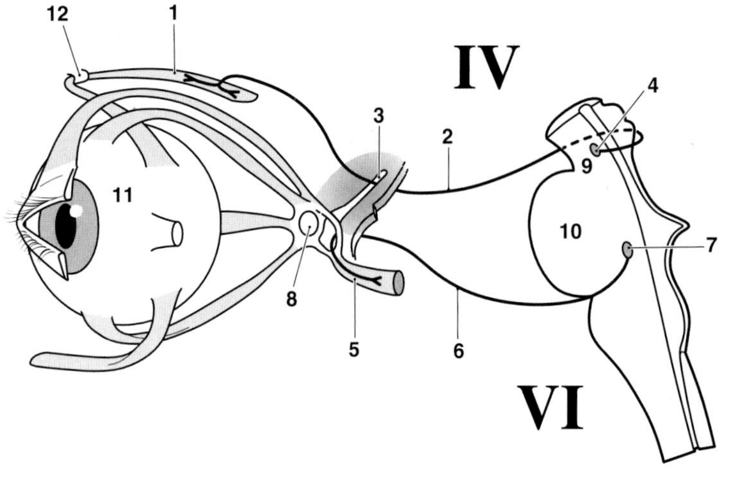

Figure 21-5: Lateral schematic of the trochlear (CN-IV) and abducens (CN-VI) nerve pathways on the left. (The lateral rectus has been cut, and the lateral aspect of the eyelid has been removed.)

1 Superior oblique muscle
2 Trochlear nerve (CN-IV)
3 Superior orbital fissure
4 Trochlear nucleus
5 Lateral rectus muscle
6 Abducens nerve (CN-VI)
7 Abducens nucleus
8 Aperture for optic nerve/sheath complex
9 Midbrain
10 Pons
11 Left globe
12 Fibrocartilaginous trochlea

THE TRIGEMINAL NERVE (CN-V)

1. The trigeminal nerve is a mixed cranial nerve with sensory as well as motor fibers.
2. The trigeminal nerve (CN-V) has one motor nucleus and three sensory nuclei.
   a. The trigeminal nerve motor nucleus is located in the midpontine region. Its fibers innervate muscles of mastication, two tensor muscles, and two muscles in the floor of the mouth (see later discussion).
   b. The three trigeminal sensory nuclei include the trigeminal mesencephalic nucleus, the chief trigeminal sensory nucleus, and the trigeminal spinal nucleus.
      i. The mesencephalic nucleus is situated in the lateral aspect of the midbrain and upper pons, between the superior colliculus and the motor nucleus of the trigeminal nerve. The afferent fibers terminating in the mesencephalic nucleus are mainly proprioceptive, with nerve endings originating in muscles of mastication and the temporomandibular joint.
      ii. The chief sensory nucleus is located lateral to the motor nucleus in the midpons. It contains fibers concerned primarily with pressure and touch.
      iii. The spinal nucleus is located laterally, between the chief sensory nucleus and the dorsal horn (laminae I–IV) gray matter of the cervical spinal cord. Its main function is the relay of pain and temperature sensation.
3. The trigeminal nerve exits the middle portion of the pons and forms the trigeminal ganglion (gasserian/semilunar ganglion) within Meckel's cave.
4. The nerve fibers then immediately divide into three divisions, including the first division, or ophthalmic nerve (CN-V1); the second division, or maxillary nerve (CN-V2); and the third division, or mandibular nerve (CN-V3).

The Ophthalmic Nerve (CN-V1)

1. The ophthalmic nerve (CN-V1) carries sensory fibers only.
2. It travels within the lateral wall of the cavernous venous sinus and enters the orbit via the superior orbital fissure.
3. There the ophthalmic nerve divides into three terminal branches: the lacrimal, frontal, and nasociliary nerves. It is a branch of the frontal nerve—the supraorbital nerve—that exits the orbit via the supraorbital notch or foramen. These fibers supply the upper facial region, including the upper eyelid, the cornea, the eyeball, the forehead, the frontal half of the scalp, the skin and mucosa of the nose, and the mucosa of the frontal, ethmoid, and sphenoid sinuses.
4. Via a recurrent meningeal branch of the ophthalmic nerve (tentorial nerve), CN-V1 also supplies a portion of the dura mater of the tentorium cerebelli.

The Maxillary Nerve (CN-V2)

1. The maxillary nerve (CN-V2) carries only sensory fibers.
2. The maxillary nerve travels within the lateral wall of the cavernous venous sinus and exits the cranial cavity through the foramen rotundum to enter the pterygopalatine fossa. There it gives off a few branches before continuing forward to exit the orbit through the infraorbital canal and foramen. Upon exiting, it then becomes the infraorbital nerve.
3. The maxillary nerve primarily supplies the midfacial region, including the skin over the cheek and zygomatic areas, the side of the nose, the lower eyelid, the upper lip, the upper teeth and gum, the nasal septum, the soft and hard palates, the nasopharynx, and the maxillary sinus. It also sends meningeal branches to the middle cranial fossa.

The Mandibular Nerve (CN-V3)

1. The mandibular nerve (CN-V3) carries both sensory and motor fibers.
2. The mandibular nerve exits the cranial cavity through the foramen ovale and soon divides into the various branches that supply the lower facial region.

3. Its sensory fibers supply the lower gum and teeth, the lower lip, the side of the scalp in the temporal region, the external ear and external auditory meatus, the external side of the eardrum, the temporomandibular joint, the mastoid air cells, the mucosa over the cheek, the anterior two-thirds of the tongue, and the floor of the mouth. It also supplies the dura mater of the anterior and middle cranial fossae.
4. The motor fibers of the mandibular nerve supply four muscles of mastication (masseter, temporalis, and lateral and medial pterygoid muscles), the two tensor muscles (tensor tympani and tensor veli palatini), and the two muscles in the floor of the mouth (mylohyoid muscle and the anterior belly of the digastric muscle).

Parasympathetic Fibers Associated with the Trigeminal Nerve (CNV)

1. The main trunk of the trigeminal nerve does not carry parasympathetic fibers as it leaves the brain stem. However, the divisions of the trigeminal nerve pick up postganglionic parasympathetic fibers emanating from the regional parasympathetic ganglia. The ophthalmic division (CN-V1) receives neural fibers from the ciliary ganglion, the maxillary division (CN-V2) from the pterygopalatine ganglion, and the mandibular division (CN-V3) from the submandibular and otic ganglia.
2. Preganglionic fibers to the ciliary ganglion are carried by branches of the oculomotor nerve (CN-III) originating from the Edinger-Westphal nucleus in the midbrain. Postganglionic parasympathetic fibers from this ganglion are carried by ciliary branches of the ophthalmic nerve (CN-V1) to supply the ciliary muscles and papillary sphincter muscles.
3. Preganglionic fibers arising from the lacrimal nucleus in the lower pons travel to the pterygopalatine ganglion via the greater petrosal branch of the facial nerve (CN-VII). From there some of the postganglionic parasympathetic fibers are distributed with branches of the maxillary nerve (CN-V2) to glands of the nasal mucosa, palate, and pharynx. The rest of the fibers then "hitchhike" with lacrimal branches of the ophthalmic nerve (CN-V1) to supply the lacrimal gland.
4. The superior salivatory nucleus, located at the pontomedullary junction, provides the parasympathetic supply to the submandibular and sublingual salivary glands. The preganglionic parasympathetic fibers first travel with the chorda tympani branch of the facial nerve (CN-VII) and then with the lingual nerve, a branch of the mandibular nerve (CN-V3), to reach the submandibular ganglion. Subsequently, postganglionic axons innervate the submandibular and sublingual salivary glands via the terminal branches of the lingual nerve.
5. The preganglionic parasympathetic fibers from the inferior salivatory nucleus, located at the pontomedullary junction, immediately inferior to the superior salivatory nucleus, travel first with the tympanic branch of the glossopharyngeal nerve (CN-X) and subsequently with the lesser petrosal nerve to reach the otic ganglion. Postganglionic fibers from this ganglion are then distributed to the parotid gland via the auriculotemporal branch of the mandibular nerve (CN-V3). (see also The Parasympathetic Neural Supply to the Head and Neck, pp. 212–213.)

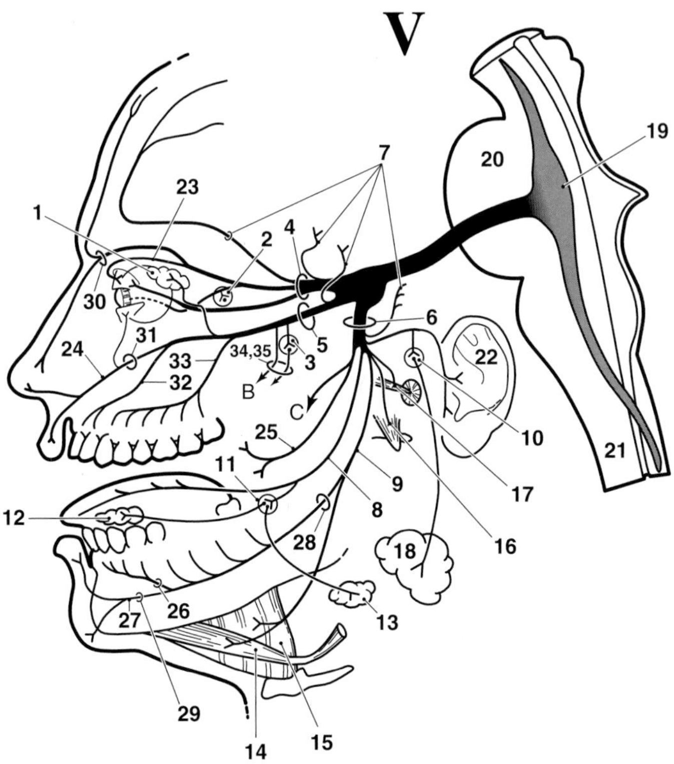

A

Figure 2I-6A: Lateral schematic of the trigeminal nerve pathway (CN-V).

1 Lacrimal gland
2 Ciliary ganglion (parasympathetic supply from CN-III)
3 Pterygopalatine ganglion (parasympathetic supply from CN-VII)
4 Ophthalmic nerve: first division of fifth cranial nerve (CN-V1)
5 Maxillary nerve: second division of fifth cranial nerve (CN-V2)
6 Mandibular nerve: third division of fifth cranial nerve (CN-V3)
7 Dural (meningeal) branches
8 Lingual nerve (parasympathetic supply from CN-VII)
9 Inferior alveolar nerve
10 Ganglion (parasympathetic supply from CN-X)
11 Submandibular ganglion (parasympathetic supply from CN-VII)
12 Sublingual gland
13 Submandibular gland
14 Digastric muscle
15 Mylohyoid muscle
16 Tensor veli palatini muscle
17 Tensor tympani muscle
18 Parotid gland
19 Trigeminal nerve nuclei
20 Pons
21 Upper cervical spinal cord
22 Auricle
23 Supraorbital nerve
24 Infraorbital nerve
25 Buccal nerve (to buccinator muscle)
26 Incisive branch of inferior alveolar nerve
27 Mental branch of inferior alveolar nerve
28 Mandibular foramen
29 Mental foramen
30 Supraorbital notch/foramen
31 Infraorbital foramen
32 Anterior–superior alveolar nerve
33 Posterior–superior alveolar nerve
34 Nasopalatine nerve
35 Greater and lesser palatine nerves

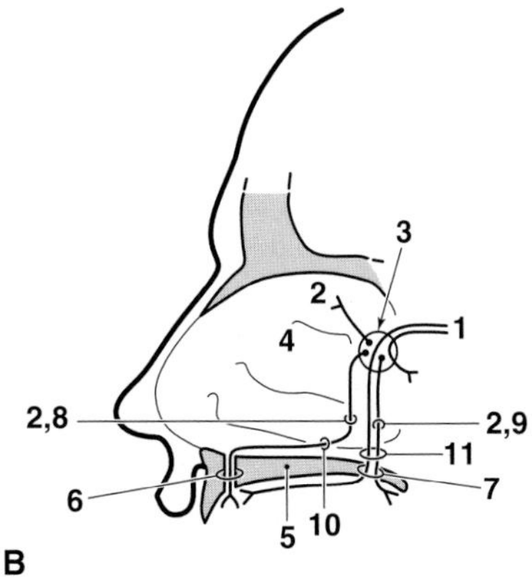

B

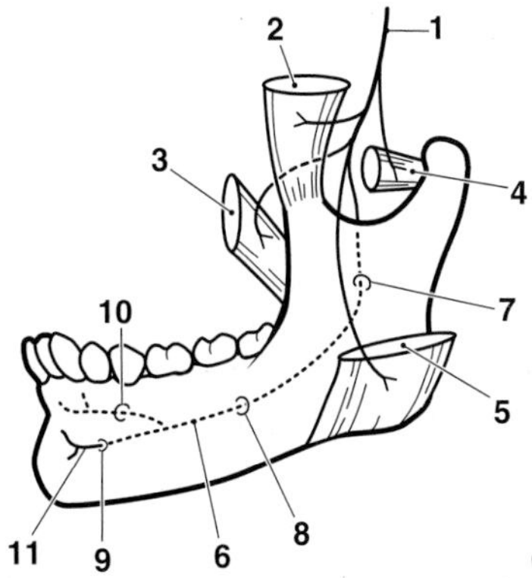

C

Figure 2I-6B: Lateral schematic of sensory and parasympathetic neural supply to nasal and palatal mucosa associated with the trigeminal nerve (CN-V) on the left side.

1 Sensory fibers
2 Parasympathetic fibers (postganglionic)
3 Pterygopalatine ganglion
4 Nasal mucosa
5 Palate
6 Incisive canal
7 Greater and lesser palatine foramena
8 Postganglionic parasympathetic fibers to anterior palatal mucosa
9 Postganglionic parasympathetic fibers to posterior palatal mucosa
10 Nasopalatine nerve
11 Greater and lesser palatine nerves

Figure 2I-6C: Lateral schematic of trigeminal nerve (CN-V) motor supply to muscles of mastication on the left side.

1 Mandibular nerve (CN-V3)
2 Temporalis muscle
3 Medial pterygoid muscle
4 Lateral pterygoid muscle
5 Masseter muscle
6 Mandible
7 Mandibular foramen
8 Mandibular canal (inferior alveolar nerve)
9 Mental foramen
10 Incisive branch of inferior alveolar nerve
11 Mental nerve

THE FACIAL NERVE (CN-VII)

1. The facial nerve consists of two roots: the facial nerve proper (motor root) and the intermediate root of the facial nerve (nervus intermedius: sensory root).
2. These two facial nerve roots leave the anterolateral aspect of brain stem at the pontomedullary junction to unite and enter the internal auditory meatus.
3. The combined facial nerve then passes into the facial nerve canal in the petrous portion of the temporal bone.
4. Within the facial canal, the facial nerve makes a bend, or genu, at the level of the geniculate ganglion anterior to the labyrinth of the inner ear.
5. The facial nerve then runs posteriorly just beneath the lateral semicircular canal to reach the posterior part of the middle ear cavity. This is the horizontal portion of the facial nerve.
6. Subsequently, the facial nerve turns sharply downward to pass vertically through the mastoid process to exit the cranium via the stylomastoid foramen.
7. The facial nerve then passes through the substance of the parotid gland, where it terminates by dividing into five terminal motor branches.

The Motor Nucleus and Roots of the Facial Nerve (CN-VII)

1. The motor nucleus of the facial nerve is located in the dorsal aspect of the lower pons.
2. The motor fibers course superiorly to loop around the abducens nucleus (CN-VI) and exit the brain stem anterolaterally as the motor root.
3. The motor root supplies the muscles of facial expression, the stylohyoid muscle, the posterior belly of the digastric muscle, the buccinator muscle, the stapedius muscle of the middle ear, and the muscles serving the scalp and auricle.

The Sensory Nuclei and Parasympathetic/Somatosensory Nerve Branches of the Facial Nerve (CN-VII)

1. The lacrimal and superior salivatory nuclei supply the parasympathetic components of the facial nerve.
2. The solitary nucleus (nucleus solitarius) in the rostral medulla oblongata supplies the gustatory and somatosensory components of the facial nerve.
3. The preganglionic efferent parasympathetic, somatosensory, and gustatory (taste) fibers of the facial nerve are initially carried by the intermediate root of the facial nerve (nervus intermedius).
4. The parasympathetic fibers are carried by two branches of the facial nerve: the greater petrosal nerve and the chorda tympani nerve.
   a. Parasympathetic fibers from the lacrimal nucleus are distributed by the greater petrosal nerve following a synapse in the pterygopalatine ganglion. The postganglionic fibers then supply the nasal and palatal mucosal glands and the lacrimal glands.
   b. Fibers from the superior salivatory nucleus travel with the chorda tympani nerve. Following a synapse in the submandibular ganglion, the postganglionic fibers supply the submandibular and sublingual salivary glands. There is some anatomic evidence to suggest that fibers from the chorda tympani nerve also form synapses in the otic ganglion and that these postganglionic fibers supply the parotid gland.
5. Visceral sensory (gustatory) fibers innervating the palate and nasal passageways are carried by the greater petrosal nerve; those gustatory sensory fibers innervating the anterior two-thirds (presulcal area) of the tongue are carried by the chorda tympani nerve.
6. The facial nerve transmits somatic sensory (somatosensory) fibers via the auricular branch of the vagus nerve (CN-X). These somatosensory fibers supply the skin overlying the auricle and the external auditory meatus. Their central projections are on the trigeminal nerve spinal nucleus (CN-V) in the medulla oblongata and upper cervical spinal cord. (see also The Parasympathetic Neural Supply to the Head and Neck, pp. 212–213.)

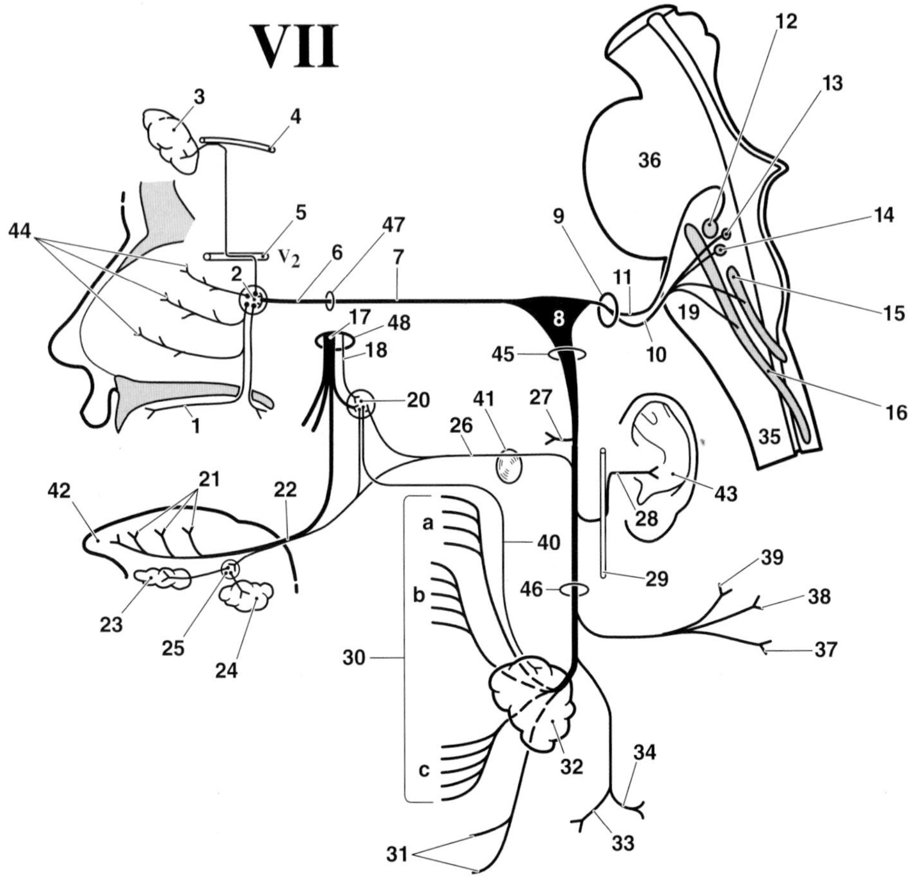

Figure 2I-7: Lateral schematic of the facial nerve pathway (CN-VII) on the left side.

1 Postganglionic fibers supplying the palatal mucosal glands
2 Pterygopalatine ganglion
3 Lacrimal gland
4 Lacrimal nerve (branch of ophthalmic nerve [CN-V1])
5 Maxillary nerve (CN-V2)
6 Nerve of the pterygoid canal (vidian nerve)
7 Greater petrosal nerve
8 Geniculate ganglion
9 Internal auditory canal with combined facial nerve (CN-VII)
10 Sensory root of the facial nerve
11 Motor root of the facial nerve
12 Facial nerve motor nuclei
13 Lacrimal nucleus
14 Superior salivatory nucleus
15 Solitary nucleus (nucleus solitarius)
16 Spinal nucleus of the trigeminal nerve (CN-V)
17 Mandibular nerve (CN-V3)
18 Lesser petrosal nerve
19 Medulla oblongata
20 Otic ganglion
21 Somatosensory (CN-V3) and taste (CN-VII) fibers of the facial nerve
22 Lingual nerve
23 Sublingual gland
24 Submandibular gland
25 Submandibular ganglion
26 Chorda tympani nerve
27 Nerve to stapedius muscle
28 Auricular branch of vagus nerve (CN-X)
29 Vagus nerve (CN-X)
30 Zygomatic (a), buccal (b), and mandibular (c) neural branches serving the muscles of facial expression
31 Neural branch serving the platysma muscle
32 Parotid gland
33 Neural branch serving the stylohyoid muscle
34 Neural branch serving the digastric muscle (posterior belly)
35 Upper cervical spinal cord
36 Pons
37 Temporal branch serving the auricularis anterior and superior muscles
38 Posterior auricular neural branch to the auricularis posterior muscle
39 Neural branch serving the occipital muscle
40 Neural branch to parotid gland
41 Tympanic membrane (and middle ear)
42 Tongue
43 Auricle
44 Postganglionic fibers supplying the nasal mucosal glands
45 Facial nerve canal
46 Stylomastoid foramen
47 Vidian (pterygoid) canal
48 Foramen ovale

THE VESTIBULOCOCHLEAR NERVE (CN-VIII)

1. The vestibulocochlear nerve consists of two components: the vestibular and cochlear nerves.
2. The vestibular nerve is the nerve of equilibrium, whereas the cochlear nerve is the auditory nerve.
3. The vestibulocochlear nerve consists of the central fibers from the ampullae of the semicircular canals and the utricle and saccule.
   a. The vestibular nerve passes through the internal auditory canal together with the cochlear nerve and the motor and sensory divisions of the facial nerve.
   b. The vestibular nerve then enters the brain stem at the pontomedullary junction to terminate in the vestibular nuclei (medial, lateral, superior, and inferior).
   c. The vestibular nuclei are located in the dorsal part of the upper medulla oblongata.
   d. Some fibers of the vestibular nerve also terminate in the cerebellum and the reticular formation of the brain stem.
4. Fibers forming the cochlear nerve receive auditory information from the organ of Corti located within the cochlea in the inner ear.
   a. The cell bodies of the cochlear nerve lie within the spiral ganglion.
   b. The cochlear nerve proper then passes alongside the vestibular nerve through the internal auditory canal to reach the medulla oblongata and subsequently terminate in the dorsal and ventral cochlear nuclei.
   c. The dorsal and ventral cochlear nuclei are located in the medulla oblongata immediately ventral to the vestibular nucleus.

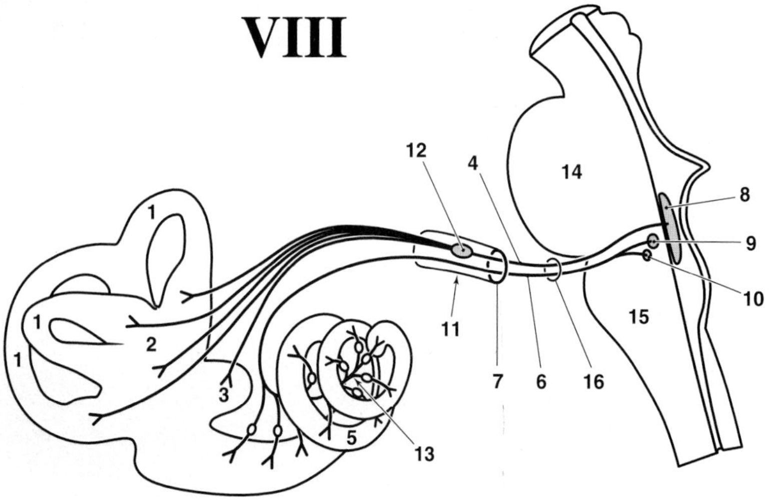

Figure 2I-8: Schematic of the vestibulocochlear nerve pathway (CN-VIII).
1 Semicircular canals (lateral, superior, posterior)
2 Utricle
3 Saccule
4 Vestibular nerve (branch of CN-VIII)
5 Cochlea
6 Cochlear nerve (branch of CN-VIII)
7 Internal auditory meatus
8 Vestibular nuclei (medial, lateral, superior, inferior)
9 Dorsal cochlear nucleus
10 Ventral cochlear nucleus
11 Internal auditory canal
12 Vestibular ganglion
13 Spiral ganglion
14 Pons
15 Medulla oblongata
16 Combined vestibulocochlear nerve (CN-VIII)

THE GLOSSOPHARYNGEAL NERVE (CN-IX)

1. The five to six rootlets making up the glossopharyngeal nerve exit the medulla oblongata posterior to the inferior olive of the brain stem.
2. The glossopharyngeal nerve then passes through the jugular foramen to exit the cranial vault together with the vagus (CN-X) and accessory (CN-XI) nerves.
3. The glossopharyngeal nerve subsequently descends behind the styloid process to pass along the lateral pharyngeal wall. There it turns forward to terminate in the base of the tongue.
4. The motor fibers of the glossopharyngeal nerve arise in the cranial portion of the nucleus ambiguus to supply the stylopharyngeus muscle and perhaps varying portions of the pharyngeal constrictor muscle(s). The nucleus ambiguus is located laterally in the medulla oblongata.
5. The parasympathetic fibers of the glossopharyngeal nerve arise in the inferior salivatory nucleus.
   a. The inferior salivatory nucleus is located above the dorsal motor nucleus of the vagus nerve (CN-X) in the medulla oblongata.
   b. After leaving the glossopharyngeal nerve, the parasympathetic fibers are carried initially by the tympanic nerve to form synapses in the otic ganglion.
   c. From there the postganglionic fibers travel with the lesser petrosal nerve to supply the parotid gland.
   d. There is also evidence to suggest that some parasympathetic fibers from the glossopharyngeal nerve hitchhike with the facial nerve (CN-VII) to the otic and submandibular ganglia.
      i. These parasympathetic fibers of the glossopharyngeal nerve travel via a connecting branch to reach the facial nerve (CN-VII).
      ii. The fibers then travel with the chorda tympani of the facial nerve to form synapses with the otic ganglion and with the submandibular ganglion to subsequently supply the submandibular and sublingual glands, respectively.
   e. Visceral sensory fibers from the glossopharyngeal nerve innervate the pharyngeal mucosa, soft palate, tonsils, posterior one-third of the tongue, mucosa of the tympanic cavity, eustachian (auditory) tube, and mastoid air cells. A small branch also innervates the carotid sinus and body. Their central projection is onto the solitary nucleus (nucleus solitarius) in the dorsal medulla oblongata.
6. A small contribution from the glossopharyngeal nerve joins the auricular branch of the vagus nerve (CN-X) to provide somatic sensory (somatosensory) supply to the skin overlying the auricle and the external auditory meatus. Their central projections end in the trigeminal nerve spinal nucleus in the medulla oblongata and upper cervical spinal cord.
7. Taste (gustatory) fibers innervating the posterior one-third of the tongue are carried by the terminal branches of the glossopharyngeal nerve. Their central processes terminate in the solitary nucleus (nucleus solitarius) in the dorsal medulla oblongata (see also The Parasympathetic Neural Supply to the Head and Neck, pp. 212–213.)

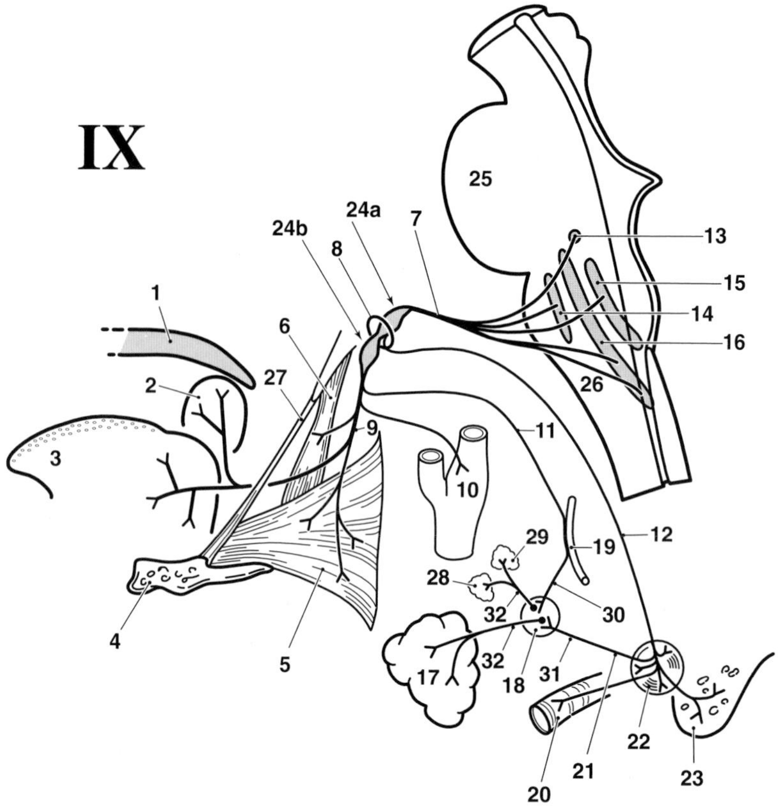

Figure 2I-9: Schematic of the glossopharyngeal nerve pathway (CN-IX) on the left side.

1 Soft palate
2 Tonsil
3 Tongue
4 Hyoid bone
5 Pharyngeal constrictor muscles
6 Stylopharyngeus muscle
7 Glossopharyngeal nerve (CN-IX)
8 Jugular foramen
9 Pharyngeal neural branch
10 Carotid sinus and body
11 Connecting neural branch to facial nerve (CN-VII)
12 Tympanic nerve
13 Inferior salivatory nucleus
14 Ambiguous nucleus (nucleus ambiguus)
15 Solitary nucleus (nucleus solitarius)
16 Spinal nucleus of the trigeminal nerve (CN-V)
17 Parotid gland
18 Otic ganglion
19 Facial nerve (CN-VII)
20 Eustachian (auditory) tube
21 Lesser petrosal nerve
22 Tympanic neural plexus
23 Mastoid process and air cells
24 Superior (a) and inferior (b) sensory ganglia (somatic and visceral afferent neurons) of glossopharyngeal nerve
25 Pons
26 Medulla oblongata
27 Stylohyoid ligament
28 Sublingual gland
29 Submandibular gland
30 Preganglionic parasympathetic fibers en route to otic (and submandibular ganglion [not shown]) ganglion after coursing with the facial nerve (CN-VII)
31 Preganglionic parasympathetic fibers en route to otic ganglion directly from the glossopharyngeal nerve
32 Postganglionic parasympathetic fibers

THE VAGUS NERVE (CN-X)

1. The vagus nerve exits from the medulla oblongata below the glossopharyngeal nerve and behind the inferior olive as 8 to 10 rootlets.
2. The vagus nerve proper leaves the cranium through the jugular foramen together with, but separate from, the glossopharyngeal (CN-IX) and accessory (CN-XI) nerves.
3. After emerging from the jugular foramen, the vagus nerve is joined by the cranial root of the accessory nerve (CN-XI), which provides motor innervation of the larynx through the recurrent laryngeal branch of the vagus nerve (CN-X).
4. The vagal trunk then passes downward in the neck within the carotid sheath between the carotid artery and the internal jugular vein.
5. At the base of the neck, the vagus nerve enters the thorax. At this point the left and right vagus nerves differ in their course.
   a. The right vagus nerve passes behind the right main bronchus and the posterior aspect of the esophagus.
   b. The left vagus nerve passes anterior to the aortic arch and behind the left main bronchus to reach the anterior aspect of the esophagus.
   c. Both vagal nerves then enter the abdomen through the esophageal hiatus of the diaphragm to diverge into their terminal branches.
6. The motor fibers of the vagus nerve arise from the intermediate portion of the nucleus ambiguus located in the lateral medulla oblongata. These motor fibers travel initially with the cranial root of the accessory nerve (CN-XI). With minor exceptions, these fibers innervate all of the muscles of the pharynx (except the stylopharyngeus muscle, which is innervated by the glossopharyngeal nerve [CN-IX]), the palate (except the tensor veli palatini muscle, which is innervated by the trigeminal nerve [CN-V]), and the larynx (except the cricothyroid muscle, which is innervated by the external laryngeal nerve, itself a true motor branch of the vagus nerve). The muscles supplied and the terminal neural motor branches innervating them include:
   a. The pharyngeal muscles, innervated by the pharyngeal branch of the vagus nerve (superior and middle pharyngeal constrictor muscles), the external laryngeal nerve (inferior constrictor muscle), and the recurrent laryngeal nerves (inferior constrictor muscle), the latter two of which are also branches of the vagus nerve.
   b. The muscles of the soft palate, innervated by the pharyngeal branch of the vagus nerve.
   c. The laryngeal muscles, innervated by the two recurrent laryngeal nerves, both branches of the vagus nerves.
7. The parasympathetic fibers of the vagus nerve arise from the dorsal motor nucleus of the vagus nerve. The dorsal motor nucleus is located in the medulla oblongata on the floor of the fourth ventricle, between the nucleus ambiguus and the hypoglossal nucleus.
   a. These preganglionic fibers form synapses with small ganglia located in the target organs in the thorax and abdomen.
   b. Specifically, the vagus nerve provides parasympathetic fibers to all of the thoracic and abdominal viscera down to the level of the splenic flexure of the colon.
8. Visceral sensory fibers of the vagus nerve innervate the mucosa of the inferior pharynx, the entire larynx, and part of the soft palate. A small branch also innervates the carotid sinus and the aortic body. Their central axons terminate in the solitary nucleus (nucleus solitarius) in the dorsal medulla oblongata.
9. The auricular branch of the vagus nerve is joined by small branches from the facial (CN-VII) and glossopharyngeal (CN-IX) nerves and provides somatic sensory (somatosensory) supply to the skin overlying the auricle and the external auditory meatus canal. A small meningeal neural branch of the vagus nerve supplies the dura of the posterior cranial fossa. Their central projections terminate in the trigeminal nerve spinal nucleus in the medulla oblongata and upper cervical spinal cord.
10. The vagus nerve also provides taste (gustatory) fibers to a small number of taste buds on the epiglottis. Their central axons synapse in the solitary nucleus in the dorsal medulla oblongata.

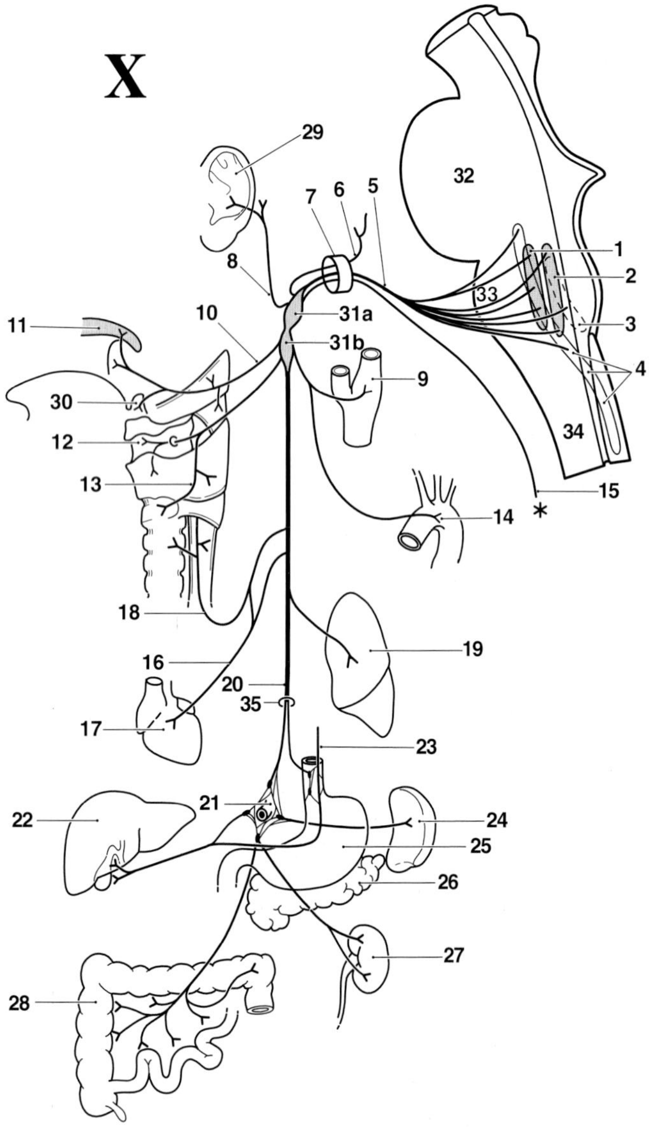

Figure 2I-10: Schematic of the vagus nerve pathway (CN-X) (*asterisk*, motor fibers from accessory nerve [CN-XI]).

1 Nucleus ambiguus (ambiguous nucleus)
2 Dorsal motor nucleus of vagus nerve
3 Nucleus solitarius (solitary nucleus)
4 Spinal nucleus of trigeminal nerve (CN-V)
5 Vagus nerve (CN-X)
6 Meningeal branch
7 Jugular foramen
8 Auricular branch
9 Carotid sinus
10 Pharyngeal branch
11 Soft palate
12 Internal laryngeal nerve
13 External laryngeal nerve
14 Aortic body
15 Cranial root of accessory nerve (CN-XI) to vagus nerve
16 Cardiac branch of vagus nerve
17 Heart
18 Recurrent laryngeal nerve
19 Lung
20 Distal right vagus nerve
21 Celiac plexus
22 Liver
23 Distal left vagus nerve
24 Spleen
25 Stomach
26 Pancreas
27 Kidney
28 Small bowel and colon through the splenic flexure
29 Auricle
30 Epiglottis
31 Superior (a) and inferior (b) sensory ganglia (somatic and visceral afferent neurons)
32 Pons
33 Medulla oblongata
34 Upper cervical spinal cord
35 Esophageal hiatus in diaphragm

THE ACCESSORY NERVE (CN-XI)

1. The accessory nerve consists of two parts: the cranial accessory and spinal accessory nerves.
2. The cranial accessory nerve consists of motor fibers supplied by the caudal part of the nucleus ambiguus in the lateral medulla oblongata.
   a. The cranial accessory nerve joins the spinal accessory nerve at the jugular foramen.
   b. After emerging from the jugular foramen, the cranial accessory nerve leaves the main trunk of the accessory nerve to join the vagus nerve (CN-X), subsequently to innervate the muscles of the larynx via the recurrent laryngeal branch of the vagus nerve.
   c. The cranial root of the accessory nerve may be considered to be aberrant fibers of the vagus nerve.
3. The spinal accessory nerve consists of motor fibers from the spinal accessory nucleus located in the dorsal–lateral aspect of the lower medulla oblongata and the upper five cervical spinal cord segments.
   a. A series of nerve rootlets join to form a single spinal accessory nerve trunk between the dorsal and ventral roots of the upper cervical nerves.
   b. The spinal accessory nerve passes upward in the spinal canal and through the foramen magnum to enter the cranium.
   c. The spinal accessory nerve then courses obliquely forward in the posterior cranial fossa to exit the cranium via the jugular foramen together with the glossopharyngeal (CN-IX) and vagus (CN-X) nerves.
   d. Extracranially, the spinal accessory nerve separates from the cranial accessory nerve to travel downward and backward through the substance of the sternocleidomastoid muscle.
   e. The spinal accessory nerve is the motor supply to two muscles of the neck: the sternocleidomastoid and trapezius muscles.

XI

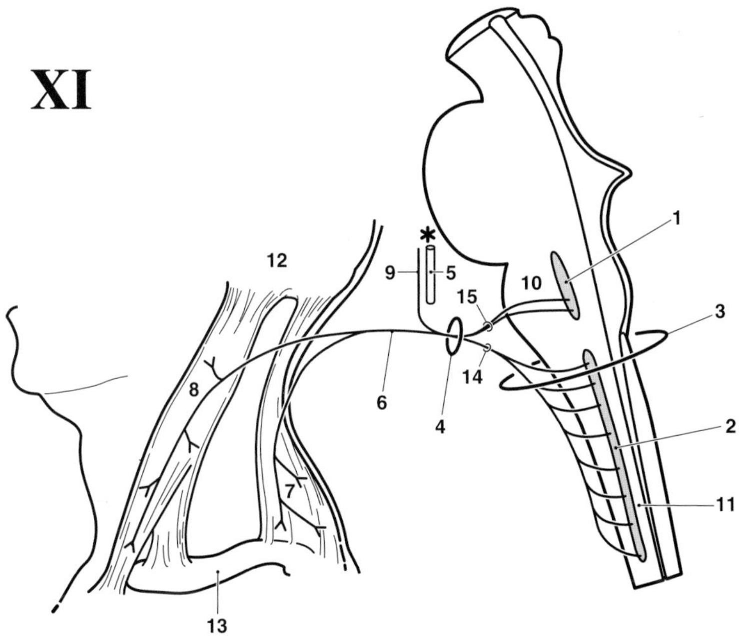

Figure 2I-11: Schematic of the accessory nerve pathway (CN-XI) on the left side. The *asterisk* indicates the place where the cranial accessory nerve leaves the spinal accessory nerve to join the vagus nerve (CN-X).

1 Nucleus ambiguus (ambiguous nucleus)
2 Spinal accessory nucleus
3 Foramen magnum
4 Jugular foramen with combined cranial and spinal accessory nerve (CN-XI)
5 Vagus nerve (CN-X)
6 Spinal accessory nerve (CN-XI) (extracranial part)
7 Trapezius muscle
8 Sternocleidomastoid muscle
9 Cranial accessory nerve (CN-XI) (extracranial part)
10 Medulla oblongata
11 Cervical spinal cord
12 Temporal and occipital bones of base of skull
13 Clavicle
14 Spinal accessory nerve (intracranial part)
15 Cranial accessory nerve (intracranial part)

THE HYPOGLOSSAL NERVE (CN-XII)

1. The hypoglossal nucleus is situated in the medulla oblongata near the midline in the floor of the fourth ventricle.
2. The hypoglossal nerve exits the brain stem as a series of rootlets anterior to the inferior olive and behind the medullary pyramid.
3. These rootlets unite to form a single hypoglossal nerve trunk, which exits the cranium through the hypoglossal canal in the occipital bone.
4. The hypoglossal nerve then descends in the neck deep to the carotid sheath to the level of the hyoid bone. There it turns forward to terminate in the body of the tongue.
5. The hypoglossal nerve provides motor fibers to intrinsic tongue muscles (longitudinal, transverse, and vertical muscles) and extrinsic tongue muscles (styloglossus, hypoglossus, and genioglossus muscles).
6. The hypoglossal nerve also receives connecting mixed sensory and motor fibers from the first and second cervical segmental spinal nerves. These connecting branches provide sensory supply to the dura of the posterior cranial fossa and motor fibers to the thyrohyoid and geniohyoid muscles and give rise to the superior root of the cervical neural plexus, called the ansa cervicalis.
7. The hypoglossal nerve also has connections proximally with the sympathetic trunk and the vagus nerve (CN-X) and distally with the lingual nerve (a branch of the mandibular [third] division of the fifth cranial nerve: CN-V3).

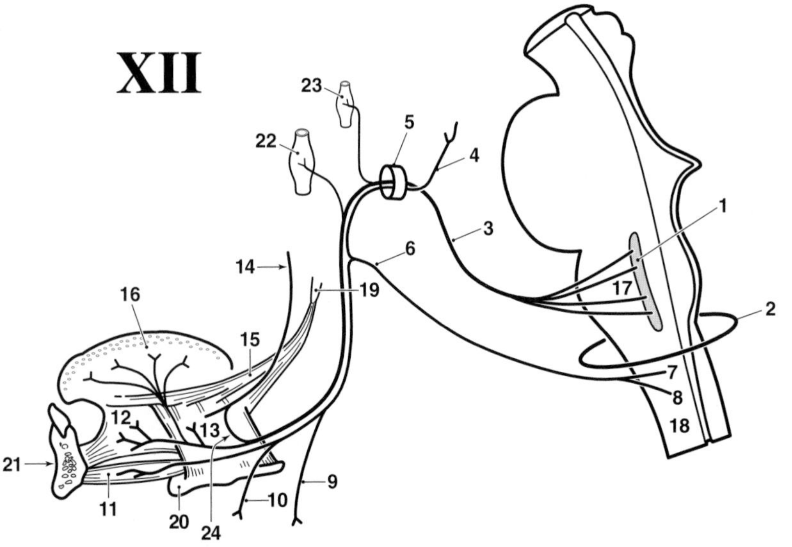

Figure 21-12: Schematic of the hypoglossal nerve pathway (CN-XII) on the left side.

1 Hypoglossal nucleus
2 Foramen magnum
3 Hypoglossal nerve (CN-XII)
4 Meningeal branch of hypoglossal nerve (CN-XII)
5 Hypoglossal canal
6 Connecting fibers from C-1 and C-2 spinal nerves
7 C-1 spinal nerve
8 C-2 spinal nerve
9 Superior neural root of ansa cervicalis
10 Neural branch serving thyrohyoid muscle
11 Geniohyoid muscle
12 Genioglossus muscle
13 Hyoglossus muscle
14 Lingual nerve
15 Styloglossus muscle
16 Intrinsic muscles of tongue
17 Medulla oblongata
18 Upper cervical spinal cord
19 Styloid process
20 Hyoid bone
21 Anterior aspect of mandible
22 Superior cervical ganglion (sympathetic)
23 Vagal (CN-X) sensory ganglion
24 Distal connection with lingual nerve

TABLE 2I-1 Summary of the Nuclei, Pathways, Exiting Cranial Apertures, and Functions of the Cranial Nerves

Cranial nerve	Type of fibers	Nucleus or structure of origin or termination	Location of nucleus	Cisternal pathway	Skull base aperture	Function
Olfactory (CN-I)	SVA	Anterior olfactory nucleus	Olfactory bulb	Olfactory groove below gyrus rectus of frontal lobe	Cribriform plate foramina	Smell
Optic (CN-II)	SSA	Lateral geniculate body	Dorsal thalamus	Enters optic canal and travels through suprasellar cistern to lateral geniculate ganglion	Optic canal	Vision
Oculomotor (CN-III)	GSE	Oculomotor nucleus	Rostral midbrain, at ventral edge of periaqueductal gray matter	Exits interpeduncular fossa of midbrain and travels through prepontine cistern to lateral wall of cavernous venous sinus	Superior orbita fissure	Motor: upper lid elevation; upward, medial, and downward globe movements
	GVE	Edinger-Westphal	Rostral midbrain, just rostral to oculomotor nucleus			Pupillary constriction accommodation
Trochlear (CN-IV)	GSE	Trochlear nucleus	Midbrain, just caudal to the oculomotor nucleus	Exits above lateral inferior colliculus, travels around midbrain in perimesence-phalic cistern and through prepontine cistern to lateral wall of cavernous sinus	Superior orbital fissure	Motor: inward torsion of globe (inward rotation) with downward lateral movement
Trigeminal (CN-V)	GSA	CN-V1: Spinal trigeminal nucleus		Exits lateral aspect of pons, travels through prepontine cistern and Mackel's cave to the trigeminal ganglion	Superior orbital fissure (ophthalmic nerve: CN-V1)	Sensory (forehead, scalp, eyelids, cornea, nose, mucous membranes of paranasal sinuses and nasal cavity)

continued

TABLE 2I-1 (continued)

Cranial nerve	Type of fibers	Nucleus or structure of origin or termination	Location of nucleus	Cisternal pathway	Skull base aperture	Function
		CN-V2: Primary sensory trigeminal nucleus	Dorsal pons, situated between middle and superior cerebellar peduncle		Foramen rotundum (maxillary nerve: CN-V2)	Sensory (cheeks, upper teeth, palate)
		CN-V2: Meshecephalic trigeminal nucleus	Dorsal pons, just dorsal to main sensory trigeminal nucleus		Foramen ovale (mandibular nerve: CN-V3)	Sensory (skin over mandible, lower teeth, mucous membranes of mouth and lower teeth)
	SVE	Trigeminal motor-nucleus	Dorsal pons just medial to main sensory trigeminal nucleus		Foramen ovale (mandibular nerve: CN-V3)	Motor: mastication
Abducens (CN-VI)	GSE	Abducens nucleus	Caudal pons, in the floor of the fourth ventricle	Exits at junction of pons and medulla (just above pyramid) and travels superiorly in prepontine cistern to enter cavernous sinus	Superior orbital fissure	Motor: temporal rotation of eyeball
Facial (CN-VII)	SVE	Facial motor nucleus	Caudal pons, ventrolateral to pontine reticular formation; fibers of facial nerve course superiorly around the abducens nucleus ("internal genu")	Exits just lateral to cranial nerve VI and travels through cerebellopontine angle cistern to the internal auditory canal	Internal auditory meatus, facial canal, stylomastoid foramen	Motor: (muscles of facial expression)
	GVE	(Superior) salivatory nucleus	Rostral medulla oblongata, dorsolateral reticular formation			Parasympathetic secretomotor (submandibular and sublingual salivary glands, lacrimal gland)

TABLE 2I-1 *(continued)*

Cranial nerve	Type of fibers	Nucleus or structure of origin or termination	Location of nucleus	Cisternal pathway	Skull base aperture	Function
	SVA	Nucleus solitarius	Rostral dorsolateral medulla, lateral to dorsal motor nucleus of vagus			Sensory (taste, anterior two-thirds of tongue)
	GSA	Principal sensory trigeminal nucleus (tactile)	Dorsal pons			Sensory (skin of auricle, external acoustic meatus)
Vestibulocochlear nerve (CN-VIII)	SSA	Cochlear nuclei (dorsal and ventral)	Caudal pons dorsolateral and lateral to inferior cerebellar peduncle	Exits lateral to cranial nerve VI and travels through cerebellopontine angle cistern to the internal auditory canal	Internal auditory meatus	Hearing (organ of Corti)
		Vestibular nuclear complex: superior–inferior, medial, and lateral vestibular nuclei	Dorsolateral caudal pons extending into rostral medulla oblongata			Equilibrium (transduces linear and angular head movements, coordinates movements)
Glossopharyngeal (CN-IX)	GVE	Inferior salivatory nucleus	Rostral medulla oblongata, dorsal lateral to reticular formation, medial to nucleus solitarius	Exits medulla between olive and inferior cerebellar peduncle and travels to pars nervosa of jugular venous bulb	Jugular foramen	Parasympathetic secretomotor (parotid gland)
	SVE	Nucleus ambiguus	Medulla oblongata ventrolateral to reticular formation, between spinal trigeminal nucleus and inferior olivary nuclei			Motor (stylopharyngeus muscle): elevation of pharynx

continued

TABLE 2I-1 *(continued)*

Cranial nerve	Type of fibers	Nucleus or structure of origin or termination	Location of nucleus	Cisternal pathway	Skull base aperture	Function
	GVA	Nucleus solitarius	Rostral dorsolateral medulla oblongata			Sensory from carotid body and carotid sinus and sensation from tongue and pharynx
	SVA	Nucleus solitarius	Rostral dorsolateral medulla oblongata			Taste of posterior one-third of tongue
	GSA	Main sensory trigeminal nucleus (tactile)	Dorsal pons			General sensation from posterior one-third of tongue
		Spinal trigeminal nucleus (thermal pain)	Pons and upper cervical spinal cord			Sensory, from external acoustic meatus and external ear
Vagus (CN-X)	GVA	Dorsal motor nucleus	Dorsal medulla oblongata in floor of the fourth ventricle	Exits medulla oblongata between inferior cerebellar peduncle and jugular bulb	Jugular foramen	Parasympathetic: innervation of thoracic and abdominal viscera
	SVE	Nucleus ambiguus	Medulla oblongata ventrolateral to reticular formation between spinal trigeminal nucleus and inferior olivary nuclei			Motor: innervation of laryngeal musculature
	GVA	Nucleus solitarius	Rostral dorsolateral medulla oblongata			Sensation from larynx, trachea, thoracic and abdominal viscera
	SVA	Nucleus solitarius	Rostral dorsolateral medulla oblongata			Taste from the epiglottis (fetus and newborn)

TABLE 2I-1 *(continued)*

Cranial nerve	Type of fibers	Nucleus or structure of origin or termination	Location of nucleus	Cisternal pathway	Skull base aperture	Function
	GSA	Main trigeminal sensory nucleus, spinal nucleus, trigeminal nerve (thermal, pain)	Dorsal pons			Sensory from skin at back of ear and in external auditory meatus
Accessory (spinal root) (CN-XI)	GSE	Spinal nucleus of accessory nerve	Anterior gray column of spinal cord	A series of cervical nerve rootlets join together and pass upward through the spinal canal and through the foramen magnum to exit the jugular foramen	Jugular foramen	Motor: head rotation (sternocleidomastoid muscle) and shoulder elevation (trapezius muscle)
Accessory (cranial root) (CN-XI)	SVE	Nucleus ambiguus	Medulla oblongata	Exits medulla oblongata between olive and inferior cerebellar peduncle and travels to pars nervosa of jugular bulb		Motor: skeletal muscle of palate and larynx
	GVA	Dorsal motor nucleus of vagus nerve	Dorsal medulla oblongata			Cardiac muscle (through myocardial branches of vagus nerve)
Hypoglossal (CN-XII)	GSE	Hypoglossal nucleus	Rostral medulla oblongata, paramedian, in floor of fourth ventricle	Exits medulla oblongata between olive and pyramid (postolivary sulcus) and travels to hypoglossal canal	Hypoglossal canal	Motor: control of tongue muscle

GSA, general somatic afferent; GVA, general visceral afferent; GSE, general somatic efferent; GVE, general visceral efferent; SSA, special somatic afferent; SVA, special visceral afferent; SVE, special visceral efferent.

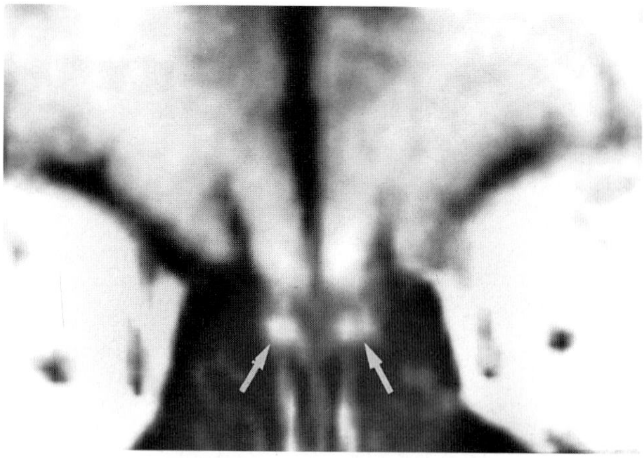

Figure 21-13A: Olfactory nerve (CN-I). Coronal T1-weighted MR image showing the olfactory tracts (*arrows*).

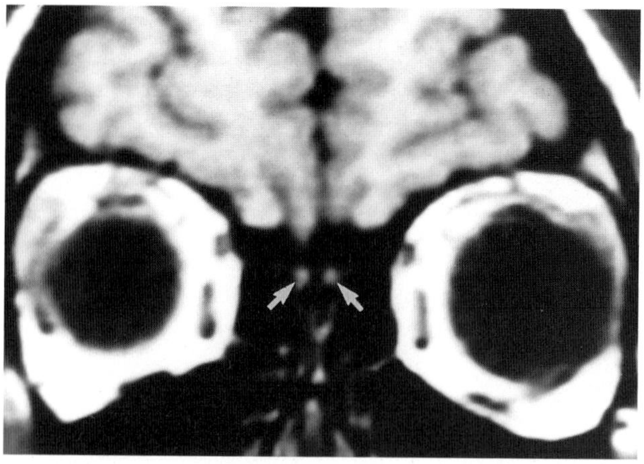

Figure 21-13B: The olfactory bulbs. Coronal T1-weighted MR image showing the olfactory bulbs (*arrows*) bilaterally.

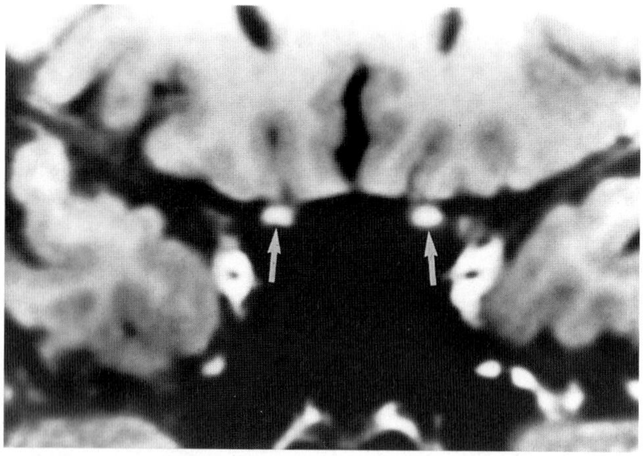

Figure 21-14A: The visual apparatus (CN-II): the cisternal segment of the optic nerves. Coronal T1-weighted MR image showing the optic nerves (*arrows*).

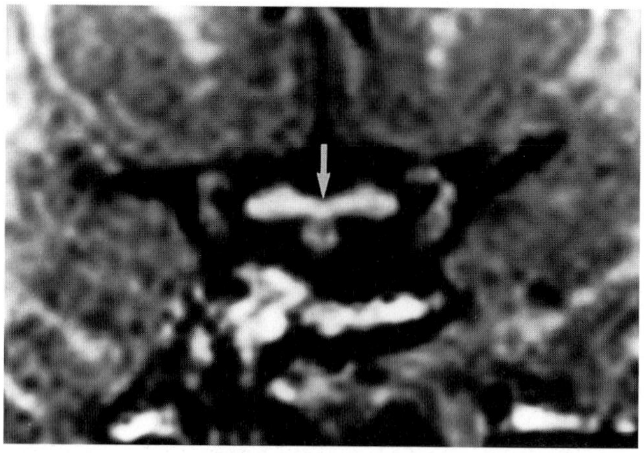

Figure 21-14B: The optic chiasm. Coronal T1-weighted MR image showing the optic chiasm.

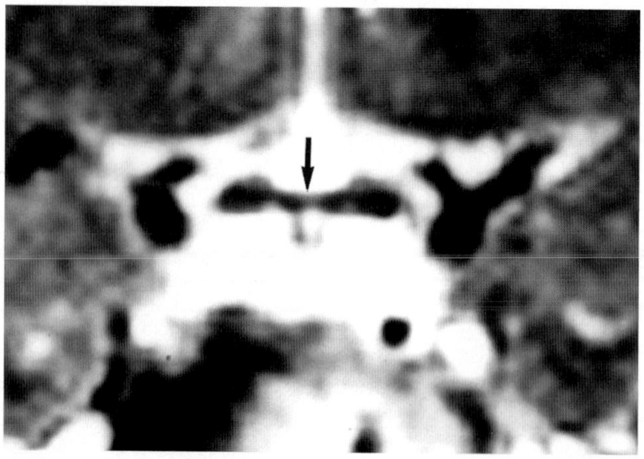

Figure 21-14C: The optic chiasm. Coronal T2-weighted MR image showing the optic chiasm (*arrow*).

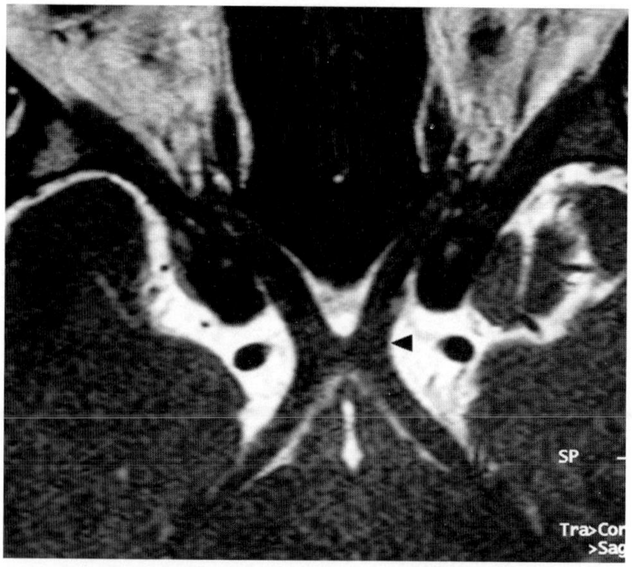

Figure 21-14D: The optic chiasm. Axial T2-weighted (three-dimensional Fourier transformation constructive interference in the steady state) MR image showing the optic chiasm (*arrowhead*) (courtesy of Indra and Tarek A. Yousry, M.D.)

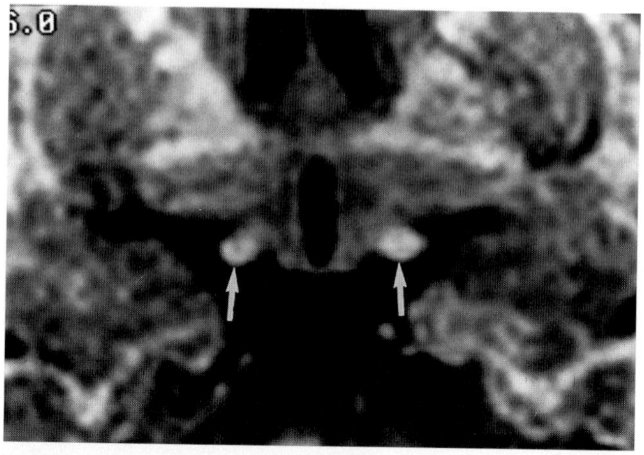

Figure 2I-14E: The optic tracts. Coronal T1-weighted MR image showing the optic tracts (*arrows*).

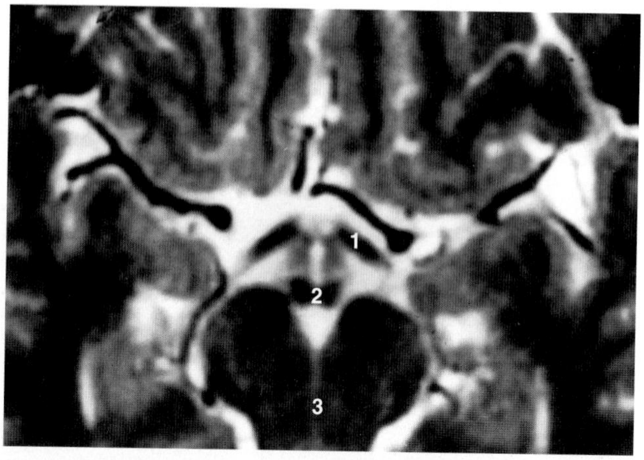

Figure 2I-14F: Magnified axial T2-weighted MR image showing the following:
1 Optic tract
2 Mammillary bodies
3 Midbrain

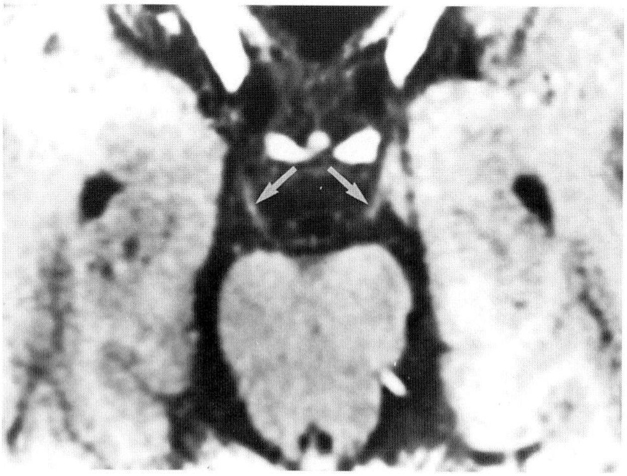

Figure 21-15A: The oculomotor nerves (CN-III). Axial T1-weighted MR image showing the oculomotor nerves (*arrows*).

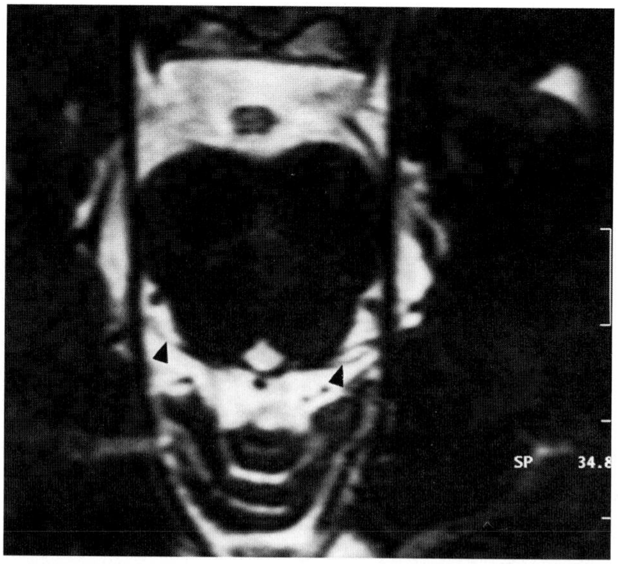

Figure 21-15B: The trochlear nerves (CN-IV). T2-weighted (three-dimensional Fourier transformation constructive interference in the steady state) MR image showing the trochlear nerves (CN-IV) (*arrowheads*) (courtesy of Indra and Tarek A. Yousry, M.D.).

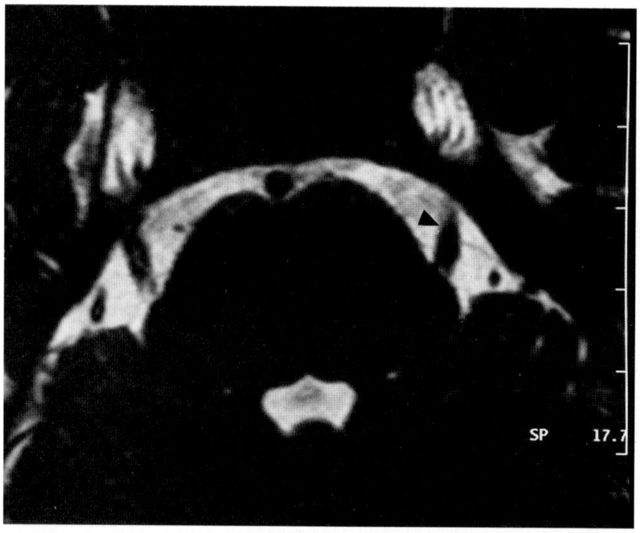

Figure 21-16A: The trigeminal nerves (CN-V). Axial T2-weighted (three-dimensional Fourier transformation constructive interference in the steady state) MR image showing the trigeminal and abducens nerves (*arrowheads*) (courtesy of Indra and Tarek A. Yousry, M.D.).

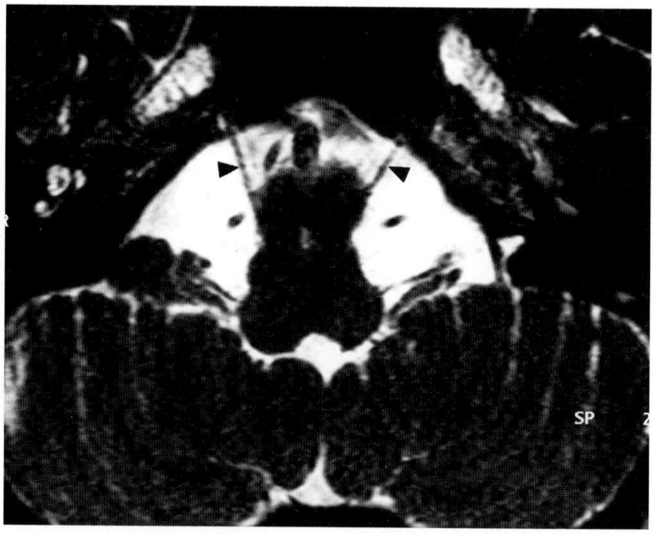

Figure 21-16B: The abducens nerves (CN-VI). Coronal T2-weighted (three-dimensional Fourier transformation constructive interference in the steady state) MR image showing the abducens nerves (*arrowheads*) (CN-VI) (courtesy of Indra and Tarek A. Yousry, M.D.).

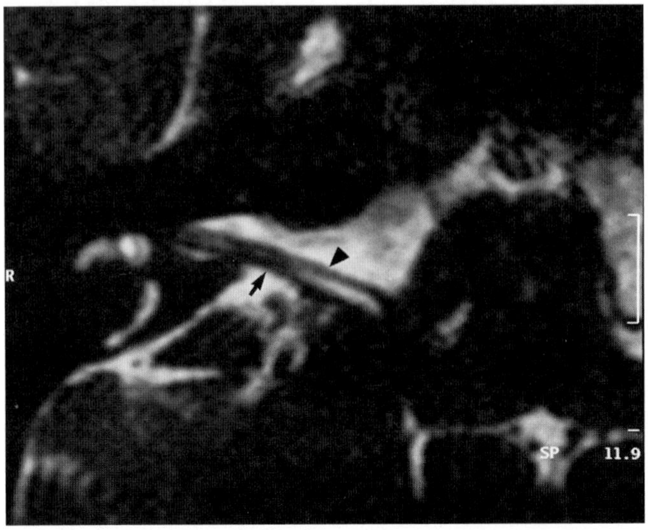

Figure 2I-17A: Facial (CN-VII) and superior vestibular (CN-VIII) nerves. Axial T2-weighted (three-dimensional Fourier transformation constructive interference in the steady state) MR image showing the facial (CN-VII: *arrowhead*) and the superior vestibular (CN-VIII: *arrow*) cranial nerves on the right side (courtesy of Indra and Tarek A. Yousry, M.D.).

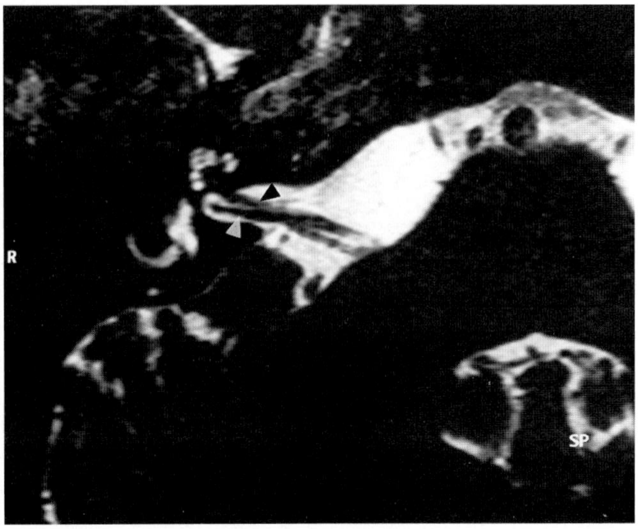

Figure 2I-17B: The cochlear and inferior vestibular nerves (CN-VIII). Axial T2-weighted (three-dimensional Fourier transformation constructive interference in the steady state) MR image with fat suppression, showing the cochlear nerve (CN-VIII: *black arrowhead*) and the inferior vestibular nerve (CN-VIII: *white arrowhead*) (courtesy of Indra and Tarek A. Yousry, M.D.).

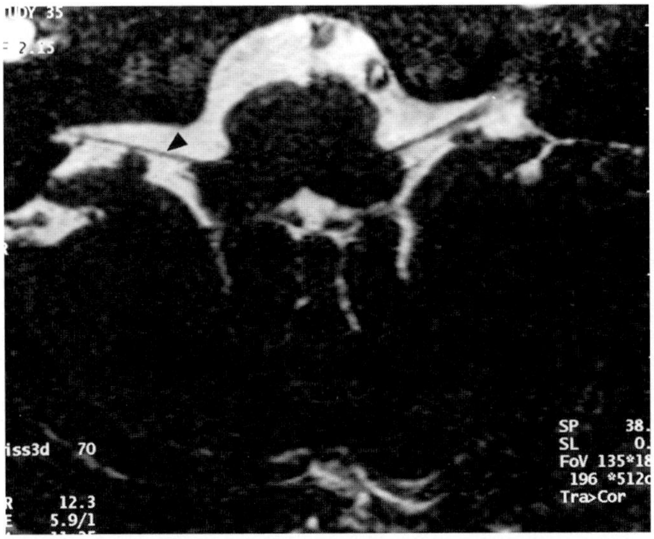

Figure 2I-18A: The remaining lower cranial nerves (CN-IX–XI). Magnified axial T2-weighted (three-dimensional Fourier transformation constructive interference in the steady state) MR image showing some of the lower cranial nerves (*arrowheads*). The glossopharyngeal (CN-IX), vagus (CN-X), and accessory (CN-XI) nerves normally cannot be distinguished from one another (courtesy of Indra and Tarek A. Yousry, M.D.).

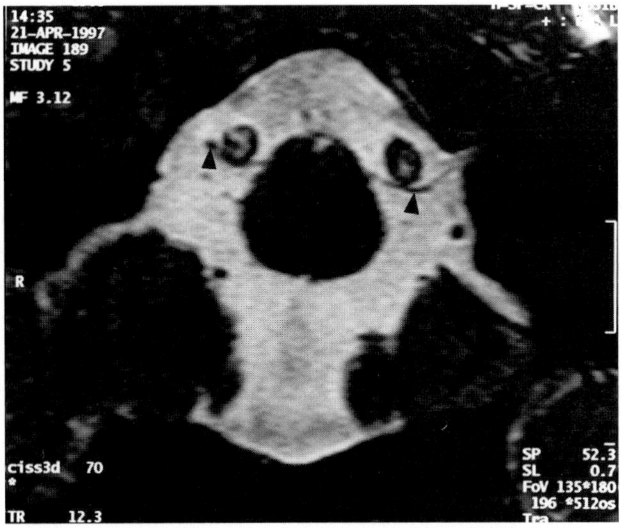

Figure 2I-18B: The hypoglossal nerves (CN-XII). Axial T2-weighted (three-dimensional Fourier transformation constructive interference in the steady state) MR image showing the hypoglossal nerves (CN-XII) (*arrowheads*) (courtesy of Indra and Tarek A. Yousry, M.D.).

THE SYMPATHETIC NEURAL SUPPLY TO THE HEAD AND NECK

1. Sympathetic neural supply to the head and neck originates from three cervical sympathetic ganglia: the superior, middle, and inferior cervical (cervicothoracic or stellate) ganglia.
2. Preganglionic sympathetic fibers come from the spinal cord primarily at the T-1 to T-4 levels, with a small contribution from the T-5 level.

The Superior Cervical Sympathetic Ganglion

1. The superior cervical sympathetic ganglion is located at the C2-3 vertebral level.
2. The superior cervical ganglion is spatially the biggest and provides the largest supply of sympathetic fibers to the head and neck.
3. The superior cervical sympathetic ganglion has the following head and neck branches.
   a. The internal carotid artery sympathetic nerve that gives rise to the proximal internal carotid artery sympathetic neural plexus
      i. The internal carotid artery plexus follows the internal carotid artery into the cranium.
      ii. The internal carotid artery plexus divides into medial and lateral branches at the level of the petrous portion of the internal carotid artery.
         - The lateral branch of the internal carotid artery sympathetic plexus is distributed along the carotid artery to form the distal internal carotid artery sympathetic neural plexus, predominantly on the lateral aspect of the artery. It supplies a) the communicating sympathetic branches to the trigeminal (CN-V) and abducens (CN-VI) cranial nerves; b) the deep petrosal nerve, which joins the greater petrosal nerve (from the facial nerve [CN-VII]) to form the nerve of the pterygoid canal (vidian nerve); this nerve passes through to the pterygopalatine ganglion without forming synapses, to supply the lacrimal gland and the mucosa of the nasal cavities, palates, and pharynx; c) the caroticotympanic nerves, which join the tympanic plexus on the promontory of the middle ear to supply the mucosa and membranes of the tympanic cavity, and small branches to the internal carotid artery itself.
         - The medial branch of the internal carotid artery sympathetic plexus forms the cavernous sympathetic neural plexus in the cavernous portion of the internal carotid artery, to supply a) the communicating branches with the oculomotor (CN-III), trochlear (CN-IV), and ophthalmic (CN-I) and abducens (CN-VI) cranial nerves; b) a branch that passes through the ciliary ganglion to supply the dilator pupillae muscle; and a branch to supply the pituitary gland and small branches to the internal carotid artery itself (carotid nervi vasorum).
         - Terminal branches of the internal carotid and cavernous sinus sympathetic neural plexi follow the anterior and middle cerebral arteries intracranially and the ophthalmic artery into the orbit. Sympathetic ramifications along these vessels are extensive.
   b. External carotid artery sympathetic neural plexus
      i. The external carotid artery sympathetic plexus consists of two to three nerves that supply sympathetic neural fibers to the common carotid artery bifurcation and the external carotid artery and its branches.
      ii. Sympathetic branches accompanying the facial artery pass through the submandibular ganglion to supply the submandibular and sublingual glands.
      iii. Sympathetic branches accompanying the middle meningeal artery pass through the otic ganglion (without synapsing) to supply the parotid gland.
      iv. Communicating sympathetic branches are present between the external carotid artery plexus and the cervical spinal nerves C-1 to C-4 (and possibly C-5) and the glossopharyngeal (CN-IX), vagus (CN-X), and hypoglossal (CN-XII) cranial nerves.

v. Pharyngeal sympathetic branches form the pharyngeal neural plexus supplying the pharyngeal mucosa.
vi. An external carotid artery sympathetic branch to the internal carotid artery plexus supplies the carotid body and carotid sinus.
vii. Terminal branches of the external carotid artery sympathetic plexus supply blood vessels of the skin, erector pilli muscles, and sweat glands of the head and neck region.

The Middle Cervical Sympathetic Ganglion

1. The middle cervical sympathetic ganglion is located at the C-6 vertebral level.
2. The middle cervical sympathetic ganglion has the following branches.
   a. Communicating branches to cervical spinal nerves C-5 and C-6.
   b. Communicating branches to the common carotid artery sympathetic neural plexus.
   c. The thyroid nerve, which forms a plexus on the surface of the inferior thyroid artery to supply the thyroid and parathyroid glands.

The Inferior Cervical (Cervicothoracic or Stellate) Sympathetic Ganglion

1. The inferior cervical sympathetic ganglion is located at the C-7 to T-1 vertebral level.
2. The inferior cervical ganglion has the following branches.
   a. There are communicating branches to cervical spinal nerves C-6 and C-8.
   b. The vertebral nerve forms a plexus accompanying the vertebral artery to supply the posterior cranial fossa. There is evidence to suggest that the vertebrobasilar vascular system is less well innervated with sympathetic fibers than is the internal carotid vascular system.

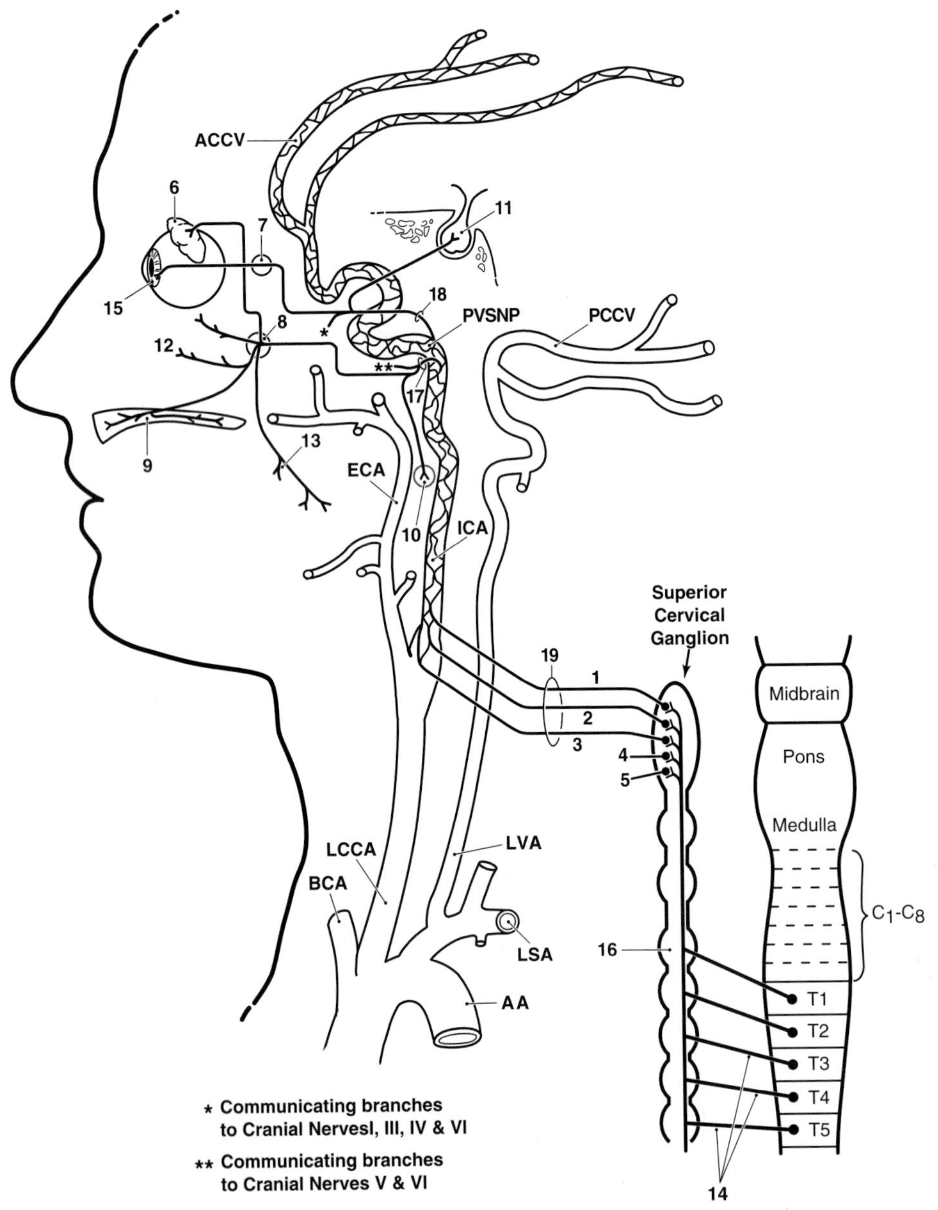

Figure 21-19A: Lateral schematic of the superior cervical sympathetic ganglion supply to the internal carotid artery sympathetic neural plexus and head and neck tissues. Note that the sympathetic fibers pass through but do not synapse within the head and neck autonomic ganglia (e.g., ciliary, pterygopalatine ganglia). *ACCV*, cerebral vessels; *PCCV*, posterior circulation cerebral vessels; *ICA*, internal carotid artery; *ECA*, external carotid artery; *BCA*, brachiocephalic artery; *LCCA*, left common carotid artery; *PVSNP*, perivascular sympathetic neural plexus; *LVA*, left vertebral artery; *LSA*, left subclavian artery; *AA*, aortic arch; *C1-8*, cervical spinal cord segments; *T1-5*, thoracic spinal cord segments.

1–5 Postganglionic sympathetic fibers arising from the superior cervical ganglion originating from T-1 to T-5 spinal cord segments
6 Lacrimal gland
7 Ciliary ganglion
8 Pterygopalatine ganglion
9 Palate
10 Tympanic plexus
11 Pituitary gland
12 Neural branches to nasal mucosa
13 Neural branches to pharyngeal mucosa
14 Thoracic white rami communicantes
15 Dilator papillae muscle (dilates pupil)
16 Sympathetic chain
17 Lateral branch of the internal carotid artery sympathetic plexus
18 Medial branch of the internal carotid artery sympathetic plexus
19 Internal carotid nerve (sympathetic postganglionic fibers)

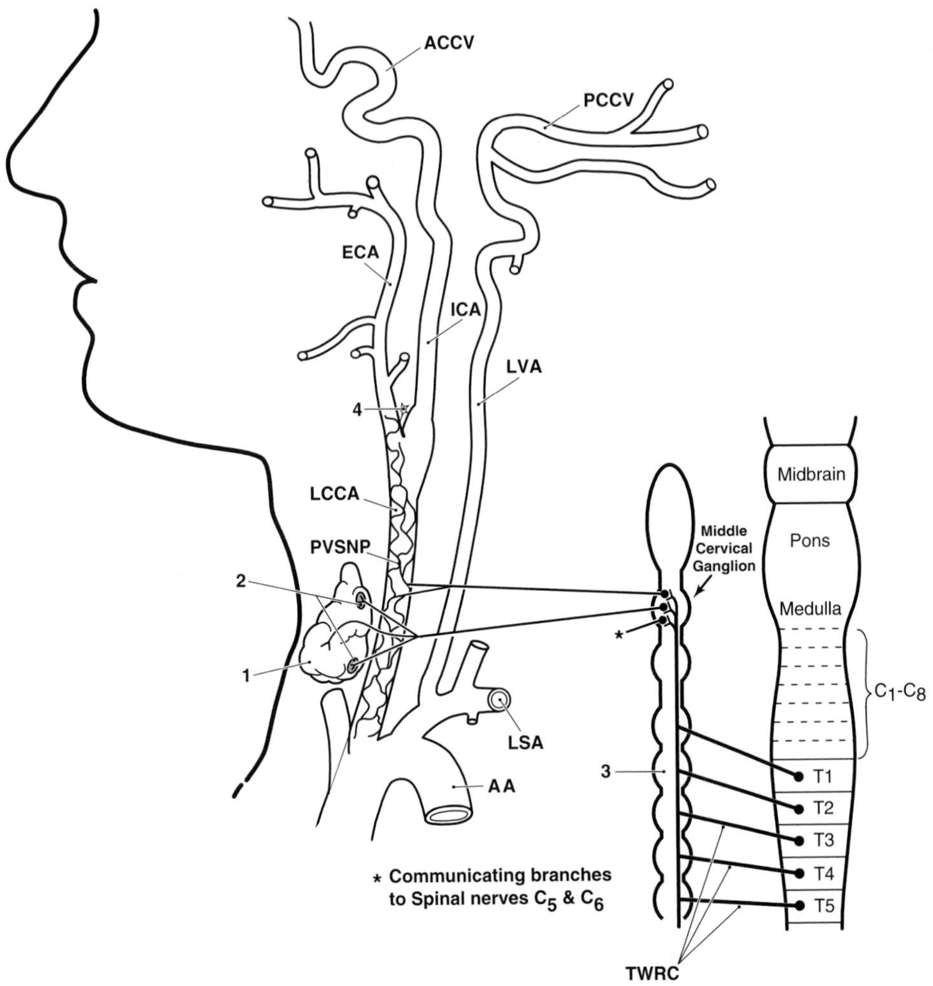

Figure 2I-19B: Lateral schematic of the middle cervical sympathetic ganglion supply to the common carotid artery sympathetic neural plexus and neck tissues. *ACCV*, anterior circulation cerebral vessels; *PCCV*, posterior circulation cerebral vessels; *ICA*, internal carotid artery; *ECA*, external carotid artery; *LCCA*, left common carotid artery; *LVA*, left vertebral artery; *LSA*, left subclavian artery; *AA*, aortic arch; *PVSNP*, perivascular sympathetic neural plexus; *TWRC*, thoracic white rami communicantes; *C1-8*, cervical spinal cord segments; *T1-5*, thoracic spinal cord segments.

1 Thyroid gland
2 Parathyroid glands
3 Sympathetic chain
4 Carotid body and sinus

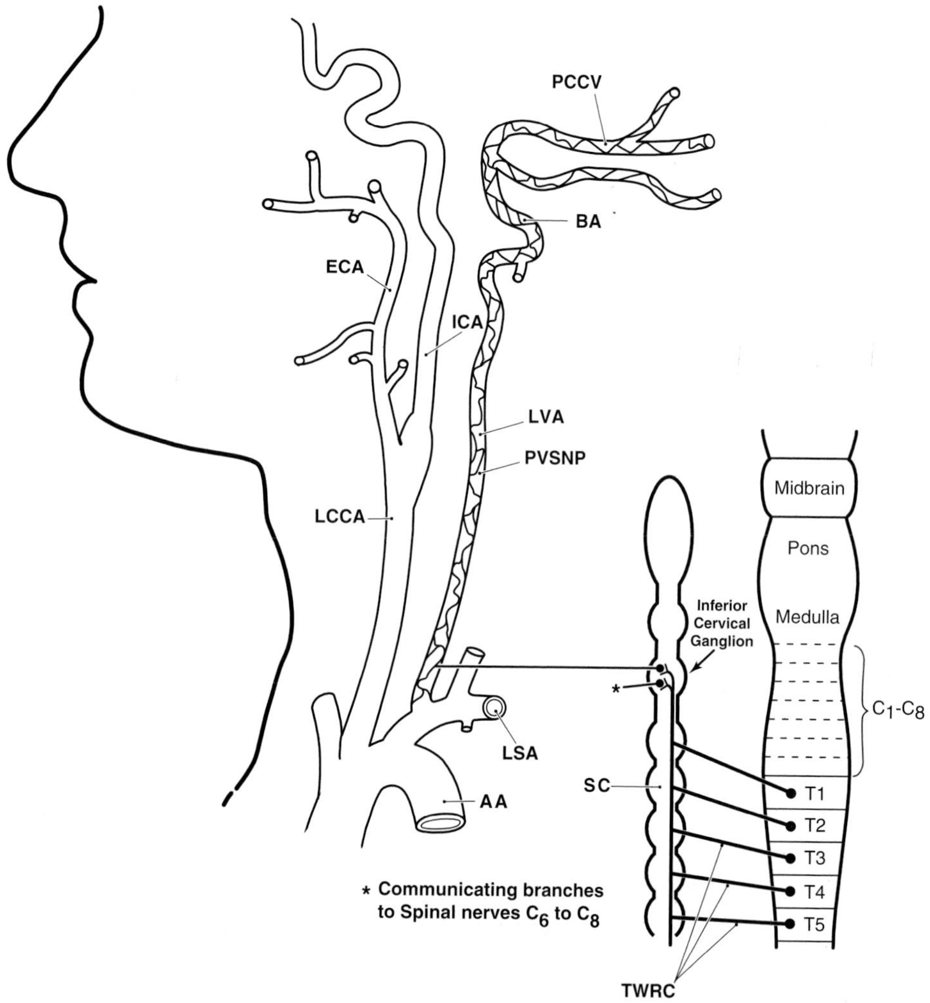

Figure 2I-19C: Lateral schematic of the inferior cervical sympathetic ganglion supply to vertebrobasilar arterial sympathetic neural plexus and neck tissues. *PCCV*, posterior circulation cerebral vessels; *ICA*, internal carotid artery; *ECA*, external carotid artery; *LCCA*, left common carotid artery; *LVA*, left vertebral artery; *LSA*, left subclavian artery; *AA*, aortic arch; *PVSNP*, perivascular sympathetic neural plexus; *TWRC*, thoracic white rami communicantes; *BA*, basilar artery; *SC*, sympathetic chain; *C1-8*, cervical spinal cord segments; *T1-5*, thoracic spinal cord segments.

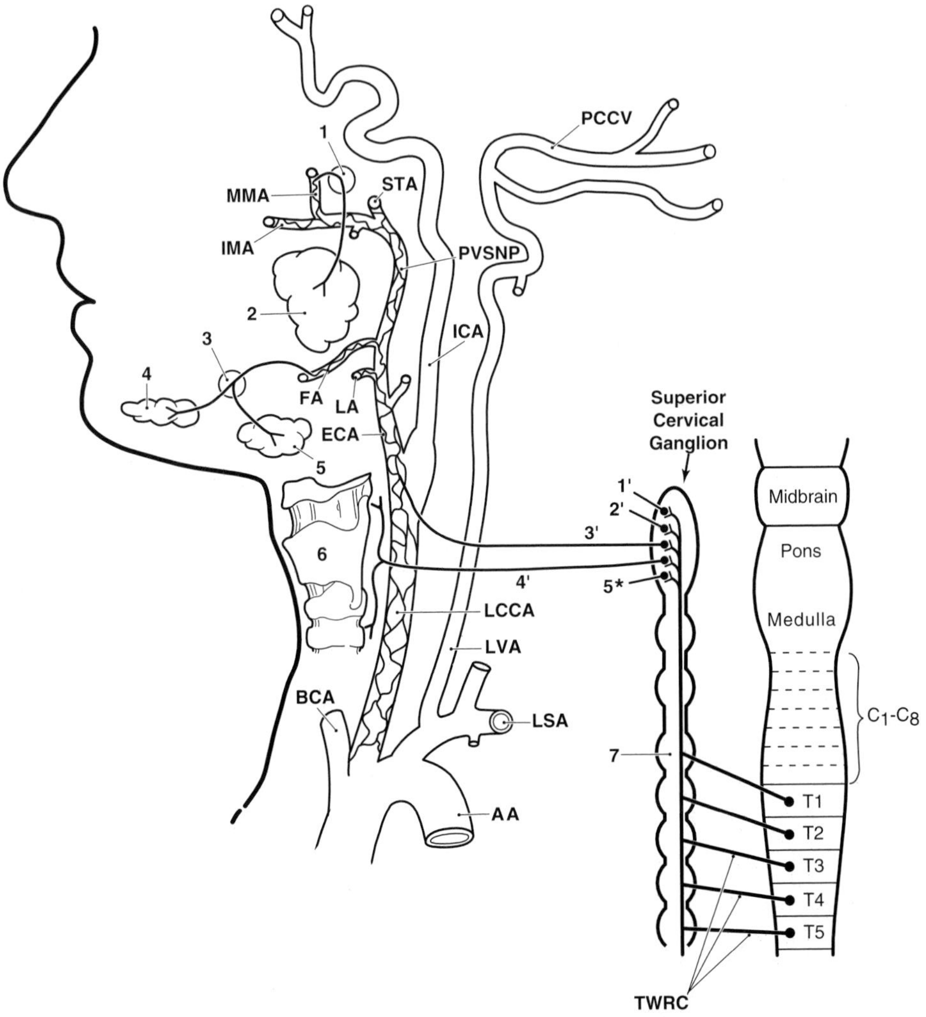

Figure 2I-19D: Lateral schematic of the superior cervical sympathetic ganglion supply to the common and external carotid artery sympathetic plexi and neck tissues. Note that the sympathetic fibers pass through but do not synapse within the head and neck autonomic ganglia (e.g., otic, submandibular ganglia). *PCCV*, posterior circulation cerebral vessels; *BCA*, brachiocephalic artery; *ICA*, internal carotid artery; *MMA*, middle meningeal artery; *ECA*, external carotid artery; *FA*, facial artery; *LCCA*, left common carotid artery; *LA*, lingual artery; *LVA*, left vertebral artery; *IMA*, internal maxillary artery; *LSA*, left subclavian artery; *STA*, superficial temporal artery; *AA*, aortic arch; *TWRC*, thoracic white rami; *PVSNP*, perivascular sympathetic neural plexus communicantes; *C1-8*, cervical spinal cord segments; *T1-5*, thoracic spinal cord segments; 1'–5', postganglionic sympathetic fibers arising from the superior cervical ganglion originating from T-1 to T-5 spinal cord segments.

1 Otic ganglion
2 Parotid gland
3 Submandibular ganglion
4 Sublingual gland
5 Submandibular gland
6 Pharynx, larynx, upper trachea
7 Sympathetic chain

THE PARASYMPATHETIC NEURAL SUPPLY TO THE HEAD AND NECK

1. There are four parasympathetic ganglia in the head and neck region, including the ciliary, pterygopalatine, otic, and submandibular parasympathetic ganglia.
2. The cranial nerves containing preganglionic parasympathetic fibers include the oculomotor (CN-III), the facial (CN-VII), the glossopharyngeal (CN-IX), and the vagus (CN-X) nerves.
3. The one cranial nerve containing postganglionic parasympathetic fibers is the trigeminal nerve (CN-V) (see later discussion of the trigeminal nerve).

Oculomotor Nerve (CN-III) Parasympathetic Supply

1. Preganglionic fibers from Edinger-Westphal nucleus in the midbrain travel with the oculomotor nerve to the ciliary ganglion.
2. Postganglionic fibers travel with the ciliary nerve of the abducens nerve (CN-VI) to supply the sphincter and ciliary muscles of eye.

Facial Nerve (CN-VII) Parasympathetic Supply

1. Preganglionic fibers from the lacrimal nucleus in the lower pons travel with the greater petrosal nerve from the facial nerve to the pterygopalatine ganglion. Postganglionic fibers then travel with branches of the maxillary nerve (CN-V2) to supply the nasal and palatal mucosal glands and with branches of the ophthalmic nerve (CN-V1) to supply the lacrimal gland.
2. Preganglionic fibers from the superior salivatory nucleus in the lower pons travel with the chorda tympani nerve of the facial nerve to synapse in the submandibular ganglion. Postganglionic fibers then travel with the lingual branch of the mandibular nerve (CN-V3) to supply the submandibular and sublingual glands.
3. There is evidence to suggest that some fibers from the facial nerve (CN-VII) also synapse in the otic ganglion to subsequently supply the parotid gland.

Glossopharyngeal Nerve (CN-IX) Parasympathetic Supply

1. Preganglionic fibers from the inferior salivatory nucleus in the lower pons travel with the glossopharyngeal nerve (tympanic and lesser petrosal branches) to reach the otic ganglion. Postganglionic fibers then travel with the auriculotemporal branch of the mandibular nerve (CN-V3) to supply the parotid gland.
2. There is evidence to suggest that some parasympathetic fibers hitchhike with branches of the facial nerve (CN-VII) to form synapses in the otic ganglion, to subsequently supply the parotid gland and, in the submandibular ganglion, to eventually supply the submandibular and sublingual glands.

Vagus Nerve (CN-X) Parasympathetic Supply

1. Preganglionic fibers from the dorsal motor nucleus of the vagus nerve travel with the vagus nerve to supply all the thoracic and abdominal viscera down to the splenic flexure of the colon.
2. The vagus nerve provides no parasympathetic supply in the head and neck region.

Trigeminal Nerve (CN-V) Parasympathetic Supply

1. The main trunk of the trigeminal nerve does not carry parasympathetic fibers as it leaves the brain stem.
2. However, the divisions of the trigeminal nerve pick up postganglionic parasympathetic fibers via its connections with the various parasympathetic ganglia.
3. The ophthalmic division (CN-V1) has connections with the ciliary ganglion, the maxillary division (CN-V2) with the pterygopalatine ganglion, and the mandibular division (CN-V3) with the submandibular and otic ganglia.

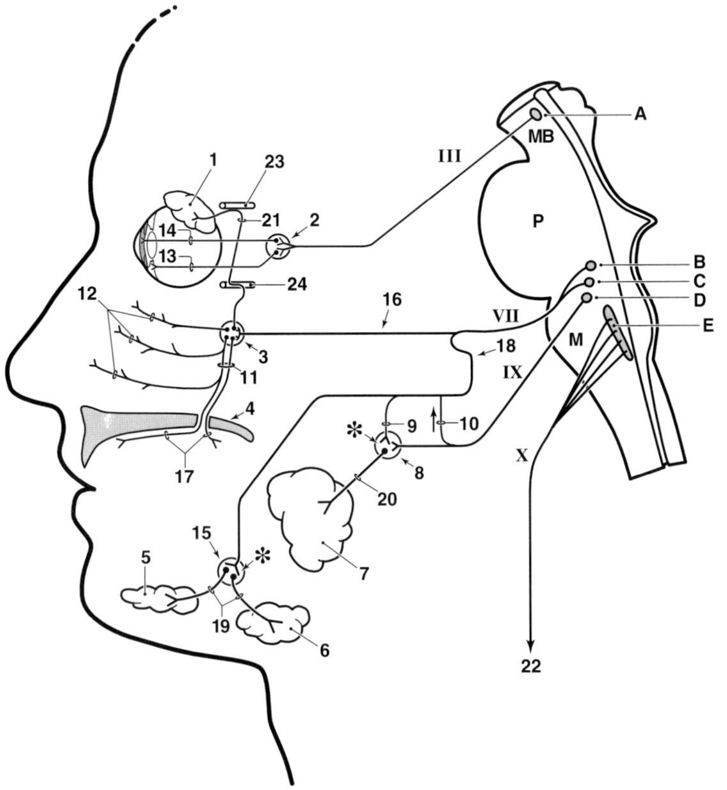

Figure 2I-20: Lateral schematic of the parasympathetic neural supply to head and neck tissues. Note that the preganglionic parasympathetic fibers do synapse within the head and neck autonomic ganglia. A: Edinger-Westphal nucleus (CN-III); B: lacrimal nucleus supplying the greater petrosal nerve (CN-VII); C: superior salivatory nucleus supplying the chorda tympani nerve (CN-VII); D: inferior salivatory nucleus (CN-IX); E: dorsal motor nucleus of the vagus nerve (CN-X). CN-III, CN-VII, CN-IX, CN-X: cranial nerves supplying paraganglionic neural fibers to the head and neck tissues. *Asterisk*, unnamed small branches of the third division of the trigeminal nerve directly transmitting postganglionic neural fibers to the submandibular and otic ganglia; *MB*, midbrain; *P*, pons; *M*, medulla oblongata.

1 Lacrimal gland
2 Ciliary ganglion
3 Pterygopalatine ganglion
4 Palate
5 Lingual gland
6 Submandibular gland
7 Parotid gland
8 Otic ganglion
9 Neural branch of the chorda tympani nerve (CN-VII) to the otic ganglion
10 Connecting neural branch of the glossopharyngeal nerve (CN-IX) to the otic and submandibular ganglia
11 Postganglionic neural branches in maxillary nerve (CN-V2)
12 Postganglionic neural branches to nasal mucosa
13 Postganglionic branch in ciliary nerve (CN-VI) to ciliary muscles of the eye
14 Postganglionic neural branch in ciliary nerve (CN-VI) to the sphincter muscles of the eye (constrictor pupillae muscle)
15 Submandibular ganglion
16 Greater petrosal nerve
17 Postganglionic neural branches to mucosa of palate
18 Chorda tympani nerve (CN-VII)
19 Postganglionic neural branches to the sublingual and submandibular glands
20 Postganglionic neural branches to the parotid gland
21 Postganglionic neural branches to the lacrimal gland
22 Peripheral distribution of vagus nerve (CN-X) (thoracic and abdominal viscera)
23 Lacrimal nerve, a branch of the ophthalmic nerve (CN-V1) transmitting hitchhiking postganglionic neural fibers
24 Maxillary nerve (CN-V1) transmitting hitchhiking postganglionic neural fibers

2J. Commissures and Association and Projection Systems of the Cerebrum

OVERVIEW

1. The projection fibers interconnect the cerebral cortex with the corpus striatum, diencephalon, brain stem, and spinal cord.
2. The association, or arcuate, fibers interconnect different cerebral cortical areas in the same hemisphere.
3. The commissural fibers interconnect the same (homotopic) or different (heterotopic) areas between the right and left cerebral hemispheres.

THE ASSOCIATION (ARCUATE) FIBERS

1. Association, or arcuate, fibers are nerve fibers that interconnect cortical regions of the same cerebral hemisphere. Collections of the fibers are often termed fasciculi.
2. The association fibers are generally classified as either short or long.
3. The short association (arcuate) fibers interconnect adjacent gyri within the same hemisphere. They may be entirely intracortical or subcortical in transit.
4. The long association (arcuate) fibers interconnect distant gyri within the same hemisphere. Several distinct groups of association fibers can be distinguished.
   a. The cingulum is a band of association fibers that interconnect the subcallosal, cingulate, and parahippocampal gyri and the adjacent temporal lobe; it forms a crucial part of the limbic system. Its main pathway is in the cingulate gyrus.
   b. The uncinate fasciculus interconnects the motor speech area and orbital gyri of the frontal lobe and the cortex in the temporal lobe. Its course is sharply curved around the stem of the Sylvian fissure.
   c. The superior longitudinal fasciculus primarily interconnects the frontal with the occipital and temporal lobes and is situated lateral to the corona radiata.
   d. The inferior longitudinal fasciculus interconnects the temporal lobe and the occipital lobe and is situated lateral to the optic radiations.
   e. The superior frontooccipital fasciculus interconnects the frontal and insular cortex with the occipital and temporal lobes, passing lateral to the lateral ventricle and medial to the fibers of the internal capsule and corpus callosum.
   f. The inferior frontooccipital fasciculus runs along the margin of the extreme capsule and interconnects the frontal cortex with the occipital lobe.

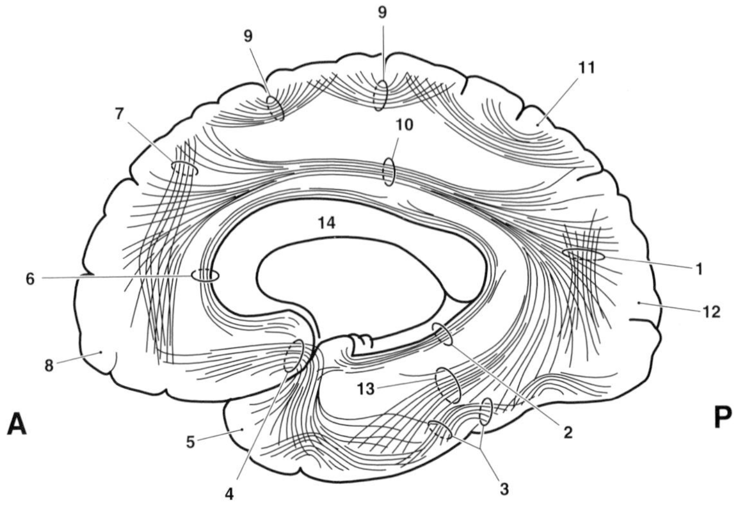

Figure 2J-1: Parasagittal schematic of a cerebral hemisphere showing some of the major association fiber pathways (fasciculi). *A*, anterior; *P*, posterior.

1 Posterior transverse fasciculi
2 Cingulum (anterosuperior aspect)
3 Inferior arcuate cascade
4 Uncinate fasciculus
5 Temporal lobe
6 Cingulum (postero-inferior aspect)
7 Anterior transverse fasciculi
8 Frontal lobe
9 Superior arcuate fasciculi
10 Superior longitudinal fasciculus
11 Parietal lobe
12 Occipital lobe
13 Inferior longitudinal fasciculus
14 Corpus callosum

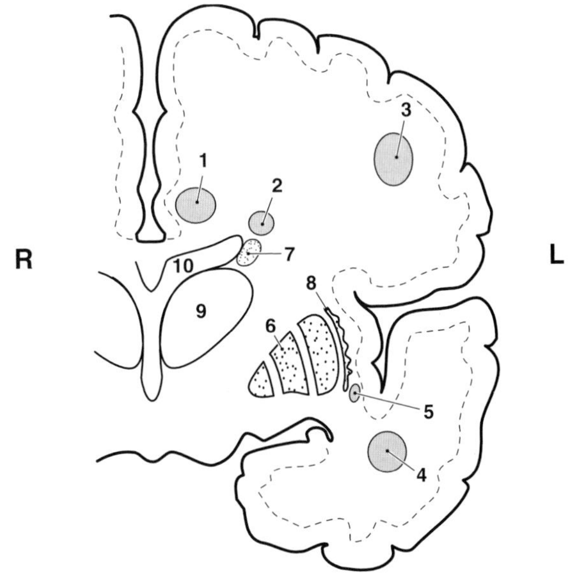

Figure 2J-2: Coronal schematic of some of the major hemispheric association fiber fasciculi on the left side. *R*, right; *L*, left.

1 Cingulum
2 Superior frontooccipital fasciculus
3 Superior longitudinal fasciculus
4 Inferior longitudinal fasciculus
5 Inferior frontooccipital fasciculus
6 Lentiform nucleus
7 Caudate nucleus
8 Claustrum
9 Thalamus
10 Lateral ventricle

THE INTERNAL, EXTERNAL, AND EXTREME CAPSULES

The Internal Capsule

1. The internal capsule fibers extend from the crus cerebri directly into the corona radiata. This structure conveys the afferent and efferent fibers, which project toward or away from the cerebral cortex. This includes the fibers of two systems.
   a. The cortical efferent motor fibers that project to the thalamus, the brain stem, and the spinal cord, which include the corticothalamic, corticopontine, corticobulbar, and corticospinal tracts
   b. The afferent thalamic peduncles, which include the thalamocortical radiation fibers to all the regions of the brain
2. Some fibers of the internal capsule are arranged into a longitudinal axis and others into a transverse axis.
3. The main longitudinal fibers of the internal capsule are those radiating to or from the cerebral cortex; they include the corticobulbar fibers, the corticospinal fibers, and the majority of the corticothalamic/thalamocortical fibers.
4. The main transverse fibers running across the internal capsule consist of the following.
   a. A minority of the corticothalamic/thalamocortical connections, including the auditory and optic radiations
   b. The fasciculus lenticularis, which arises from the inner portion of the medial segment of the globus pallidus and ultimately enters the thalamic fasciculus
   c. The subthalamic fasciculus, which projects ventrolaterally in the internal capsule to enter and end in the medial segment of the globus pallidus
   d. The connections with the claustrum and the insular cortex
5. In the axial plane, the internal capsule has an anterior limb, genu, posterior limb, and retrolentiform and sublentiform parts.
6. The internal capsule is located between the caudate nucleus, which lies anteromedially; the thalamus, which lies posteromedially; and the lentiform nucleus (globus pallidus and putamen), which lies laterally.
7. The anterior limb of the internal capsule contains the fibers of the frontopontine tract and the anterior thalamic radiation, which connects the frontal lobe with the opposite cerebellar hemisphere via the nucleus pontis (pontine nuclei). The anterior thalamic radiation also connects the medial and anterior thalamic nuclei, hypothalamic nuclei, and limbic structures with the frontal lobe.
8. The genu of the internal capsule is directed medially and contains the fibers of the corticobulbar tract projecting to the motor nuclei of the cranial nerves. The anterior part of the thalamic radiation to the cerebral cortex also passes through the genu.
9. The posterior limb of the internal capsule contains the fibers of the corticospinal tract and the corticorubral tract (pyramidal tract).
10. A retrolentiform part of the internal capsule extends caudally behind the lentiform nucleus. This area contains the parietopontine, occipitopontine, occipitocollicular, occipitotectal, and posterior thalamic radiations. The optic radiation is included, as well as connections between the occipital/parietal lobes and the pulvinar.
11. The sublentiform part of the internal capsule contains temporopontine and parietopontine fibers, the acoustic radiation, and connections between the thalamus and temporal lobe/insula.
12. The blood supply of the internal capsule:
    a. The anterior and posterior limbs of the internal capsule are normally supplied in part by the lateral lenticulostriate arteries.
    b. The medial lenticulostriate arteries supply parts of the anterior limb.
    c. The genu is usually supplied by direct unnamed branches from the internal carotid artery.
    d. The retrolentiform portion, including the optic radiation and inferior parts of the posterior limb of the internal capsule, are supplied by branches of the anterior choroidal artery.

The External Capsule

1. The external capsule is the layer of white matter lateral to the lentiform nucleus and medial to the claustrum.
2. The external capsule together with the extreme capsule connects the insula with the remainder of the cerebrum.

The Extreme Capsule

1. The extreme capsule is the layer of white matter between the claustrum and the insular cortex.
2. The extreme capsule together with the external capsule connects the insula with the remainder of the cerebrum.

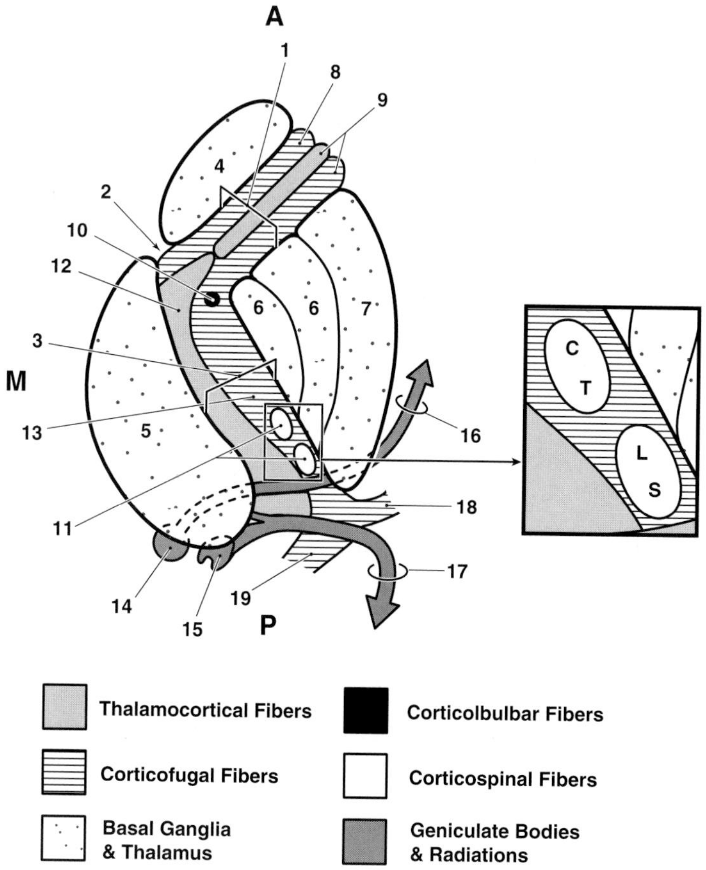

Figure 2J-3: Axial section schematic of the internal capsule at the level of the mid-thalamus and lentiform nucleus on the left side. Inset shows the general somatotopic organization of the corticospinal fibers within the caudal aspect of the posterior limb of the internal capsule. *M*, medial; *A*, anterior; *P*, posterior; *C*, cervical; *T*, thoracic; *L*, lumbar; *S*, sacral fibers of corticospinal tracts.

1 Anterior limb of internal capsule
2 Genu of internal capsule
3 Posterior limb of internal capsule
4 Head of caudate nucleus
5 Thalamus
6 Globus pallidus
7 Putamen
8 Frontopontine fibers
9 Anterior thalamic radiation
10 Corticobulbar fibers
11 Corticospinal fibers
12 Superior thalamic radiation
13 Parietopontine fibers
14 Medial geniculate body
15 Lateral geniculate body
16 Auditory radiation
17 Optic radiation
18 Tempopontine fibers
19 Occipitopontine fibers

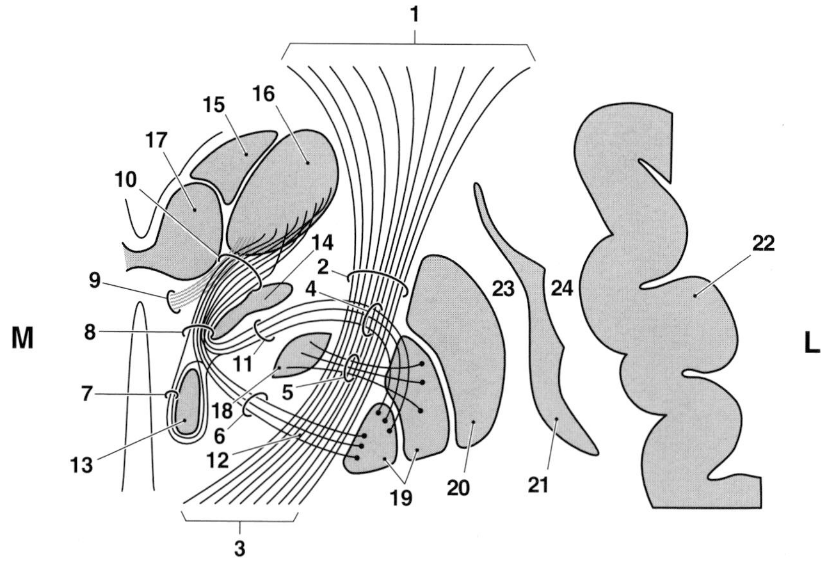

Figure 2J-4: Coronal sectional schematic of the mid-internal capsule and related structures. *M*, medial; *L*, lateral.

1 Corona radiata
2 Internal capsule
3 Crus cerebri
4 Fasciculus lenticularis
5 Fasciculus subthalamicus
6 Ansa lenticularis
7 Pallidohypothalamic fasciculus
8 Prerubral field (field H of Forel)
9 Dentothalamic, rubrothalamic, and thalamostriate fibers
10 Thalamic fasciculus (field H of Forel)
11 Field H2 of Forel (continuation)
12 Endopeduncular nucleus of the ansa lenticularis
13 Column of fornix
14 Zona incerta
15 Anterior nuclear group of thalamus
16 Lateral nuclear group of thalamus
17 Medial nuclear group of thalamus
18 Nucleus subthalamicus
19 Internal and external parts of globus pallidus
20 Putamen
21 Claustrum
22 Cortex of insula
23 External capsule
24 Extreme capsule

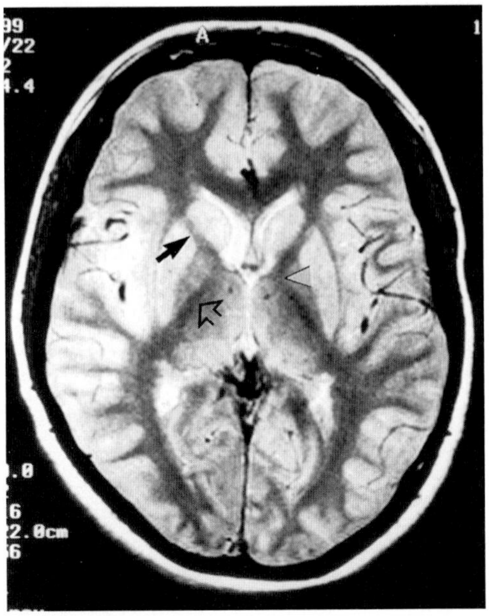

Figure 2J-5A: The internal capsule. Axial intermediate-weighted MR image showing the sectors of the internal capsule, including the anterior limb (*solid arrow*), the genu (*arrowhead*), and the posterior limb (*open arrow*).

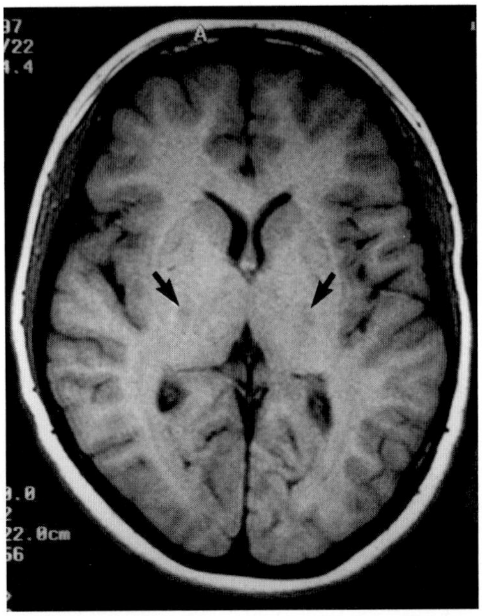

Figure 2J-5B: The internal capsule. Axial T1-weighted MR image showing the typical focal area of normal hypointensity within the distal posterior limb of the internal capsule (*arrows*).

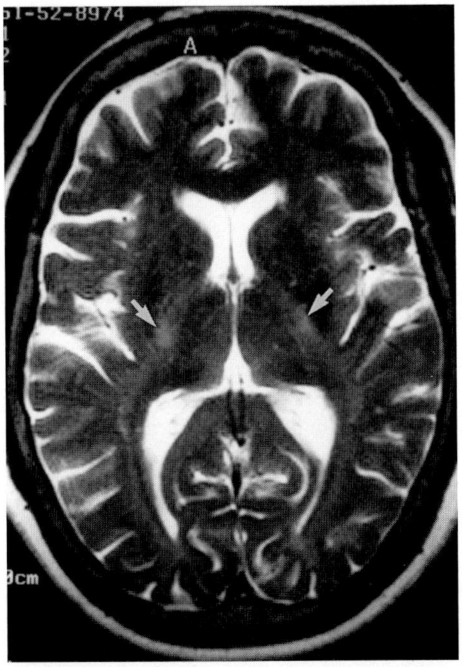

Figure 2J-5C: The internal capsule. Axial T2-weighted MR image showing that the typical area in the distal aspect of the internal capsule observed in Fig. 2J-5A is normally hyperintense (*arrows*) on this acquisition.

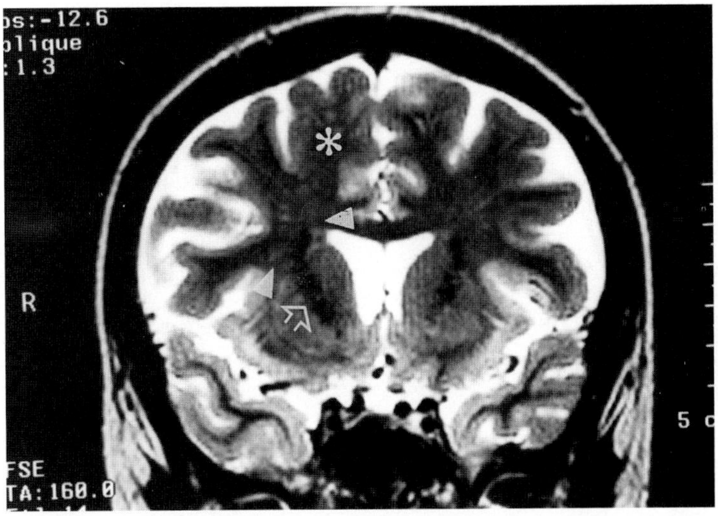

Figure 2J-5D: The internal capsule. Coronal T2-weighted MR image showing the upper extent of the internal capsule (*open arrow*), corona radiata (*arrowheads*), and centrum semiovale (*asterisk*).

THE COMMISSURAL FIBERS

1. Commissural fibers are nerve fibers that cross the midline and interconnect similar (homotopic) and occasionally dissimilar (heterotopic) regions of the two cerebral hemispheres.
2. There are four cerebral commissural groups that initially develop from the region of the anterior wall of the third ventricle: the corpus callosum, the anterior commissure, the hippocampal commissure, and the supraoptic commissures.
3. Two commissures develop in the posterior wall of the third ventricle: the posterior commissure and the habenular commissure.
4. The floor of the third ventricle contains two very small commissural bundles, the subthalamic and hypothalamic commissures.

The Corpus Callosum

1. The corpus callosum is the largest of all the cerebral commissures.
2. The corpus callosum interconnects parts of the frontal, parietal, temporal, and occipital lobes.
3. The corpus callosum consists of four parts.
   a. Genu of the corpus collosum: knee-shaped anterior extent, connecting the lateral and medial surfaces of the frontal lobes
   b. Splenium: bulbous posterior extent, connecting the occipital lobes
   c. Body of the corpus collosum: the region extending between the genu and the splenium, connecting wide neocortical regions of the cerebral hemispheres
   d. Rostrum of the corpus collosum: the thin ventral tapering portion extending from the genu to the lamina terminalis, connecting the orbital surfaces of the frontal lobes
      i. The genu together with the fibers interconnecting the frontal lobes form the forceps minor.
      ii. The splenium together with the fibers interconnecting the occipital lobes form the forceps major.
      iii. Some of the fibers from the body and splenium of the corpus callosum that cover the roofs of the lateral ventricle further extend to cover the lateral aspect of the temporal horns of the lateral ventricles on each side, thereby forming the tapetum.
      iv. Several structures are intimately related to the corpus callosum.
         - The indusium grisium is a thin layer of neurons covering the superior surface of the corpus callosum. Traversing the indusium grisium are two pairs of longitudinal bundles of fibers, the medial and lateral longitudinal striae. These structures are continuous anteriorly with the paraterminal gyrus and posteriorly through the gyrus fasciolaris with the dentate gyrus and hippocampus.
         - The crura and columns of the paired fornices underlie the inferior surface of the splenium and body of the corpus callosum.

The Anterior Commissure

1. The anterior commissure is located rostral to the foramina of Monro and the columns of the fornix. It is embedded in the lamina terminalis.
2. The fibers of the anterior commissure pass through the globus pallidus.
3. The smaller anterior portion or bundle of the anterior commissure interconnects olfactory structures, whereas the larger posterior portion or bundle of the anterior commisure interconnects the temporal lobes and a small portion of the frontal lobes.

The Hippocampal Commissure (Forniceal Commissure, or Psalterium)

1. The hippocampal commissure interconnects the hippocampal formation of both sides.
2. The hippocampal commissure fibers pass from the crus of one fornix to the opposite fornix beneath the posterior part of the body of the corpus callosum.

The Supraoptic Commissures

Three small commissural bundles are found immediately dorsal to the optic chiasm in the anterior wall of the third ventricle.

1. The anterior hypothalamic commissure of Ganser interconnects the gray matter around the third ventricle and the subthalamic region.
2. The dorsal supraoptic commissure of Meynert interconnects the subthalamic nuclei, the lateral geniculate bodies, the superior colliculi of the quadrigeminal plate, and the globus pallidus.
3. The ventral supraoptic commissure of Gudden interconnects the medial geniculate bodies.

The Posterior Commissure

1. Located immediately below the stalk of the pineal gland, the posterior commissure forms the roof of the cerebral aqueduct and anchors the ventral lip of the third ventricular pineal recess.
2. The posterior commissure interconnects the pretectal nuclei, superior colliculi, tectal nuclei, habenular nuclei, dorsal thalamic nuclei, and posterior commissural nuclei. The latter include the interstitial nuclei of the posterior commissure, the dorsal nuclei of the posterior commissure, the nucleus of Darkschewitsch, and the interstitial nucleus of Cajal.

The Habenular Commissure

1. The habenular commissure forms part of the posterosuperior wall of the third ventricle and anchors the dorsal lip of the third ventricular pineal recess.
2. The habenular commissure interconnects the bilateral habenular nuclei of the epithalamus, the amygdaloid nuclear complexes, and the hippocampal cortices; crossed tectohabenular fibers also traverse this commissure.

The Subthalamic and Hypothalamic Commissures

The subthalamic and hypothalamic commissures interconnect the subthalamic and hypothalamic nuclei of both sides.

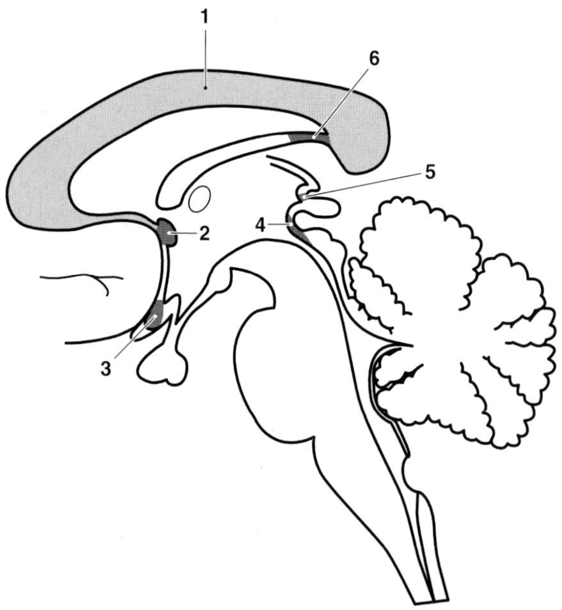

Figure 2J-6: Sagittal and coronal schematics of the commissures.
1 Corpus callosum
2 Anterior commissure
3 Optic chiasm
4 Posterior commissure
5 Habenular commissure
6 Hippocampal commissure (psalterium)

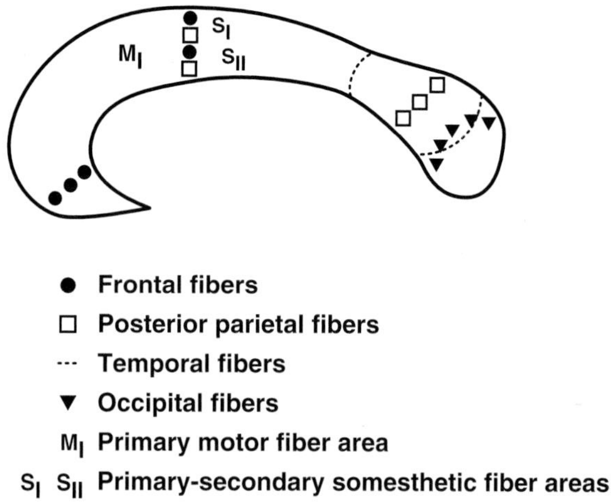

Figure 2J-7: Midline sagittal schematic of the hemispheric representation of the corpus callosum (fibers denoted inclusive between geometric symbols or at the point of the following symbols: M_I, S_I, S_{II}).

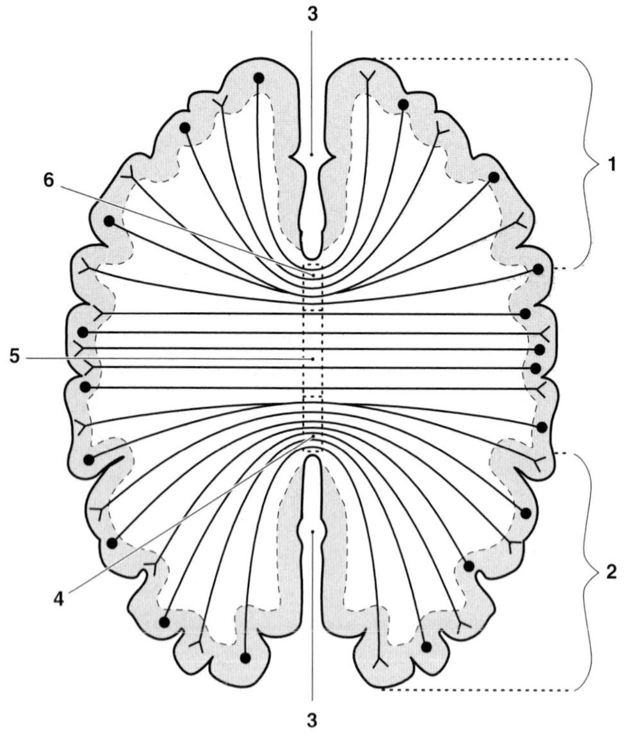

Figure 2J-8: Axial cross section schematic through the cerebral hemisphere and body of the corpus callosum, showing the general pattern of the distribution of homotropic callosal nerve fibers.
1 Forceps minor (anterior forceps)
2 Forceps major (posterior forceps)
3 Interhemispheric fissure
4 Splenium of corpus callosum
5 Body of corpus callosum
6 Genu of corpus callosum

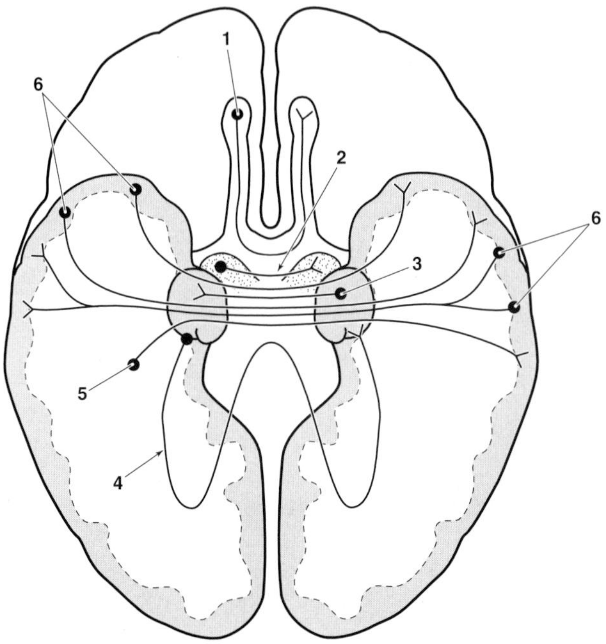

Figure 2J-9: Axial cross section schematic of the cerebral hemispheres inferiorly, showing the pattern of distribution of the fibers of the anterior commissure.
1 Interbulbar component
2 Intertubercular components (anterior interperforated substance)
3 Interamygdaloid component
4 Stria terminalis ("long" interamygdaloid component)
5 Interparahippocampal gyrus component
6 Ectocortical component

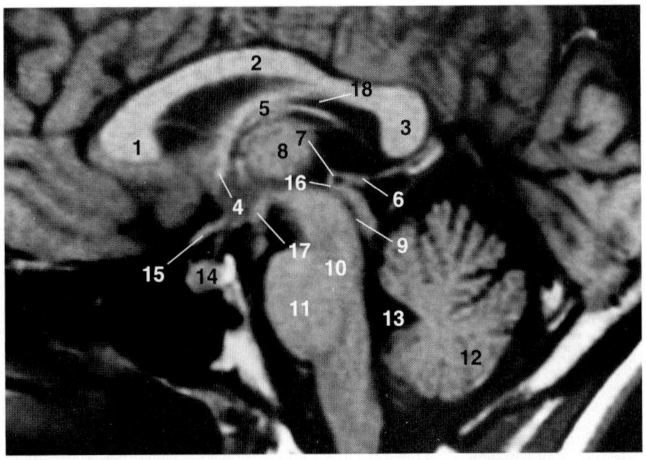

Figure 2J-10A: The cerebral commissures. Sagittal T1-weighted MR image of the cerebral commissures and surrounding structures.
1 Genu of corpus callosum
2 Body of corpus callosum
3 Splenium of corpus callosum
4 Anterior commissure
5 Fornix
6 Pineal gland
7 Habenular commissure
8 Thalamus
9 Cerebral aqueduct
10 Midbrain
11 Pons
12 Cerebellum
13 Fourth ventricle
14 Pituitary gland
15 Optic chiasm
16 Posterior commissure
17 Mammillary body
18 Posterior body of fornix

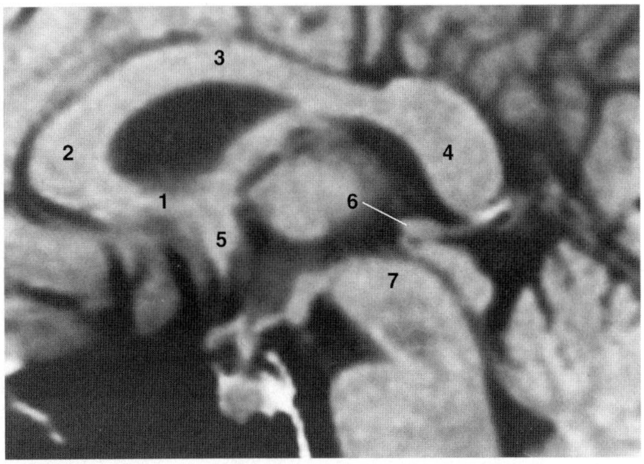

Figure 2J-10B: The cerebral commissures. Magnified sagittal midline T1-weighted MR image shows the following.
1 Rostrum of the corpus callosum
2 Genu
3 Body
4 Splenium of the corpus callosum
5 Anterior commissure
6 Habenular commissure
7 Posterior commissure

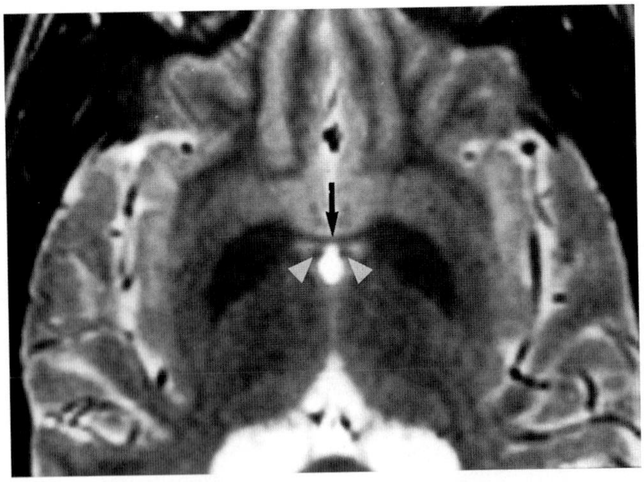

Figure 2J-10C: The cerebral commissures. Axial midline section of the anterior commissure (*arrows*). The anterior columns of the fornices are also identified (*arrowheads*).

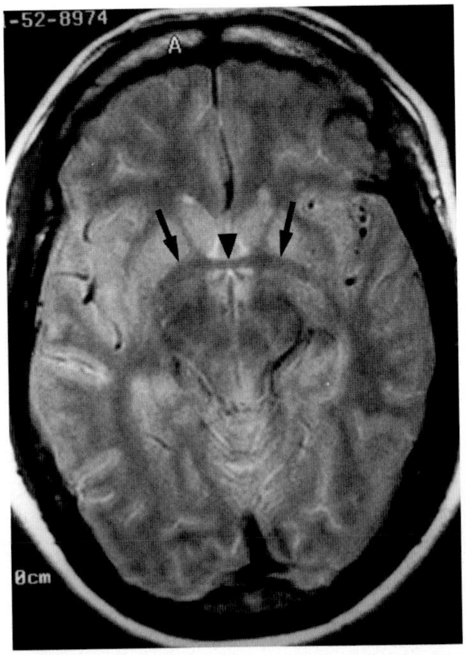

Figure 2J-10D: The cerebral commissures. Axial intermediate-weighted MR image showing the anterior commissure (*arrows*) crossing the midline (*arrowhead*).

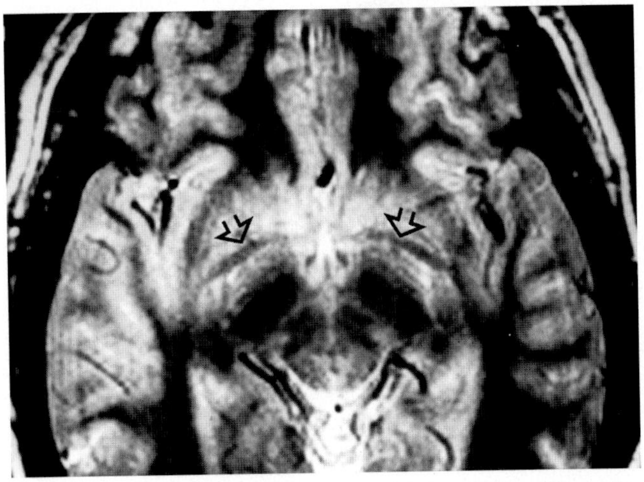

Figure 2J-10E: The cerebral commissures. Axial T2-weighted MR image showing the lateral extension of the anterior commissure (*arrows*).

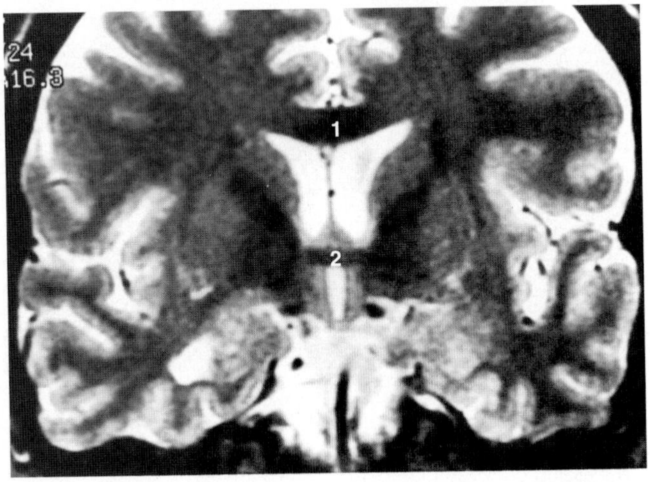

Figure 2J-10F: The cerebral commissures. Coronal T2-weighted MR image showing the corpus callosum and midline anterior commissure.

1 Corpus callosum
2 Anterior commissure

CEREBRAL COMMISSURE VARIANTS

Normal variations in commissural size

- Agenesis/hypogenesis of corpus collosum
- Hypoplastic corpus callosum, anterior commissure
- Hypertrophic corpus callosum, anterior commissure
- Agenesis, hypogenesis, hypoplasia, or hypertrophy of other cerebral commissures (theoretical)

Commissural calcification

- Habenular commissure calcification

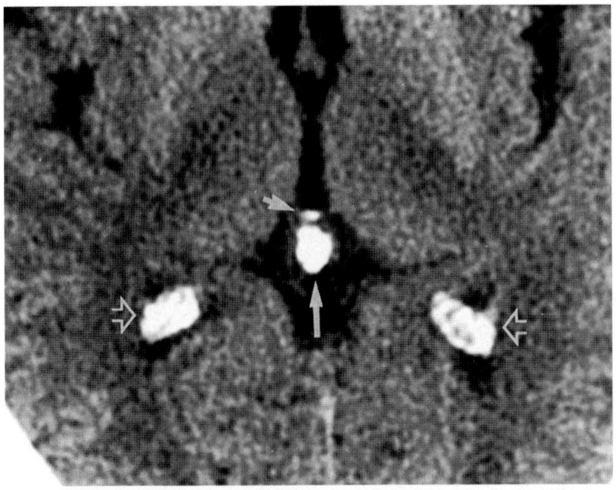

Figure 2J-11A: Habenular commissure calcification. Unenhanced axial CT image showing pineal calcification (*long arrow*), habenular commissure calcification (*short arrow*), and choroid plexus calcification (*open arrows*).

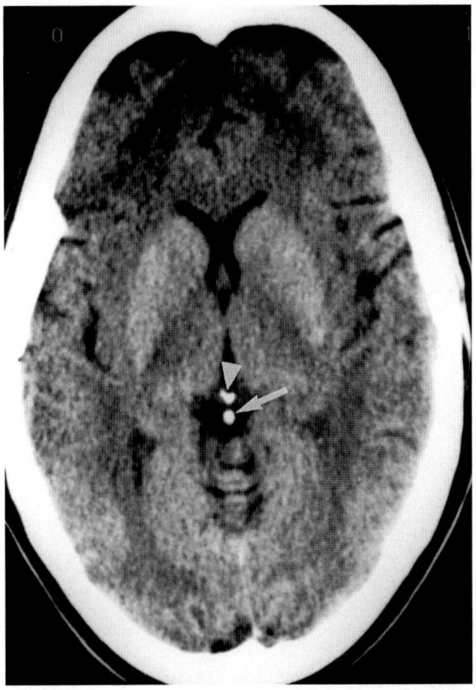

Figure 2J-11B: Habenular commissure calcification. Pineal/habenular commissure calcifications. Axial CT showing calcification of the pineal gland (*arrow*) and the adjacent habenular commissure (*arrowhead*).

2K. Cerebral Ventricular System, Choroid Plexi, and Arachnoid Granulations

THE CEREBRAL VENTRICULAR SYSTEM

1. The cerebrospinal fluid (CSF)–filled cerebral ventricular system comprises the ependymally lined paired lateral ventricles communicating via the foramina of Monro with the unpaired midline third and the fourth ventricles, which, in turn, are joined together by the cerebral aqueduct of Sylvius.
2. The C shape of the lateral ventricle is a result of the phylogenetic expansion of the human brain, causing the developmental displacement of the temporal lobe anteroinferiorly in relationship to the remainder of the brain (frontal, parietal, occipital lobes).

The Lateral Ventricles

1. The paired lateral ventricles consist of an anterior horn, body, occipital horn, and temporal horn. The triangular area where the body, occipital horn, and temporal horn join is termed the atrium, or collateral trigone.
2. The bodies of the lateral ventricles are separated by the paired septi pellucidi. The paired septi pellucidi may harbor a CSF-containing space, the cavum septi pellucidi anteriorly, and its posterior extent, the cavum vergae.
3. The choroid plexus of the lateral ventricle is located anteromedially in the body and superiomedially in the temporal horn; the two are continuous through the atrium, which also contains a large component of the plexus. The anterior horn and occipital horn do not contain elements of the choroid plexus.
4. The lateral ventricles communicate with the third ventricles via the paired foramina of Monro at the junction of the anterior horn and body of the lateral ventricles inferiorly. The choroid plexus of each lateral ventricle extends through the foramen of Monro on both sides to directly join the choroid plexus in the roof of the third ventricle.

The Third Ventricle

1. The borders of the third ventricle include the hypothalamus inferiorly, the thalami laterally, the lamina terminalis anteriorly, the midbrain tegmentum posteriorly, and the choroidal fissure and choroid plexus of the third ventricle superiorly .
2. In the sagittal plane, several recesses of the third ventricle are visible, including the preoptic recess adjacent to the optic chiasm, the infundibular recess extending into the base of the pituitary infundibulum, the suprapineal recess above the pineal gland, and the pineal recess ending in the base of the pineal gland.
3. The third ventricle communicates with the fourth ventricle via the cerebral aqueduct of Sylvius.
4. A band of tissue principally composed of gray matter, the interthalamic adhesion (massa intermedia), joins the two dorsal thalami across the midline traversing the cavity of the third ventricle. While the two cerebral hemispheres are joined at the midline at the massa intermedia, few, if any, axons cross the midline to connect areas between the two thalami. The massa intermedia is absent in 25% to 30% of cases; when present, it forms the medial central nucleus of the thalamus.
5. The area beneath the roof of the third ventricle may harbor a CSF-containing space, the cavum velum interpositum.

The Cerebral Aqueduct of Sylvius

1. The cerebral aqueduct links the third and fourth ventricles.
2. The cerebral aqueduct traverses the midbrain.

The Fourth Ventricle

1. The roof of the fourth ventricle is formed by the combination of the superior medullary velum and the inferior medullary velum joined at the posteriorly directed apex, the fastigium.
2. The floor of the fourth ventricle, or rhomboid fossa, is composed of the caudal midbrain, the pons, and the medulla oblongata. The floor has a midline median sulcus dividing the floor into two halves; each half, in turn, is divided by the sulcus limitans into two parts, the medial eminence and the vestibular area.
3. The tela choroidea in the inferior medullary velum gives rise to the choroid plexus of the fourth ventricle. This choroid plexus extends directly through the paired lateral apertures of the fourth ventricle, the foramina of Luschka, into the basal subarachnoid cisterns. The single midline fourth ventricle aperture, the foramen of Magendie, does not transmit choroid plexus.
4. The foramina of Luschka and Magendie communicate directly with the basal subarachnoid cisterns.
5. The obex is the apex of the inferior termination of the fourth ventricle at the cranial end of the central canal of the spinal cord. The obex forms the barrier between the CSF-filled space of the ventricular system and the potential space of the central canal of the spinal cord.

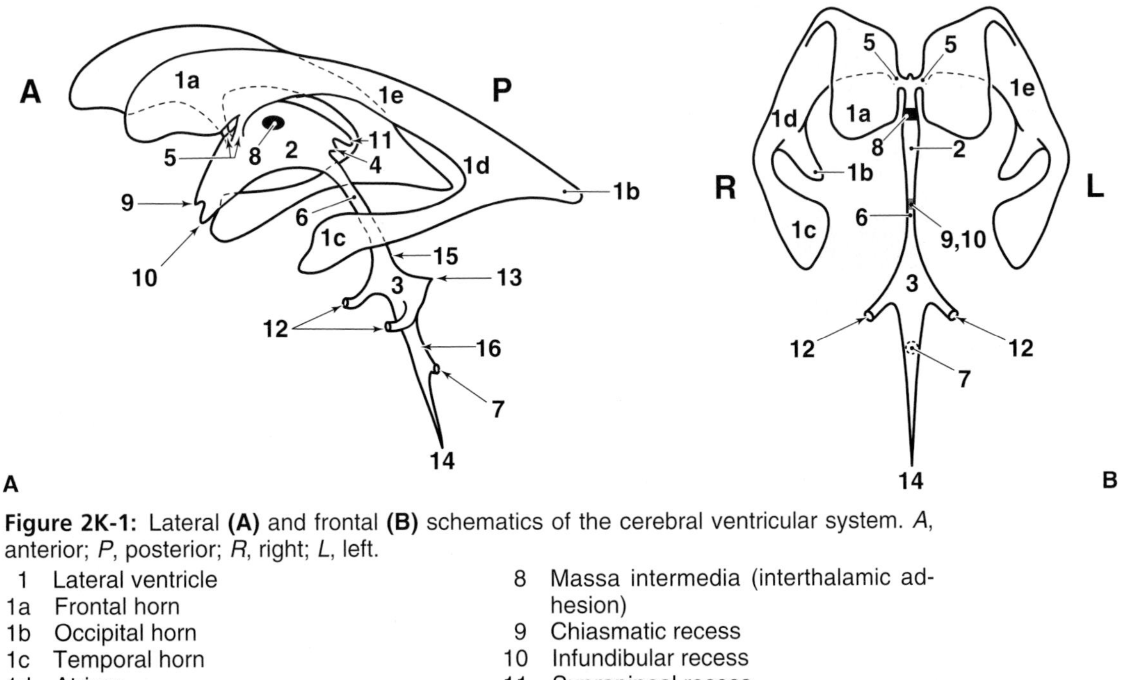

Figure 2K-1: Lateral **(A)** and frontal **(B)** schematics of the cerebral ventricular system. *A*, anterior; *P*, posterior; *R*, right; *L*, left.

1 Lateral ventricle
1a Frontal horn
1b Occipital horn
1c Temporal horn
1d Atrium
1e Body
2 Third ventricle
3 Fourth ventricle
4 Pineal recess
5 Foramina of Monro
6 Cerebral aqueduct of Sylvius
7 Foramen of Magendie
8 Massa intermedia (interthalamic adhesion)
9 Chiasmatic recess
10 Infundibular recess
11 Suprapineal recess
12 Foramina of Luschka
13 Fastigium
14 Obex
15 Superior medullary velum
16 Inferior medullary velum

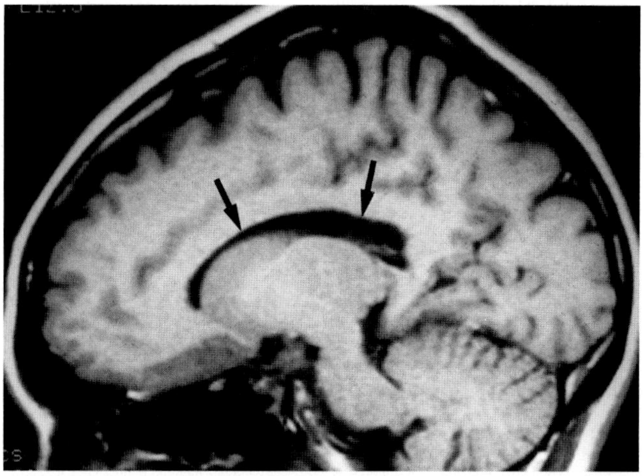

Figure 2K-2A: The lateral ventricles. Sagittal T1-weighted MR image showing the body of the lateral ventricle (*arrows*).

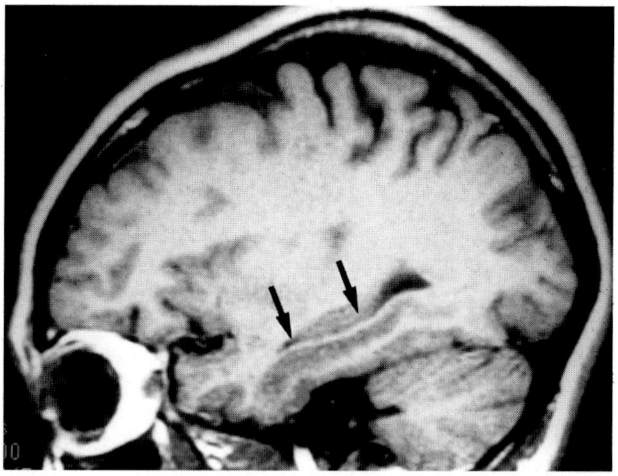

Figure 2K-2B: The temporal horn of the lateral ventricle. Sagittal T1-weighted MR image showing the temporal horn (*arrows*) of the lateral ventricle.

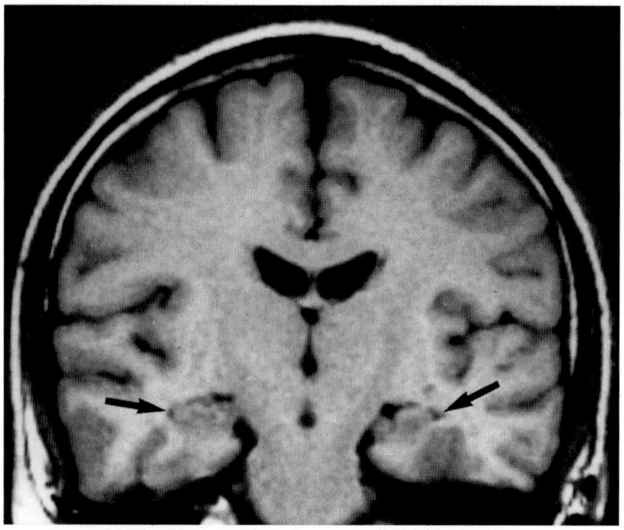

Figure 2K-2C: The temporal horns of the lateral ventricles. Axial T1-weighted MR image showing the typically "collapsed" temporal horns (*arrows*) of the lateral ventricles.

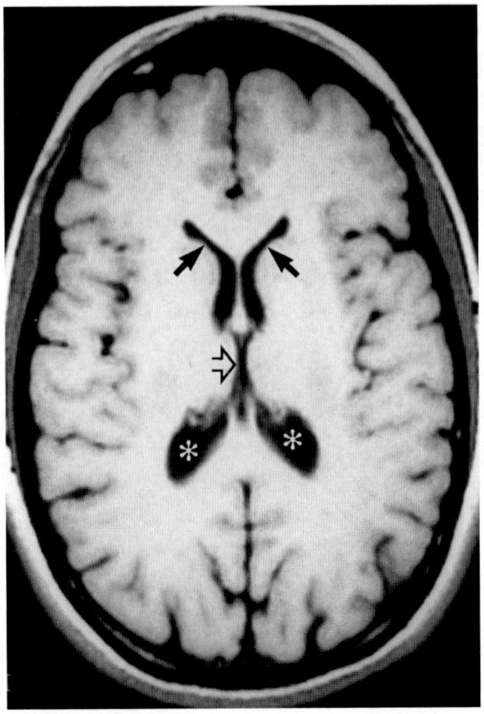

Figure 2K-2D: The lateral and third ventricles. Axial T1-weighted MR image showing the anterior horns (*solid arrows*) and atria (*asterisks*) of the lateral ventricles and the midline third ventricle (*open arrow*).

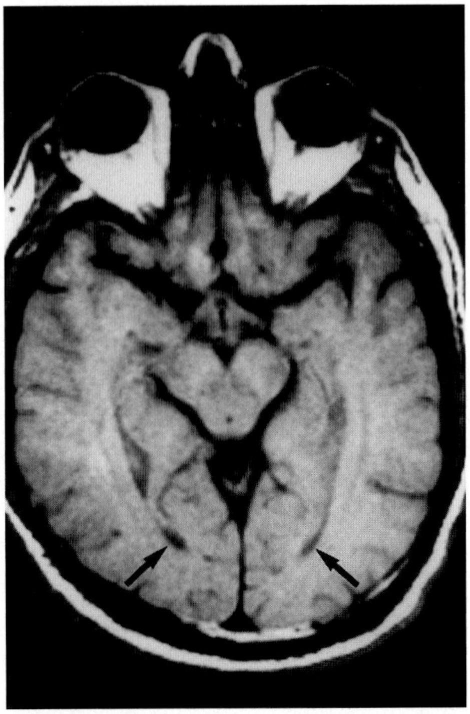

Figure 2K-2E: The occipital horns of the lateral ventricle. Axial T1-weighted MR image showing the typically "collapsed" occipital horns (*arrows*) of the lateral ventricles.

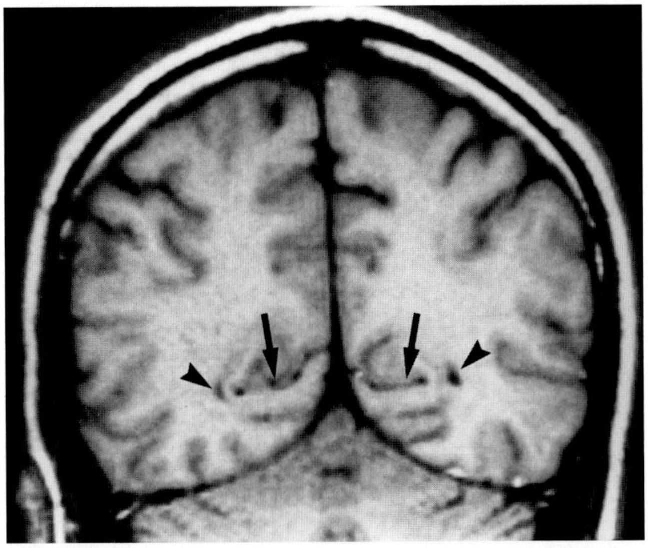

Figure 2K-2F: The calcarine fissure and occipital horns. Coronal T1-weighted MR image showing the calcarine fissures (*arrows*) bilaterally. Also note the small occipital horns (*arrowheads*) of the lateral ventricles.

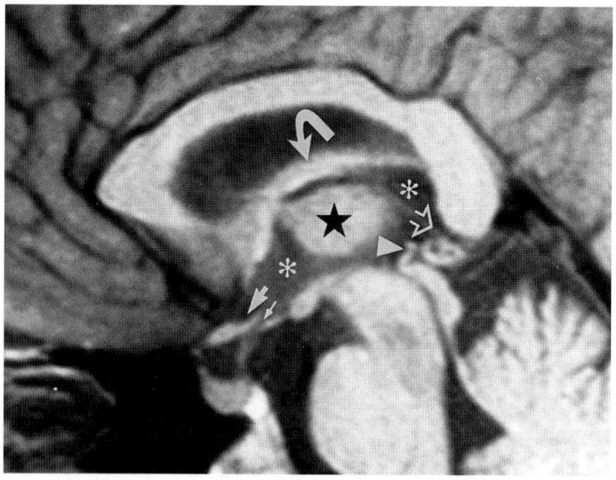

Figure 2K-3A: The third ventricle. Midline sagittal MR image showing the third ventricle (*asterisks*), the infundibular recess (*small solid arrow*), the chiasmatic recess (*large solid arrow*), the suprapineal recess (*open arrow*), the pineal recess (*arrow-head*), the fornix(ices) (*large curved arrow*) in the roof of the third ventricle, and the thalami (*star*) protruding into the third ventricle.

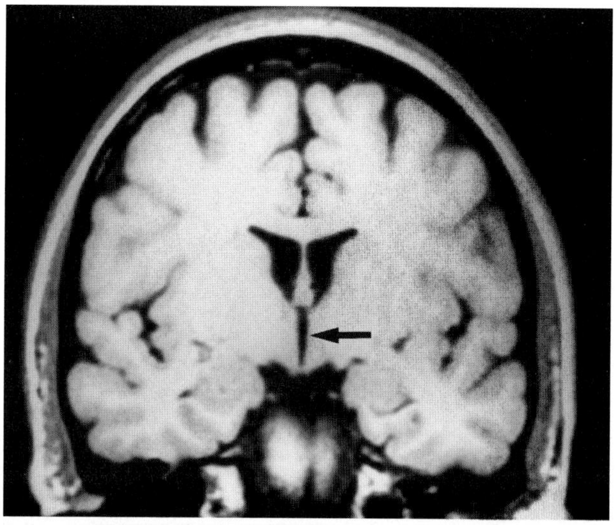

Figure 2K-3B: The third ventricle. Coronal T1-weighted MR image showing the central portion of the third ventricle (*arrow*).

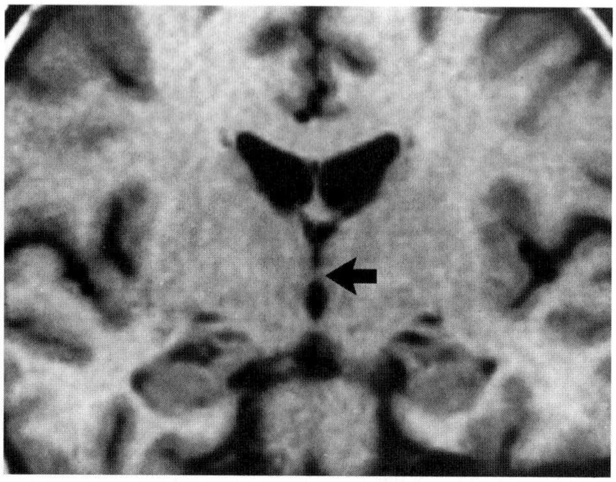

Figure 2K-3C: The massa intermedia. Coronal T1-weighted MR image showing the massa intermedia (*arrow*, interthalamic adhesion) traversing the lumen of the third ventricle.

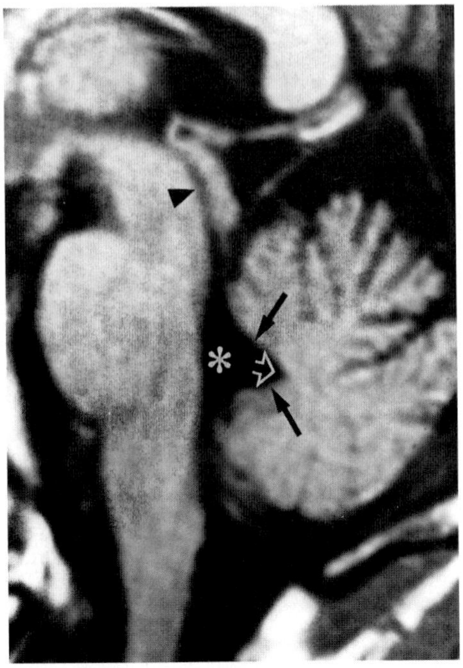

Figure 2K-4A: The fourth ventricle. Sagittal T1-weighted MR image showing the lumen of the fourth ventricle (*asterisk*), the superior medullary velum (*upper solid arrow*), the inferior medullary velum (*lower solid arrow*), the fastigium (*open arrow*), and the aqueduct of Sylvius (*arrowhead*).

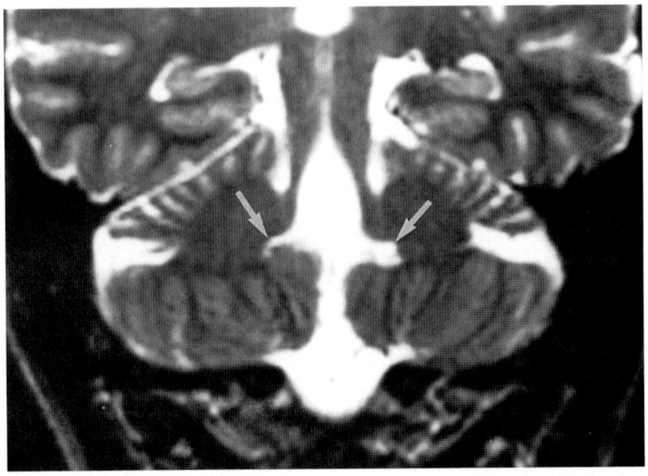

Figure 2K-4B: The fourth ventricle. Coronal T2-weighted MR image showing the lateral wings (ala) (*arrows*) of the fourth ventricle.

THE CHOROID PLEXI AND ARACHNOID GRANULATIONS

The Ventricular Ependyma, Choroid Plexi, and Arachnoid Granulations

1. The ependyma lining the ventricular cavities of the brain consists of cuboidal epithelium. Fine microvilli cover the ventricular surface of these modified epithelial cells.
2. During the development of the brain and the choroid fissure of the lateral ventricles, the ependymal layer of certain areas of the ventricles comes in contact with the meninges to form the tela choroidea. These ependymal cells differentiate into a secretory epithelium that, in combination with the meningeal vessels, forms the choroid plexi.
3. The choroid plexi are located in the two lateral and the third and fourth ventricles; the choroid plexi of the lateral and third ventricles are directly continuous via the foramina of Monro and via the shared tela choroidea for these plexi.
4. The surface of the choroid plexus is thrown into small folds, or arachnoid villi. The surface epithelium is a modified type of cuboidal epithelium that is similar to, and continuous with, the ventricular ependyma.
5. This plexal cuboidal epithelium has microvilli over its apical surface and infoldings over its basal surface; the basal surface is further covered by a prominent basement membrane.
6. The small folds of the choroid plexus are filled with connective tissue and fenestrated capillaries.
7. The blood–CSF barrier of the choroid plexus is found at the level of the intercellular tight junctions in the plexal cuboidal epithelium. These epithelial cells have the characteristics of active transport and secretion and possibly of absorption as well.
8. The choroid plexus cuboidal epithelium is responsible for producing the majority of the CSF. According to estimates, the choroid plexi of the lateral, third, and fourth ventricles produces over 70% of the CSF. The remainder is produced from unidentified sites within the central nervous system but probably originates from the ventricular ependyma and pia mater, coming directly from the brain, spinal cord, and subarachnoid segments of the cranial and spinal nerve roots.
9. The combined rate of CSF secretion by the choroid plexi is believed to be approximately 0.35 to 0.4 ml/min. The choroid plexi can continuously secrete CSF at a rate of approximately 20 ml per hour, or nearly 500 ml per day. Since the total volume of CSF in the ventricles and subarachnoid spaces is approximately 150 ml, an estimated threefold turnover of CSF occurs daily.
10. CSF resorption takes place through the arachnoid granulations (villi) in the cranial dural venous sinuses and within venous lacunae near the dural venous sinuses.
11. These granulations function as passive, pressure gradient–dependent one-way valves between the CSF and the venous blood that are readily permeable to fluids and even large solutes (e.g., proteins).

Choroid Plexus Blood Supply

1. The blood supply to the choroid plexus in the tela choroidea of the third and lateral ventricles is from the anterior choroidal branch of the internal carotid artery and from choroidal branches of the posterior cerebral artery. Anastomoses exist between the distal branches of these vessels.
2. The blood supply to the fourth ventricular choroid plexus arises from the inferior cerebellar arteries.
3. Capillaries drain into a venous plexus that subsequently empties into a single choroidal vein leaving the tela choroidea.
4. There is one choroidal vein each draining the choroid plexus in the right and left lateral ventricles, the third ventricle, and the fourth ventricle.

5. The choroidal veins of the lateral and third ventricles drain into the internal cerebral veins.
6. The choroidal vein of the fourth ventricle drains into the inferior vermian vein.

Anatomy of the Arachnoid Granulations

1. Microscopic arachnoid villi composing macroscopic arachnoid granulations provide the major pathway for bulk flow drainage of CSF from the subarachnoid space of the central nervous system into the venous bloodstream.
2. These granulations are most commonly associated with the superior sagittal and transverse venous sinuses, although they may be seen in association with other venous sinuses and even in the spinal region.
3. The arachnoid villi and granulations are specialized extensions of the subarachnoid space. The specialized arachnoid extends through a gap in the dura to provide an extensive exchange surface with the venous endothelium.
4. The arachnoid granulation communicates directly with the subarachnoid space proper via a narrow channel at the neck of the granulation.
5. The subarachnoid space in the core of the arachnoid granulation is traversed by a fine network of collagenous trabeculae that contain fenestrae allowing intercommunication among the spaces of the arachnoid granulation, the drainage channel(s) at the neck of the granulation, and the subarachnoid space proper.
6. At the apex of the arachnoid granulation, there is an apical cap composed primarily of arachnoid apical cap cells. This cap is traversed by microchannels that transmit the CSF to the potential subendothelial (interstitial) space of the arachnoid granulation.
7. The movement of subarachnoid space CSF from this point into the venous system is believed to be effected by active macro- or microvesicular transport across the venous endothelium covering the arachnoid granulation.

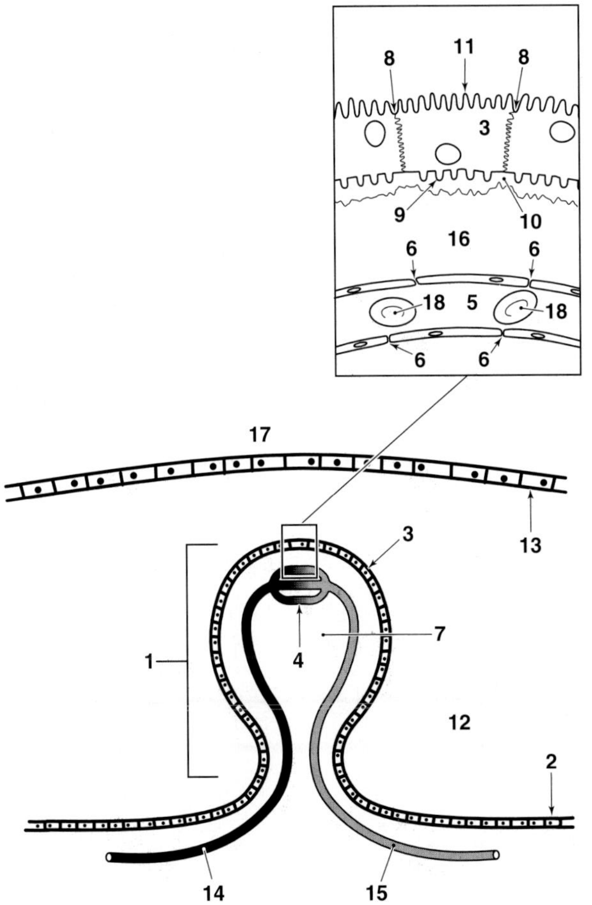

Figure 2K-5: Schematic of the microstructure of an arachnoid villus of the choroid plexus.

1 Arachnoid villus of choroid plexus
2 Ventricular ependyma along margins of choroid plexus
3 Apical plexal cell–modified cuboidal epithelium over surface of choroid plexus (plexal cuboidal epithelium)
4 Arachnoid villus (choroid plexus) capillary system
5 Choroid plexus capillary lumen
6 Intercellular fenestra in choroid plexus capillary endothelium (fenestrated capillaries)
7 Fibrous vascular core of tela choroidea of choroid plexus
8 Epithelial plexal cell intercellular tight junctions (level of blood–CSF barrier)
9 Interdigitations on basal surface of plexal epithelial cells
10 Basement membrane along inner surface of infolded plexal epithelium
11 Apical microvilli on apical surface of plexal epithelium
12 Cerebral ventricular lumen (cerebrospinal fluid)
13 Parietal ependyma of cerebral ventricular system
14 Arteriole of arachnoid villus
15 Venule of arachnoid villus
16 Apical interstitial space of arachnoid villus
17 Brain parenchyma
18 Red blood cell in choroid plexus capillary

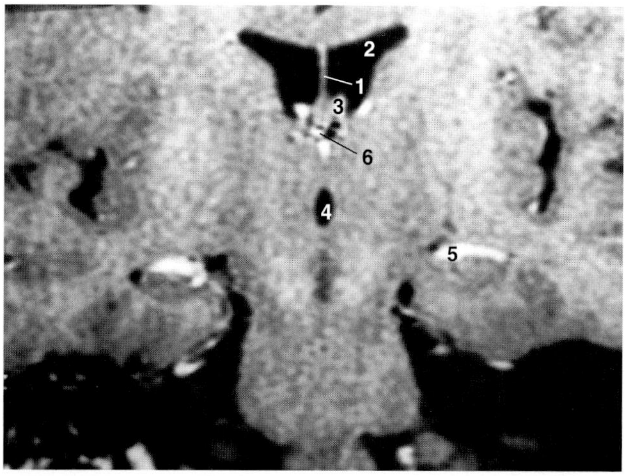

Figure 2K-6A: The choroid plexi. Magnified, enhanced T1-weighted MR image in the coronal plane, showing the choroid plexi within the bodies and distal temporal horns of the lateral ventricles.

1. Septum pellucidum
2. Body of lateral ventricle
3. Choroid plexus in lateral ventricle
4. Third ventricle
5. Choroid plexus in temporal horn of lateral ventricle
6. Choroid plexus in roof of third ventricle

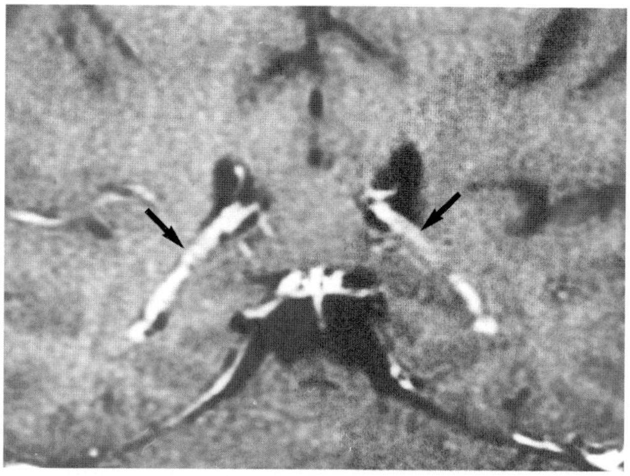

Figure 2K-6B: The choroid plexi. Magnified, enhanced T1-weighted MR image in the coronal plane, showing the choroid plexi (*arrows*) within the atria and proximal temporal horns of the lateral ventricles.

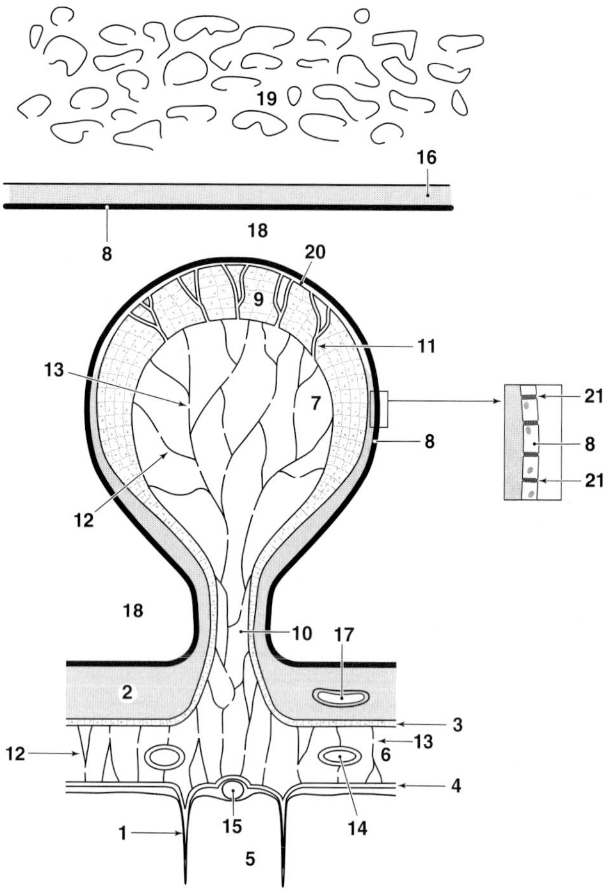

Figure 2K-7: Cross section schematic of an arachnoid granulation.

1 Cerebral sulcus
2 Meningeal layer of cranial dura mater
3 Arachnoid mater
4 Pia mater
5 Cerebrum
6 Subarachnoid space over cerebrum
7 Subarachnoid space of arachnoid granulation
8 Venous endothelium
9 Arachnoid granulation apical cap and arachnoid apical cap cells
10 Subarachnoid space channel in neck of arachnoid granulation
11 Subarachnoid space microchannel of arachnoid granulation cap
12 Arachnoid trabeculations
13 Communicating fenestra in arachnoid trabeculations
14 Subarachnoid space blood vessels
15 Subpial cortical blood vessels
16 Periosteal layer of cranial dura mater
17 Meningeal blood vessels
18 Venous vascular lumen of dural venous sinus/lacuna (venous blood)
19 Calvarium
20 Subendothelial space of apex of arachnoid granulation
21 Intercellular endothelial tight junctions

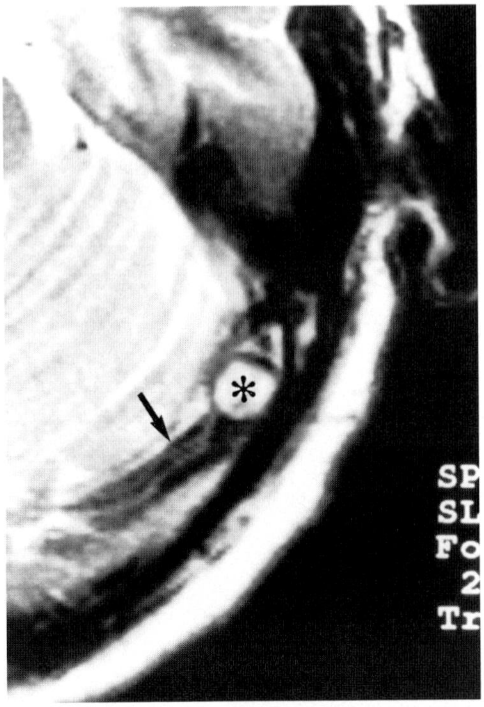

Figure 2K-8A: Arachnoid granulation. Magnified axial T2-weighted MR image showing a hyperintense arachnoid granulation (*asterisk*) surrounded by the flow void of the transverse venous sinus (*arrow*).

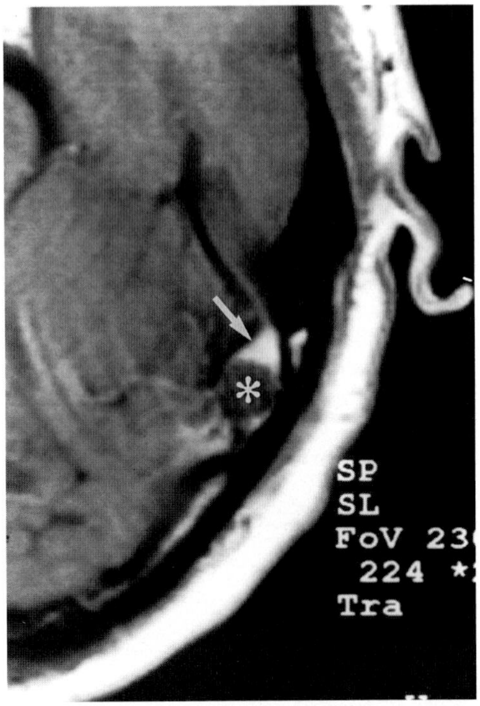

Figure 2K-8B: Arachnoid granulation. Magnified, contrast-enhanced axial T1-weighted MR image showing a nonenhancing arachnoid granulation (*asterisk*) surrounded by the enhancement within the transverse venous sinus (*arrow*).

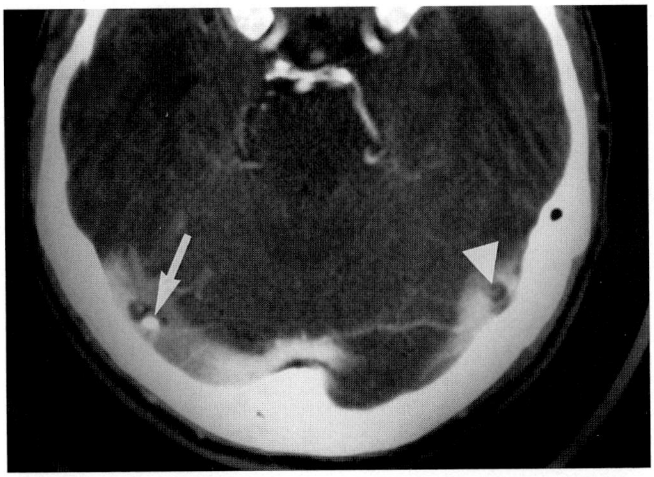

Figure 2K-8C: Calcified and noncalcified arachnoid granulations within the transverse venous sinuses. Bolus contrast-enhanced axial CT image showing a calcified arachnoid granulation (*arrow*) within the opacified right transverse venous sinus and a noncalcified arachnoid granulation (*arrowhead*) within the left transverse venous sinus, resulting in bilateral venous channel-filling defects.

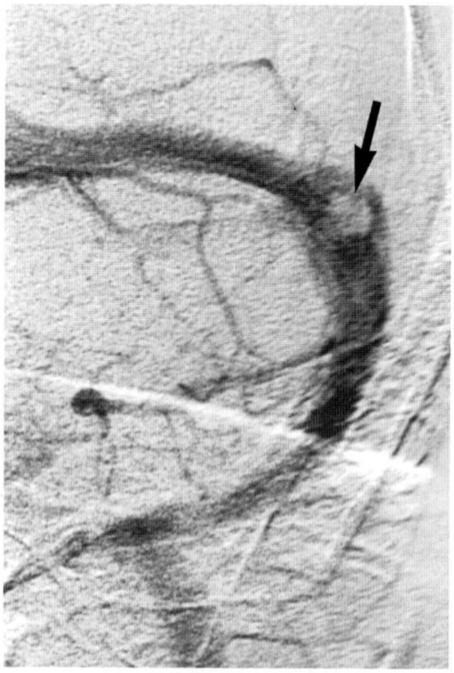

Figure 2K-8D: Left internal carotid angiogram in the venous phase, showing a filling defect in an expanded section of the left transverse venous sinus (*arrow*) corresponding to an arachnoid granulation.

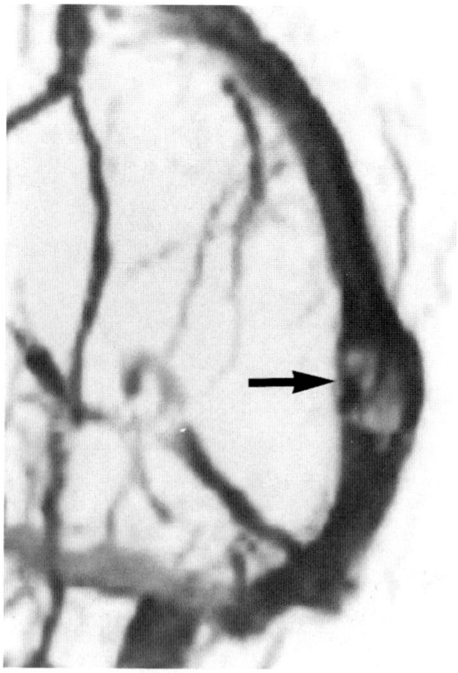

Figure 2K-8E: Magnetic resonance angiogram (venogram) of a different patient shows a signal void in the expanded distal superior sagittal sinus (*arrow*) representing an arachnoid granulation.

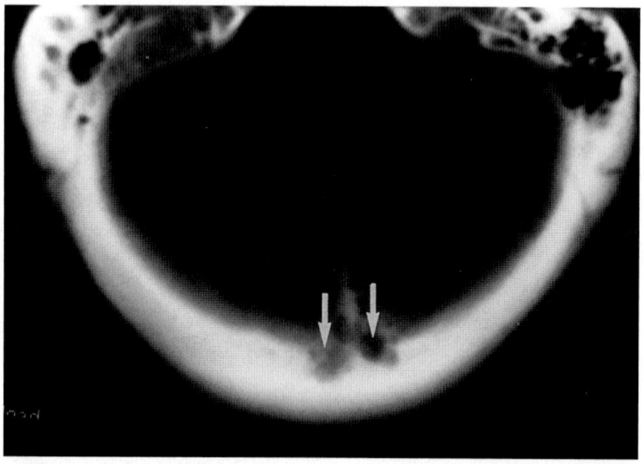

Figure 2K-8F: Calvarial excavations of arachnoid granulations. Magnified axial CT image showing large arachnoid granulation impressions (excavations) in the occipital bone (*arrows*) on either side of the midline.

THE CIRCUMVENTRICULAR ORGANS

1. The eight circumventricular organs are areas of specialized tissue located at strategic positions in the midline cerebral ventricular system. These organs are the following.
   a. Subforniceal organ
   b. Organum vasculosum of the lamina terminalis (supraoptic crest)
   c. Medial eminence
   d. Neurohypophysis
   e. Pineal body
   f. Subcommissural organ
   g. Area postrema (paired)
2. Only the area postrema located in the caudal margin of the fourth ventricle is paired; the remaining six circumventricular organs are unpaired.
3. All of the circumventricular organs are highly vascularized, with the exception of the subcommissural organ.
4. All of the circumventricular organs lack a blood–brain barrier, with the exception of the subcommissural organ.
5. The subforniceal organ is located between the interventricular foramina of Monro and functionally probably regulates body fluids.
6. The organum vasculosum located in the lamina terminalis is probably a vascular outlet for luteinizing hormone–releasing hormone and somatostatin.
7. The medial eminence of the tuber cinereum (the portion of the hypothalamic floor lying between the optic chiasm and the mammillary bodies), in the floor of the third ventricle serves as a neuroendocrine transducer. The hypothalamus stimulates the neurosecretory neurons of the medial eminence to discharge hormone-releasing factors into the hypophyseal portal system.
8. The neurohypophysis (i.e., posterior lobe of the pituitary gland, pars nervosa) receives neural fibers from the paraventricular and supraoptic nuclei of the hypothalamus. These are terminal fibers that contain neurophysin, a carrier protein, and vasopressin and oxytocin, which are stored in the posterior lobe of the hypophysis. These hormones are released into the bloodstream upon specific hypothalamic stimulation.
9. Pineal gland
   a. The pineal gland or body is an unpaired, midline endocrine organ attached to the diencephalon by the pineal stalk, or infundibulum.
   b. The pineal stalk is invaginated by the pineal recess, an ependymally lined recess extending directly from the posterior aspect of the third ventricle. The pineal stalk is split into the superior and inferior infundibular laminae. The pineal stalk also contains the habenular (superior lamina) and posterior (inferior lamina) commissures.
   c. The pineal gland principally contains pinealocytes and neuroglial cells. Afferent and efferent neural ramifications are also present.
   d. The pineal gland is highly vascularized and lacks a blood–brain barrier.
   e. Postganglionic sympathetic fibers from the superior cervical sympathetic ganglion enter the pineal gland as a single or paired nervus conarii. These adrenergic fibers are associated with both parenchymal pineal cells and pineal blood vessels. Postganglionic fibers from the nervus conarii also reach the habenular nuclei; in turn, these nuclei may give rise to the habenulopineal tracts innervating the pineal gland and the ganglion conarii in the apex of the gland.
   f. In the fetus, certain innervations to and from the pineal may or may not persist into adulthood; they may be only phylogenetic vestiges. These fetal innervations include the nervus pinealis, which connects the pineal to the posterior commissure. This nerve might be involved with light impulse transmission and/or fetal pineal differentiation. Another described neural structure, which may be parasympathetic, includes the intrapineal ganglion.
   g. A great deal of research has attempted to elucidate the functional aspects of this neuroendocrine gland. Among other constituents, the pineal contains serotonin and

norepinephrine and possibly also thyrotropin-releasing hormone, luteinizing hormone–releasing hormone, and somatostatin. In addition, melatonin is a major hormonal product of the pineal gland. Melatonin is a product of metabolism of the indole amino acid, tryptophan, which is released into the bloodstream in a classic circadian manner. The production of melatonin in the pineal gland is confined almost exclusively to the "daily dark period" (i.e., night). Blood levels of melatonin in all animal species, including the human being, are higher at night than during the day. In the mammalian brain, this is a result of light perceived by the lateral (orbital) eyes, which limits the production of melatonin by the pineal gland to periods of darkness. Serum melatonin levels also correlate with the length of darkness and exhibit seasonal changes; for example, longer nights in winter correlate with more prolonged elevated nighttime melatonin levels. That the human pineal gland readily responds to light perceived by the lateral eyes is amply demonstrated by the experiments in which the suppression of high circulating melatonin levels was achieved when individuals are deliberately exposed to light at nighttime.

Among other features, melatonin is believed to exert some control over the reproductive system, possibly including the determination of onset of puberty in the human being. Conditions such as seasonal affective disorder, jet lag, and aberrant sleep patterns have been reported to be related to altered melatonin levels. With aging, serum melatonin levels have been observed to decline progressively. Since melatonin is a potent free radical scavenger, the reduction of melatonin with age may be a contributory factor in a variety of diseases (e.g., neurodegenerative conditions) as well as in aging itself.

h. Overall, the pineal seems to be a neuroendocrine transducer that receives neural signals primarily via sympathetic neurons and converts this input into an endocrine output, melatonin.

10. The subcommissural organ is located at the junction of the third ventricle and the cerebral aqueduct. Cells of the subcommissural organ secrete a mucopolysaccharide into the CSF, but the actual function of this structure and the secreted mucopolysaccharide are not known.
11. The (paired) area postrema is located along the caudal margins of the fourth ventricle. The area postrema is considered to be a chemoreceptor that triggers vomiting in response to circulating emetic substances.

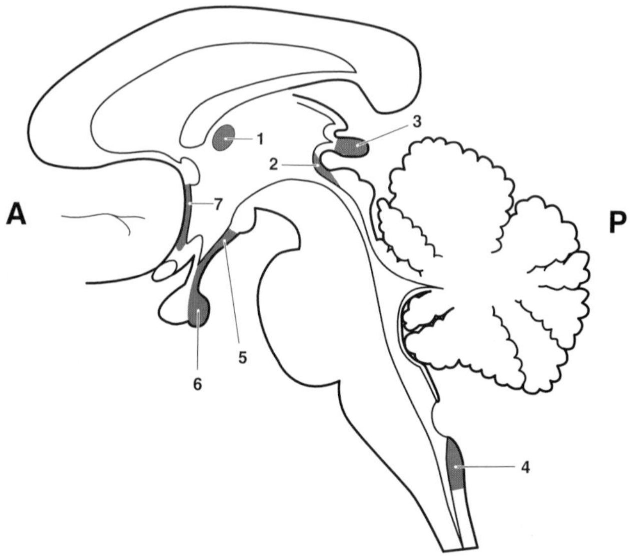

Figure 2K-9: Midsagittal schematic of the circumventricular organs. *A*, anterior; *P*, posterior.

1 Subforniceal organ
2 Subcommissural organ
3 Pineal
4 Area postrema
5 Medial eminence
6 Neurohypophysis
7 Organum vasculosum

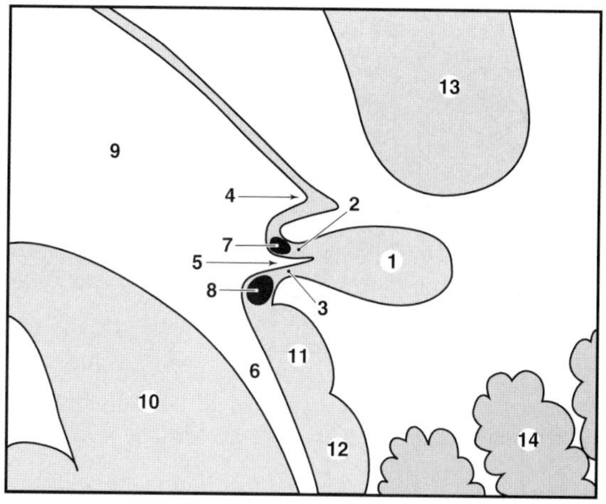

Figure 2K-10A: Sagittal schematic of the pineal gland and related structures. *A*, anterior; *P*, posterior.

1 Pineal gland
2 Superior lamina of pituitary stalk
3 Inferior lamina of pituitary stalk
4 Suprapineal recess of third ventricle
5 Pineal recess of third ventricle
6 Cerebral aqueduct of Sylvius
7 Habenular commissure
8 Posterior commissure
9 Third ventricle
10 Midbrain
11 Superior colliculae
12 Inferior colliculae
13 Splenium of corpus callosum
14 Cerebellar vermis

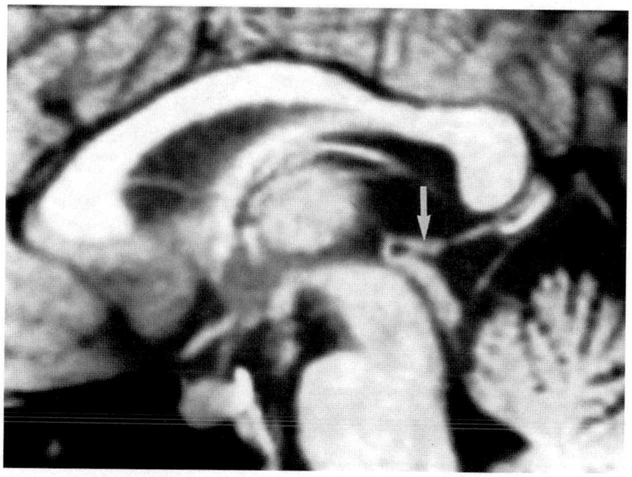

Figure 2K-10B: The pineal gland. Sagittal T1-weighted MR image showing the pineal gland (*arrow*).

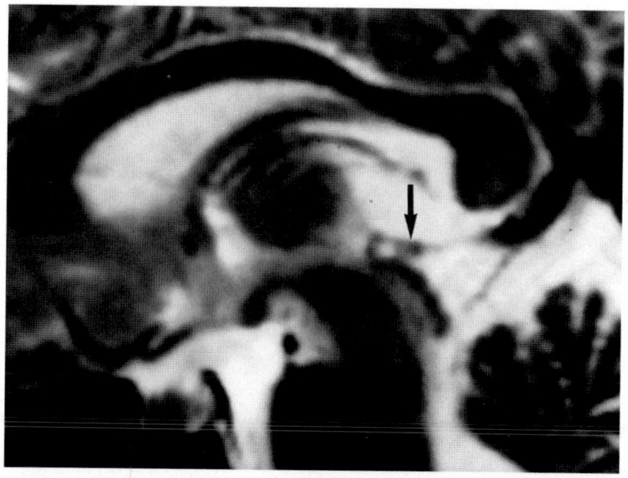

Figure 2K-10C: The pineal gland. Sagittal T2-weighted MR image showing the pineal gland (*arrow*).

PINEAL GLAND VARIANTS

- Absence of pineal calcification
- Pineal calcification
- Pineal cyst formation

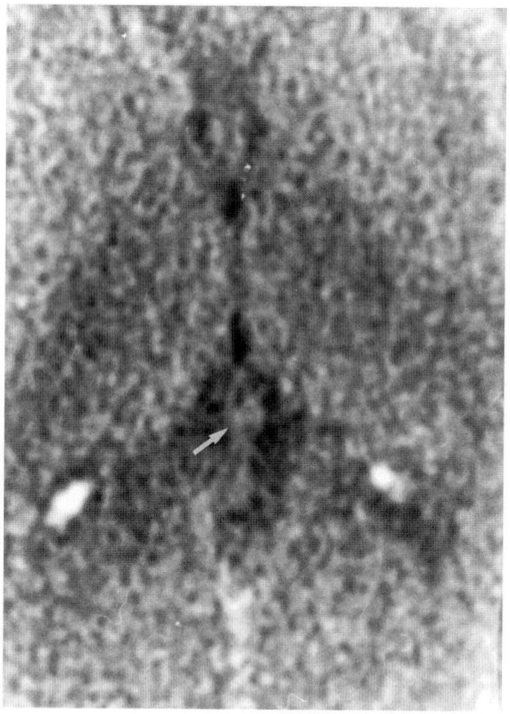

Figure 2K-11A: Noncalcified pineal gland. Unenhanced axial CT image showing noncalcification of the pineal gland (*arrow*).

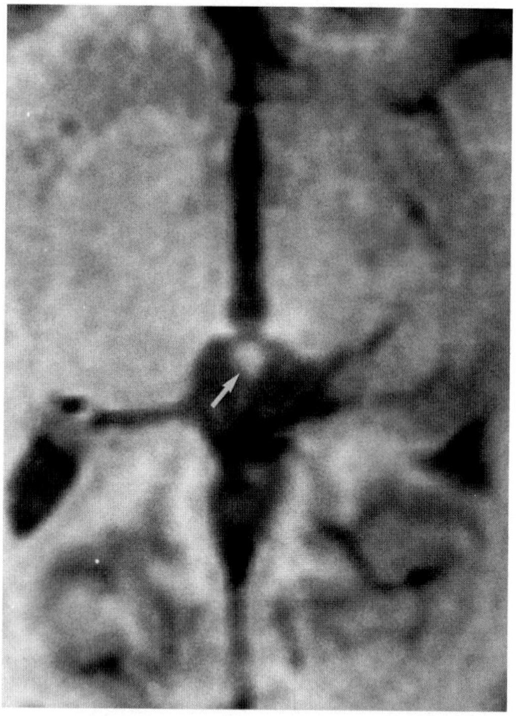

Figure 2K-11B: Unenhanced axial T1-weighted MR image showing the pineal gland (*arrow*) to be isointense compared with the cerebrum.

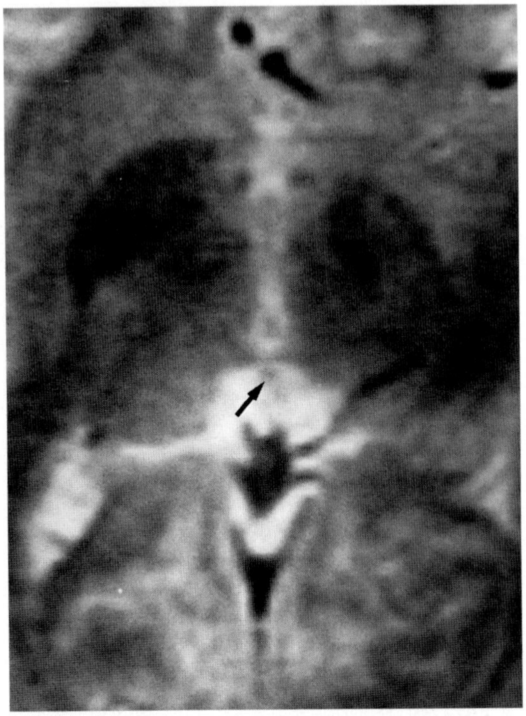

Figure 2K-11C: Axial T2-weighted MR image showing the pineal gland (*arrow*) to be isointense as compared with the cerebral gray matter.

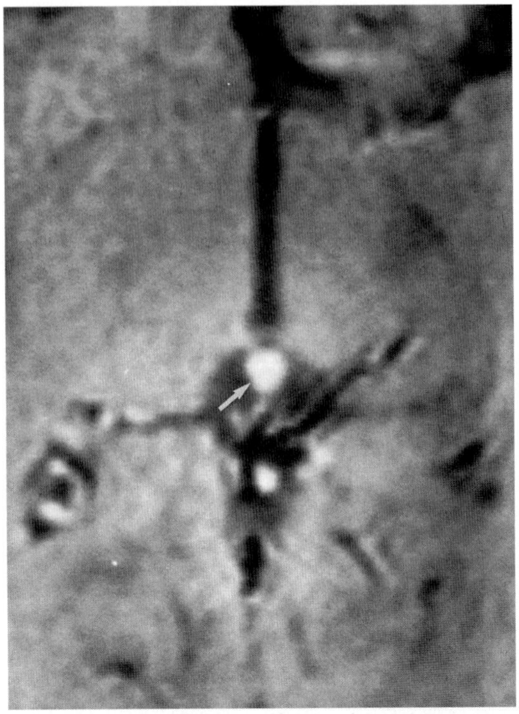

Figure 2K-11D: Enhanced T1-weighted MR image showing generalized homogeneous enhancement of the pineal gland (*arrow*), indicating an absent blood–brain barrier. This is a normal characteristic of the pineal body (gland).

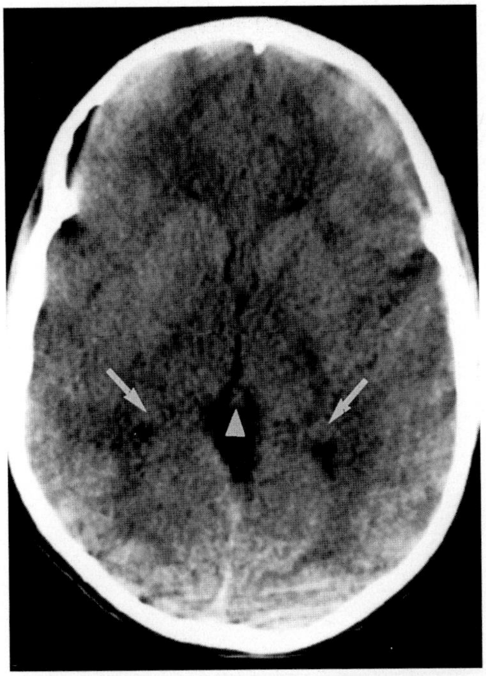

Figure 2K-11E: Absence of pineal calcification. Axial CT image in a seven-year-old boy showing absence of calcification of the pineal gland (*arrowhead*) and choroid plexi (*arrows*) of the lateral ventricles.

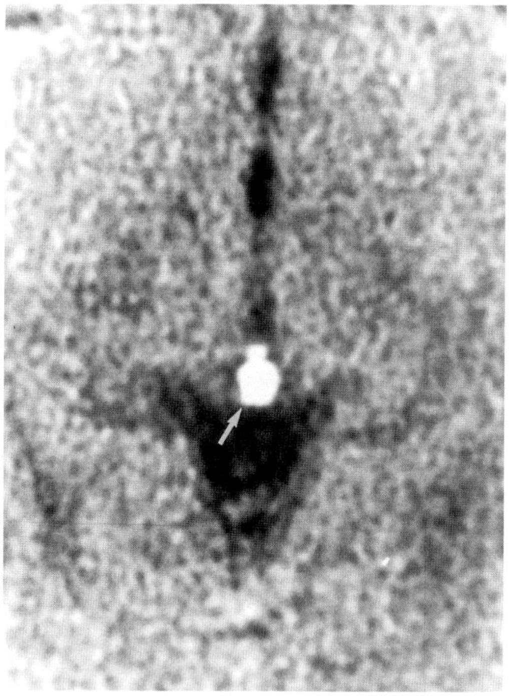

Figure 2K-12A: Pineal gland calcification. Unenhanced axial CT image showing a solid pineal calcification (*arrow*).

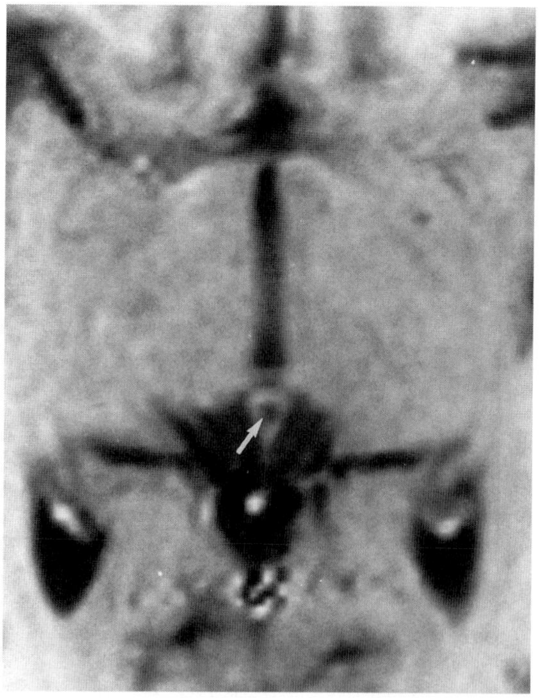

Figure 2K-12B: Unenhanced axial T1-weighted MR image showing the central hypointensity (*arrow*) within the pineal gland, representing a signal void due to the calcification observed in Fig. 2K-12A and not representing a pineal cyst.

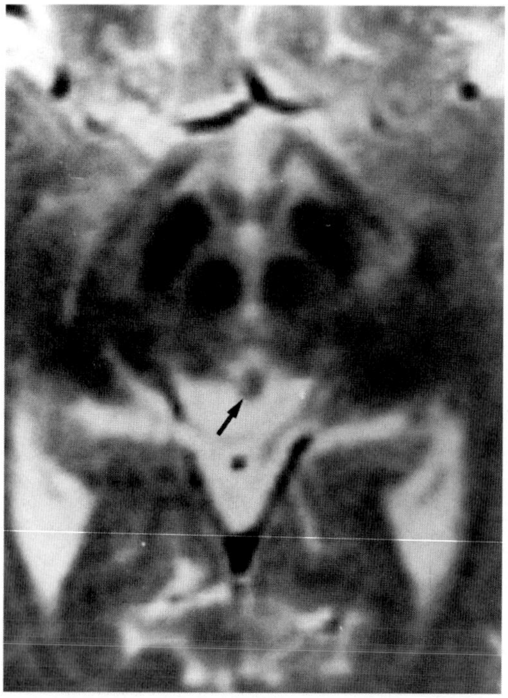

Figure 2K-12C: Axial T2-weighted MR image showing marked hypointensity (*arrow*) of the central pineal gland caused by the dense calcification; a pineal cyst would be hyperintense instead of hypointense.

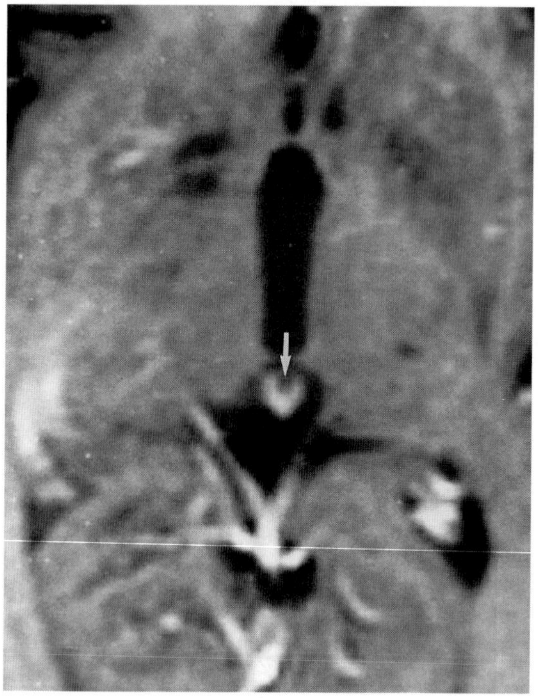

Figure 2K-12D: Enhanced axial T1-weighted MR image showing rim enhancement surrounding the nonenhancing central pineal calcification (arrow).

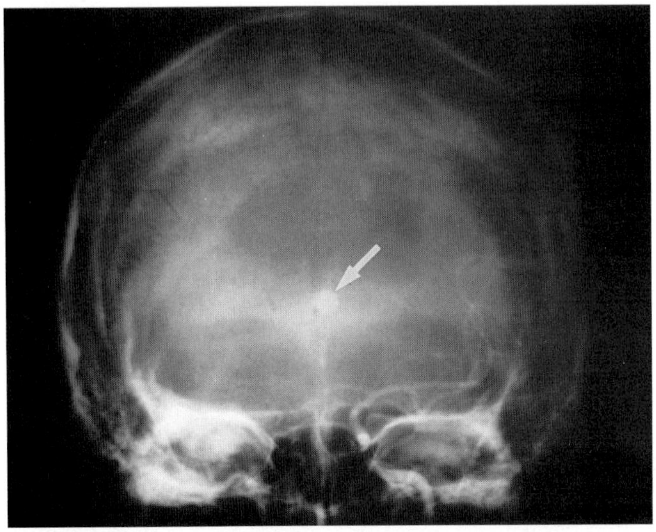

Figure 2K-12E: Dense pineal calcification. Skull radiograph in the frontal projection from the early phase of a carotid angiogram, showing a dense pineal calcification (*arrow*).

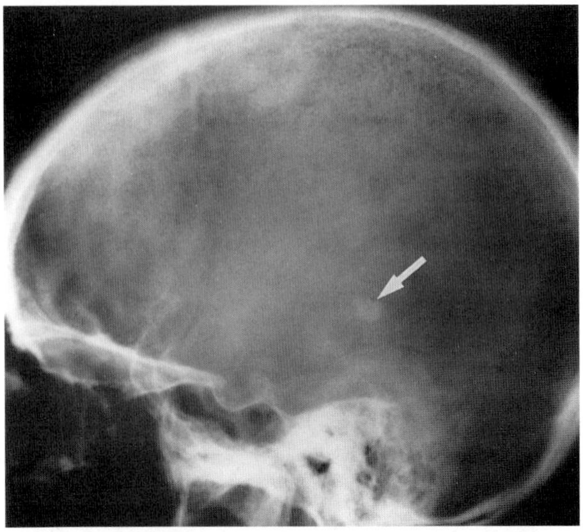

Figure 2K-12F: Skull radiograph in the lateral projection showing dense pineal calcification (*arrow*).

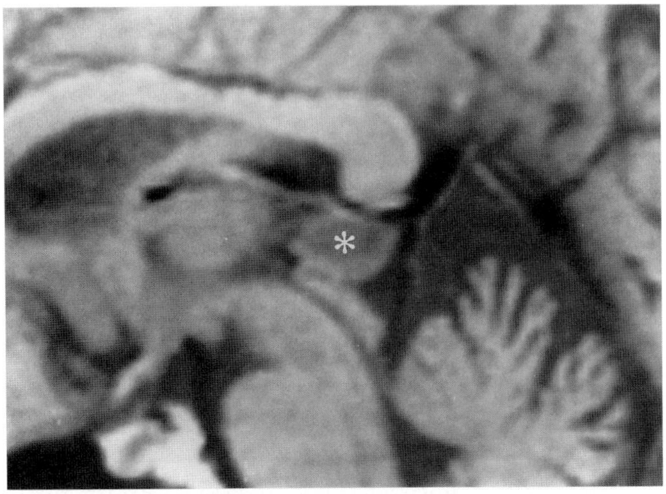

Figure 2K-13A: Pineal cyst. Sagittal T1-weighted MR image showing a large pineal cyst (*asterisk*).

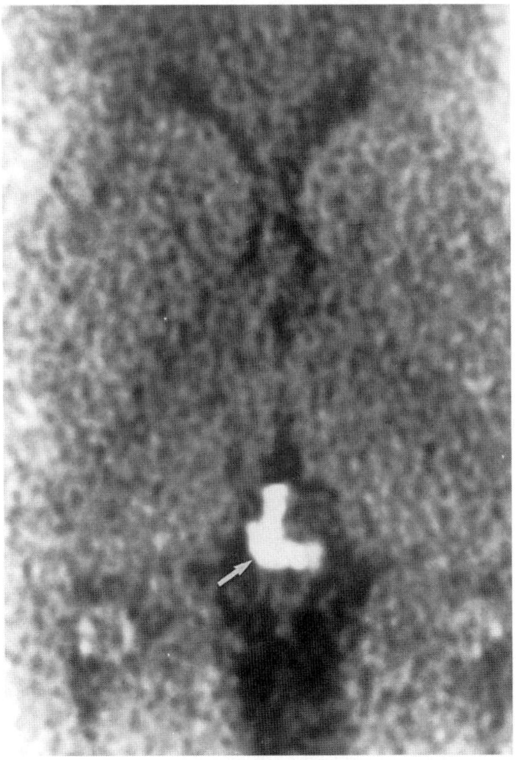

Figure 2K-13B: Pineal cyst. Unenhanced axial CT image showing cresenteric calcification (*arrow*) within the wall of the pineal cyst.

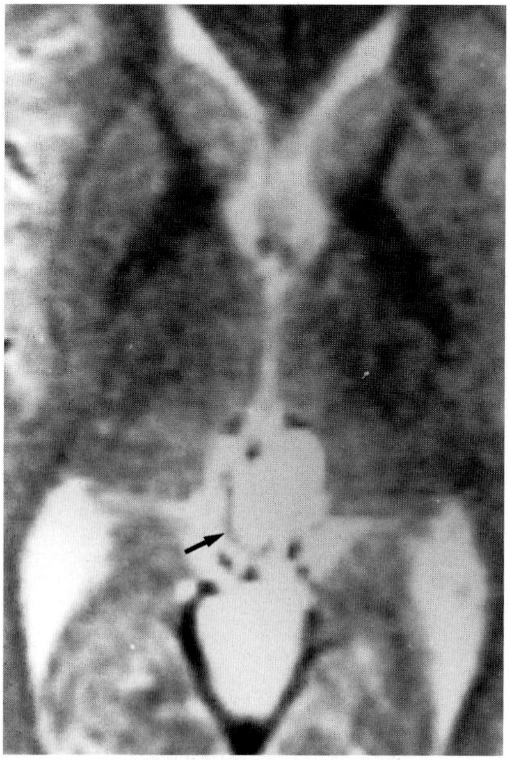

Figure 2K-13C: Pineal cyst. Axial T2-weighted MR image showing cresenteric hypointensity (*arrow*) within the calcification in the wall of the pineal cyst.

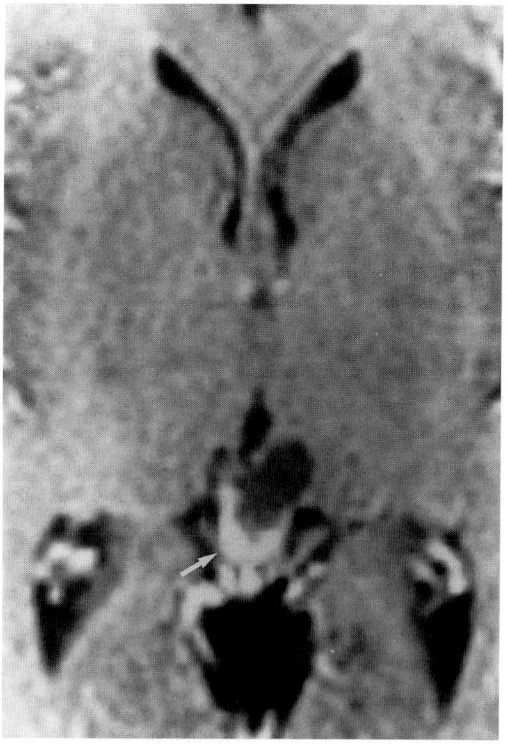

Figure 2K-13D: Pineal cyst. Enhanced T1-weighted MR image showing cresenteric enhancement (*arrow*) within the wall of the pineal cyst.

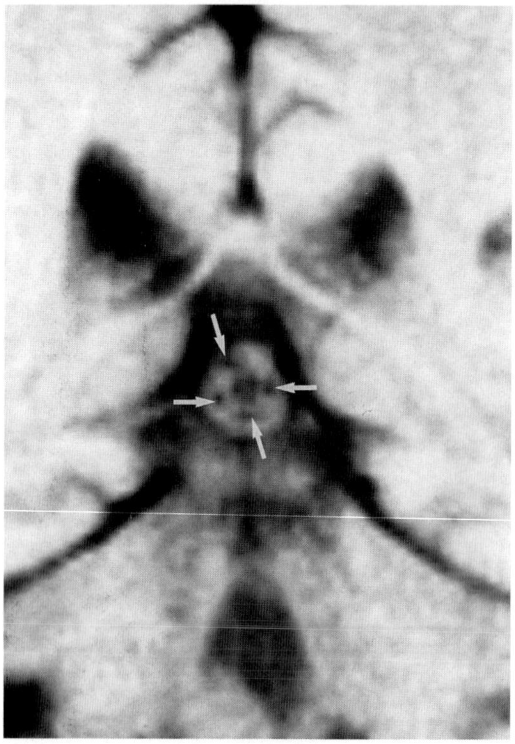

Figure 2K-13E: Multiple pineal cysts. Coronal T1-weighted MR image showing multiple pineal cysts (*arrows*).

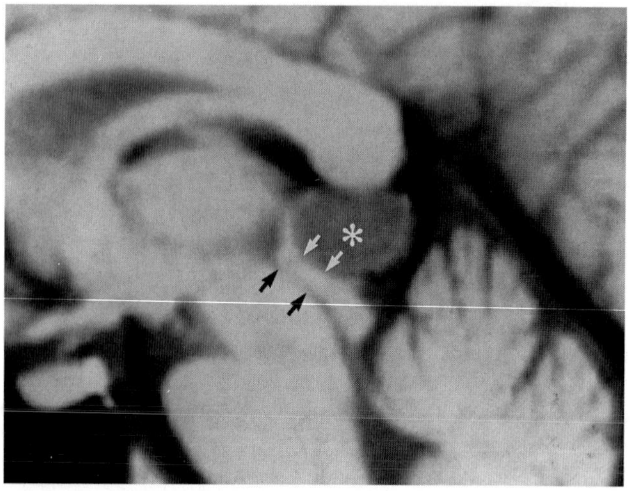

Figure 2K-14: Large pineal cyst with regional mass effect. Unenhanced sagittal T1-weighted MR image showing mass effect of the pineal cyst (*asterisk*) on the quadrigeminal plate (*white arrows*) and the aqueduct of Sylvius (*black arrows*). No hydrocephalus was present.

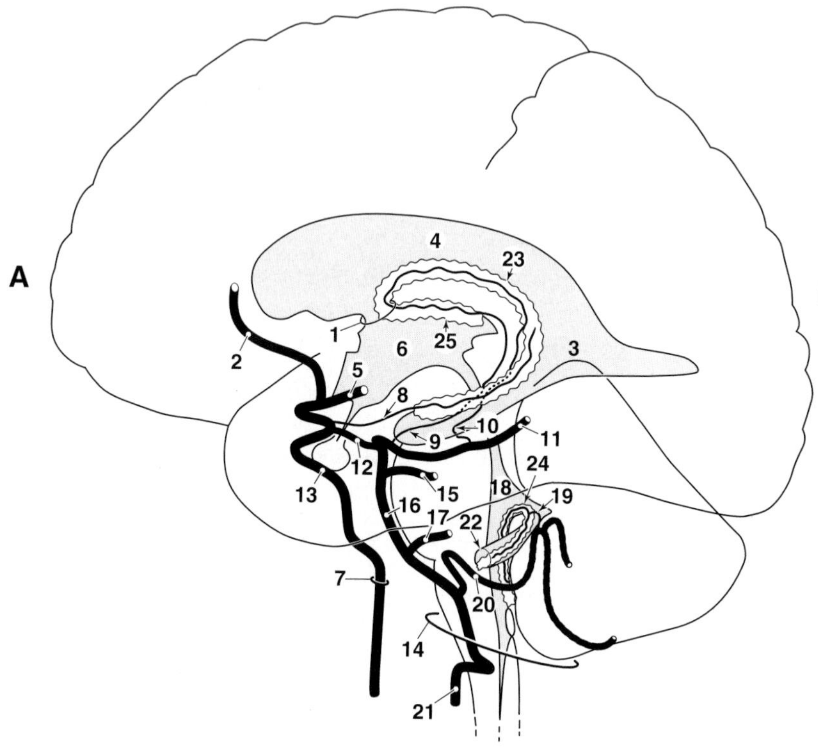

Figure 2K-15: Lateral schematic of the arterial supply to the choroid plexi. *A*, anterior; *P*, posterior.
1 Interventricular foramen of Monro
2 Anterior cerebral artery
3 Atrium of lateral ventricle
4 Body of lateral ventricle
5 Middle cerebral artery
6 Third ventricle
7 Carotid canal
8 Anterior choroidal artery
9 Medial posterior choroidal artery
10 Lateral posterior choroidal artery
11 Posterior cerebral artery
12 Posterior communicating artery
13 Internal carotid artery
14 Foramen magnum
15 Superior cerebellar artery
16 Basilar artery
17 Anterior–inferior cerebellar artery
18 Fourth ventricle
19 Choroidal artery to fourth ventricular choroid plexus
20 Posterior–inferior cerebellar artery
21 Vertebral artery
22 Foramen of Luschka
23 Choroid plexus of lateral ventricle
24 Choroid plexus of fourth ventricle
25 Choroid plexus of third ventricle

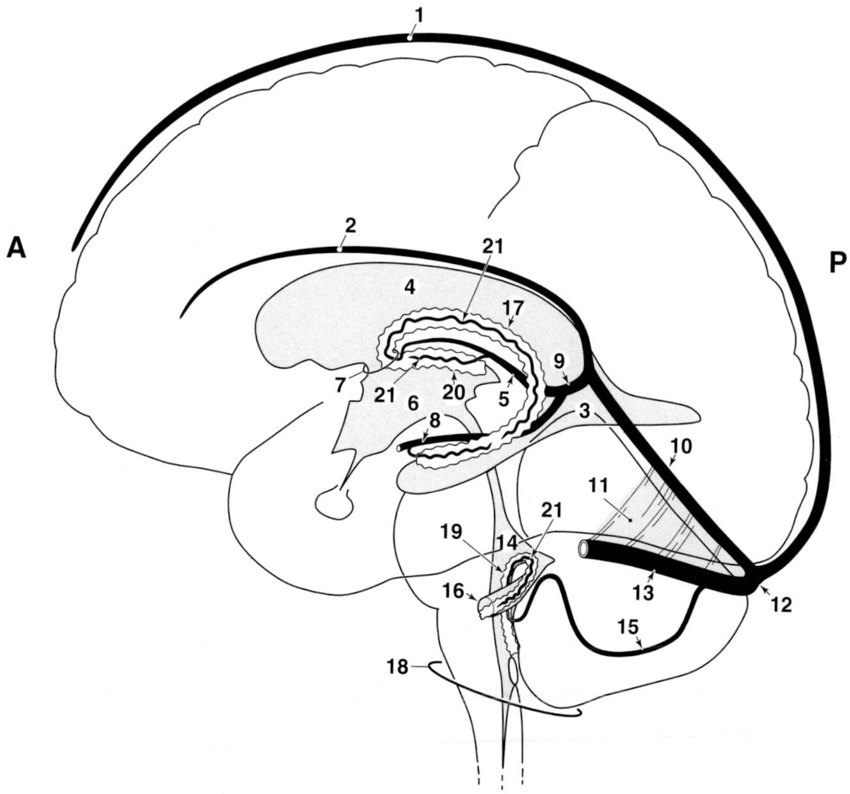

Figure 2K-16: Lateral schematic of venous drainage of choroid plexi. *A, anterior; P, posterior.*
1 Superior sagittal venous sinus
2 Inferior sagittal venous sinus
3 Atrium of lateral ventricle
4 Body of lateral ventricle
5 Internal cerebral vein
6 Third ventricle
7 Interventricular foramen of Monro
8 Basilar vein of Rosenthal
9 Vein of Galen
10 Straight venous sinus
11 Tentorium cerebelli
12 Torcular herophili
13 Transverse venous sinus
14 Fourth ventricle
15 Inferior vermian vein
16 Foramen of Luschka
17 Choroid plexus of lateral ventricle
18 Foramen magnum
19 Choroid plexus of fourth ventricle
20 Choroid plexus of third ventricle
21 Choroid plexi veins

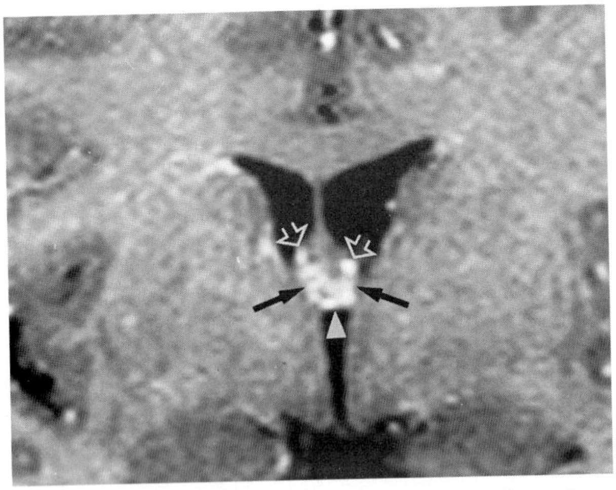

Figure 2K-17A: Choroid plexi traversing the foramina of Monro. Enhanced coronal T1-weighted MR image showing the choroid plexi of the lateral ventricles (*open arrows*) traversing the foramina of Monro (*solid arrows*) to continue contiguously into the third ventricle choroid plexus (*arrowhead*).

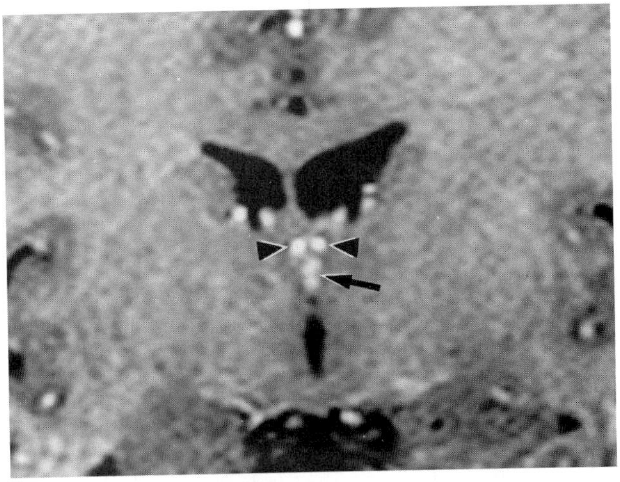

Figure 2K-17B: Third ventricle choroid plexus. Enhanced T1-weighted coronal MR image showing the enhancing choroid plexus (*arrow*) in the superior aspect of the third ventricle. The internal cerebral veins (*arrowheads*) are seen in the roof of the third ventricle.

CEREBRAL VENTRICULAR SYSTEM, ARACHNOID GRANULATION, AND CHOROID PLEXI VARIANTS

- Cavum septi pellucidi
- Cavum vergae
- Cavum velum interpositum (roof of third ventricle)
- Lateral ventricular size asymmetry
- Massa intermedia (interthalamic adhesion: third ventricle)
- Coarctation of the frontal horn(s)
- Coarctation of the occipital horn(s)
- Absence of choroid plexus calcification (lateral, third, fourth ventricles)
- Choroid plexus calcification (lateral, third, fourth ventricles)
- Asymmetric lateral ventricle choroid plexus calcification
- Fat in choroid plexus (lateral ventricle)
- Choroid plexus cyst
- Intraluminal dural venous sinus arachnoid granulation
- Inner table calvarial arachnoid granulation impression/excavation

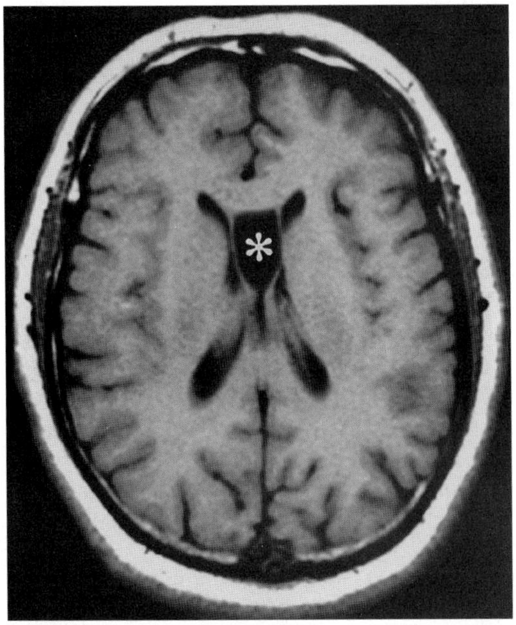

Figure 2K-18A: Cavum septi pellucidi et vergae. Enhanced axial T1-weighted MR image showing a cavum septi pellucidi (*asterisk*).

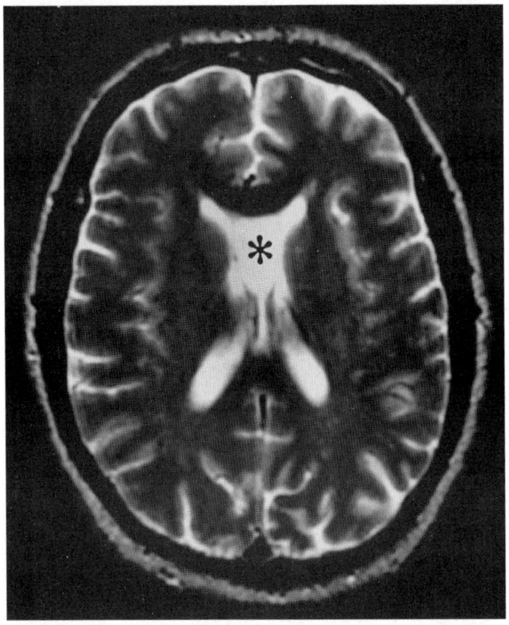

Figure 2K-18B: Cavum septi pellucidi et vergae. Axial T2-weighted MR image showing a cavum septi pellucidi (*asterisk*).

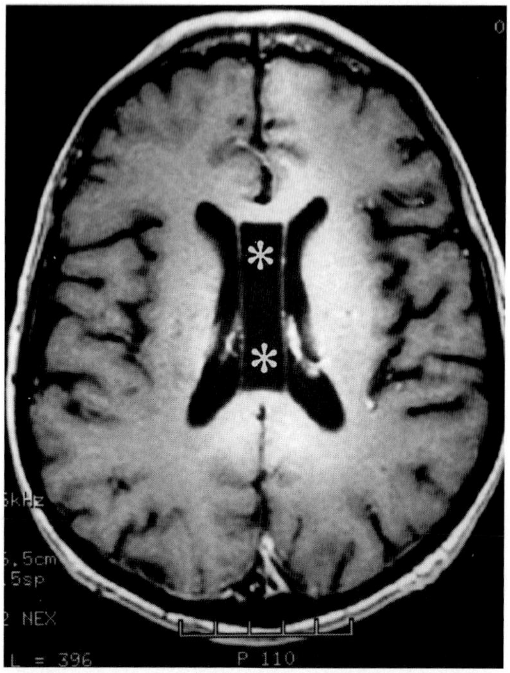

Figure 2K-18C: Cavum septi pellucidi et vergae. Enhanced axial Tl-weighted MR image at a higher level than Fig. 2K-18A and Fig. 2K-18B, showing a cavum septi pellucidi et vergae (*asterisks*).

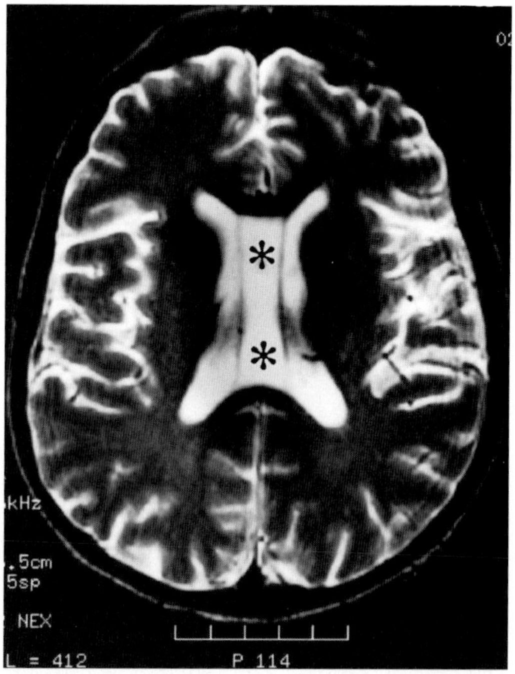

Figure 2K-18D: Cavum septi pellucidi et vergae. Axial T2-weighted MR image showing a cavum septi pellucidi et vergae (*asterisks*).

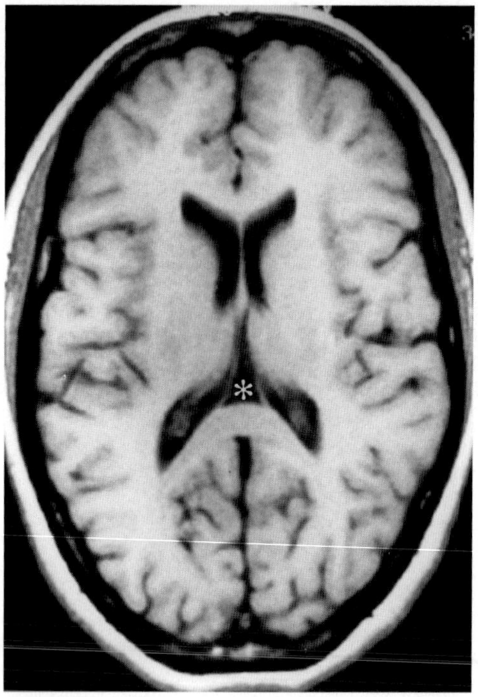

Figure 2K-19A: Cavum velum interpositum. Unenhanced axial Tl-weighted MR image showing a cavum velum interpositum (*asterisk*).

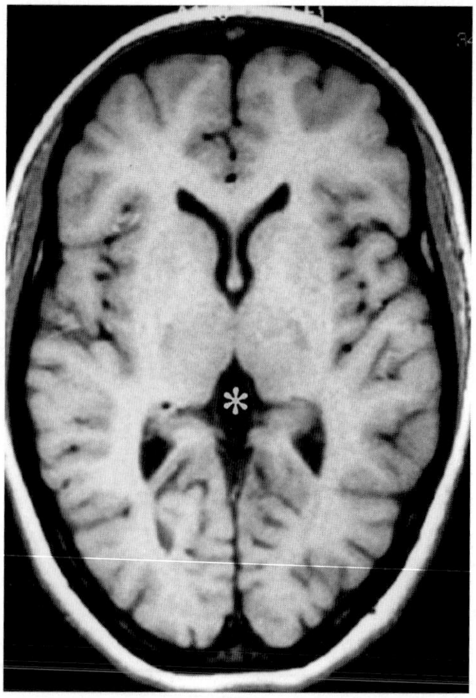

Figure 2K-19B: Cavum velum interpositum. Unenhanced axial Tl-weighted MR image at a level below that of Fig. 2K-19A, showing a cavum velum interpositum (*asterisk*).

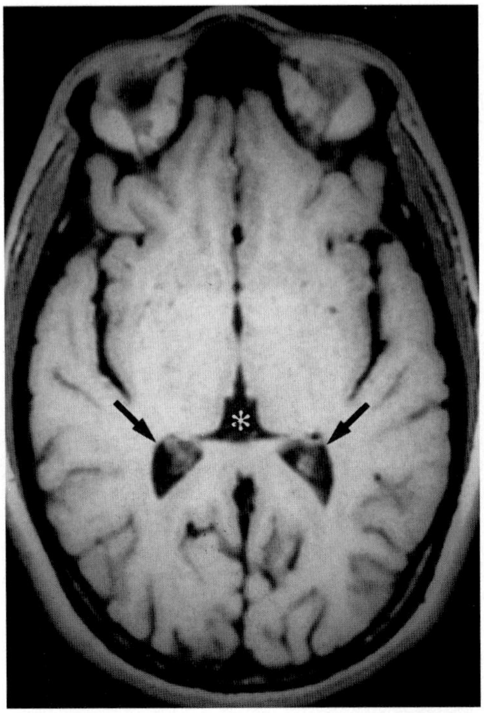

Figure 2K-19C: Cavum velum interpositum. Axial TI-weighted MR image showing the atria of the lateral ventricles (*arrows*) and the cavum velum interpositum (*asterisk*).

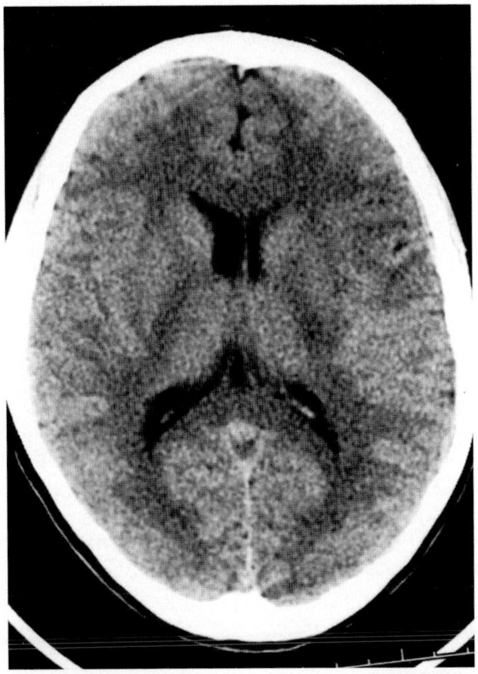

Figure 2K-20A: Lateral ventricular asymmetry. Unenhanced axial CT image showing asymmetric lateral ventricles (larger on the right side).

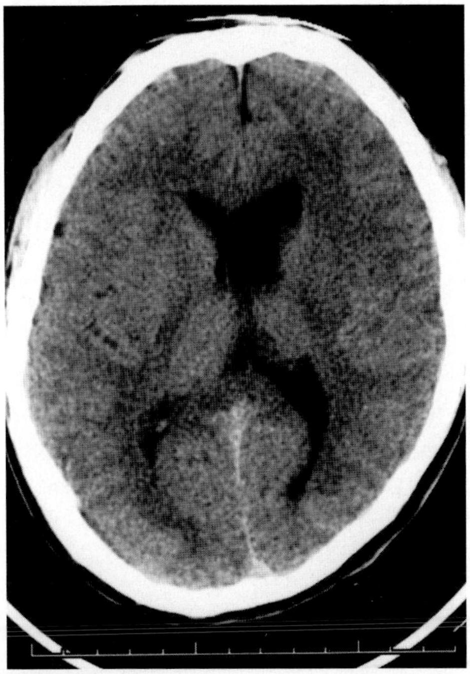

Figure 2K-20B: Lateral ventricular asymmetry. Unenhanced axial CT image in a different patient, showing lateral ventricular asymmetry (larger on the left side).

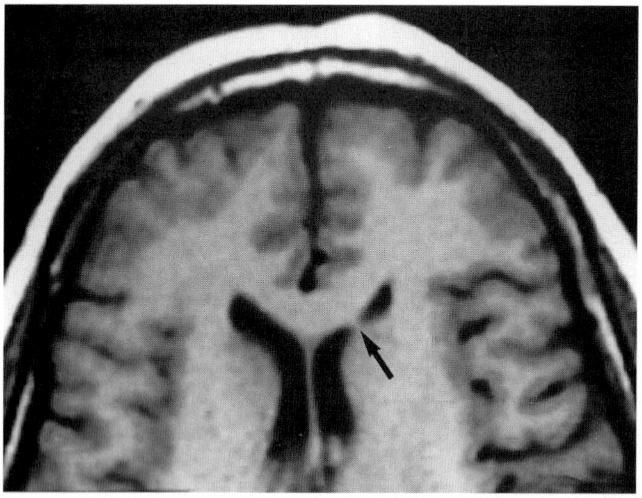

Figure 2K-21A: Coarctation of the frontal horn. Magnified axial T1-weighted MR image showing coarctation of the frontal horn (*arrow*) of the lateral ventricle.

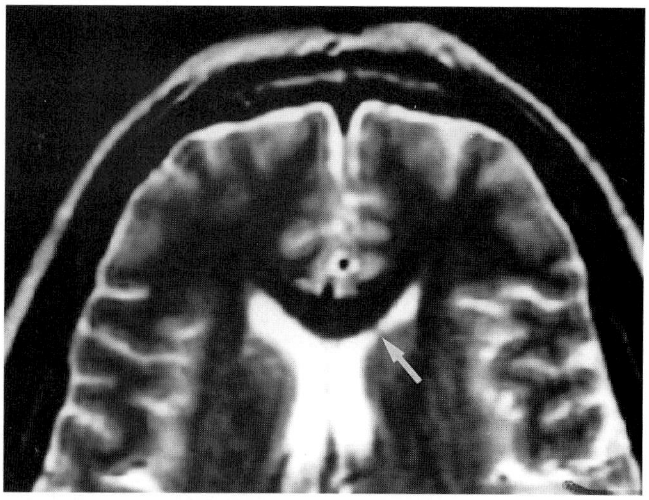

Figure 2K-21B: Coarctation of the frontal horn. Magnified axial T2-weighted MR image showing coarctation of the frontal horn (*arrow*) of the lateral ventricle.

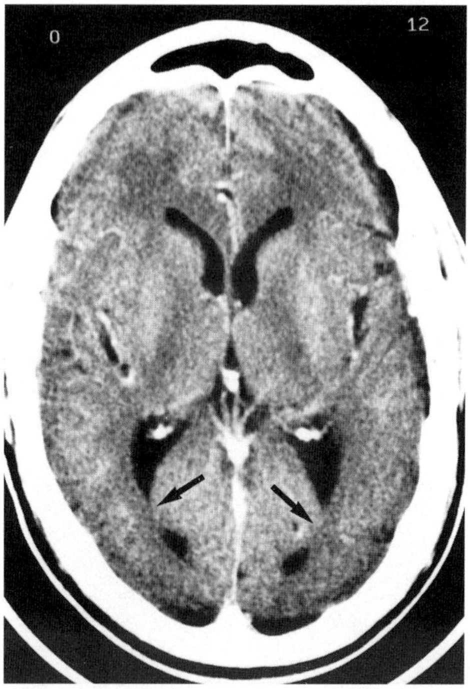

Figure 2K-22: Coarctation of the occipital horn. Enhanced axial CT image showing bilateral coarctation (*arrows*) of the occipital horns of the lateral ventricles.

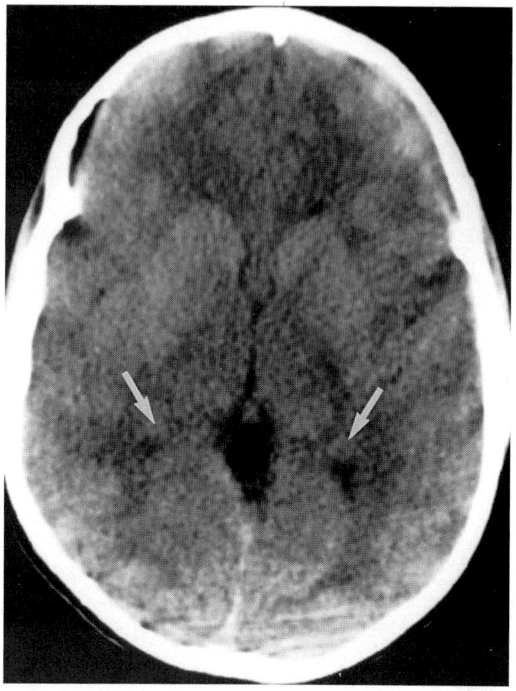

Figure 2K-23: Absence of choroid plexus calcification. Axial CT image in a seven-year-old boy shows no lateral ventricular choroid plexus calcification (*solid arrows*). The pineal gland is also noncalcified.

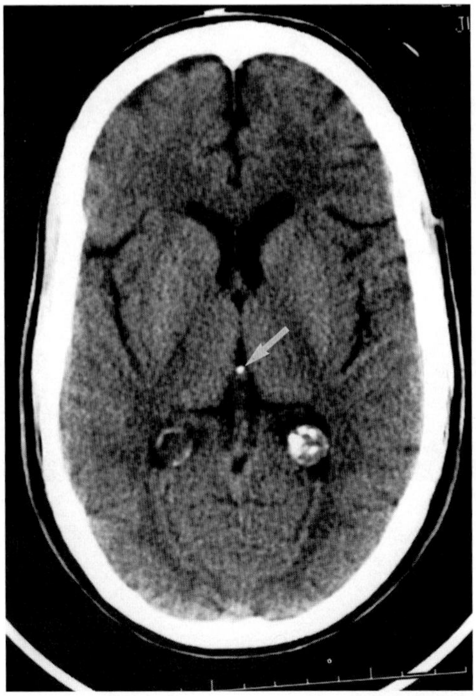

Figure 2K-24A: Choroid plexus calcification. Axial CT image shows asymmetric calcification of the choroid plexi of the lateral ventricles and calcification within the choroid plexus of the third ventricle (*arrow*).

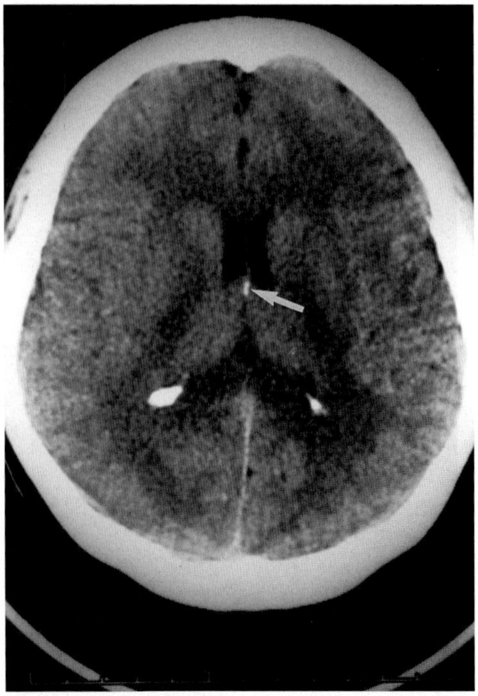

Figure 2K-24B: Choroid plexus calcification. Axial CT image showing calcification (*arrow*) within the choroid plexus of the third ventricle.

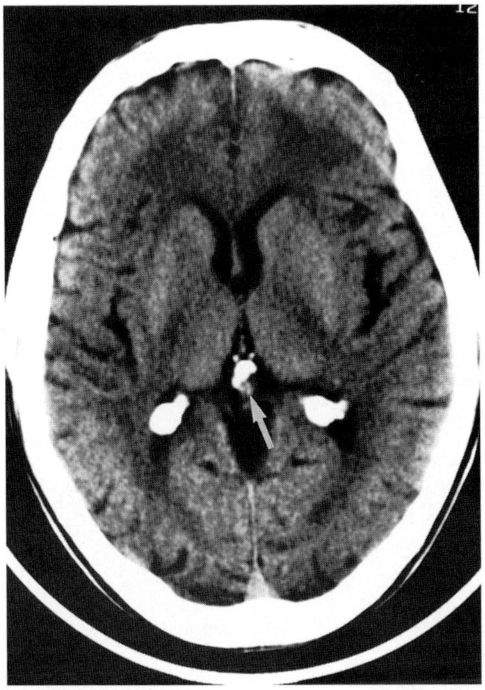

Figure 2K-24C: Choroid plexus calcification. Unenhanced axial CT image showing dense calcification of the choroid plexi in the atria of the lateral ventricles. Note also the pineal gland calcification (*arrow*).

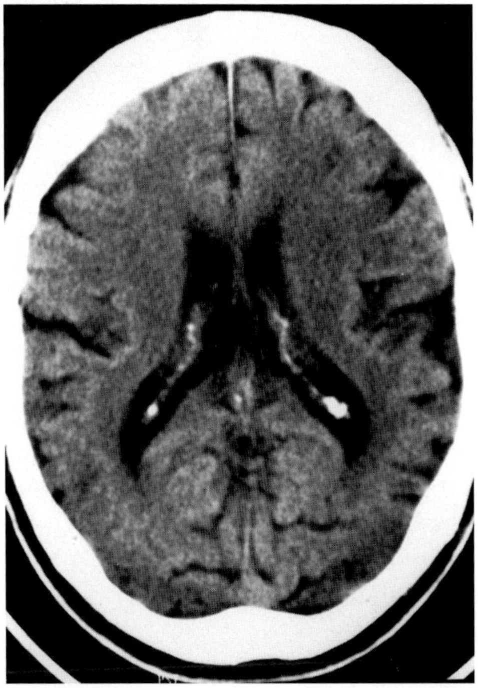

Figure 2K-24D: Choroid plexus calcification. Axial CT image showing calcification of the choroid plexi in the bodies of the lateral ventricles.

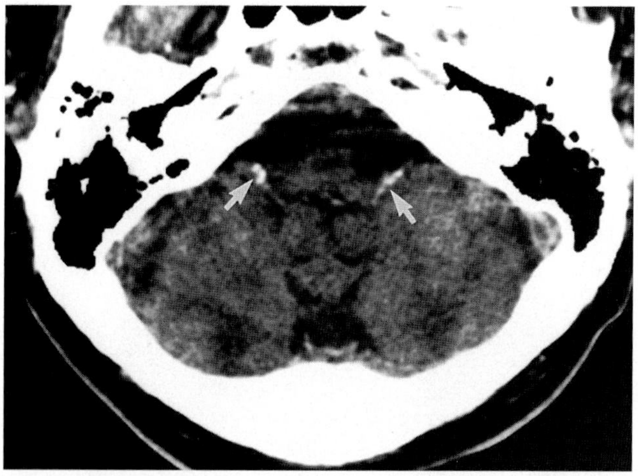

Figure 2K-24E: Choroid plexus calcification. Unenhanced axial CT image showing calcifications extending through the foramina of Luschka (*arrows*), representing cisternal fourth ventricle choroid plexus calcification.

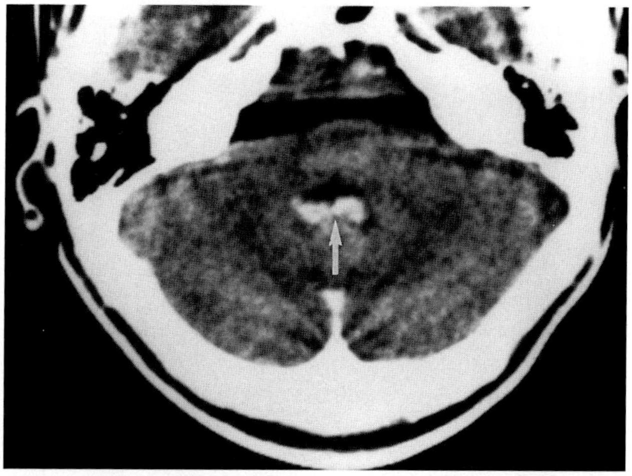

Figure 2K-24F: Choroid plexus calcification. Unenhanced axial CT image showing calcification (*arrow*) within the intraluminal fourth ventricle choroid plexus.

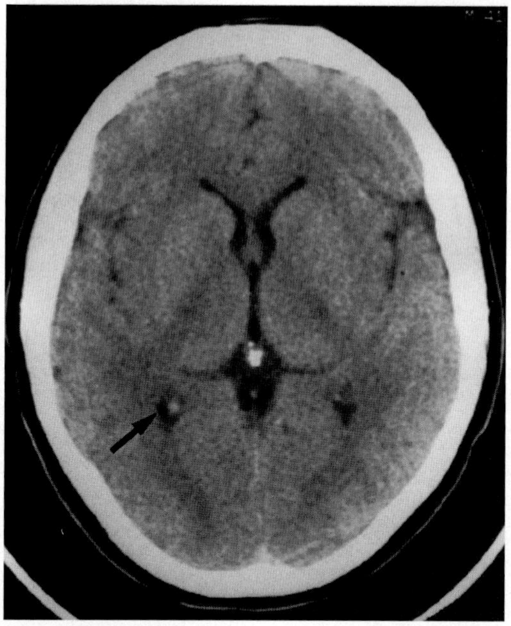

Figure 2K-25: Fat in choroid plexus. Unenhanced axial CT image showing hypodense fat (*arrow*) in the lateral ventricle.

2L Meninges and Subarachnoid Pathways

OVERVIEW

1. The brain and spinal cord are enveloped by three membranes, or meninges, named from the outermost layer inward the dura mater, the arachnoid mater, and the pia mater.
2. In the cranium the dura mater has two layers surrounding the brain: an inner, or meningeal, cranial dural layer and an outer, or periosteal (endosteal), cranial dural layer. In the spine there is a single dural layer, the spinal dura mater.
3. In the cranium the dura mater is adherent to the inner table of the skull. This union is especially strong at sutural sites and the cranial base and around the borders of the foramen magnum.
4. The inner, or meningeal, layer of the cranial dura mater is closely applied to the underlying arachnoid mater. This meningeal layer of the cranial dura mater is continuous with the spinal dura mater.
5. The two layers of the cranial dura mater are united, except where they separate to form the dural venous sinuses.
6. The potential space between the inner table of the skull and the periosteal layer of the cranial dura mater is the cranial epidural space. The potential space between the spinal dura mater and the spinal column (ligaments, periosteum) is the spinal epidural space.
7. The spinal dura mater forms a tube that extends from the edge of the foramen magnum to the dorsal aspect of the coccyx to blend with the coccygeal periosteum as the coccygeal ligament. The thecal space of this dural tube typically ends at the level of the second sacral vertebra, at which point the spinal dura mater invests the distal filum terminale.
8. The spinal dura mater has small, blind-ending tubular extensions (dural root sleeves) that surround the spinal nerve roots for a short distance as they exit through the intervertebral neural foramina.
9. The arachnoid mater is a nonvascular membrane that invests the brain and spinal cord. The arachnoid mater does not enter the cerebral sulci or fissures, with the exception of the midline sagittal fissure between the cerebral hemispheres.
10. The arachnoid membrane also extends along the cranial and spinal nerve roots.
11. The potential space between the dura mater and the arachnoid mater is the subdural space. This subdural space contains a number of bridging veins.
12. The pia mater is intimately attached to the brain, spinal cord, cranial nerves, and spinal nerve roots. The pia mater follows every surface contour, including the sulci and fissures of the brain and spinal cord.
13. The arachnoid mater and pia mater together constitute the *leptomeninges*. These two membranes are separated by the cerebrospinal fluid (CSF)–filled subarachnoid space and are joined together by numerous fibrous trabeculae.
14. The *pachymeninges* consist of the dual meningeal and periosteal layers of the dura mater in the cranium and the single layer of dura mater in the spine.

THE DURAL FOLDS/REFLECTIONS

1. The meningeal layer of the cranial dura is folded inward to form four septa, or reflections, which divide the cranial cavity into various compartments.
2. The largest dural reflection is the sickle-shaped falx cerebri, which descends vertically in the midline sagittal fissure between the cerebral hemispheres. It extends from the crista galli/foramen cecum junction to the internal occipital protuberance and blends in the posterior midline with the tentorium cerebelli. It is narrow in ventrodorsal width anteriorly and relatively broad posteriorly.
3. The tentorium cerebelli is a crescent-shaped transverse dural reflection separating the cerebellum from the occipital lobes of the cerebral hemispheres. It is attached posteriorly to the inner table of the occipital bone and anteriorly to the superior border of the

petrous portion of the temporal bone and the anterior/posterior clinoid processes of the sphenoid bone.

4. Between the concave, anterior, free border of the tentorium cerebelli and the dorsum sellae is a large hiatus, or tentorial incisura; this hiatus is the only opening between the supratentorial and infratentorial cranial compartments. The brain stem passes through the tentorial incisura.
5. The falx cerebri and tentorium cerebelli divide the cranial cavity into a paired supratentorial compartment and a single infratentorial compartment, respectively.
6. A small midline, sagittally oriented crescentic fold of dura below the tentorium cerebelli posteriorly forms the falx cerebelli, which partially separates the cerebellar hemispheres dorsally. The falx cerebelli may be duplicated or triplicated.
7. The diaphragma sellae is a small, horizontal dural fold that forms the roof over the sella turcica as an extension of the tentorium cerebelli and the regional parasellar dura mater. The diaphragma sellae transmits the pituitary infundibulum through a circular hiatus of varying diameter. In this way, the pituitary fossa directly communicates with the suprasellar subarachnoid cistern.

TABLE 2L-1: The Cranial Layers and Interspaces from Outward to Inward

Layers	Space
Bone (calvarium)	
	Potential epidural space
Outer dura mater (periosteal layer)	
	None (dural venous sinuses)
Inner dura mater (meningeal layer)	
	Subdural space
Arachnoid mater	
	Subarachnoid space
Pia mater	
	Potential subpial space
Brain/cranial nerves	

TABLE 2L-2: The Spinal Layers and Interspaces from Outward to Inward

Layers	Space
Bone (spine)	
	Potential subperiosteal space
Periosteum	
	Potential epidural space
Dura mater	
	Subdural space
Arachnoid mater	
	Subarachnoid space
Pia mater	
	Potential subpial space
Spinal cord/spinal nerve roots	

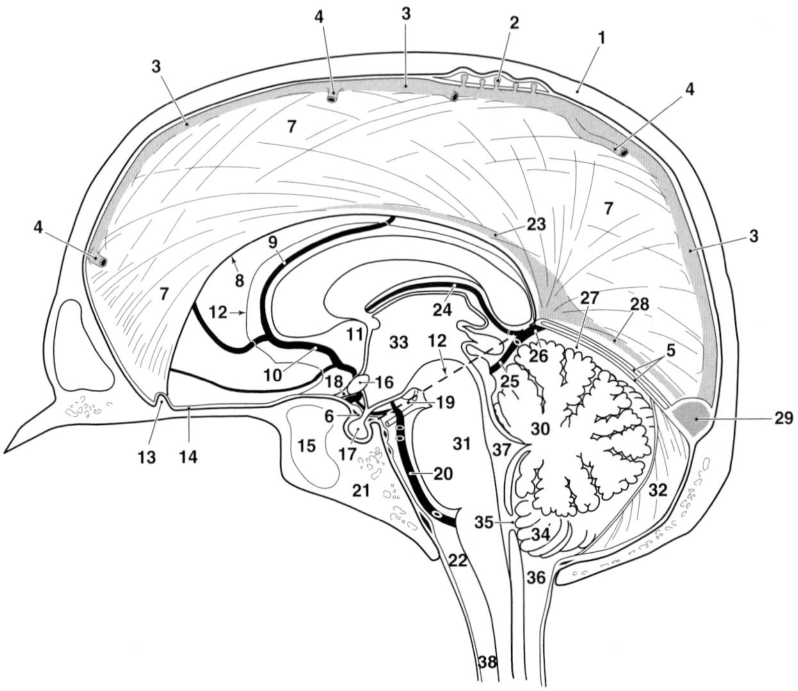

Figure 2L-1: Lateral schematic of the falx cerebri, tentorium cerebelli, and surrounding structures.

1 Calvarium
2 Arachnoid granulations
3 Superior sagittal venous sinus
4 Superficial cerebral veins
5 Cut edge of tentorium cerebelli
6 Diaphragma sellae
7 Falx cerebri
8 Free margin of falx cerebri
9 Pericallosal cistern and artery
10 Anterior cerebral artery
11 Cistern of the laminae terminalis
12 Plane of tentorial hiatus
13 Crista galli
14 Lamina cribrosa
15 Sphenoid sinus
16 Optic chiasm
17 Pituitary gland
18 Chiasmatic cistern
19 Interpeduncular cistern
20 Pontine cistern and basilar artery
21 Clivus
22 Medullary cistern
23 Inferior sagittal venous sinus
24 Internal cerebral vein
25 Basal vein of Rosenthal
26 Vein of Galen
27 Superior cerebellar cistern
28 Sinus rectus (straight venous sinus)
29 Torcular Herophili
30 Cerebellum
31 Pons
32 Falx cerebelli
33 Third ventricle
34 Cerebellar tonsil
35 Foramen of Magendie
36 Cisterna magna
37 Fourth ventricle
38 Spinal subarachnoid space

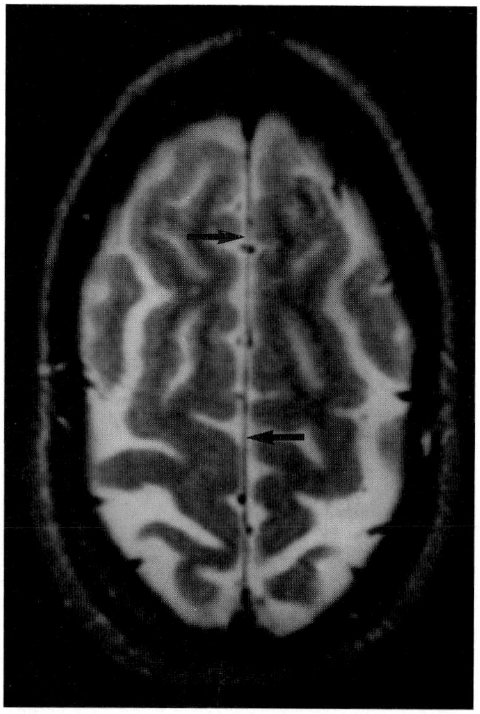

Figure 2L-2A: The falx cerebri. Axial T2-weighted MR image showing the falx cerebri (*arrows*) within the interhemispheric fissure.

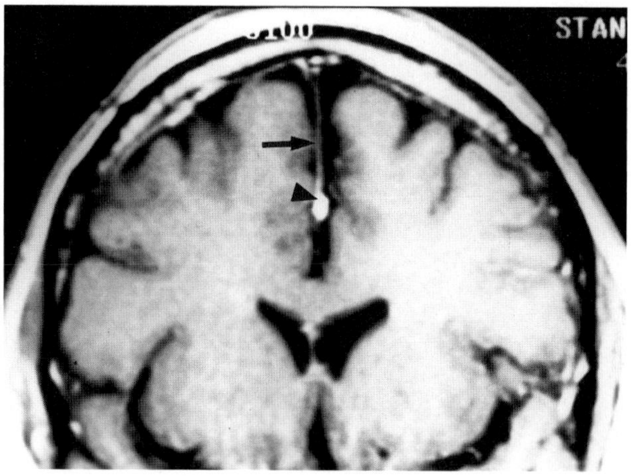

Figure 2L-2B: The falx cerebri. Enhanced coronal T1-weighted MR image shows the falx cerebri (*straight arrow*) terminating inferiorly in the inferior sagittal sinus (*arrowhead*).

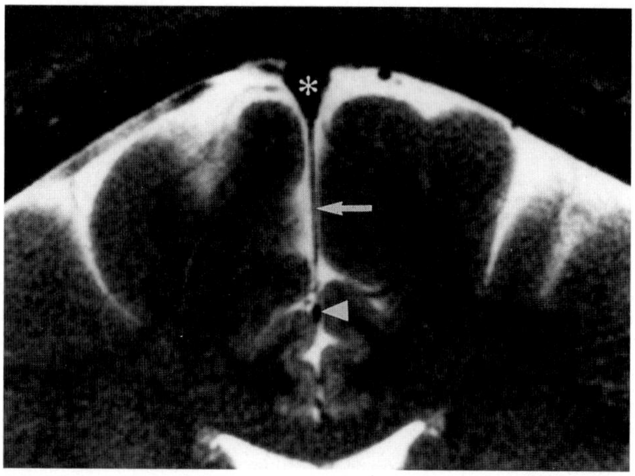

Figure 2L-2C: The falx cerebri. Coronal T2-weighted MR image showing the falx cerebri (*arrow*), the superior sagittal venous sinus (*asterisk*), and the inferior sagittal venous sinus (*arrowhead*).

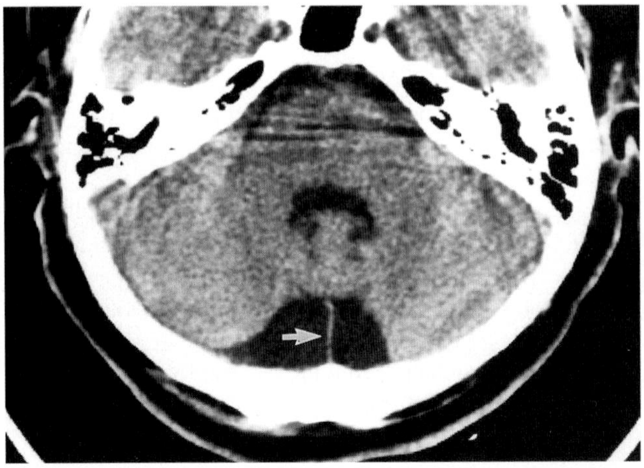

Figure 2L-3A: The falx cerebelli. Unenhanced axial CT image showing the falx cerebelli (*arrow*).

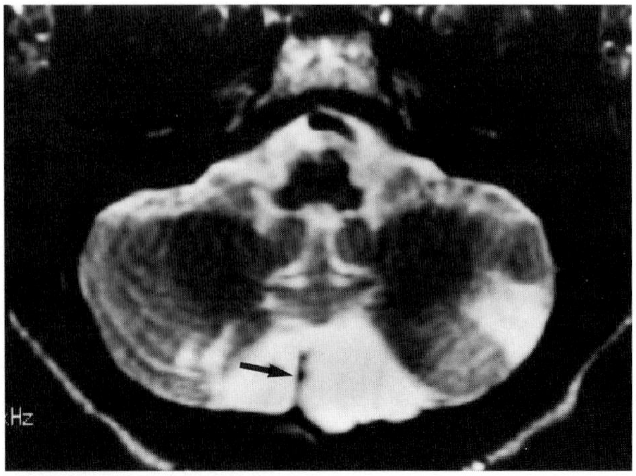

Figure 2L-3B: The falx cerebelli. Axial T2-weighted MR image showing the falx cerebelli (*arrow*).

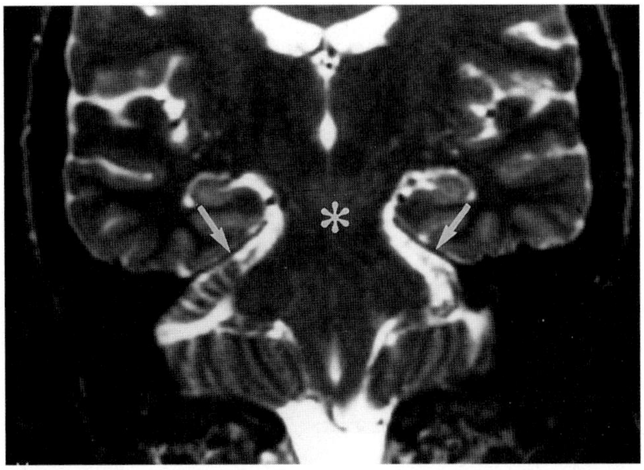

Figure 2L-4: Tentorium cerebelli. Coronal T2-weighted MR image showing the anterior aspect of the tentorium cerebelli (*arrows*) traversed by the brain stem (*asterisk*) through the tentorial hiatus.

THE CEREBROSPINAL FLUID PATHWAYS

1. CSF is primarily produced by the villi of the choroid plexi located in the lateral, third, and fourth ventricles. Some CSF is also formed by the cerebral parenchyma and possibly the spinal cord parenchyma. The potential CSF contribution of the cranial and spinal nerve roots as they traverse the subarachnoid space is unknown.
2. The total volume of CSF in the cerebral ventricles and cranial extraventricular subarachnoid spaces is approximately 125 to 150 mL (25 mL in the ventricles and 100 mL in the cranial subarachnoid space).
3. CSF flows from the lateral ventricles through the paired foramina of Monro into the third ventricle.
4. CSF subsequently passes through the aqueduct of Sylvius into the fourth ventricle.
5. CSF then exits the ventricular system through the single median dorsal foramen of Magendie and the paired lateral foramina of Luschka to empty into the posterior fossa basal subarachnoid cisterns.
6. The CSF then circulates within the subarachnoid spaces surrounding both the brain and the spinal cord.
7. CSF is returned to the venous system primarily via the arachnoid granulations (Pacchionian bodies) that are intimately associated with the dural venous sinuses and the spinal nerve roots. Arachnoid granulations are specialized protrusions of arachnoid mater through the meningeal layer of the dura into the dural venous sinuses and other regional venous structures.
8. Other sites of CSF absorption are the walls of the vasculature of the brain and spinal cord via the extracellular (i.e., interstitial) fluid of the central nervous system (CNS) parenchyma and perhaps through the extra-CNS lymphatic channels in or adjacent to the CNS dura mater (in theory).

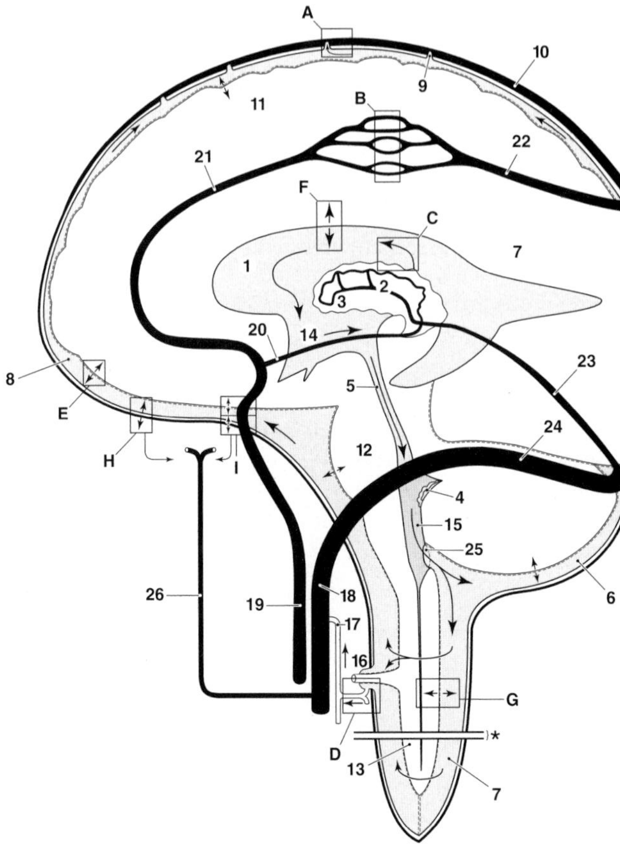

Figure 2L-5: Lateral schematic of the CSF pathways and CNS barriers/interfaces. A: CSF–blood barrier at an arachnoid granulation. B: Blood–brain barrier at the parenchymal capillary level. C: Blood–CSF barrier at the choroid plexus. D: CSF–lymphatic barrier/interface at the spinal nerve root/sheath complex (theoretical in human beings). E: CSF–brain interface at the pial surface of the brain. F: CSF–brain interface at the ependymal surface of the ventricular system. G: CSF–spinal cord interface at the pial surface of the cord. H: CSF–lymphatic barrier/interface at the cribriform plate (theoretical in human beings). I: Perivascular lymphatic barrier/interface in the region of the cranial penetrating vessels (theoretical in human beings). *Asterisk*, break in diagram; *arrows*, CSF flow, secretion, and absorption.

1 Lateral ventricle
2 Choroid plexi of the lateral ventricles
3 Choroid plexus of the third ventricle
4 Choroid plexus of the fourth ventricle (vascular supply and drainage not shown)
5 Aqueduct of Sylvius
6 Posterior fossa subarachnoid space
7 Spinal subarachnoid space
8 Supratentorial subarachnoid space
9 Arachnoid granulation
10 Superior sagittal venous sinus
11 Cerebral hemisphere
12 Brain stem
13 Spinal cord
14 Third ventricle
15 Fourth ventricle
16 Spinal nerve
17 Paraspinal lymphatics
18 Internal jugular vein
19 Internal carotid artery
20 Anterior choroidal artery
21 Cerebral artery
22 Cerebral vein
23 Straight venous sinus
24 Transverse venous sinus
25 Foramina of Luschka and Magendie
26 Craniocervical lymphatics

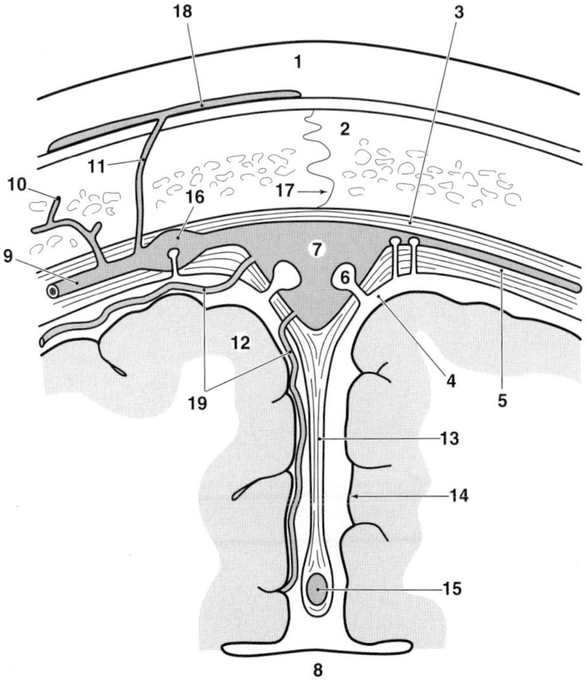

Figure 2L-6: Coronal sectional schematic of the cranial meningeal coverings and dural venous sinuses over the cranial convexity.

1 Scalp
2 Calvarium
3 Dura mater (periosteal and meningeal layers)
4 Subarachnoid space
5 Arachnoid mater
6 Arachnoid granulation
7 Superior sagittal venous sinus
8 Corpus callosum
9 Meningeal vein
10 Diploic vein
11 Emissary vein
12 Cerebral cortex
13 Falx cerebri
14 Pia mater
15 Inferior sagittal venous sinus
16 Venous lacuna (lake)
17 Calvarial suture
18 Scalp vein
19 Cerebral vein(s)

THE SUBARACHNOID CISTERNS, FISSURES, AND SPACES

1. The cranial subarachnoid cisterns are expansions of the subarachnoid spaces situated between the pia mater and the arachnoid mater.
2. The cranial subarachnoid cisterns are filled with CSF and are traversed by numerous fenestrated trabeculae that connect the pia mater and arachnoid mater but do not inhibit the free flow of CSF.
3. The cranial and spinal nerves and blood vessels are invested by a thin layer of the leptomeninges as they traverse the subarachnoid cisterns.

TABLE 2L-3: The Cranial Subarachnoid Cisterns, Fissures, and Spaces

Ventral spaces
Median
Perimedullary cistern
Prepontine cistern
Interpeduncular cistern
Suprasellar cistern
Paramedian
Cerebellopontine angle cisterns
Retropulvinar cisterns
Sylvian fissures/cisterns
Dorsal spaces
Median
Superior cerebellar cistern
Quadrigeminal plate cistern
Pericallosal cistern
Cistern of the lamina terminalis
Cisterna magna
Interhemispheric fissure/cistern
Cistern of the velum interpositum
Paramedian
Ambient cisterns

Modified from Hayman LA, Hinck VC. In: *Clinical brain imaging*. St. Louis: Mosby, 1992: 311.

TABLE 2L-4: The Contents of the Cranial Subarachnoid Cisterns, Fissures, and Spaces

Subarachnoid cistern	Location/borders	Contents
Cisterna magna	Between the medulla, roof of the fourth ventricle, and the inferior surface of cerebellum	PICA
Perimedullary cistern	Anterior and lateral to medulla	VA, PICA, CN IX–XII
Prepontine cistern	Anterior to pons	BA, AICA, CN–V, CN–VI
Cerebellopontine angle cistern	Between the petrous portion of the temporal bone, cerebellum, pons, and tentorium	AICA, PICA, CN-V–VIII
Interpeduncular cistern	Between the cerebral peduncles, anterior to the midbrain	SCA, PCA, PCOM, AchA, CN–III
Ambient cistern	Around midbrain: connects the suprasellar pontine and quadrigeminal cisterns	PCA, SCA, AchA, PchA, CN-IV, BVR
Quadrigeminal plate cistern	Posterior to midbrain/pineal gland: connects the ambient and superior cerebellar cisterns	PCA, SCA, PChA, BVR, VG
Superior cerebellar cistern	Between the tentorium and superior surface of vermian vein cerebellum: connects with the quadrigeminal cistern anterosuperiorly	SCA, superior
Suprasellar cistern	Superior to the sella turcica/optic chiasm	ICA, ACA, MCA, PCOM, AChA, CN-II, BVR, pituitary infundibulum
Retropulvinar cistern (wings of the ambient cistern)	Behind the thalamus	PchA, BVR
Cistern of the Sylvian fissure	Between the insula and opercula: connects medially with the suprasellar cistern	MCA, superfical middle cerebral veins
Cistern of the transverse fissure (cistern of the thalamus: velum interpositum)	Between the corpus callosum, roof of the third ventricle, and anterior continuation of the quadrigeminal cistern	ICV, AchA, PchA
Pericallosal cistern	Between the corpus callosum and the inferior free edge of the falx cerebri	PA
Interhemispheric fissure (the medial surface of the cerebral hemisphere)	Between the falx cerebri and cerebral arteries, veins	Cerebral arteries and veins
Cistern of lamina terminalis	Anterior to lamina terminalis and anterior commissure: connects the suprasellar cistern with the pericallosal cistern	ACA, ACOM
Convexity (subarachnoid space)	Over the surfaces of the cerebral hemispheres	Cerebral arteries, veins

ACA, anterior cerebral artery; ICA, internal carotid artery; PCOM, posterior communicating artery; AChA, anterior choroidal artery; MCA, middle cerebral artery; PICA, posterior inferior cerebellar artery; ACOM, anterior communicating artery; PCA, posterior cerebral artery; SCA, superior cerebellar artery; AICA, anterior–inferior cerebellar artery; PchA, posterior choroidal artery; VA, vertebral artery; CN, cranial nerve; BA, basilar artery; BVR, basal vein of Rosenthal; VG, vein of Galen; ICV, internal cerebral vein; PA, pericallosal artery.

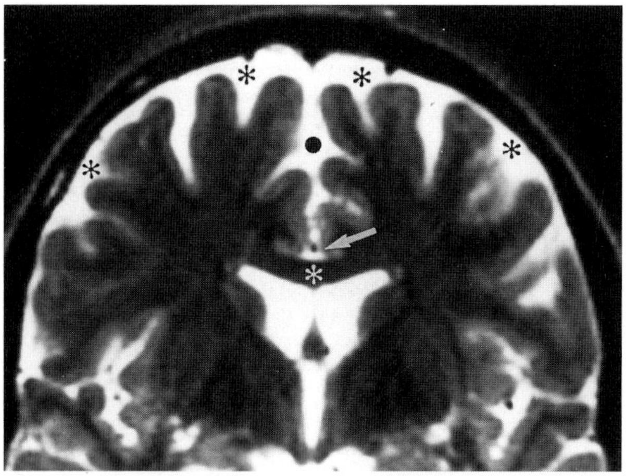

Figure 2L-7A: Pericallosal cistern: convexity subarachnoid space and interhemispheric fissure/cistern. Coronal T2-weighted MR image showing the pericallosal cistern (*arrow*) above the corpus callosum (*white asterisk*), the convexity subarachnoid space (*black asterisks*), and the interhemispheric fissure/cistern (*dot*).

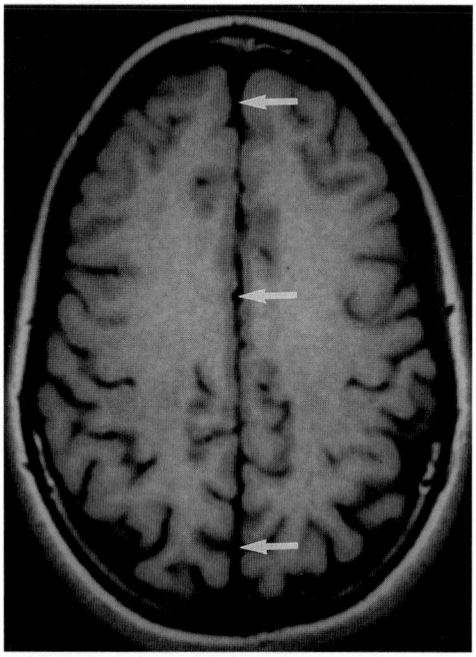

Figure 2L-7B: Interhemispheric fissure/cistern. Axial T1-weighted MR image showing the interhemispheric fissure/cistern (*arrows*).

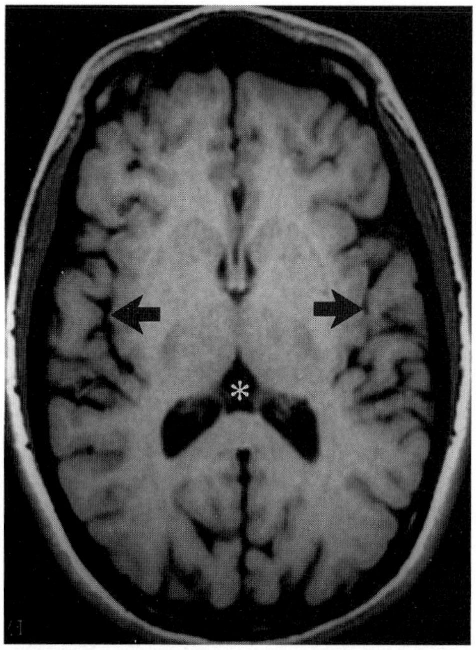

Figure 2L-7C: Sylvian fissures and cistern of the velum interpositum. Axial T1-weighted MR image shows the upper aspect of the Sylvian fissures (arrows) and the cistern of the velum interpositum (asterisk).

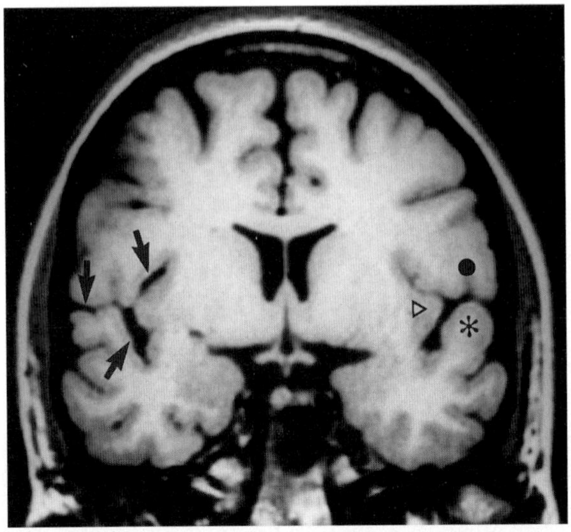

Figure 2L-8A: The Sylvian fissure. Coronal T1-weighted MR image showing the central portion of the Sylvian fissure (*arrows*), the insula (*arrowhead*), the parietal operculum (*dot*), and the temporal operculum (*asterisk*).

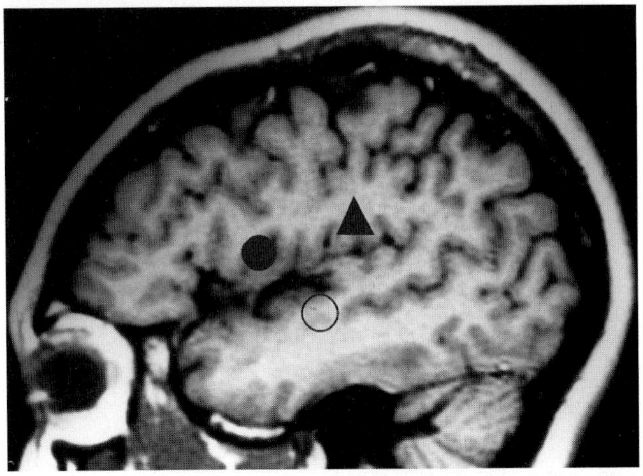

Figure 2L-8B: The Sylvian fissure. Parasagittal T1-weighted MR image showing the Sylvian fissure surrounded by the frontal (*black dot*), temporal (*open circle*), and parietal (*triangle*) opercula.

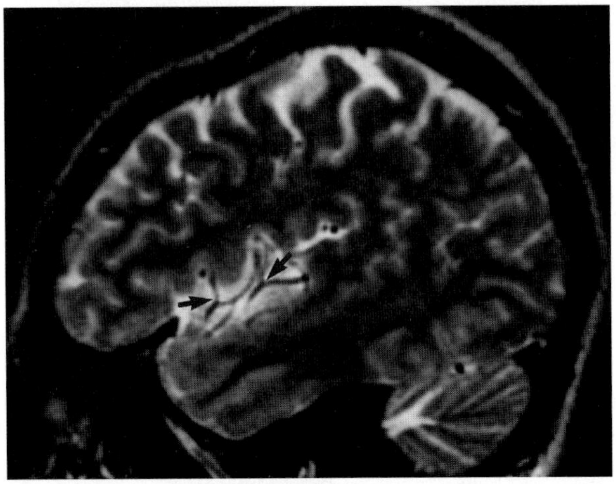

Figure 2L-8C: The Sylvian fissure. Parasagittal T2-weighted MR image showing the middle cerebral vessels (*arrows*: flow voids) within the Sylvian fissure.

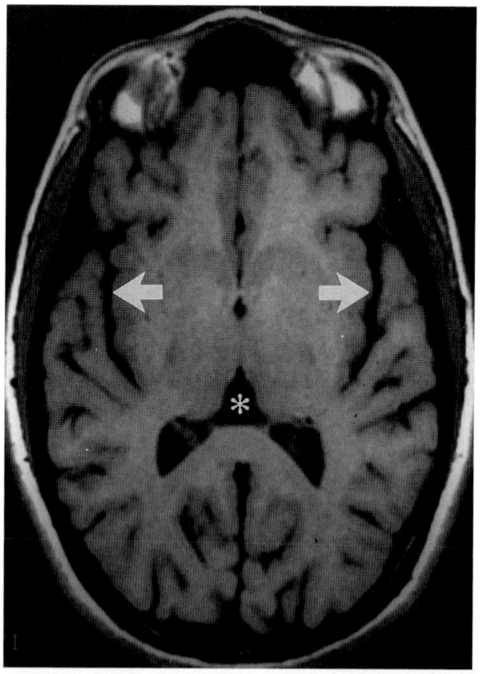

Figure 2L-9: Cistern of the velum interpositum and Sylvian fissures. Axial T1-weighted MR image showing the middle aspect of the Sylvian fissures (*arrows*) and the cistern of the velum interpositum (*asterisk*).

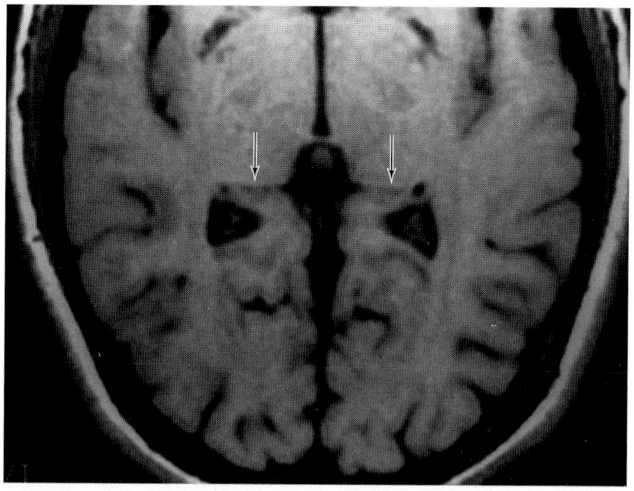

Figure 2L-10: Retropulvinar cisterns. Axial T1-weighted MR image showing the retropulvinar cisterns (*arrows*).

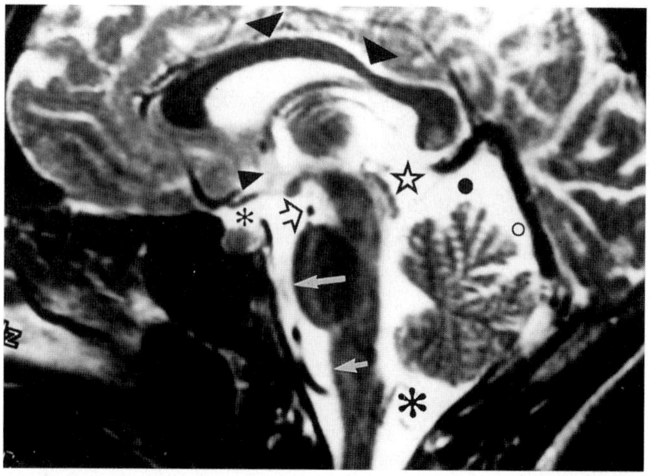

Figure 2L-11: Basal subarachnoid cisterns. Sagittal T2-weighted MR image showing the suprasellar cistern (*small asterisk*), the interpeduncular cistern (*open arrow*), the premedullary (perimedullary) cistern (*short arrow*), the prepontine cistern (*long arrow*), the cistern (*short arrow*), the cisterna magna (*large asterisk*), the quadrigeminal cistern (*star*), the superior cerebellar cistern (*dot*), the superior (peri-) vermian cistern (*circle*), the cistern of the lamina terminalis (*small arrowhead*), and the pericallosal cistern (*large arrowheads*).

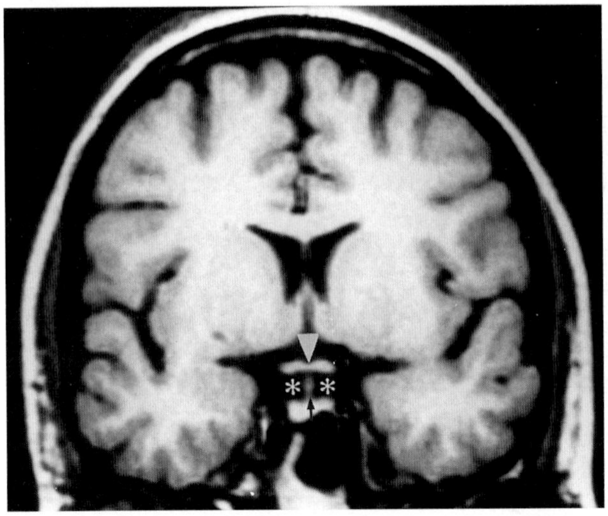

Figure 2L-12A: Suprasellar cistern. Coronal T1-weighted MR image showing the suprasellar cistern (*asterisks*) containing the pituitary infundibulum (*arrow*) and the optic chiasm (*arrowhead*).

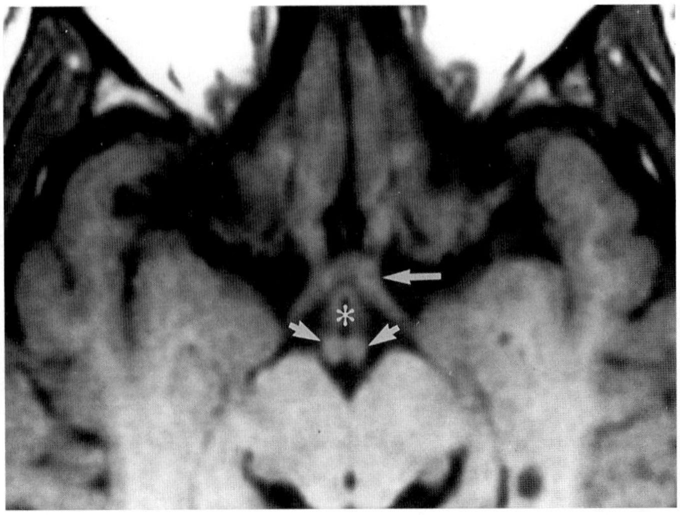

Figure 2L-12B: The upper suprasellar cistern. Axial T1-weighted MR image showing the suprasellar cistern containing the optic chiasm (*large arrow*), the inferior hypothalamus (*asterisk*), and the mammillary bodies (*small arrows*).

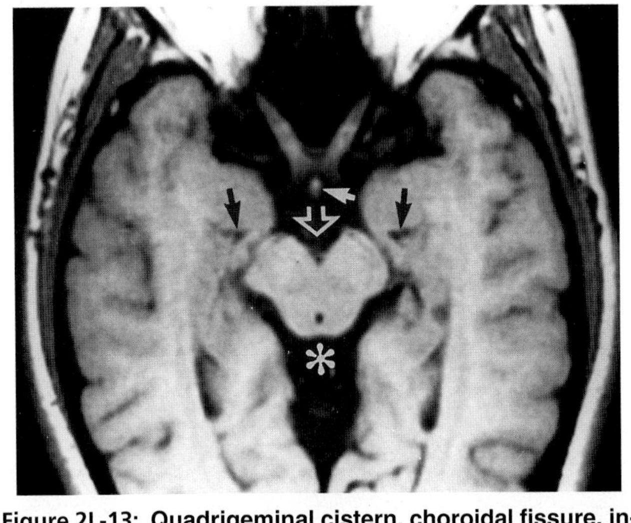

Figure 2L-13: Quadrigeminal cistern, choroidal fissure, interpeduncular cistern, and lower suprasellar cistern. Axial T1-weighted MR image showing the quadrigeminal cistern (*asterisk*), the choroidal fissures (*black arrows*), and the interpeduncular cistern (*open arrow*). Note the pituitary infundibulum (*white arrow*) traversing the suprasellar cistern.

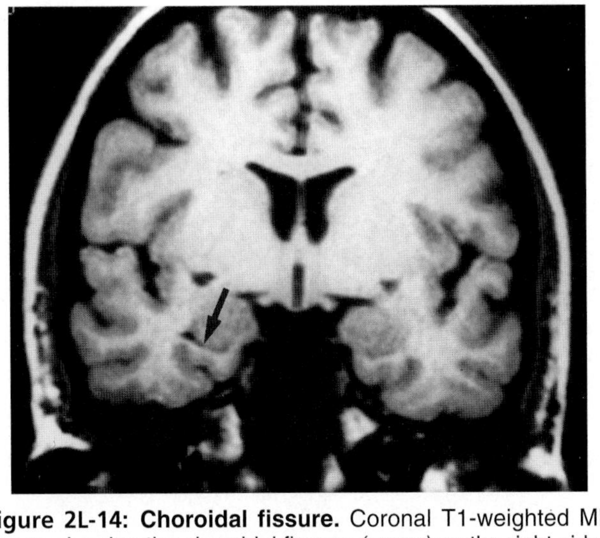

Figure 2L-14: Choroidal fissure. Coronal T1-weighted MR image showing the choroidal fissure *(arrow)* on the right side.

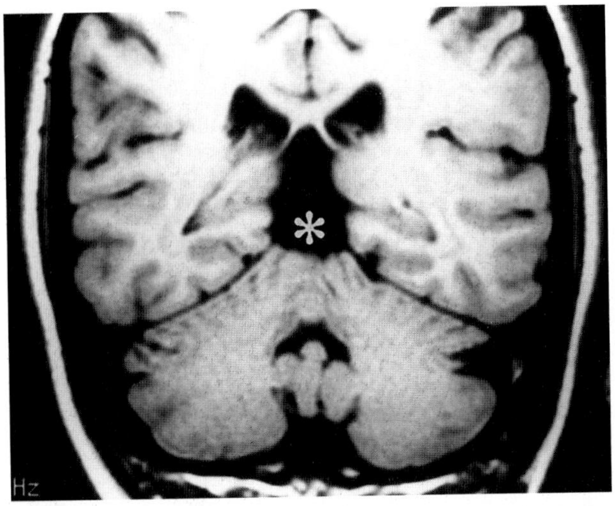

Figure 2L-15: Superior cerebellar/quadrigeminal cistern. Coronal T1-weighted MR image showing the junction between the superior cerebellar and the quadrigeminal cisterns (*asterisk*).

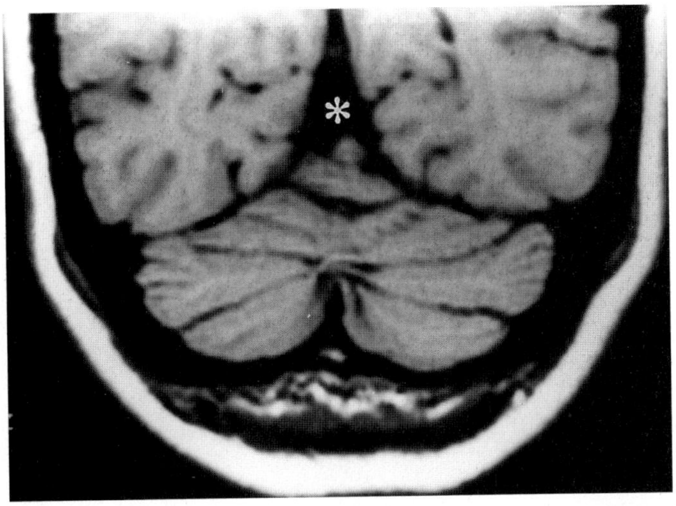

Figure 2L-16: Superior vermian cistern. Coronal T1-weighted MR image showing the superior vermian cistern (*asterisk*).

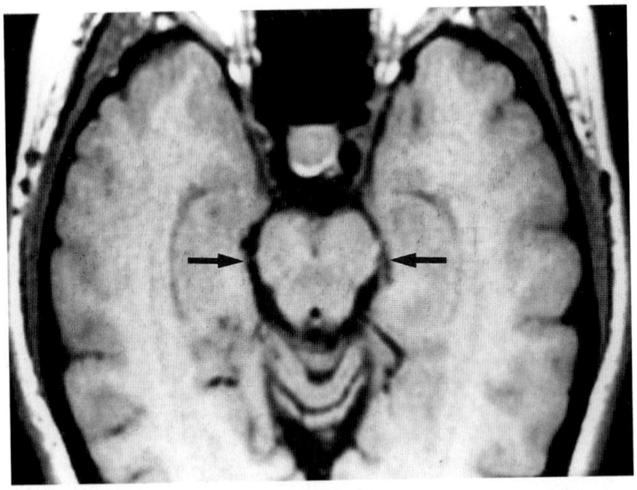

Figure 2L-17: Ambient cistern. Axial T1-weighted MR image showing the ambient cistern (*arrows*) surrounding the upper brain stem.

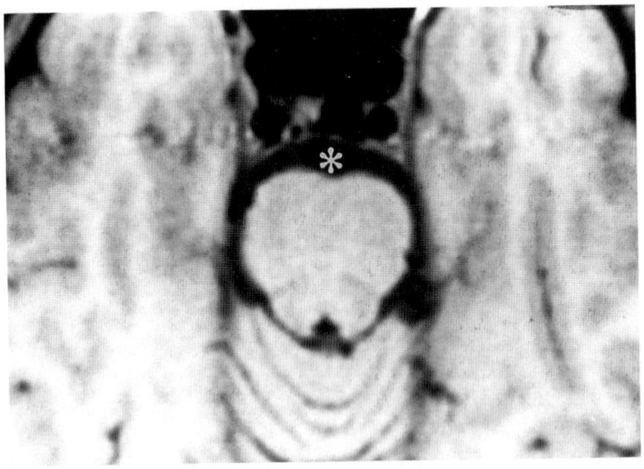

Figure 2L-18: Prepontine cistern. Axial T1-weighted MR image showing the prepontine cistern (*asterisk*).

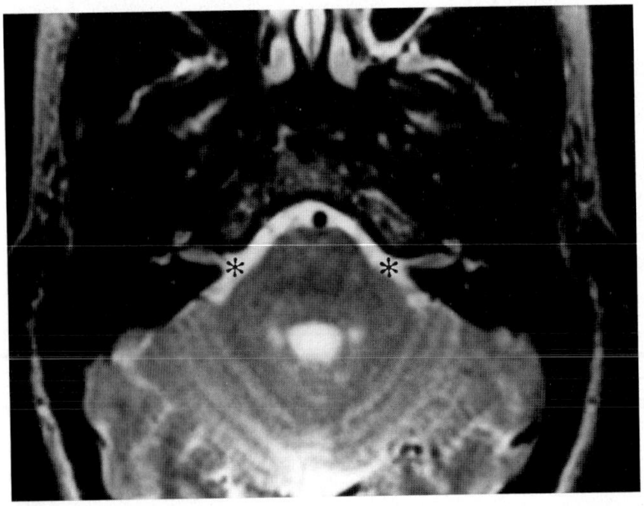

Figure 2L-19A: Cerebellopontine angle cisterns. Axial T2-weighted MR image showing the cerebellopontine angle cisterns (*asterisks*).

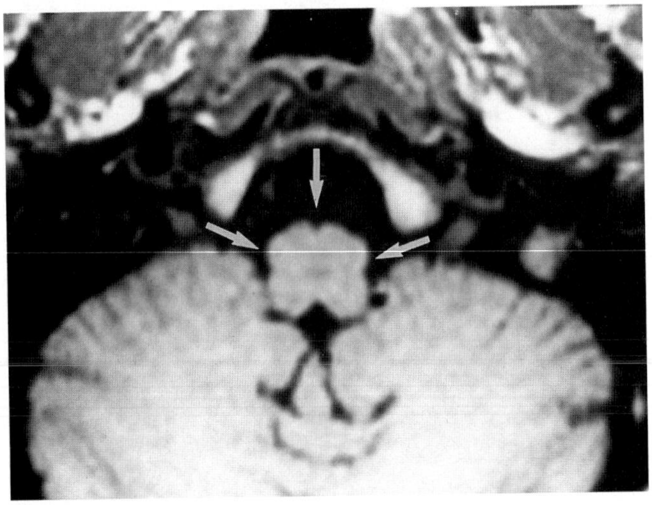

Figure 2L-19B: Perimedullary cistern. Axial T1-weighted MR image showing the perimedullary cistern (*arrows*).

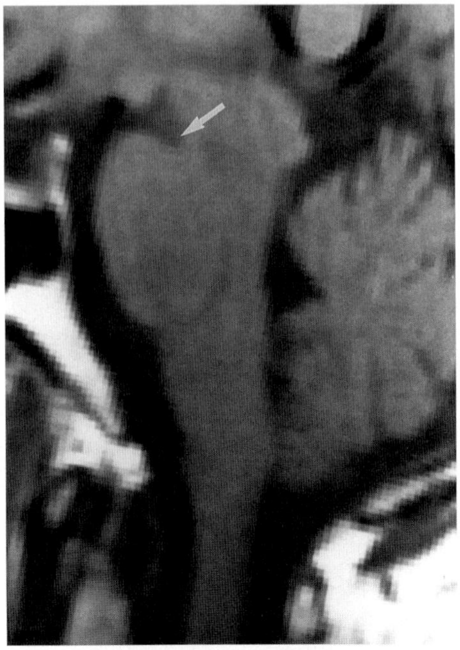

Figure 2L-20A: Inferior recess of the interpeduncular cistern. Sagittal T1-weighted MR image showing the inferior recess (*arrow*) of the interpeduncular cistern.

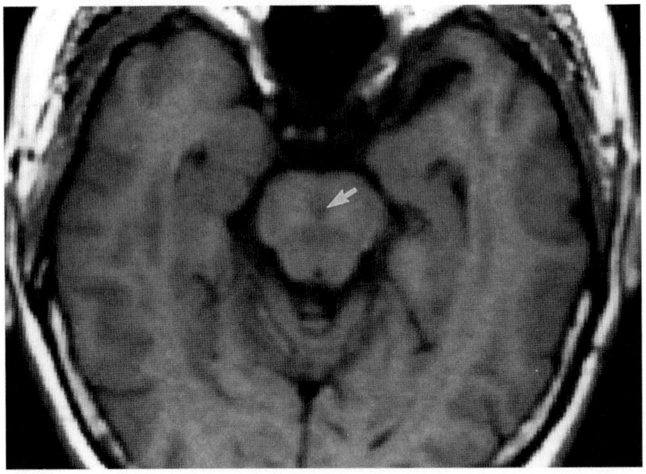

Figure 2L-20B: Inferior recess of the interpeduncular cistern. Axial T1-weighted MR image showing the inferior recess (*arrow*) of the interpeduncular cistern.

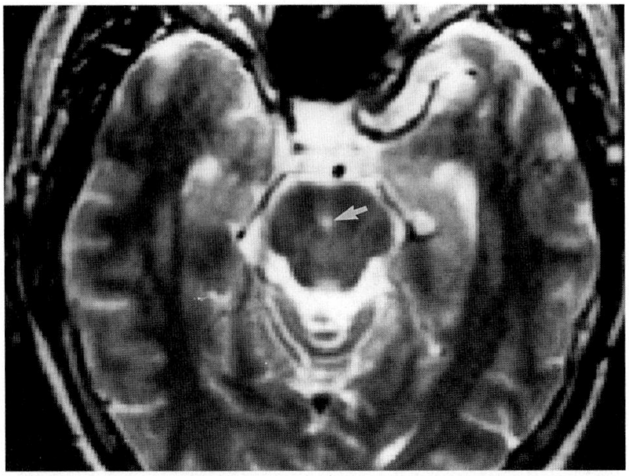

Figure 2L-20C: Inferior recess of the interpeduncular cistern. Axial T2-weighted MR image showing the inferior recess (*arrow*) of the interpeduncular cistern.

THE PERIVASCULAR, OR VIRCHOW-ROBIN, SPACES

1. The perivascular, or Virchow-Robin, spaces are the spaces between a vessel entering the CNS parenchyma (perforating vessel) and the layer of pia mater cells over the surface of the cerebrum and spinal cord.
2. Detailed electron microscope analysis scans show that the pia mater has outer and inner layers that are reflected from the surface of the brain onto the surface of arteries in the subarachnoid space to form their outer coating. This sheath of pia mater is either incomplete or absent around the penetrating portions of the veins. In this anatomical arrangement, the subarachnoid space is therefore separated from the CNS *epipial perivascular space* (Jinkins) by this thin layer of perivascular pia mater that in turn is surrounded by the potential subpial perivascular space.
3. There is a second potential *intrapial perivascular space* (Jinkins) lying between the two layers of the pia mater. Some authors believe that it is this perivascular space that may become dilated, leading to enlarged perivascular spaces.
4. Finally, there is a third potential *subpial perivascular space* (Jinkins)—between the outer (parenchymal) layer of the pia mater and the CNS parenchyma surrounding the penetrating vessel.
5. The layer of pia mater that accompanies CNS perforating vessels gradually becomes fenestrated and discontinuous and eventually disappears as the vessel approaches the capillary stage.
6. It seems to be true that the parenchymal subpial space directly communicates with the epipial perivascular space of penetrating vessels via fenestre.
7. Apparently, then, the subarachnoid space does not theoretically communicate freely with the perivascular spaces in most or all instances. Therefore, the subarachnoid space seems to be a relatively closed envelope, open only through the relative barriers of the pia mater, the choroid plexi, and the arachnoid granulations.
8. Perivascular space dilatations result hypothetically from a form of aberrant connection of the subarachnoid space with one or more of the epi-, intra-, or subpial perivascular spaces.

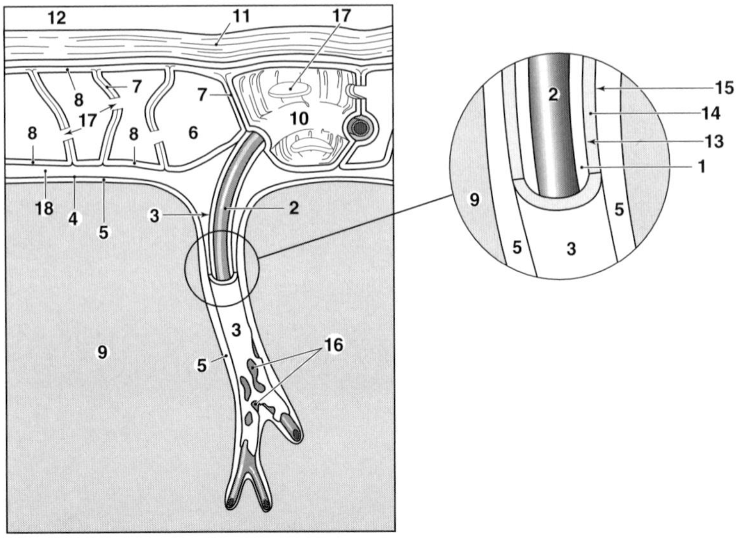

Figure 2L-21: Cross-sectional schematic of the perivascular (Virchow-Robin) spaces. Note the manner in which the pia mater becomes discontinuous and ends as the vessel penetrates deeper into the CNS parenchyma. Also note that the subarachnoid space does not freely communicate with the perivascular space (theoretically).

1 Epipial perivascular space
2 Penetrating blood vessel
3 Perivascular pia mater
4 Pia mater over cerebral surface
5 Subpial perivascular/parenchymal space
6 Subarachnoid space
7 Collagenous trabeculae traversing subarachnoid space
8 Arachnoid mater
9 Cerebral parenchyma
10 Blood vessel traversing subarachnoid space
11 Dura mater
12 Calvarium
13 Inner perivascular layer of pia mater
14 Intrapial perivascular space
15 Outer parenchymal layer of pia mater
16 Pial fenestrae
17 Arachnoid fenestrae
18 Epipial space

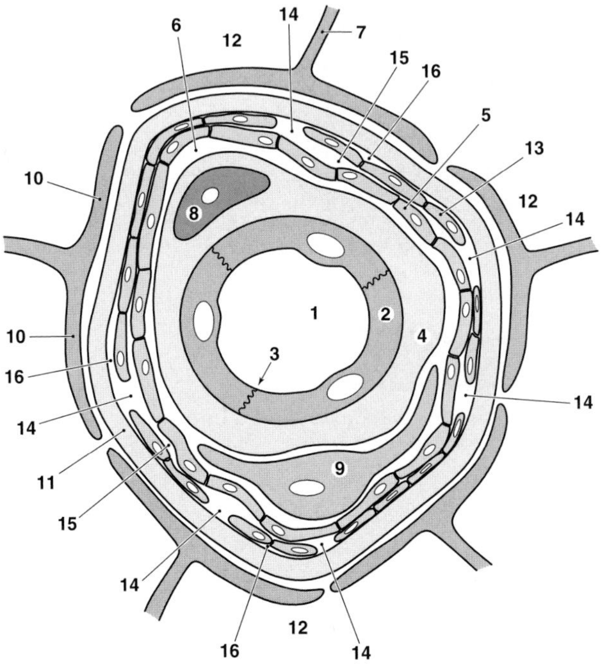

Figure 2L-22: Magnified cross-sectional schematic of a CNS arteriole, showing the relationship of the vascular endothelium to the perivascular space and overlying CNS parenchyma.

1 Arteriole lumen
2 Endothelial cell of arteriole with nucleus
3 Intercellular endothelial tight junction
4 Endothelial basement membrane (basal lamina)
5 Pial cells in inner layer of pia mater
6 Epipial perivascular space
7 Astrocyte processes
8 Pericyte
9 Perivascular cell (macrophage)
10 Astrocyte end feet
11 Astrocytic basement membrane
12 CNS parenchyma
13 Pial cells in outer layer of pia mater
14 Pial fenestrae
15 Intrapial perivascular space
16 Subpial perivascular space

MENINGES, SUBARACHNOID PATHWAY, AND RELATED TISSUE VARIANTS

- Dural calcification
- Dural ossification
- Duplicated/triplicated falx cerebelli
- Hypoplastic falx cerebri/falx cerebelli
- Fenestrations in falx cerebri/tentorium cerebelli
- Hypoplastic tentorium cerebelli with large tentorial hiatus
- Mega cisterna magna
- Posterosuperior diverticulum of midline tentorium cerebelli
- Dilated Virchow-Robin (perivascular) spaces
- Arachnoid webs, pouches, and cysts.

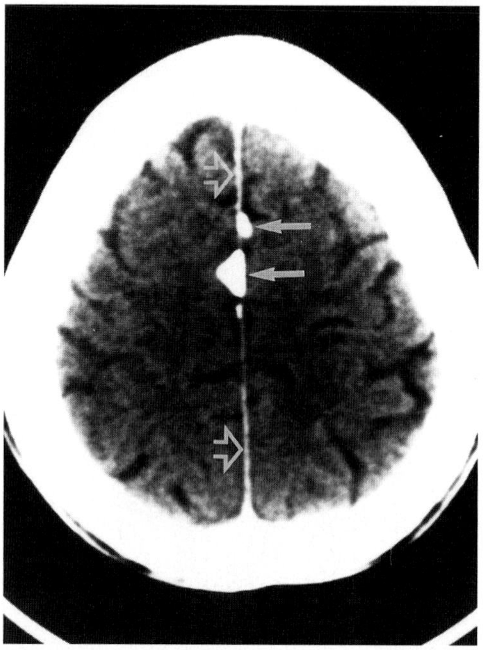

Figure 2L-23: Dural calcification. Enhanced axial CT image showing calcification/ossification (*closed arrows*) of the falx cerebri (*open arrows*).

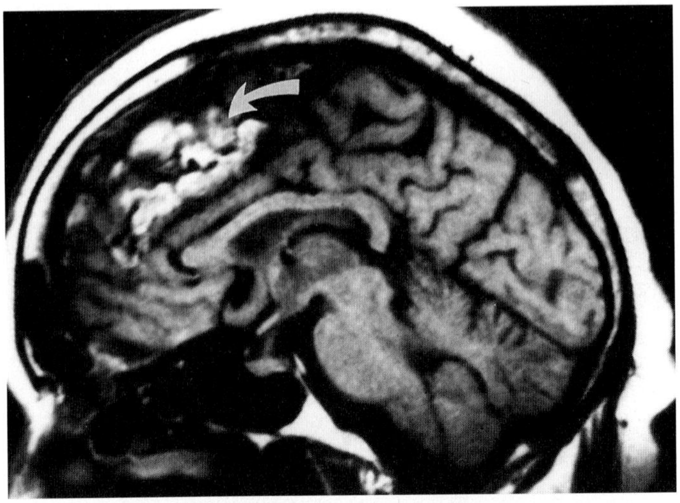

Figure 2L-24A: Dural ossification. Unenhanced sagittal Tl-weighted MR image showing the hyperintensity within fatty marrow in an ossified falx cerebri (*arrow*).

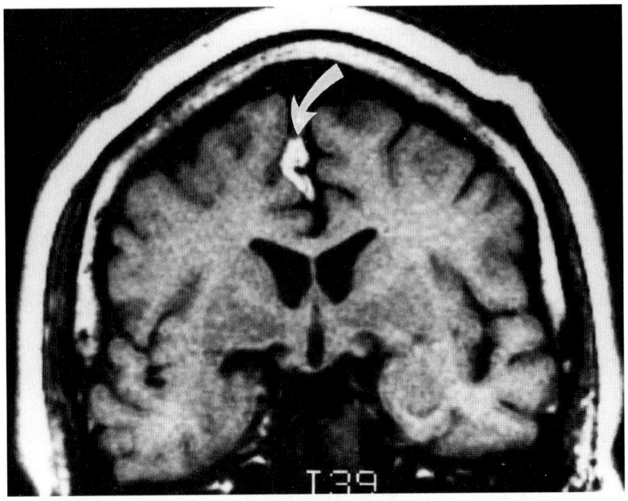

Figure 2L-24B: Dural ossification. Unenhanced coronal T1-weighted MR image showing the hyperintense marrow fat within the ossified falx cerebri (*arrow*) in the interhemispheric fissure.

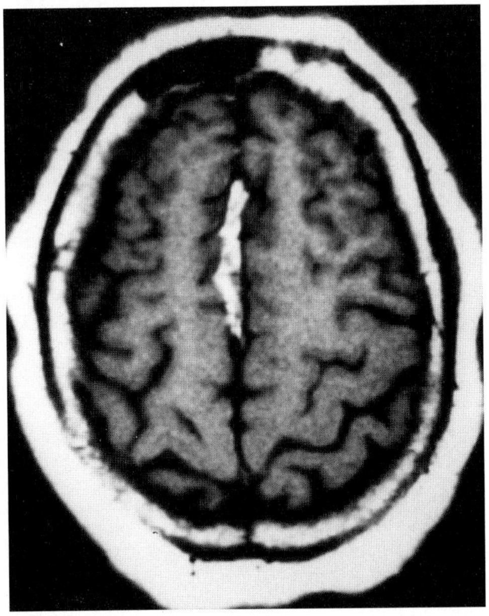

Figure 2L-24C: Dural ossification. Unenhanced axial T1-weighted MR image showing the hyperintense marrow in the ossified falx cerebri.

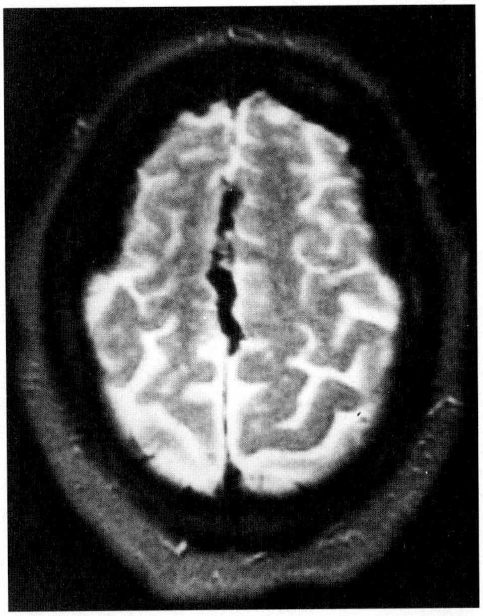

Figure 2L-24D: Dural ossification. Axial T2-weighted MR image showing the marrow fat to be typically hypointense (i.e., suppressed) on this sequence.

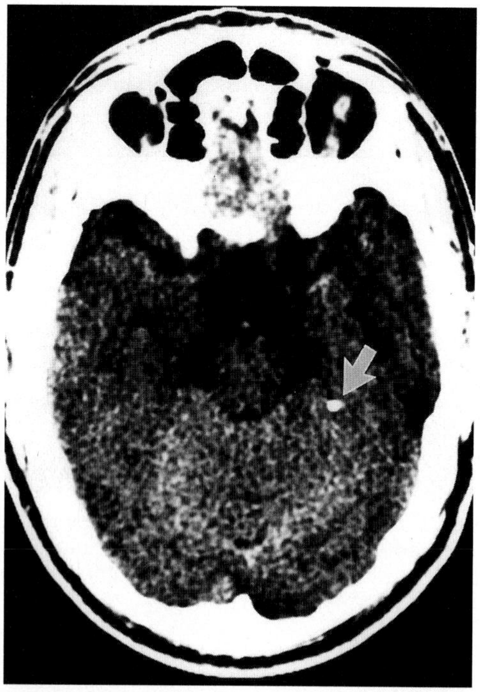

Figure 2L-25A: Calcification in the tentorium cerebelli. Enhanced axial CT image showing a calcification of the tentorium cerebelli (*arrow*).

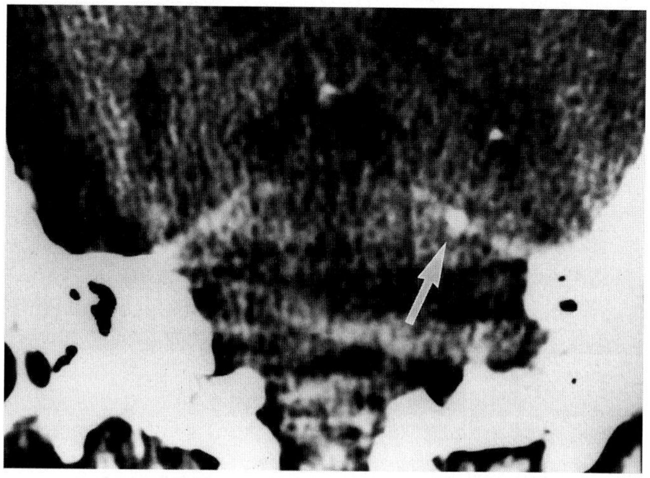

Figure 2L-25B: Calcification in the tentorium cerebelli. Enhanced coronal CT image showing tentorial calcification (*arrow*).

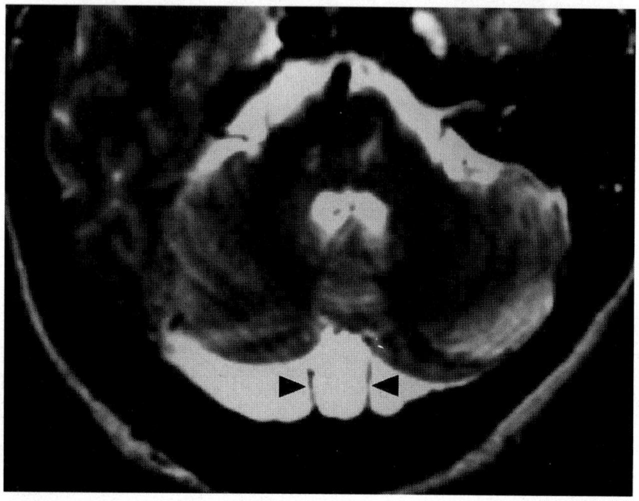

Figure 2L-26: Duplicated falx cerebelli. Axial T2-weighted MR image showing a duplicated falx cerebelli (*arrowheads*).

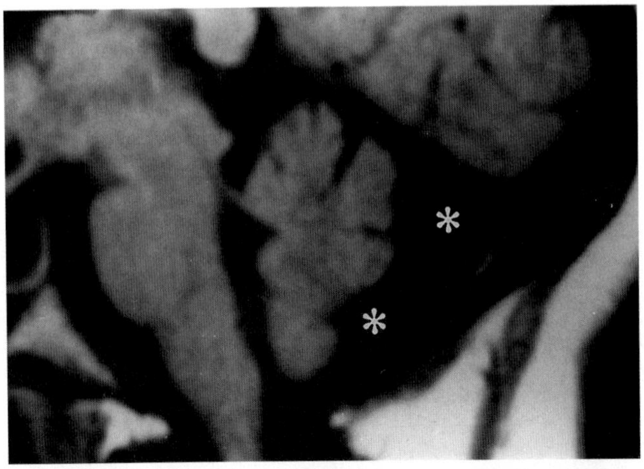

Figure 2L-27A: Mega cisterna magna. T1-weighted MR image showing a mega cisterna magna (*asterisks*). Note the absence of pressure mass effect on the cerebellum, fourth ventricle, and brain stem.

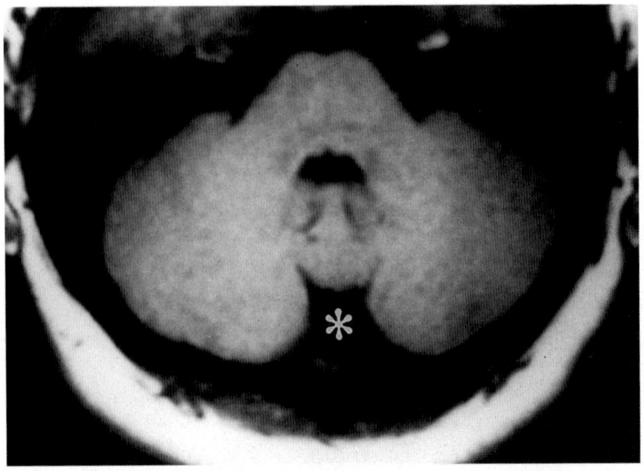

Figure 2L-27B: Mega cisterna magna. Axial MR image showing a mega cisterna magna (*asterisk*).

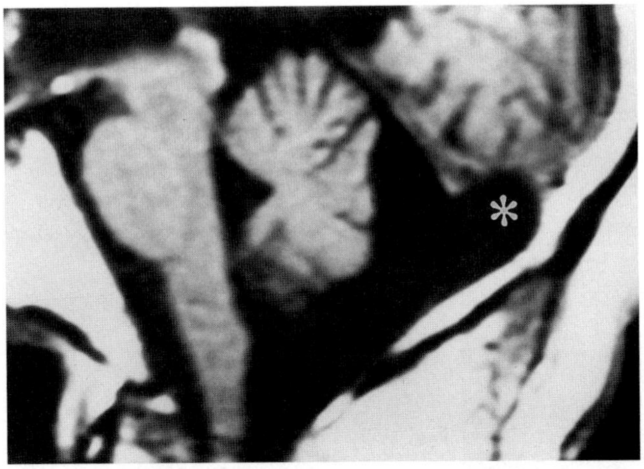

Figure 2L-28: Posterosuperior diverticulum of midline tentorium cerebelli. Sagittal T1-weighted MR image showing an upward extension of the superior vermian subarachnoid cistern at the level of the posterior tentorium cerebelli (*asterisk*).

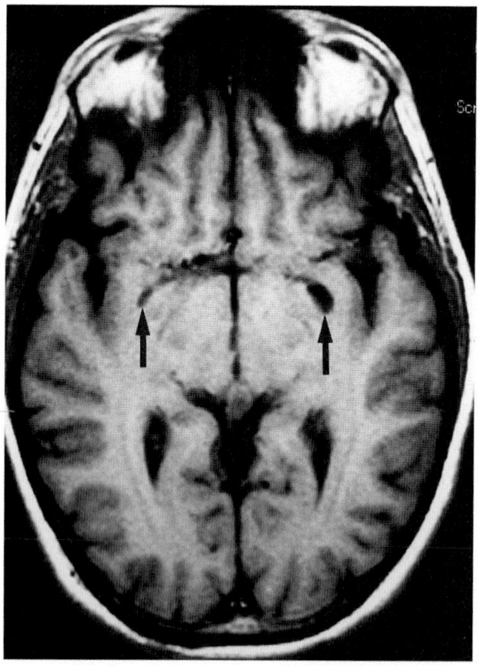

Figure 2L-29A: Enlarged Virchow-Robin (perivascular) spaces. Unenhanced axial Tl-weighted MR image showing dilated Virchow-Robin (perivascular) spaces (*arrows*) in the regions of the lenticulostriate arteries bilaterally. Incidentally identified is a pineal cyst.

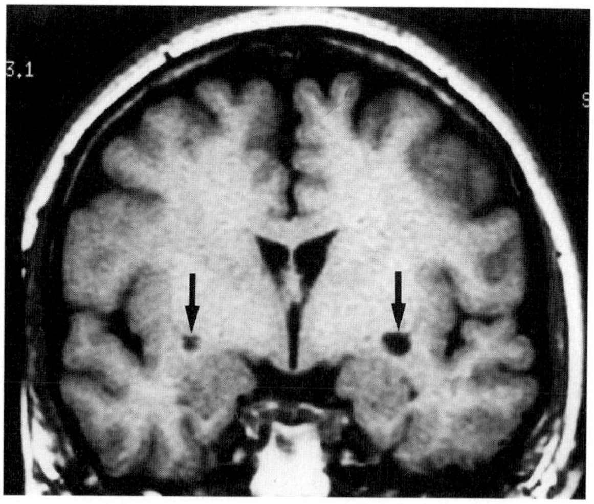

Figure 2L-29B: Enlarged Virchow-Robin spaces. Unenhanced coronal Tl-weighted MR image showing the dilated Virchow-Robin spaces (*arrows*).

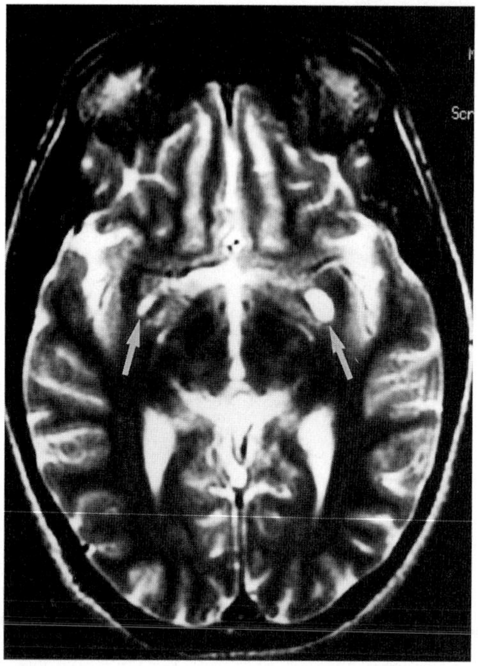

Figure 2L-29C: Enlarged Virchow-Robin spaces. Axial T2-weighted MR image showing that the dilated Virchow-Robin spaces (*arrows*) typically have the same intensity as the regional CSF.

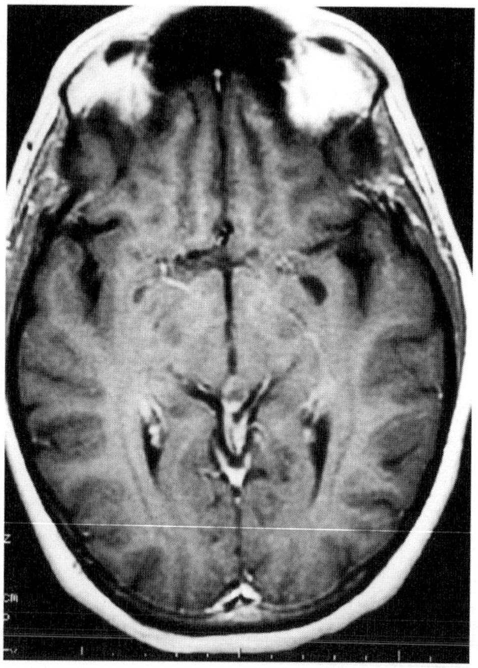

Figure 2L-29D: Enlarged Virchow-Robin spaces. Enhanced axial Tl-weighted MR image showing no abnormal enhancement associated with the dilated Virchow-Robin spaces.

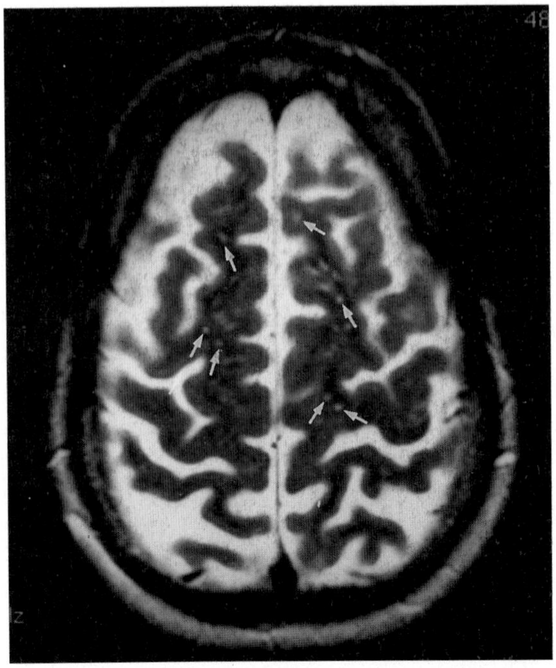

Figure 2L-30A: Prominent Virchow-Robin perivascular space. Axial T2-weighted MR image showing hyperintense areas in the cerebral cortex over the convexity representing the perivascular space (*arrows*) and the parent vessel in cross section.

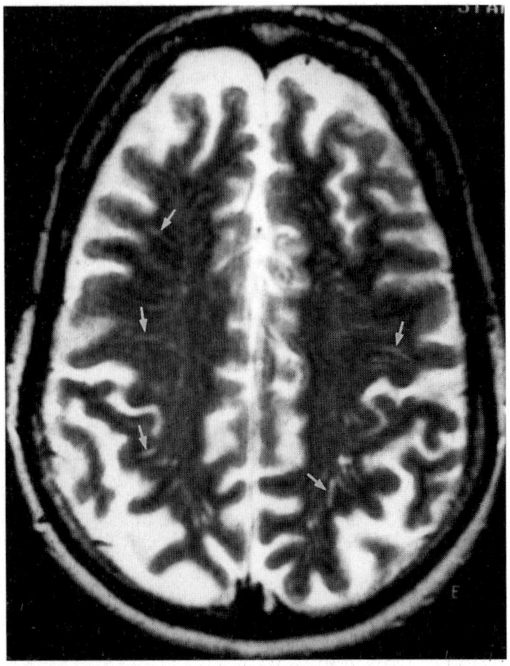

Figure 2L-30B: Prominent Virchow-Robin perivascular space. Axial T2-weighted MR image showing the hyperintense perivascular spaces (*arrows*) in longitudinal section.

2M Aortic Arch

THE LEFT AORTIC ARCH

1. The normal left-sided aortic arch lies in the superior mediastinum and is a continuation of the ascending aorta.
2. The left aortic arch courses from right to left in front of the trachea.
3. The left aortic arch curves posteroinferiorly above the left main-stem pulmonary bronchus, finally descending to the left of the trachea and esophagus and continuing as the descending thoracic aorta.
4. Most commonly, three branches originate from the superior convex aspect of the left aortic arch. This branching pattern is termed Type A.
   a. The brachiocephalic trunk (innominate artery) is usually the first branch from the aortic arch. Shortly after its origin, it divides into the right subclavian and the right common carotid artery. The right vertebral artery arises from the right subclavian artery distal to the right common carotid origin.
   b. The second aortic branch is the left common carotid artery.
   c. The last branch arising from the aortic arch is the left subclavian artery. The first branch of the left subclavian vessel is the left vertebral artery. Other branches originating from the subclavian artery distal to the left vertebral artery include the thyrocervical and costocervical trunks and the internal mammary (thoracic) artery.

LEFT AORTIC ARCH VARIANTS

Note: Although they are statistically more rare, identical anomalies and variants may involve the right aortic arch.

- Type A: The innominate artery and the left common carotid artery arise separately from the aortic arch.
- Type B: The left common carotid artery arises at a common origin from the aortic arch with the innominate artery or from the trunk of the innominate artery.
- Type C: The left vertebral artery arises from the aortic arch independently between the aortic origins of the left common carotid and left subclavian arteries.
- Type D: The left common carotid artery arises from the aortic arch with or from the innominate artery, and the left vertebral artery arises from the aortic arch independently between the aortic origins of the left common carotid/innominate arterial combination and the left subclavian artery (combination of types B and C).
- Type E: The left vertebral artery arises independently from the aortic arch distal to the origin of the left subclavian artery.
- Type F: There is a low bifurcation of the right common carotid artery, sometimes to the degree that the internal and external carotid arteries arise independently from the innominate artery.
- Type G: The right subclavian artery originates from the aortic arch distal to the origin of the left subclavian artery and passes behind the esophagus. In this case, both the right and left common carotid arteries arise from the aortic arch independently as the first and second branch vessels from the arch, respectively.

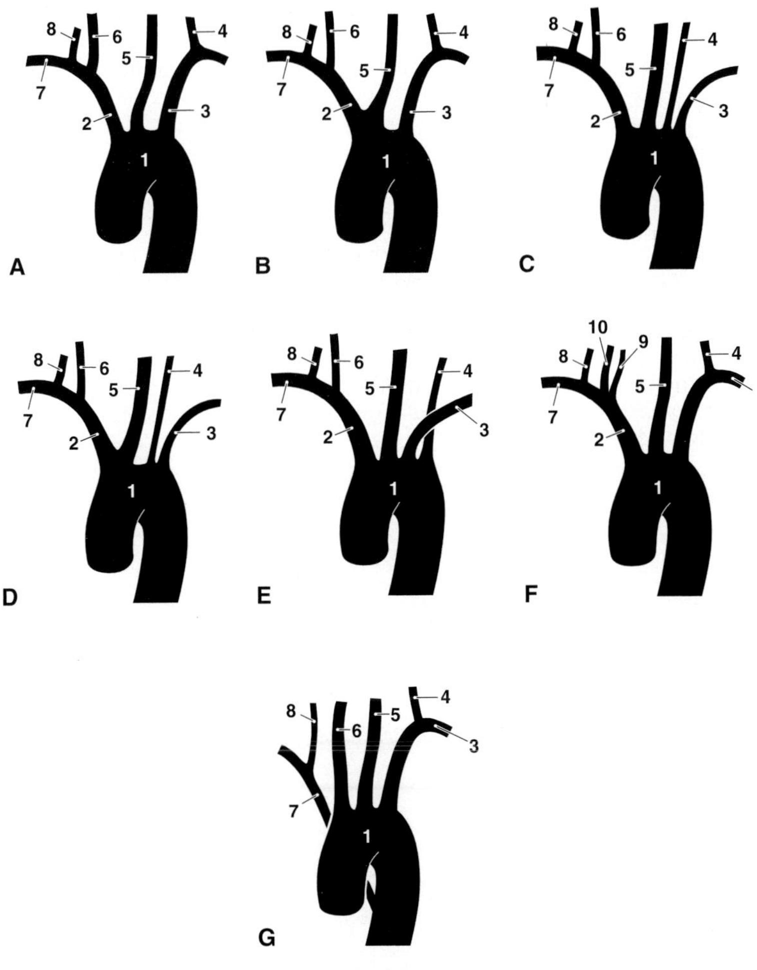

Figure 2M-1: Schematic of the variations of the left-sided aortic arch.
Type A: Three major branches originating from the left aortic arch.
Type B: Common origin of the innominate artery (brachiocephalic trunk) and left common carotid artery.
Type C: Separate origin of left vertebral artery from aortic arch.
Type D: Combination of types B and C.
Type E: Independent origin of left vertebral artery from arch distal to left subclavian artery origin.
Type F: Low or separate origins of right external and internal carotid arteries from the innominate artery (brachiocephalic trunk).
Type G: Aberrant right subclavian artery from left aortic arch.

1 Left aortic arch
2 Innominate artery (brachiocephalic trunk)
3 Left subclavian artery
4 Left vertebral artery
5 Left common carotid artery
6 Right common carotid artery
7 Right subclavian artery
8 Right vertebral artery
9 Right internal carotid artery
10 Right external carotid artery

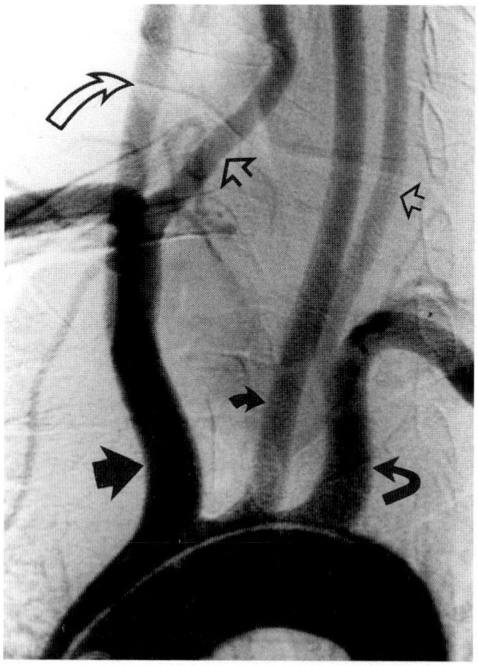

Figure 2M-2: Normal left aortic arch: type A. Angiogram of left aortic arch in the oblique projection (type A). *Large solid black arrow*, innominate artery (brachiocephalic trunk); *large solid curved arrow*, left subclavian artery; *large open arrow*, right vertebral artery; *small open arrow*, left vertebral artery; *small solid curved arrow*, left common carotid artery; *open curved arrow*, right common carotid artery.

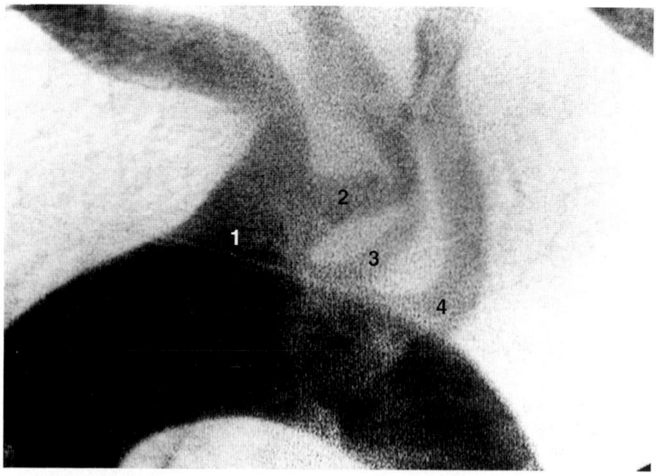

Figure 2M-3: Common origin of brachiocephalic trunk and left common carotid artery and origin of left vertebral artery from the aortic arch (type D). Aortic arch angiogram shown.

1 Common origin of the brachiocephalic trunk (innominate artery) and left common carotid artery from the aortic arch
2 Left common carotid artery originating from the innominate artery
3 Left vertebral artery originating from the aortic arch
4 Left subclavian artery

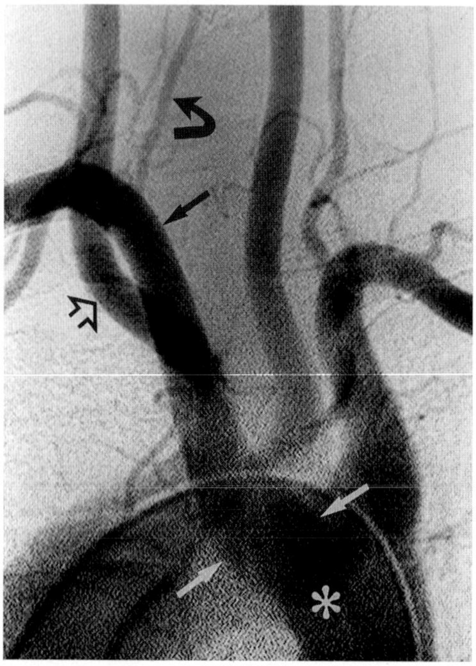

Figure 2M-4: Aberrant right subclavian artery. Arch aortogram shows an aberrant right subclavian artery (*closed black arrow*) associated with a left aortic arch (type G). Note its proximal course (*white arrows*), originating (*asterisk*) as the most distal major vessel from the aortic arch, and the right vertebral artery (*curved black arrow*) arising from it proximally. The first vessel originating from the aortic arch in this circumstance is the right common carotid artery (*open black arrow*). Because of overlap, the vascular origins are somewhat difficult to discern.

THE RIGHT AORTIC ARCH

1. The right aortic arch results from a persistence of the fourth embryonic aortic arch on the right.
2. The most common configuration of the right aortic arch is that associated with an aberrant left subclavian artery. In this situation, the left common carotid artery arises as the first aortic branch, followed, in order, by the right common carotid artery, the right subclavian artery, and, finally, the aberrant left subclavian artery.
3. The second most common configuration of the right aortic arch is a mirror image of the normal left aortic arch. The left innominate artery (brachiocephalic trunk) originates first, followed by the right common carotid artery and, finally, the right subclavian artery.
4. The remaining variant configurations of the right aortic arch show a great variety of patterns and are less frequently encountered. They are usually mirror images of the normal variations of the left-sided aortic arch.

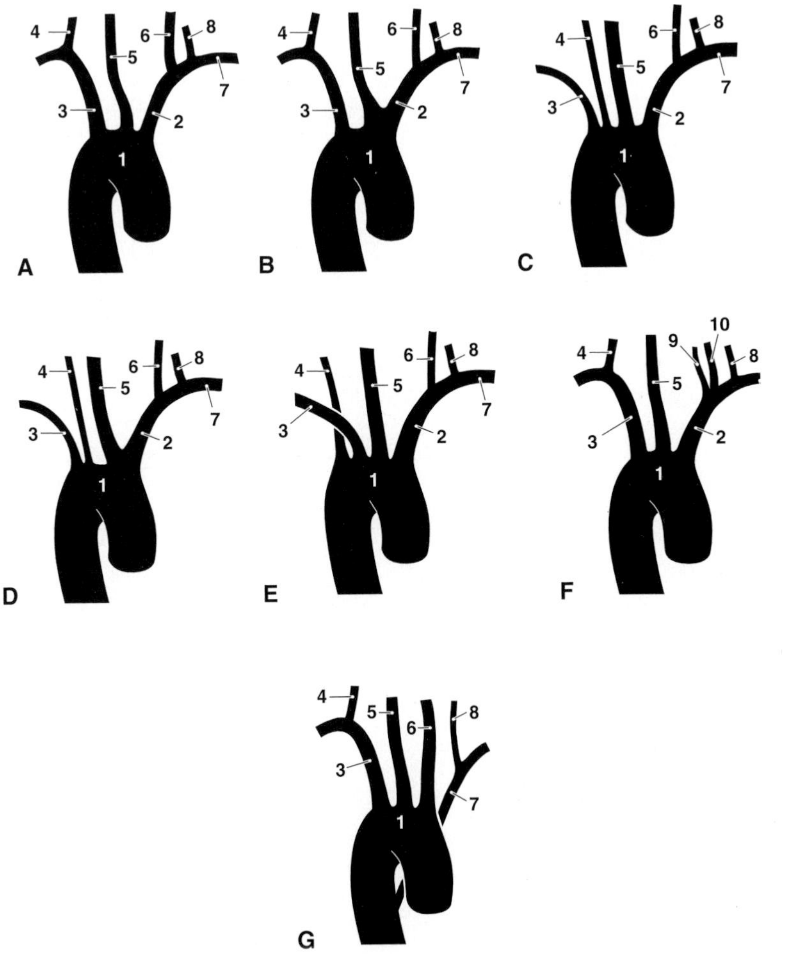

Figure 2M-5: Schematic of the variations of the right aortic arch.
Type A: Three major branches originating from right aortic arch.
Type B: Common origin of left innominate artery (left brachiocephalic trunk) and right common carotid artery.
Type C: Separate origin of right vertebral artery from aortic arch.
Type D: Combination of types B and C.
Type E: Independent origin of right vertebral artery from arch proximal to right subclavian artery origin and distal to left common carotid artery.
Type F: Low or separate origins of left external and internal carotid arteries from left innominate artery (left brachiocephalic trunk).
Type G: Aberrant left subclavian artery from right aortic arch.

1 Right aortic arch
2 Left brachiocephalic trunk (left innominate artery)
3 Right subclavian artery
4 Right vertebral artery
5 Right common carotid artery
6 Left common carotid artery
7 Left subclavian artery
8 Left vertebral artery
9 Left internal carotid artery
10 Left external carotid artery

2N Subclavian Arteries

OVERVIEW

1. The right subclavian artery arises from the innominate artery (brachiocephalic trunk), whereas the left subclavian artery originates directly from the aortic arch.
2. There are five main branches of the subclavian artery, including the vertebral artery, the internal mammary (thoracic) artery, the thyrocervical trunk (TCT), the costocervical trunk (CTC), and the dorsal scapular artery. The arterial branching patterns have many variations.
3. The three subclavian branches that pertain to the central nervous system are the vertebral artery and the thyrocervical and costocervical trunks. Of these branches, the latter two are discussed here, together with the branch variations of the subclavian artery.

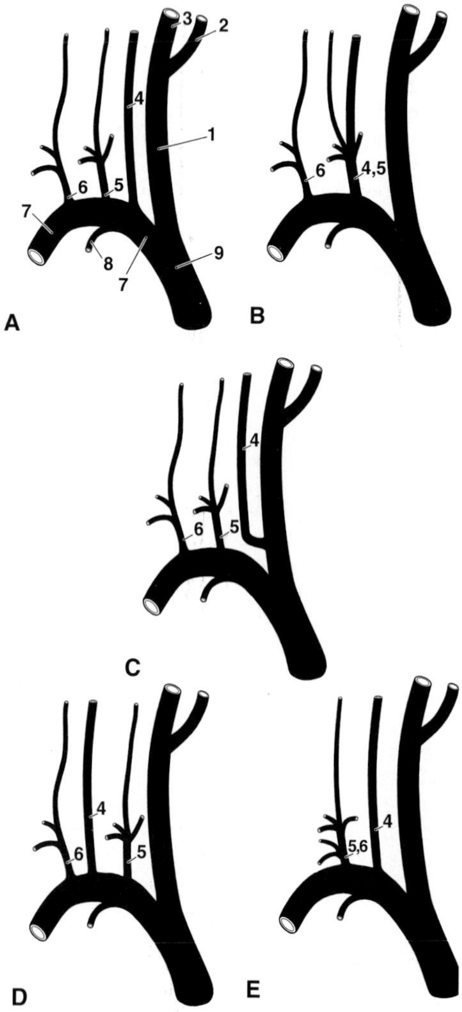

Figure 2N-1: Frontal schematics of some of the variations in branching of the proximal right subclavian artery. **A:** Classic configuration, where the vertebral artery is the first branch arising from the subclavian artery (following the common carotid artery), followed in order by the internal mammary (thoracic) artery, the thyrocervical trunk, and the costocervical trunk. **B:** The vertebral artery and thyrocervical trunk share a common origin. **C:** The vertebral artery arises from the proximal common carotid artery. **D:** The vertebral artery arises distal to the thyrocervical trunk. **E:** The thyrocervical and costocervical trunks share a common origin.

1 Right common carotid artery
2 Right external carotid artery
3 Right internal carotid artery
4 Right vertebral artery
5 Thyrocervical trunk
6 Costocervical trunk
7 Proximal right subclavian artery
8 Internal mammary (thoracic) artery
9 Innominate artery (brachiocephalic trunk)

THE THYROCERVICAL TRUNK

1. The thyrocervical trunk divides into three main branches: the inferior thyroid, suprascapular, and transverse (superficial) cervical arteries.
2. The inferior thyroid artery consists of the following.
   a. An arterial branch to the inferior aspect of the thyroid gland
   b. Muscular arterial branches of the TCT supplying the infrahyoid, longus colli, scalenus anterior, and inferior pharyngeal constrictor muscles
   c. The ascending cervical artery supplying regional muscles and one or more spinal branches (radiculomedullary arteries) of the TCT that enter the central spinal canal via the spinal neural foramen(ina) to supply the vertebrae, meninges, spinal nerve root, and spinal cord
   d. The inferior laryngeal artery supplying the laryngeal muscles and mucosa
   e. Pharyngeal branches supplying the trachea, esophagus, posteroinferior aspect of the thyroid gland, and the parathyroid gland(s)
3. The suprascapular artery consists of branches that supply the supraspinatus, sternocleidomastoid, subclavius, and infraspinatus muscles and the skin over the upper thorax and shoulder.
4. The transverse (superficial) cervical artery supplies the trapezius and adjoining muscles and the regional cervical lymph nodes.
5. There are many variations of arterial pattern.

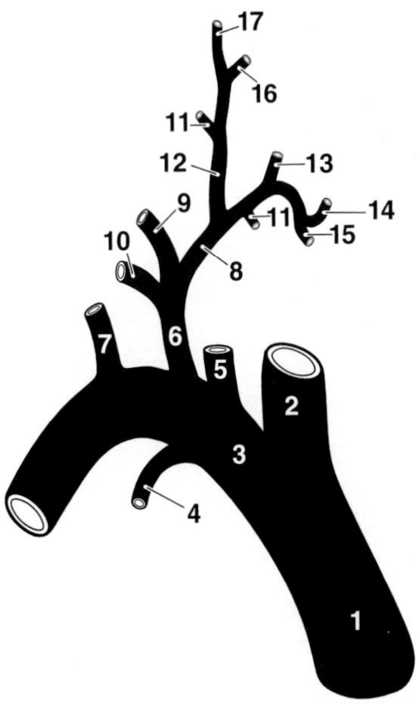

Figure 2N-2: Frontal schematic of the branches of the thyrocervical trunk on the right side.
1 Innominate artery (brachiocephalic trunk)
2 Right common carotid trunk
3 Proximal right subclavian artery
4 Internal mammary (thoracic) artery trunk
5 Right vertebral artery trunk
6 Thyrocervical trunk
7 Costocervical trunk
8 Inferior thyroid artery
9 Transverse (superficial) cervical artery
10 Suprascapular artery
11 Muscular branch(es)
12 Ascending cervical artery
13 Inferior laryngeal artery
14 Pharyngeal arterial branches
15 Glandular arterial branches to the inferior aspect of the thyroid gland and parathyroid gland(s)
16 Spinal (radiculomedullary) arterial branch
17 Anastomotic branch of ascending cervical artery

THE COSTOCERVICAL TRUNK

1. The costocervical trunk divides into two main branches: the superior intercostal artery and the deep cervical artery.
2. The superior intercostal artery anastomoses with the third posterior intercostal artery and gives off the first posterior intercostal artery in the first intercostal space. It terminates in the second posterior intercostal artery (inconstant). When the latter is absent, it is replaced by a direct branch from the aorta.
3. The deep cervical artery gives off a spinal branch (radiculomedullary artery) of the TCT that typically enters the central spinal canal at the C-7 to T-1 vertebral level. The deep cervical artery then ascends to the second cervical level, where it anastomoses with the descending branch of the ipsilateral occipital artery and vertebral artery branches to supply regional muscles.
4. There are many variations of arterial pattern.

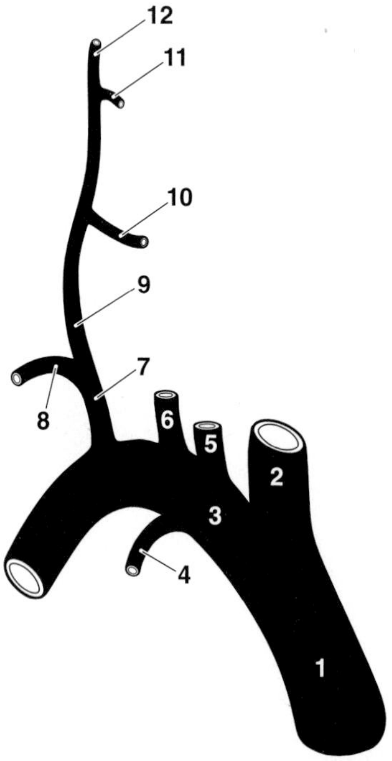

Figure 2N-3: Frontal schematic of the branches of the costocervical trunk on the right side.
1 Innominate artery (brachiocephalic trunk)
2 Right common carotid trunk
3 Proximal right subclavian artery
4 Internal mammary (thoracic) artery trunk
5 Right vertebral artery trunk
6 Thyrocervical trunk
7 Costocervical trunk
8 Superior intercostal artery
9 Deep cervical artery
10 Spinal (radiculomedullary) arterial branch
11 Muscular branch(es)
12 Anastomotic branch of deep cervical artery

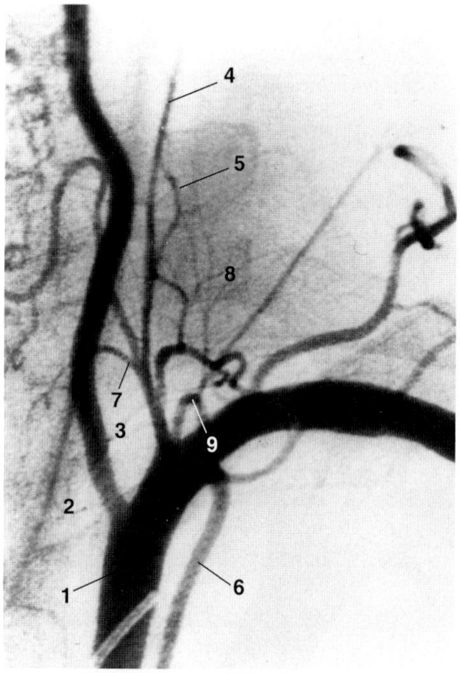

Figure 2N-4: Left subclavian artery branches. Left subclavian arteriogram in the oblique projection, showing some of the major branches of the proximal subclavian artery.
1 Left subclavian artery
2 Left vertebral artery
3 Common origin of thyrocervical trunk and costocervical trunk
4 Ascending cervical artery
5 Deep cervical artery
6 Internal mammary (thoracic) artery
7 Inferior thyroid artery
8 Transverse cervical suprascapular artery
9 Superior intercostal artery

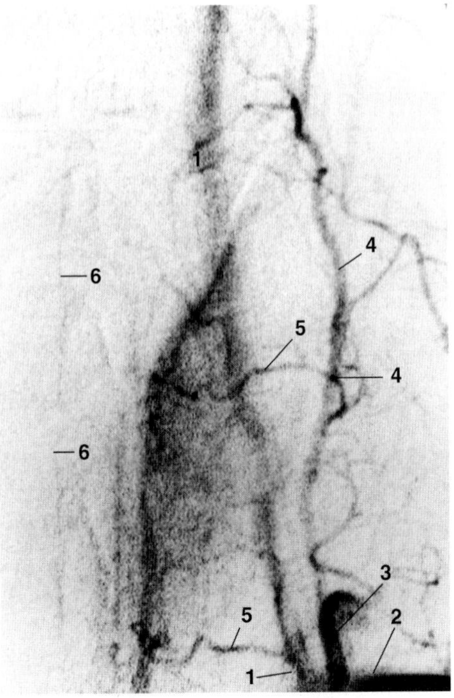

Figure 2N-5: Radiculomedullary arterial branches. Left subclavian artery angiogram in the frontal projection in the late arterial phase, showing radiculomedullary branches of the ascending cervical artery supplying the anterior spinal artery of the spinal cord.

1 Left vertebral artery
2 Left subclavian artery
3 Left thyrocervical trunk
4 Left ascending cervical artery
5 Radiculomedullary arterial branches arising from the left ascending cervical artery
6 Anterior spinal artery

20 Common Carotid Artery

COMMON CAROTID ARTERY ORIGIN VARIANTS

1. The right common carotid artery may arise from the right innominate artery (right brachiocephalic trunk) or separately from the aortic arch.
2. The right common carotid artery may arise as the first brachiocephalic vessel of the aortic arch in association with an aberrant right subclavian artery. In this situation, the aberrant right subclavian artery arises as the last brachiocephalic branch from the aortic arch.
3. The left common carotid artery may arise separately from the aortic arch, from the left subclavian artery, or from the right innominate artery (right brachiocephalic trunk).

COMMON CAROTID ARTERY BIFURCATION VARIANTS

1. Any variation in the pattern of common carotid bifurcation is usually bilateral.
2. The level of bifurcation of the common carotid artery varies from the first cervical vertebra to the second thoracic vertebra, but the most common (normal) site is between the levels of the C2-4 vertebrae.
3. Very rarely, the right carotid artery terminates solely in either the external or the internal carotid artery; this is usually seen in combination with an aberrant right subclavian artery.
4. Rarely, the common carotid artery is replaced by separate external and internal carotid arteries arising directly from the aorta on one side or bilaterally; these vessels may also originate separately from the right innominate artery (right brachiocephalic trunk).

DEVELOPMENTAL ANOMALIES OF THE COMMON CAROTID ARTERY

In rare instances the common carotid artery may be hypoplastic or aplastic.

VARIANT OR ANOMALOUS BRANCHES OF THE COMMON CAROTID ARTERY

1. The common carotid artery usually has no major branches.
2. Branches occasionally arising from the common carotid artery include the following.
   a. The vertebral artery
   b. The superior thyroid artery or its laryngeal branch
   c. The ascending pharyngeal artery
   d. The inferior thyroid artery
   e. The occipital artery

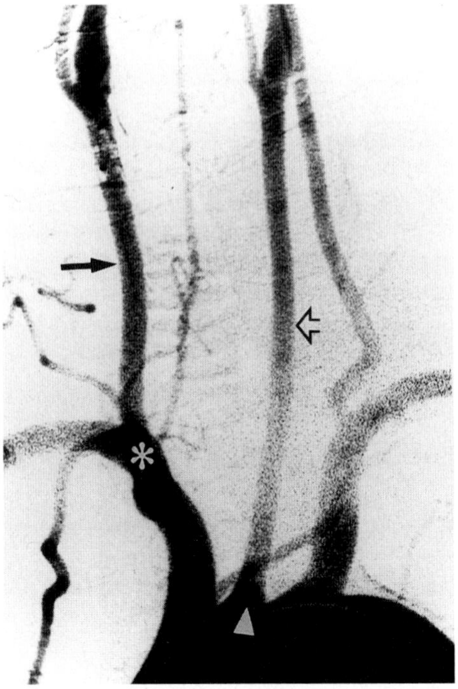

Figure 2O-1A: Common carotid arteries. Arch aortogram in the oblique projection, showing the right common carotid artery (*solid arrow*) originating from the brachiocephalic (innominate) artery (*asterisk*) and the left common carotid artery (*open arrow*) arising directly from the aortic arch (*arrowhead*).

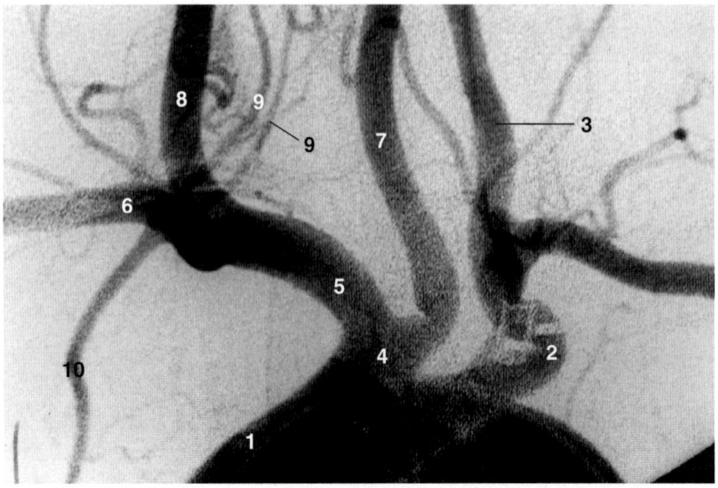

Figure 2O-1B: Common carotid arteries. Aortic arteriogram showing a common origin of the right brachiocephalic artery and the left common carotid artery. There is some vascular tortuosity present in this older person and marked dominance of the vertebral artery on the left side.

1 Aortic arch
2 Left subclavian artery
3 Left vertebral artery
4 Common origin of brachiocephalic trunk and left common carotid artery
5 Brachiocephalic trunk
6 Right subclavian artery
7 Left common carotid artery
8 Right common carotid artery
9 Right vertebral artery
10 Internal mammary (thoracic) artery

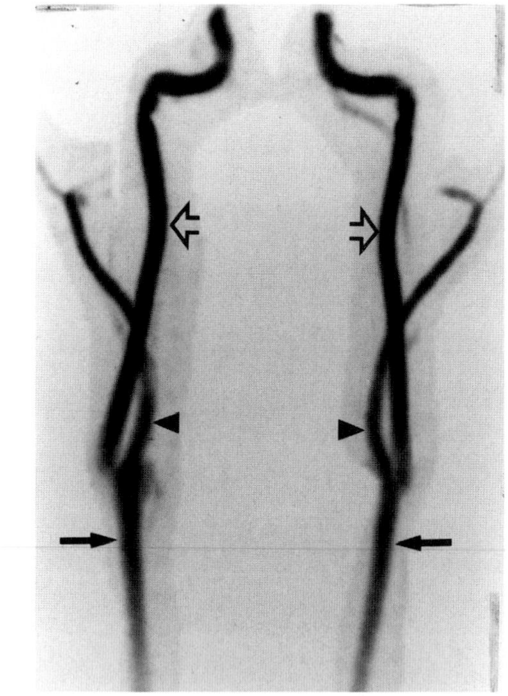

Figure 20-2A: Cervical carotid arteries. Phase-contrast MR angiogram in the frontal projection, showing the common carotid arteries (*straight arrows*), the external carotid arteries (*arrowheads*), and the cervical internal carotid arteries (*open arrows*).

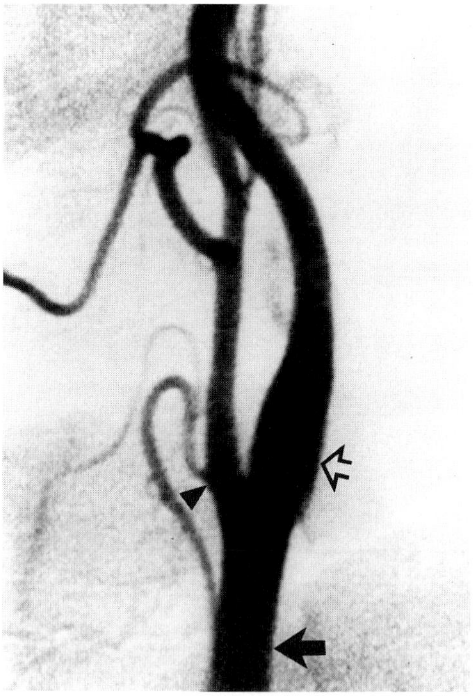

Figure 20-2B: Left cervical carotid artery. Left common carotid arteriogram in the oblique projection, showing the distal common carotid artery (*solid arrow*), the proximal internal carotid artery (*open arrow*: carotid bulb), and the external carotid artery trunk (*arrowhead*).

COMMON CAROTID ARTERY VARIANTS

Variants in the Origin of the Common Carotid Artery

- Origin of the left common carotid artery directly from the aortic arch
- Origin of the left common carotid artery from the innominate artery (right brachio-cephalic trunk)

Variants in Common Carotid Artery Bifurcation/Termination

- Bifurcation level varying from C1 to T2
- Separate internal and external carotid arteries arising from the aorta or innominate artery (brachiocephalic trunk)
- Termination in solely the external or internal carotid artery

Anomalies of the Common Carotid Artery

- Hypoplasia/aplasia of the common carotid artery
- Anomalous branches of the common carotid artery
    - Vertebral artery
    - Superior thyroid artery or its laryngeal branch
    - Ascending pharyngeal artery
    - Inferior thyroid artery
    - Occipital artery

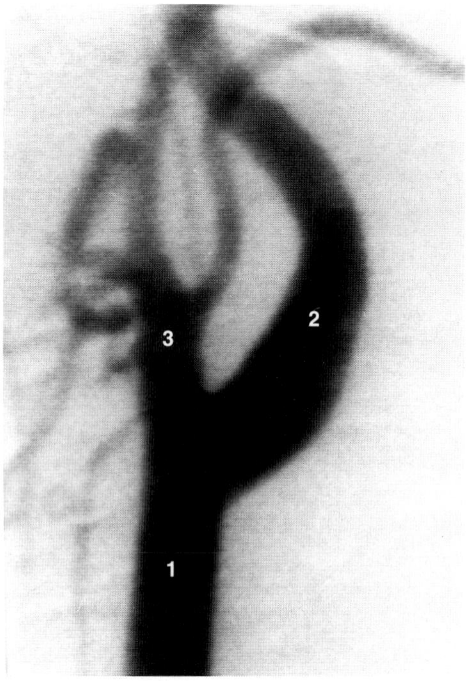

Figure 20-3A: Right common carotid artery bifurcation. Common carotid angiogram in the oblique projection, showing a normal common carotid artery bifurcation on the right side.
1 Distal common carotid artery
2 Cervical internal carotid artery
3 External carotid artery trunk

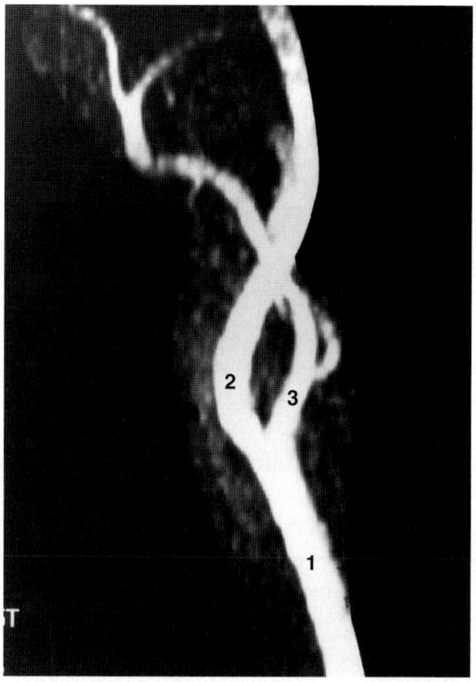

Figure 20-3B: Left common carotid artery bifurcation. MR angiogram showing the normal common carotid artery bifurcation on the left side.
1 Distal common carotid artery
2 Cervical internal carotid artery
3 External carotid artery trunk

2P External Carotid Artery

OVERVIEW

1. The external carotid artery normally originates at the common carotid artery bifurcation lateral to the upper level of the thyroid cartilage or at the level of the disc space between the third and fourth cervical vertebrae (C3-4).
2. The external carotid artery ascends first craniad and then laterally to pass midway between the angle of the mandible and the mastoid process tip.
3. At its origin, the external carotid artery lies anteromedial to the internal carotid artery, but as it ascends it becomes anterior and then lateral to this vessel.

THE BRANCHES OF THE EXTERNAL CAROTID ARTERY

The Superior Thyroid Artery

1. The superior thyroid artery is usually the first branch arising from the external carotid artery; rarely, it may arise from the distal common carotid artery.
2. The superior thyroid artery may arise as a common trunk with other external carotid artery branches.
3. The superior thyroid artery supplies the larynx, the superior pole of the thyroid gland, and the (superior) parathyroid glands.

The Ascending Pharyngeal Artery

1. The ascending pharyngeal artery arises from the posterior aspect of the external carotid artery or, less commonly, from the distal common carotid artery, the occipital artery, or the internal carotid artery.
2. The ascending pharyngeal artery supplies portions of the basal meninges and the lower cranial and upper cervical spinal nerves and their respective foramina (the neuromeningeal trunk), the middle ear (the inferior tympanic artery), the nasopharynx and oropharynx (the pharyngeal trunk), and the cervical musculature, the accessory nerve (CN-XI), and the superior sympathetic ganglion (musculospinal branch).
3. Terminal vessels of the ascending pharyngeal artery feed the bone, dura mater, and traversing nerves associated with the foramen lacerum, the jugular foramen, and the hypoglossal canal.
4. A larger posterior meningeal artery may arise from the ascending pharyngeal artery to traverse the jugular foramen to supply the meninges of the posterior fossa.
5. A major anastomotic pathway between the internal and the external carotid arteries is at the foramen lacerum, via the carotid branch of the superior pharyngeal branch of the ascending pharyngeal artery, and the recurrent artery of the foramen lacerum, the latter being a branch of the inferolateral trunk of the internal carotid artery.

The Lingual Artery

1. The lingual artery frequently arises as a common branch with the facial artery.
2. The lingual artery courses superomedially, then inferolaterally.
3. The lingual artery supplies the floor of the mouth and hyoid muscles as well as the submandibular and sublingual glands and the tongue (the terminal dorsal artery).
4. The lingual artery shares rich anastomoses with the facial artery, as well as the territory bordering it.

The Facial Artery

1. Although it may arise independently, the facial artery frequently originates as a common trunk with the lingual artery.
2. The facial artery then ascends and passes forward to supply the submandibular gland, the mandible, the cheek, and the nose.
3. The lingual and facial arteries are said to be "hemodynamically balanced:" hypoplasia of one arterial territory is compensated by hyperplasia of the other.

The Occipital Artery

1. The occipital artery courses posterosuperiorly between the occipital bone and the first cervical vertebra (C-1).
2. The occipital artery anastomoses with muscular branches of the vertebral artery, the deep cervical artery, and the ascending pharyngeal artery.
3. The occipital artery supplies the musculocutaneous structures of the neck and scalp and provides arterial rami to the posterior fossa meninges. Two typical endocranial branches to the posterior fossa meninges include the stylomastoid artery, passing via the stylomastoid canal, and the transmastoid branch (artery of the mastoid foramen), passing via the mastoid foramen. Other meningeal branches that may arise from the occipital artery include the posterior meningeal artery proper and the artery of the falx cerebelli; these meningeal branches enter the cranial cavity via the foramen magnum.

The Posterior Auricular Artery

1. The posterior auricular artery may arise independently from the external carotid artery or as a common trunk with the occipital artery.
2. The posterior auricular artery courses posterosuperiorly.
3. The posterior auricular artery supplies the parotid gland, the regional scalp, the pinna of the ear, and the tympanic cavity.
4. The posterior auricular artery may give rise to the stylomastoid artery.

The Superficial Temporal Artery

1. The superficial temporal artery is one of two terminal branches of the external carotid artery, the other being the internal maxillary artery.
2. Major facial arterial branches include the zygomatic orbital arterial branch to the orbicularis oculi muscle, the transverse facial artery to the parotid gland and duct and the masseter muscle, the posterior deep temporal artery to the temporalis muscle, the frontal arterial branch to the frontal scalp and underlying muscles, and the parietal arterial branch to the parietal scalp and underlying muscles.
3. The anterior auricular artery is a branch of the superficial temporal artery that anastomoses with the terminal branches of the posterior auricular artery to supply the anterior aspect of the auricle and the external auditory canal.

The Internal Maxillary Artery

1. The internal maxillary artery is the larger of the two terminal branches of the external carotid artery (see The Superficial Temporal Artery); it arises behind the neck of the mandible.

2. The internal maxillary artery lies initially within the matrix of the parotid gland and then runs obliquely forward and anteromedially within the infratemporal fossa.
3. The first portion of the internal maxillary artery runs along the inferior aspect of the lateral pterygoid muscle and gives rise to the deep auricular artery, the anterior tympanic artery, the middle meningeal artery, the accessory meningeal artery, the inferior alveolar artery, and the middle deep temporal artery.
4. The second portion of the internal maxillary artery runs in the infratemporal fossa and gives rise to the buccal and masseteric arteries, branches that supply the muscles of mastication, and the anterior deep temporal arteries that supply the temporalis muscle.
5. The third, or pterygopalatine, portion of the internal maxillary artery branches within the pterygopalatine fossa. The distal branches of the third portion of the internal maxillary artery are divided into posterior and anterior groups.
   a. The posterior branches of the third portion of the internal maxillary artery include the following:
      i. The artery of the foramen rotundum, which passes through this foramen and then anastomoses with the artery of the inferior cavernous venous sinus
      ii. The vidian artery (i.e., the artery of the pterygoid canal) may arise from the internal maxillary artery; it passes through the pterygoid canal toward the foramen lacerum to anastomose in the roof of the oropharynx with the branches of the accessory meningeal and ascending pharyngeal arteries
      iii. The pharyngeal artery, which supplies parts of the choanae, the pharynx, and the eustachian (auditory) tube and anastomoses with the ascending pharyngeal artery, the vidian artery, and the cavernous arterial branches of the internal carotid artery
   b. The anterior branches of the third portion of the internal maxillary artery include the following:
      i. The posterior–superior alveolar artery, which supplies the mucosa of the cheek, the buccinator muscle, the maxillary antrum, and the maxillary alveolar ridge and teeth
      ii. The infraorbital artery traversing the inferior orbital fissure, which is a major source of blood supply to the orbit and maxilla
      iii. The greater palatine artery, which descends from the pterygopalatine fossa in the pterygopalatine canal and supplies the soft and hard palates
      iv. The sphenopalatine artery—the terminal branch of the internal maxillary artery—which supplies the nasal turbinates and nasal septum and the tissues surrounding the maxillary, ethmoid, and sphenoid sinuses

EXTERNAL CAROTID ARTERY VARIANTS

- When the common carotid artery is absent on either side, both the external and internal carotid arteries originate separately from the respective subclavian artery(ies).
- In cases of a persistent third embryonic aortic arch (i.e., instead of the normally persistent fourth), the internal and external carotid arteries originate separately from the innominate artery (brachiocephalic trunk) or from a right cervical aortic arch.
- When the internal carotid artery is aplastic, only the external carotid artery is present.
- The external carotid artery may originate from the common carotid artery at any point from the first cervical to the second thoracic vertebral level (C-1 to T-2).
- The external carotid artery usually originates from the anteromedial aspect of the common carotid artery, but, on occasion, it may arise from the lateral or posterolateral aspect.
- The external carotid artery branching pattern and branch origins have many variations.

  The superior thyroid artery may originate directly from the common carotid artery.

  The ascending pharyngeal artery may originate from the proximal part of the occipital artery.

  The occipital artery occasionally arises directly from the posterior aspect of the internal carotid artery.

  The occipital artery may arise in a common trunk with the posterior auricular artery.

  The middle meningeal artery or one of its branches may arise from the ophthalmic artery or, rarely, as a direct branch of the distal portion of the internal carotid artery.

  There is a variable point of origin of the middle meningeal artery along the anteroposterior length of the main trunk of the internal maxillary artery.

  The accessory meningeal artery, which usually arises directly from the internal maxillary artery and enters the middle cranial fossa through the foramen ovale, may arise from the extracranial portion of the middle meningeal artery proper.

  The lingual artery may originate in a common trunk with the facial artery (common).

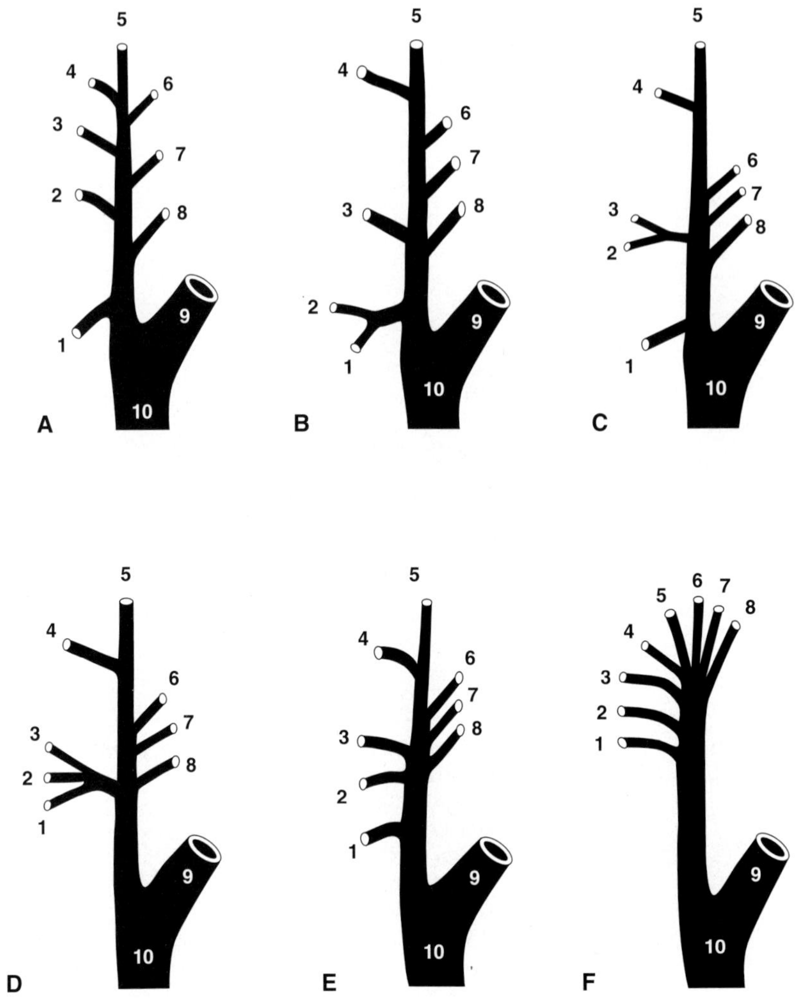

Figure 2P-1: Frontal schematic of some of the variations in the branching pattern of the external carotid artery (arterial branches caliber not to scale). **A:** Pattern of evenly dispersed branches. **B:** Common trunk of superior thyroid and lingual arteries. **C:** Common trunk of lingual and facial arteries. **D:** Common trunk of lingual, facial, and superior thyroid arteries. **E:** Intermediately close grouping of vascular origins. **F:** Markedly close grouping of vascular origins.

1 Superior thyroid artery
2 Lingual artery
3 Facial artery
4 Internal maxillary artery
5 Superficial temporal artery
6 Posterior auricular artery
7 Occipital artery
8 Ascending pharyngeal artery
9 Internal carotid artery trunk
10 Common carotid artery trunk

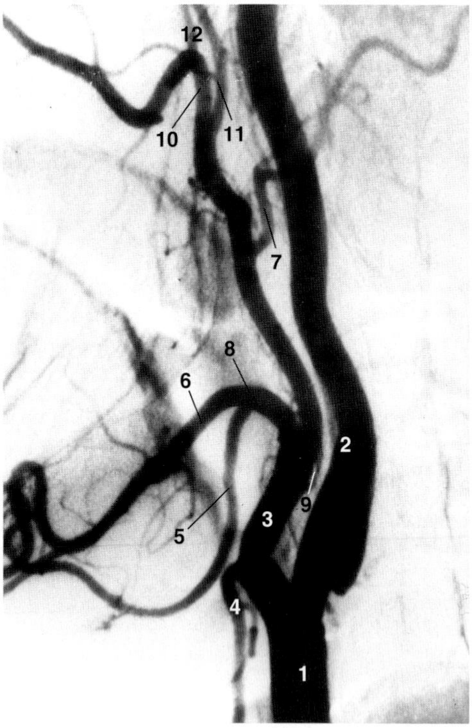

Figure 2P-2A: Major external carotid artery branches. Common carotid angiogram in the oblique projection, showing many of the major external carotid artery branches.

1 Common carotid artery
2 Cervical internal carotid artery
3 External carotid artery trunk
4 Superior thyroid artery
5 Lingual artery
6 Facial artery
7 Occipital artery
8 Common trunk of lingual and facial arteries
9 Ascending pharyngeal artery
10 Internal maxillary artery
11 Superficial temporal artery
12 Middle meningeal artery

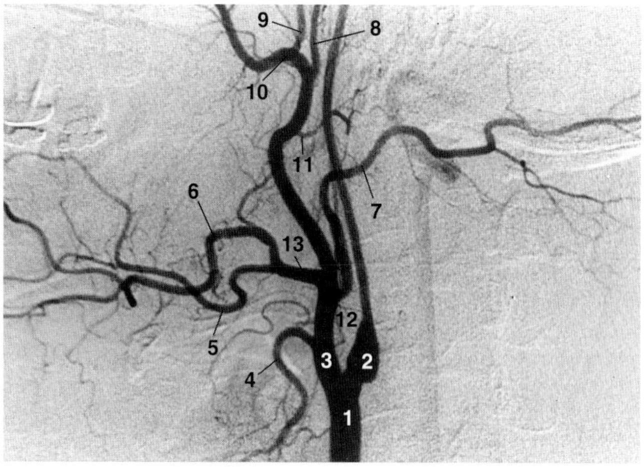

Figure 2P-2B: Major external carotid artery branches. Angiogram in the lateral projection, showing the major proximal branches of the external carotid artery.

1 Common carotid artery
2 Cervical internal carotid artery (with a stenotic segment)
3 External carotid artery trunk
4 Superior thyroid artery
5 Lingual artery
6 Facial artery
7 Occipital artery
8 Superficial temporal artery
9 Middle meningeal artery
10 Internal maxillary artery
11 Posterior auricular artery
12 Ascending pharyngeal artery
13 Common trunk of lingual and facial arteries

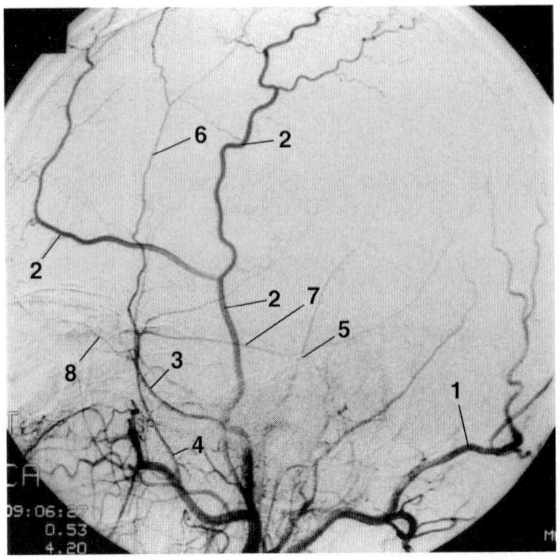

Figure 2P-2C: Major external carotid artery branches. Right external carotid angiogram in the lateral projection, showing some of the distal branches of the external carotid artery.

1 Occipital artery
2 Superficial temporal artery
3 Middle meningeal artery trunk
4 Deep temporal artery
5 Posterior meningeal artery branch arising from the posterior auricular artery
6 Frontal branch of middle meningeal artery
7 Squamous branch of middle meningeal artery
8 Lacrimal branch of middle meningeal artery

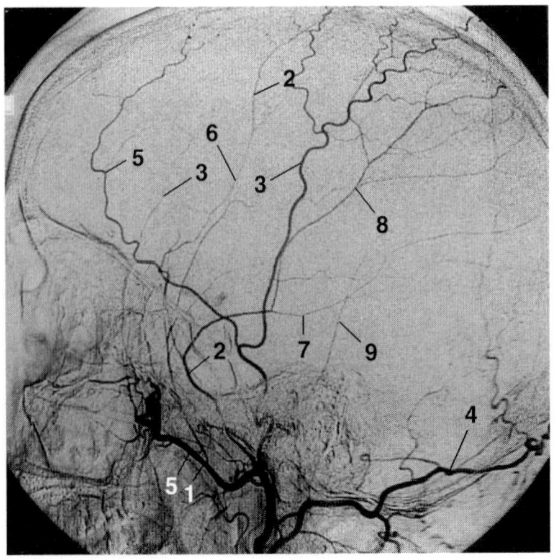

Figure 2P-2D: Major external carotid artery branches. Right external carotid angiogram in the lateral projection shows some of the distal branches of the external carotid artery.

1 Internal maxillary artery
2 Middle meningeal artery trunk
3 Parietal branch of superficial temporal artery
4 Occipital artery
5 Frontal branch of superficial temporal artery
6 Frontal branch of middle meningeal artery
7 Squamous branch of middle meningeal artery
8 Parietal branch of middle meningeal artery
9 Posterior deep temporal artery

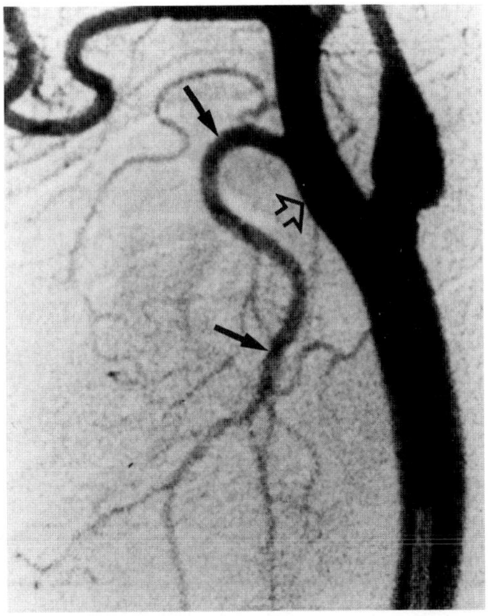

Figure 2P-3: Superior thyroid artery. Common carotid arteriogram in the lateral projection, showing the superior thyroid artery (*solid arrows*) originating from the external carotid artery trunk (*open arrow*).

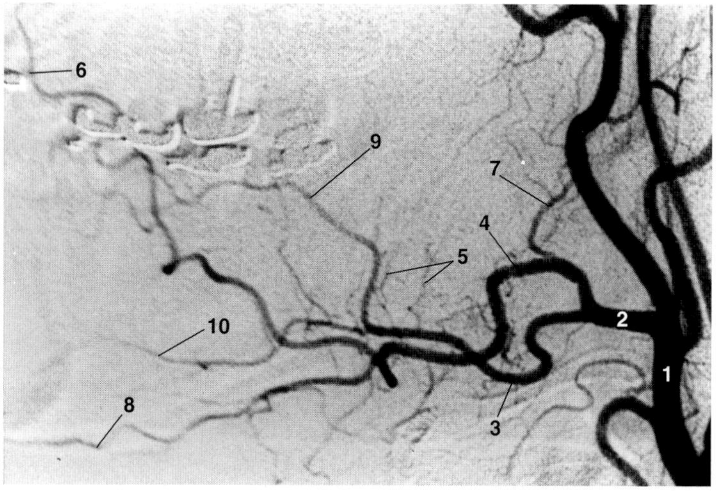

Figure 2P-4: External carotid angiogram in the lateral projection, showing the major branches of the lingual and facial arteries.

1 External carotid artery
2 Common linguofacial trunk
3 Lingual artery trunk
4 Facial artery trunk
5 Arterial branches to tongue
6 Angular artery
7 Ascending palatine artery
8 Inferior mental artery
9 Superior labial artery arising from lingual artery
10 Inferior labial artery arising from fascial artery

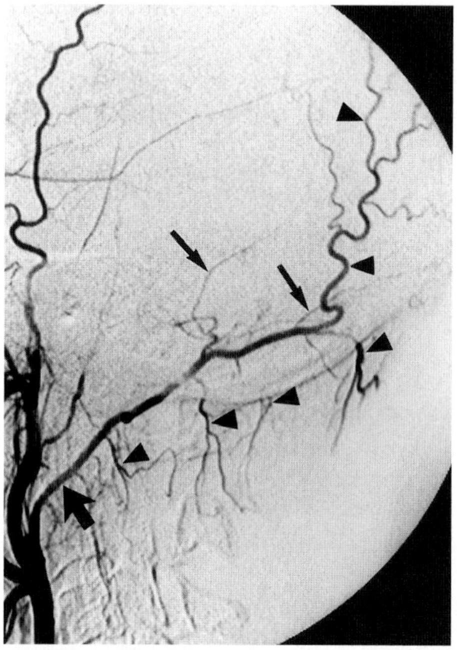

Figure 2P-5A: The occipital artery. External carotid angiogram in the lateral projection, showing the occipital artery trunk (*large arrow*) and musculocutaneous branches (*arrowheads*). Also noted is a small posterior meningeal branch (*small arrows*) arising from the occipital artery.

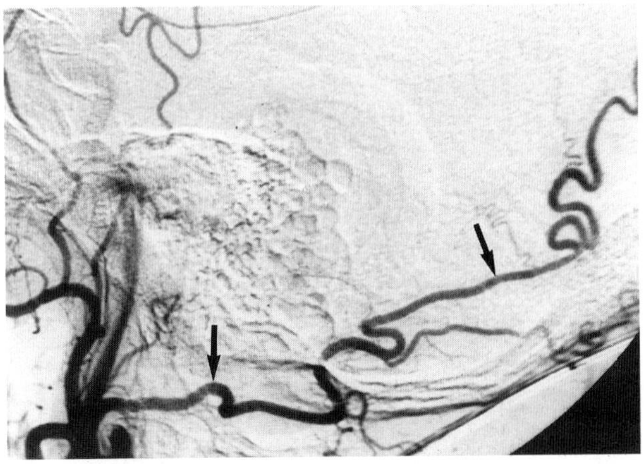

Figure 2P-5B: The occipital artery. External carotid angiogram in the lateral projection, showing the normal anatomy of the occipital artery (*arrows*).

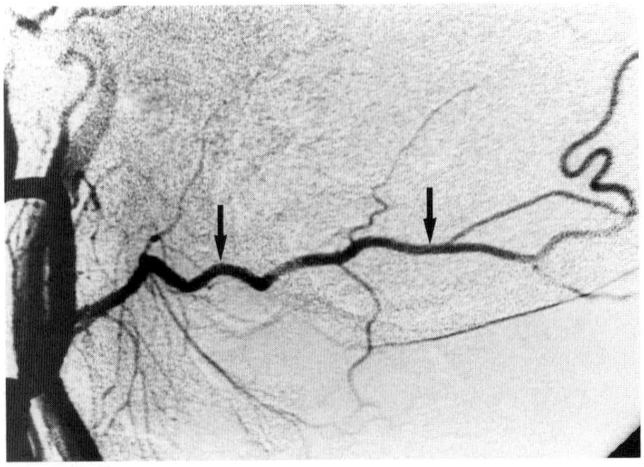

Figure 2P-5C: The occipital artery. External carotid artery angiogram in the lateral projection, showing the extracranial branches from the trunk of the occipital artery (*arrows*).

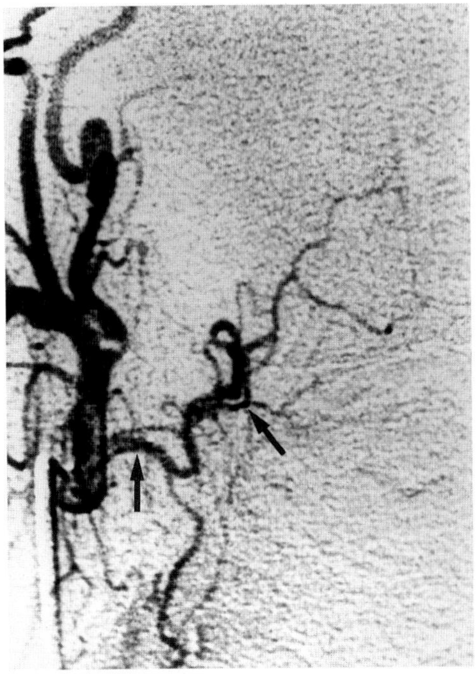

Figure 2P-6: External carotid angiogram in the lateral projection, showing the posterior auricular artery (*arrows*).

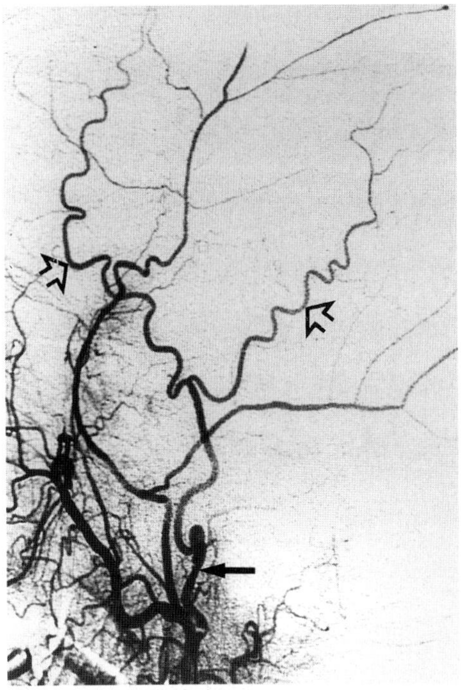

Figure 2P-7: External carotid angiogram in the lateral projection, showing the superficial temporal artery trunk (*solid arrow*) and its main anterior and posterior branches (*open arrows*).

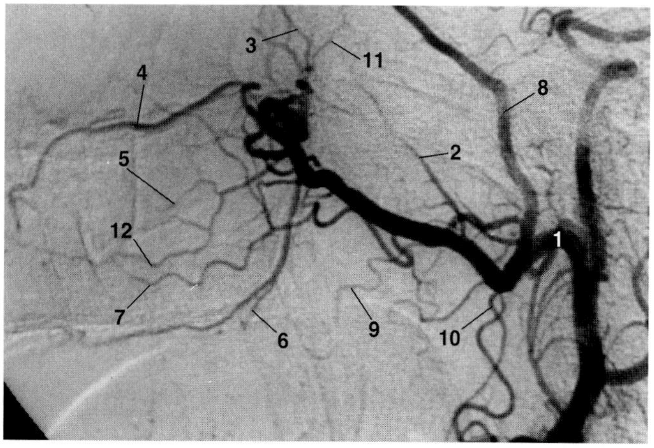

Figure 2P-8: External carotid angiogram in the lateral projection, showing the main branches of the internal maxillary artery.

1 Internal maxillary artery trunk
2 Middle deep temporal artery
3 Anterior deep temporal artery
4 Superior orbital artery
5 Sphenopalatine artery(ies)
6 Greater descending palatine artery
7 Superior alveolar artery
8 Middle meningeal artery
9 Buccal artery
10 Inferior alveolar artery
11 Artery of the foramen rotundum connecting with the inferolateral trunk
12 Antral artery

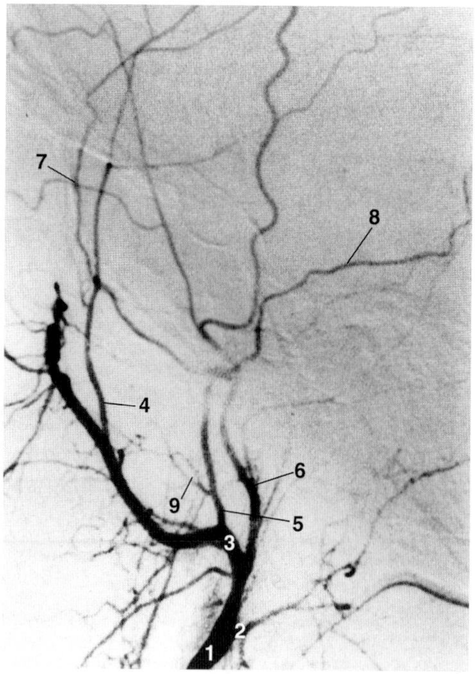

Figure 2P-9: External carotid angiogram in the lateral projection, showing some of the distal branches of the external carotid artery.

1 Distal external carotid artery trunk
2 Posterior auricular artery
3 Internal maxillary artery trunk
4 Deep temporal artery
5 Middle meningeal artery trunk
6 Superficial temporal artery trunk
7 Anterior branch of middle meningeal artery
8 Posterior branch of middle meningeal artery
9 Accessory meningeal artery

2Q Internal Carotid Artery

THE INTERNAL CAROTID ARTERY

The Origin of the Internal Carotid Artery

1. The common carotid artery (CCA) may bifurcate into the internal and external carotid arteries at any level from C-1 to T-2, but bifurcation usually occurs at or near the fourth cervical vertebral body level.
2. In adults the CCA bifurcates at the C-4/C-5 level in 48% and at the C-3/C-4 level in 34% of patients. In children the CCA bifurcation is usually slightly higher than in adults, often occurring at the C-2/C-3 or C-3/C-4 level. The CCA typically bifurcates at the same level on both sides.
3. Proximally, the internal carotid artery (ICA) is directed laterally, dorsally, and upward, medially to the sternomastoid muscle. Distally, it runs upward, medially, and posteriorly to the stylopharyngeal aponeurosis.
4. The ICA enters the skull base through the bony carotid canal and terminates at the bifurcation of the anterior and middle cerebral arteries just above the anterior clinoid process of the sella turcica.

The Segments of the Internal Carotid Artery

1. The cervical segment of the ICA
   a. The cervical (i.e., neck) segment extends from the origin of the ICA at the level of the CCA bifurcation to the base of the skull. The cervical segment runs in the carotid sheath and is accompanied by the internal jugular vein and the vagus nerve (CN-X). The vagus nerve is usually located posterior to both arterial and venous vascular structures. Rarely, the cervical ICA may form a complete loop in its course.
2. The petrous segment of the ICA
   a. The vertical and horizontal portions of the petrous segment begin as the ICA enters the bony carotid canal and end at a point just lateral to the sella turcica, near the apex of the petrous portion of the temporal bone.
3. The precavernous segment of the ICA
   a. The short precavernous ICA segment passes upward, forward, and medially, from the apex of the petrous bone to a point below, lateral, and posterior to the sella at the level at which it enters the cavernous venous sinus.
4. The juxtasellar, or intracavernous, segment of the ICA
   a. The intracavernous ICA segment passes upward in the posterior part of the cavernous venous sinus, turns anteriorly to run in the carotid sulcus, and comes to lie inferior and medial to the anterior clinoid process of the sella turcica.
   b. The final part of the intracavernous ICA segment turns superiorly and penetrates the dura mater medial to the anterior clinoid process.
   c. The intracavernous and the supraclinoid ICA segments are jointly termed the carotid siphon.
5. The supraclinoid segment of the ICA
   a. The supraclinoid ICA segment passes upward, posteriorly, and laterally to bifurcate into the anterior and middle cerebral arteries.

The Branches of the Internal Carotid Artery

1. Cervical ICA segment branches
   a. The cervical ICA ordinarily has no branches.

2. Petrous ICA segment branches
   a. The caroticotympanic artery arises from the vertical portion of the petrous ICA laterally and supplies the tympanic cavity after passing through a small foramen.
   b. The artery of the pterygoid canal (vidian artery) usually arises from the horizontal segment of the petrous ICA segment and courses into the pterygoid canal (vidian canal) to anastomose with a branch of the internal maxillary artery.
3. Pre- and intracavernous ICA segment branches
   a. The meningohypophyseal (dorsal main-stem) artery
      i. The meningohypophyseal artery arises from the dorsal aspect of the precavernous ICA segment and divides into three branches: the basal and marginal tentorial branch(es), the inferior hypophyseal artery, and the dorsal meningeal artery.
         - The basal tentorial artery diverges laterally along the insertion of the tentorium cerebelli into the petrous ridge of the temporal bone.
         - The marginal tentorial artery (artery of Bernasconi and Cassinari) ascends and extends posteriorly along the free margin of the tentorium cerebelli to supply this structure.
         - The inferior (postero-inferior) hypophyseal artery runs superiorly and medially to reach the lateral surface of the hypophysis (pituitary gland) and predominantly supplies the posterior lobe of the pituitary gland (neurohypophysis). It may also supply the periphery of the anterior lobe (adenohypophysis).
         - The dorsal meningeal (lateral clival) artery supplies the dura overlying the clivus and dorsum sellae and may extend inferiorly to the foramen magnum.
   b. The inferolateral trunk (lateral main-stem artery)
      i. The inferolateral trunk arises anterior to the meningohypophyseal artery from the inferolateral aspect of the cavernous ICA segment. It has many small branches that supply portions of the tentorium cerebelli, the orbit via the superior orbital fissure where it anastomoses with branches of the ophthalmic artery, the maxillary division of the fifth cranial nerve (CN-V2) in the foramen rotundum, the gasserian ganglion (ganglion of CN-V), the foramen ovale and the mandibular division of the fifth cranial nerve (CN-V3), and the foramen lacerum via the recurrent artery of the foramen lacerum that anastomoses with the carotid branch of the superior pharyngeal branch of the ascending pharyngeal artery.
   c. MacConnell's capsular arteries
      i. MacConnell's capsular arteries are the most distal branches of the cavernous ICA segment. They supply the inferior and peripheral aspect of the adenohypophysis (anterior lobe of the pituitary gland) and the dura of the diaphragma sellae.
4. Supraclinoid ICA segment branches
   a. The ophthalmic artery
      i. The ophthalmic artery arises from the junction of the intracavernous and supraclinoid ICA segments, just after the ICA perforates the dura mater to enter the subdural space.
      ii. The ophthalmic artery has many branches that supply the orbital, ocular, and periorbital structures.
   b. The posterior communicating artery
      i. The posterior communicating artery arises from the posterior aspect of the supraclinoid ICA segment above the anterior clinoid process.
      ii. The posterior communicating artery passes posteromedially to join the posterior cerebral artery on the same side; it constitutes a part of the circle of Willis.
      iii. The posterior communicating artery gives off many small perforating arteries that supply diencephalic and mesencephalic structures.
   c. The anterior choroidal artery

i. The anterior choroidal artery arises from the posterior wall of the supraclinoid ICA segment just above the posterior communicating artery origin, either as a single trunk or as one or more smaller vessels (4%).
ii. The anterior choroidal artery originates from the middle cerebral artery trunk or posterior communicating artery in 2% to 11% of cases.
iii. The anterior choroidal artery supplies the choroid plexus of the lateral ventricle and individually varying areas of the temporal lobe, the visual system, the posterior aspect of the internal capsule, the basal ganglia, the diencephalon, and the midbrain.

d. The superior hypophyseal arteries
  i. The superior hypophyseal arteries may arise from the posterior communicating artery or the supraclinoid ICA segment to supply the pituitary infundibulum and portions of the anterior lobe (adenohypophysis) of the pituitary gland.
e. Anterolateral lenticulostriate arteries
  i. Multiple small lenticulostriate arteries arise directly from the distal supraclinoid ICA segment.
f. The terminal arterial branches of the ICA
  i. The anterior cerebral artery.
  ii. The middle cerebral artery.
  iii. Rarely, anterior cerebral artery branches may originate directly from the supraclinoid ICA.

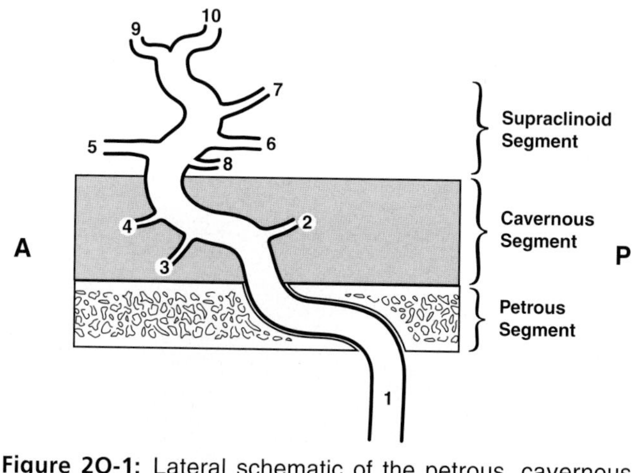

Figure 2Q-1: Lateral schematic of the petrous, cavernous, and supraclinoid segments of the internal carotid artery and the main arterial branches. *A*, anterior; *P*, posterior.
1 Internal carotid artery—distal cervical segment
2 Meningohypophyseal trunk
3 Inferolateral trunk
4 MacConnell's capsular artery(ies)
5 Ophthalmic artery
6 Posterior communicating artery
7 Anterior choroidal artery
8 Superior hypophyseal artery(ies)
9 Anterior cerebral artery
10 Middle cerebral artery

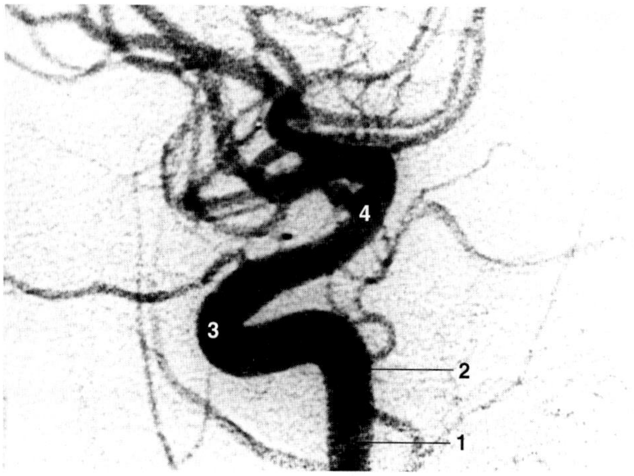

Figure 2Q-2A: Internal carotid artery siphon and bifurcation. Internal carotid angiogram in the lateral projection, showing the internal carotid artery (ICA) siphon.
1 Ascending cervical segment of the ICA
2 Petrous segment of the ICA
3 Cavernous segment of the ICA
4 Supraclinoid segment of the ICA

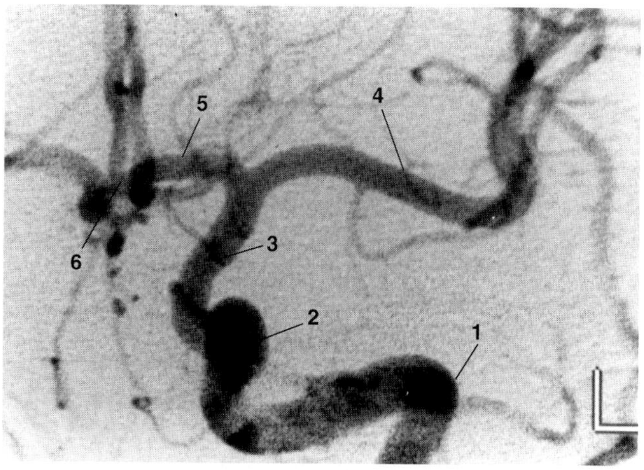

Figure 2Q-2B: Internal carotid artery siphon and bifurcation. Internal carotid angiogram in the frontal projection, showing the internal carotid siphon and the proximal segments of the anterior and middle cerebral arteries.
1 Petrous segment of the internal carotid artery
2 Cavernous segment of the internal carotid artery
3 Supraclinoid segment of the internal carotid artery
4 M1 segment of the middle cerebral artery
5 A1 segment of the anterior cerebral artery
6 Anterior communicating artery

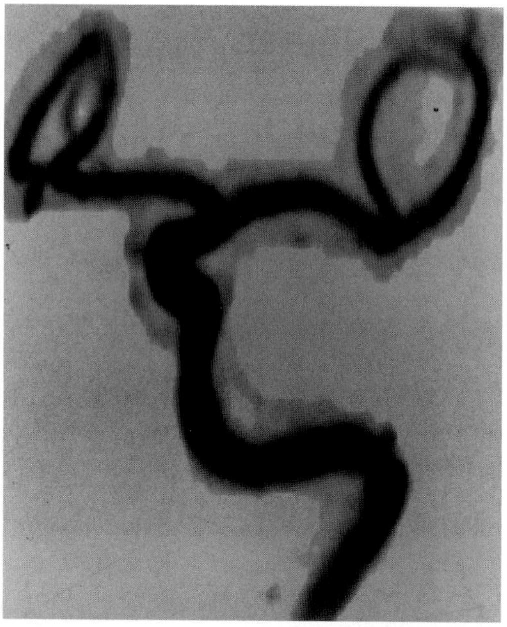

Figure 2Q-2C: Internal carotid artery siphon and bifurcation. MR angiogram showing the distal internal carotid artery, the carotid artery bifurcation, and the proximal middle and anterior cerebral arteries.

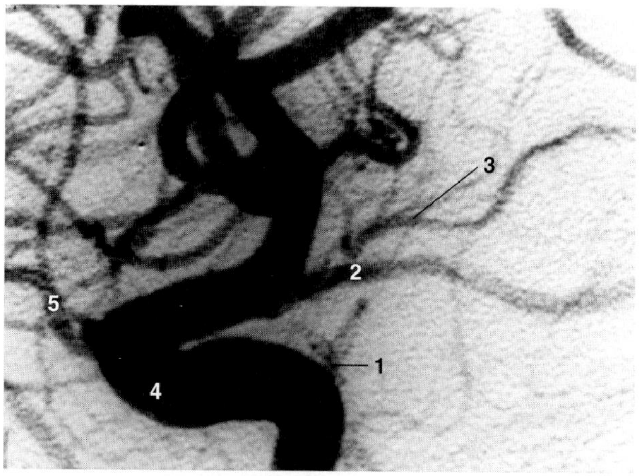

Figure 2Q-2D: Internal carotid artery siphon and bifurcation. Internal carotid angiogram in the lateral projection, showing the major cranial internal carotid artery branches proximal to the supraclinoid bifurcation.
1 Meningohypophyseal trunk
2 Posterior communicating artery
3 Anterior choroidal artery
4 Internal carotid artery siphon
5 Ophthalmic artery

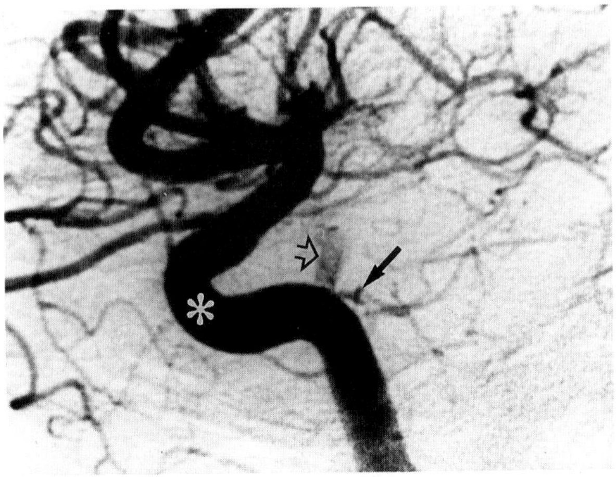

Figure 2Q-2E: Internal carotid artery siphon. Arterial phase of magnified right internal carotid angiogram in the lateral projection, showing the carotid siphon (*asterisk*), the meningohypophyseal trunk (*closed arrow*), and an associated posterior pituitary (posterior hypophyseal) blush (*open arrow*).

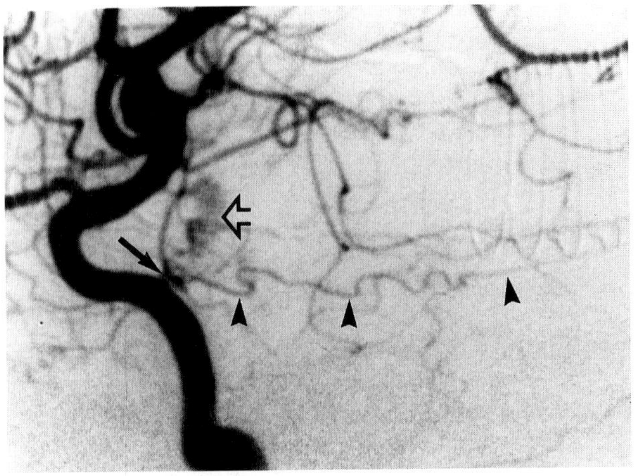

Figure 2Q-2F: Meningohypophyseal trunk and posterior pituitary gland vascular blush. Internal carotid arteriogram in the lateral projection, showing the base of the meningohypophyseal trunk (*closed arrow*), the posterior pituitary gland vascular blush (*open arrow*), and the tentorial artery of Bernasconi and Cassinari (*arrowheads*).

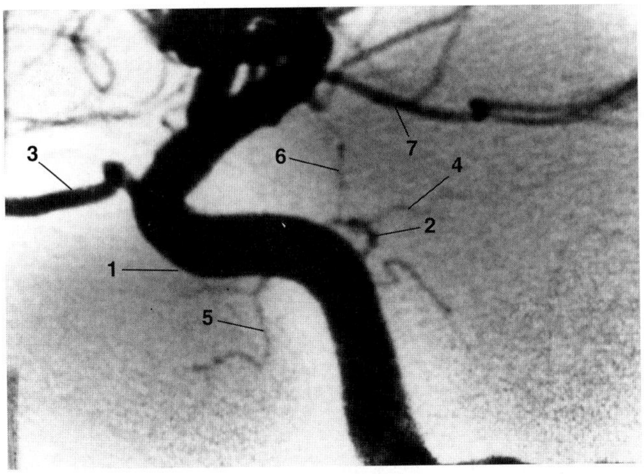

Figure 2Q-2G: Internal carotid angiogram showing additional branches of the distal internal carotid artery.
1 Cavernous segment of the internal carotid artery
2 Meningohypophyseal trunk
3 Ophthalmic artery
4 Tentorial branch
5 Vidian artery
6 Hypophyseal branch
7 Posterior communicating artery

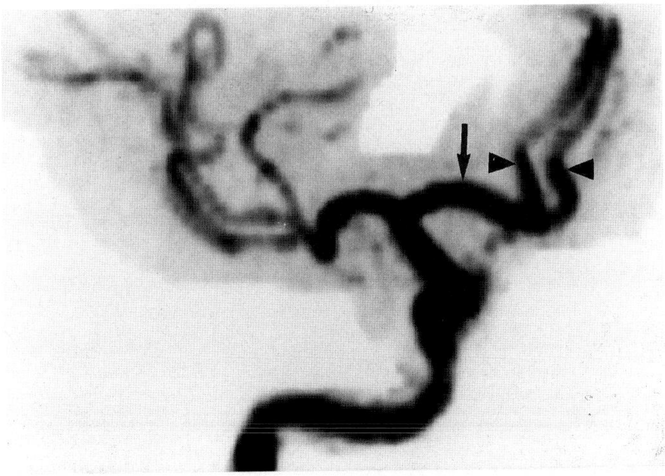

Figure 2Q-2H: Functionally hypoplastic internal carotid artery secondary to A1 segment atresia. MR angiogram in the frontal projection, showing functionally enlarged A1 segment (*arrow*) on the right side, the result of both anterior cerebral arteries (*arrowheads*) being supplied by the right internal carotid artery.

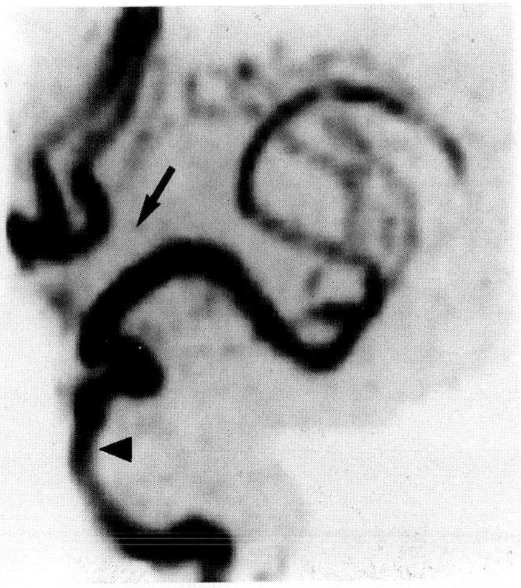

Figure 2Q-2I: MR angiogram in the frontal projection in same patient as Figure 2Q-2H, showing an atretic A1 segment (*arrow*) and a functionally hypoplastic internal carotid artery (*arrowhead*) on the left due to the sole supply of this artery to the left middle cerebral artery (compare with Fig. 2Q-2H).

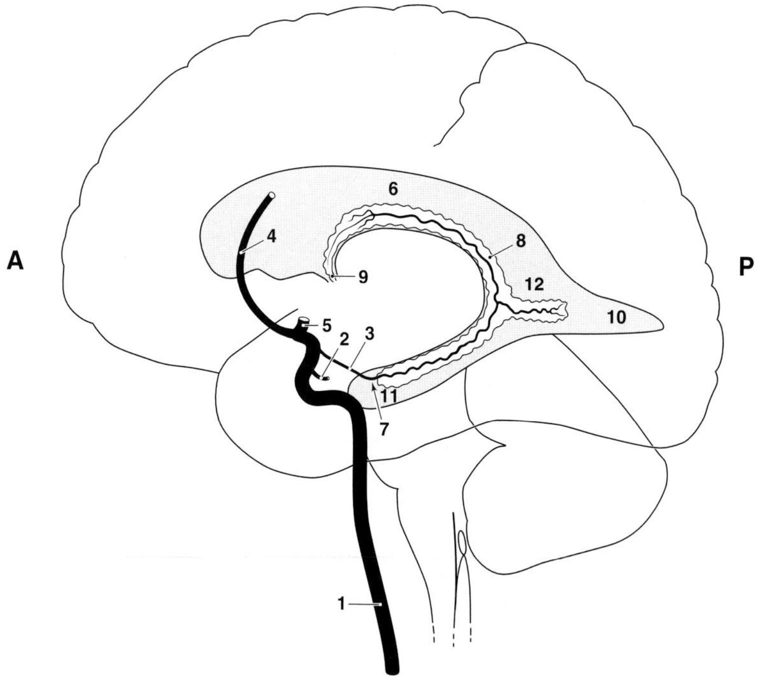

Figure 2Q-3: Lateral schematic of the anterior choroidal artery. *A,* anterior; *P,* posterior.
1 Internal carotid artery
2 Posterior communicating artery
3 Anterior choroidal artery
4 Anterior cerebral artery
5 Middle cerebral artery
6 Body of lateral ventricle
7 Plexal point (choroidal fissure)
8 Choroid plexus of lateral ventricle
9 Foramen of Monro
10 Occipital horn of lateral ventricle
11 Temporal horn of lateral ventricle
12 Atrium of lateral ventricle

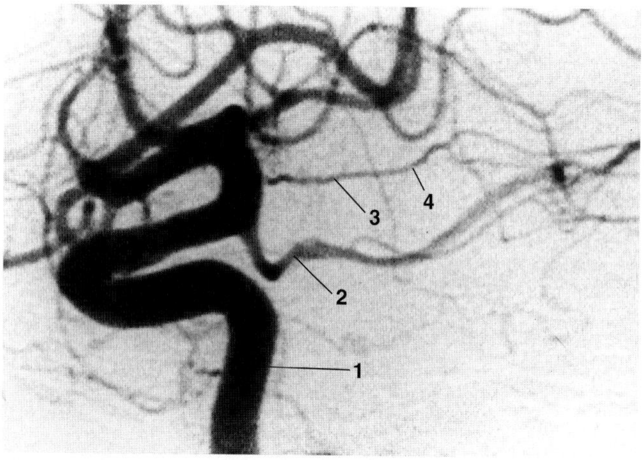

Figure 2Q-4: Internal carotid angiogram in the lateral projection, showing the anterior choroidal artery.
1 Internal carotid artery
2 Posterior communicating artery
3 Anterior choroidal artery
4 Plexal point

THE ANTERIOR CEREBRAL ARTERY

The Origin of the Anterior Cerebral Artery

1. The anterior cerebral artery originates at the bifurcation of the supraclinoid ICA into the anterior and middle cerebral arteries.
2. The anterior cerebral artery is normally the smaller of the two terminal branches (i.e., anterior vs. middle cerebral artery) of the ICA.

The Segments of the Anterior Cerebral Artery

1. The anterior cerebral artery has two main segments, and each main segment has many smaller branches.
   a. The A1, or horizontal anterior cerebral artery segment
      i. The A1 segment extends medially from the anterior cerebral artery origin to its junction with the anterior communicating artery.
      ii. The A1 segments of the right and left anterior cerebral arteries share in the formation of the circle of Willis.
   b. The A2, postcommunicating, or vertical anterior cerebral artery segment
      i. The A2 segment of the anterior cerebral artery begins at the junction of the horizontal segment of the anterior cerebral artery with the anterior communicating artery.
      ii. The A2 segment extends around the genu of the corpus callosum until it bifurcates into the pericallosal and callosomarginal arteries.
   c. The A3 anterior cerebral artery segment
      i. The A3 segment consists of the genu of the main anterior cerebral artery.
   d. The A4 and A5 anterior cerebral artery segments
      i. Some anatomists further divide the supracallosal ramifications of the anterior cerebral artery into A4 and A5 segments.
      ii. The A4 segment extends from the genu of the anterior cerebral artery to the region of the central sulcus; the A5 segment extends backward from the central sulcus to the terminal branches of the anterior cerebral artery.
2. The anterior cerebral artery supplies the anterior two-thirds of the medial aspect of the cerebral hemisphere and several centimeters of the contiguous superior medial surface of the brain convexity.

The Branches of the Anterior Cerebral Artery

1. Variation is the rule in the arrangement of the branches of the anterior cerebral vessels.
2. The main branches of the A1 segment of the anterior cerebral artery include the medial lenticulostriate arteries, the anterior communicating artery, and the recurrent artery of Heubner.
   a. The medial lenticulostriate arteries
      i. The medial lenticulostriate arteries arise from the A1 segment of the anterior cerebral artery as small branches that pierce the brain in the region of the anterior perforated substance.
      ii. The medial lenticulostriate arteries supply part of the basal ganglia (e.g., the head of the caudate nucleus) and the anterior limb of the internal capsule.
   b. The anterior communicating artery
      i. The anterior communicating artery extends between and connects the most distal A1 segments of the right and left anterior cerebral arteries and shares in the formation of the circle of Willis.
      ii. Anteromedial perforating arterial branches originating from the anterior communicating artery supply the anterior corpus callosum, the head of the caudate

nucleus, other portions of the basal ganglia anteriorly, and parts of other regional structures, such as the hypothalamus.

c. The recurrent artery of Heubner
   i. The recurrent artery of Heubner most commonly (49%–78%) arises from the A2 segment of the anterior cerebral artery. The A1 segment of the anterior cerebral artery is the second most common source, and the anterior communicating artery is the third most common origin. Rarely, it may arise from regional cortical branches of the anterior cerebral artery.
   ii. The recurrent artery of Heubner is absent in 3% or duplicated in 12% of the population.
   iii. The recurrent artery of Heubner supplies the antero-inferior aspect of the head of the caudate nucleus, the rostral part of the globus pallidus, the paraterminal gyrus, and the anterior limb of the internal capsule.

3. The main branches of the A2 segment of the anterior cerebral artery include the following:
   a. The orbitofrontal arteries
      i. The orbitofrontal branches of the A2 segment of the anterior cerebral artery are two or three in number.
      ii. The orbitofrontal branches supply the orbital surface of the ipsilateral frontal lobe.
   b. The frontopolar artery
      i. The frontopolar artery originates from the A2 segment of the anterior cerebral artery near the genu of the corpus callosum and extends to the anterior pole of the frontal lobe; at this point it divides into two or three smaller branches.
      ii. The frontopolar artery supplies the anterior border of the frontal lobe and portions of the lateral convexity of the cerebral hemisphere.
   c. The callosomarginal artery
      i. The callosomarginal artery is one of the two major bifurcation branches of the anterior cerebral artery.
      ii. The callosomarginal artery usually originates distal to the frontopolar artery and passes upward and backward to give off the anterior, the middle, and the posterior internal frontal branches.
      iii. The callosomarginal artery supplies the anterior two-thirds of the medial hemisphere surface and a small area that extends superiorly for a short distance over the lateral convexities of the cerebral hemisphere.
   d. The pericallosal artery
      i. The pericallosal artery is the terminal branch of the anterior cerebral artery.
      ii. The pericallosal artery terminates as the precuneal branch, which supplies the precuneus, and/or as a posterior callosal branch, which terminates as the splenial artery, which supplies the posterior aspect of the corpus callosum.

TABLE 2Q-1: Main Segments and Branches of the Anterior Cerebral Artery

A1: horizontal segment (precommunicating) branches
- Medial lenticulostriate arteries
- Recurrent artery of Heubner (≈25% of cases)
- Anterior communicating artery

A2: distal segment (postcommunicating) branches
- Anteromedial striate arteries
- Recurrent artery of Heubner (≈75% of cases)
- Orbitofrontal artery
- Frontopolar artery
- Callosomarginal artery
- Pericallosal trunk

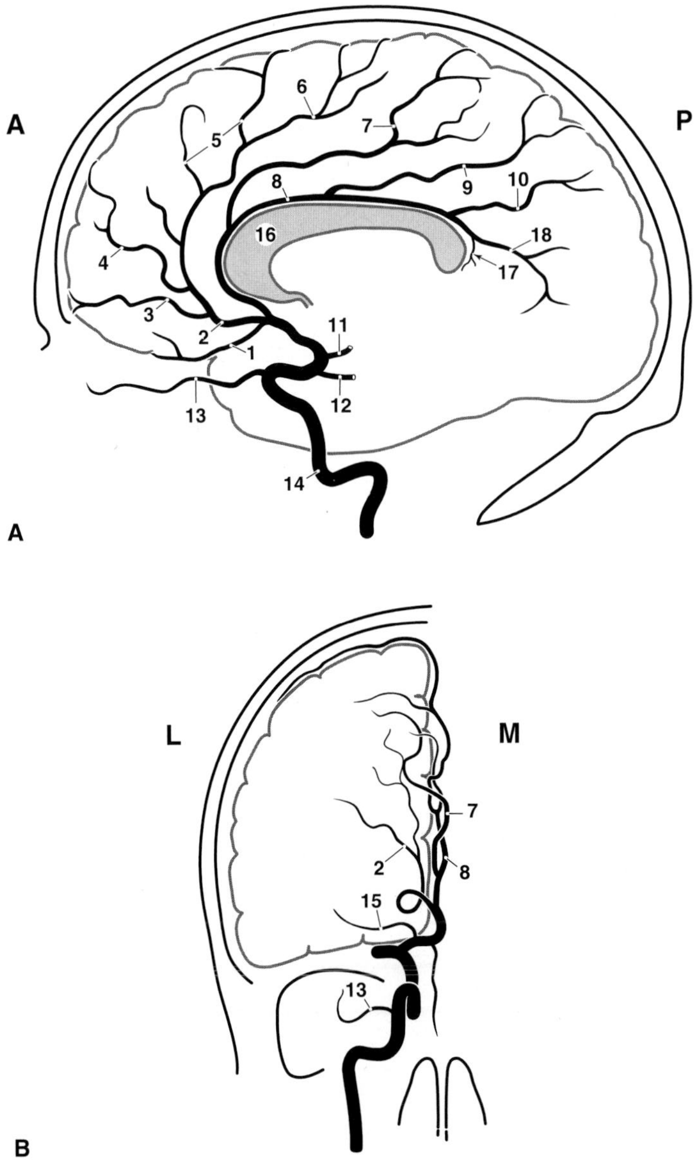

Figure 2Q-5: A: Lateral schematic of the major branches of the anterior cerebral artery. **B:** Frontal schematic of the major branches of the anterior cerebral artery. *A,* anterior; *P,* posterior; *M,* medial; *L,* lateral.

1 Orbitofrontal artery
2 Callosomarginal artery
3 Frontopolar artery
4 Anterior internal frontal artery
5 Middle internal frontal artery(ies)
6 Posterior internal frontal artery
7 Central sulcus artery(ies)
8 Pericallosal artery
9 Superior internal parietal artery
10 Inferior internal parietal artery
11 Anterior choroidal artery
12 Posterior communicating artery
13 Ophthalmic artery
14 Internal carotid artery
15 Recurrent artery of Heubner
16 Corpus callosum
17 Splenial artery
18 Precuneal branch

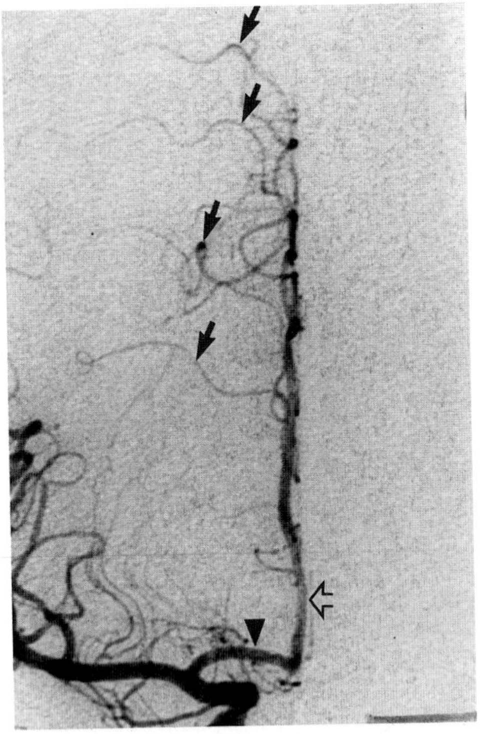

Figure 2Q-6A: Anterior cerebral artery. Carotid angiogram in the frontal projection, showing the A1 segment (*arrowhead*), the A2 segment (*open arrow*), and hemisphere branches (*solid arrows*) of the anterior cerebral artery on the right side.

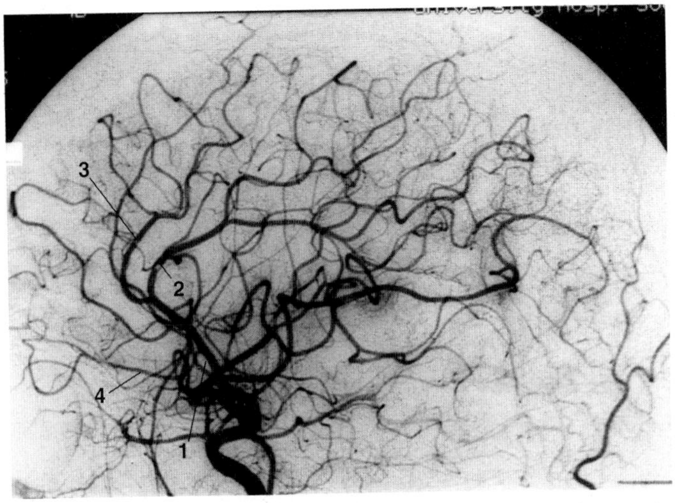

Figure 2Q-6B: Anterior cerebral artery. Carotid arteriogram in the lateral projection, showing the normal arterial anatomy.
1 A2 segment of anterior cerebral artery
2 Pericallosal artery
3 Callosomarginal artery
4 Frontopolar artery

THE MIDDLE CEREBRAL ARTERY

The Origin of the Middle Cerebral Artery

1. The middle cerebral artery is a continuation of the ICA. It is the larger of the two terminal branches of the ICA.
2. As the middle cerebral artery extends laterally from the bifurcation of the ICA, it is situated between the temporal lobe and the lower aspect of the insula (i.e., island of Reil).

The Segments of the Middle Cerebral Artery

1. The horizontal, or M1, segment of the middle cerebral artery courses laterally from its origin at the bifurcation of the ICA to the point of the major branching of the middle cerebral artery. The middle cerebral artery divides into two or more branches at the end of the M1 segment.
2. The insular, or M2, segment of the middle cerebral artery extends from the termination of the M1 segment and runs deep in the Sylvian fissure looping over the insula. The M2 segment ends as the vessels exit the Sylvian fissure.
3. The opercular, or M3, segment of the middle cerebral artery begins as the branches of the middle cerebral artery emerge from the Sylvian fissure to ramify over the cortical surface and ends at the origination of the terminal branching of the middle cerebral artery.
4. The supra-Sylvian terminal, or M4 segment of the middle cerebral artery represents the terminal branching of this artery; it consists of two groups of arterial branches.
   a. The superior group supplies portions of the frontal and parietal lobes.
   b. The inferior group supplies portions of the temporal lobe.

The Branches of the Middle Cerebral Artery

1. The lateral lenticulostriate arterial branches
   a. The lateral lenticulostriate branches arise from the M1 segment of the middle cerebral artery.
   b. The lenticulostriate arteries are represented by two groups of three to six small branches each, which penetrate the brain after arising almost at right angles from the M1 segment of the middle cerebral artery.
   c. The lenticulostriate arteries supply the body and head of the caudate nucleus, the lateral part of the globus pallidus, the entire anteroposterior length of the upper (dorsal) part of the internal capsule, and the lateral portion of the anterior commissure.
2. The temporopolar arterial branch
   a. The temporopolar branch of the middle cerebral artery arises near the origin of the anterior temporal artery (discussed later herein).
   b. The temporopolar branch supplies the most anterior portion of the temporal lobe.
3. The frontobasal (orbitofrontal) arterial branch
   a. The frontobasal (orbitofrontal) branch of the middle cerebral artery arises from the M1 segment of the middle cerebral artery.
   b. The frontobasal branch supplies the middle and inferior frontal gyri on the lateral surface of the frontal lobe.
4. The operculofrontal arterial branches
   a. The operculofrontal branches of the middle cerebral artery arise from the M3 segment.
   b. The operculofrontal branches of the middle cerebral artery loop around the insula

within the Sylvian fissure and include all branches of the superior group of the M4 segment of the middle cerebral artery anterior to the arteries of the central sulcus.
   c. The operculofrontal arteries supply Broca's (speech) area and the premotor area.
5. The precentral and postcentral sulcal arterial branches
   a. The precentral and postcentral sulcal branches (Rolando's arteries) of the middle cerebral artery arise near Rolando's fissure as two branches that encircle the operculum.
   b. The precentral and postcentral sulcal branches supply the precentral and postcentral gyri.
6. The posterior parietal artery
   a. The posterior parietal artery of the middle cerebral artery varies in origin between the superior or inferior trunk of the M4 segment of the middle cerebral artery.
   b. The posterior parietal artery supplies the posterior part of the first and second parietal gyri and the supramarginal gyrus.
7. The angular artery
   a. The angular artery of the middle cerebral artery emerges at or near the posterior end of the Sylvian fissure to course over the superior temporal gyrus.
   b. The angular artery is the largest branch of the middle cerebral artery.
   c. The angular artery supplies the posterior part of the superior temporal gyrus, the supramarginal gyrus, the angular gyrus, and the first two occipital gyri.
8. The anterior temporal artery
   a. The anterior temporal artery of the middle cerebral artery arises distal to the lenticulostriate arteries and passes downward over the outer surface of the temporal lobe.
   b. The anterior temporal artery supplies the anterior portion of the temporal lobe.
9. The middle temporal artery
   a. The middle temporal artery arises from the inferior trunk of the M4 segment of the middle cerebral artery.
   b. The middle temporal artery varies in size but is frequently small and supplies the temporal gyri anterior to the territory of supply of the posterior temporal artery branches (see later discussion).
10. The posterior temporal artery branches
   a. The posterior temporal artery branches of the middle cerebral artery usually arise from the inferior trunk of the M4 segment of the middle cerebral artery.
   b. The posterior temporal artery branches of the middle cerebral artery supply the middle and posterior parts of the superior temporal gyrus, the posterior third of the middle temporal gyrus, and the posterior part of the inferior temporal gyrus.

The Sylvian Triangle

1. The Sylvian triangle is a set of angiographic landmarks that are used to localize cerebral mass lesions.
2. The Sylvian triangle is formed by the middle cerebral artery branches as they loop over the insula deep within the Sylvian fissure.
3. As the branches of the middle cerebral artery enter the Sylvian fissure, they are situated against the outer surface of the insula; the Sylvian branches are directed upward or upward and backward.
4. As the Sylvian branches reach the uppermost part of the outer surface of the insula (Sylvian point), they reverse their direction and course downward toward the margin of the frontoparietal operculum.
5. At the margin of the frontoparietal operculum, five to eight Sylvian arterial branches are directed laterally to emerge from the Sylvian fissure.
6. After emerging, the majority of the middle cerebral artery branches extend upward and backward over the outer surface of the cerebral hemisphere.

7. The borders and points of the Sylvian triangle
   a. The anterior–superior point of the Sylvian triangle is the top of the most anterior identifiable opercular branch.
   b. The posterior–superior point of the Sylvian triangle is the top of the most posterior identifiable opercular branch.
   c. The anterior–inferior point of the Sylvian triangle is represented by the most anterior aspect of the trunk of the middle cerebral artery or, alternatively, the inferior aspect of the most anterior opercular branch.
   d. By connecting the upper points of reversal of the course of each Sylvian artery, a straight line is formed, which is the upper border of the Sylvian triangle (superior insular line).
   e. The inferior border of the Sylvian triangle is formed by connecting the anterior–inferior point with the posterior point (inferior insular line).
   f. The anterior border of the Sylvian triangle is formed by connecting the anterior–superior point with the anterior–inferior point (anterior insular line).

TABLE 2Q-2: Main Segments and Branches of the Middle Cerebral Artery

MI: Proximal horizontal segment branches
Lateral lenticulostriate arteries
Temporopolear branch
Frontobasal branch
Anterior temporal artery
M2: Insular segment
M3: Opercular segment branches
Operculofrontal arteries
M4: Terminal cortical branches
Central sulcus arteries (Rolandic group)
Anterior parietal artery
Posterior parietal artery
Angular artery
Middle temporal artery
Posterior temporal artery branches

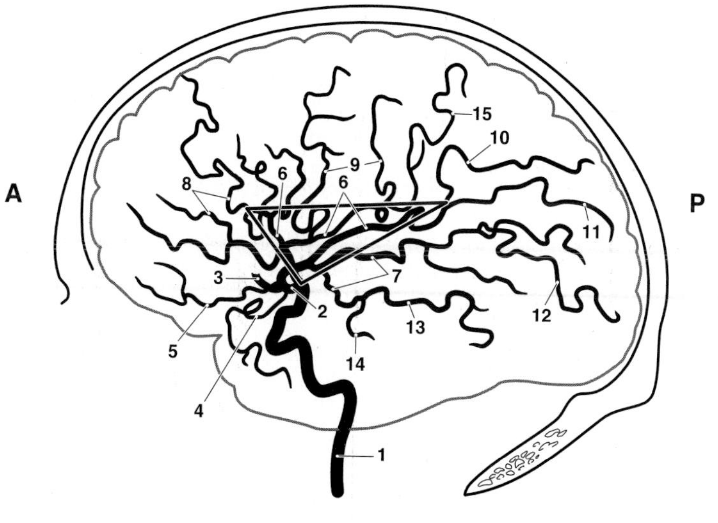

Figure 2Q-7: Lateral schematic of the branches of the middle cerebral artery. Note the overlay of the Sylvian triangle. *A,* anterior; *P,* posterior.
1 Internal carotid artery
2 Middle cerebral artery trunk
3 Cut edge of anterior cerebral artery
4 Temporal polar artery
5 Frontobasal (orbitofrontal) artery
6 Insular arteries
7 Temporal arterial branches
8 Operculofrontal arteries
9 Central sulcus arteries
10 Posterior parietal artery
11 Angular artery
12 Posterior temporal artery
13 Middle temporal artery
14 Anterior temporal artery
15 Anterior parietal artery

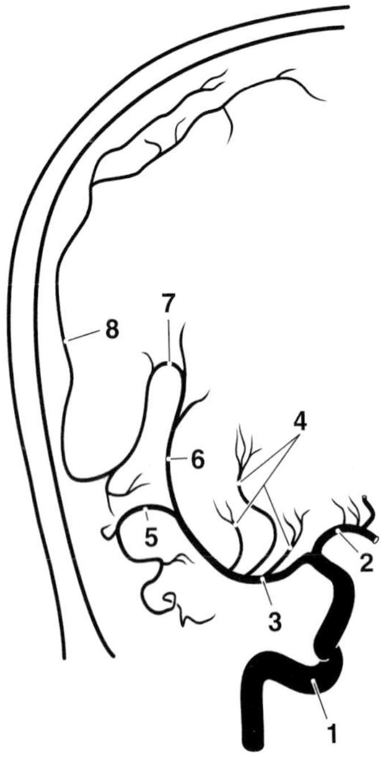

Figure 2Q-8: Frontal schematic of the branches of the right middle cerebral artery. Only one Sylvian segment and one opercular segment (M2 and M3) branch are shown, for simplification. *M,* medial; *L,* lateral.
1 Internal carotid artery
2 Trunk of anterior cerebral artery
3 Middle cerebral artery—horizontal segment (M1)
4 Lateral lenticulostriate arteries
5 Anterior temporal artery
6 Sylvian segments of middle cerebral artery (M2)
7 Sylvian point
8 Opercular middle cerebral artery branches (M3)

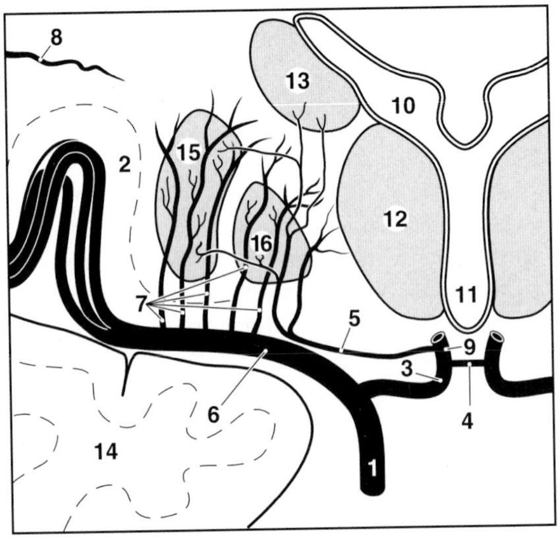

Figure 2Q-9: Frontal schematic of the perforating branches of the anterior and middle cerebral artery(ies) (not to scale).
1 Supraclinoid internal carotid artery
2 Insula
3 A1 segment of anterior cerebral artery
4 Anterior communicating artery
5 Recurrent artery of Heubner shown originating from most common site (approximately 75%: A2 segment of the anterior cerebral artery)
6 M1 (horizontal) segment of middle cerebral artery
7 Lateral lenticulostriate arteries
8 Cortical perforating branches
9 A2 segment of anterior cerebral artery
10 Right lateral ventricle
11 Third ventricle
12 Thalamus
13 Head of caudate nucleus
14 Temporal lobe
15 Putamen
16 Globus pallidus

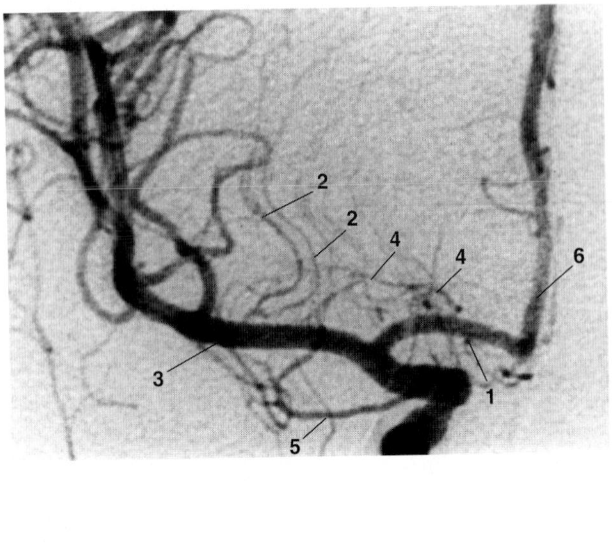

Figure 2Q-10: Right common carotid angiogram in the frontal projection, showing the lenticulostriate arteries and the recurrent artery of Heubner on the right side. In this case, the recurrent artery of Heubner arises from the A1 segment of the anterior cerebral artery.
1 A1 segment of the anterior cerebral artery
2 Lenticulostriate arteries
3 M1 segment of the middle cerebral artery
4 Recurrent artery of Heubner arising from the A1 segment of the anterior cerebral artery
5 Ophthalmic artery
6 A2 segment of the anterior cerebral artery

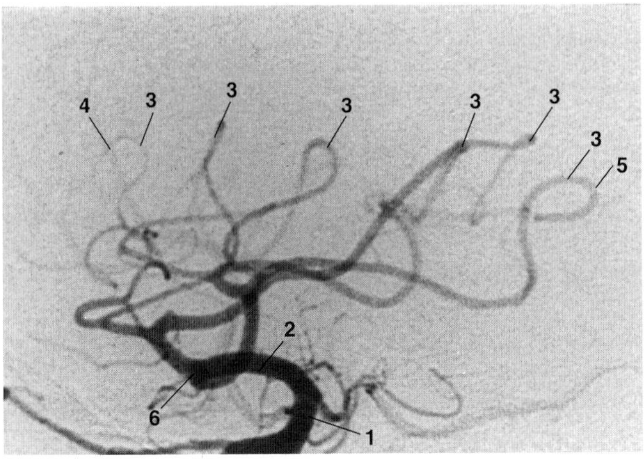

Figure 2Q-11: The Sylvian triangle. Left internal carotid arteriogram in the lateral projection in a patient with an atretic A1 segment of the ipsilateral anterior cerebral artery, showing the arteries of the Sylvian triangle.

1 Internal carotid artery
2 M1 segment of the middle cerebral artery
3 Uppermost extent of middle cerebral vessels defining superior border of Sylvian triangle
4 Anterosuperior extent of Sylvian triangle
5 Posterosuperior extent of Sylvian triangle
6 Antero-inferior extent of Sylvian triangle

A

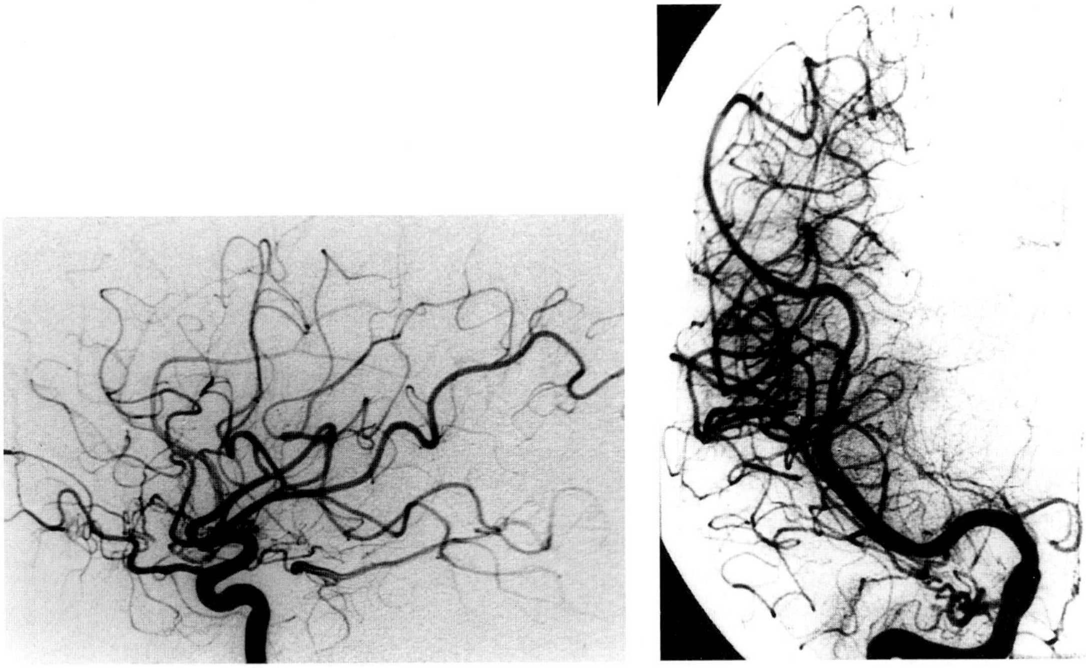

B

Figure 2Q-12: The middle cerebral artery. Right internal carotid angiogram showing the arterial phases of filling of the right middle cerebral artery in the lateral projection **(A)** and the late arterial phase in the frontal projection **(B)**. The A1 segment of the anterior cerebral artery is developmentally atretic on the right, resulting in poor filling of that vessel.

INTERNAL CAROTID ARTERY VARIANTS

1. The caliber of the ICA will generally vary, in part according to the volume of brain supplied.
2. True ICA agenesis/aplasia (unilateral or bilateral) is very rare and is usually accompanied by a hypoplastic carotid canal in the skull base. Enlarged intercarotid anastomotic vessels at the base of the brain (e.g., circle of Willis) are almost always seen in such cases.
3. The cavernous segments of the ICAs may interconnect by transverse collaterals arising from these vessels (i.e., intercavernous ICA anastomoses).
4. Anomalous branches arising from the ICA include the following:
   a. External carotid artery branches arise from the cervical segment of the ICA (e.g., occipital, ascending pharyngeal, and superior thyroid arteries); very rarely all branches of the external carotid artery may originate directly from the carotid artery.
   b. Persistent mandibular artery arising from the cervical segment of the ICA
   c. The persistent stapedial artery arises from the petrous segment of the ICA. This is an anomalous derivation of the hyoid–stapedial artery that usually regresses to become the caroticotympanic branch of the petrous ICA. For this reason, it passes through the middle ear to supply the middle ear itself and the territory of the middle meningeal artery, resulting in an absence or diminution in size of the ipsilateral foramen spinosum. Less frequently, the persistent stapedial artery may supply branches to the ipsilateral orbit and to the maxillomandibular distribution of the internal maxillary artery.
   d. ICA origin of various posterior fossa vessels (e.g., superior, anterior–inferior, and posterior–inferior cerebellar arteries; posterior meningeal artery)
   e. Fetal configuration of the posterior cerebral artery arising directly from the ICA (approximately 20%).
   f. Persistent fetal carotid-vertebrobasilar arterial anastomoses (e.g., persistent trigeminal, otic, and hypoglossal arteries; proatlantal intersegmental artery)
   g. Rarely, the upper portion of the ICA may be replaced by a branch or branches of the internal maxillary artery entering the skull through the foramen rotundum and foramen ovale; if multiple, these vessels typically join intracranially to form a single vessel, before branching into the anterior and middle cerebral arteries.
   h. Rarely, anterior or middle cerebral arterial vessels may originate directly from the supraclinoid ICA.
5. Anomalous course of the ICA
   a. Aberrant course of the cervical ICA traversing the retropharyngeal soft tissues may physically have the appearance of a submucosal mass.
   b. The cervical ICA may form a partial or complete loop.
   c. The petrous ICA may take an aberrant course within the middle ear. When the bony canal wall separating the petrous ICA from the middle ear is incomplete, the petrous segment of the ICA may buckle laterally into the middle ear.
   d. The intracavernous ICAs may course more medially than usual and produce enlargement and deepening of the carotid groove (i.e., carotid sulcus) of the sella turcica. If this occurs bilaterally, the ICAs may approximate in the midline, producing so-called "kissing carotids" ("kissing ICAs").

INTERNAL CAROTID ARTERY (ICA) VARIANTS

- ICA hypoplasia
- ICA aplasia (agenesis)
- Abnormal course of the ICA (e.g., submucosal-retropharyngeal ICA, ICA loop)
- Intercavernous anastomosis of the ICAs
- Anomalous branches arising from the ICA
  - External carotid artery branches
  - Persistent mandibular artery
  - Persistent stapedial artery
  - Posterior fossa artery branches
  - Posterior cerebral artery (fetal configuration)
  - Persistent fetal carotid-vertebrobasilar arterial anastomoses
  - ICA replacement by a branch(es) of the internal maxillary artery
  - Anterior or middle cerebral artery branches

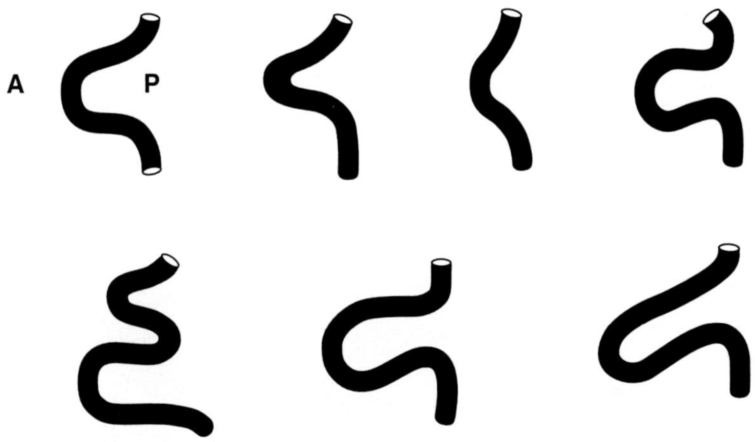

Figure 2Q-13: Lateral schematic of some variations of the carotid artery siphon. *A*, anterior; *P*, posterior.

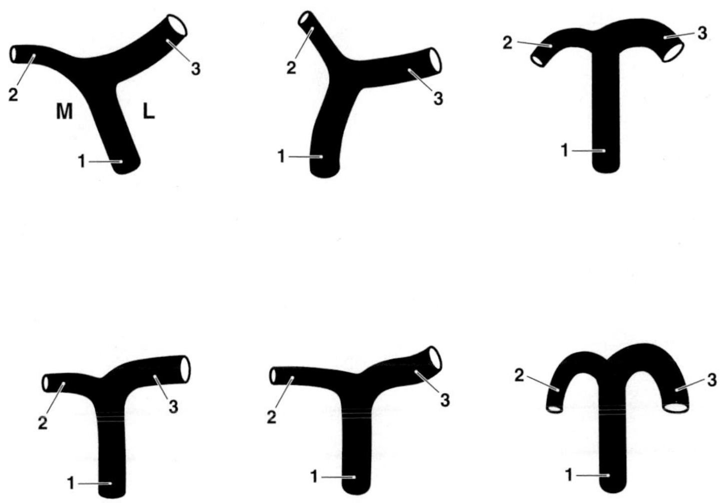

Figure 2Q-14: Frontal schematics of some variations in the bifurcation of the right supraclinoid internal carotid artery *(1)* into the anterior *(2)* and middle *(3)* cerebral arteries. *M,* medial; *L,* lateral.

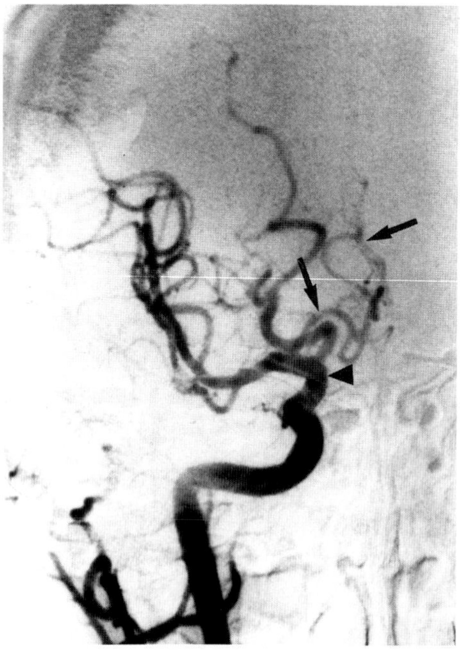

Figure 2Q-15A: Right common carotid angiogram in the frontal projection, showing orbitofrontal and frontopolar branches (*arrows*) arising from the supraclinoid internal carotid artery (*arrowhead*).

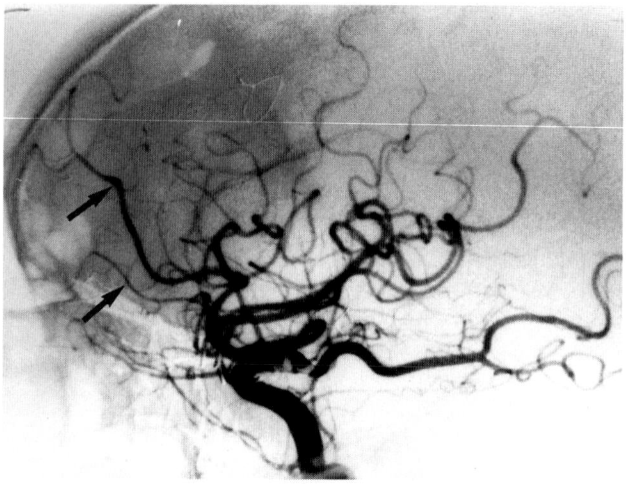

Figure 2Q-15B: Right common carotid artery angiogram in the lateral projection, showing the orbitofrontal and frontopolar branches (*arrows*).

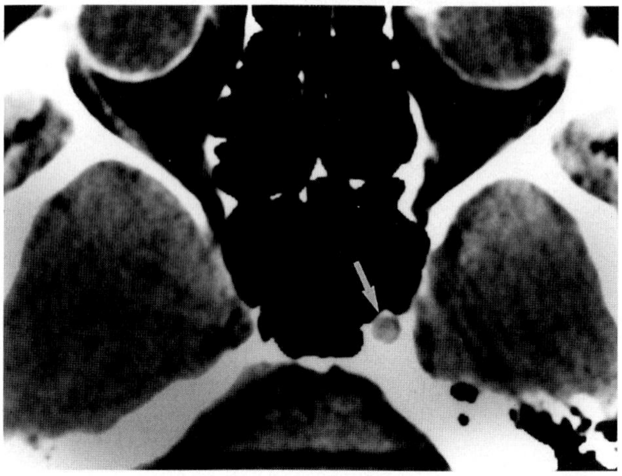

Figure 2Q-16A: Course of internal carotid artery through the sphenoid sinus. Axial CT showing a "naked" left internal carotid artery traversing the well-aerated sphenoid sinus (*arrow*).

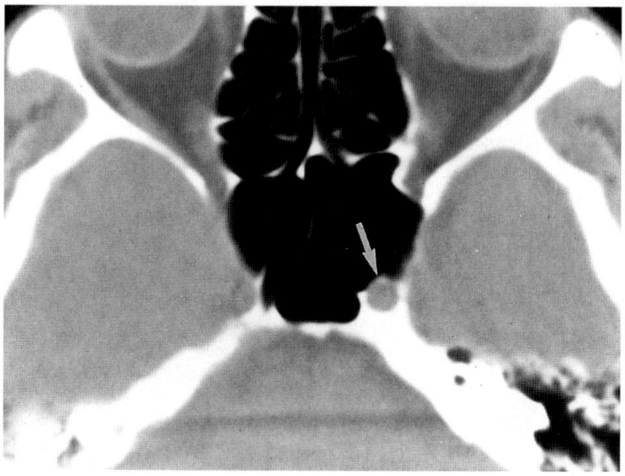

Figure 2Q-16B: Course of internal carotid artery through the sphenoid sinus. Axial CT with bone window filming shows partial absence of bone between the left internal carotid artery and the sphenoid sinus (*arrow*).

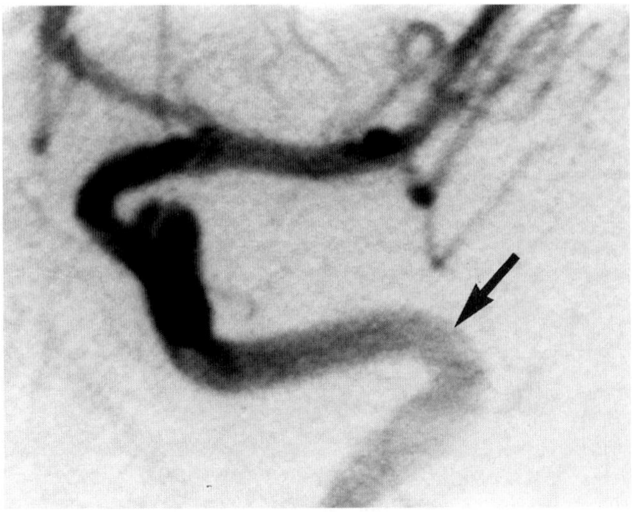

Figure 2Q-17A: Ectopic course of the petrous internal carotid artery. Left internal carotid arteriogram in the frontal projection, showing the laterally ectopic left petrous internal carotid artery (*arrow*). (Compare with Figure 2Q-17B.)

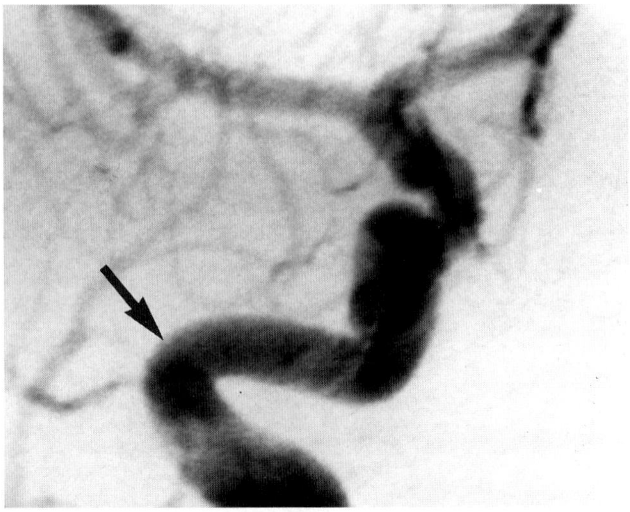

Figure 2Q-17B: Right internal carotid artery angiogram in the frontal projection shows the normal course of the right internal carotid artery (*arrow*) in the same patient, for comparison (case courtesy of Jose Guilherme Caldas, M.D., São Paulo, Brazil).

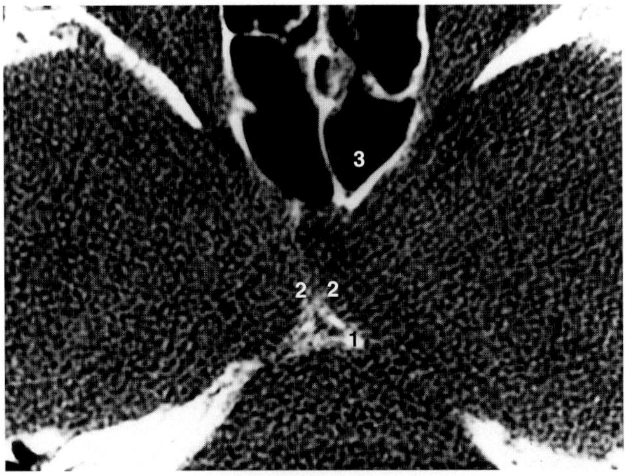

Figure 2Q-18A: "Kissing" internal carotid arteries. Noncontrast axial CT scan acquired at the level of the sella turcica, showing distal "kissing carotids" (artery canals/sulci) approximating in the midline.

1 Dorsum sella
2 Cavernous segment of the internal carotid arteries. Note the close approximation of both carotid artery sulci: "kissing carotids"
3 Sphenoid sinus

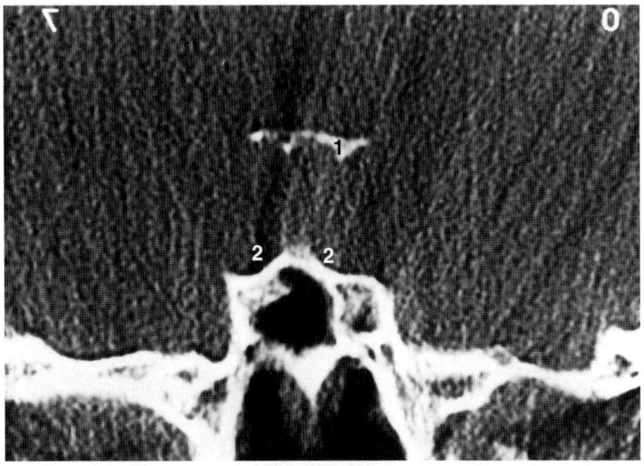

Figure 2Q-18B: "Kissing" internal carotid arteries. Coronal CT scan acquired at the level of the sella turcica, showing "kissing carotid" artery sulci.

1 Dorsum sella
2 Sulci for the internal carotid arteries within the sphenoid bone. Note the close approximation of the carotid artery grooves, indicating so-called kissing carotids.

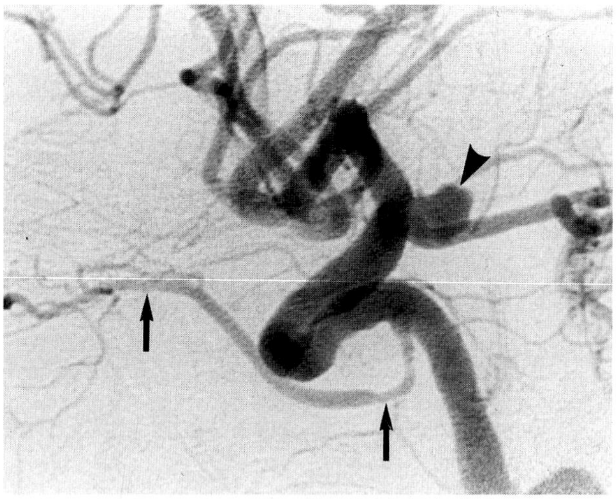

Figure 2Q-19: Ophthalmic artery originating from the cavernous segment of the internal carotid artery. Right internal carotid angiogram in the lateral projection shows the ophthalmic artery (*arrows*) originating from the cavernous segment of the internal carotid artery. Note also an aneurysm (*arrowhead*) at the posterior communicating artery origin.

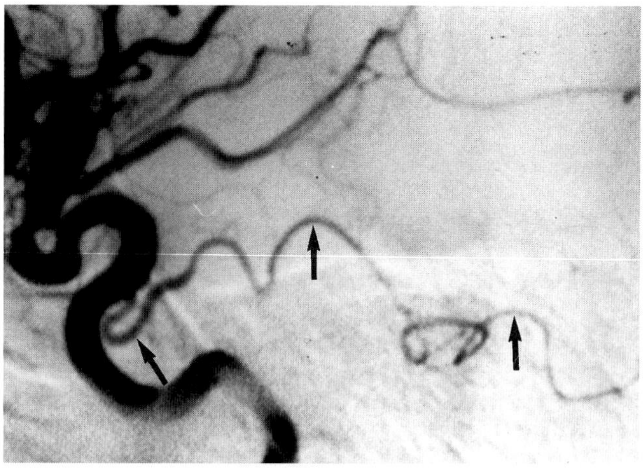

Figure 2Q-20: Cerebellar artery originating from the cavernous segment of the internal carotid artery. Left internal carotid artery angiogram in the lateral projection showing a cerebellar artery (*arrows*) originating from the cavernous/precavernous segment of the left internal carotid artery.

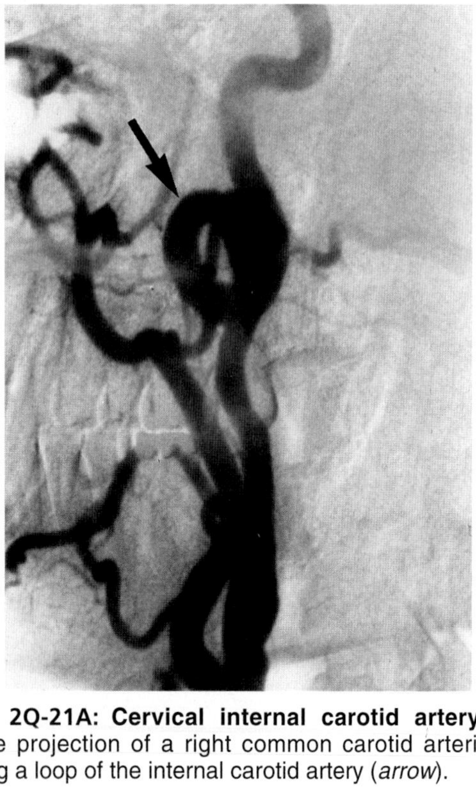

Figure 2Q-21A: Cervical internal carotid artery loop. Oblique projection of a right common carotid arteriogram, showing a loop of the internal carotid artery (*arrow*).

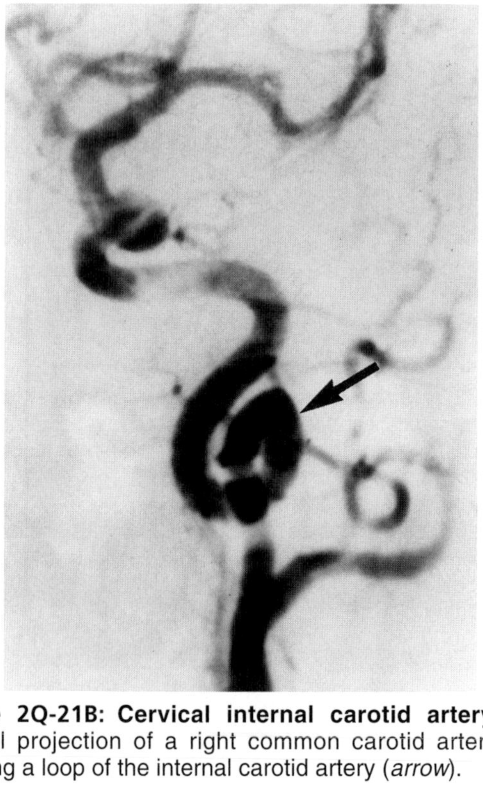

Figure 2Q-21B: Cervical internal carotid artery loop. Frontal projection of a right common carotid arteriogram, showing a loop of the internal carotid artery (*arrow*).

ANTERIOR CEREBRAL ARTERY VARIANTS

1. Developmental anomalies and variants of the anterior cerebral artery include the following.
   a. Complete absence of the anterior cerebral artery (rare).
   b. Anomalous origins of the anterior cerebral artery are uncommon. Rarely, the anterior cerebral artery arises from the intradural ICA near the ophthalmic artery origin. In such cases, it passes inferiorly to the optic nerve and then ascends in front of the optic chiasm.
   c. The A1 segment of the anterior cerebral artery may be hypoplastic or absent in up to 10% of cases; in both instances (absence or hypoplasia), the A1 segment of the contralateral anterior cerebral artery supplies the anterior cerebral artery distal to the hypoplastic or absent segment via the anterior communicating artery.
   d. There may be an accessory (i.e., third) or duplicated anterior cerebral artery. This accessory or duplicated vessel arises from the anterior communicating artery. An accessory or duplicated A2 segment of one of the anterior cerebral arteries occurs in about 4% of cases.
   e. A common (i.e., azygous) or single trunk of the proximal anterior cerebral arteries may be encountered, but it is uncommon. In this circumstance, the A1 (horizontal) segments of both the anterior cerebral arteries join at the midline and ascend as a common trunk until they reach the falx, where they bifurcate to supply both cerebral hemispheres.
   f. Although two anterior cerebral arteries are present in the case of a bihemispheric anterior cerebral artery, one nevertheless gives rise to vessels supplying both cerebral hemispheres. Partial bihemispheric supply of one or both anterior cerebral arteries is not uncommon.
   g. The middle meningeal artery originates from the anterior cerebral artery in 0.5% of cases.
2. Pericallosal and callosomarginal artery variants
   a. Dominance of the callosomarginal artery is a common normal variant wherein the anterior cerebral artery ends in a large callosomarginal artery.
   b. Hypoplasia of the callosomarginal artery is also encountered; in this case, a large (dominant) pericallosal artery supplies the usual area of distribution of the callosomarginal artery.
   c. In cases of agenesis of the corpus callosum, the anterior cerebral artery branches are seen to wander in a haphazard fashion within the large midline space between the cerebral hemispheres resulting from the absent callosum.
   d. In cases of pericallosal lipoma, the pericallosal artery may reveal displacement and an irregular luminal diameter as the vessel traverses around and/or through the lipoma.

ANTERIOR CEREBRAL ARTERY VARIANTS

- Anterior cerebral artery hypoplasia
- Anterior cerebral artery aplasia (agenesis)
- Anomalous origin of the anterior cerebral artery
- A1 segment anterior cerebral artery hypoplasia/aplasia
- Accessory/duplicated anterior cerebral artery
- Common (azygous) trunk of the anterior cerebral artery
- Bihemispheric anterior cerebral artery
- Origin of the middle meningeal artery from the anterior cerebral artery
- Pericallosal or callosomarginal artery hypoplasia

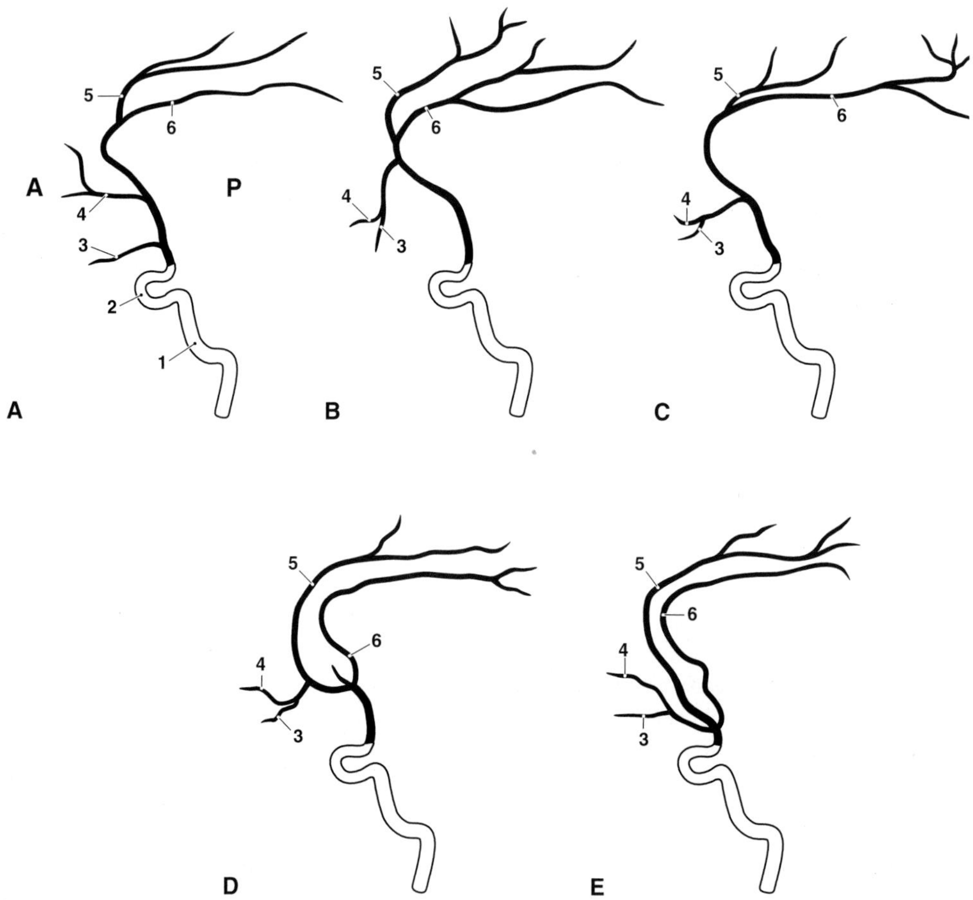

Figure 2Q-22: Lateral schematic of some of the variations in the configuration of the anterior cerebral artery branches. **A:** Typical balanced branching pattern. **B:** Dominant callosomarginal artery. The orbitofrontal and frontopolar branches have a common trunk. **C:** Dominant pericallosal artery. **D:** Moderately low pericallosal–callosomarginal artery bifurcation. **E:** Markedly low pericallosal–callosomarginal artery bifurcation. *A,* anterior; *P,* posterior.

1 Internal carotid artery
2 Carotid siphon
3 Orbitofrontal artery
4 Frontopolar artery
5 Callosomarginal artery
6 Pericallosal artery

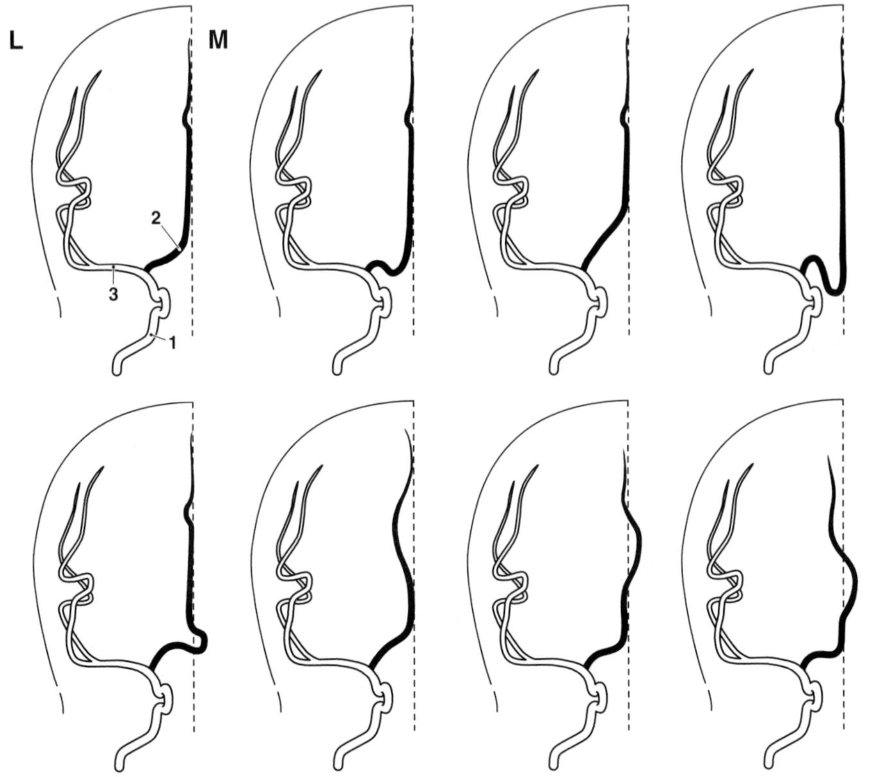

Figure 2Q-23: Frontal schematics of some of the variations in the configuration of the A1 segment of the right anterior cerebral artery. *M,* medial; *L,* lateral.

1 Internal carotid artery
2 Anterior cerebral artery
3 Middle cerebral artery

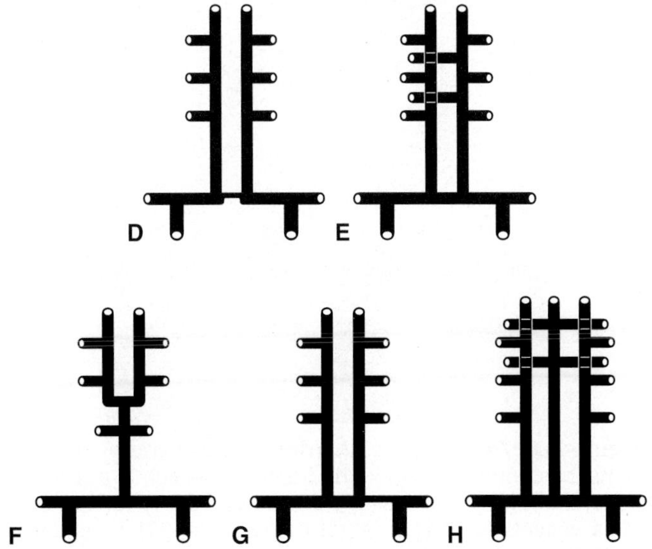

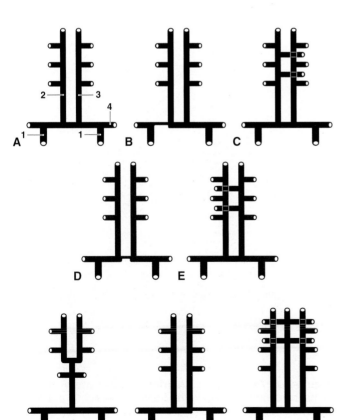

Figure 2Q-24: Frontal schematic of some of the variations of the anterior cerebral artery branches. **A:** Idealized balanced configuration. **B:** Atretic right A1 segment. **C:** Bihemispheric right anterior cerebral artery. **D:** Atretic anterior communicating artery. **E:** Bihemispheric left anterior cerebral artery. **F:** Azygous anterior cerebral artery. **G:** Atretic left A1 segment. **H:** Accessory or duplicated anterior cerebral artery.

1 Internal carotid artery
2 Right anterior cerebral artery
3 Left anterior cerebral artery
4 Middle cerebral artery

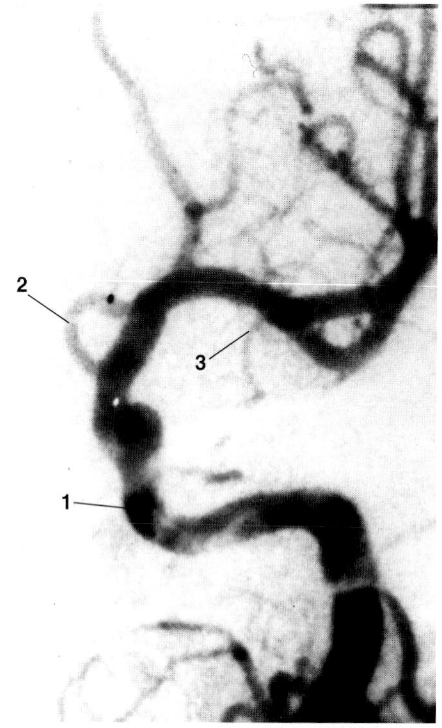

Figure 2Q-25: A1 segment anterior cerebral artery atresia. Left internal carotid angiogram in the frontal projection, showing an atretic A1 segment (nonfilling) of the left anterior cerebral artery.

1 Internal carotid artery
2 Posterior cerebral artery originating from internal carotid artery
3 Middle cerebral artery

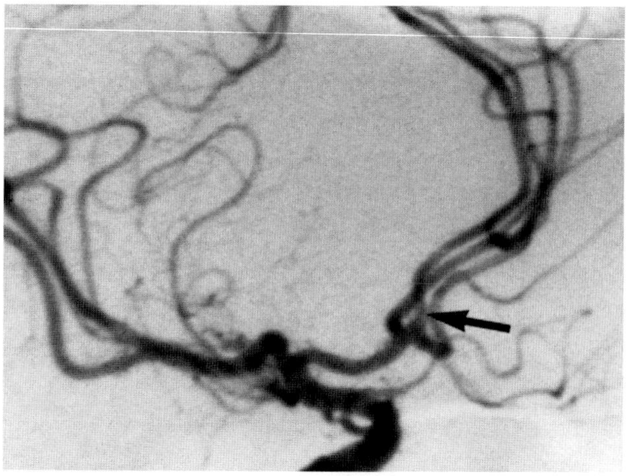

Figure 2Q-26: Accessory or duplicated anterior cerebral artery. Right internal carotid angiogram in the oblique projection, showing three anterior cerebral arteries. The central of the three vessels (*arrow*) is the accessory or duplicated anterior cerebral artery that may contribute vessels to one or both cerebral hemispheres.

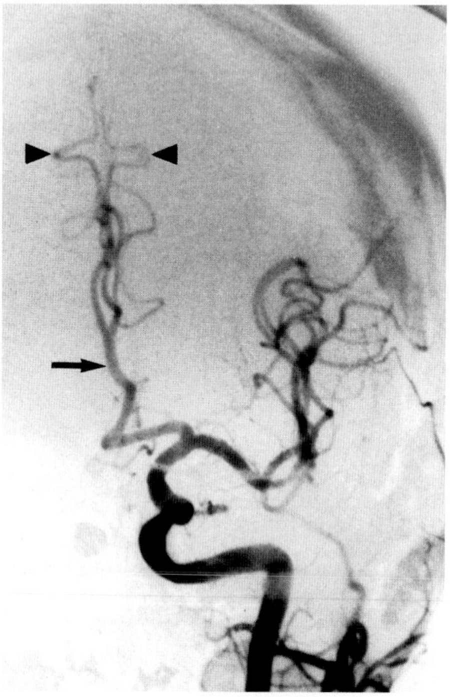

Figure 2Q-27A: Azygous anterior cerebral artery. Left common carotid angiogram in the frontal plane, showing a single anterior cerebral artery trunk (*arrow*) supplying major branches to both cerebral hemispheres (*arrowheads*).

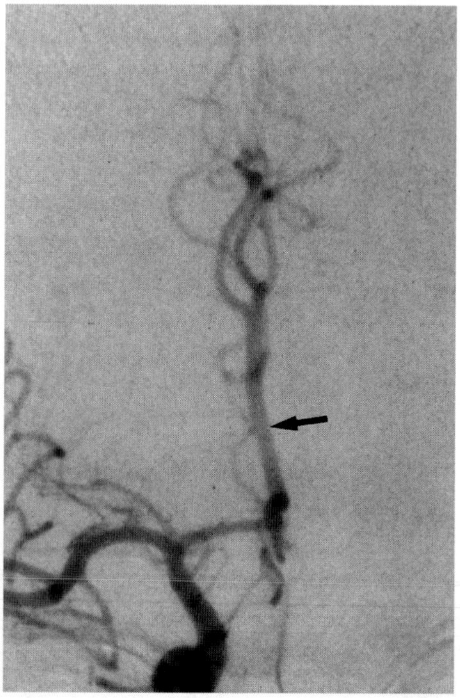

Figure 2Q-27B: Azygous anterior cerebral artery. Right internal carotid angiogram in the frontal projection in a different patient, showing that a single pericallosal artery (*arrow*) supplies vessels to both cerebral hemispheres. This variant is termed an azygous anterior cerebral artery.

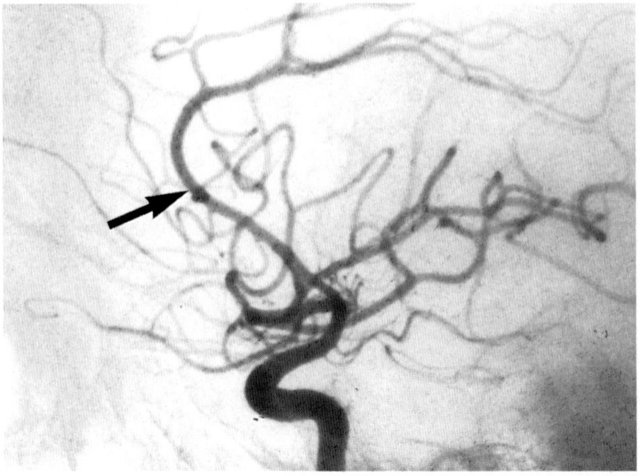

Figure 2Q-27C: Azygous anterior cerebral artery. Right internal carotid angiogram in the lateral projection (same case as that shown in Figure 2Q-27B), showing an azygous (single) proximal anterior cerebral artery (*arrow*).

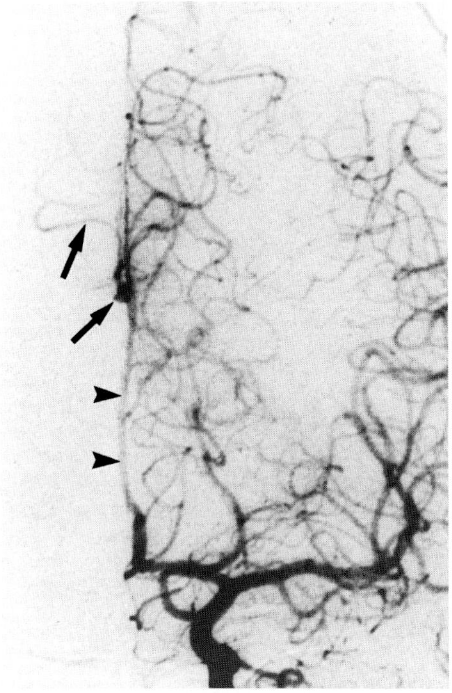

Figure 2Q-28: Bihemispheric anterior cerebral artery distribution. Conventional angiogram in the frontal projection, showing filling of the left anterior cerebral artery (*arrowheads*) and opacification of anterior cerebral artery branch(es) (*arrows*) crossing the midline to supply the right cerebral hemisphere.

MIDDLE CEREBRAL ARTERY VARIANTS

1. Major variants of the middle cerebral artery are uncommon and occur less frequently than do those of the other major intracranial vessels.
2. Fenestration of the M1 (horizontal) segment of the middle cerebral artery occurs in approximately 1% of patients.
3. The M1 segment of the middle cerebral artery may be accompanied by a small additional artery coursing laterally. This artery is called either the accessory middle cerebral artery (0.3%–4.0%) (when it originates from the proximal or distal A1 segment of the anterior cerebral artery) or a duplicated middle cerebral artery (0.2%–2.9%) (when it arises directly from the supraclinoid portion of the ICA).
4. Minor variations are common in the manner in which the middle cerebral artery branches originate from the common trunk (M1) as well as in the number of middle cerebral artery branches formed. The M1 segment of the middle cerebral artery terminates in a bifurcation in approximately 64% to 90% of cases, in a trifurcation in 12% to 29% of cases, and in other branching patterns in the remainder.
5. An anterior temporal artery branch may arise from the M1 segment of the middle cerebral artery independently, in combination with the orbitofrontal branch, or as one of the vessels making up a middle cerebral trifurcation.

MIDDLE CEREBRAL ARTERY VARIANTS

- Fenestration of the M1 (horizontal) segment of the middle cerebral artery
- Accessory or duplicated middle cerebral artery
- Bifurcation/trifurcation of the M1 segment of the middle cerebral artery
- Origin of an anterior temporal artery branch from the M1 segment

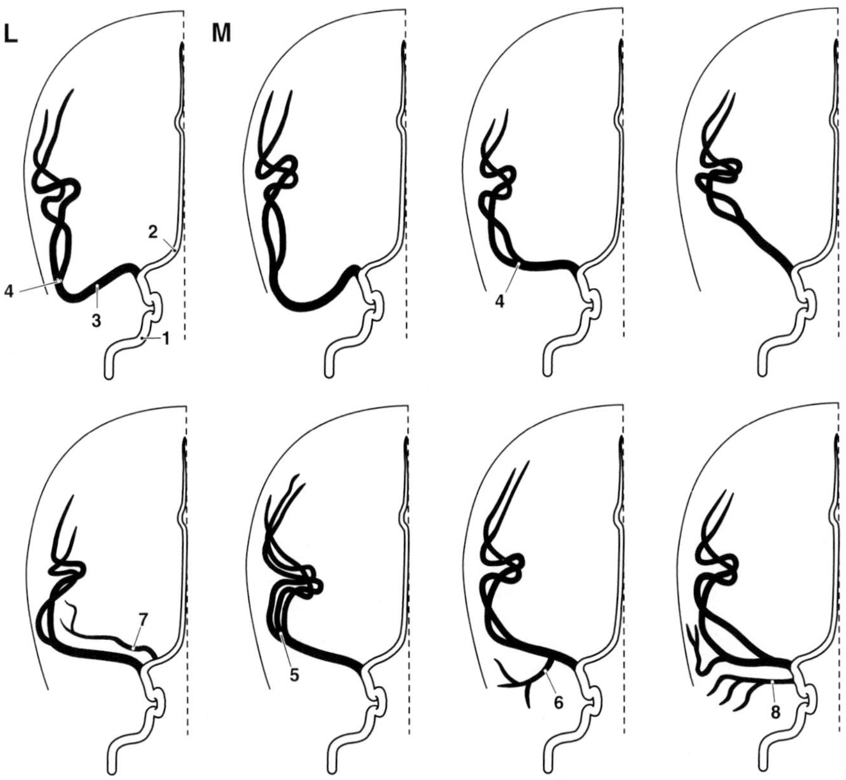

Figure 2Q-29: Frontal schematics of some variants in the configuration of the right middle cerebral artery. *M,* medial; *L,* lateral.

1 Internal artery
2 Anterior cerebral artery
3 Middle cerebral artery
4 Bifurcation of middle cerebral artery
5 Trifurcation of middle cerebral artery
6 Anterior temporal artery branch arising from M1 segment
7 Accessory middle cerebral artery
8 Duplicated middle cerebral artery

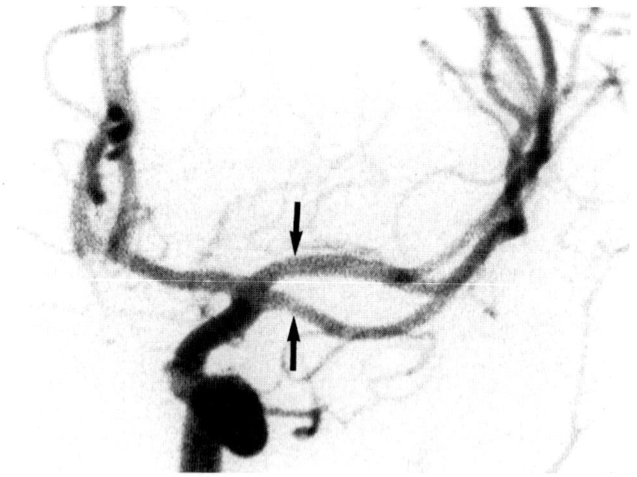

Figure 2Q-30: Duplicated middle cerebral artery. Left common carotid artery angiogram in the frontal projection, showing a duplicated middle cerebral artery (*arrows*) on the left side. Note that both arise from the supraclinoid internal carotid artery.

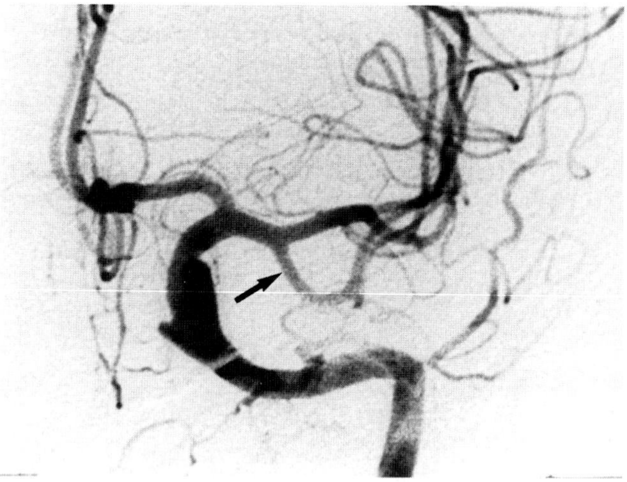

Figure 2Q-31: Anterior temporal artery branch originating from the M1 segment of the middle cerebral artery. Left internal carotid angiogram in the frontal projection shows an anterior temporal artery branch (*arrow*) originating from the proximal M1 segment of the middle cerebral artery on the left side.

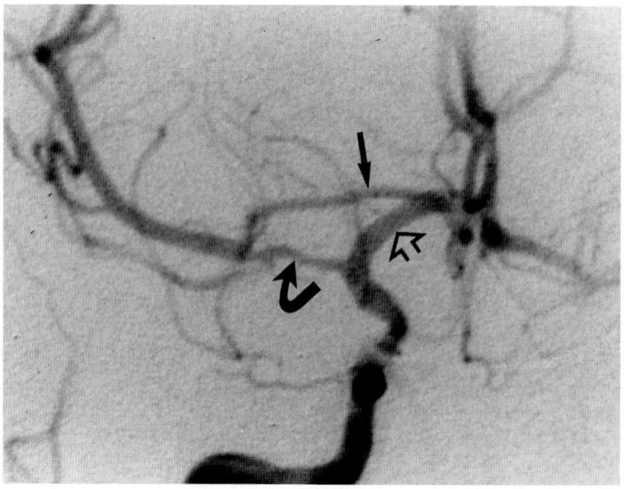

Figure 2Q-32: Accessory middle cerebral artery. Right internal carotid angiogram in the frontal projection, showing an accessory middle cerebral artery (*solid straight arrow*) originating from the A1 segment (*open arrow*) of the anterior cerebral artery on the right side. Note the atretic M1 segment (*curved arrow*) of the middle cerebral artery.

ANTERIOR COMMUNICATING ARTERY VARIANTS

- Atresia of the anterior communicating artery
- Duplication or triplication of the anterior communicating artery
- Fenestrated anterior communicating artery
- Accessory or duplicated anterior cerebral artery arising from the anterior communicating artery
- Other vessel originating from anterior communicating artery (e.g., artery of Heubner)

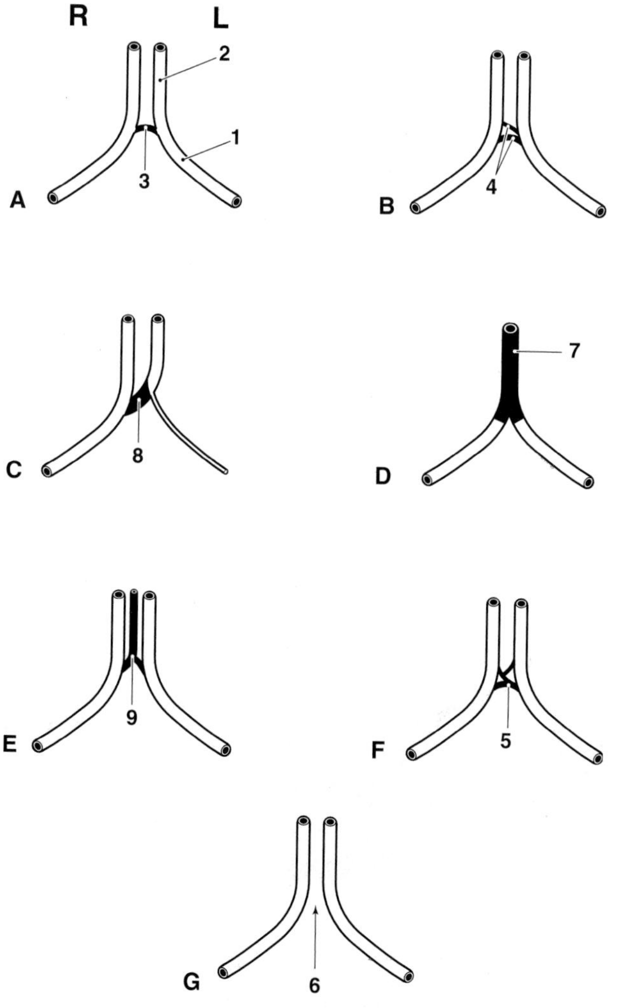

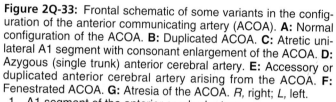

Figure 2Q-33: Frontal schematic of some variants in the configuration of the anterior communicating artery (ACOA). **A:** Normal configuration of the ACOA. **B:** Duplicated ACOA. **C:** Atretic unilateral A1 segment with consonant enlargement of the ACOA. **D:** Azygous (single trunk) anterior cerebral artery. **E:** Accessory or duplicated anterior cerebral artery arising from the ACOA. **F:** Fenestrated ACOA. **G:** Atresia of the ACOA. *R,* right; *L,* left.

1 A1 segment of the anterior cerebral artery
2 A2 segment of the anterior cerebral artery
3 ACOA (normal appearance)
4 Duplicated ACOA
5 Triplicated ACOA
6 Atretic/hypoplastic/aplastic ACOA
7 Azygous (single) anterior cerebral artery with aplastic ACOA
8 Hyperplastic ACOA associated with atretic unilateral A1 segment anterior cerebral artery
9 Accessory or duplicated anterior cerebral artery originating from ACOA
10 Duplicated (triple) anterior cerebral artery(ies)

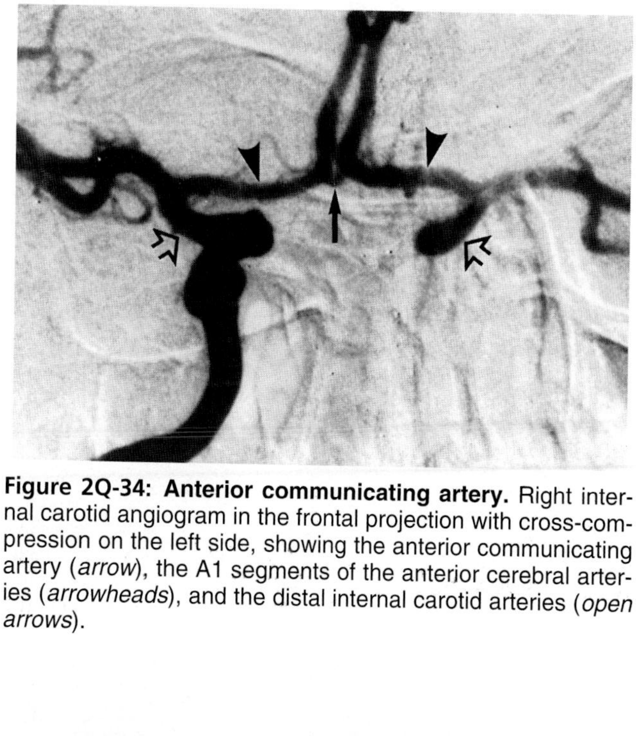

Figure 2Q-34: Anterior communicating artery. Right internal carotid angiogram in the frontal projection with cross-compression on the left side, showing the anterior communicating artery (*arrow*), the A1 segments of the anterior cerebral arteries (*arrowheads*), and the distal internal carotid arteries (*open arrows*).

POSTERIOR COMMUNICATING ARTERY VARIANTS

- Atresia of the posterior communicating artery
- Differing length and course of the posterior communicating artery
- Fetal configuration of the posterior cerebral communicating artery originating directly from the ICA
- Vessel originating from the posterior communicating artery (e.g., anterior choroidal artery)

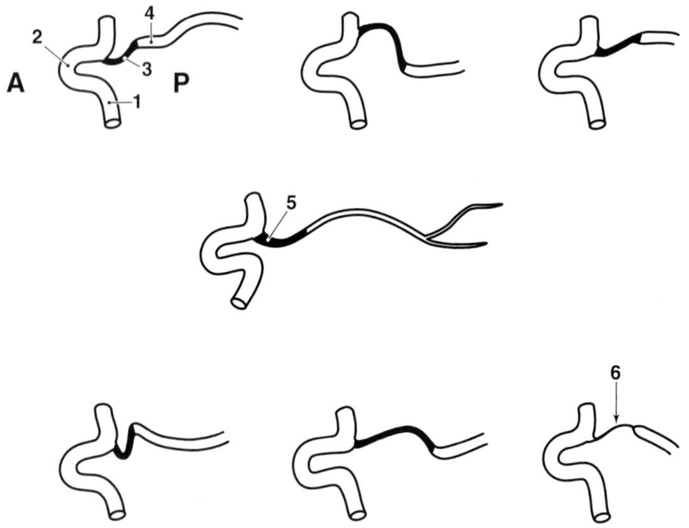

Figure 2Q-35: Lateral schematic of some variants in the configuration of the posterior communicating artery. *A*, anterior; *P*, posterior.
1 Internal carotid artery
2 Carotid siphon
3 Posterior communicating artery
4 Posterior cerebral artery
5 Fetal origin of posterior cerebral artery directly from internal carotid artery
6 Atresia of posterior communicating artery

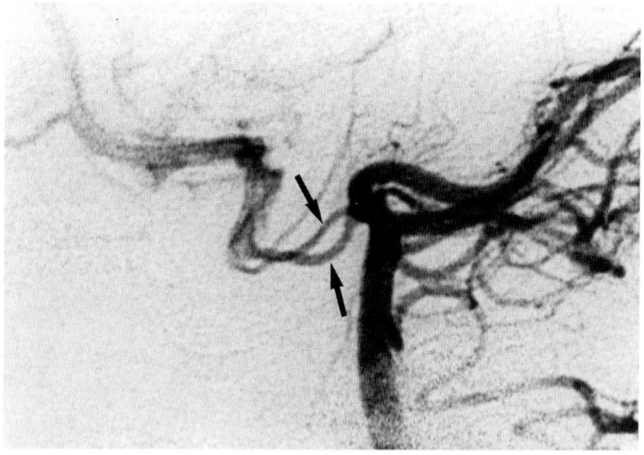

Figure 2Q-36: Posterior communicating arteries. Arterial phase of a vertebral angiogram in the lateral projection, showing the posterior communicating arteries bilaterally (*arrows*).

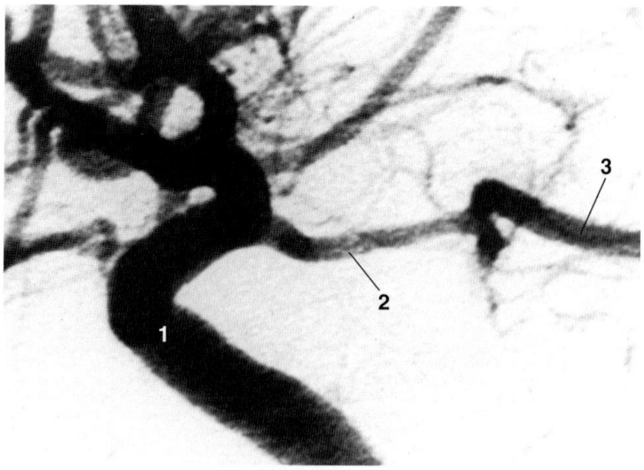

Figure 2Q-37: Posterior communicating artery. Right internal carotid artery angiogram in the lateral projection, showing the posterior communicating artery.
1 Internal carotid artery
2 Posterior communicating artery
3 P2 (post communal) segment, posterior cerebral artery

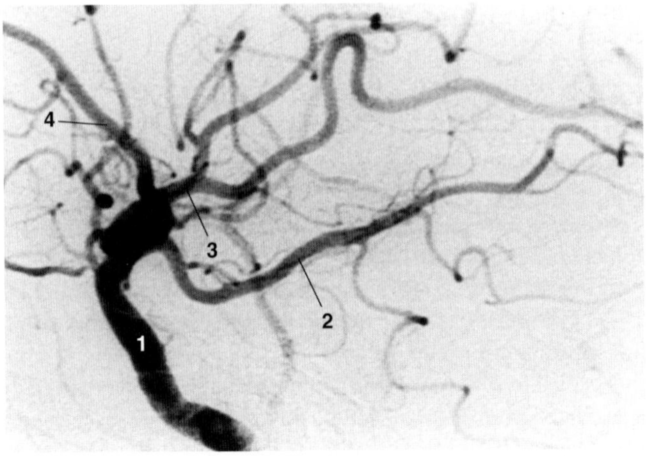

Figure 2Q-38: Fetal configuration of the posterior communicating artery. Internal carotid angiogram in the lateral projection, showing a fetal configuration of the origin of the posterior cerebral artery directly from the internal carotid artery.

1 Internal carotid artery
2 Fetal configuration of the origin of the posterior cerebral artery directly from the internal carotid artery
3 Middle cerebral artery
4 Anterior cerebral artery

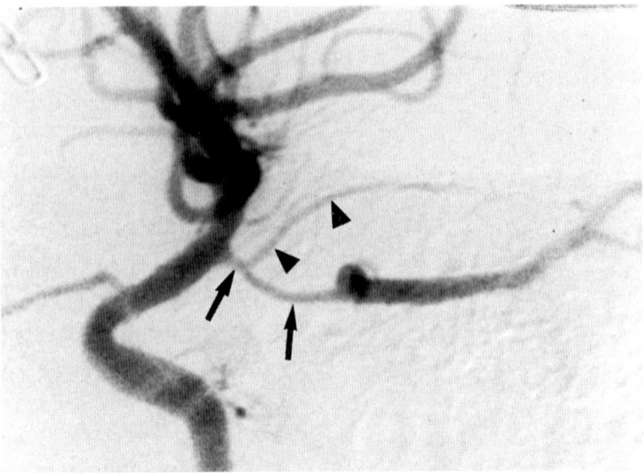

Figure 2Q-39: Anterior choroidal artery originating from the posterior communicating artery. Internal carotid angiogram in the lateral projection, showing the anterior choroidal artery (*arrowheads*) originating from the posterior communicating artery (*arrows*).

2R Vertebrobasilar Arterial System

THE VERTEBROBASILAR ARTERIAL VASCULAR SYSTEM

The Cervical Vertebral Artery

1. There are four segments of the cervical vertebral artery.
   a. The first segment originates from the subclavian artery on either side. Although it is somewhat variable, in the majority of cases, the vertebral artery enters the foramen transversarium at the C-6 vertebral level. When the left vertebral artery originates directly from the aortic arch proximal to the left subclavian artery, it commonly ascends to the C-4 level before first entering the foramina transversaria.
   b. The second segment ascends from the C-6 level, traveling within the cervical foramina transversaria of each vertebra from C-6 to C-1.
   c. The third segment extends from the C-1 foramen transversarium posteriorly and horizontally over the superior surface of the posterior bony arch of C-1; the posterior bony arch of C-1 may have a groove on its superior surface for the vertebral artery or, alternatively, a complete bony ring (the arcuate foramen).
   d. The fourth segment extends through the atlantooccipital membrane and dura mater to ascend within the subarachnoid space into the intracranial cavity through the foramen magnum.
2. The branches of the cervical vertebral artery include:
   a. The segmental radiculomedullary arteries supply the cervical spinal nerves at each level, on each side; they are numbered for the exiting spinal nerve root that they accompany.
   b. The radiculomedullary artery(ies) with medullary components supplies the artery of the cervical spinal cord enlargement (cervical anterior spinal artery of the cervical spinal cord). This radiculomedullary artery(ies) may arise at any level from the vertebral artery. Furthermore, this arterial supply is not infrequently seen to be bilateral.
   c. The paired posterior cervical spinal cord arteries may also receive radiculomedullary arteries either directly or via the anastomoses of the arterial vasocorona of the spinal cord.
   d. A major medullary branch often originates from one or both distal (cranial) vertebral arteries at or near their junction with the basilar artery, to directly supply the cervical anterior spinal artery.
   e. Muscular arterial branches to the paraspinal muscles
   f. The posterior meningeal artery proper (common) and an accessory middle meningeal arterial branch (uncommon)
   g. The posterior–inferior cerebellar artery (PICA), which is a branch of the most distal vertebral artery originating after it pierces the dura mater.

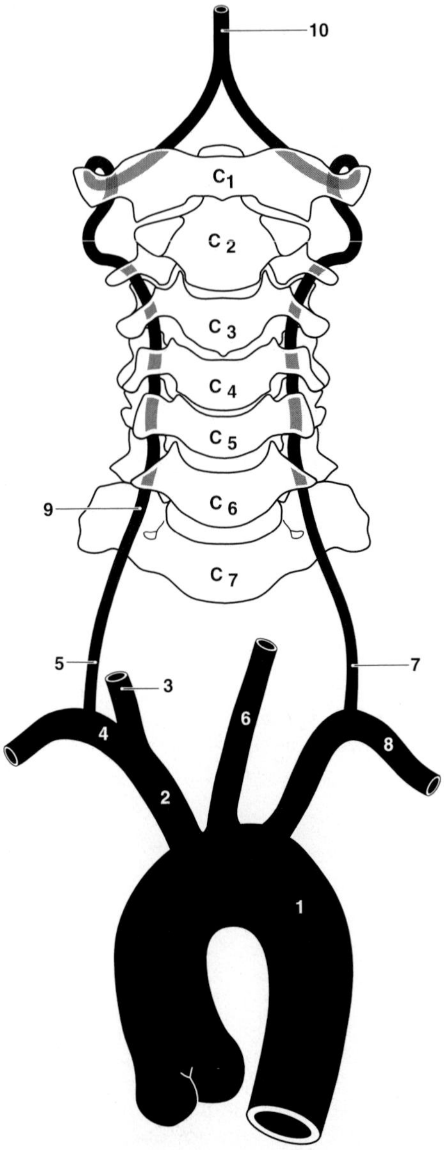

Figure 2R-1A: Frontal schematic of the cervical vertebral arteries, showing varying origins and courses. The typical arterial course is when both vertebral arteries originate from their respective subclavian arteries. *C1–7,* numbered cervical vertebrae.

1 Aortic arch
2 Brachiocephalic trunk (innominate artery)
3 Right common carotid artery
4 Right subclavian artery
5 Right vertebral artery originating from subclavian artery
6 Left common carotid artery
7 Left vertebral artery originating from subclavian artery
8 Left subclavian artery
9 Typical entry of vertebral artery into cervical foramina transversaria at the C-6 level
10 Basilar artery

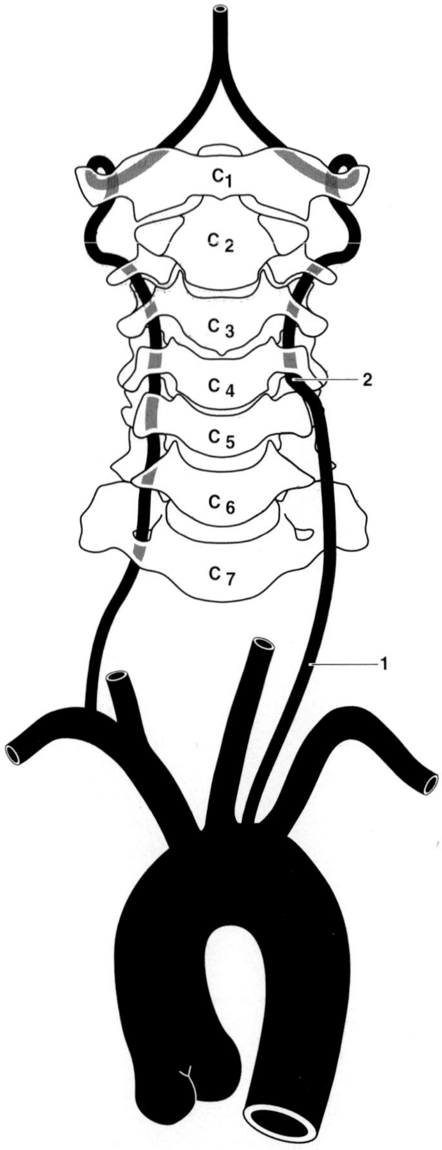

Figure 2R-1B: Schematic arterial course when the left vertebral artery originates from the aortic arch. *C1–7,* numbered cervical vertebrae.

1 Left vertebral artery originating from aortic arch
2 Entry of vertebral artery into the foramina transversaria at the C-4 level, when left vertebral artery originates directly from the aortic arch

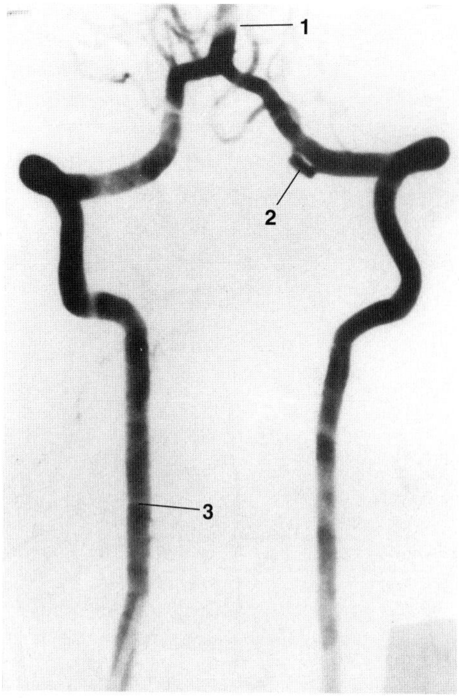

Figure 2R-2: Cervical vertebrobasilar arterial system. Vertebral angiogram in the frontal projection, showing the cervical vertebrobasilar system.
1 Basilar artery
2 Posterior–inferior cerebellar artery (PICA)
3 Right vertebral artery

THE CRANIAL VERTEBROBASILAR ARTERIAL SYSTEM

The Cranial Vertebral Artery

1. After piercing the dura mater at the level of C-1, the vertebral artery enters the cranium via the foramen magnum.
2. At the level of the lower pons, the vertebral artery on one side joins its counterpart on the opposite side to form the basilar artery.
3. Before joining the basilar artery, the vertebral artery typically gives off the PICA and an arterial branch to the anterior spinal artery of the cervical spinal cord.
4. The PICA
   a. The PICA is the largest branch of the vertebral artery. It originates from the vertebral artery at a distance of 15 to 65 mm below the origin of the basilar artery. Approximately 80% of the time, the PICA originates above the foramen magnum; 20% of the time it arises below the foramen magnum, as far caudally as C-2.
   b. The segments and branches of the PICA include the following.
      i. Anterior medullary segment. After its origin from the vertebral artery, the PICA courses posteriorly within the medullary cistern and winds around the lower end of the olive of the medulla oblongata.
      ii. Lateral medullary segment. The PICA continues posteriorly in the cerebellomedullary fissure around the lateral aspect of the medulla as the lateral medullary segment. This segment corresponds to the caudal loop of the PICA. The caudal loop often curves around the anterior margin of the lower pole of the cerebellar tonsil.
      iii. Posterior medullary segment. On reaching the posterior margin of the medulla oblongata, the PICA ascends behind the roots of the glossopharyngeal and vagus nerves (CN-IX and CN-X) to the anterior aspect of the superior pole of the tonsil, behind the posterior medullary velum.
      iv. Supratonsillar segment. The PICA continuation over the posterior aspect of the superior pole of the tonsil is called the supratonsillar segment. After giving off medullary arterial branches, the PICA extends onto the inferior surface of the cerebellum to supply the inferior portion of the cerebellar vermis, the tonsil, the inferolateral surface of the cerebellar hemisphere, and the choroid plexus of the fourth ventricle.
      v. Perforating branches. Small arterial branches from the anterior, lateral, and posterior medullary segments and the supratonsillar segment of the PICA supply the dorsolateral region of the medulla from the level of the inferior olive to the medullopontine angle. When the PICA is absent, these branches originate directly from the vertebral artery.

The Basilar Artery

1. The basilar artery is formed by the union of the terminal ends of the two vertebral arteries.
2. The basilar artery runs cranially through the pontine cistern and into the interpeduncular cistern; it follows a serpentine course in the majority of cases.
3. Major branches of the basilar artery include:
   a. Pontine perforating arteries
   b. The anterior–inferior cerebellar artery (AICA)
   c. The SCA
   d. The PCA
   e. The artery of the internal auditory meatus may occasionally originate directly from the basilar artery (see next section).

4. The AICA
   a. The AICA, the smallest of the three cerebellar arteries, arises from the first or middle third of the basilar artery and courses laterally and inferiorly over the belly of the pons. During its proximal course, the AICA sends off numerous penetrating branches that supply the lower two-thirds of the pons and the upper part of the medulla oblongata.
   b. Bulbar branches of the AICA supply most of the pontine tegmentum in the lower pons. The cerebellar portion swings around the lateral margin of the pons toward the cerebellopontine angle. Near the facial (CN-VII) and vestibulocochlear (CN-VIII) nerves, it turns laterally above the flocculus and spreads over the inferior surface of the cerebellar hemisphere. Superficial branches supply the flocculus, the inferior surface of the cerebellar hemisphere, and portions of the vermis; deep penetrating branches supply the ipsilateral dentate nucleus of the cerebellar hemisphere.
   c. Subsequently, the AICA divides into rostrolateral and caudomedial trunks within the cerebellopontine angle cistern. The lateral branch courses laterally and curls around the flocculus. It then runs within the horizontal fissure between the superior and inferior semilunar lobules of the cerebellum, at the same time sending arterial branches to these structures. The distal hemispheric branches form a rich anastomotic network with distal branches of the SCA and PICA. The medial branch of the AICA courses downward toward the medial anterior border of the cerebellum, supplying primarily the biventral lobule. This branch also supplies the middle cerebellar peduncle, the lower lateral aspect of the pons, and the cisternal portion of the fourth ventricular choroid plexus.
   d. The artery of the internal auditory meatus most commonly originates from the proximal portion of the AICA; less frequently, it arises directly from the basilar artery distal to the origin of the AICA. This artery supplies the nerve roots within the internal auditory canal and the sensory structures of the inner ear.
5. The superior cerebellar artery (SCA)
   a. The SCA on each side originates from the basilar artery a few millimeters proximal to the origin of the posterior cerebral arteries (PCAs). The SCAs course posteriorly to encircle the upper pons and lower mesencephalon (midbrain).
   b. The cisternal segments of the SCA are designated the anterior pontine and the ambient segments.
      i. The anterior pontine segment courses laterally over the anterior aspect of the upper pons. Anterolaterally, it lies inferior to the oculomotor nerve, which separates it from the superiorly positioned PCA.
      ii. The ambient segment begins at the lateral border of the pons running posteriorly over the brachium pontis. It then courses posteriorly in the infratentorial portion of the ambient cistern.
   c. Cortical branches of the SCA are designated the lateral marginal, hemispheric, and vermian branches:
      i. Within the horizontal fissure, the lateral marginal branch is an anatomical landmark that separates the superior and inferior cerebellar lobes. This lateral branch supplies the tissue bordering on the horizontal fissure, the superolateral aspects of the cerebellar hemispheres, the superior cerebellar peduncle, the superior aspect of the dentate nucleus, and parts of the middle and superior cerebellar peduncles.
      ii. The medial SCA and vermian branches supply the superior surface of the cerebellar hemisphere and the superior vermis, respectively.

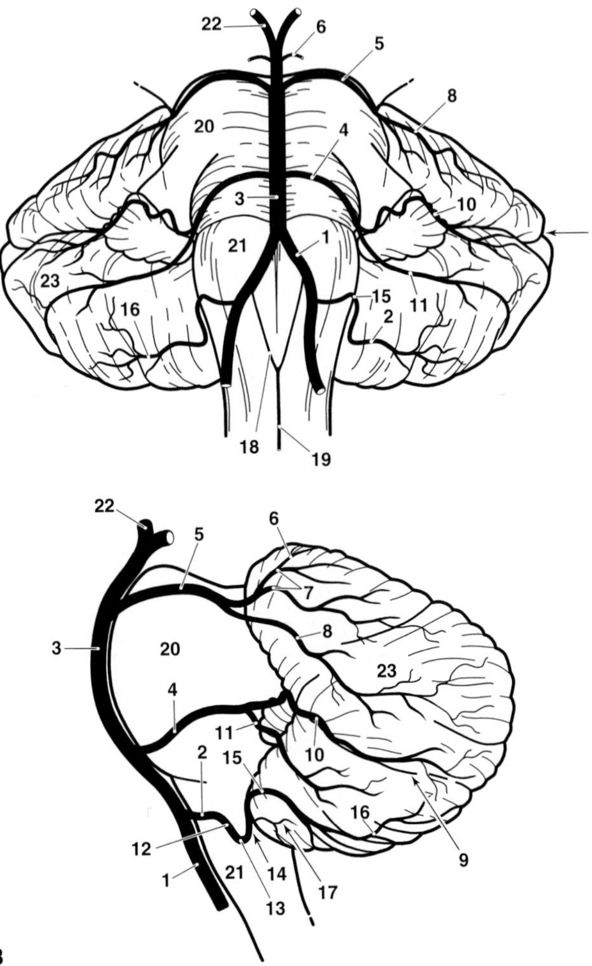

A

B

Figure 2R-3: Frontal **(A)** and lateral **(B)** schematics of the intracranial vertebrobasilar arterial system.

1 Vertebral artery
2 Posterior–inferior cerebellar artery (PICA)
3 Basilar artery
4 Anterior–inferior cerebellar artery (AICA)
5 Superior cerebellar artery (SCA)
6 Superior vermian branch of SCA
7 Hemispheric branch of SCA
8 Lateral marginal branch of SCA
9 Horizontal fissure
10 Rostrolateral branch of AICA
11 Caudomedial branch of AICA
12 Anterior medullary segment of PICA
13 Lateral medullary segment of PICA (caudal loop)
14 Posterior medullary segment of PICA
15 Supratonsillar segment of PICA
16 Hemispheric and vermian branches of PICA
17 Tonsillar branches of PICA
18 Vertebral artery branch to cervical anterior spinal artery
19 Upper cervical anterior spinal (cord) artery
20 Pons
21 Medulla oblongata
22 Posterior cerebral artery
23 Cerebellar hemisphere

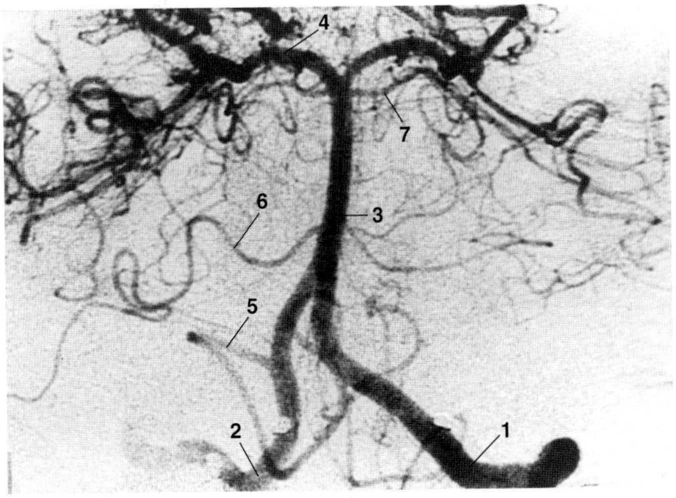

Figure 2R-4A: The vertebrobasilar arterial system. Left vertebral angiogram in the transfacial projection, showing normal anatomic branching.

1 Left vertebral artery
2 Right vertebral artery
3 Basilar artery
4 Posterior cerebral artery
5 Posterior–inferior cerebellar artery (PICA)
6 Anterior–inferior cerebellar artery (AICA)
7 Superior cerebellar artery (SCA)

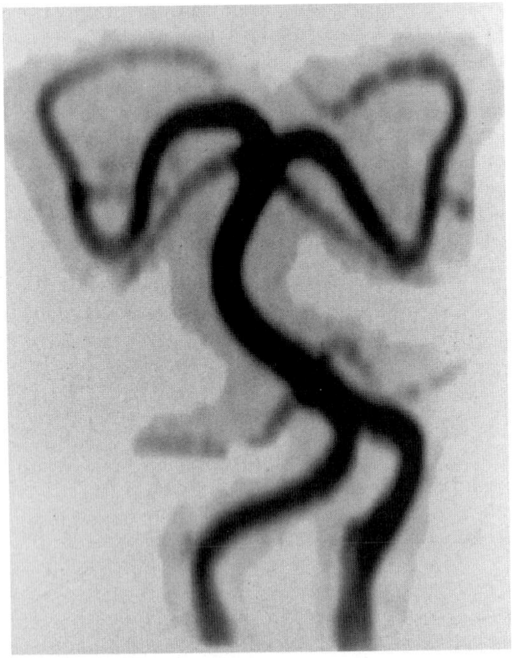

Figure 2R-4B: The vertebrobasilar arterial system. Normal magnetic resonance angiogram of the vertebrobasilar arterial system (2D time-of-flight) in the frontal projection.

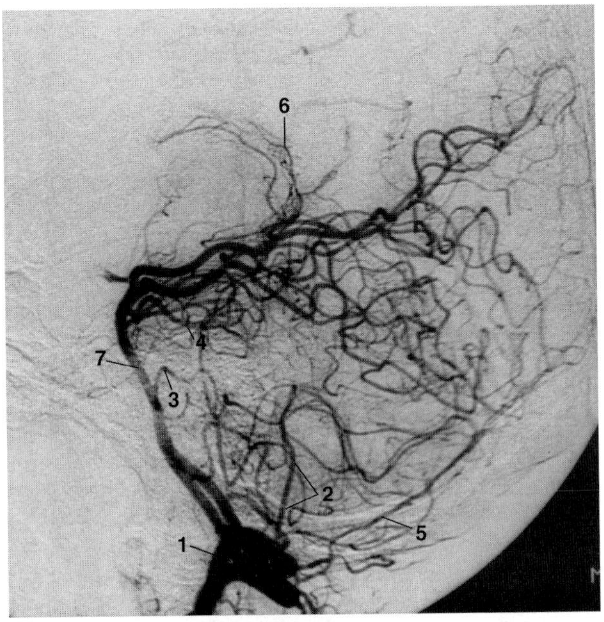

Figure 2R-4C: The vertebrobasilar arterial system. Right vertebral angiogram in the lateral projection, showing the normal anatomy of the vertebrobasilar system.

1 Vertebral artery(ies)
2 Posterior–inferior cerebellar artery
3 Anterior–inferior cerebellar artery
4 Superior cerebellar artery
5 Posterior meningeal artery arising from vertebral artery
6 Posterior choroidal arteries
7 Basilar artery

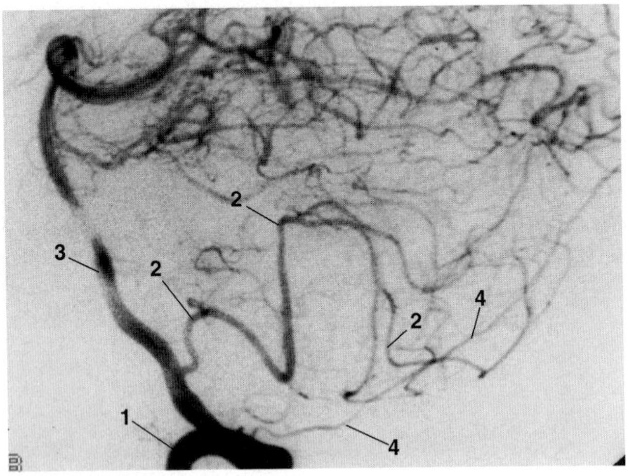

Figure 2R-4D: The vertebrobasilar arterial system. Vertebral angiogram in the lateral projection, showing the posterior–inferior cerebellar artery (PICA).

1 Vertebral artery
2 PICA
3 Basilar artery
4 Posterior meningeal artery arising from vertebral artery

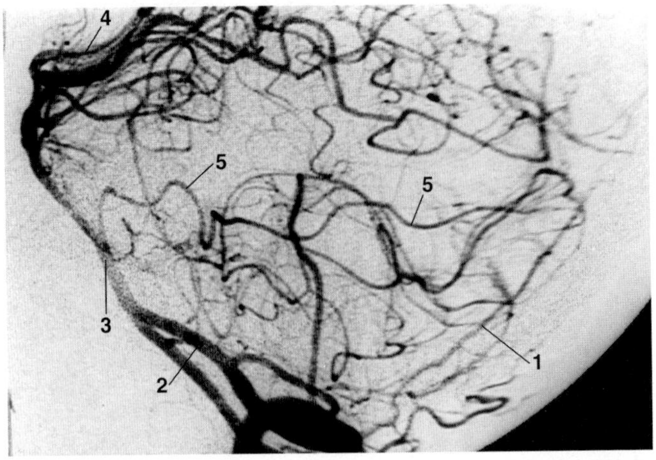

Figure 2R-4E: The vertebrobasilar arterial system. Vertebral angiogram in the lateral projection, showing the anterior–inferior cerebellar artery (AICA).

1 Posterior meningeal artery arising from vertebral artery
2 Vertebral artery
3 Basilar artery
4 Posterior cerebral artery
5 AICA

THE POSTERIOR CEREBRAL ARTERY

1. The PCAs arise from the rostral end of the basilar artery within the interpeduncular cistern. They course posteriorly in the perimesencephalic cisterns to encircle the midbrain (mesencephalon). The proximal trunk of the PCA may be divided into peduncular, ambient, and quadrigeminal segments corresponding to the subarachnoid cisterns through which the vessel passes.
2. The P1, or the peduncular segment, is the most proximal portion of the PCA arising from the basilar artery. The posterior communicating artery originates/terminates in the midportion of the peduncular segment. Numerous mesencephalic and thalamic perforating arterial branches arise directly from the proximal peduncular segment of the PCA.
   a. The mesencephalic arterial branches of these vessels supply the oculomotor and trochlear nuclei (CN-III and CN-IV) and the paramedian mesencephalic reticular formation.
   b. The thalamic branches or thalamoperforating arteries may be divided into anterior and posterior groups. The anterior branches arise from the posterior communicating artery to supply the posterior chiasm, optic tract, and posterior hypothalamus. Some posterior thalamoperforating arteries arise from the proximal peduncular segment of the PCA and supply the thalamus and geniculate bodies.
3. The P2, or the ambient segment of the PCA, gives rise to the following.
   a. Perforating branches arise from the ambient segment of the PCA, the so-called thalamogeniculate perforating arterial branches. These small vessels supply portions of the thalamus as well as the lateral geniculate bodies.
   b. The medial and lateral posterior choroidal arteries
      i. The medial posterior choroidal artery arises from the proximal segment of the PCA. It then enters the quadrigeminal cistern, where it contributes to the blood supply of the quadrigeminal plate. Multiple small branches from the medial posterior choroidal artery subsequently supply the choroid plexus of the third ventricle.
      ii. The lateral posterior choroidal artery originates from the ambient segment of the PCA. Branches of the lateral posterior choroidal artery supply the choroid plexus of the temporal horn, the trigone, and the body of the lateral ventricle.
   c. Other arterial branches of the ambient segment of the PCA include unnamed hippocampal and meningeal branches and the posterior pericallosal (perisplenial) artery.
4. After traversing the quadrigeminal cistern, the P3 or the quadrigeminal segment of the PCA terminates in cortical branches. The cortical branches of the PCA include the hippocampal, anterior temporal, middle temporal, posterior temporal, parietooccipital, and calcarine arteries.
   a. The hippocampal artery is the most proximal temporal lobe branch to arise from the PCA. It supplies the uncus, hippocampal gyrus, and dentate gyrus.
   b. The anterior temporal artery supplies the inferior and anterior surfaces of the temporal lobe.
   c. The middle temporal artery, when present, serves the temporal lobe between the vascular distribution of the anterior and posterior temporal arteries.
   d. The posterior temporal artery supplies the posterior undersurface of the temporal and occipital lobes. It may also contribute collateral vessels to the calcarine fissure.
   e. The parietooccipital artery supplies the uncus and portions of the precuneus and lateral occipital gyrus. It may also give off an accessory calcarine artery.
   f. The calcarine artery supplies the visual cortex within the calcarine fissure. It may originate from the main PCA trunk, the posterior temporal artery, or the parietooccipital artery.
   g. The posterior pericallosal (perisplenial) artery supplies the posterior corpus callosum and is an important route of collateral supply to the anterior pericallosal arte-

rial system. The posterior pericallosal artery most commonly arises from the parietooccipital artery. It may also originate from the main trunk of the PCA, from a common trunk with the medial posterior choroidal artery, or from the temporal or calcarine branches of the PCA.

TABLE 2R-1: Posterior Cerebral Artery Segments

P1: Peduncular or precommunicating segment branches
Thalamoperforating arteries
Peduncular perforating branches
P2: Ambient segment branches
Thalamogeniculate arteries
Medial posterior choroidal artery(ies)
Lateral posterior choroidal artery(ies)
Hippocampal artery
Unnamed meningeal branches
P3: Distal segment (quadrigeminal) branches
Parietooccipital artery
Calcarine artery
Posterior pericallosal (perisplenial) artery
Anterior temporal artery
Posterior temporal artery

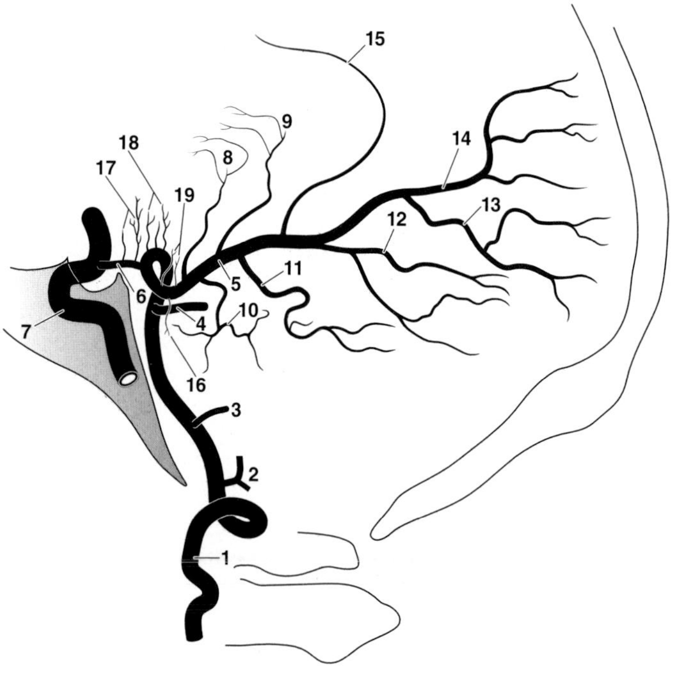

Figure 2R-5: Lateral schematic of the posterior cerebral artery and regional branches.
1 Vertebral artery
2 Posterior–inferior cerebellar artery (PICA)
3 Anterior–inferior cerebellar artery (AICA)
4 Superior cerebellar artery
5 Posterior cerebral artery
6 Posterior communicating artery
7 Internal carotid artery
8 Medial posterior choroidal artery
9 Lateral posterior choroidal artery
10 Anterior temporal artery
11 Middle temporal artery
12 Posterior temporal artery
13 Calcarine artery
14 Parietooccipital artery
15 Posterior pericallosal (perisplenial) artery
16 Hippocampal artery
17 Anterior thalamoperforating arteries
18 Posterior thalamoperforating arteries
19 Thalamogeniculate arteries

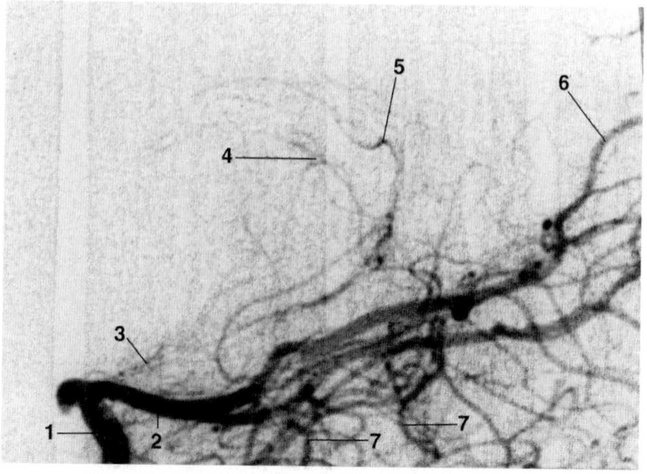

Figure 2R-6: Left vertebral angiogram in the lateral projection, showing some of the major branches of the posterior cerebral artery.
1 Basilar artery
2 Posterior cerebral artery
3 Thalamoperforating arteries
4 Medial posterior choroidal artery(ies)
5 Lateral posterior choroidal artery(ies)
6 Parietooccipital artery
7 Temporal arteries

THE CHOROIDAL POINT

1. The posterior medullary segment of the PICA continues in a posterior course over the superior pole of the cerebellar tonsil as the supratonsillar segment.
2. At the junction of the posterior medullary and supratonsillar segments of the PICA, small branches are sent out to the anterior aspect of the cerebellar tonsil and the choroid plexus of the fourth ventricle. This junction of the PICA is designated the *choroidal point*.
3. The choroidal point is normally located 1 to 2 mm behind a perpendicular line drawn through the junction of the anterior and middle thirds of a line connecting the anterior margin of the foramen magnum (i.e., basion) and the torcular Herophili.
4. The choroidal point is an important landmark in the angiographic diagnosis of masses in the posterior fossa.

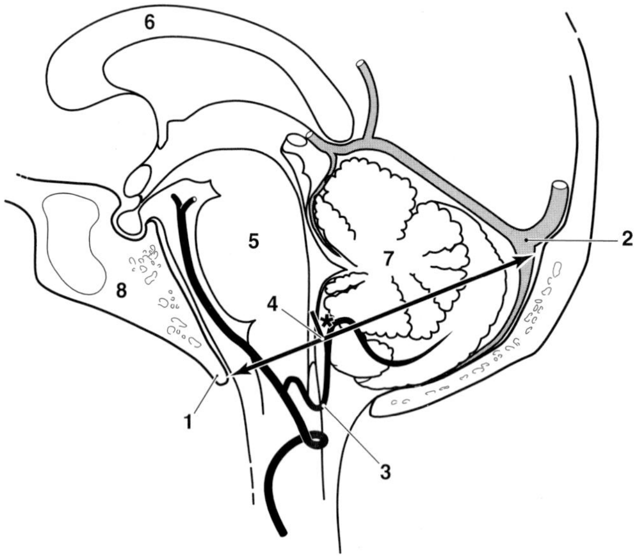

Figure 2R-7: Schematic showing the determination of the choroidal point (*asterisk*).
1 Basion
2 Torcular Herophili
3 Posterior–inferior cerebellar artery (PICA)
4 Junction of anterior and middle thirds of line connecting 1 and 2
5 Pons
6 Corpus callosum
7 Cerebellum
8 Clivus

VERTEBRAL ARTERY VARIANTS

1. The left vertebral artery is larger in caliber than the right in 42% of cases, the right and left vertebral arteries are approximately of the same caliber in 26% of cases, and the right side is larger than the left in 32% of cases.
2. One vertebral artery, usually the right, may be hypoplastic.
3. The vertebral artery may terminate in the PICA.
4. Both vertebral arteries may be mildly or moderately hypoplastic when there is a reduced flow demand, such as that seen in bilateral fetal-type PCAs or in cases of fetal carotid–basilar arterial anastomoses (e.g., persistent trigeminal artery).

POSTERIOR–INFERIOR CEREBELLAR ARTERY VARIANTS

1. The PICA may be unilaterally absent (10%–20%) or bilaterally absent (2%). In these instances, the AICA usually supplies the PICA territory. The right and left PICAs are often asymmetric in size.
2. The PICA can be hypoplastic in 5% of cases. Rarely, two (duplicated) PICAs can arise from one vertebral artery. Anastomoses between the PICA and AICA are common.
3. The PICA has the most variable origin of any of the arteries of the posterior fossa. It may originate from a persistent hypoglossal artery, a persistent proatlantal artery, a posterior meningeal artery, the basilar artery, or the extracranial segment of the vertebral artery. Anomalous origin of the PICA from the internal carotid artery has been reported.
4. The PICA may supply the area normally supplied by the AICA when the latter is hypoplastic or absent.

ANTERIOR–INFERIOR CEREBELLAR ARTERY VARIANTS

1. The size of the AICA is usually inversely related to the size of the PICA. When the PICA is hypoplastic or absent, the ipsilateral AICA is usually larger and supplies the area of the missing or hypoplastic PICA.
2. The left and right AICAs may be asymmetric in size.

SUPERIOR CEREBELLAR ARTERY VARIANTS

1. Duplication of one SCA is seen in 28% of cases. Both SCAs are duplicated in 8%, and triplication of one SCA is seen in 2% of cases.
2. The horizontal fissure of the cerebellum may be supplied by the AICA. In these instances, SCA size is usually smaller than that of the ipsilateral AICA.
3. In 4% of cases, the SCA arises from the proximal PCA.

VERTEBROBASILAR ARTERIAL SYSTEM VARIANTS

- Variations in size between the two vertebral arteries
- Vertebral artery hypoplasia
- Termination of the vertebral artery in the PICA
- PICA hypoplasia
- PICA aplasia
- Duplication of the PICA
- Variable origin of the PICA (e.g., from the extracranial segment of the vertebral artery, the proximal basilar artery)
- PICA supply of the AICA region when the latter is absent
- Duplication of the AICA
- Duplication/triplication of the SCA
- AICA supply of the PICA territory when the latter is absent
- Lateral asymmetry of the PICAs, AICAs, and SCAs
- Variable origin of the SCA (e.g., from the PCA)
- Arterial fenestration: vertebral artery, basilar artery, PCA

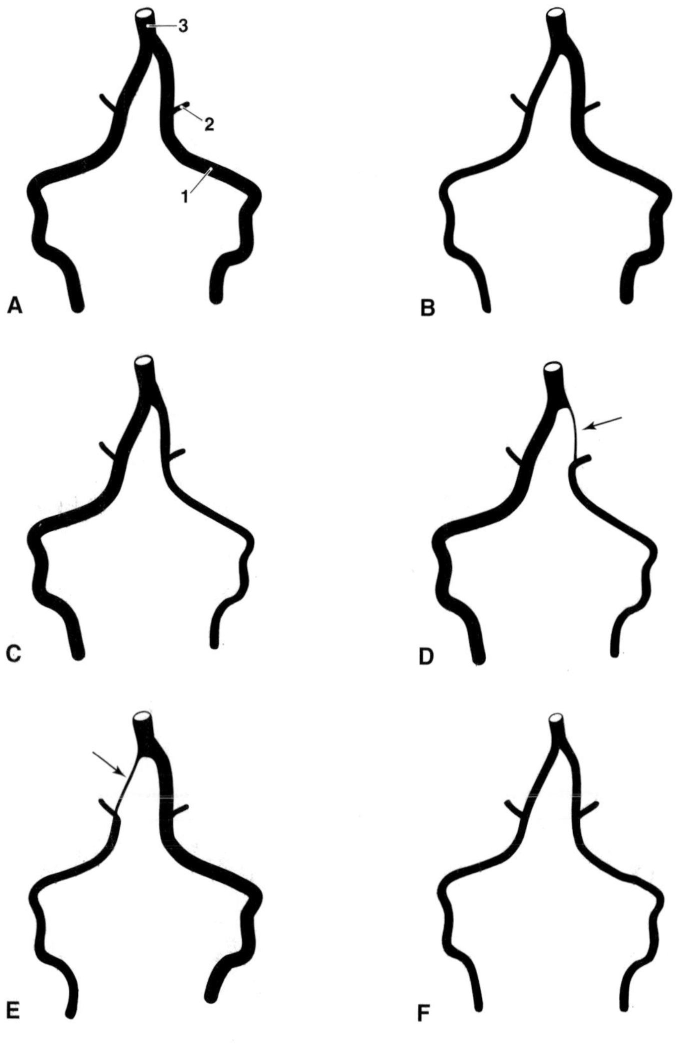

Figure 2R-8: Frontal schematics of some of the variants of the distal vertebral arteries. **A:** Balanced/symmetric system. **B:** Hypoplastic right vertebral artery. **C:** Hypoplastic left vertebral artery. **D:** Atretic distal left vertebral artery (*arrow*) terminating in the left posterior–inferior cerebellar artery (PICA). **E:** Atretic distal right vertebral artery (*arrow*) terminating in the right PICA. **F:** Bilateral hypoplastic vertebral and proximal basilar arteries as seen in bilateral fetal-type posterior cerebral arteries or fetal carotid–basilar arterial anastomoses (e.g., persistent trigeminal artery).

1 Vertebral artery
2 PICA
3 Basilar artery

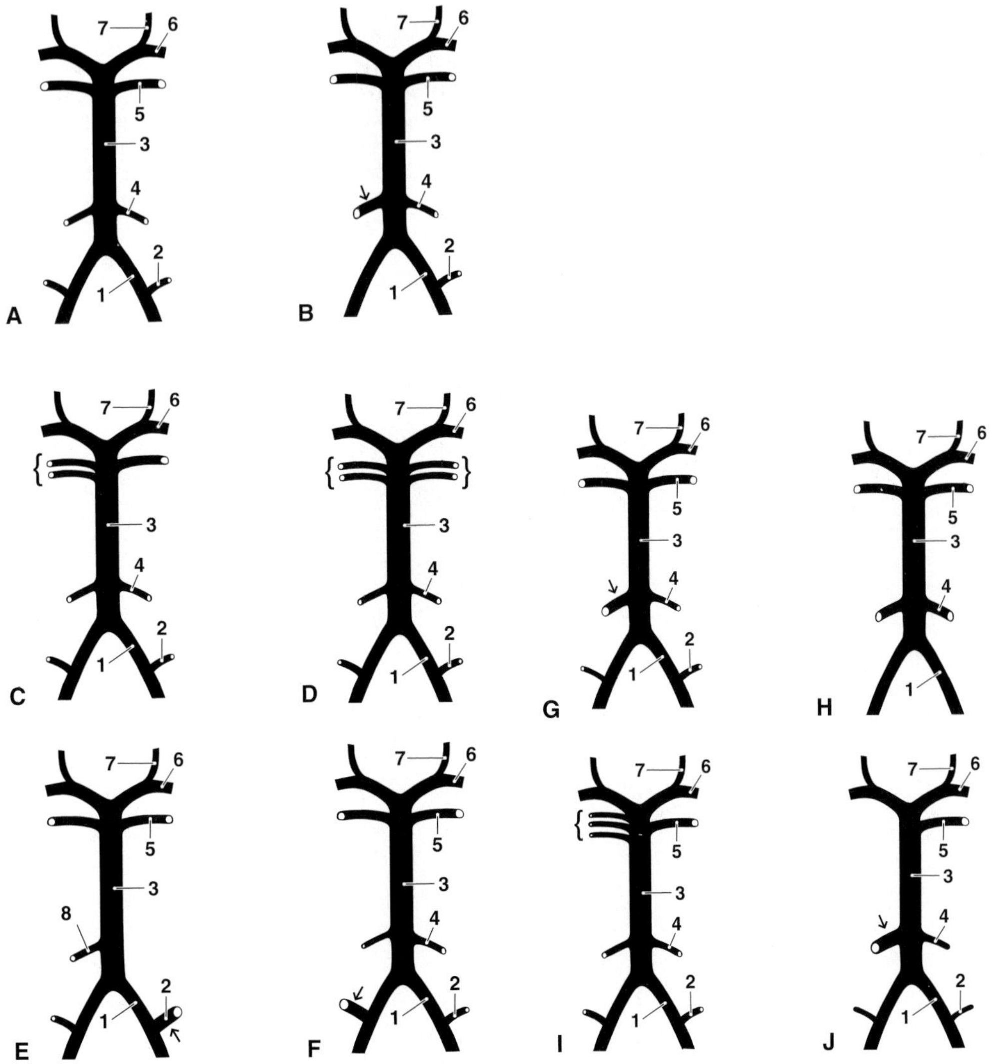

Figure 2R-9: Frontal schematic of some of the variants of the vertebrobasilar system. **A:** Balanced/symmetric configuration. **B:** Large anterior–inferior cerebellar artery (AICA) on one side (right: *arrow*) due to absent ipsilateral posterior–inferior cerebellar artery (PICA). **C:** Two superior cerebellar arteries (SCAs) (*bracket*: duplication) branching from the basilar artery on one side. **D:** Two SCAs on both sides (*brackets*: duplications) branching from the basilar artery. **E:** Large PICA on one side (left: *arrow*) due to absent ipsilateral AICA. **F:** Small AICA on one side (right) associated with large (dominant) ipsilateral PICA (right: *arrow*). **G:** Small PICA on one side (right) associated with large (dominant) ipsilateral AICA (*arrow*). **H:** Absent PICAs associated with large AICAs bilaterally. **I:** Triple SCA (*bracket*) arising from one side of basilar artery. **J:** Absent SCA on one side (right) associated with a large (dominant) ipsilateral AICA (*arrow*).

1 Left vertebral artery
2 Left PICA
3 Basilar artery
4 Left AICA
5 Left SCA
6 Left PCA
7 Left posterior communicating artery
8 Right AICA

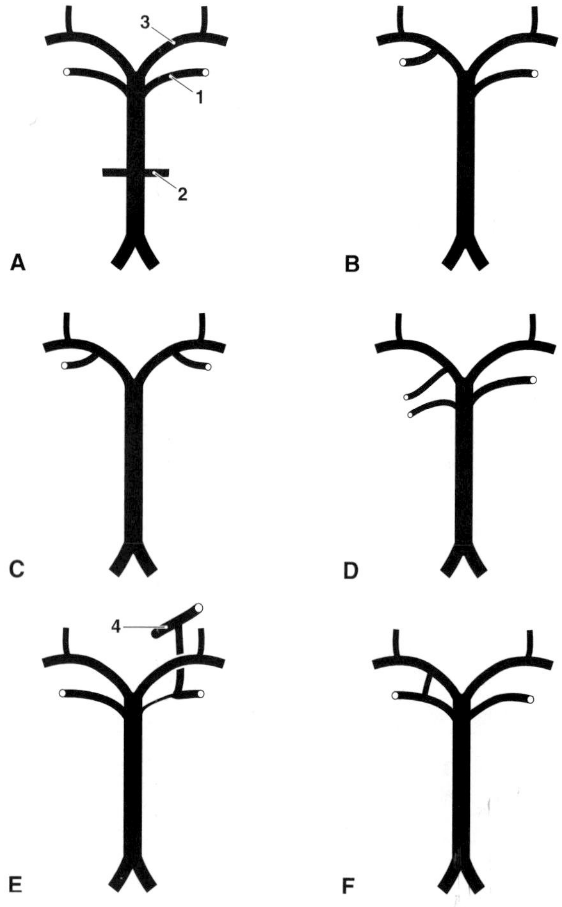

Figure 2R-10: Frontal schematic of the variants of the origin of the superior cerebellar artery (SCA). **A:** Balanced/symmetric origins of the SCAs from the distal basilar artery. **B:** Origin of SCA from P1 segment of the posterior cerebral artery (PCA). **C:** Bilateral P1 segment SCA origin from the PCAs. **D:** Duplicated SCAs with one originating from the basilar artery and the other from the P1 segment of the PCA. **E:** Origin of the SCA from the internal carotid artery (ICA) with atretic proximal SCA segment. **F:** Fenestration of the SCA and proximal PCA.

1 SCA
2 Anterior–inferior cerebellar artery (AICA)
3 PCA
4 ICA

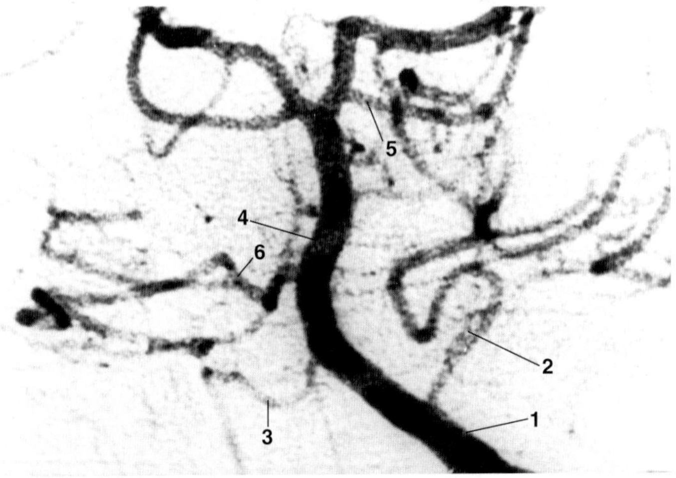

Figure 2R-11A: Vertebrobasilar system variants. Left vertebral arteriogram in the frontal projection, showing a hypoplastic right vertebral artery, hypoplasia of the left anterior–inferior cerebellar artery (AICA) with dominance of the left posterior–inferior cerebellar artery (PICA), and aplasia of the right PICA with dominance of the right AICA. Note also that the superior cerebellar arteries (SCA) on both sides originate from the proximal posterior cerebral arteries (PCAs).

1 Left vertebral artery
2 Dominant left PICA
3 Hypoplastic right vertebral artery
4 Basilar artery
5 SCA arising from the PCA
6 Dominant right AICA

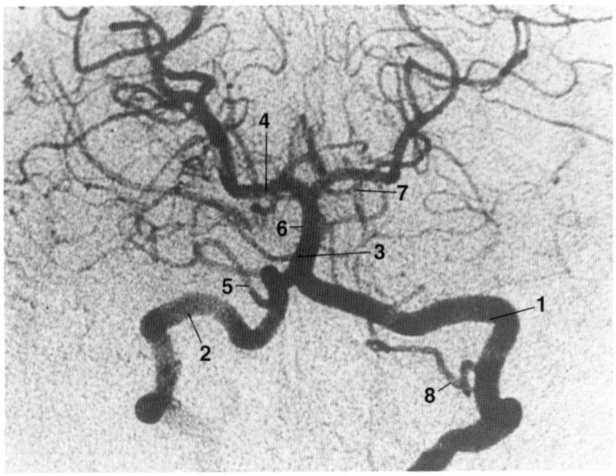

Figure 2R-11C: Left vertebral arteriogram acquired in the Towne projection, showing the left posterior–inferior cerebellar artery (PICA) arising from the left vertebral artery below the foramen magnum. Note the more typical origin of the PICA on the right.

1 Left vertebral artery
2 Right vertebral artery
3 Basilar artery
4 Posterior cerebral artery
5 Right PICA
6 Anterior–inferior cerebellar artery (AICA)
7 Superior cerebellar artery (SCA)
8 Left PICA arising from vertebral artery below foramen magnum

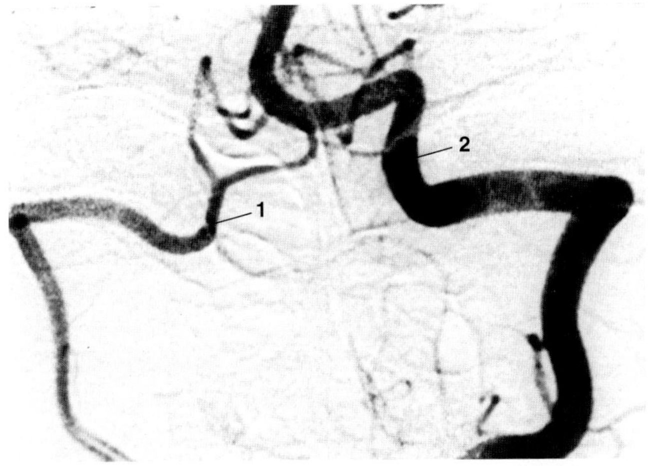

Figure 2R-11B: Vertebral artery asymmetry. Vertebral angiogram showing asymmetry of the vertebral arteries.

1 Hypoplastic right vertebral artery
2 Hypertrophic left vertebral artery

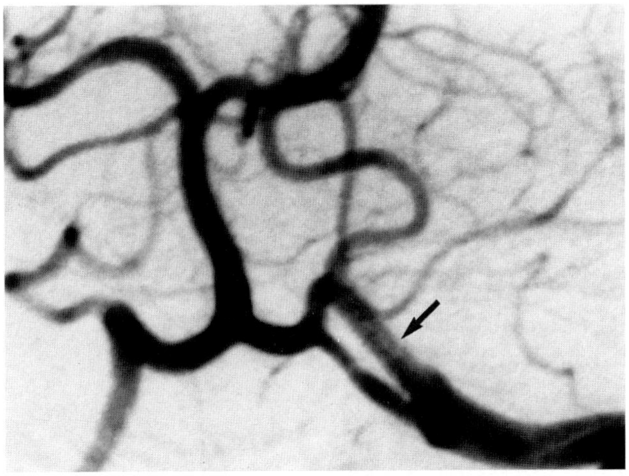

Figure 2R-11D: Fenestrated distal vertebral artery. Left vertebral angiogram in the frontal projection demonstrates fenestration of the distal left vertebral artery (*arrow*) (case courtesy of Jose Guilherme Caldas, M.D., São Paulo, Brazil).

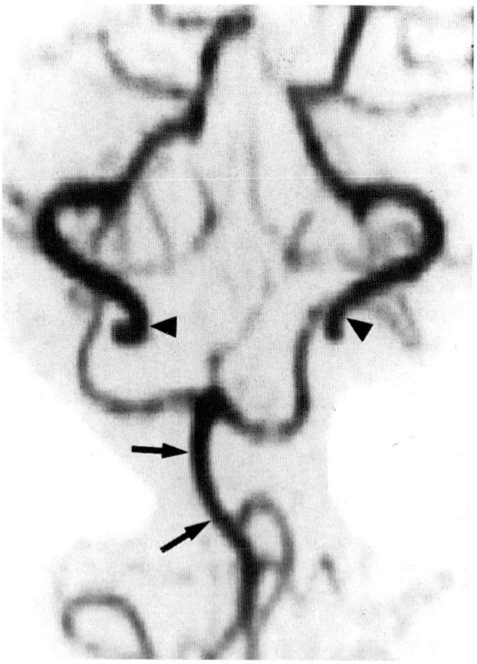

Figure 2R-11E: Hypoplastic basilar artery. MR angiogram in the frontal projection, showing hypoplasia of the basilar artery (*arrows*) stemming from reduced demand, which is the result of the bilateral fetal origin of the posterior cerebral arteries (*arrowheads*: trunks) from the internal carotid arteries (not shown because of segmentation of image).

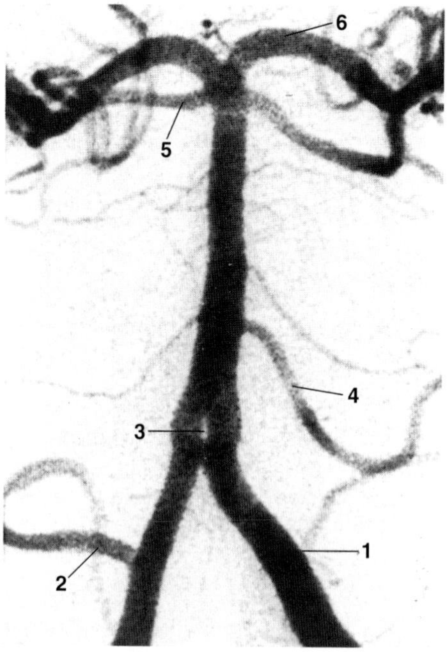

Figure 2R-11F: Fenestration of the basilar artery. Vertebral artery angiogram in the frontal projection, showing a proximal fenestration of the basilar artery.

1 Left vertebral artery
2 Right posterior–inferior cerebellar artery
3 Fenestration of the basilar artery
4 Left anterior–inferior cerebellar artery
5 Right superior cerebellar artery
6 Left posterior cerebral artery

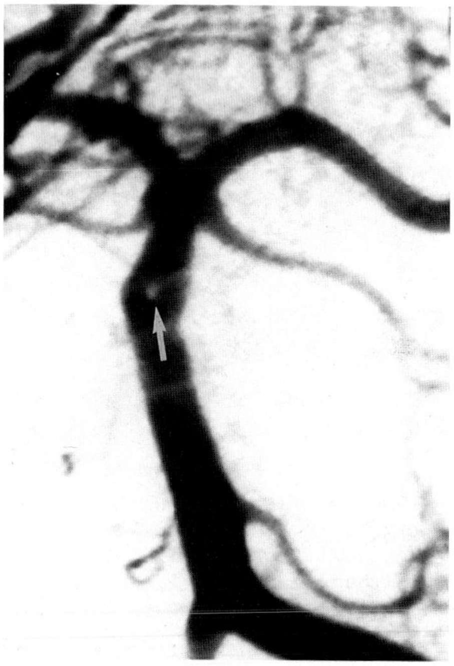

Figure 2R-11G: Fenestration of the basilar artery. Left vertebral angiogram in the frontal projection, showing distal fenestration (*arrow*) of the basilar artery.

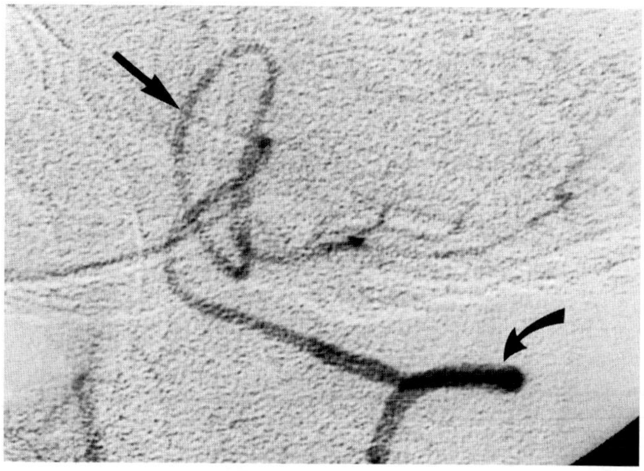

Figure 2R-11H: Termination of vertebral artery in the posterior-inferior cerebellar artery. Left vertebral angiogram in the oblique projection, showing that the distal left vertebral artery (*curved arrow*) terminates in the left posterior–inferior cerebellar artery (*straight arrow*).

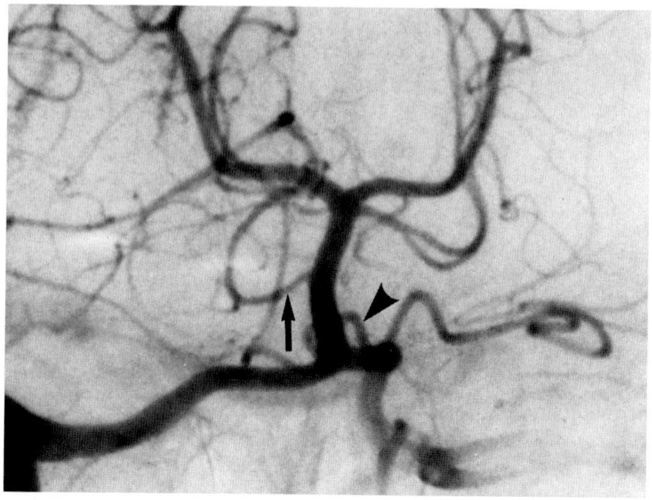

Figure 2R-11I: Right vertebral arteriogram in the frontal projection, showing absence of the anterior–inferior cerebellar artery (AICA) on the left. Note the normal AICA on the right side (*arrow*) and the compensatorily enlarged left posterior–inferior cerebellar artery (*arrowhead*).

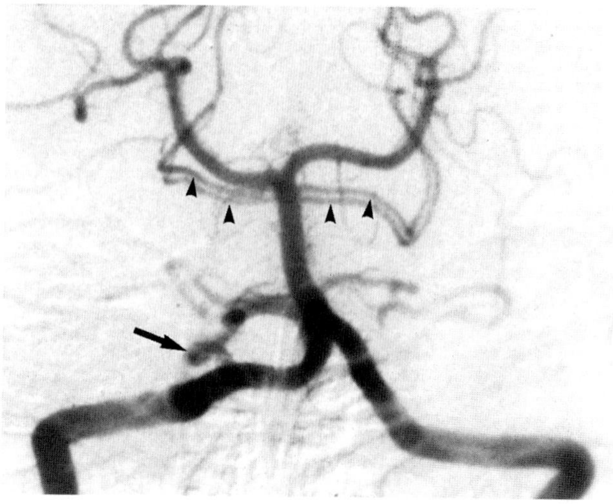

Figure 2R-11J: Right vertebral artery angiogram in the anteroposterior projection, showing accessory (duplicated) superior cerebellar arteries bilaterally (*arrowheads*). Note also that the left posterior–inferior cerebellar artery (PICA) is absent, the right anterior–inferior cerebellar artery is absent, and the right PICA (*arrow*) is compensatorily hypertrophied.

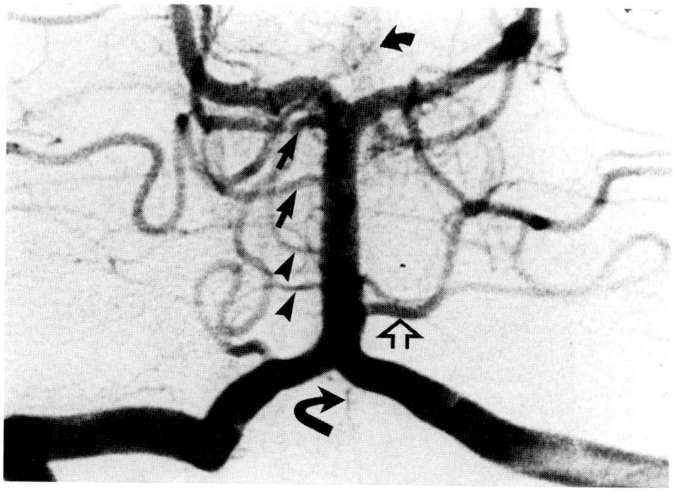

Figure 2R-11K: Arterial phase of a vertebral angiogram in the frontal projection, showing duplication of the anterior–inferior cerebellar arteries (*arrowheads*) on the right and the superior cerebellar arteries (*arrows*) on the right. Note also the displacement of the posterior–inferior cerebellar artery (*open arrow*) on the left side onto the proximal basilar artery, the anterior spiral artery (*large curved arrow*) arising from the distal left vertebral artery, and thalamostriate arterial branches (*small curved arrow*).

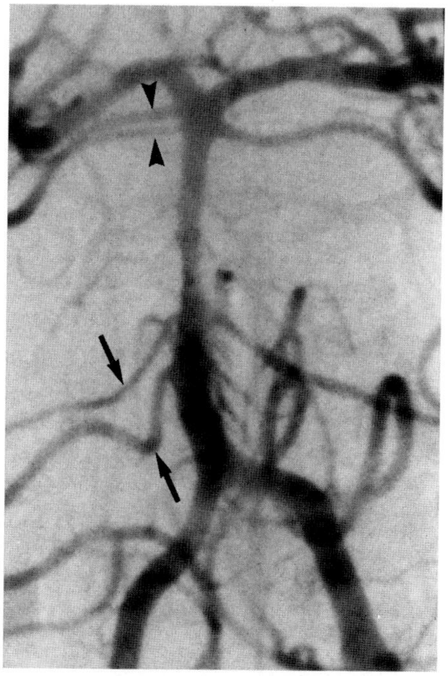

Figure 2R-11L: Right vertebral artery angiogram in the anteroposterior projection, showing duplicated superior cerebellar arteries on the right (*arrowheads*), duplicated anterior–inferior cerebellar arteries (AICAs) on the right (*arrows*), and an absent posterior–inferior cerebellar artery (PICA) on the right. The lower AICA on the right is, in effect, perhaps a PICA displaced onto the basilar artery.

2S Arterial Vascular Territories of the Cerebrum, Brain Stem, and Cerebellum

OVERVIEW

1. The blood supply of the brain is normally derived entirely from the paired internal carotid and vertebral arteries.
2. There is considerable variability in the territories of the brain supplied by the various branches of the carotid and vertebral arteries.
3. The major cerebral arteries are end arteries.
4. The smaller branches of the major cerebral arteries as well as the central branches supplying the brain stem, diencephalon, basal ganglia, and internal capsules are also end arteries.
5. The junctions between the various end arteries between vascular territories represent vascular watersheds.
6. Major and minor collateral vascular connections link the internal intracranial vascular system with itself and the internal and external cranial vascular systems.

THE INTERNAL CAROTID ARTERY SYSTEM

1. The internal carotid arterial system includes the two internal carotid arteries and their branches. The regions supplied encompass parts of the diencephalon and most of the cerebral hemispheres.
2. The internal carotid artery territories
   a. The territory of the cavernous internal carotid arteries includes the trigeminal cranial nerve ganglia and the basal meningeal dura mater.
   b. The territory of the hypophyseal arteries includes the posterior lobe of the pituitary gland and the dura mater surrounding the sella turcica and the cavernous venous sinus.
   c. The ophthalmic artery territory includes the eye, the tissues of the orbit, and part of the basal meninges.
   d. The anterior choroidal artery territory includes the hypothalamus, the cerebral peduncles, the anterior medial temporal lobes, the optic tracts, the lateral geniculate bodies of the thalamus, the retrolenticular and inferior parts of the internal capsule, and portions of the basal ganglia.
   e. The posterior communicating artery territory includes parts of the midbrain and diencephalon.
   f. The anterior cerebral artery territory includes the superomedial aspect of the frontal and parietal lobes of the cerebral hemispheres, the substantia innominata, parts of the basal ganglia (i.e., the anteroinferior part of the globus pallidus, the head of the caudate nucleus, and parts of the putamen), the anterior limb of the internal capsule, the hypothalamus, the optic chiasm, the septal region, and the anterior columns of the fornices.
   g. The middle cerebral artery territory includes most of the cortex and underlying white matter of the superolateral surface of the cerebral hemispheres, the insula, and the temporal pole of the temporal lobe and parts of the internal capsule and basal ganglia.
   h. The territory of the striate arteries includes parts of the basal ganglia and the internal capsule.

THE VERTEBROBASILAR ARTERIAL SYSTEM

1. The vertebrobasilar arterial system includes the paired vertebral arteries, the basilar artery, and their branches. The regions supplied include the whole of the brain stem,

the cerebellum, most of the diencephalon, and the postero-inferior parts of the cerebral hemispheres.

2. The vertebrobasilar arterial territories
   a. The vertebrobasilar meningeal artery territory includes the tentorium cerebelli and the bones of the posterior fossa bony structures.
   b. The proximal anterior spinal (cord) artery territory includes the medial parts of the medulla oblongata (e.g., the hypoglossal nucleus, the medial longitudinal fasciculus, the medial lemniscus, the pyramids, the solitary nucleus, the dorsal motor nucleus of the vagus nerve [CNX], and the medial accessory olive).
   c. The territory of the proximal posterior spinal (cord) artery(ies) includes a small dorsal sector of the medulla oblongata (gracile and cuneate fasciculi and nuclei) and the dorsal portions of the inferior cerebellar peduncles.
   d. The posterior–inferior cerebellar artery territory includes a large dorsolateral segment of the craniad part of the medulla oblongata, the inferior and caudal parts of the cerebellum, the dentate nucleus, and the choroid plexus of the fourth ventricle.
   e. The territory of the medullary arteries or bulbar arteries of the vertebral arteries (minute arteries that arise from the vertebral arteries and their branches) includes the intermediate part of the medulla oblongata.
   f. The territory of the paramedian and short and long circumferential bulbar arteries of the basilar artery includes major portions of the pons and the midbrain.
   g. The anterior–inferior cerebral artery territory includes the anterolateral region of the inferior cerebellar surface, the lateral part of the middle cerebellar peduncle, the tegmental parts of the pons, and, occasionally, the craniad part of the medulla oblongata.
   h. The superior cerebellar artery territory includes the anterior part of the cerebellum, the dorsal parts of the pons and the midbrain, the pineal body, and the choroid plexus of the third ventricle.
   i. The territory of the left and right posterior cerebral arteries includes the inferior surface of the temporal lobe (including the uncus and hippocampal formation, but excluding the temporal pole); the whole of the occipital lobe, including the visual cortex and neighboring areas of the parietal lobe; the medial part of the diencephalon; the pineal body; the posterior thalamus; and part of the midbrain, including the colliculi.
   j. The territory of the posterior choroidal arteries includes the third and lateral ventricle choroid plexi, the tectum, the superior and medial surface of the thalamus, and the fornices.

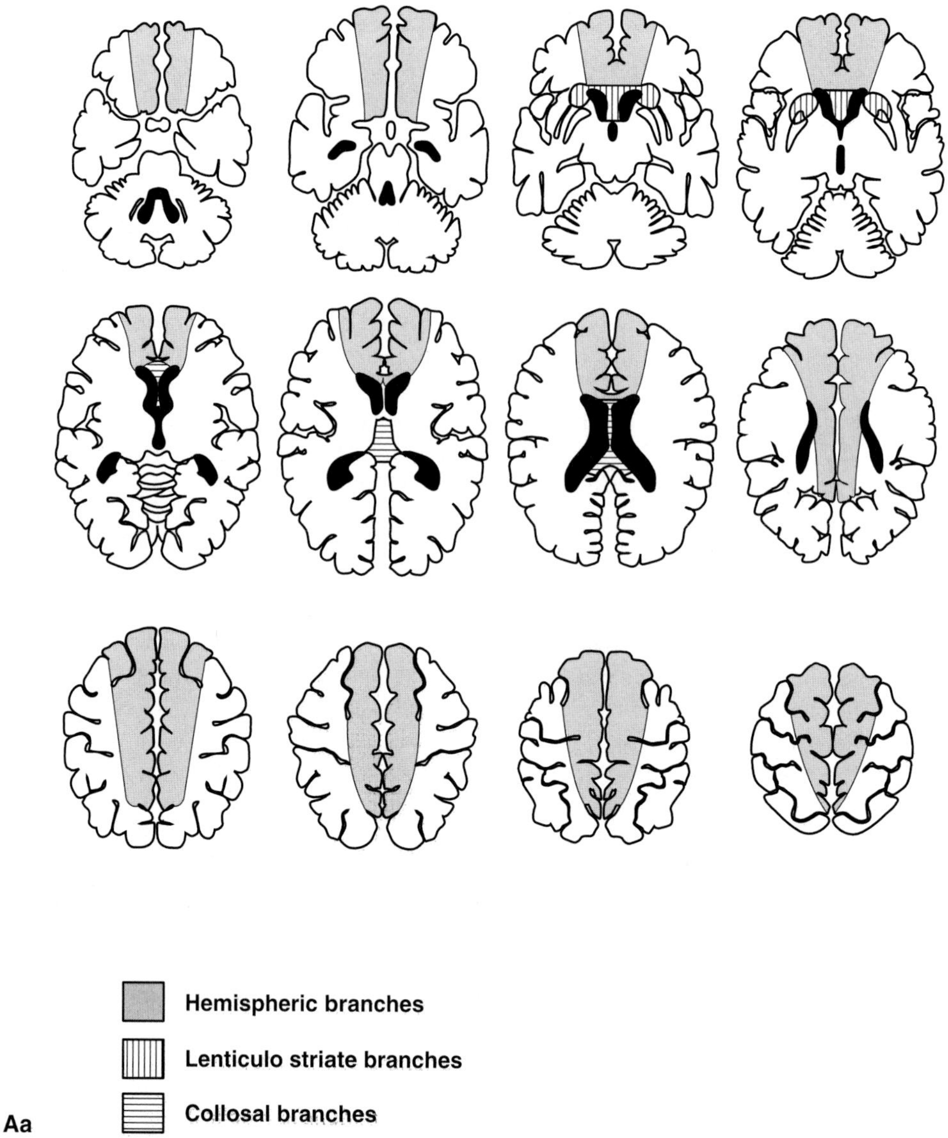

Figure 2S-1A: Schematics of the distribution of the arterial vascular territories (*shaded area*) of anterior, middle, and posterior cerebral arteries in the axial plane (**left to right/top to bottom:** inferior to superior). **a:** Anterior cerebral artery distribution.

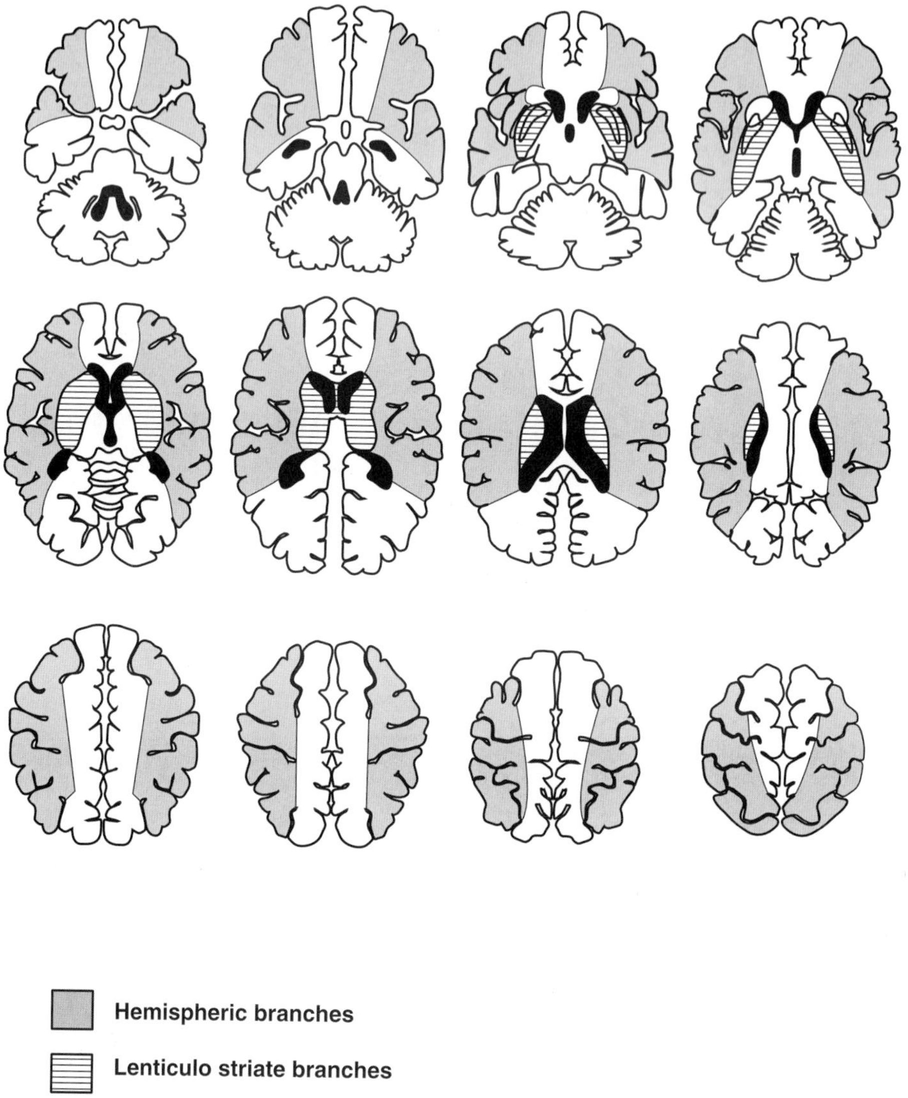

b

Figure 2S-1A *(continued)*: **b:** Middle cerebral artery distribution.

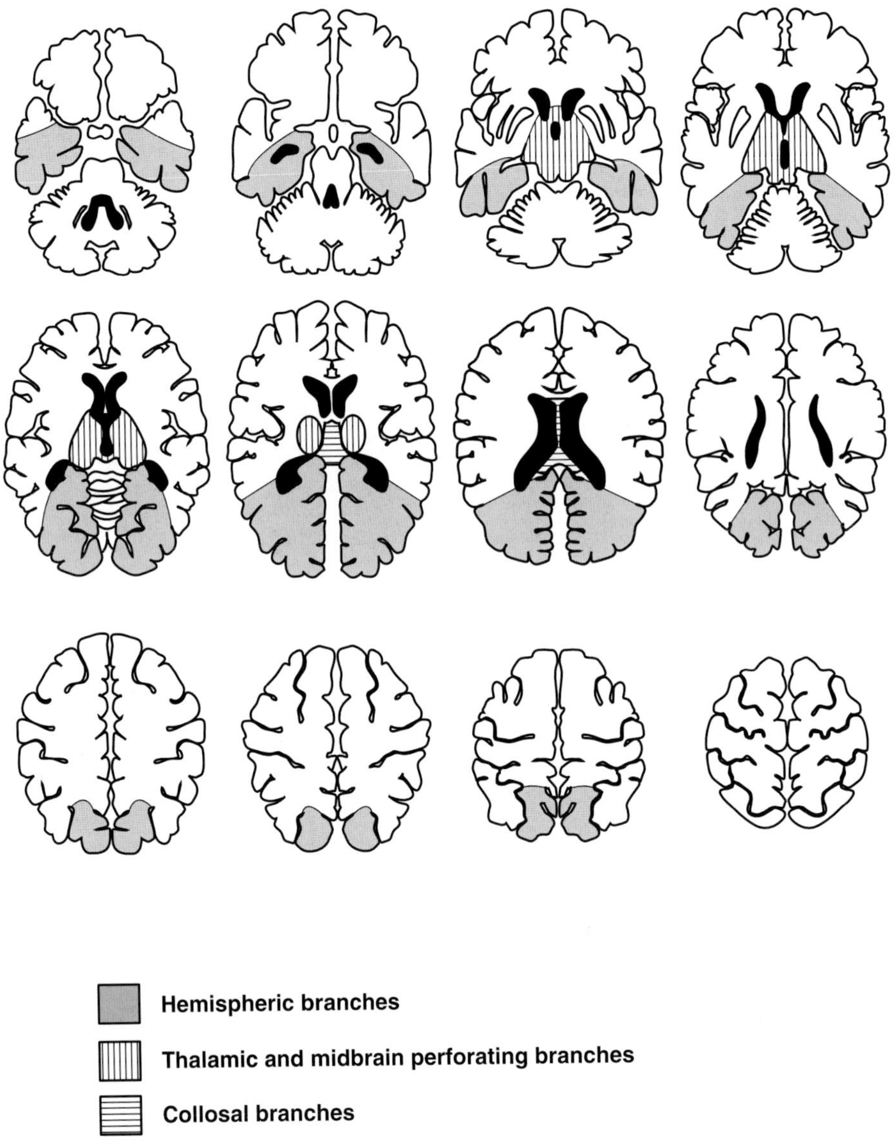

c

Figure 2S-1A *(continued)*: **c:** Posterior cerebral artery distribution.

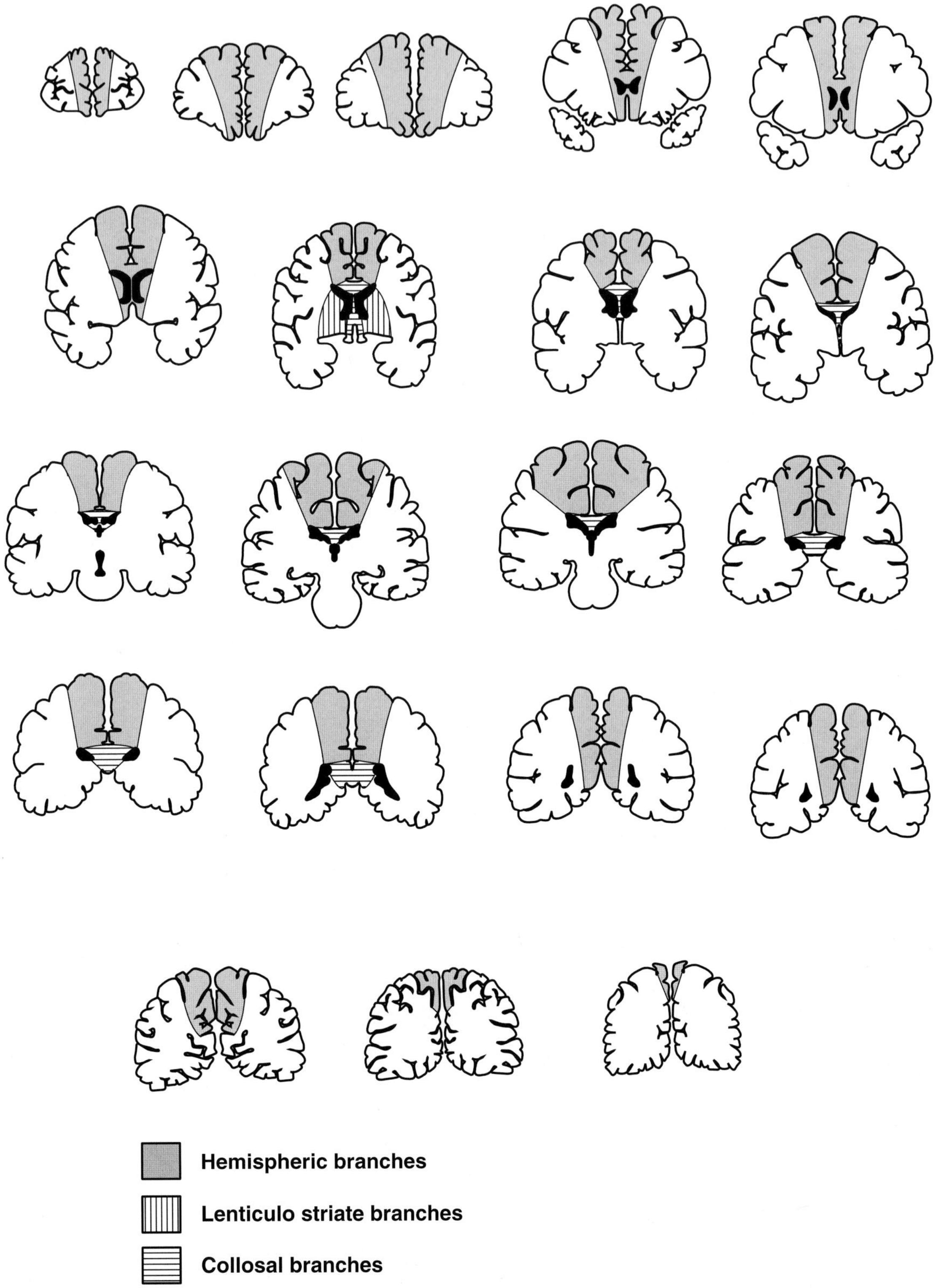

Ba

Figure 2S-1B: Schematics of the distribution of the arterial vascular territories (*shaded areas*) of anterior, middle, and posterior cerebral arteries in the coronal plane (**left to right/top to bottom:** front to back). **a:** Anterior cerebral artery distribution.

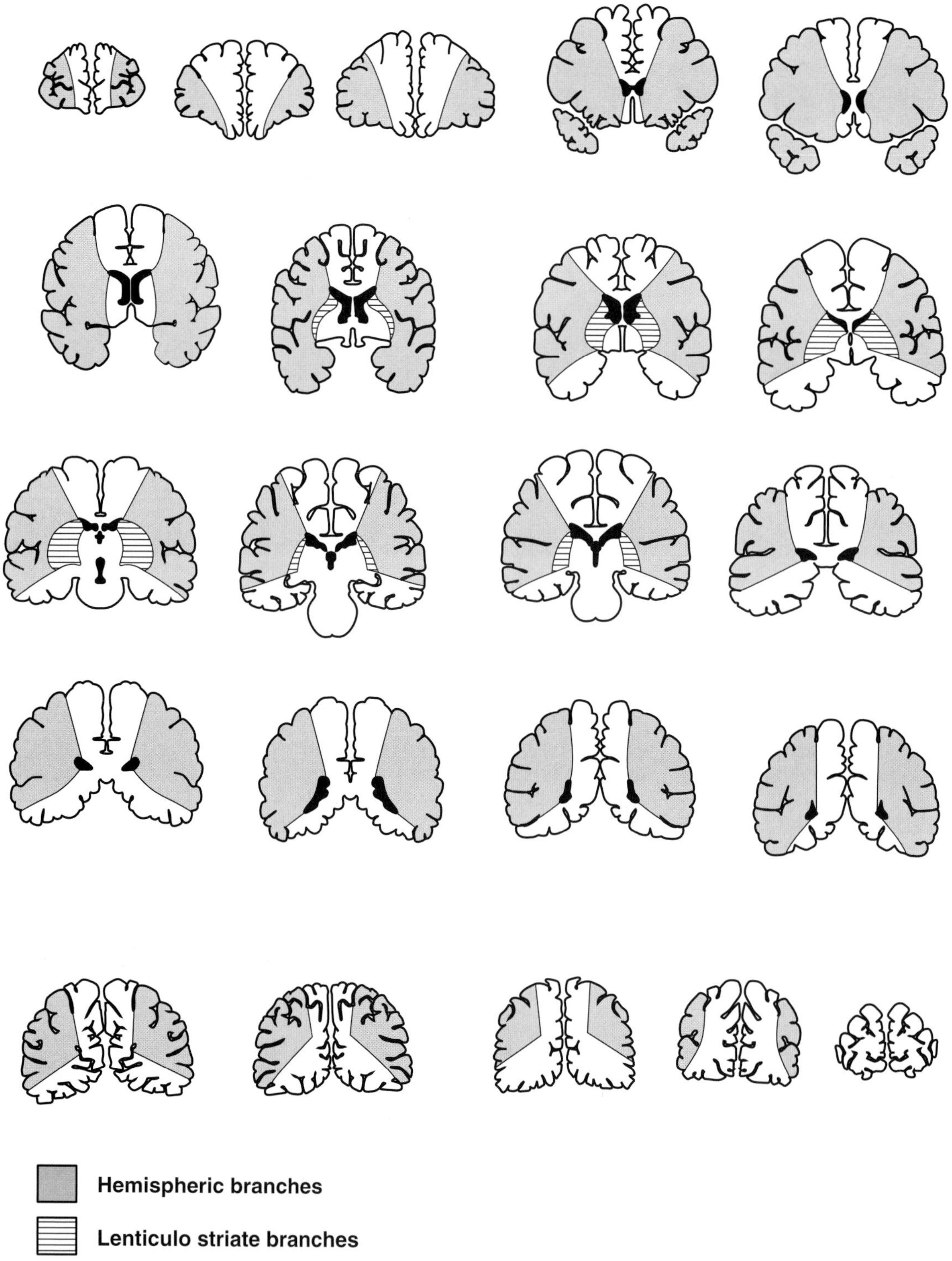

b

Figure 2S-1B *(continued)*: **b:** Middle cerebral artery distribution.

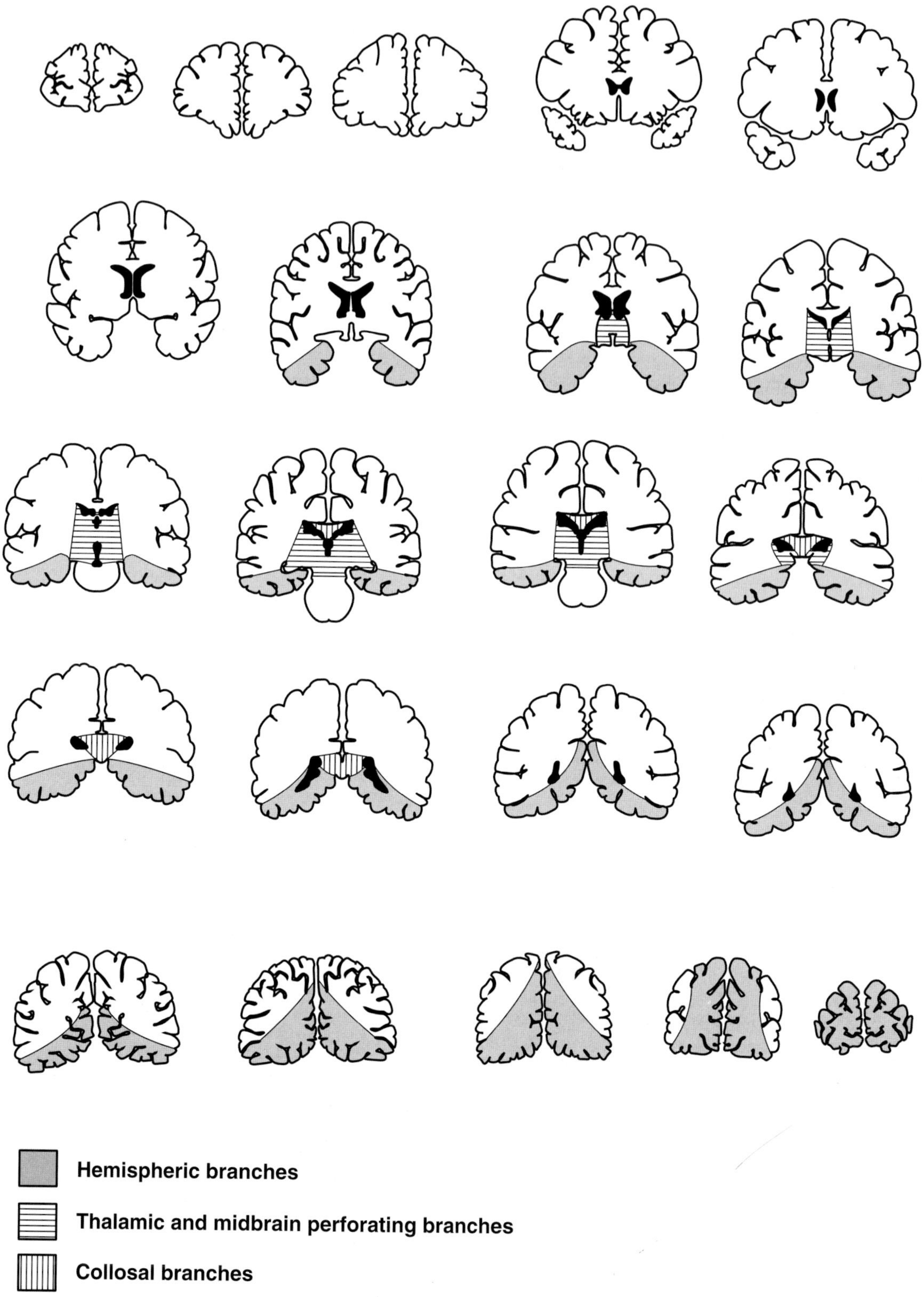

c

Figure 2S-1B *(continued)*: c: Posterior cerebral artery distribution.

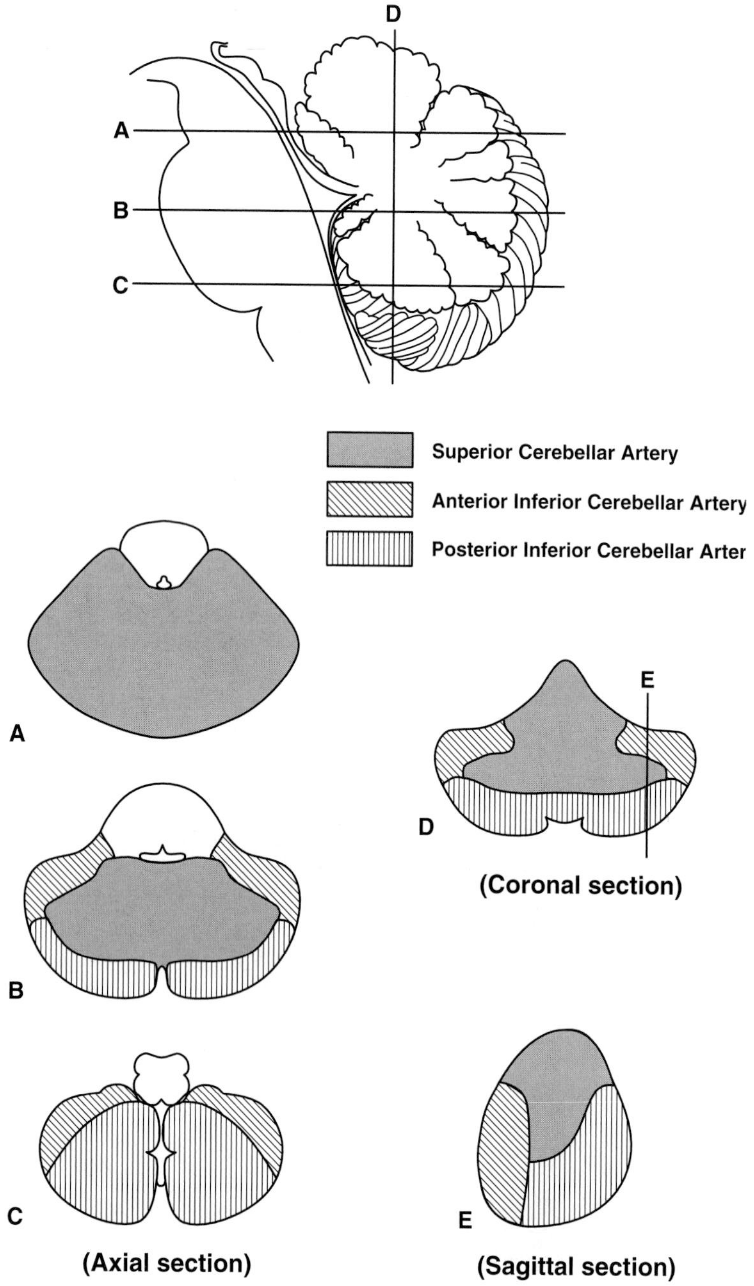

Figure 2S-2A–E: Schematics of the major arterial territories of the cerebellum. *A–D*, levels and planes of section in parts **A–D**.

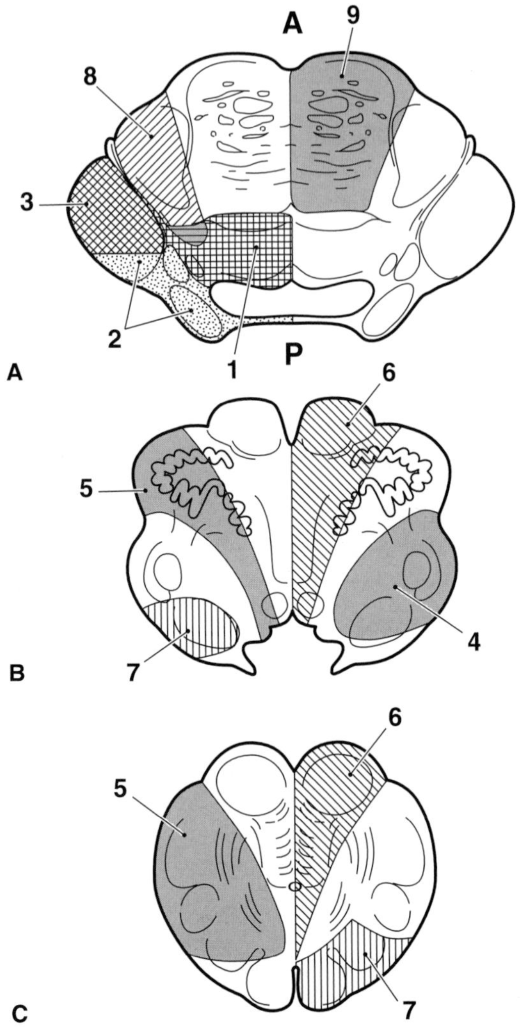

Figure 2S-3: Schematics of the vascular territories of the pons and medulla oblongata of the brain stem. **A:** Pons. **B:** Upper medulla oblongata. **C:** Lower medulla oblongata.

1 Long circumferential branches of basilar artery
2 Superior cerebellar artery
3 Anterior–inferior cerebellar artery
4 Posterior–inferior cerebellar artery
5 Bulbar branches of the vertebral artery
6 Anterior spinal artery
7 Posterior spinal artery
8 Short circumferential branches of basilar artery
9 Paramedian branches of basilar artery

2T Cerebral Vascular Anastomotic Patterns

THE ARTERIAL CIRCLE OF WILLIS

1. The circle of Willis is an interconnecting arterial polygon that lies along the ventral surface of the diencephalon adjacent to the optic nerves and tracts.
2. Some 20% to 40% of individuals have the classic configuration of the circle of Willis, in which no segment is hypoplastic or absent.

The Components of the Circle of Willis

1. The right and left supraclinoid internal carotid arteries
2. The horizontal (A1) segments of the right and left anterior cerebral arteries
3. The anterior communicating artery
4. The right and left posterior communicating arteries
5. The horizontal (P1) segments of the right and left posterior cerebral arteries
6. The basilar artery tip

The Branches of the Circle of Willis

1. The medial, anteromedial, and anterolateral lenticulostriate arteries
   a. The medial lenticulostriate arteries arise from the A1 segments of the anterior cerebral arteries.
   b. The anteromedial striate arteries arise from the anterior communicating artery.
   c. The anterolateral striate arteries arise from the internal carotid arteries.
   d. The medial and anteromedial lenticulostriate arteries supply parts of the basal ganglia, the internal capsule, the hypothalamus, the septum pellucidum, the anterior commissure, the pillars of the fornices, the anterior striatum, and the optic chiasm.
2. The posteromedial striate and thalamoperforating arteries
   a. The thalamoperforating arteries arise from the basilar tip and/or the P1 segment of the posterior cerebral artery on each side.
   b. The posteromedial striate arteries arise from the posterior communicating arteries.
   c. The thalamoperforating and posteromedial striate arteries supply parts of the thalamus, the posterior limb of the internal capsule, the optic chiasm, the hypothalamus, and the midbrain.
3. The thalamogeniculate arteries
   a. The thalamogeniculate arteries arise from the proximal part of the P2 segment of the posterior cerebral artery and therefore are not true branches of the circle of Willis.
   b. The thalamogeniculate arteries supply the lateral aspect of the thalamus, the geniculate bodies, the optic tracts, and the internal capsule.
4. The lateral striate (lenticulostriate) arteries
   a. The lateral striate arteries arise from the M2 segment of the middle cerebral artery and therefore are not true branches of the circle of Willis.
   b. The vascular supply of these vessels is discussed elsewhere.
5. The recurrent artery of Heubner
   a. Occasionally (<25%), the recurrent artery of Heubner arises from the A1 segment of the anterior cerebral artery or the anterior communicating artery (more common origin: A2 segment).
   b. The peripheral vascular supply of this vessel is discussed elsewhere.

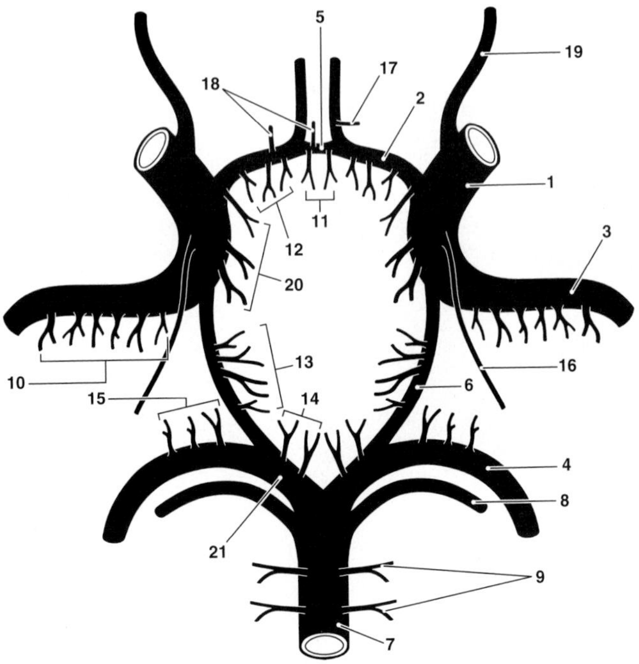

Figure 2T-1: Schematic of the components of the arterial circle of Willis and the origins of the perforating branches of the circle of Willis from below.

1 Internal carotid artery
2 Anterior cerebral artery (A1 segment)
3 Middle cerebral artery (M1 segment)
4 Posterior cerebral artery (P2 segment)
5 Anterior communicating artery
6 Posterior communicating artery
7 Basilar artery
8 Superior cerebellar artery
9 Perforating pontine rami
10 Lateral lenticulostriate arteries
11 Anteromedial lenticulostriate arteries
12 Medial lenticulostriate arteries
13 Posteromedial lenticulostriate arteries
14 Thalomoperforating arteries
15 Thalamogeniculate arteries
16 Anterior choroidal artery
17 Recurrent artery of Heubner (most common origin)
18 Recurrent artery of Heubner (alternate origins)
19 Ophthalmic artery
20 Anterolateral striate arteries
21 Posterior cerebral artery (P1 segment)

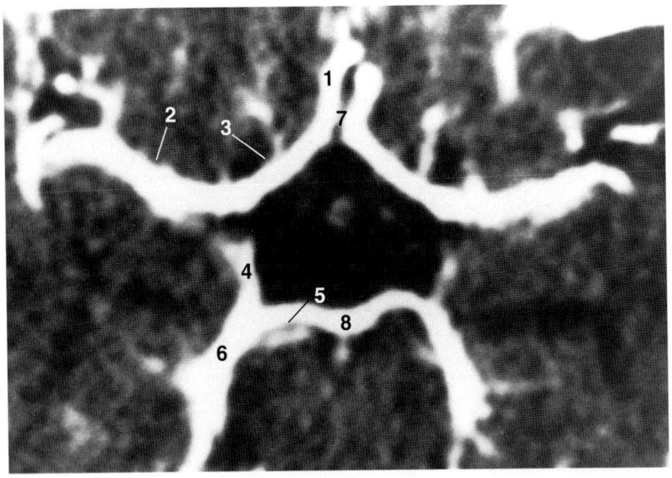

Figure 2T-2A: The arterial circle of Willis. Intravenous bolus, contrast-enhanced axial CT image showing the circle of Willis.

1 A2 segment of the right anterior cerebral artery
2 M1 segment of the right middle cerebral artery
3 A1 segment of the right anterior cerebral artery
4 Right posterior communicating artery
5 P1 segment of the right posterior cerebral artery
6 P2 segment of the right posterior cerebral artery
7 Anterior communicating artery
8 Tip of the basilar artery

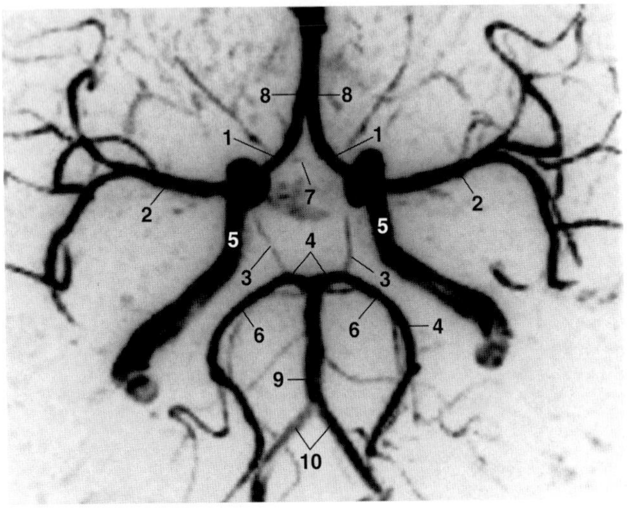

Figure 2T-2B: MR angiogram viewed from above, showing the normal anatomy of the circle of Willis.

1 A1 segments of the anterior cerebral arteries
2 M1 segments of the middle cerebral arteries
3 Left and right posterior communicating arteries
4 P1 segments of the posterior cerebral arteries
5 Left and right supraclinoid internal carotid arteries
6 P2 segments of the posterior cerebral arteries
7 Anterior communicating artery
8 A2 segments of the anterior cerebral arteries
9 Basilar artery
10 Vertebral arteries

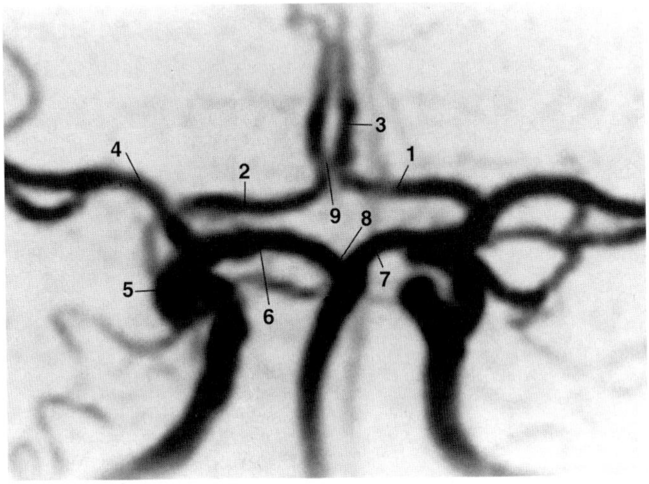

Figure 2T-2C: MR angiogram shows the normal appearance of the circle of Willis in the frontal projection.

1 A1 segment of left anterior cerebral artery
2 A1 segment of right anterior cerebral artery
3 A2 segment of left anterior cerebral artery
4 M1 segment of right middle cerebral artery
5 Supraclinoid right internal carotid artery
6 P1 segment of right posterior cerebral artery
7 P1 segment of left posterior cerebral artery
8 Basilar artery tip
9 Region of anterior communicating artery

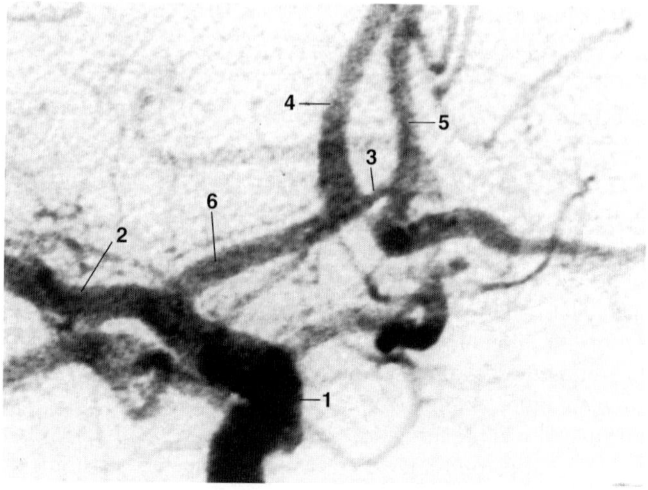

Figure 2T-2D: Internal carotid artery angiogram in the oblique projection, showing the anterior communicating artery.

1 Right internal carotid artery
2 M1 segment, right middle cerebral artery
3 Anterior communicating artery
4 A2 segment, right anterior cerebral artery
5 A2 segment, left anterior cerebral artery
6 A1 segment, right anterior cerebral artery

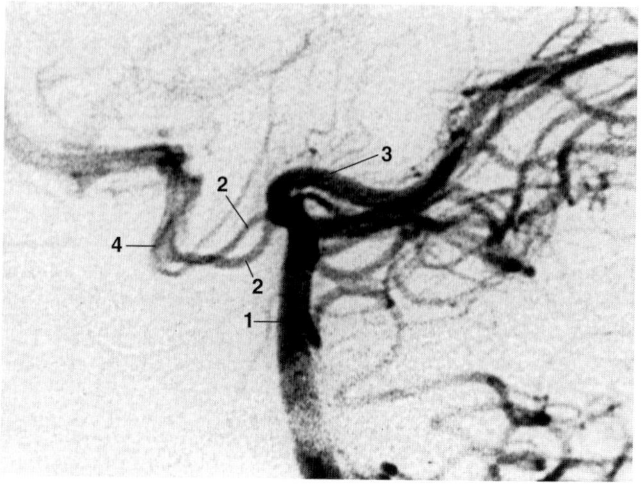

Figure 2T-2E: Vertebral angiogram in the lateral projection, showing both posterior communicating arteries.

1 Basilar artery
2 Posterior communicating arteries
3 Posterior cerebral artery
4 Supraclinoid internal carotid artery(ies)

ANASTOMOSES BETWEEN THE EXTRACRANIAL AND THE INTRACRANIAL ARTERIES

Anastomoses Between the Internal Carotid and the External Carotid Arteries

There are many anastomoses between the internal carotid and the external carotid arteries and their branches. The most important anastomoses include the following.

1. The ascending pharyngeal artery, which is a branch of the external carotid artery, anastomoses with intracavernous branches of the internal carotid artery.
2. The inferolateral trunk (i.e., lateral main-stem artery or artery of the inferior cavernous sinus), which is a branch of the internal carotid artery, has numerous small anastomoses with the external carotid artery through the foramen ovale, the foramen rotundum, the foramen spinosum, and the superior orbital fissure.
3. The vidian artery (i.e., the artery of the pterygoid canal), seen in 25% of cases, is a branch of the intrapetrous internal carotid artery. The vidian artery has anastomoses with the external carotid artery via branches of the internal maxillary artery.
4. The ophthalmic artery, which is a branch of the internal carotid artery, has many anastomoses with the external carotid artery via branches of the facial, the internal maxillary, and the middle meningeal arteries. The most important anastomoses are the following.
   a. The internal maxillary artery anastomoses with the ophthalmic artery via the ethmoidal branches of the maxillary and the ophthalmic arteries
   b. The facial artery anastomoses with the ophthalmic artery via the angular branch of the facial artery
   c. The middle meningeal artery anastomoses directly with the meningeal branch of the ophthalmic artery or indirectly via the lacrimal branch of the ophthalmic artery

Anastomoses Between the Vertebral Artery and the External Carotid Artery

1. The occipital artery, which is a branch of the external carotid artery, anastomoses either directly or through its muscular branches with the ipsilateral vertebral artery.
2. The ascending pharyngeal artery, which is a branch of the external carotid artery, anastomoses through its meningeal branches with the ipsilateral vertebral artery.

ANASTOMOSES BETWEEN THE INTRACRANIAL ARTERIES

There are many anastomoses between the intracranial vessels and their branches. The most important anastomoses include:

1. Intrinsic anastomoses of the arterial circle of Willis
2. Leptomeningeal anastomoses between terminal vascular territories at the level of small branches of both the pia mater and the arachnoid mater
3. Anterior choroidal artery anastomoses with branches of the posterior choroidal, the posterior communicating, the posterior cerebral, and the middle cerebral arteries
4. Anomalous internal carotid–vertebrobasilar arterial anastomoses occur via persistent embryonic circulatory connections. The main persistent embryonic anastomoses include the following.
   a. The persistent trigeminal artery
      i. The persistent trigeminal artery is the most common of the persistent embryonic carotid–vertebrobasilar arterial anastomoses (85%).
      ii. The persistent trigeminal artery originates just proximal to the intracavernous segment of the internal carotid artery.
      iii. The persistent trigeminal artery joins directly with the upper part of the basilar artery.

b. The persistent otic (acoustic) artery
   i. The persistent otic artery is very rare.
   ii. The persistent otic artery arises from the petrous portion of the internal carotid artery.
   iii. The persistent otic artery joins the basilar artery just caudal to the origins of the anterior–inferior cerebellar arteries.
c. The persistent hypoglossal artery
   i. The persistent hypoglossal artery is the second most common of the persistent embryonic carotid–vertebrobasilar arterial anastomoses.
   ii. The persistent hypoglossal artery arises from the upper portion of the cervical internal carotid artery.
   iii. The persistent hypoglossal artery joins the vertebrobasilar circulation at or near the junction of the vertebral arteries to form the basilar artery; the ipsilateral vertebral artery is often hypoplastic.
d. The persistent proatlantal intersegmental artery
   i. The persistent proatlantal intersegmental artery arises from the uppermost cervical internal carotid artery or, less commonly, the external carotid artery.
   ii. The type 1 persistent proatlantal intersegmental artery courses between the arch of C-l and the occiput to join the distal ipsilateral vertebral artery. The type 2 proatlantal intersegmental artery courses between the C1-2 interspace to join the ipsilateral vertebral artery.
   iii. One or both vertebral arteries may be absent in up to 50% of cases.
   iv. The vascular anomaly may originate from a malformation of the occipital artery. For this reason, the persistent proatlantal artery may give rise to the ipsilateral occipital artery.

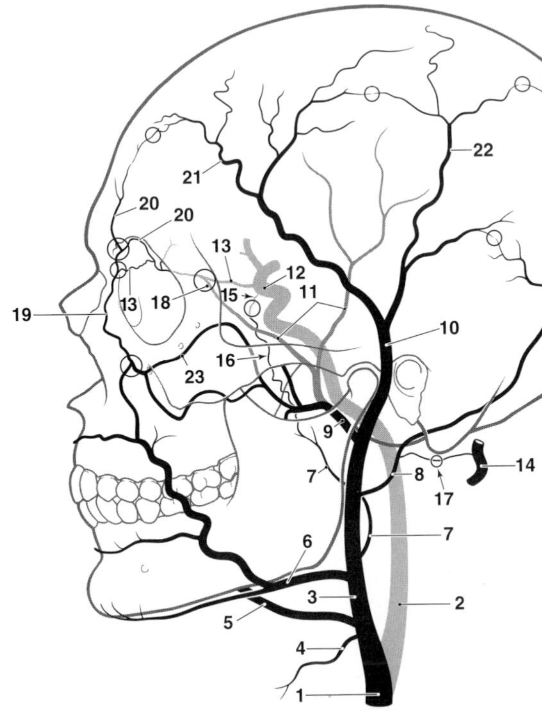

Figure 2T-3: Lateral schematic of the external carotid artery and its branches and common anastomotic pathways (the intracranial vessels are shaded gray). Note some of the common points of anastomosis in circles (not to scale).

1 Common carotid artery
2 Internal carotid artery
3 External carotid artery trunk
4 Superior thyroid artery
5 Lingual artery
6 Facial artery
7 Ascending pharyngeal artery
8 Occipital artery
9 Internal maxillary artery
10 Superficial temporal artery
11 Middle meningeal artery
12 Carotid siphon
13 Ophthalmic artery
14 Vertebral artery
15 Recurrent artery of the foramen lacerum, a branch of the inferolateral trunk of the internal carotid artery
16 Carotid branch of the superior pharyngeal branch of the ascending pharyngeal artery that enters the cranium via the foramen lacerum
17 Anastomosing muscular branches of vertebral and occipital arteries
18 Recurrent meningeal artery anastomosing with orbital branch of middle meningeal artery
19 Angular artery
20 Supraorbital artery
21 Frontal branch of superficial temporal artery
22 Parietal branch of superficial temporal artery
23 Infraorbital artery

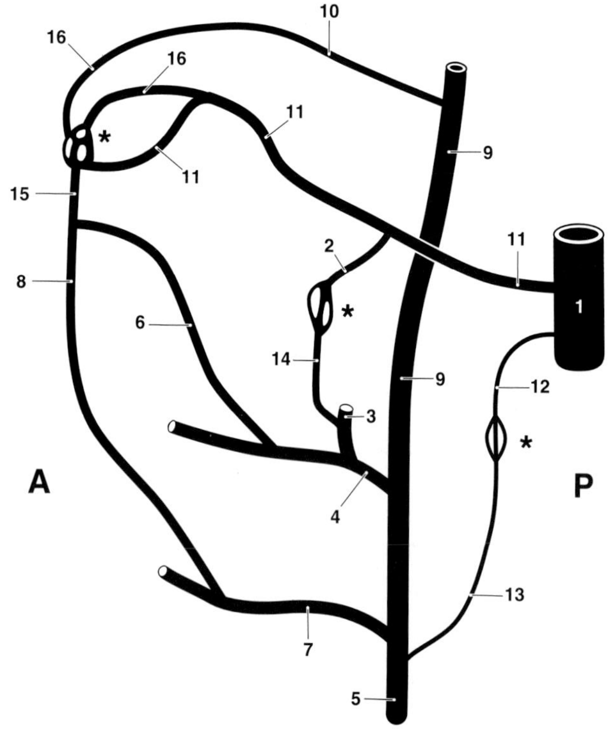

Figure 2T-4: Lateral schematic of some of the external carotid artery–internal carotid artery anastomotic pathways. Note some of the major anastomotic sites indicated by asterisks. *A,* anterior; *P,* posterior.

1 Internal carotid artery
2 Recurrent meningeal artery branch of lacrimal artery from ophthalmic artery
3 Middle meningeal artery
4 Internal maxillary artery
5 External carotid artery
6 Infraorbital artery
7 Facial artery
8 Facial artery branch
9 Superficial temporal artery
10 Frontal branch of superficial temporal artery
11 Ophthalmic artery
12 Recurrent artery of the foramen lacerum, a branch of the inferolateral trunk of the internal carotid artery
13 Carotid branch of the superior pharyngeal branch of the ascending pharyngeal artery entering the cranium via the foramen lacerum
14 Orbital branch of the middle meningeal artery
15 Angular artery
16 Supraorbital artery

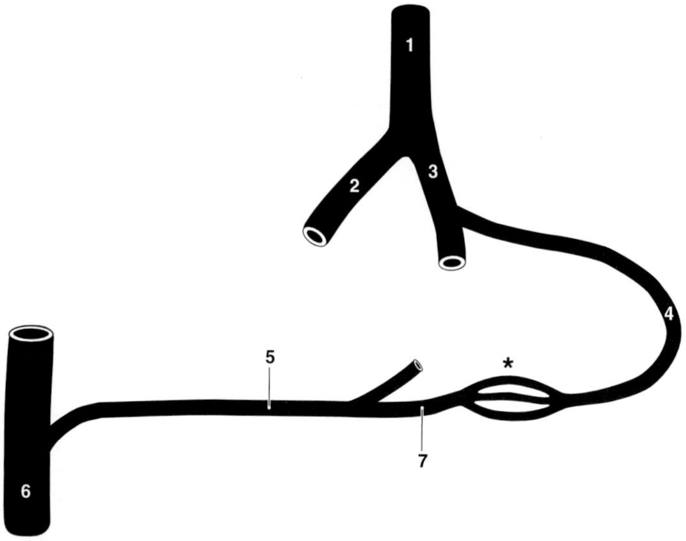

Figure 2T-5: Simplified schematic of some of the major external carotid artery–vertebrobasilar system anastomoses. Note anastomotic site at the *asterisk.*

1 Basilar artery
2 Right vertebral artery
3 Left vertebral artery
4 Muscular branch of vertebral artery
5 Occipital artery
6 External carotid artery
7 Muscular branch of occipital artery

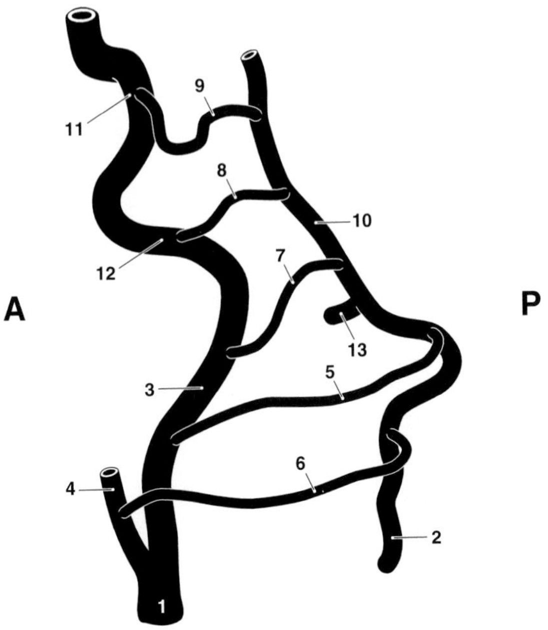

Figure 2T-6: Lateral schematic of potential persistent embryonic carotid–vertebrobasilar arterial anastomoses (not to scale). *A,* anterior; *P,* posterior.
1 Common carotid artery
2 Ipsilateral distal vertebral artery
3 Upper cervical internal carotid artery
4 External carotid artery
5 Persistent proatlantal intersegmental artery, type 1
6 Persistent proatlantal intersegmental artery, type 2
7 Persistent hypoglossal artery
8 Persistent otic artery
9 Persistent trigeminal artery
10 Basilar artery
11 Precavernous segment, internal carotid artery
12 Petrous segment, internal carotid artery
13 Contralateral vertebral artery

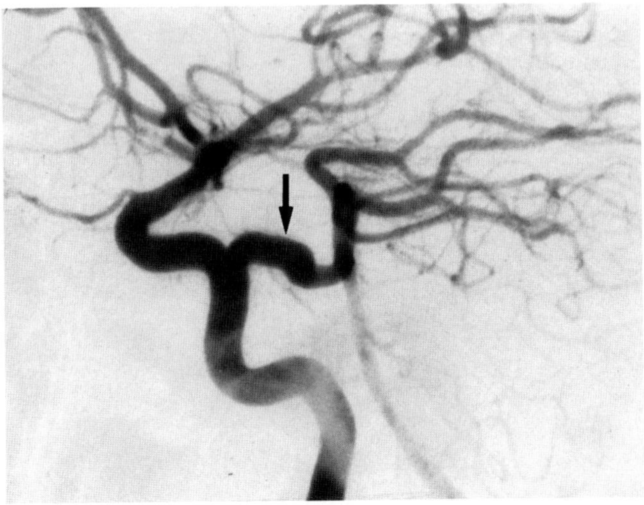

Figure 2T-7A: Persistent trigeminal artery. Right internal carotid angiogram in the lateral projection, showing filling of the basilar arterial system through a persistent trigeminal artery (*arrow*).

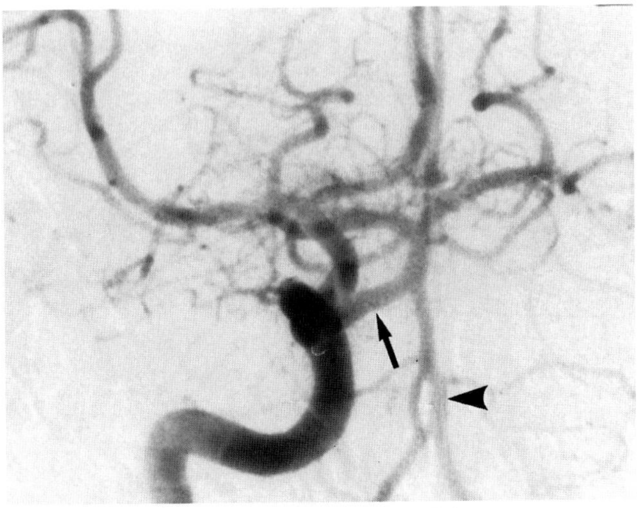

Figure 2T-7B: Persistent trigeminal artery. Right internal carotid artery angiogram in the frontal projection, showing the persistent trigeminal artery (*arrow*) filling the basilar arterial system. The proximal basilar artery is noted to be fenestrated (*arrowhead*).

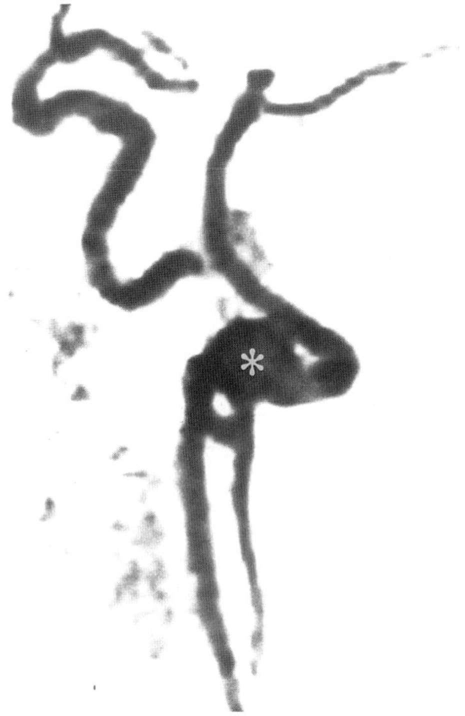

Figure 2T-8: Persistent hypoglossal artery. MR angiogram in the lateral projection, showing a low carotid–basilar anastomosis representing a persistent hypoglossal artery. Note the aneurysmal dilation (*asterisk*) of the anastomosis. (Courtesy of P. Corr, M.D.)

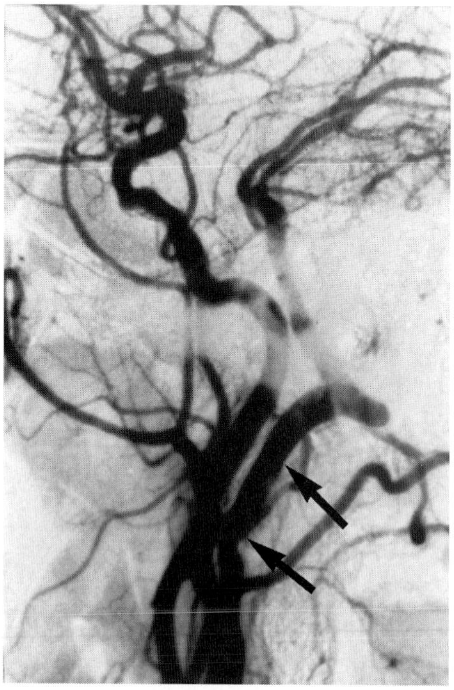

Figure 2T-9A: Type 1 persistent proatlantal intersegmental artery. Left common carotid angiogram in the lateral projection shows a type 1 persistent proatlantal intersegmental artery (*arrows*) originating from the internal carotid artery.

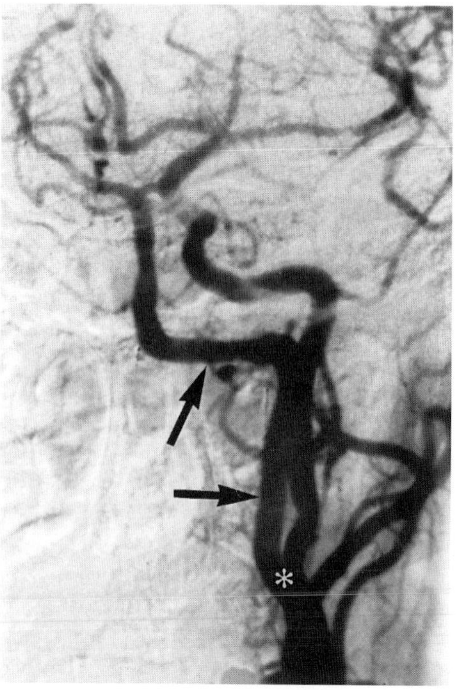

Figure 2T-9B: Type 1 persistent proatlantal intersegmental artery. Left common carotid angiogram in the anteroposterior projection, showing a persistent proatlantal intersegmental artery (*arrows*). Note the site of origin of this anomalous vessel from the internal carotid artery (*asterisk*).

ARTERIAL CIRCLE OF WILLIS VARIANTS

- Asymmetric shape of the circle of Willis, with one side of smaller caliber than the other (type 1: 18%)
- Symmetric circle of Willis, but with all the components of rather small caliber (type 2: 6%)
- Unilateral hypoplasia of the A1 (horizontal) segment of the anterior cerebral artery (type 3: 25%)
- Unilateral hypoplasia of the P1 segment of the posterior cerebral artery (type 4: 16%)
- Bilateral hypoplasia of the P1 segment of the posterior cerebral artery (type 5: 11%)
- Unilateral hypoplasia of the P1 segment of the posterior cerebral artery, with unilateral segment (A1) hypoplasia of the anterior cerebral artery on the same side (type 6: 8%)
- Unilateral P1 segment hypoplasia of the posterior cerebral artery, with contralateral A1 segment hypoplasia of the anterior cerebral artery (type 7: 8%)
- Bilateral P1 segment hypoplasia of the posterior cerebral artery, with A1 segment hypoplasia of the anterior cerebral artery (type 8: 8%)
- Hypoplasia of the posterior communicating artery occurs in 34% of cases.
- A fetal configuration of the posterior cerebral artery arising directly from the internal carotid artery is seen in 20% of cases. In this situation, the posterior communicating artery provides the major blood supply to the posterior cerebral artery. In such cases, the P1 or precommunicating segment of the ipsilateral posterior cerebral artery is smaller than the posterior communicating artery or is even atretic.
- The A1 segment of the anterior cerebral artery is hypoplastic in 10% of cases. Complete absence of the horizontal A1 segment of the anterior cerebral artery is unusual.
- Multiple (i.e., double or triple) anterior communicating arteries may be seen rarely.
- Anterior communicating artery hypoplasia is seen in 15% of cases. Absence of the anterior communicating artery may occur in 4% of cases.

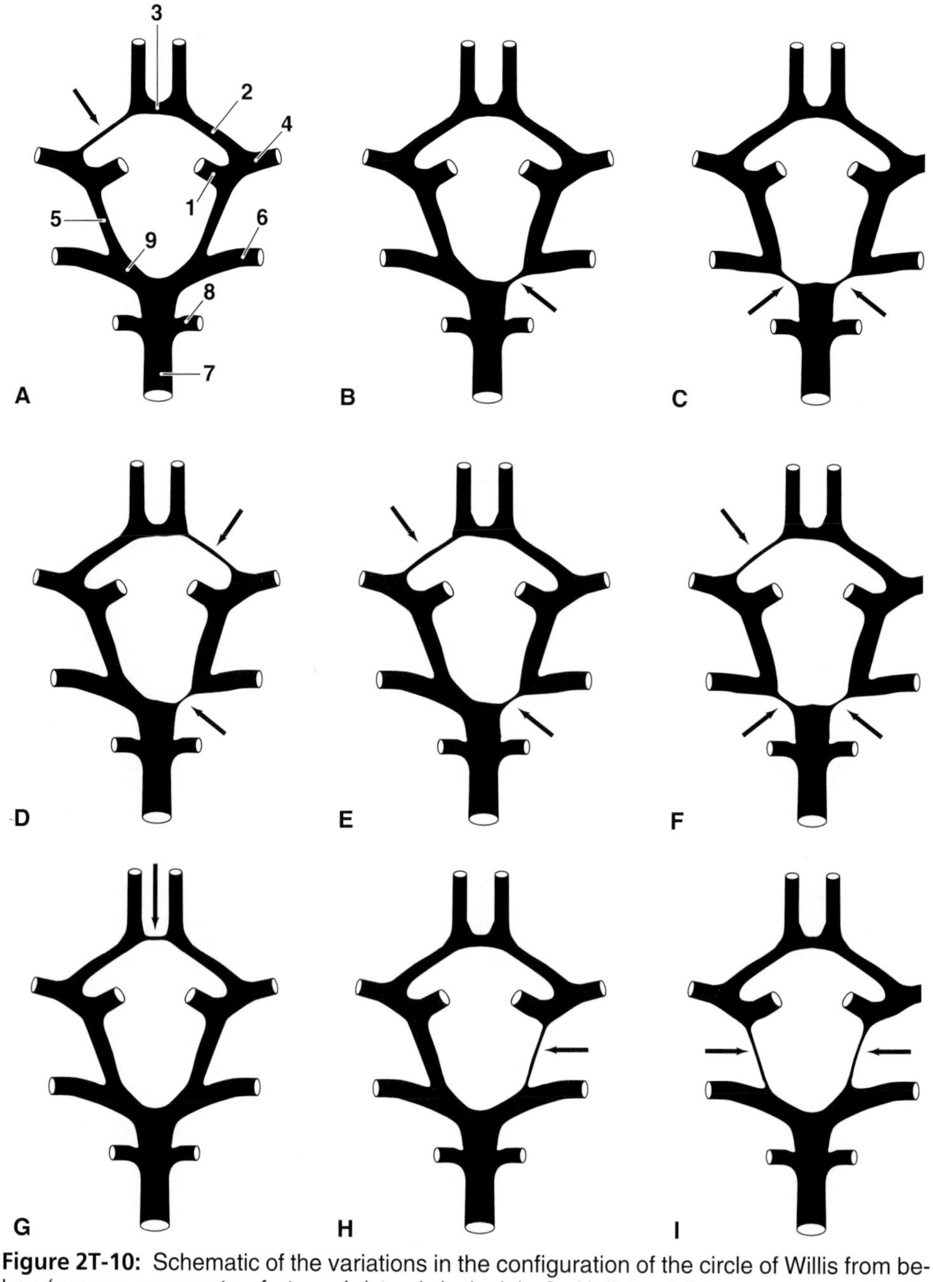

Figure 2T-10: Schematic of the variations in the configuration of the circle of Willis from below (*arrows*: segments of stenosis/atresia/aplasia). **A:** Unilateral A1 segment atresia. **B:** Unilateral P1 segment atresia. **C:** Bilateral P1 segment atresia. **D:** Ipsilateral A1 and P1 segment atresia. **E:** Contralateral A1 and P1 segment atresia. **F:** Unilateral A1 and bilateral P1 segment atresia. **G:** Anterior communicating artery atresia. **H:** Unilateral posterior communicating artery atresia. **I:** Bilateral posterior communicating artery atresia.

1 Internal carotid artery
2 P1 segment of the anterior cerebral artery
3 Anterior communicating artery
4 M1 segment of the middle cerebral artery
5 P2 segment of the posterior communicating artery
6 P2 segment of the posterior cerebral artery
7 Basilar artery
8 Superior cerebellar artery
9 P1 segment of the posterior cerebral artery

2U Venous Drainage of the Cranium

THE SUPRATENTORIAL VEINS

The cerebral veins are divided into deep and superficial groups. The superficial and deep groups of veins are interconnected by numerous anastomotic channels; the cerebral veins are devoid of valves.

The Superficial Cerebral Veins

1. The superficial cerebral veins arise from the cerebral cortex and the subcortical white matter.
2. The small veins that emerge from the brain substance form the pial venous plexi, which then drain into the cerebral veins proper.
3. The superficial cerebral veins anastomose freely in the pia mater to form larger veins that pass through the subarachnoid space to empty into the dural venous sinuses.
4. The superficial cerebral veins are extremely variable in size, position, number, and configuration. In addition, there is great bilateral asymmetry within the superficial cerebral venous system.
5. The lateral superficial cerebral veins
   a. The superior superficial cerebral veins
      i. The superior superficial cerebral veins collect blood from the medial and convex surfaces of the cerebral hemisphere.
      ii. The superior superficial cerebral veins generally number 10 to 15 on each side.
      iii. The superior superficial cerebral veins drain into the superior sagittal venous sinus.
   b. The superficial middle cerebral (Sylvian) vein
      i. The superficial middle cerebral vein courses along the Sylvian fissure.
      ii. The superficial middle cerebral vein anastomoses with the superior anastomotic (i.e., Trolard) and inferior anastomotic (i.e., Labbé) veins.
      iii. The superficial middle cerebral vein receives drainage from the opercular areas adjacent to the Sylvian fissure and drains into the cavernous venous sinus.
6. The inferior superficial cerebral veins
   a. The inferior superficial cerebral veins drain the basal surfaces and ventral aspects of the lateral surfaces of the cerebral hemispheres.
   b. The inferior superficial cerebral veins on the basal surface of the cerebral hemispheres drain into the basal venous sinuses. Rostrally these superficial cerebral veins empty into the cavernous and sphenoparietal venous sinuses, and caudally they drain into the petrosal and transverse venous sinuses.
7. The medial superficial cerebral veins
   a. The medial superficial cerebral veins draining toward the convexity are named for the lobe of drainage: medial frontal, parietal, and occipital hemispheric veins. These veins drain into the superior sagittal venous sinus.
   b. The medial superficial cerebral veins of the frontal and parietal regions draining centrally are unnamed and empty into the inferior sagittal sinus.
   c. The medial superficial cerebral veins of the occipital region draining centrally empty into the straight venous sinus.
   d. The medial superficial cerebral vein(s) draining the anterior cingulate gyrus and paraterminal gyrus empty into the anterior pericallosal vein. This vein, in turn, drains into the deep middle cerebral vein.
   e. The inferior striate and posterior thalamic veins drain into the deep middle cerebral vein.
   f. The superior thalamic veins drain into the internal cerebral vein.

The Deep Cerebral Veins

1. The deep cerebral veins draining the choroid plexi of the third and lateral ventricles, the periventricular region of the cerebral hemispheres, the diencephalon, the basal ganglia, and the deep hemispheric white matter empty into the great cerebral vein of Galen.
2. Large cortical areas along the inferior and medial surfaces of the cerebral hemisphere are also drained by a number of veins that empty into the great cerebral vein of Galen.

The Internal Cerebral Veins

1. The paired internal cerebral veins are located near the midline in the tela choroidea of the choroid plexus in the roof of the third ventricle.
2. The internal cerebral veins extend caudally from the interventricular foramina of Monro and course over the superior medial surfaces of the thalami.
3. The internal cerebral veins join in the rostral part of the quadrigeminal cistern to drain into the great cerebral vein of Galen.
4. The internal cerebral vein on each side receives the following.
   a. The thalamostriate vein, which drains the anterior terminal vein and numerous transverse caudate veins
   b. The choroidal vein, which extends distally into the temporal horn of the lateral ventricle
   c. The anterior septal vein, which drains the septum pellucidum and portions of the corpus callosum
   d. The epithalamic vein, which drains the dorsal part of the diencephalon
   e. The lateral ventricular vein, which extends over the surface of the thalamus and the tail of the caudate nucleus and drains the white matter of the parahippocampal gyrus and part of the choroid plexus of the lateral ventricle

The Basal Vein of Rosenthal

1. The basal vein of Rosenthal arises in the medial aspect of the anterior part of the temporal lobe.
2. The basal vein of Rosenthal is formed by the confluence of the deep anterior and middle cerebral veins.
3. The basal vein of Rosenthal receives the following:
   a. The deep anterior cerebral vein (posterior orbitofrontal vein), which accompanies the anterior cerebral artery and drains the orbital surface of the frontal lobe and rostral portions of the corpus callosum and cingulate gyrus
   b. The deep middle cerebral vein, which is located in the depths of the Sylvian fissure and drains the insular cortex and the opercular cortices
   c. The inferior striate veins, which drain the ventral portions of the striatum, emerge through the anterior perforated substance, and empty into the deep middle cerebral vein
   d. Tributaries from the insula and the cerebral peduncles

The Great Cerebral Vein of Galen

1. The single great cerebral vein of Galen receives the paired internal cerebral veins, the paired basal veins of Rosenthal, the paired occipital veins, and the posterior callosal vein.
2. The paired occipital veins are superficial cerebral veins that drain the inferior and medial surfaces of the occipital lobe and adjacent parietal regions.
3. The posterior callosal vein drains the splenium of the corpus callosum and adjacent surfaces of the brain.
4. The great cerebral vein of Galen is a short vein that passes caudally beneath the splenium of the corpus callosum and empties into the straight venous sinus.

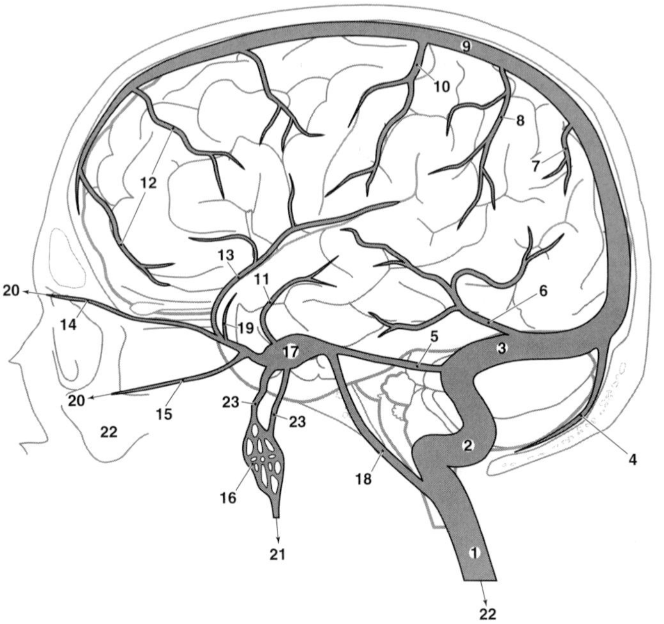

Figure 2U-1: Schematic of a "balanced-pattern" superficial venous system over the lateral aspect of the left cerebral hemisphere and the primary drainage.

1 Internal jugular vein
2 Sigmoid venous sinus
3 Transverse venous sinus
4 Occipital venous sinus
5 Superior petrous venous sinus
6 Inferior anastomotic vein of Labbé
7 Lateral occipital hemispheric vein(s)
8 Lateral parietal hemispheric vein(s)
9 Superior sagittal venous sinus
10 Superior anastomotic vein of Trolard
11 Temporal (uncal) vein
12 Lateral frontal hemispheric vein(s)
13 Superficial middle cerebral (Sylvian) vein
14 Superior ophthalmic vein
15 Inferior ophthalmic vein
16 Pterygoid venous plexus
17 Cavernous venous sinus
18 Inferior petrosal venous sinus
19 Sphenoparietal venous sinus
20 Drainage into facial venous system
21 Drainage into the deep facial vein
22 Drainage into the subclavian/brachiocephalic vein
23 Cavernous venous sinus/pterygoid venous plexus emissary veins

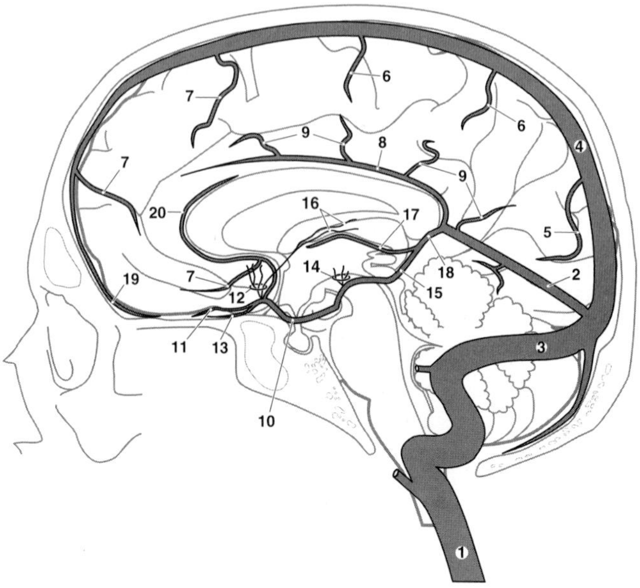

Figure 2U-2: Schematic of a "balanced-pattern" superficial cerebral venous system over the medial aspect of the left cerebral hemisphere and the primary drainage.

1 Internal jugular vein
2 Straight venous sinus
3 Transverse venous sinus
4 Superior sagittal venous sinus
5 Medial occipital hemispheric veins
6 Medial parietal hemispheric veins
7 Medial frontal hemispheric veins
8 Inferior sagittal venous sinus
9 Medial hemispheric veins draining into inferior sagittal venous sinus or straight venous sinus
10 Deep middle cerebral vein
11 Olfactory vein
12 Inferior striate vein(s)
13 Posterior frontoorbital vein
14 Inferior thalamic vein(s)
15 Basal vein of Rosenthal
16 Superior thalamic veins
17 Internal cerebral vein
18 Vein of Galen
19 Anterior frontoorbital vein
20 Anterior pericallosal vein

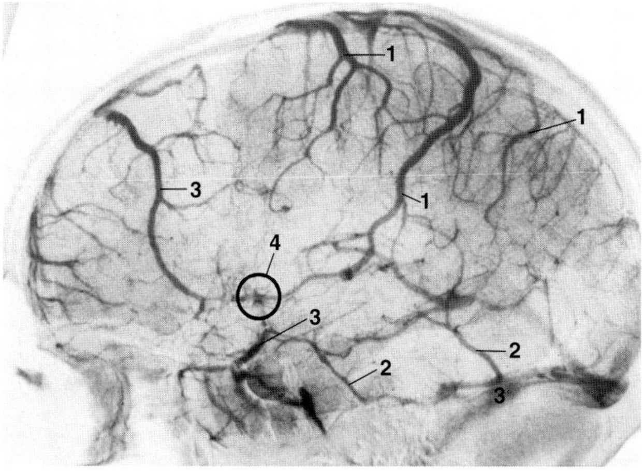

Figure 2U-3: Superficial cerebral veins. Cerebral angiogram in the venous phase in the lateral projection shows the superficial cerebral veins with balanced drainage.
1 Superior superficial cerebral veins
2 Inferior superficial cerebral veins
3 Superficial middle cerebral (Sylvian) vein
4 *Circle*: superficial venous watershed

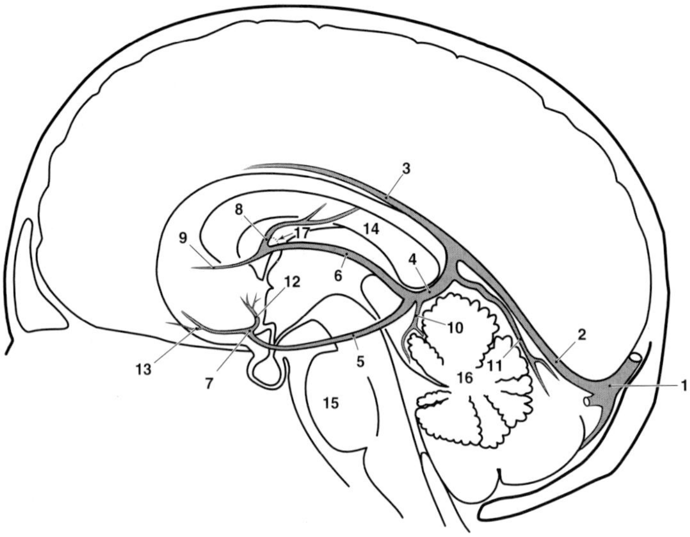

Figure 2U-4: Lateral schematic of the deep cerebral venous system.
1 Confluent venous sinus (torcular Herophili)
2 Straight venous sinus
3 Inferior sagittal venous sinus
4 Vein of Galen
5 Basal vein of Rosenthal
6 Internal cerebral vein
7 Deep middle cerebral vein
8 Thalamostriate vein
9 Anterior septal vein
10 Precentral cerebellar vein
11 Superior vermian vein
12 Inferior striate vein(s)
13 Deep anterior cerebral vein (posterior frontoorbital vein)
14 Corpus callosum
15 Pons
16 Cerebellum
17 Venous angle

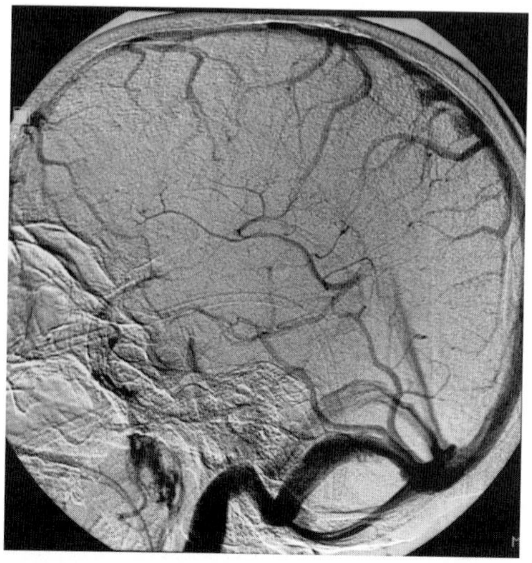

Figure 2U-5A: **Deep cerebral veins.** Subtraction film from the venous phase of a right internal carotid angiogram in the lateral projection, showing the relationship of the deep cerebral venous system to the other cerebral veins.

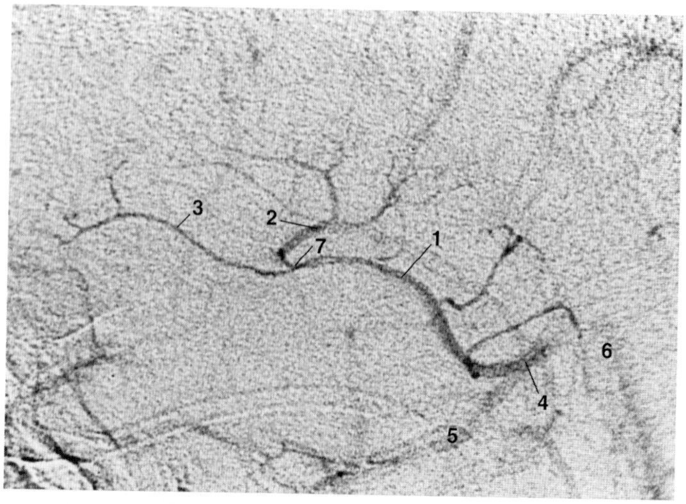

Figure 2U-5B: Deep cerebral veins. Magnified image from Fig. 2U-5A, showing the following.

1 Internal cerebral vein
2 Thalamostriate vein
3 Anterior septal vein
4 Vein of Galen
5 Basal vein of Rosenthal
6 Straight venous sinus
7 Venous angle

THE INFRATENTORIAL VEINS

1. The venous system of the posterior fossa, in particular and in general, is remarkably variable.
2. The veins of the posterior fossa primarily drain into three principal structures: the petrosal venous sinuses, the vein of Galen, and the dural venous sinuses bordering on the posterior fossa.

Venous Drainage of the Brain Stem

1. Inferior thalamic veins drain via the posterior perforated substance into small mesencephalic veins in the region of the interpeduncular fossa. These medullary veins, in turn, empty into the peduncular vein that runs around the lateral aspect of the peduncle to join the posterior mesencephalic vein.
2. The lateral mesencephalic (pontomesencephalic) vein runs longitudinally, connecting the posterior mesencephalic vein superiorly with the petrosal vein inferiorly.
3. The anterior pontomesencephalic vein is an unpaired midline structure that connects with the posterior mesencephalic vein superiorly and the anterior medullary vein inferiorly. It typically is linked with the petrosal vein by the transverse pontine vein.
4. The petrosal vein ultimately drains into the superior petrosal sinus.
5. The anterior medullary vein drains inferiorly into the anterior spinal vein at the junction of the medulla oblongata and the cervical spinal cord.
6. The lateral anterior medullary vein runs longitudinally along the lateral surface of the medulla oblongata.

Venous Drainage of the Cerebellum

The venous system of the cerebellum drains primarily in three directions: anteriorly, superiorly, and inferiorly.

Anterior Venous Drainage of the Cerebellum

1. Major cerebellar venous drainage occurs in the anterior direction through the brachial vein related to the brachium pontis and brachium conjunctivum. This vessel subsequently empties into the superior petrosal vein draining into the superior petrosal sinus.
2. The precentral cerebellar vein lies within the cerebellomesencephalic fissure and drains superiorly into the vein of Galen. This vessel receives superior hemispheric and vermian venous branches.
3. The vein of the lateral recess (vein of the cerebellomedullary fissure) lies within the cerebellomedullary fissure and drains small veins related to the inferior vermis, lower fourth ventricle, inferior cerebellar peduncle, and cerebellar tonsils. This vein subsequently drains into the superior petrosal vein.

Superior (Tentorial Surface) Drainage of the Cerebellum

1. The medial-superior surface of the cerebellum is drained by superior cerebellar hemispheric and superior vermian veins.
   a. The medial superior cerebellar hemispheric veins may drain into the superior petrosal vein, the superior vermian vein, and the brachial vein.
   b. The various medial superior vermian vein(s) drain into the vein of Galen, the straight venous sinus, and the torcular Herophili.
2. The lateral hemispheric cerebellar veins drain into the transverse venous sinus and torcular Herophili.

Inferior (Suboccipital) Drainage of the Cerebellum

1. The inferior surface is drained by the inferior cerebellar hemispheric and inferior vermian veins.
   a. The inferior hemispheric veins drain primarily into the transverse venous sinus. Drainage may also occur into the vein of the lateral recess.
   b. The inferior vermian veins drain the superior and inferior tonsillar veins, which subsequently anastomose directly with the superior vermian venous system.

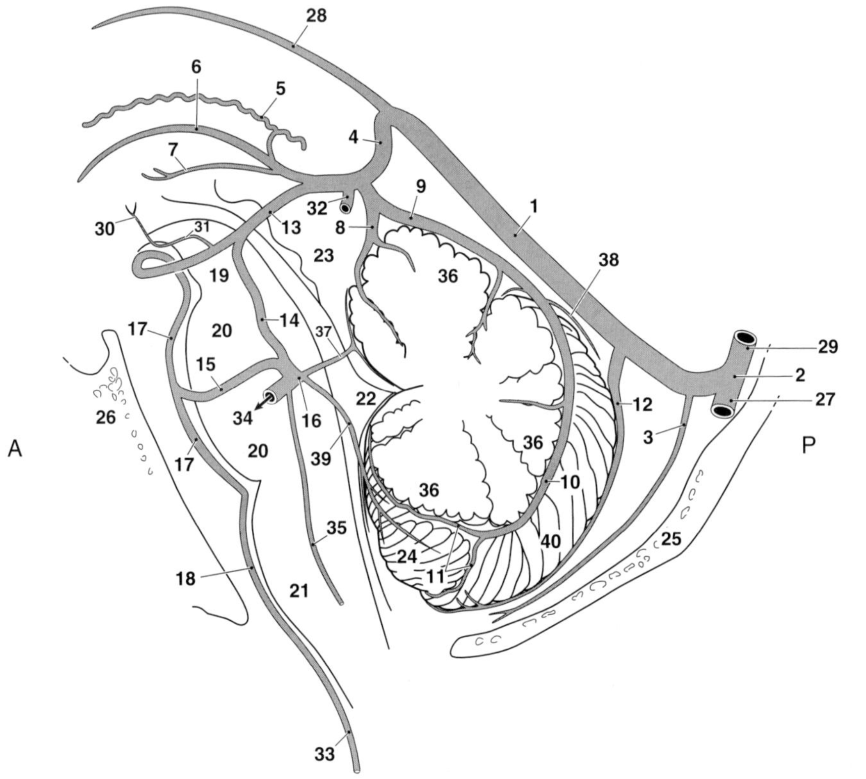

Figure 2U-6: Lateral schematic of the infratentorial (posterior fossa) veins. *A*, anterior; *P*, posterior.

1 Straight venous sinus
2 Confluent venous sinus (torcular Herophili)
3 Occipital venous sinus
4 Vein of Galen
5 Superior choroidal vein
6 Internal cerebral vein
7 Superior thalamic vein
8 Precentral cerebellar vein
9 Superior vermian vein
10 Inferior vermian vein
11 Tonsillar veins
12 Inferior hemispheric vein
13 Posterior mesencephalic vein
14 Lateral mesencephalic (pontomesencephalic) vein
15 Transverse pontine vein
16 Cut-edge superior petrosal vein (drains into superior petrosal sinus)
17 Anterior pontomesencephalic vein
18 Anterior medullary vein
19 Midbrain (mesencephalon)
20 Pons
21 Medulla oblongata
22 Fourth ventricle
23 Quadrigeminal cistern
24 Cerebellar tonsils
25 Occipital bone
26 Clivus
27 Cut edge of transverse venous sinus
28 Inferior sagittal venous sinus
29 Cut-edge superior sagittal venous sinus
30 Inferior thalamic veins
31 Peduncular vein
32 Cut edge of basal vein of Rosenthal
33 Anterior spinal vein
34 Final drainage into superior petrosal sinus
35 Lateral anterior medullary vein
36 Cerebellar vermis
37 Brachial vein
38 Superior hemispheric veins
39 Vein of the lateral recess (vein of the cerebellomedullary fissure)
40 Cerebellar hemisphere

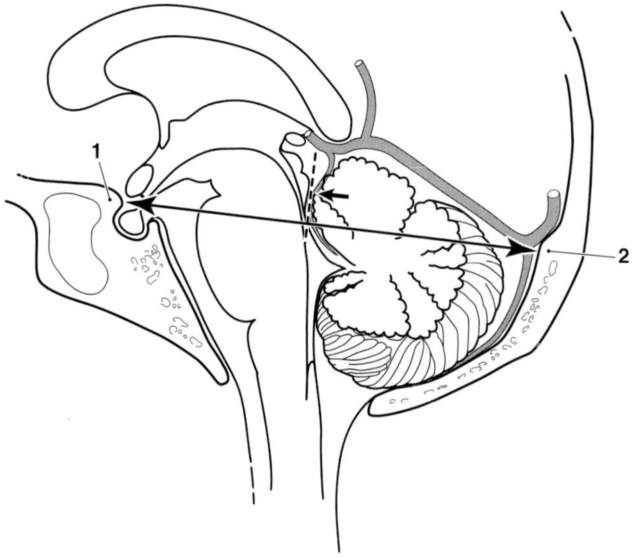

Figure 2U-7: Lateral schematic showing the determination of the colliculocentral point. The most anterior point of the precentral cerebellar vein, where the vein lies between the inferior colliculi and precentral lobe, is called the colliculocentral point (*arrow*). The perpendicular line (*dashed line*) from the colliculocentral point to a line (*solid line with double-ended arrowheads*) extending from the tuberculum sella *(1)* to the internal occipital protuberance *(2)* should be within 5% of the midpoint of that line when the colliculocentral point is displaced. It is used to locate posterior fossa masses on angiography.

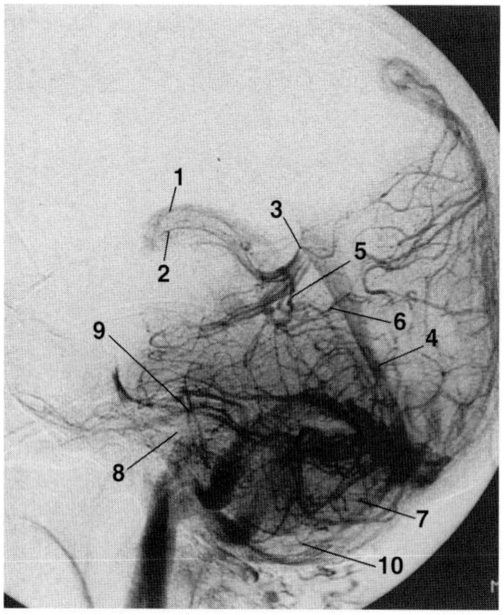

Figure 2U-8A: Infratentorial (posterior fossa) venous system. Venous phase of a right vertebral angiogram in the lateral projection, showing the posterior fossa venous system.

1 Superior choroidal veins
2 Internal cerebral vein
3 Vein of Galen
4 Straight venous sinus
5 Precentral cerebellar vein
6 Superior vermian vein
7 Inferior vermian vein
8 Anterior pontomesencephalic vein
9 Transverse pontine vein
10 Occipital venous sinus

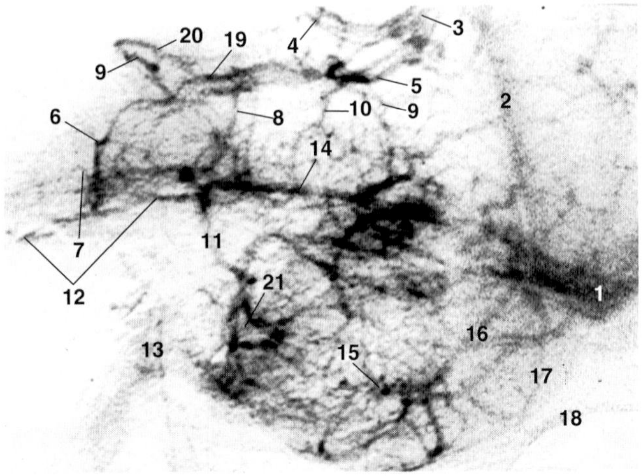

Figure 2U-8B: Venous phase of a magnified vertebral angiogram in the lateral projection, showing the cerebellar and brain stem venous system.

1 Torcular Herophili
2 Straight venous sinus
3 Proximal vein of Galen
4 Distal internal cerebral vein(s)
5 Posterior mesencephalic vein
6 Anterior pontomesencephalic vein
7 Transverse pontine vein(s)
8 Lateral mesencephalic (pontomesencephalic) vein
9 Superior vermian vein
10 Precentral cerebellar vein
11 Lateral anterior medullary vein
12 Drainage to superior petrosal venous sinus
13 Anterior medullary vein
14 Brachial vein
15 Tonsillar veins
16 Inferior vermian vein
17 Inferior hemispheric vein
18 Occipital venous sinus
19 Inferior thalamic vein
20 Peduncular vein
21 Vein of the lateral recess

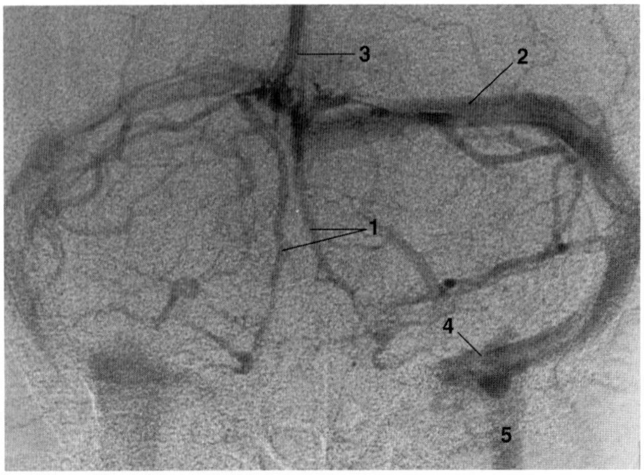

Figure 2U-8C: Venous phase of left vertebral angiogram in the frontal projection.

1 Inferior vermian veins
2 Transverse venous sinus
3 Straight venous sinus
4 Jugular bulb
5 Internal jugular vein

VENOUS VASCULAR TERRITORIES OF THE CEREBRUM

The venous vascular territories of the cerebrum are individually and laterally variable. Any systematization should serve only as a general guide.

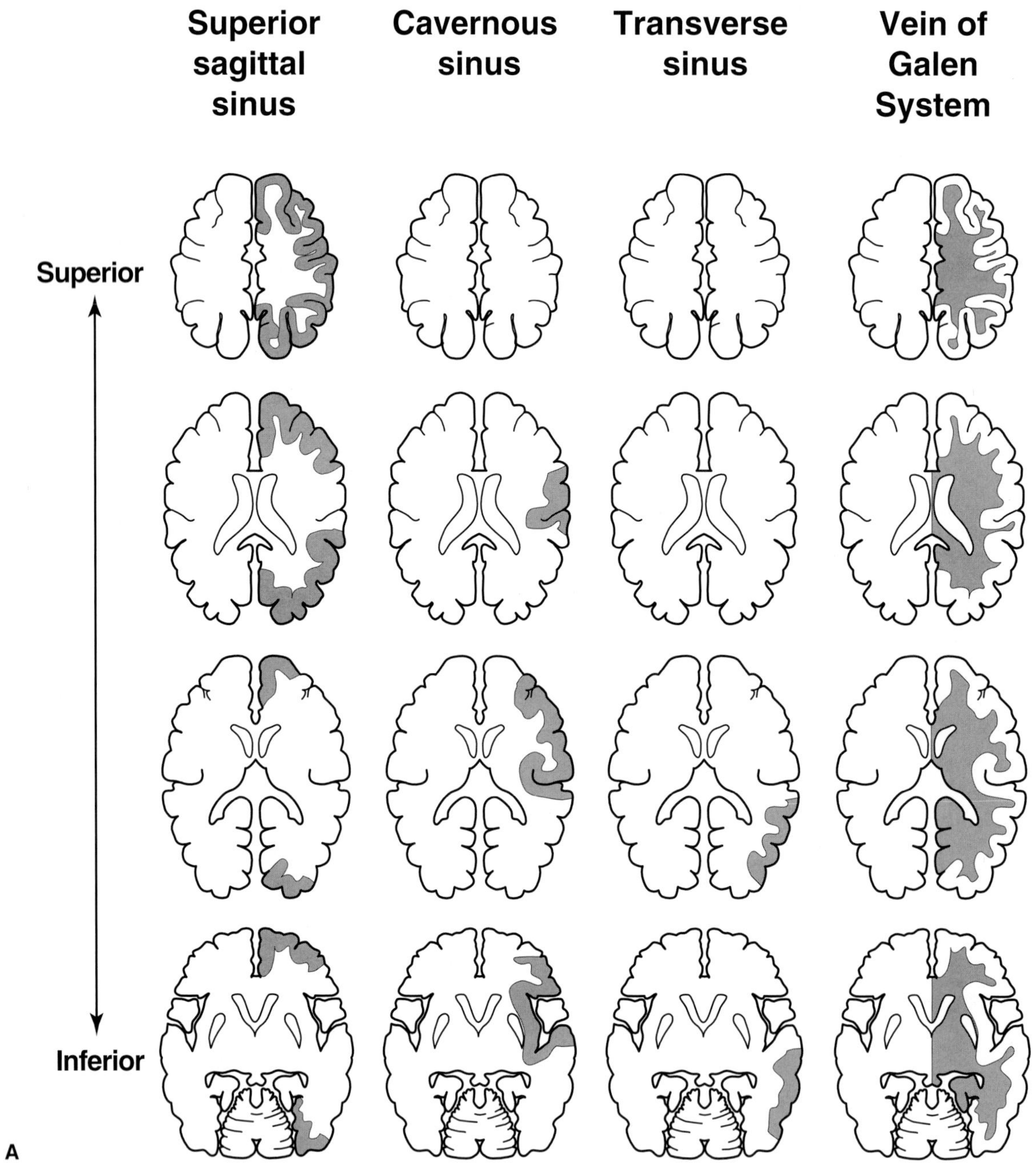

Figure 2U-9: Schematics of a generalization of the major cerebral venous territories. The individual and hemispheric variations of the venous drainage system explain why their systemization is similarly variable. These schematics should serve only as a general guide (**top to bottom:** superior to inferior). **A:** Axial plane. (*continued*)

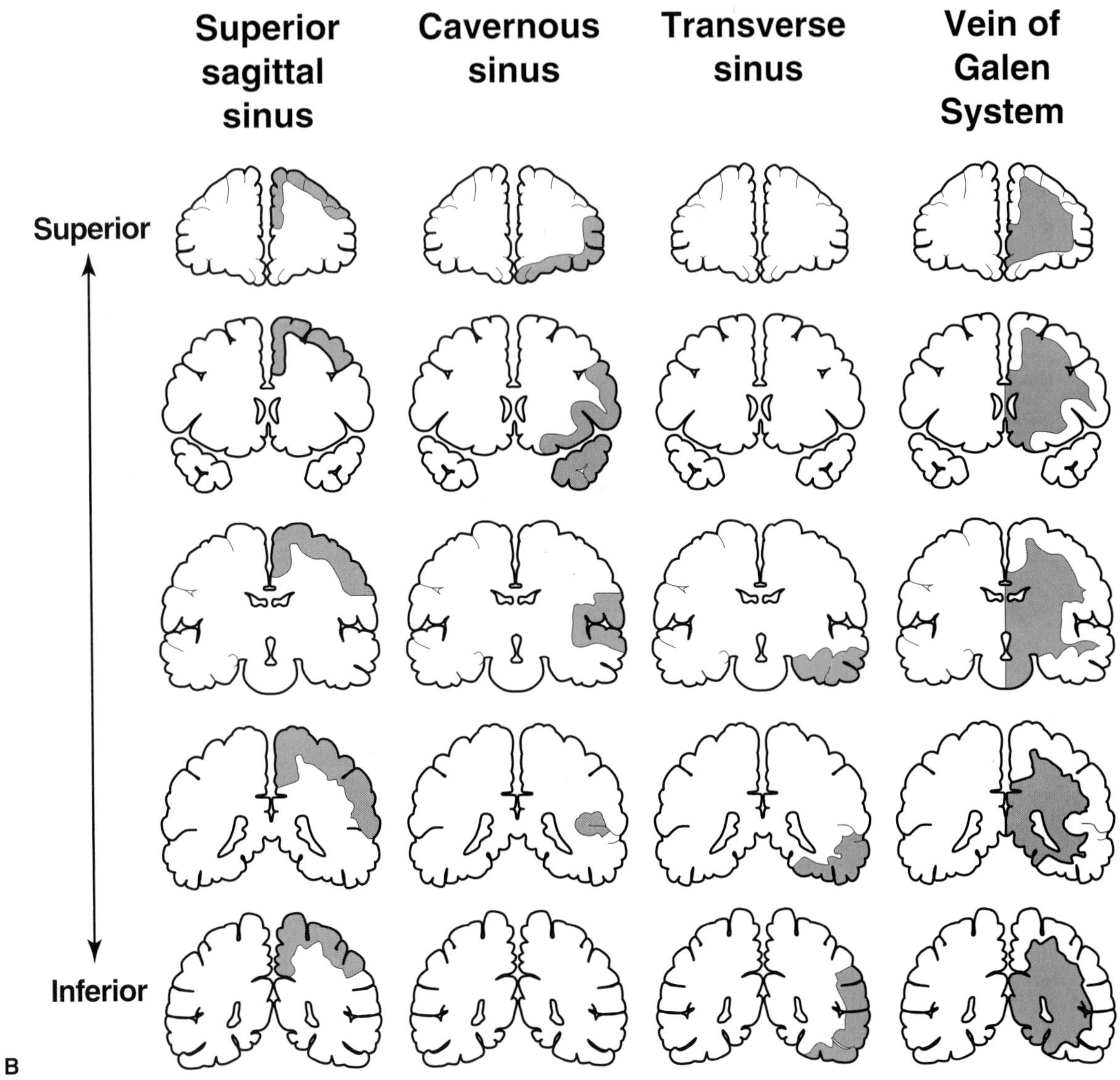

Figure 2U-9: B: Coronal plane.

THE DURAL VENOUS SINUSES

1. The cranial dural venous sinuses are located between and formed by the periosteal and meningeal layers of the cranial dura mater.
2. The dural venous sinuses are endothelium-lined, trabeculated venous channels that are devoid of valves.
3. The dural venous sinuses converge near the internal occipital protuberance to form the confluens sinuum or torcular Herophili. The torcular Herophili receives drainage from the occipital, straight, and superior sagittal venous sinuses as well as from some tentorial and cerebellar veins.
4. Arachnoid granulations draining cerebrospinal fluid from the subarachnoid space project into the lumina of the venous lacunae and dural venous sinuses.
5. The superficial veins of the scalp communicate with the dural venous sinuses via small emissary veins that perforate the skull.
6. The dural venous sinuses include the superior and inferior sagittal venous sinuses; the straight venous sinus; the occipital venous sinus; the paired transverse, sigmoid, cavernous, superior, and inferior petrosal venous sinuses; and the paired sphenopalatine venous sinuses.

The Superior Sagittal Venous Sinus

1. The superior sagittal venous sinus lies along the superior margin of the falx cerebri.
2. The superior sagittal venous sinus originates near the crista galli and extends in a posterior direction in the midline from the foramen cecum anteriorly to the torcular Herophili posteriorly.
3. The superior sagittal venous sinus increases in size as it passes posteriorly and caudally.
4. The superior sagittal venous sinus communicates anteriorly with the extracranial facial and nasal veins via emissary veins perforating the skull.

The Inferior Sagittal Venous Sinus

1. The inferior sagittal venous sinus runs posteriorly along the inferior free margin of the falx cerebri.
2. The inferior sagittal venous sinus is joined caudally by the great cerebral vein of Galen, and together they drain into the straight venous sinus.

The Straight Venous Sinus

1. The straight venous sinus is located at the junction of the falx cerebri and tentorium cerebelli.
2. The straight venous sinus receives drainage from the great cerebral vein of Galen and the inferior sagittal venous sinus and empties into the torcular Herophili.

The Occipital Venous Sinus

1. The occipital venous sinus is the smallest of the dural venous sinuses.
2. The occipital venous sinus begins at the margin of the foramen magnum.
3. The occipital sinus passes posteriorly and superiorly to drain into the torcular Herophili.
4. The occipital sinus may also communicate directly inferiorly with the extracranial internal jugular vein or vertebral venous plexus via emissary veins that perforate the skull.

The Paired Transverse Venous Sinuses

1. The two transverse venous sinuses arise from the torcular Herophili and pass laterally, forward, and downward along the inner table of the skull.
2. The two transverse venous sinuses course between the attachment of the leaves of the tentorium cerebelli to the calvarium.
3. The right transverse venous sinus is larger than the left in 25% of cases.
4. Each of the two transverse venous sinuses run in a groove or sulcus in the occipital bone; at the level of the petrous portion of the temporal bone, they drain into the paired sigmoid venous sinuses.
5. The transverse venous sinuses receive blood from the torcular Herophili and from veins of the cerebellum, the temporal lobes, and the occipital lobes draining into the transverse sinus along its course.

The Paired Sigmoid Venous Sinuses

1. The sigmoid venous sinus is the continuation of the transverse venous sinus at the occipitopetrosal junction.
2. The sigmoid venous sinus takes its name from its S shape.
3. The sigmoid venous sinus curves inferomedially toward the jugular foramen to drain into the internal jugular vein.

The Paired Cavernous Venous Sinuses

1. The two cavernous venous sinuses are paired, irregularly shaped, intercommunicating venous channels; the two lie on each side of the sella turcica.
2. On each side, the cavernous venous sinus encloses the internal carotid artery and the occulomotor, the trochlear, and the abducens cranial nerves (CN-III, CN-IV, CN-VI) in addition to the ophthalmic and maxillary divisions of the trigeminal cranial nerve (CN-V1, CN-V2).
3. The cavernous venous sinuses are connected with each other across the midline by the basal venous plexus lying on the posterior surface of the clivus and the small venous channels anterior and posterior to the hypophysis (the intercavernous venous sinuses).
4. Anteriorly, the ophthalmic veins (superior and inferior) and the sphenoparietal venous sinuses drain into the cavernous venous sinuses.
5. The cavernous venous sinuses drain in part into the internal jugular veins inferiorly via the paired inferior petrosal venous sinuses.
6. Posteriorly, the cavernous venous sinuses also communicate with the transverse venous sinuses, via the superior petrosal venous sinuses.
7. Fine venous emissary channels also connect the cavernous venous sinuses with the paired extracranial pterygoid venous plexi through the foramina ovale and other named and unnamed skull base foramina (foramina innominata).

See also Chapter 3, The Cavernous Venous Sinuses.

The Paired Superior Petrosal Venous Sinuses

1. The superior petrosal venous sinus extends from the cavernous venous sinus to the transverse venous sinus.
2. The superior petrosal venous sinus runs along the dorsal ridge of the petrous portion of the temporal bone at the dural attachment of the tentorium cerebelli.
3. In addition to the cavernous venous sinus, the superior petrosal venous sinus receives drainage from the veins of the pons, the upper medulla oblongata, the cerebellum, and the inner ear.

The Paired Inferior Petrosal Venous Sinuses

1. The paired inferior petrosal venous sinuses arise from the cavernous venous sinuses on each side.
2. Each inferior petrosal venous sinus penetrates the skull and drains into the proximal internal jugular vein.
3. The two inferior petrosal venous sinuses are interconnected rostrally via the basal venous plexus of the clivus (clival venous plexus) and the intercavernous venous sinuses.

The Paired Sphenopalatine Venous Sinuses

1. The sphenopalatine venous sinus is the anteroinferior continuation of the marginal venous sinus.
2. The sphenopalatine venous sinus receives drainage from the marginal venous sinus, some regional meningeal veins, and the superficial middle cerebral Sylvian vein.
3. The sphenopalatine venous sinus runs along the inner calvarial surface of the greater sphenoid wing to drain into the cavernous venous sinus.

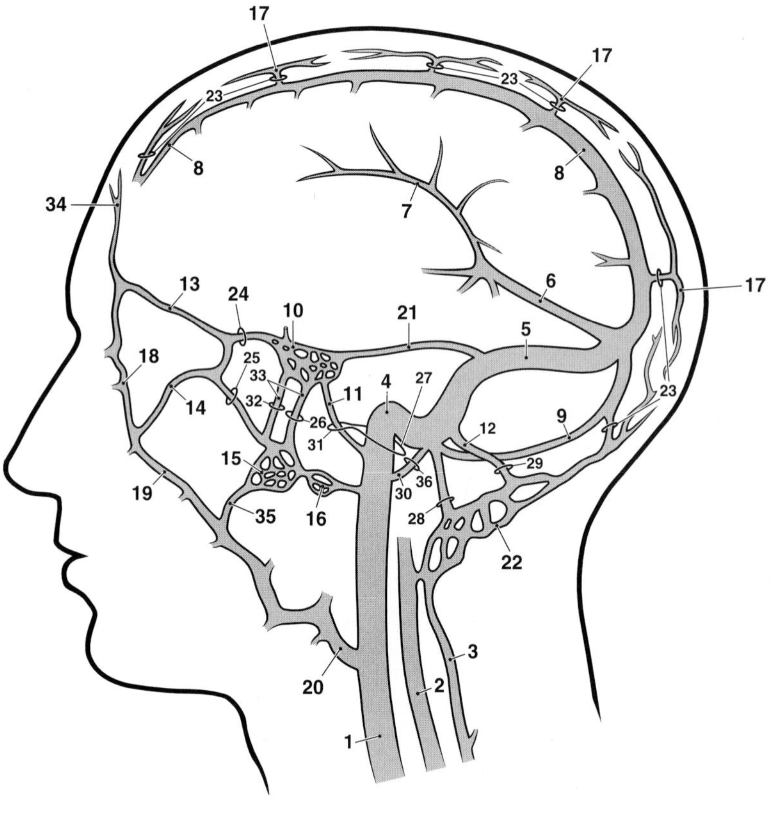

Figure 2U-10: Lateral schematic of the dural venous sinuses, craniofacial venous system, venous plexi, and cranial emissary veins.

1 Internal jugular vein
2 External jugular vein
3 Vertebral venous plexus
4 Sigmoid venous sinus
5 Transverse venous sinus
6 Straight venous sinus
7 Inferior sagittal venous sinus
8 Superior sagittal venous sinus
9 Occipital venous sinus
10 Cavernous venous sinus
11 Inferior petrosal venous sinus
12 Posterior condylar emissary vein
13 Superior ophthalmic vein
14 Inferior ophthalmic vein
15 Pterygoid venous plexus
16 Pharyngeal venous plexus
17 Scalp veins
18 Angular vein
19 Anterior facial vein
20 Common facial vein
21 Superior petrosal sinus
22 Suboccipital venous plexus
23 Frontal, parietal, and occipital calvarial emissary foramina
24 Superior orbital fissure
25 Inferior orbital fissure
26 Foramen ovale
27 Pars venosa of jugular foramen
28 Mastoid emissary venous foramen
29 Posterior condylar emissary venous foramen
30 Anterior condylar (hypoglossal) vein (plexus)
31 Pars nervosa of jugular foramen
32 Other unnamed emissary skull base foramina (foramen of Vesalius, foramen lacerum, foramina innominata)
33 Cavernous sinus–pterygoid plexus anastomotic veins
34 Supraorbital vein
35 Deep facial vein
36 Hypoglossal canal

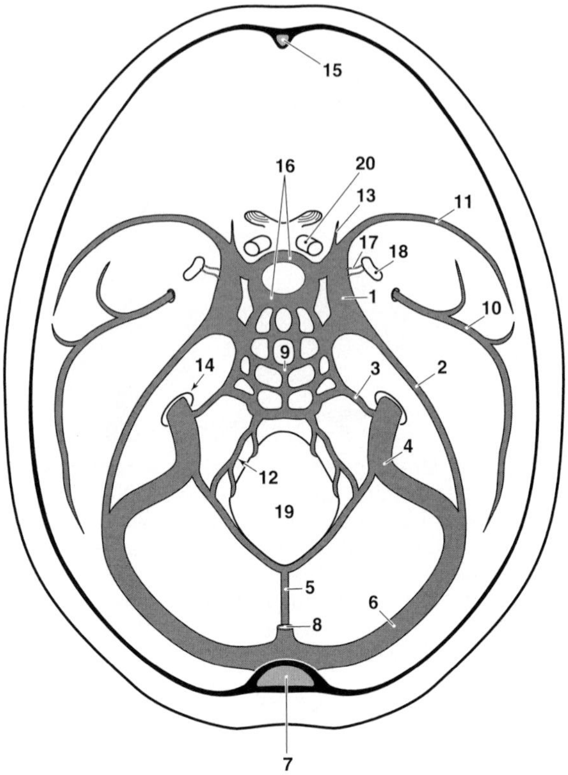

Figure 2U-11: Superior schematic of the veins of the skull base.

1 Cavernous venous sinus
2 Superior petrosal venous sinus
3 Inferior petrosal venous sinus
4 Sigmoid venous sinus
5 Occipital venous sinus
6 Transverse venous sinus
7 Confluence of venous sinuses (torcular Herophili)
8 Straight venous sinus (cut edge)
9 Clival venous plexus
10 Middle meningeal venous sinus
11 Sphenoparietal sinus
12 Marginal venous sinus
13 Superior ophthalmic vein (entering orbit)
14 Jugular foramen
15 Anterior extent of superior sagittal venous sinus
16 Anterior and posterior intercavernous venous sinuses
17 Emissary venous network connecting cavernous venous sinus with extracranial pterygoid venous plexus
18 Foramen ovale
19 Foramen magnum
20 Internal carotid artery (cut edge)

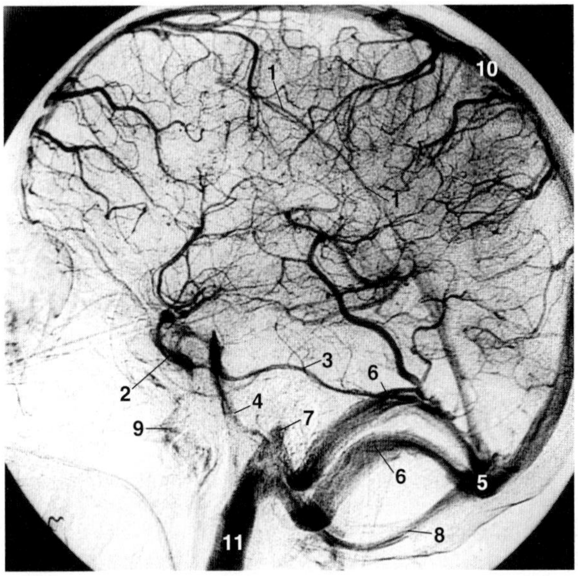

Figure 2U-12: Dural venous sinuses. Subtraction film from the venous phase of right internal carotid angiogram shows the dural venous sinuses and the drainage of the cavernous venous sinus.

1 Inferior sagittal venous sinus
2 Cavernous venous sinus
3 Superior petrosal venous sinus
4 Inferior petrosal venous sinus
5 Torcular Herophili
6 Transverse venous sinuses
7 Jugular bulb
8 Occipital venous sinus
9 Pterygoid venous plexus
10 Superior sagittal venous sinus
11 Internal jugular vein

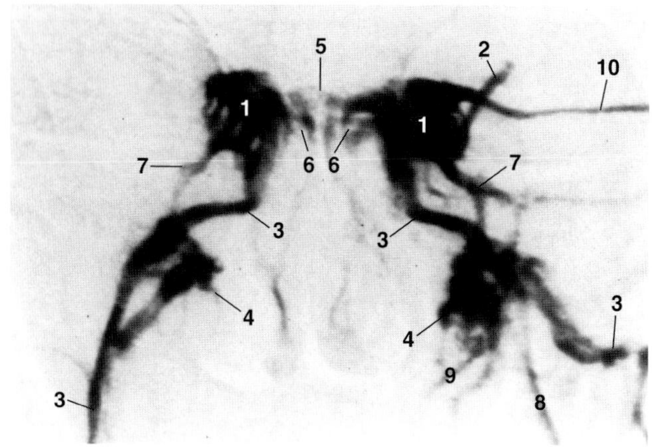

Figure 2U-13: The cavernous venous sinus. Venogram in the frontal projection, showing the cavernous venous sinus and some of its major drainage vessels.

1 Cavernous venous sinuses
2 Superior petrosal sinus
3 Inferior petrosal sinuses
4 Pterygoid venous plexi
5 Intercavernous venous plexus
6 Clival venous plexus
7 Emissary veins to pterygoid venous plexus
8 Deep facial vein
9 Vein draining to pharyngeal venous plexus
10 Sphenoparietal sinus

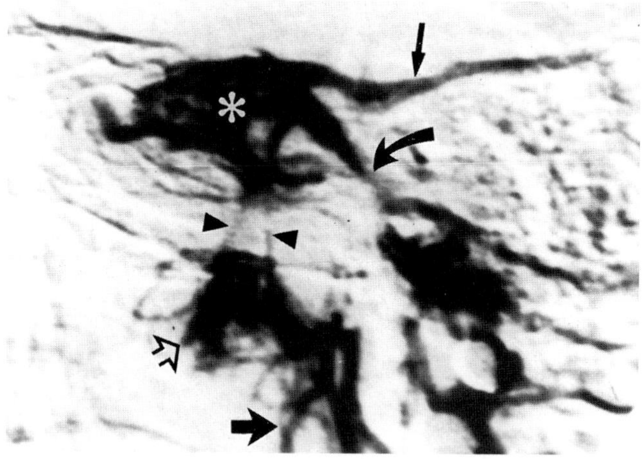

Figure 2U-14: Drainage of the cavernous venous sinuses. Venogram in the lateral projection showing the following: the cavernous venous sinus (*asterisk*), the superior petrosal venous sinus (*small straight arrow*), the inferior petrosal venous sinus (*curved arrow*), the pterygoid venous plexus (*open arrow*), emissary veins to pterygoid venous plexus (*arrowheads*), veins draining to the deep facial vein and pharyngeal venous plexus (*large straight arrow*).

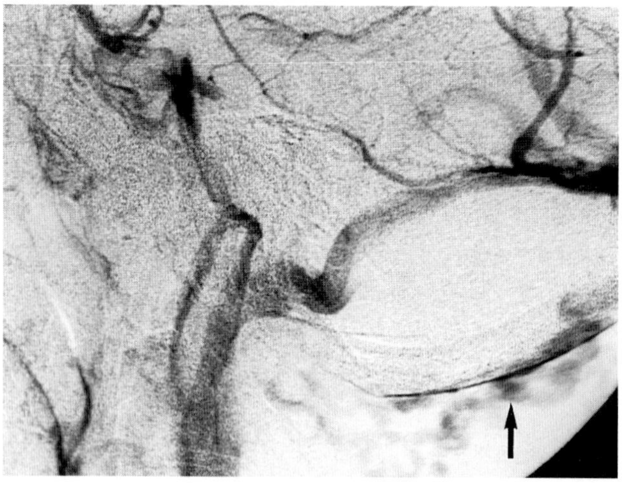

Figure 2U-15: Suboccipital venous plexus. Angiogram in the lateral projection in the venous phase, showing the suboccipital venous plexus (*arrow*).

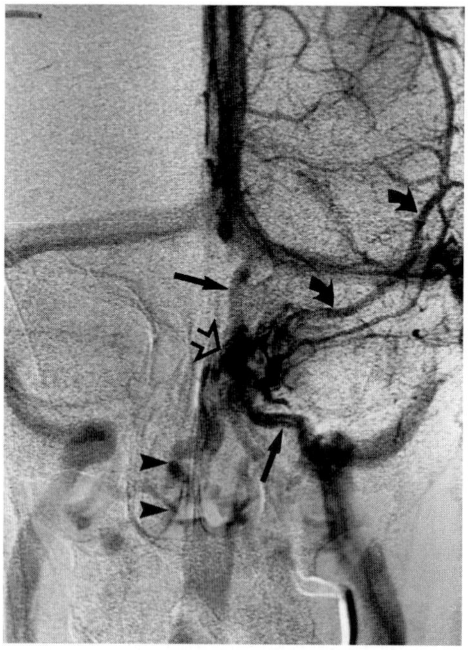

Figure 2U-16: Suboccipital venous plexus and vertebral veins. Angiogram in the frontal projection, showing the suboccipital venous plexus (*open arrow*) overlying the cavernous venous sinus. The occipital venous sinus (*solid straight arrows*) connecting the torcular Herophili with the sigmoid venous sinus, an occipital scalp vein (*curved arrows*), and the proximal vertebral veins (*arrowheads*) are also identified.

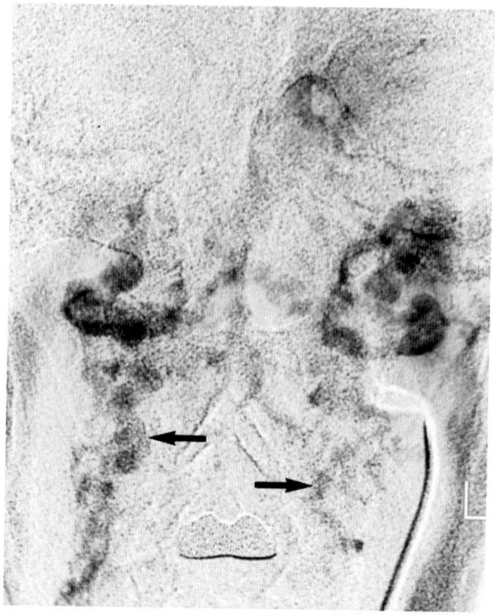

Figure 2U-17: Vertebral venous plexi. Angiogram in the frontal projection shows the vertebral venous plexi bilaterally (*arrows*).

THE MENINGEAL VEINS

In general, the meningeal veins accompany their respective meningeal arteries.

The Anterior Meningeal Vein(s)

The anterior meningeal vein joins the superficial middle cerebral (Sylvian) vein to become the sphenoparietal venous sinus, which, in turn, drains into the cavernous venous sinus.

The Middle Meningeal Vein(s)

1. The middle meningeal vein(s) communicate superiorly with the calvarial venous lacunae and the superior sagittal venous sinus.
2. Inferiorly, the many meningeal veins unite to form the frontal and parietal meningeal venous trunks that accompany the respective middle meningeal arterial branches.
3. The frontal meningeal venous trunk may drain into the pterygoid venous plexus via the foramen ovale, the sphenoparietal venous sinus, or the cavernous venous sinus.
4. The parietal meningeal venous trunk typically drains into the pterygoid venous plexus via the foramen spinosum.
5. In addition to meninges, the middle meningeal veins also drain or anastomose with small, unnamed inferior cerebral veins, diploic veins, and the superficial middle cerebral (Sylvian) vein.

The Posterior Meningeal Vein(s)

1. Little is documented regarding posterior meningeal venous drainage, given the fact that the posterior meningeal arterial supply is normally so irregular between individuals and sides.
2. Nevertheless, theoretically posterior meningeal venous drainage would logically be into veins emptying into the straight venous sinus, the transverse venous sinus, the occipital venous sinus, the sigmoid venous sinus, or one of the many posterior fossa emissary veins.

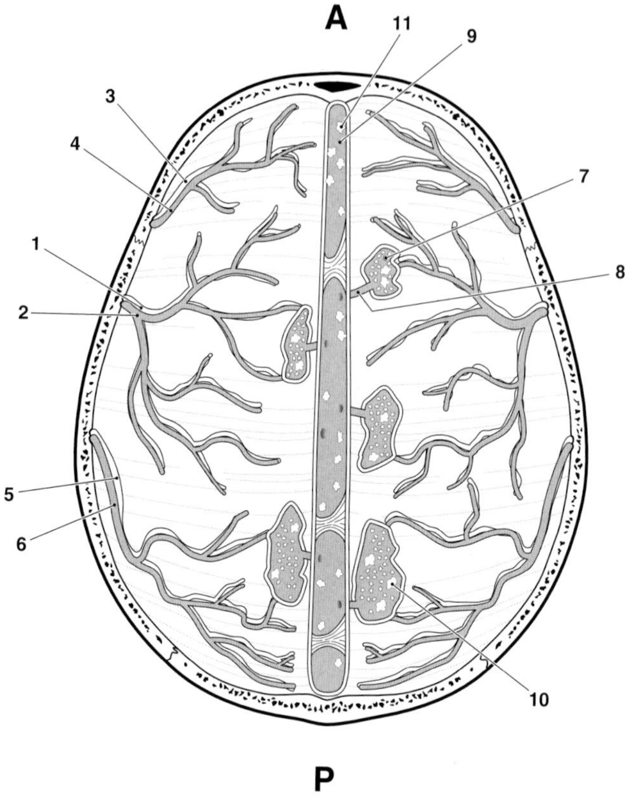

Figure 2U-18: Superior schematic of the meningeal arteries and veins. The skull has been removed. *A,* anterior; *P,* posterior.

1 Middle meningeal artery
2 Middle meningeal vein
3 Frontal meningeal artery
4 Frontal meningeal vein (trunk)
5 Parietal meningeal artery
6 Parietal meningeal vein (posterior parietal trunk)
7 Venous lacuna
8 Venous connection between venous lacuna and dural venous sinus
9 Superior sagittal venous sinus
10 Arachnoid granulation in venous lacuna
11 Arachnoid granulation in dural venous sinus

THE DIPLOIC VEINS

1. The calvarial veins are termed diploic veins.
2. The diploic veins run between the inner and outer tables of the skull.
3. The diploic veins drain outwardly into the scalp veins and inwardly into the meningeal veins and dural venous sinuses.
4. The diploic veins are devoid of valves.
5. Although irregular in anatomic configuration, typical diploic veins include the following.
   a. The frontal diploic vein drains into the supraorbital vein.
   b. The anterior temporal (parietal) diploic vein drains into the sphenoparietal venous sinus or anterior deep temporal vein.
   c. The posterior temporal (parietal) diploic vein drains into the transverse venous sinus.
   d. The occipital diploic vein drains either directly into the occipital vein(s) or into an occipital emissary vein and subsequently into an occipital vein.
   e. Many unnamed diploic veins drain into the venous lacunae connecting with the superior sagittal venous sinus.

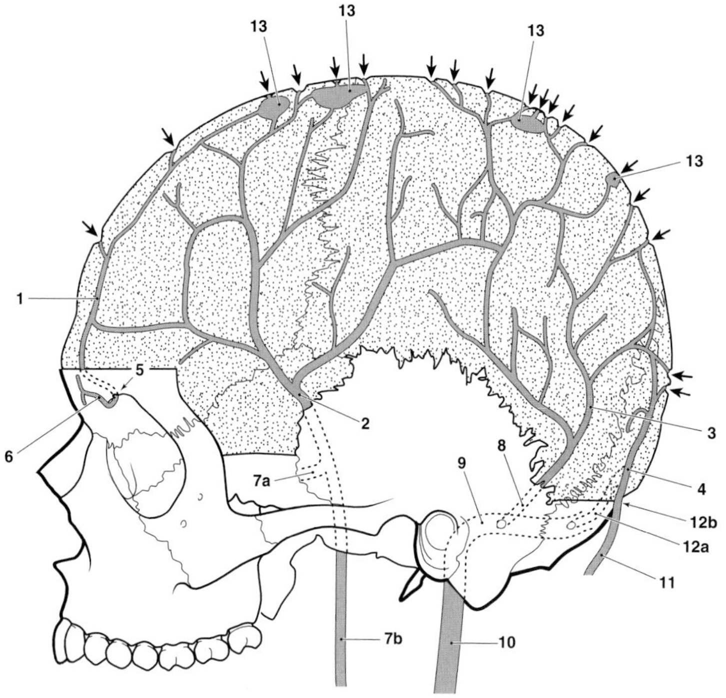

Figure 2U-19: Lateral schematic of the diploic veins. The outer cortex (table) of the skull has been partly removed (*arrows*: points of communication with contralateral side or the superior sagittal venous sinus).

1 Frontal diploic vein
2 Anterior temporal (parietal) diploic vein
3 Posterior temporal (parietal) diploic vein
4 Occipital diploic vein
5 Supraorbital notch/foramen or occipital emissary foramen
6 Supraorbital vein
7 To the sphenoparietal venous sinus (a) or anterior deep temporal vein (b)
8 Mastoid foramen
9 Transverse venous sinus
10 Internal jugular vein
11 Occipital vein
12 Occipital diploic vein draining to transverse sinus (a) or occipital vein (b)
13 Venous lacuna

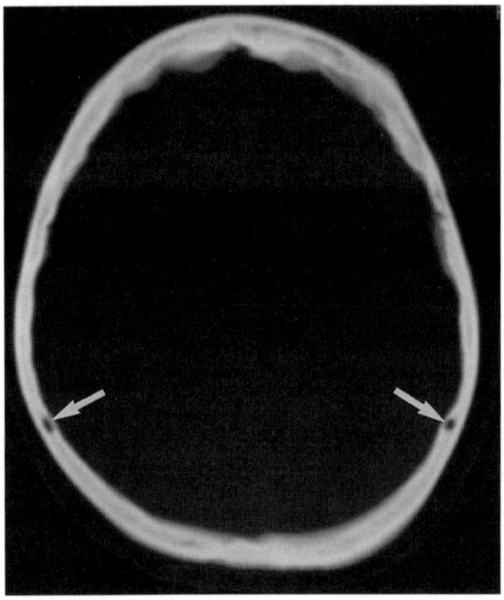

Figure 2U-20: Diploic veins. Axial CT image showing prominent calvarial diploic veins (*arrows*) in the parietal region bilaterally.

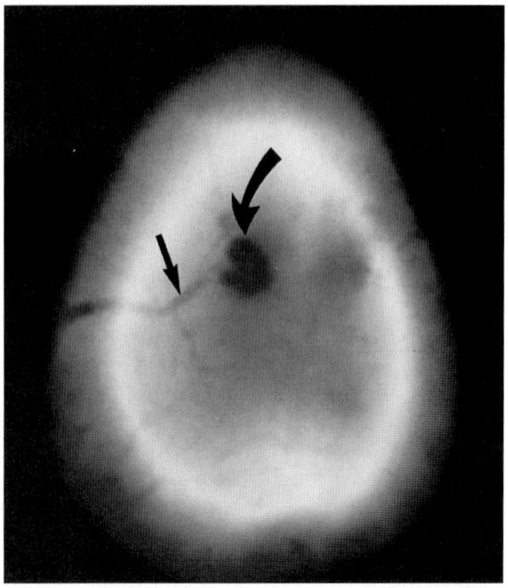

Figure 2U-21: Calvarial venous lake. Axial CT showing a well-demarcated, round, radiolucent venous lake in the calvarium (*curved arrow*) over the vertex, with a vascular channel (*straight arrow*) converging upon it.

THE CRANIAL EMISSARY VEINS, CANALS, AND FORAMINA

1. Cranial emissary veins interconnect the cranial dural venous sinuses and extracranial venous structures.
2. These interconnections take place via calvarial emissary canals and foramina.
3. Emissary veins, canals, and foramina of the skull are very variable between individuals and between sides in the same individuals.
4. Emissary veins include:
   a. The emissary vein of the foramen caecum connects the nasal veins with the anterior aspect of the superior sagittal venous sinus.
   b. The parietal emissary vein connects the veins of the scalp with the superior sagittal venous sinus in the parietal region.
   c. The occipital emissary vein connects the torcular Herophili with the occipital vein at the level of the occipital protuberance; the occipital diploic vein also drains into this emissary vein, when present.
   d. The occipital sinus emissary vein connects the occipital venous sinus with the vertebral venous plexus via the marginal venous sinus surrounding the foramen magnum.
   e. The mastoid emissary vein in the mastoid foramen connects the sigmoid venous sinus with the posterior auricular or occipital vein via the mastoid foramen in the posterior part of the mastoid part of the temporal bone.
   f. The posterior condylar emissary vein connects the sigmoid venous sinus with the internal jugular vein.
   g. The venous plexus (emissary vein) of the hypoglossal canal connects the sigmoid venous sinus with the internal jugular vein.
   h. The petrosquamous venous sinus (emissary vein) connects the transverse venous sinus with the external jugular vein.
   i. The ophthalmic veins (superior and inferior) connect the cavernous venous sinus with the facial veins.
   j. Central skull base emissary veins
      i. The internal carotid artery venous plexus (carotid emissary venous plexus) connects the cavernous venous sinus with the internal jugular vein via the carotid canal.
      ii. The venous plexus of the foramen ovale connects the cavernous venous sinus with the pterygoid venous plexus via the foramen ovale.
      iii. The venous plexus of the foramen lacerum connects the cavernous venous sinus with the pterygoid venous plexus via the foramen lacerum.
      iv. The emissary vein of the foramen of Vesalius (sphenoid emissary foramen) connects the cavernous venous sinus with the pterygoid venous plexus via the foramen of Vesalius (when present).
      v. There may be other unnamed emissary venous foramina in the skull base (i.e., foramina innominata).

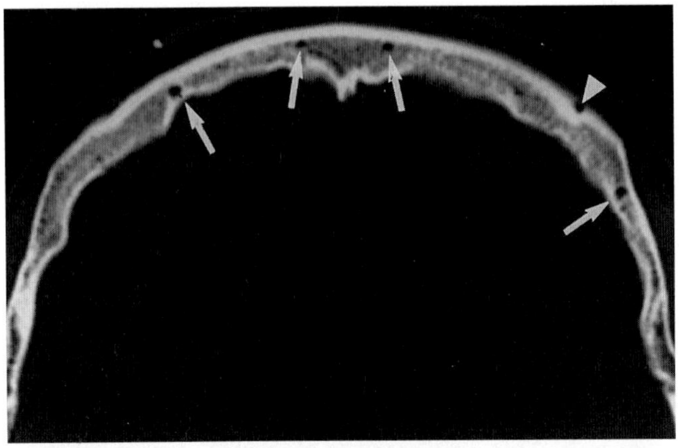

Figure 2U-22A: Diploic venous channels and emissary foramen. Axial CT image showing a frontal diploic venous channel (*arrows*) and a frontal emissary venous channel and foramen (*arrowhead*) on the left side.

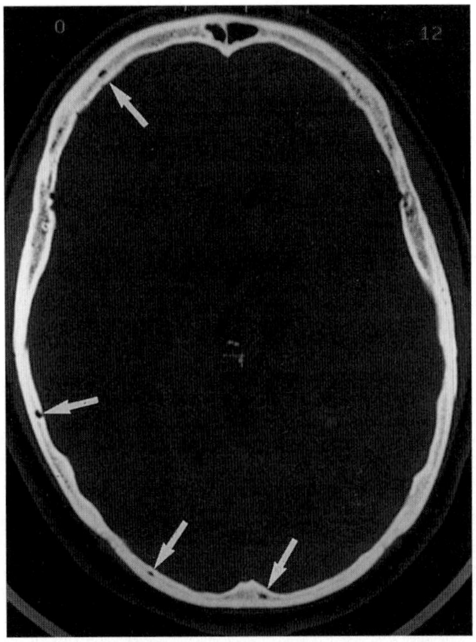

Figure 2U-22B: Diploic venous channels. Axial CT image showing frontal, parietal, and occipital diploic venous channels (*arrows*).

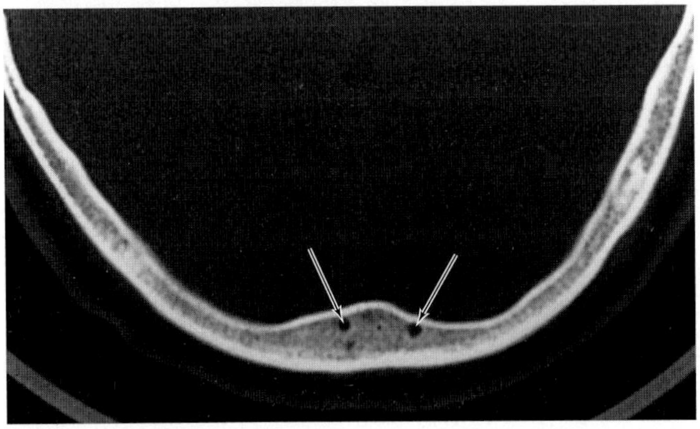

Figure 2U-22C: Axial CT image showing two diploic venous channels (*arrows*) in the occipital region.

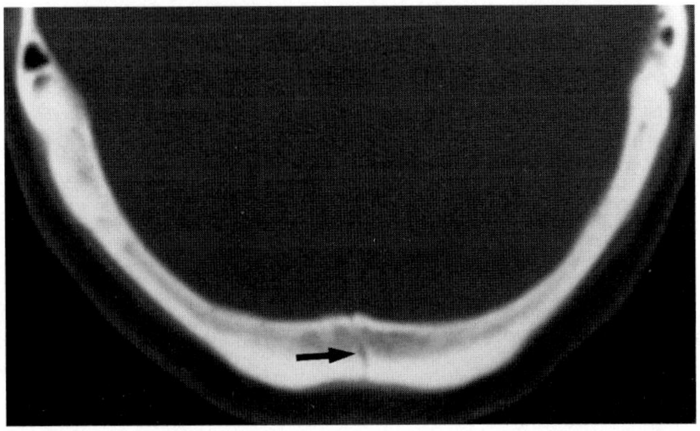

Figure 2U-22D: Magnified axial CT image showing a midline occipital diploic venous emissary channel (*arrow*).

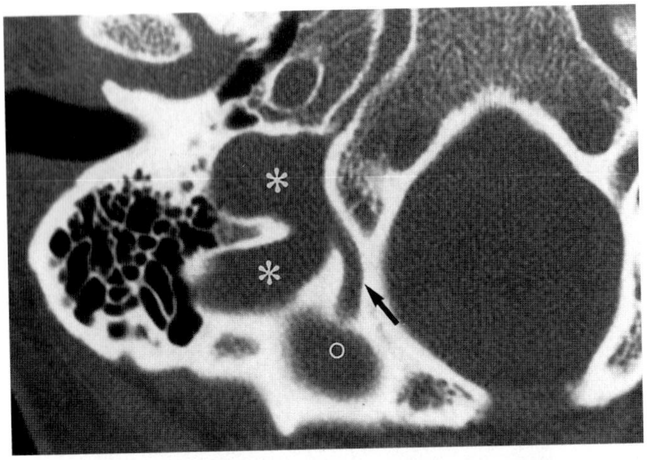

Figure 2U-23A: Posterior condylar emissary vein canal. Magnified axial CT image showing the condylar emissary vein canal on the right side (*arrow*) communicating directly with the sigmoid venous sinus canal (*asterisks*). The emissary foramen is in the occipital bone (*circle*).

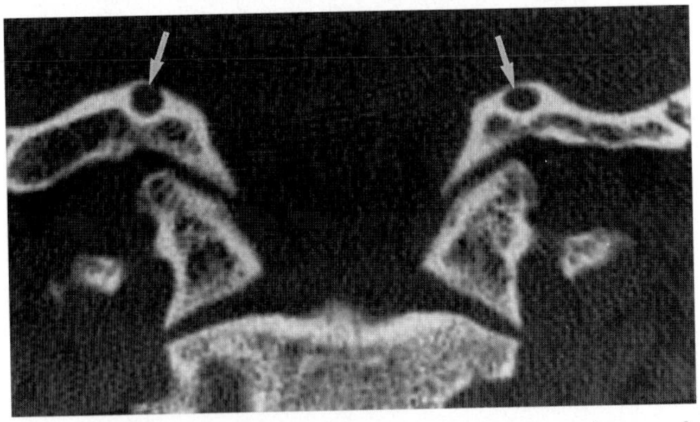

Figure 2U-23B: Posterior condylar emissary vein canal. CT image in the coronal plane showing the condylar emissary venous canals bilaterally (*arrows*).

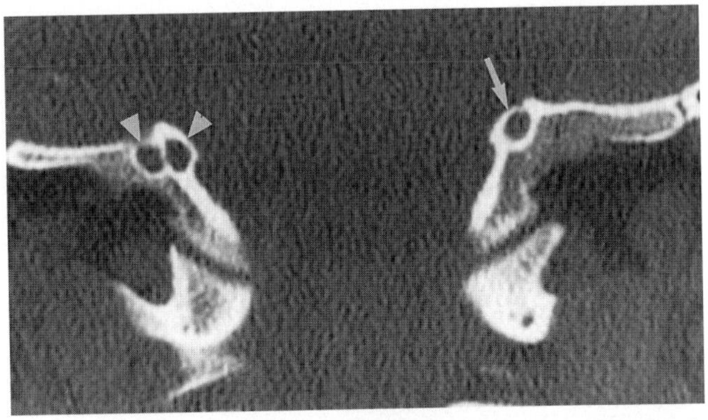

Figure 2U-23C: Posterior condylar emissary vein canal. Coronal CT image in a different patient, showing a single condylar emissary venous channel on the left (*arrow*) and a duplicated venous emissary channel on the right (*arrowheads*).

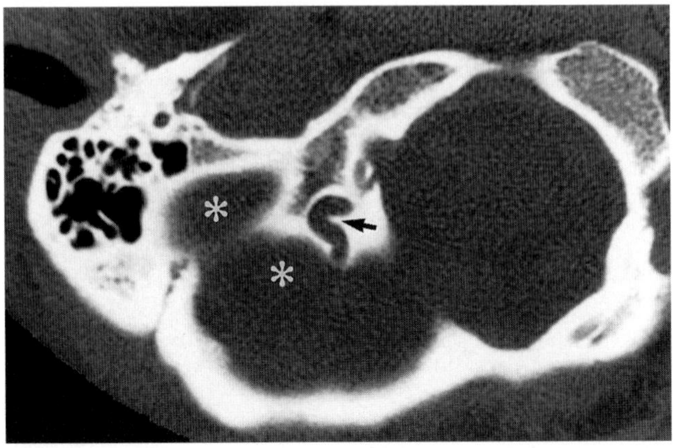

Figure 2U-24A: Posterior condylar vein draining into the hypoglossal canal. Magnified axial CT image showing the proximal part of the condylar emissary vein canal (*arrow*) communicating with the sigmoid venous sinus canal (*asterisks*).

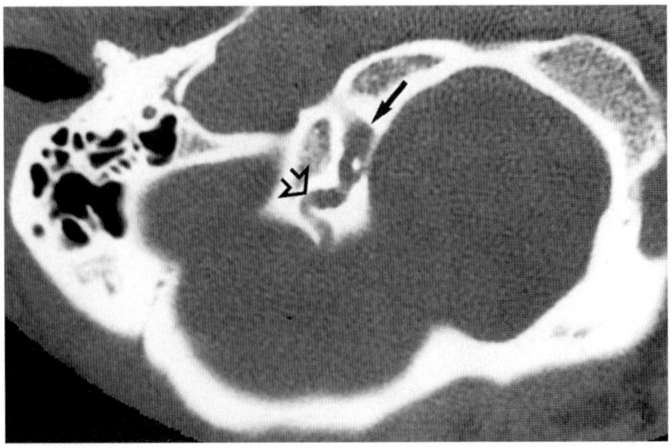

Figure 2U-24B: Posterior condylar vein draining into hypoglossal canal. Magnified CT image showing the condylar emissary vein canal (*open arrow*) draining into the hypoglossal canal (*solid arrow*).

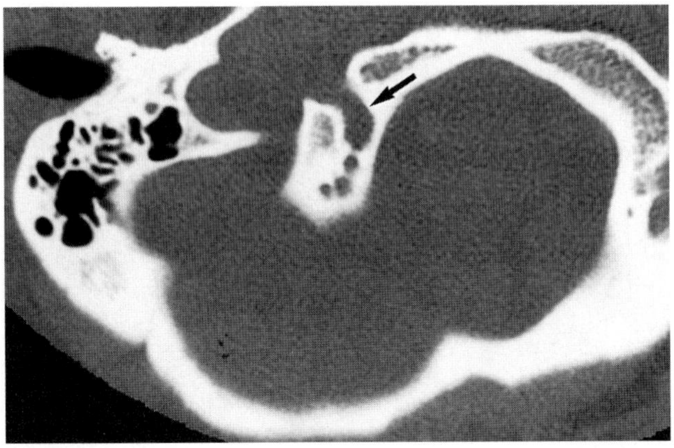

Figure 2U-24C: Posterior condylar vein draining into the hypoglossal canal. Magnified axial CT image showing the condylar emissary vein canal draining into the hypoglossal canal (*arrow*).

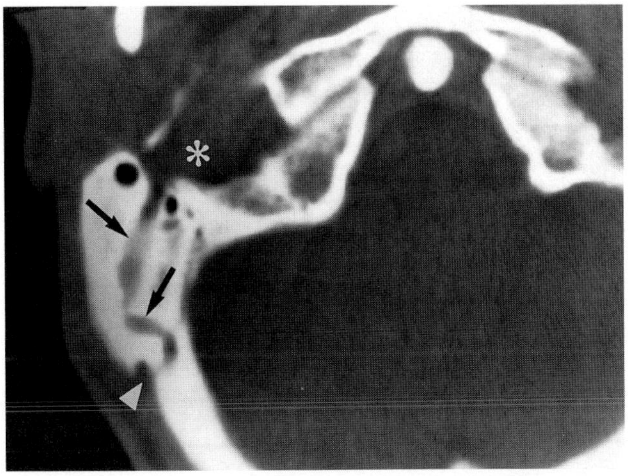

Figure 2U-25: Mastoid emissary venous channel and foramen. Axial CT showing the region of the inferior aspect of the jugular siphon (*asterisk*) and the mastoid emissary venous channel (*arrows*) and foramen (*arrowhead*) draining into the suboccipital venous plexus (not shown).

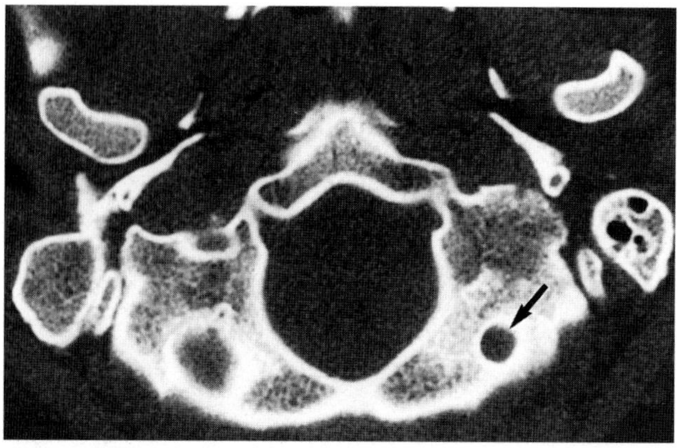

Figure 2U-26A: Occipital emissary vein foramen. Axial CT image in a different patient, showing the occipital emissary venous foramen (*arrow*) on the left side.

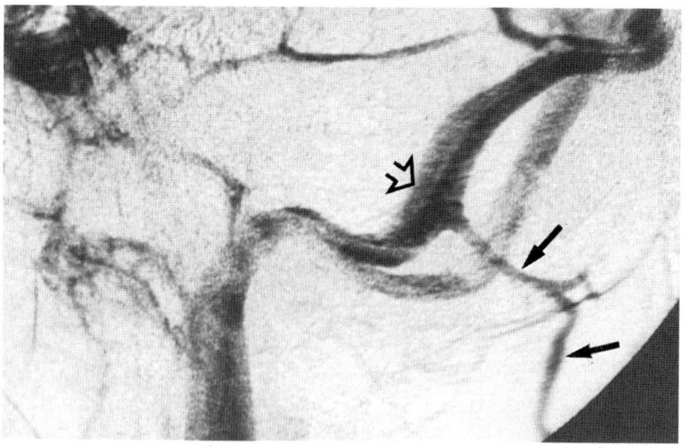

Figure 2U-26B: Occipital emissary vein. Venous phase of a right internal carotid angiogram in the lateral projection showing an occipital transcalvarial emissary vein (*solid arrows*) originating from the transverse venous sinus (*open arrow*).

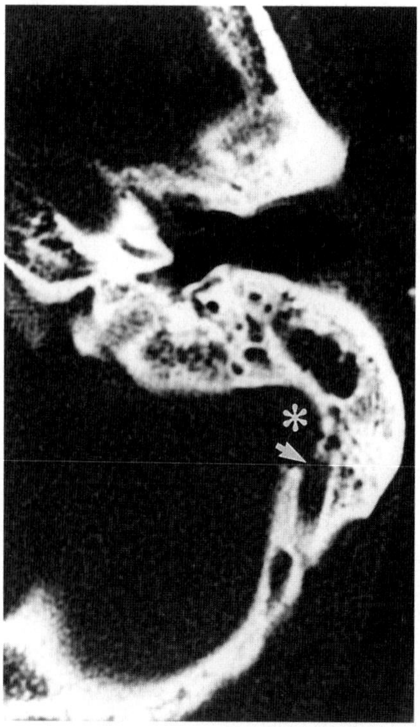

Figure 2U-26C: Occipital emissary vein foramen. Axial CT image showing a mastoid/occipital emissary venous canal (*arrow*) communicating with the sigmoid venous sinus (*asterisk*).

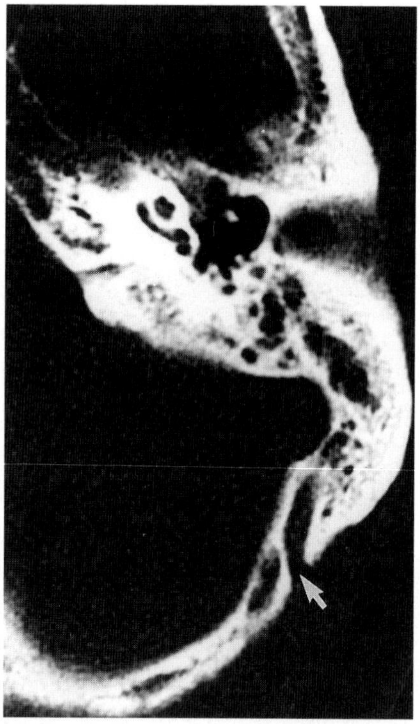

Figure 2U-26D: Occipital emissary vein canal. Axial CT image showing a mastoid/occipital emissary venous canal communicating exteriorly (*arrow*).

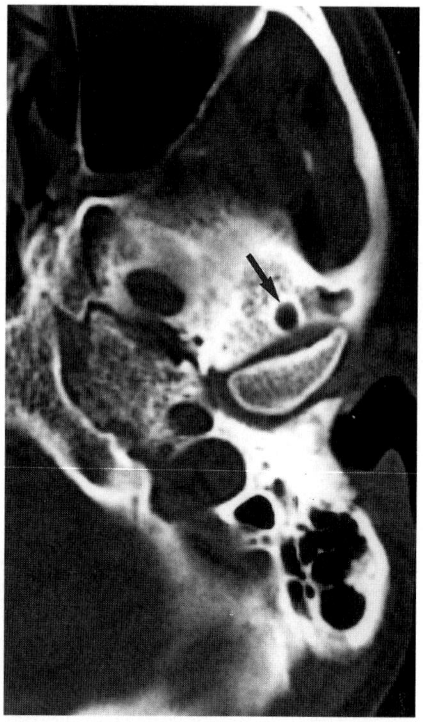

Figure 2U-26E: Accessory temporal emissary venous foramen. Axial CT image showing an accessory temporal emissary venous foramen (*arrow*) on the left side.

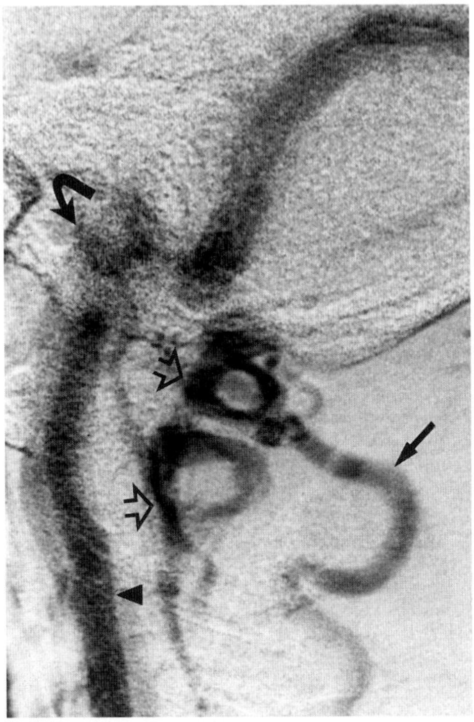

Figure 2U-27A: The suboccipital and vertebral venous plexi. Venous phase of a carotid arteriogram in the lateral projection, showing the suboccipital venous plexus (*straight arrow*), the sigmoid venous sinus (*curved arrow*), the internal jugular vein (*arrowhead*), and the vertebral venous plexus (*open arrows*).

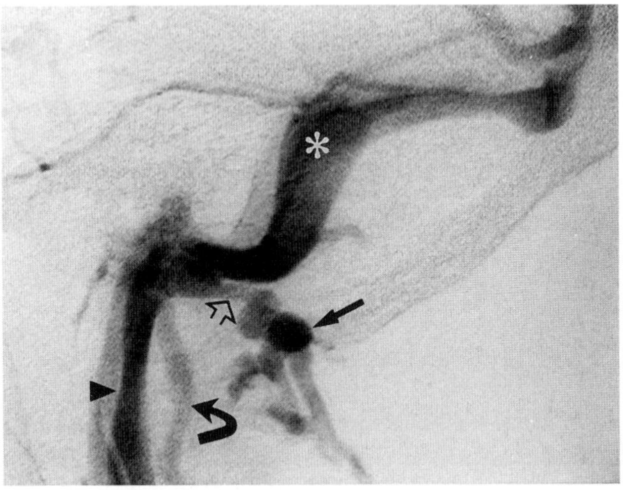

Figure 2U-27B: The suboccipital and vertebral venous plexi. Venous phase of right internal carotid arteriogram in the lateral projection in a different patient, showing the internal jugular vein(s) (*arrowhead*), the suboccipital venous plexus (*straight arrow*), the transverse venous sinus (*asterisk*), the condylar emissary vein (*open arrow*), and the vertebral venous plexus (*curved arrow*).

THE SCALP VEINS

1. The superficial temporal vein generally drains the widespread vascular territory supplied by the superficial temporal artery. The superficial temporal vein anastomoses with the supraorbital vein via its frontal tributaries and with the occipital vein via its parietal tributaries. It is also joined across the vertex via terminal anastomoses with the respective contralateral veins. The superficial temporal vein also drains the parotid veins, veins serving the temporomandibular joint, the anterior auricular veins, and the transverse facial vein. The superficial temporal vein runs inferiorly, typically to drain into either the retromandibular vein or the internal jugular vein.
2. The supratrochlear and supraorbital veins anastomose with the frontal tributaries of the superficial temporal vein and drain inferiorly into the angular vein. The angular vein also anastomoses with the superior ophthalmic vein. The angular vein drains inferiorly into the facial vein.
3. The occipital vein drains inferiorly into the deep cervical, suboccipital, or vertebral veins. It may also drain directly into the internal jugular vein, or it may join the posterior auricular and, subsequently, the external jugular veins. The occipital vein is linked with superior sagittal and transverse venous sinuses via calvarial (parietal and mastoid) emissary veins.
4. The posterior auricular vein anastomoses with the occipital and superficial temporal scalp veins and drains the parietooccipital region. The posterior auricular vein also receives tributaries from the deep aspect of the auricle and the stylomastoid region.
5. The retromandibular vein drains the superficial temporal vein. Inferiorly, the retromandibular vein branches: the posterior branch joins the posterior auricular vein to form the external jugular vein, and the anterior branch joins the facial vein proper.

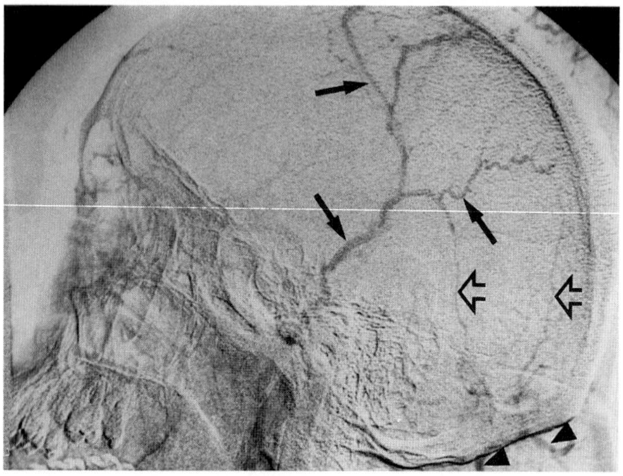

Figure 2U-28A: The scalp veins. Venous phase of carotid angiogram in the lateral projection showing the superficial temporal vein (*solid arrows*), the occipital veins (*open arrows*), and the suboccipital venous plexus (*arrowheads*).

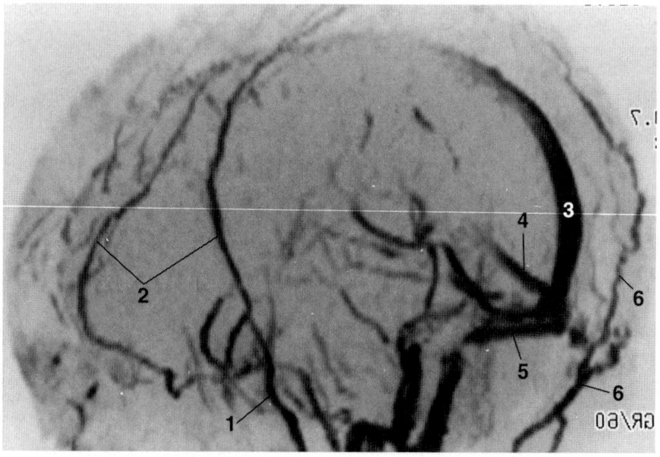

Figure 2U-28B: The scalp veins. Magnetic resonance venography in the lateral projection showing the superficial scalp veins.
1 Superficial temporal vein trunk
2 Superficial temporal vein branches
3 Superior sagittal venous sinus
4 Straight venous sinus
5 Transverse venous sinus
6 Occipital vein

THE VEINS OF THE FACE

1. The main trunk of the facial vein drains the angular vein (the uppermost segment of the facial vein), the pterygoid venous plexus via the deep facial vein, and other smaller facial veins (inferior palpebral, superior and inferior labial, buccinator, parotid, and masseteric veins above and submental, tonsillar, external palatine, and submandibular veins below), which, in turn, drain the maxillary and mandibular facial regions.
2. The main trunk of the facial vein drains inferiorly into the retromandibular vein or the internal jugular vein.
3. The facial vein has no valves.
4. The pterygoid venous plexus drains many deep veins, including the sphenopalatine, deep temporal, pterygoid, masseteric/buccal, dental, greater palatine, and middle meningeal veins. A tributary from the inferior ophthalmic vein may anastomose with the pterygoid venous plexus. Anastomoses in the pterygoid venous plexus also are present with the facial vein via the deep facial vein and with the cavernous venous sinus via many veins, including those emissary veins traversing the sphenoidal emissary foramen (foramen of Vesalius), the foramen ovale, and the foramen lacerum. The middle meningeal vein may also drain directly into the pterygoid venus plexus via diploic veins. The pterygoid venus plexus ultimately drains into the internal jugular vein, either directly or via the pharyngeal venous plexus.

THE VEINS OF THE NECK

1. The veins of the neck are markedly variable with regard to size and drainage pattern.
2. Relative to the deep cervical fascia, the veins of the neck are classified as either deep or superficial. Nevertheless, the superficial and deep venous system of the neck are usually anastomotically interconnected.
3. The main venous drainage of the neck is into two major veins: the internal jugular vein and the external jugular vein.

The Internal Jugular Veins

1. The paired internal jugular veins receive drainage from the skull, brain, superficial parts of the face, and all of the neck except the subcutaneous tissues and the areas drained by the vertebral veins.
2. The internal jugular vein runs deep in the neck in the carotid sheath together with the carotid artery and the vagus nerve (CN-X).
3. Each internal jugular vein originates at the base of the skull as a continuation of the sigmoid venous sinus on each side, after emerging from the jugular foramen.
4. The internal jugular vein drains into the subclavian vein; the two join to form the brachiocephalic vein at the level of the sternal end of the clavicle.
5. A slight dilation is seen near the origin of the internal jugular vein and another near the termination. The upper dilation is called the superior bulb of the internal jugular vein, and the lower one is termed the inferior bulb of the interal jugular vein.
6. A pair of opposed valves (i.e., two bicusp valves) are present craniad to the inferior bulb.
7. Each internal jugular vein receives drainage from the following.
   a. The inferior petrosal dural sinus, which leaves the skull through the anterior part of the jugular foramen (pars nervosa) and joins the internal jugular vein at the level of the superior bulb.
   b. The facial vein joins the anterior branch of the retromandibular vein as it emerges from the parotid gland and then drains into the internal jugular vein at the level of the greater cornu of the hyoid bone.
   c. The lingual veins are variable but usually follow two general patterns.

i. The dorsal lingual vein drains into the internal jugular vein at the level of the greater cornu of the hyoid bone.
ii. The deep lingual vein either joins a minor sublingual vein to form the vena comitans nervi hypoglossi, which drains directly into the internal jugular vein, or, alternatively, joins the facial or the lingual veins proper before draining into the internal jugular vein.

d. The pharyngeal veins arise from the pharyngeal venous plexus and usually drain directly into the internal jugular vein.
e. The superior thyroid vein usually accompanies the superior thyroid artery and receives drainage from the superior laryngeal and cricothyroid veins. The superior thyroid vein subsequently drains either directly into the internal jugular vein below the pharyngeal veins or, alternatively, into the facial vein before emptying into the internal jugular vein.
f. The middle thyroid vein(s) receives blood from the middle and lower part of the thyroid gland and drains directly into the internal jugular vein behind the superior belly of the omohyoid muscle.
g. The thoracic (left lymphatic) duct drains into the venous system near the union of the left subclavian and internal jugular veins; the right lymphatic duct drains into the venous system at the same site on the right side.

The External Jugular Veins

1. The paired external jugular veins lie superficially in the neck and drain parts of the cranial scalp and facial structures.
2. Each external jugular vein originates near the apex of the parotid gland and terminates in front of the scalenus anterior muscle in the posterior triangle of the neck.
3. The external jugular vein arises from the confluence of the posterior branch of the retromandibular vein and the posterior auricular vein.
4. The external jugular vein drains into the subclavian vein.
5. The external jugular vein has two paired sets of valves, one at the point of drainage into the subclavian vein and the other approximately 4 cm above the clavicle.
6. The external jugular vein receives drainage from the occipital vein, the superficial cervical vein, the posterior external jugular vein, the suprascapular vein, and the anterior jugular vein.

Neck Veins Primarily Related to the Cervical Spine

The Vertebral Veins

1. The paired vertebral veins receive drainage from the small tributaries of the internal vertebral venous plexi, which leave the central spinal canal above the posterior arch of the atlas, and small veins draining the regional deep muscular structures of the upper posterior neck. The vertebral veins usually anastomose superiorly.
2. Each vertebral vein enters the foramen transversarium of the atlas on its respective side and forms a plexus around the vertebral artery. It subsequently descends through successive transverse vertebral foramina and emerges inferiorly from the sixth cervical foramen transversarium.
3. The vertebral vein on each side drains inferiorly into the brachiocephalic vein of the same side.
4. The vertebral vein has a paired valve at its opening into the brachiocephalic vein.

The Anterior Vertebral Vein

The anterior vertebral vein originates in a plexus around the upper cervical transverse processes and descends between the attachments of the scalenus anterior and longus capitis to drain into the distal (inferior) end of the vertebral vein.

The Deep Cervical Vein

1. The deep cervical vein originates in the suboccipital region from communicating venous branches of the occipital and suboccipital muscles and small venous plexi immediately surrounding the cervical spine.
2. The deep cervical vein then descends to pass between the transverse process of the seventh cervical vertebra and the neck of the first rib to drain into the lower part of the vertebral vein.

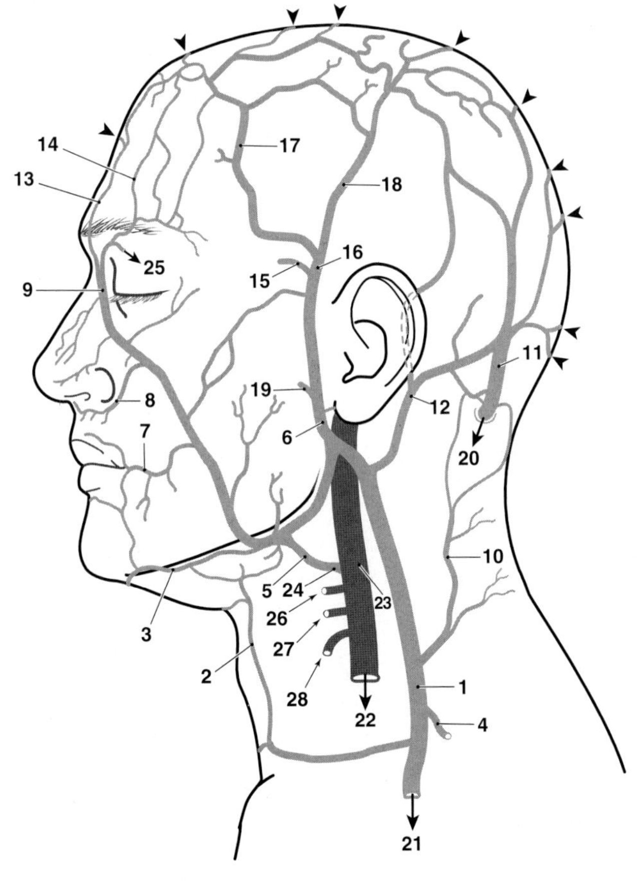

Figure 2U-29: Lateral schematic of the superficial veins of the head and neck (*arrowheads:* anastomoses with contralateral superficial veins across midline).

1 External jugular vein
2 Anterior jugular vein
3 Submental vein
4 Transverse cervical vein
5 Facial veins, lower end
6 Retromandibular vein
7 Inferior labial vein
8 Superior labial vein
9 Angular vein (upper facial vein)
10 Posterior external jugular vein
11 Occipital vein (may receive emissary branches from transverse or superior sagittal venous sinuses and occipital diploic vein[s])
12 Posterior auricular vein (sometimes anastomosing with occipital vein)
13 Supratrochlear vein
14 Supraorbital vein
15 Middle temporal vein trunk
16 Superficial temporal vein
17 Frontal branch of superficial temporal vein
18 Parietal branch of superficial temporal vein
19 Maxillary vein trunk
20 Drainage to deep cervical or occipital/vertebral venous plexus
21 Drainage to subclavian vein
22 Drainage to subclavian vein to form the brachiocephalic vein
23 Internal jugular vein
24 Anastomosis of facial vein with the internal jugular vein
25 Venous branch traversing supraorbital notch and joining the superior ophthalmic vein and the frontal diploic vein
26 Lingual vein
27 Pharyngeal vein
28 Superior thyroid vein

VENOUS DRAINAGE OF THE CRANIUM VARIANTS

- Variants in territorial venous drainage
- Variants in terminal venous drainage
- Venous (specific vein) aplasia/hypoplasia
- Venous (specific vein) hyperplasia
- Venous duplication/triplication
- Venous ectasia
- Venous diverticulum
- Venous varix
- Variants in venous trunk bifurcation/trifurcation

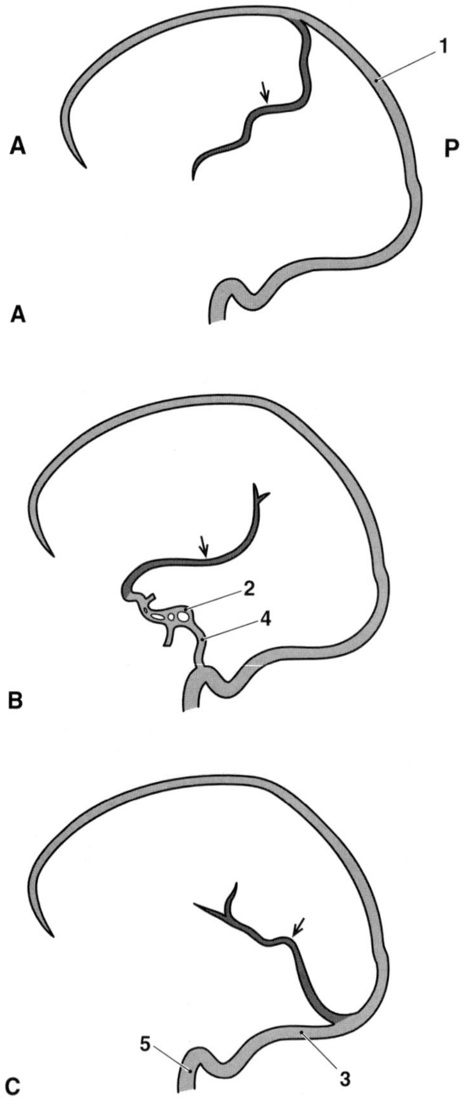

Figure 2U-30: Lateral schematic of the major superficial anastomotic cerebral veins over the lateral surface of the cerebral hemisphere. **A:** Vein of Trolard (*arrow*). **B:** Superficial middle cerebral (Sylvian) vein (*arrow*). **C:** Vein of Labbé (*arrow*). *A,* anterior; *P,* posterior.

1 Superior sagittal venous sinus
2 Cavernous venous sinus
3 Transverse venous sinus
4 Inferior petrosal venous sinus
5 Internal jugular vein

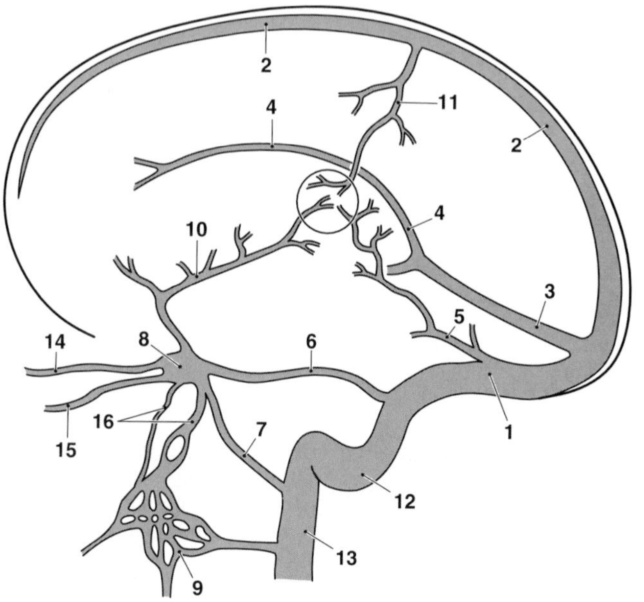

Figure 2U-31: Lateral schematic of the anastomoses of the superficial cerebral veins (venous watershed indicated by *open circle*).

1 Transverse venous sinus
2 Superior sagittal venous sinus
3 Straight venous sinus
4 Inferior sagittal venous sinus
5 Vein of Labbé
6 Superior petrosal venous sinus
7 Inferior petrosal venous sinus
8 Cavernous venous sinus
9 Pterygoid venous plexus
10 Superficial middle cerebral (Sylvian) vein
11 Vein of Trolard
12 Sigmoid venous sinus
13 Internal jugular vein
14 Superior ophthalmic vein
15 Inferior ophthalmic vein
16 Anastomotic veins between the cavernous venous sinus and the pterygoid plexus

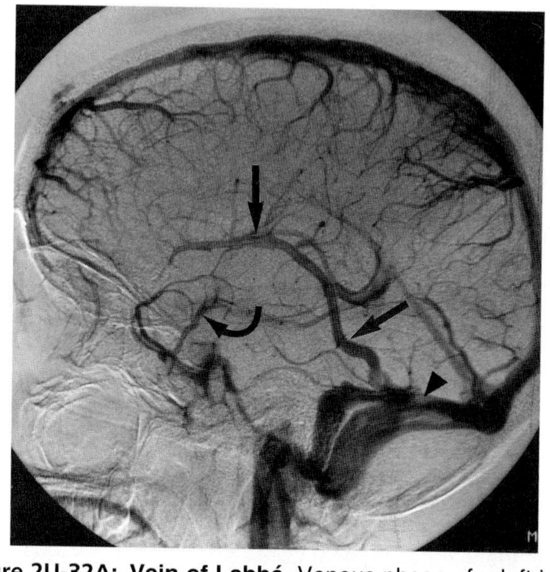

Figure 2U-32A: Vein of Labbé. Venous phase of a left internal carotid angiogram in the lateral projection, showing a prominent vein of Labbé (*solid arrows*), the superior sagittal venous sinus (*open arrow*), the transverse venous sinus (*arrowhead*), and the superficial middle cerebral (Sylvian) vein (*curved arrow*).

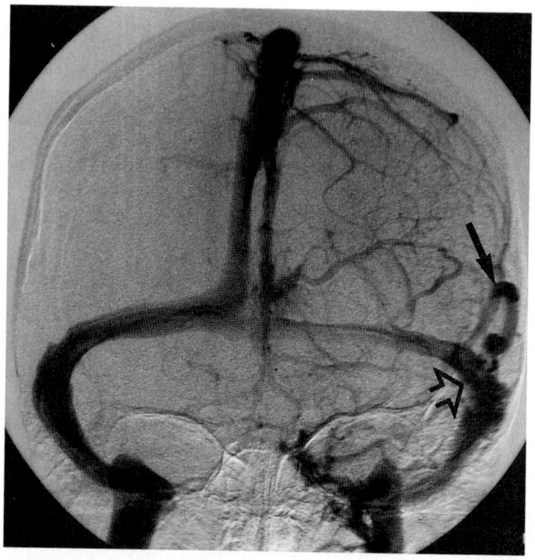

Figure 2U-32B: Vein of Labbé. Venous phase of a left internal carotid angiogram in the lateral projection shows the prominent vein of Labbé (*solid arrow*) draining into the transverse venous sinus (*open arrow*).

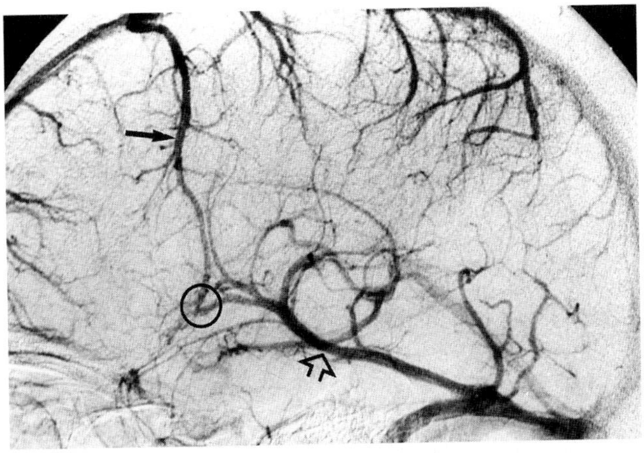

Figure 2U-33A: Superficial venous anastomoses. Venous phase of a common carotid angiogram in the lateral projection, showing an anastomosis (*circle*) between the superficial anastomotic veins of Trolard (*solid arrow*) and Labbé (*open arrow*). The superficial middle cerebral (Sylvian) vein is hypoplastic.

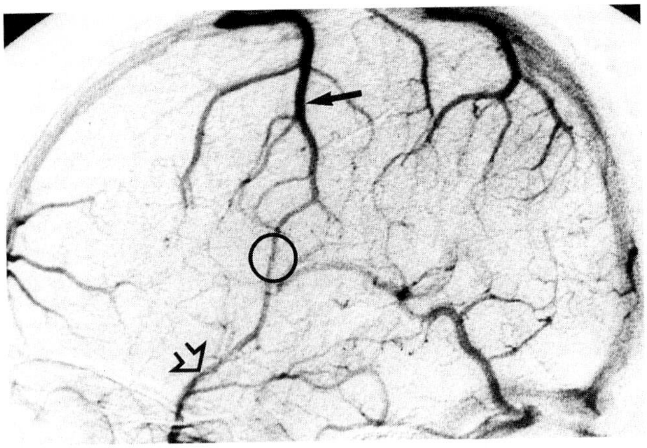

Figure 2U-33B: Superficial venous anastomoses. Venous phase of carotid angiogram in the lateral projection, showing anastomosis (*circle*) between the superior anastomotic vein of Trolard (*solid arrow*) and the superficial middle cerebral (Sylvian) vein (*open arrow*).

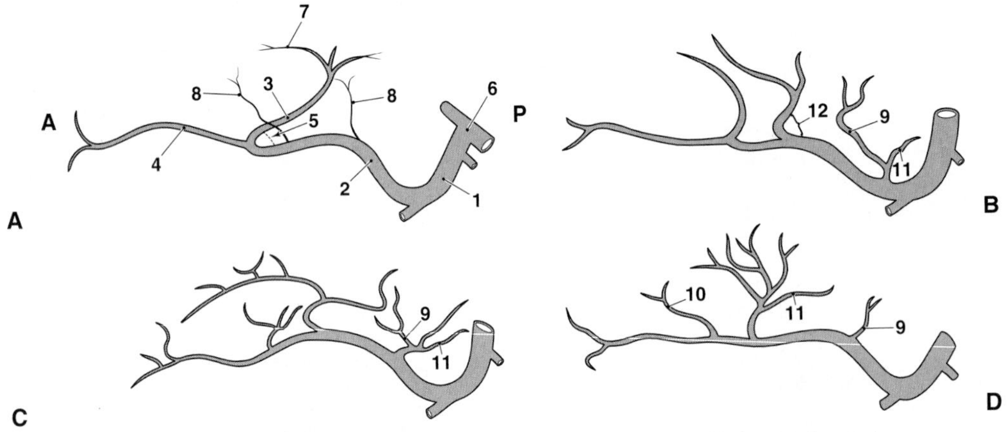

Figure 2U-34: Lateral schematic showing some of the widely varying patterns of venous drainage of the tributaries of the internal cerebral veins. **A:** Classic pattern. **B–D:** Variations. *A,* anterior; *P,* posterior.

1 Vein of Galen
2 Internal cerebral vein
3 Thalamostriate vein
4 Anterior septal vein
5 Venous angle
6 Straight venous sinus
7 Longitudinal caudate vein
8 Posterior septal veins
9 Medial atrial veins
10 Anterior caudate vein
11 Superior choroidal vein
12 False venous angle

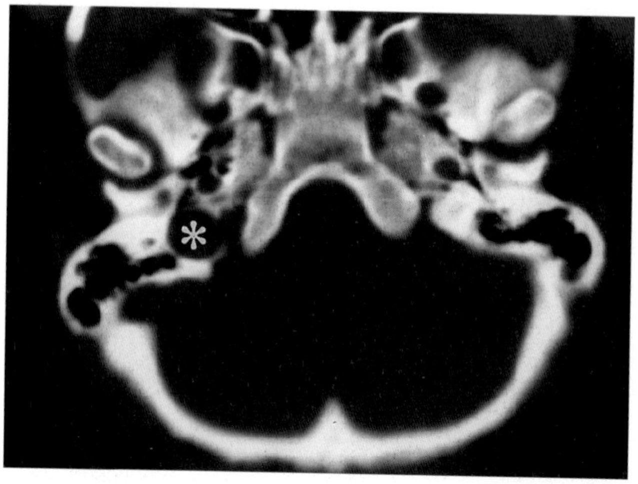

Figure 2U-35: Lateral dominance (hyperplasia) of the jugular bulb/sigmoid venous sinus. Axial CT image showing a dominant right jugular bulb (*asterisk*) on the right side.

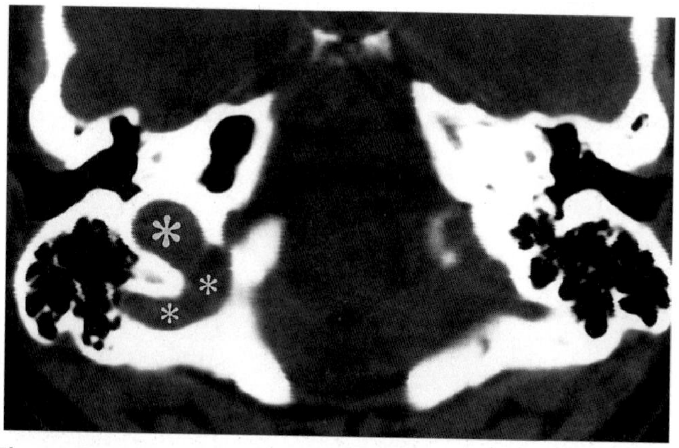

Figure 2U-36A: Jugular bulb diverticulum. Axial CT image showing a prominent jugular bulb (*large asterisk*) and a sigmoid venous sinus (*small asterisks*) on the right side.

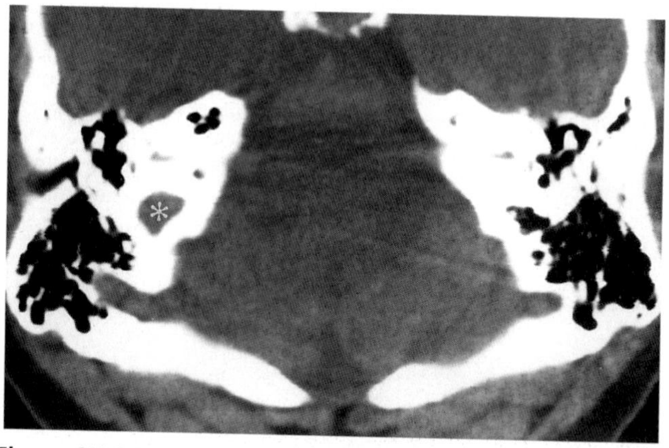

Figure 2U-36B: Jugular bulb diverticulum. Axial CT image showing superior extension of the jugular bulb (*asterisk*).

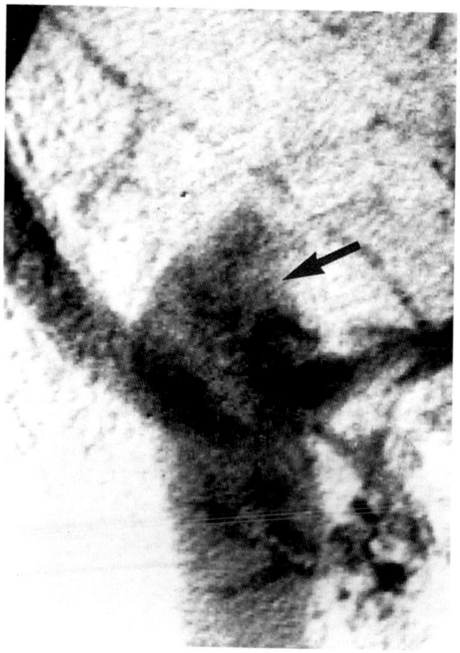

Figure 2U-36C: Jugular bulb diverticulum. Magnified venous phase of right internal carotid angiogram in the oblique projection shows the jugular bulb diverticulum (*arrow*).

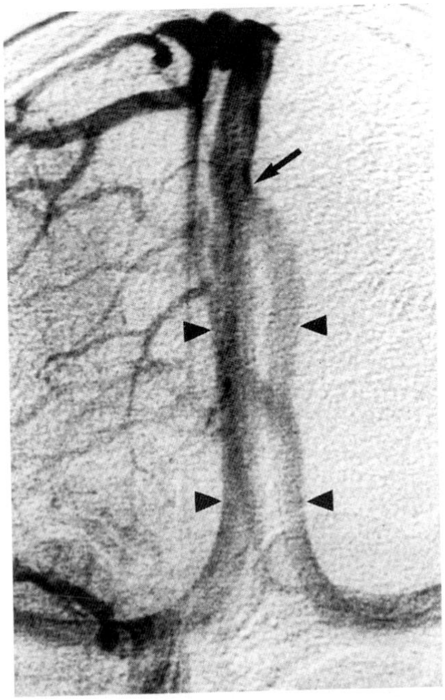

Figure 2U-37: High dural venous sinus bifurcation/partial (distal) sagittal venous sinus duplication. Venous phase of right common carotid angiogram in the frontal projection, showing a high bifurcation of the superior sagittal venous sinus (*arrow*) and the duplicated distal segments (*arrowheads*).

2v Major Arterial Vascular Supply to the Cranial Meninges

THE MAJOR ANTERIOR MENINGEAL ARTERIES

Most common origins are the anterior falcian artery (artery to the falx cerebri), arising from an anterior ethmoidal branch of the ophthalmic artery (unilateral or bilateral) to penetrate the cribriform plate; the anterior meningeal arteries, arising from the middle, posterior, and ethmoidal branches of the ophthalmic artery to penetrate the cribriform plate; the recurrent anterior meningeal artery arising from the ophthalmic artery and traversing the superior orbital fissure; and the recurrent anterior meningeal artery arising from the lacrimal artery.

THE MIDDLE MENINGEAL ARTERY

1. Common origin: the middle meningeal artery, arising from the internal maxillary artery
2. Uncommon origin: the middle meningeal artery, arising from the ophthalmic artery, ascending pharyngeal artery, inferolateral trunk, or basilar artery

THE ACCESSORY MENINGEAL ARTERY

1. Most common origin: the accessory meningeal artery, arising from the internal maxillary artery or from the external carotid artery
2. Uncommon origin: the accessory meningeal artery, arising from the ophthalmic artery or from the middle meningeal artery

THE MAJOR POSTERIOR MENINGEAL ARTERIES (POSTERIOR MENINGEAL ARTERY PROPER OR ARTERY TO THE FALX CEREBELLI)

1. Most common origin: the posterior meningeal artery, arising from the distal vertebral artery(ies) and entering the cranium via the foramen magnum.
2. Uncommon origins: posterior meningeal artery(ies), arising from a branch(es) of the external carotid artery (especially the internal maxillary artery or the occipital artery, via the jugular foramen or mastoid foramen, or the ascending pharyngeal artery, via the jugular foramen or hypoglossal canal).

MAJOR ARTERIAL SUPPLY TO DEEP/CENTRAL MENINGES (REGION OF TENTORIAL NOTCH/CENTRAL SKULL BASE)

1. Most common origin: the tentorial artery (i.e., artery of Bernasconi-Cassinari: a branch of the meningohypophyseal trunk); small, unnamed meningeal arteries arising from branches of the internal carotid artery siphon
2. Uncommon origin: central skull base meningeal arterial supply, arising from the ascending pharyngeal artery (passing via the foramen lacerum).

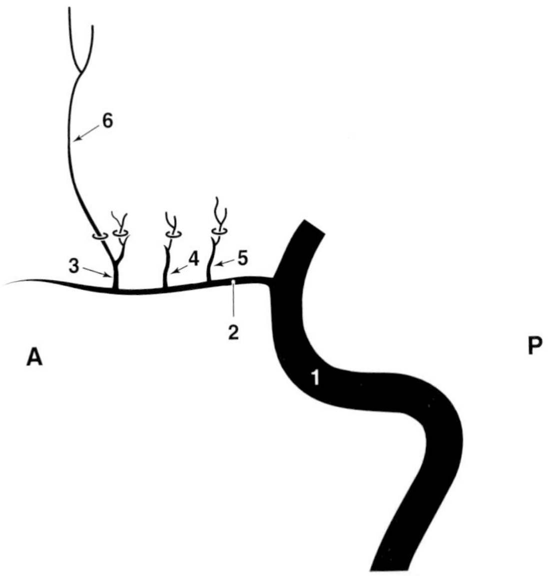

Figure 2V-1: Lateral schematic of the origins of the anterior meningeal arteries. *A,* anterior; *P,* posterior; *ovals,* points (foraminal) of perforation of cribriform plate by penetrating meningeal vessels.

1 Internal carotid artery siphon
2 Ophthalmic artery trunk
3 Anterior ethmoidal artery(ies) with penetrating meningeal branches
4 Middle ethmoidal artery(ies) with penetrating meningeal branches
5 Posterior ethmoidal artery (ies) with penetrating meningeal branches
6 Anterior falcian artery to anterior falx cerebri

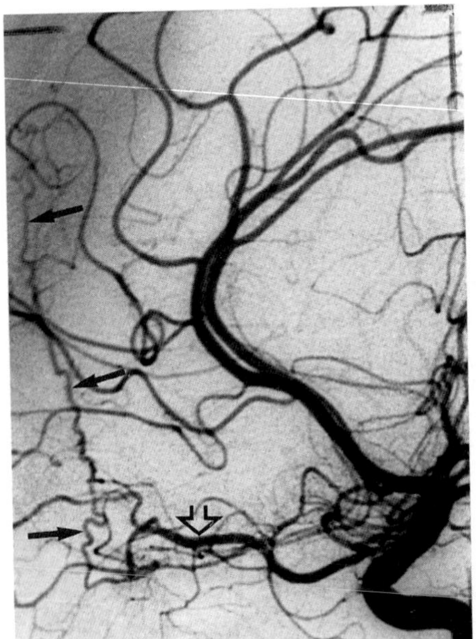

Figure 2V-2A: Carotid arteriogram in the lateral projection, showing the anterior falcian artery (*solid arrows*) originating from the ophthalmic artery (*open arrow*).

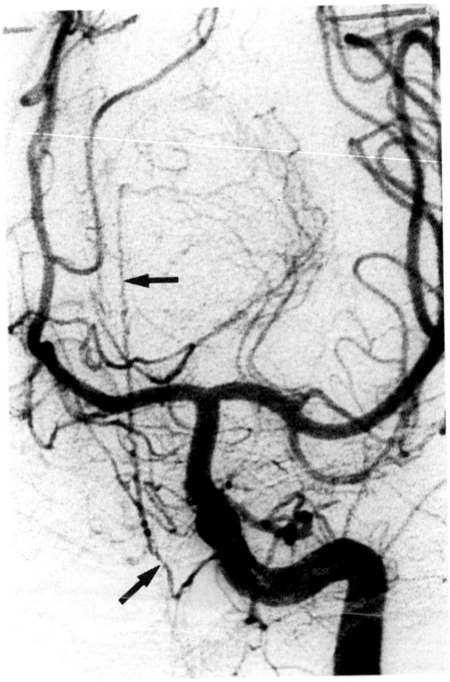

Figure 2V-2B: Carotid arteriogram in the frontal projection, showing the anterior falcian artery (*arrows*).

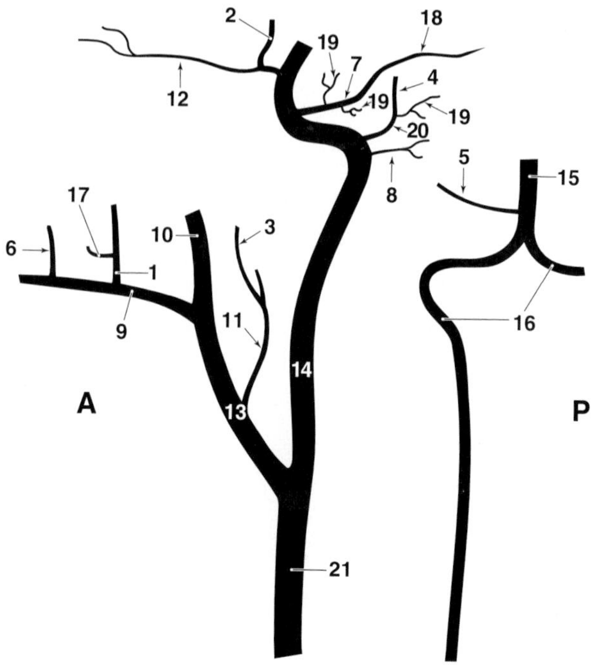

Figure 2V-3: Lateral/oblique schematic of the origin of the middle meningeal artery(ies) and some of the meningeal arteries to the central skull base (arterial branch caliber not to scale). *A,* anterior; *P,* posterior.

1 Most common origin of middle meningeal artery proper (MMAP) from the internal maxillary artery
2 MMAP origin from ophthalmic artery
3 MMAP origin from ascending pharyngeal artery
4 MMAP origin from inferolateral trunk
5 MMAP origin from basilar artery
6 Accessory middle meningeal artery origin from internal maxillary artery
7 Meningohypophyseal trunk
8 Unnamed meningeal vessels to central skull base from internal carotid artery siphon
9 Internal maxillary artery trunk
10 Superficial temporal artery trunk
11 Ascending pharyngeal artery
12 Ophthalmic artery
13 External carotid artery
14 Internal carotid artery
15 Basilar artery
16 Vertebral arteries
17 Accessory middle meningeal artery origin from MMAP
18 Tentorial artery
19 Meningeal branches
20 Inferolateral trunk
21 Common carotid artery

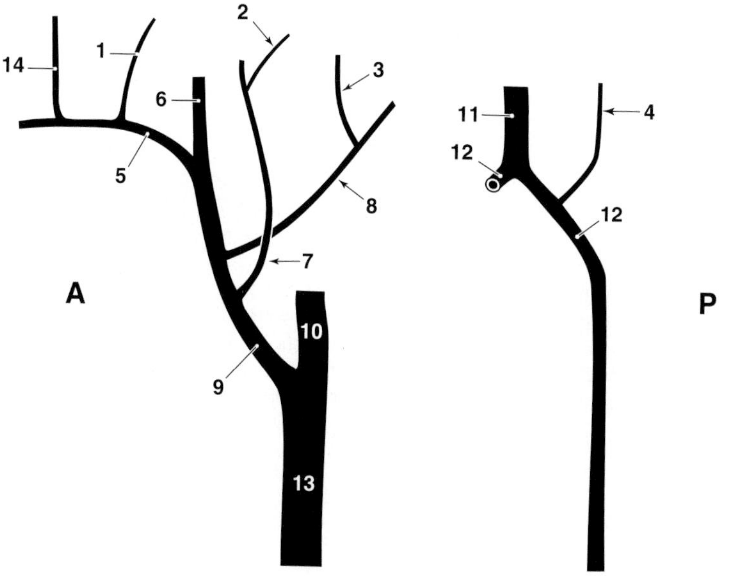

Figure 2V-4: Lateral/oblique schematic of posterior meningeal arteries. *A,* anterior; *P,* posterior.

1 Posterior meningeal artery (PMA) origin from the internal maxillary artery
2 PMA origin from the ascending pharyngeal artery
3 PMA origin from the occipital artery
4 PMA origin from distal vertebral artery
5 Internal maxillary artery trunk
6 Superficial temporal artery trunk
7 Ascending pharyngeal artery
8 Occipital artery
9 External carotid artery
10 Internal carotid artery trunk
11 Basilar artery
12 Vertebral arteries
13 Common carotid artery
14 Middle meningeal artery proper

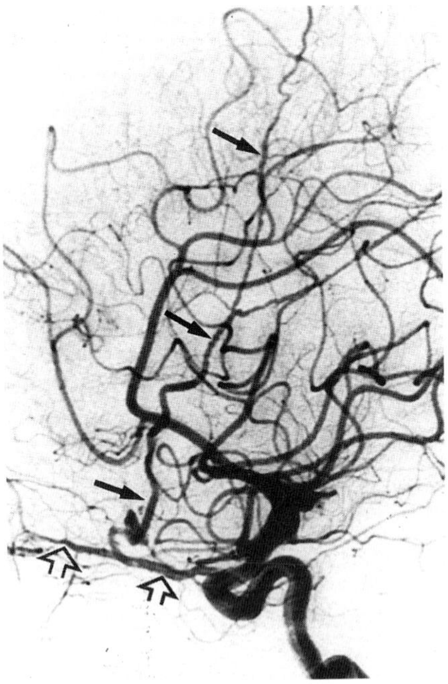

Figure 2V-5A: Middle meningeal artery origin from the ophthalmic artery. Subtraction film from a left internal carotid angiogram in the lateral projection shows the middle meningeal artery (*solid arrows*) originating directly from the ophthalmic artery (*open arrows*).

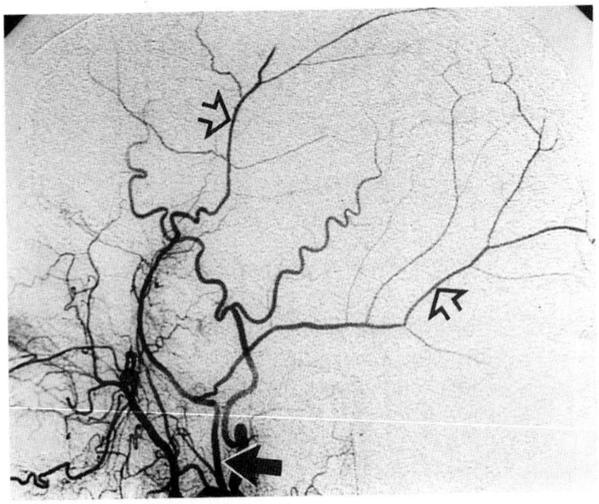

Figure 2V-5B: Middle meningeal artery origin from the ophthalmic artery. External carotid angiogram in the lateral projection, showing the middle meningeal artery trunk (*solid arrow*) as well as its main anterior and posterior branches (*open arrows*).

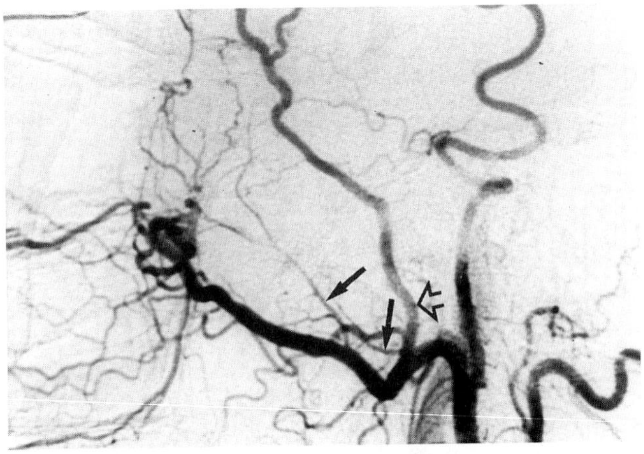

Figure 2V-5C: Accessory middle meningeal artery origin from the middle meningeal artery proper. External carotid angiogram in the lateral projection, showing the accessory middle meningeal artery (*solid arrows*) arising from the main middle meningeal artery proper (*open arrow*).

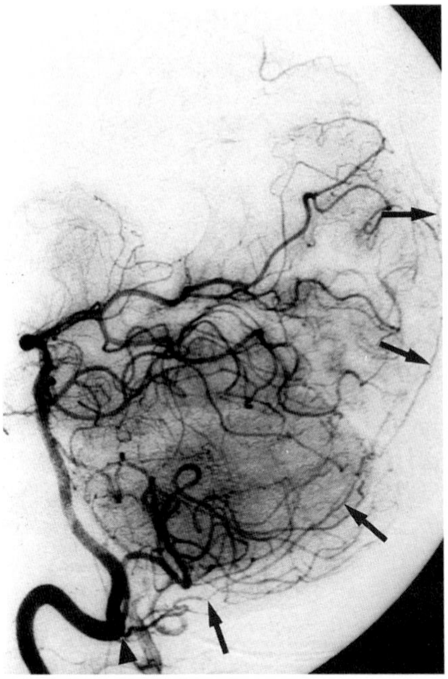

Figure 2V-6A: Posterior meningeal artery. Vertebral arteriogram in the lateral projection, showing the posterior meningeal artery (*arrows*) arising from the vertebral artery (*arrowhead*).

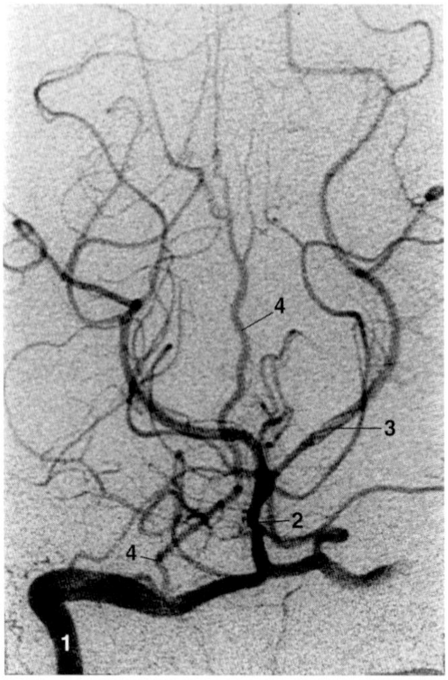

Figure 2V-6B: Posterior meningeal artery. Vertebral artery angiogram in the Towne's projection in the same case as that in Figure 2V-6A, showing the posterior meningeal artery arising from the right vertebral artery.

1 Right vertebral artery
2 Basilar artery
3 Left posterior cerebral artery
4 Posterior meningeal artery

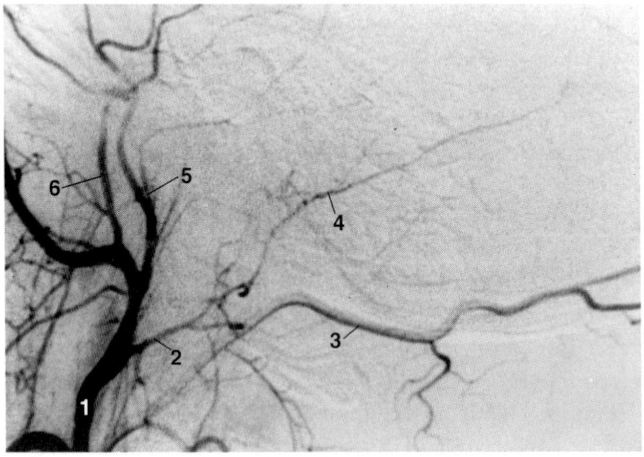

Figure 2V-6C: Posterior meningeal artery. External carotid angiogram in the lateral projection, showing the posterior meningeal artery arising from either the occipital or the posterior auricular artery.

1 External carotid artery
2 Posterior auricular artery
3 Occipital artery
4 Posterior meningeal artery arising from the posterior auricular artery
5 Superficial temporal artery trunk
6 Middle meningeal artery trunk

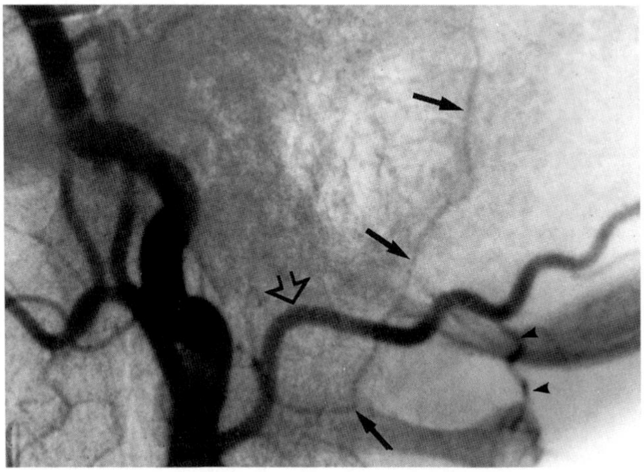

Figure 2V-6D: Posterior meningeal artery origin from occipital artery. Subtraction film from left common carotid angiogram in the lateral projection, showing the posterior meningeal artery (*solid arrows*) originating from the occipital artery (*open arrow*). Note also the muscular branches originating from the middle portion of the occipital artery (*arrowhead*).

2W Central Nervous System Barriers and Interfaces

OVERVIEW

1. Brain, spinal cord, and cranial spinal nerve capillaries are continuous capillaries; the capillary wall is composed of a layer of endothelial cells connected at the interendothelial boundaries by tight junctions.
2. There are no discontinuities in the endothelial wall; the capillary is further surrounded by a continuous basal lamina.
3. The *blood–brain/blood–cord/blood–nerve barrier(s)* (i.e., *blood–CNS barrier*) are due to these very tight interendothelial junctions combined with an absence of free transendothelial vesicular transport. The blood–cord barrier is essentially the same as the blood–brain barrier. The dorsal root ganglia of the spinal nerves are excluded from the blood–nerve barrier, and the blood–nerve barrier of the peripheral nerve is less secure than that of the proximal peripheral neural segments (e.g., intrathecal spinal nerve roots).
4. The relative affinity of a solute for lipid versus water is expressed by its oil–water partition coefficient. For example, high lipophilic solutes, such as caffeine, ethanol, and heroin, have high oil–water partition coefficients and pass the blood–brain barrier owing to their affinity for plasma membrane lipids.
5. Tight junctions between the cuboidal epithelial cells of the choroid plexi form the *blood–cerebrospinal fluid (CSF) barrier.*
6. The blood–brain and blood–CSF barriers differ greatly in surface area. The surface area of the blood–brain barrier has been estimated to be 5,000 times greater than that of the blood–CSF barrier.
7. The *CSF–brain interface* consists of the ependymal lining of the cerebral ventricles and the pial–glial membrane on the surface of the brain, spinal cord, and subarachnoid segments of the cranial spinal nerve roots. This interface does not impede the free exchange of fluid and some solutes between the CSF and the central nervous system (CNS) parenchyma.
8. The *CSF–blood barrier* is formed by the tufted prolongations of the pia-arachnoid at the level of the arachnoid granulations interfacing between the CSF and the venous blood of the cranial dural venous sinuses. These granulations function as passive, pressure gradient–dependent, one-way valves between the CSF and the venous blood that are readily permeable to fluids and even large solutes (e.g., proteins).
9. Although it has been established in a number of mammalian species, *lymphatic drainage of the CNS* in humans is at present theoretical. Several pathways in nonhuman mammals seem to progress along the perivascular spaces following cerebral arteries and veins, and the perineural (interstitial) spaces surrounding cranial-spinal nerves that penetrate the cranium and spine when traversing the intra- and extracranial and intra- and extraspinal compartments. Sites for these pathways include the cribriform plate, the perforating arteries and veins along the surface of the CNS, the spinal/cranial nerve root/sheath complexes as they exit the CNS. Once exiting the CNS via these sites, drainage would be to the craniocervical and paraspinal lymphatic system.

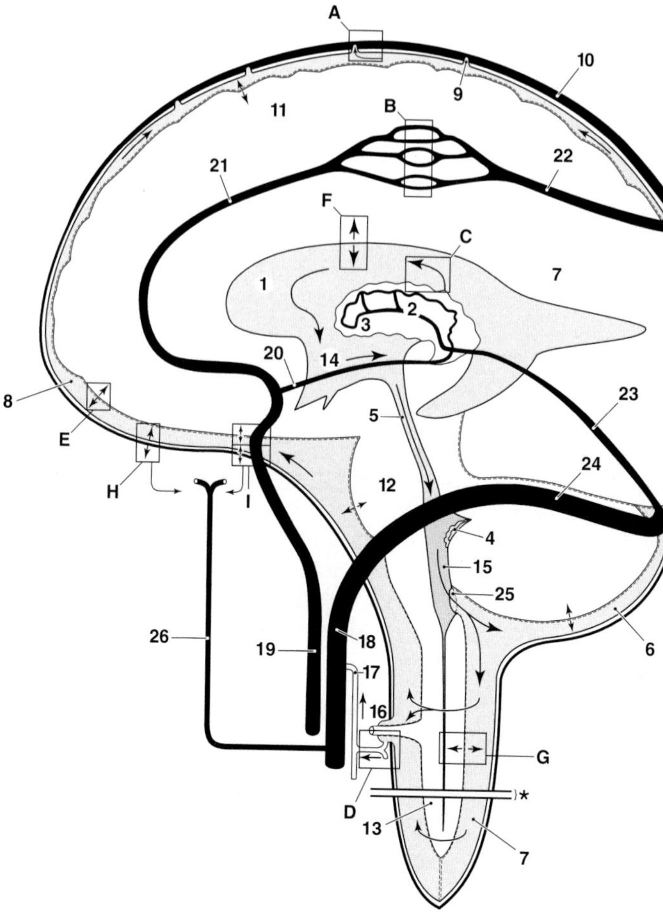

Figure 2W-1: Lateral schematic showing the general levels of the central nervous system barriers and interfaces.
A Cerebrospinal fluid (CSF)–blood barrier at an arachnoid granulation.
B Blood–brain barrier at the central nervous system parenchymal capillary level.
C Blood–CSF barrier at the cerebral ventricular choroid plexus.
D Perineural–lymphatic/interface barrier at the spinal nerve root/sheath complex (theoretical).
E CSF–brain interface at the pial surface of the brain.
F CSF–brain interface at the ependymal surface of the ventricular system.
G CSF–spinal cord interface at the pial surface of the cord.
H CSF–lymphatic barrier/interface at the foramina of the cribriform plate (theoretical).
I Perivascular–lymphatic barrier/interface in the region of the cranial penetrating vessels (theoretical). *Asterisk,* break in diagram; *arrows,* CSF flow, secretion, and absorption.
1 Lateral ventricle
2 Choroid plexus of the third ventricle
3 Choroid plexus of the third ventricle
4 Choroid plexus of the fourth ventricle (vascular supply and drainage not shown)
5 Aqueduct of Sylvius
6 Posterior fossa subarachnoid space
7 Spinal subarachnoid space
8 Supratentorial subarachnoid space
9 Arachnoid granulation
10 Superior sagittal venous sinus
11 Cerebral hemisphere
12 Brain stem
13 Spinal cord
14 Third ventricle
15 Fourth ventricle
16 Spinal nerve
17 Paraspinal lymphatics
18 Internal jugular vein
19 Internal carotid artery
20 Anterior choroidal artery
21 Cerebral artery
22 Cerebral vein
23 Straight venous sinus
24 Transverse venous sinus
25 Craniocervical lymphatics
26 Veins draining skull base

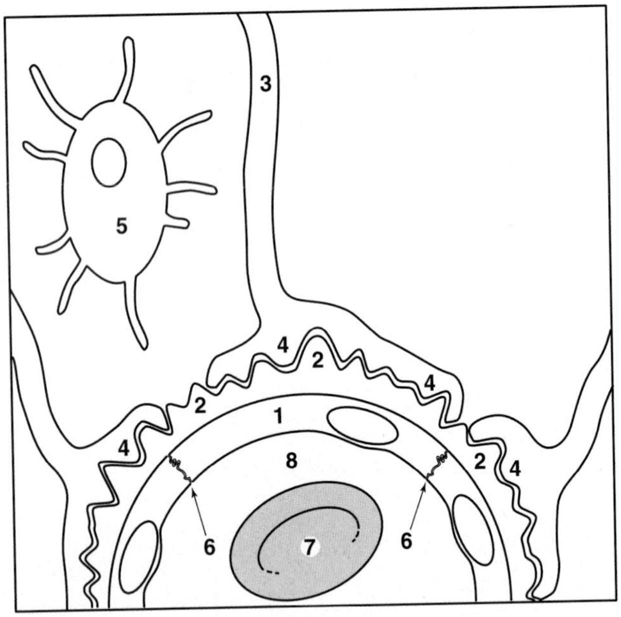

Figure 2W-2: Magnified cross-sectional schematic of a segment of a central nervous system (CNS) capillary. The level of the blood–brain/blood–cord/blood–nerve barrier (blood–CNS barrier) is at the interendothelial tight junction.

1 Endothelial cell of capillary with nucleus
2 Astrocyte basement membrane (basal lamina)
3 Astrocyte process
4 Astrocyte end-feet
5 Oligodendrocyte
6 Intercellular endothelial tight junction (site of the bloodCNS barrier)
7 Red blood cell
8 Vascular lumen

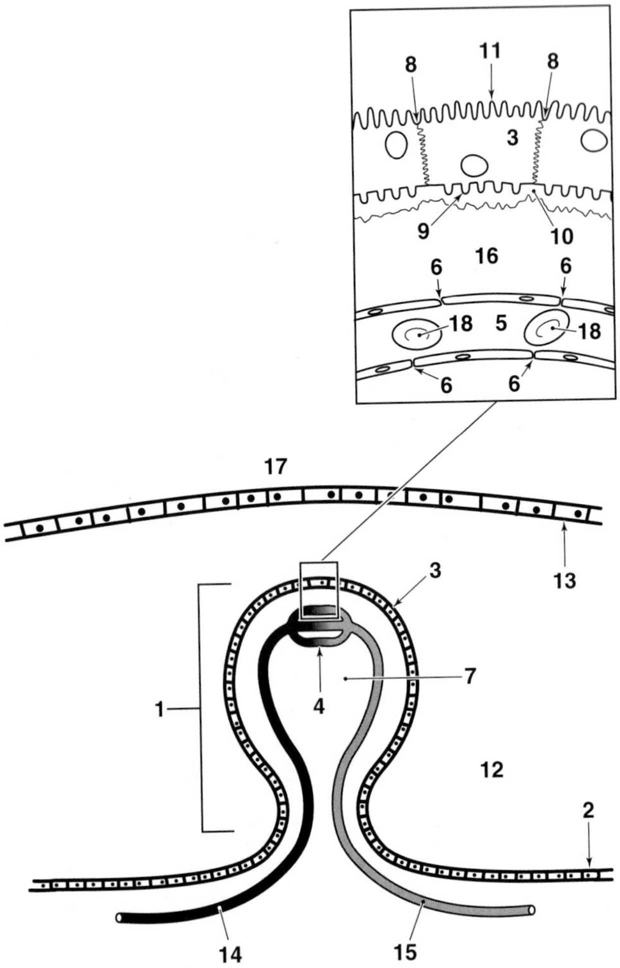

Figure 2W-3: Longitudinal schematic of the microstructure of an arachnoid villus of the choroid plexus, showing the blood-cerebrospinal fluid (CSF) barrier at the level of the epithelial plexal cell intercellular tight junction.

1 Arachnoid villus of choroid plexus
2 Ventricular ependyma along margins of choroid plexus
3 Apical plexal cell–modified cuboidal epithelium over surface of choroid plexus (plexal cuboidal epithelian)
4 Arachnoid villus (choroid plexus) capillary system
5 Choroid plexus capillary lumen
6 Intercellular fenestra in choroid plexus capillary endothelium (fenestrated capillaries)
7 Fibrous vascular core of tela choroidea of choroid plexus
8 Epithelial plexal cell intercellular tight junctions (site of the blood–CSF barrier)
9 Interdigitations on basal surface of plexal epithelial cells
10 Basement membrane along inner surface of infolded plexal epithelium
11 Apical microvilli on apical surface of plexal epithelium
12 Cerebral ventricular lumen
13 Parietal ependyma of cerebral ventricular system
14 Arteriole of arachnoid villus
15 Venule of arachnoid villus
16 Apical interstitial space of arachnoid villus
17 Brain parenchyma
18 Red blood cells in choroid plexus capillary

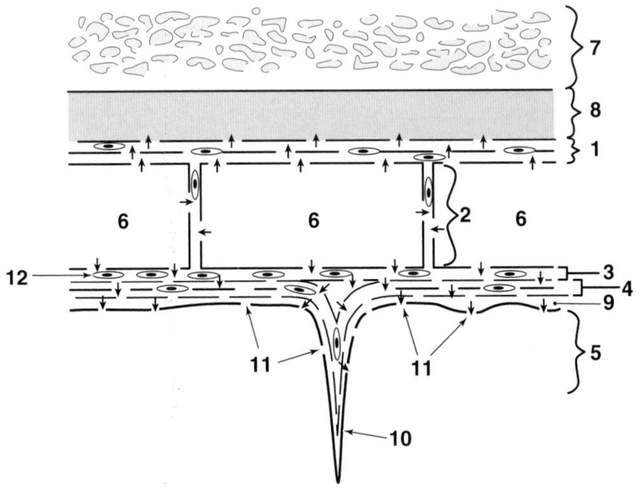

Figure 2W-4: Cross-sectional schematic of the cerebrospinal fluid–brain interface (*arrows*: intercellular fenestrae).

1 Dura mater
2 Subarachnoid septae
3 Arachnoid mater
4 Pia mater
5 Central nervous system (CNS) parenchyma (brain, spinal cord)
6 Subarachnoid space
7 Peri-CNS cancellous bone (calvarium, spine)
8 Peri-CNS cortical bone (calvarium, spine)
9 Potential subpial space
10 Fissure/sulcus in CNS parenchyma
11 Fenestrae between cells of CNS parenchyma (site of the CSF–brain interface)
12 Native meningeal cell

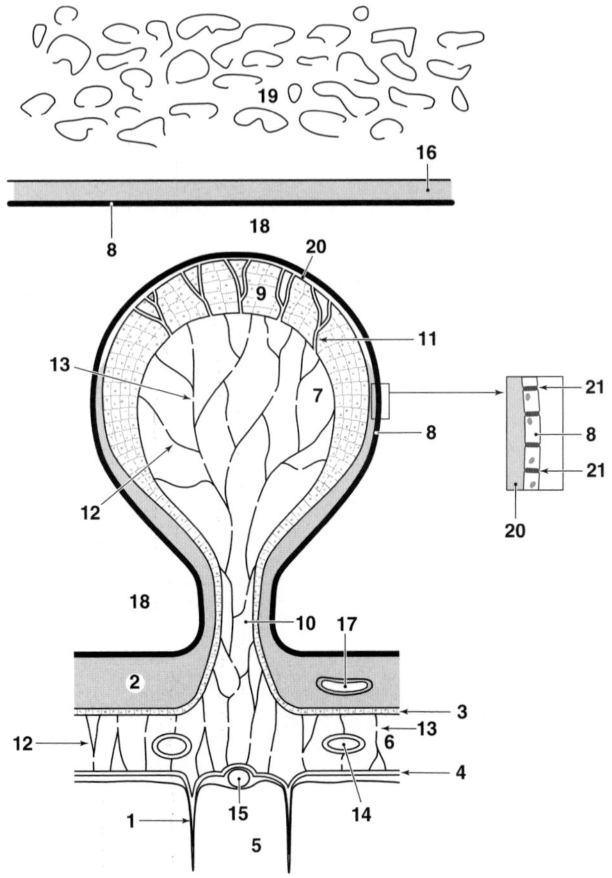

Figure 2W-5: Longitudinal schematic of an arachnoid granulation, showing the cerebrospinal fluid (CSF)–blood barrier at the level of the venous endothelium intercellular tight junctions.

1 Cerebral sulcus
2 Meningeal layer of cranial dura mater
3 Arachnoid mater
4 Pia mater
5 Cerebrum
6 Subarachnoid space over cerebrum
7 Subarachnoid space of arachnoid granulation
8 Venous endothelium
9 Arachnoid granulation apical cap and arachnoidal apical cap cells
10 Subarachnoid space channel in neck of arachnoid granulation
11 Subarachnoid space microchannel of arachnoid granulation cap
12 Arachnoid trabeculations
13 Communicating fenestra in arachnoid trabeculations
14 Subarachnoid space blood vessels
15 Subpial cortical blood vessels
16 Periosteal layer of cranial dura mater
17 Meningeal blood vessels
18 Venous vascular lumen of dural venous sinus lacuna
19 Calvarium
20 Subendothelial space of apex of arachnoid granulation
21 Intercellular endothelial tight junctions (site of CSF–blood barrier)

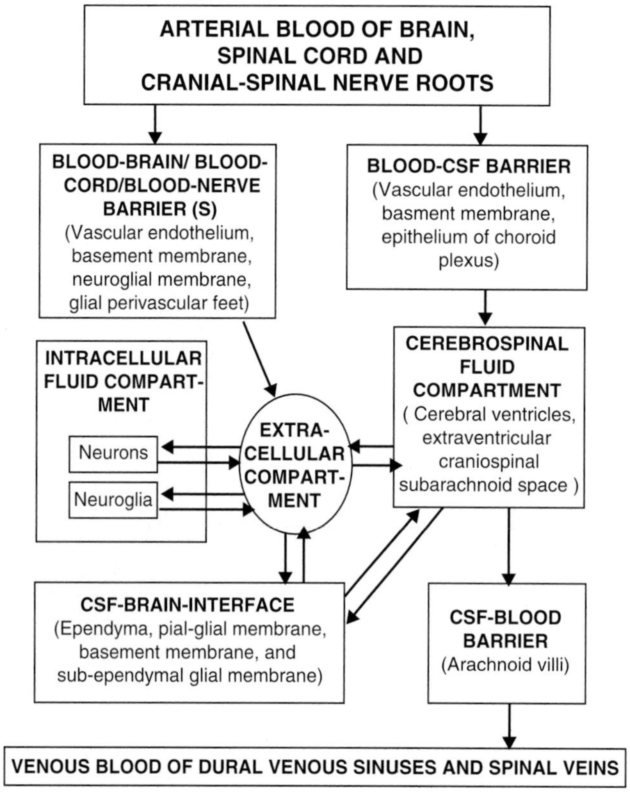

Figure 2W-6: Schematic of the blood–brain/ blood–cord/blood–nerve barrier(s), blood–cerebrospinal fluid (CSF) barrier, CSF–brain interface, and CSF–blood barrier that lie at several points between the central nervous system, the CSF pathways, and the vascular compartment.

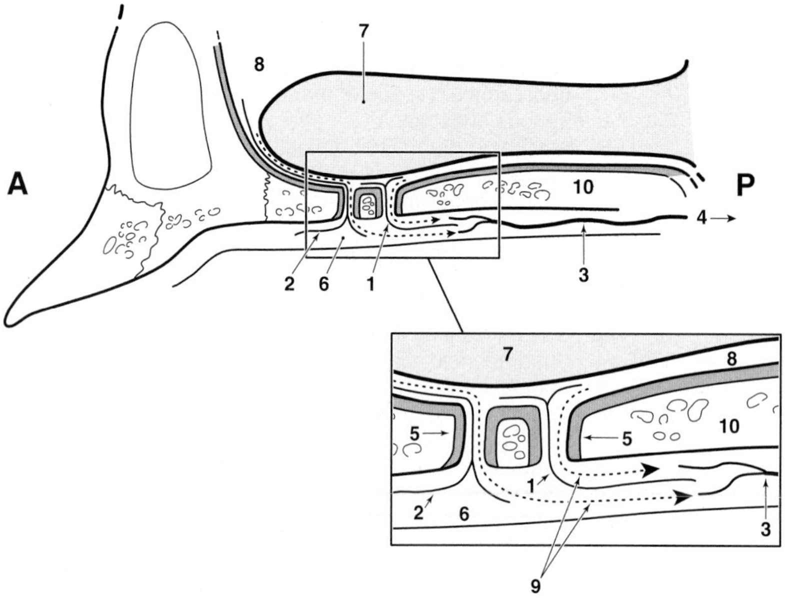

Figure 2W-7: Lateral schematic of theoretical central nervous system (CNS)–lymphatic drainage at the base of the skull. *Long dashed arrows* indicate the direction of interstitial drainage from the CNS to the lymphatics via perforating vascular/neural channels or foramina. *A*, anterior; *P*, posterior.

1 Perforating emissary vein/nerve
2 Perforating artery/nerve
3 Lymphatics of nasal mucosa
4 Submucosal lymphatic drainage to craniocervical lymphatic system
5 Foramina in cribriform plate
6 Nasal mucosa
7 Olfactory bulb (CN-I) (not to scale)
8 Cranial subarachnoid space
9 Theoretical passage of solates and fluid directly from the intracranial subarachnoid space via the perivascular/perineural interstitial space through penetrating vascular/neural foramina at the base of the skull
10 Cribriform plate

CHAPTER 3

The Sella Turcica, Pituitary Gland, and Cavernous Venous Sinuses

THE SELLA TURCICA

Bony Anatomy

1. The sella turcica is formed by the bony confines of the pituitary gland, termed the pituitary fossa. The floor of this fossa may be flat or slightly concave.
2. Posteriorly the pituitary fossa is bordered by the dorsum sellae from which project the two posterior clinoid processes.
3. Anteriorly the pituitary fossa is bordered by the tuberculum sellae; the chiasmatic groove, for the optic chiasm, is found in the midline anterior to the tuberculum sellae. The two anterior clinoid processes project posteriorly immediately lateral to the supraclinoid internal carotid artery. Ossification of the anteroposterior interclinoid ligament creates a *lateral "bridge" sella turcica.*
4. The middle clinoid processes are inconstant, paired, small, bony excrescences directed posteriorly inferomedial to the anterior clinoid processes. The internal carotid arteries pass anterolateral to the middle clinoid processes after exiting the cavernous venous sinuses. The regional dura, continuous with the outer wall of the cavernous venous sinus, interconnects the anterior and middle clinical processes on each side. Ossification of this *anterior-middle interclinoid ligament* (Jinkins) creates an *anterior "bridge" sella turcica* (Jinkins) foramen also termed the caroticoclinoid foramen.
5. The pituitary fossa varies normally in size and shape. For this reason, direct visualization of sellar contents on imaging is a more accurate means of pituitary analysis than are measurements of sellar dimensions.

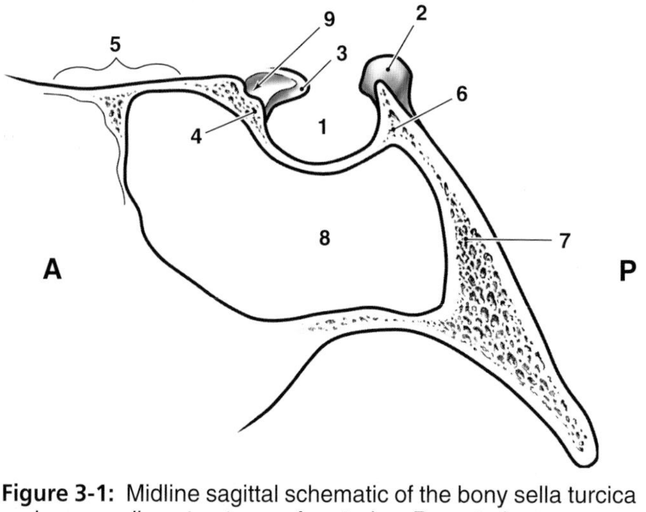

Figure 3-1: Midline sagittal schematic of the bony sella turcica and surrounding structures. *A*, anterior; *P*, posterior.
1 Pituitary fossa
2 Posterior clinoid process
3 Anterior clinoid process
4 Tuberculum sellae and middle clinoid process
5 Planum sphenoidal
6 Dorsum sellae
7 Clivus
8 Sphenoid sinus
9 Chiasmatic recess

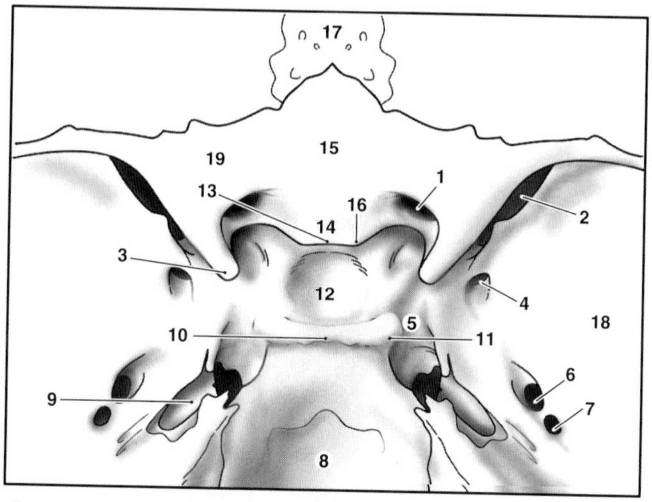

Figure 3-2: Schematic of the bony sella turcica and surrounding structures of the central skull base viewed from above.
1 Optic canal
2 Superior orbital fissure
3 Anterior clinoid process
4 Foramen rotundum
5 Carotid sulcus
6 Foramen ovale
7 Foramen spinosum
8 Clivus
9 Foramen lacerum
10 Dorsum sellae
11 Posterior clinoid process
12 Pituitary fossa
13 Tuberculum sellae
14 Chiasmatic recess
15 Planum sphenoidal
16 Middle clinoid
17 Cribriform plate
18 Middle cranial fossa
19 Greater wing of sphenoid bone

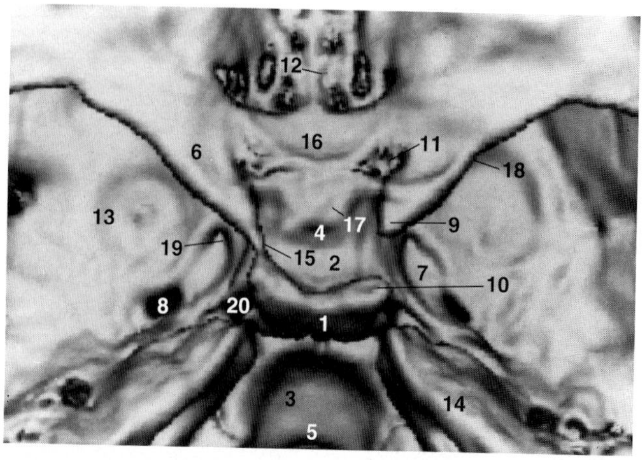

Figure 3-3: The sella turcica. Three-dimensional CT image viewed from above with the cranial vault deleted showing bony sella turcica and surrounding structures of the central skull base.
1 Dorsum sella
2 Hypophyseal fossa
3 Clivus
4 Tuberculum sella
5 Foramen magnum
6 Greater wing of the sphenoid bone
7 Carotid sulcus
8 Foramen ovale
9 Anterior clinoid process
10 Posterior clinoid process
11 Optic foramen
12 Cribriform plate
13 Middle cranial fossa
14 Medial aspect of petrous part of the temporal bone
15 Ossified anteroposterior interclinoid ligament (lateral bridge sella turcica)
16 Planum sphenoidal
17 Middle clinoid process
18 Superior orbital fissure
19 Foramen rotundum
20 Foramen lacerum

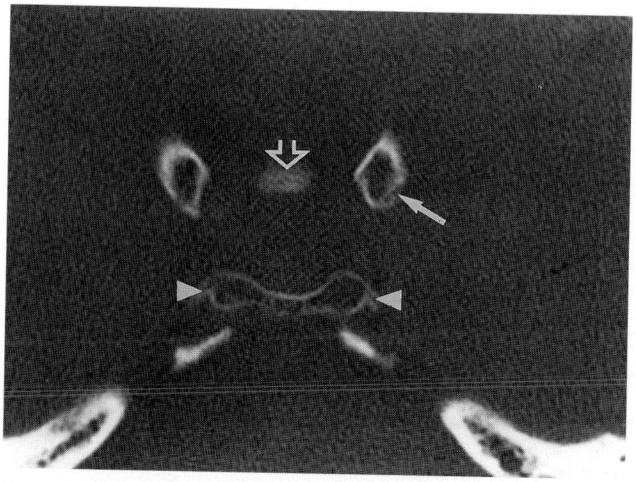

Figure 3-4A: Sella turcica. Axial CT image showing the anterior clinoid processes (*solid arrow*), the posterior clinoid processes (*arrowheads*), and the tuberculum sella (*open arrow*).

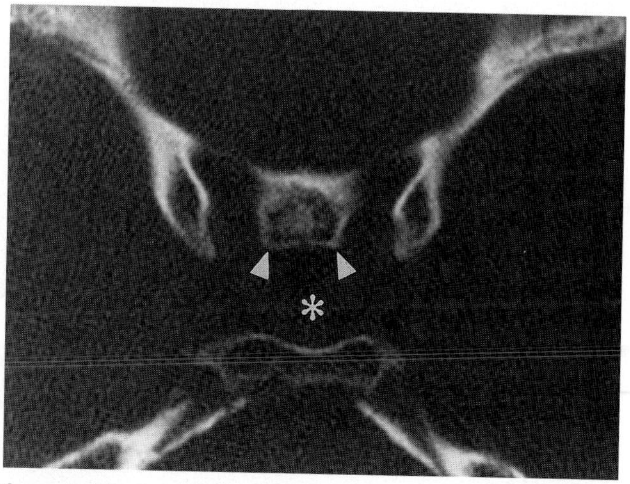

Figure 3-4B: Axial CT image at a level just below that of Figure 3-4A shows the middle clinoid processes (*arrowheads*) and the pituitary fossa (*asterisk*).

BONY SELLA TURCICA VARIANTS

- Lateral bridge sella turcica (caroticoclinoid foramen: bony bridge between the anterior and posterior clinoid processes)
- Anterior bridge sella turcica (bony bridge between the anterior and middle clinoid processes)
- Aplastic or hypoplastic sella turcica
- Enlarged, partially empty sella turcica
- Duplicated sella turcica
- Intrasellar bony spike

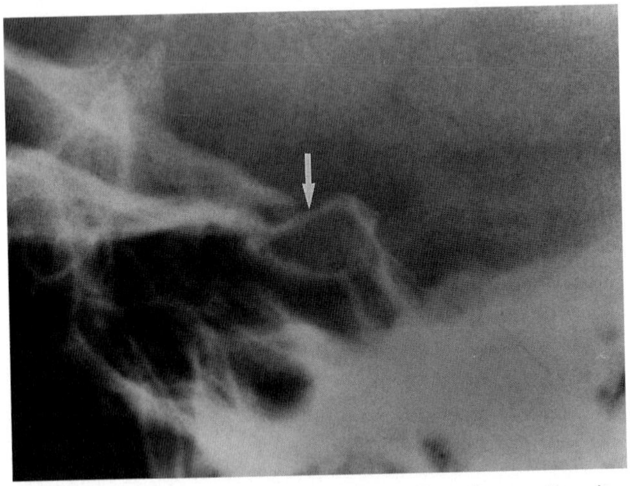

Figure 3-5A: Lateral "bridge" sella turcica. Conventional radiograph in the lateral projection showing a "bridge" sella (*arrow*) or ossification of the interclinoid ligament.

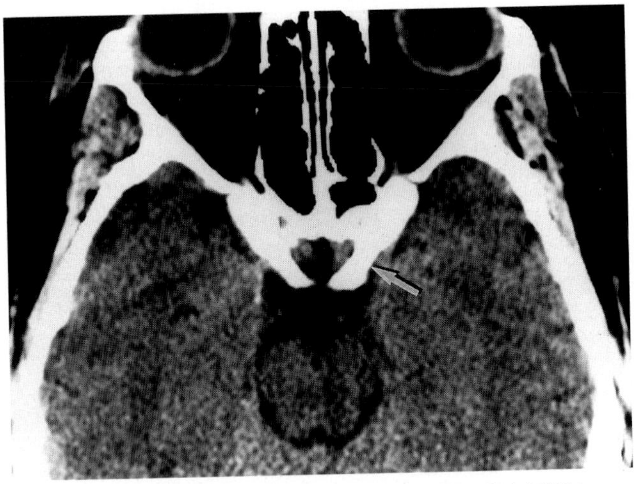

Figure 3-5B: Lateral "bridge" sella turcica. Axial CT image similarly shows a "bridge" sella (*arrow*).

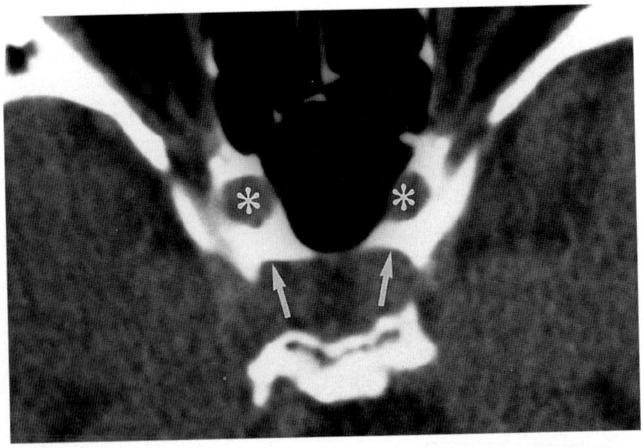

Figure 3-5C: Anterior "bridge" sella turcica (caroticoclinoid foramen). Axial CT image showing bilateral bridges that connects the anterior and middle clinoid processes (*arrows*) forming complete terminal bony carotid canals posteriorly (*asterisks*).

THE PITUITARY GLAND

Anatomy

1. The pituitary gland (hypophysis cerebri) consists of (a) the anterior lobe (adenohypophysis) and (b) the posterior lobe (neurohypophysis).
2. The anterior lobe (adenohypophysis) of the pituitary gland consists of (a) the pars tuberalis (located anterior to the medial eminence and the infundibulum), (b) the pars distalis (located in the anterior aspect of the pituitary fossa), and (c) the pars intermedia (located between the pars distalis and the pars nervosa).
3. The anterior lobe (adenohypophysis) secretes several hormones, including prolactin, growth hormone, thyroid-stimulating hormone, follicle-stimulating hormone, luteinizing hormone, adrenocorticotropic hormone (ACTH) precursor, and melanocyte-stimulating hormone.
4. The hypothalamic input controls the hormone secretions from the anterior lobe of the pituitary gland through the hypothalamic-hypophyseal portal venous system.
5. The posterior lobe (neurohypophysis) of the pituitary gland consists of (a) the medial eminence of the hypothalamus, (b) the pituitary infundibulum (pituitary stalk), and (c) the pars nervosa (located in the posterior aspect of the pituitary fossa).
6. The posterior lobe (neurohypophysis) of the pituitary gland stores and secretes the following hormones: antidiuretic hormone (ADH or vasopressin) and oxytocin.
7. The shape of the pituitary gland may be upwardly convex, flat, or concave. The upper normal limit of pituitary gland height is 12 mm.
8. The pituitary gland usually increases in size during puberty and pregnancy, and on average it is usually slightly larger in females than in males.
9. The posterior lobe of the pituitary gland is hyperintense on T1-weighted magnetic resonance imaging (MRI) in up to 90% of normal individuals. The cause of this hyperintense signal may be due to one or more of several factors (e.g., pituicyte neurosecretory granules, lipids, or phospholipid vesicles). The entire gland can be normally hyperintense during pregnancy and in infants less than 2 months of age.
10. The pituitary gland normally enhances on contrast-enhanced computed tomography (CT) and MRI because it lacks a blood–brain barrier. Following bolus injection of intravenous contrast agents, the posterior pituitary lobe enhances first because it has a direct arterial supply; the anterior pituitary lobe enhances somewhat later due to its dominant blood supply via the portal venous system from the hypothalamus.

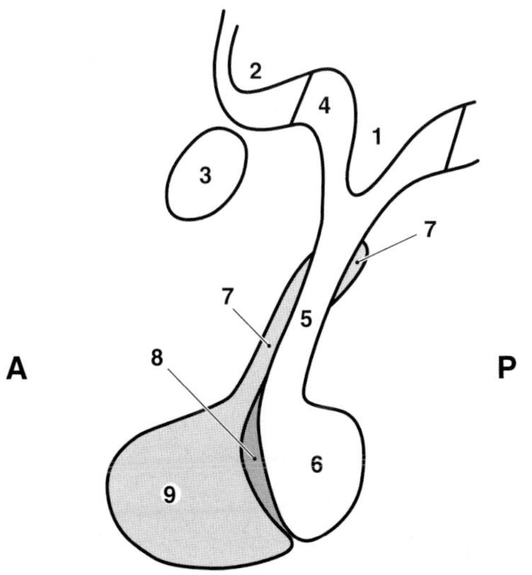

Figure 3-6: Midline sagittal schematic of the pituitary gland. *A*, anterior; *P*, posterior.

1 Infundibular recess of third ventricle
2 Chiasmatic recess of third ventricle
3 Optic chiasm
4 Medial eminence
5 Infundibulum (pituitary stalk) } posterior lobe (neurohypophysis)
6 Pars nervosa
7 Pars tuberalis
8 Pars intermedia } anterior lobe (adenohypophysis)
9 Pars distalis

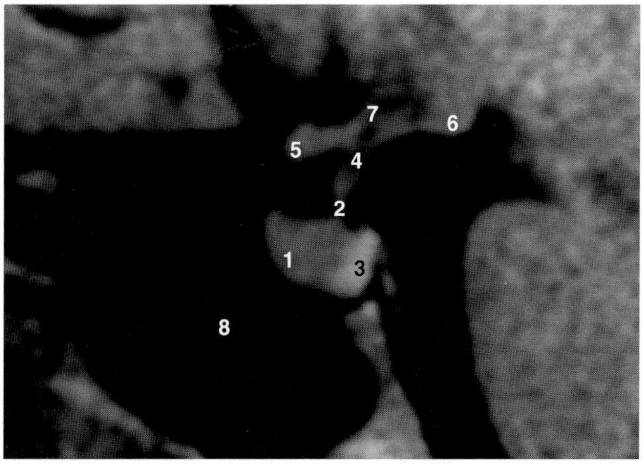

Figure 3-7A: Normal pituitary gland. Unenhanced sagittal T1-weighted MR image of the sellar region shows relative hyperintensity of the posterior lobe of the pituitary gland. The anterior lobe is relatively isointense to brain on this acquisition.

1 Anterior lobe (pars distalis)
2 Pituitary infundibulum
3 Posterior lobe (pars nervosa)
4 Medial eminence
5 Optic chiasm
6 Mamillary body(ies)
7 Infundibular recess of third ventricle
8 Sphenoid sinus

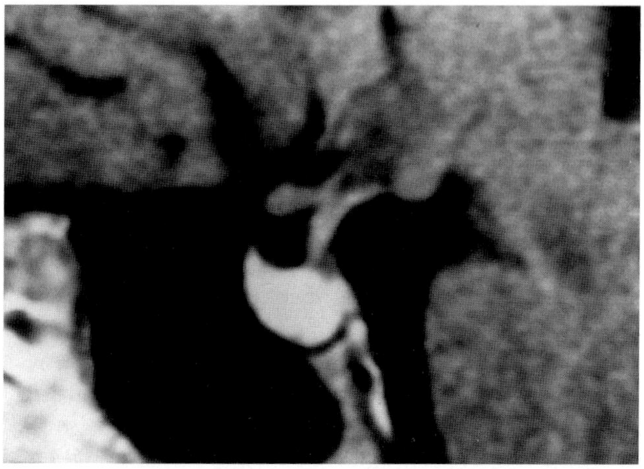

Figure 3-7B: Enhanced sagittal T1-weighted MR image showing marked generalized enhancement of the pituitary gland and a lesser degree of enhancement of the pituitary infundibulum. It may be difficult to determine neurohypophysis enhancement in some cases because the neurohypophysis may be normally hyperintense on unenhanced T1-weighted MR images (compare with Figure 3-7A).

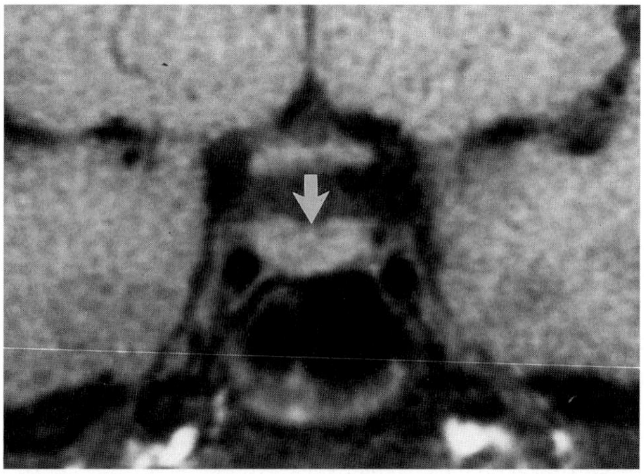

Figure 3-7C: Unenhanced coronal T1-weighted MR image showing the normally isointense (as compared to brain) anterior lobe (adenohypophysis) of the pituitary gland (*arrow*).

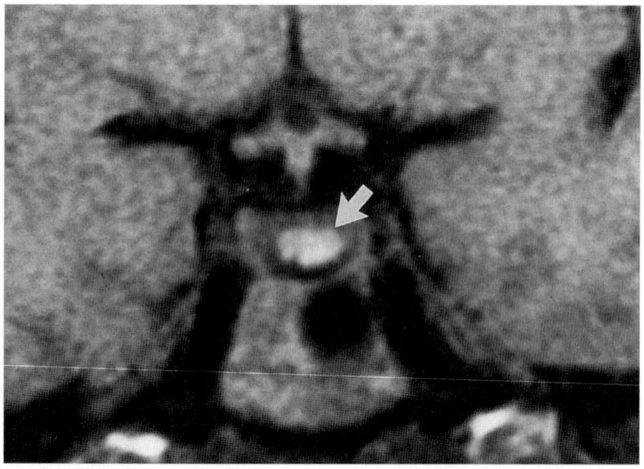

Figure 3-7D: Unenhanced coronal T1-weighted MR image showing the normally relatively hyperintense posterior lobe (neurohypophysis) of the pituitary gland (*arrow*).

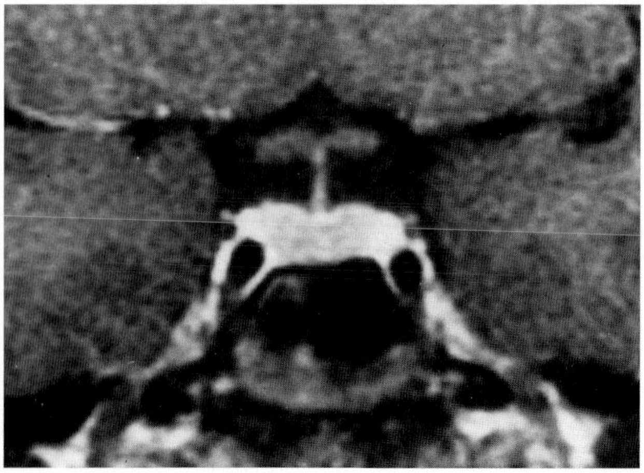

Figure 3-7E: Enhanced coronal T1-weighted MR image showing homogeneous enhancement of the pituitary gland and infundibulum.

PITUITARY GLAND VARIANTS

Size/Number Variants
- Pituitary gland hypoplasia (i.e., developmental)
- Pituitary gland hyperplasia (e.g., puberty, pregnancy)
- Partially empty sella turcica (i.e., acquired)
- Duplication of the pituitary gland

Magnetic Resonance Imaging Signal Intensity Variants
- Normally hyperintense posterior lobe
- Normally isointense posterior lobe
- Normally hyperintense anterior and posterior lobes in pregnancy
- Hyperintense pituitary gland in cirrhotic liver disease or total parenteral nutrition

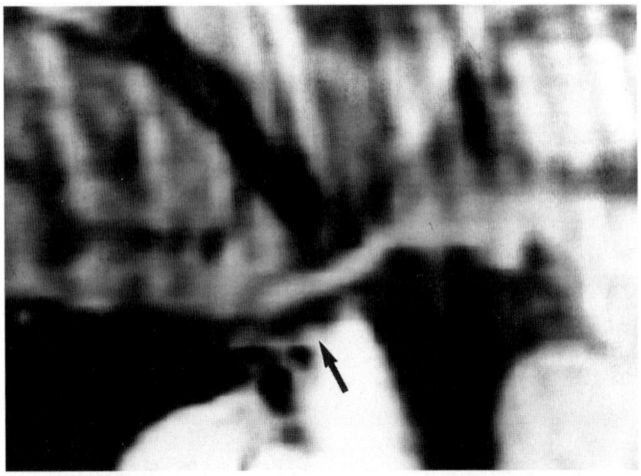

Figure 3-8A: Pituitary gland and fossa hypoplasia. Sagittal unenhanced T1-weighted MR image showing hypoplasia (*arrow*) of the pituitary gland and a shallow pituitary fossa.

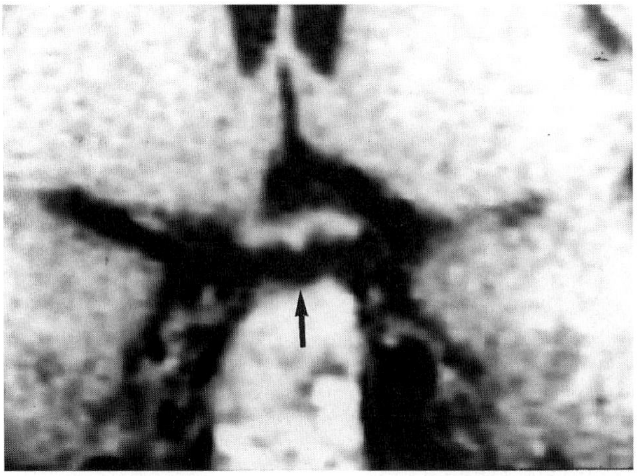

Figure 3-8B: Coronal unenhanced T1-weighted MR image showing hypoplasia of the pituitary gland, a shallow pituitary fossa (*arrow*), and nonvisualization of the infundibulum.

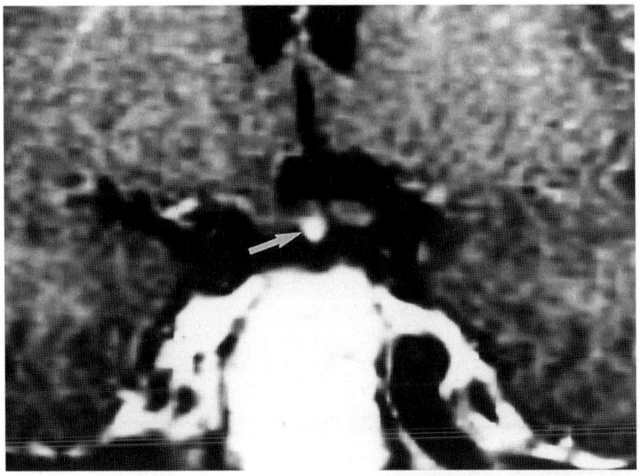

Figure 3-8C: Coronal contrast-enhanced T1-weighted MR image again showing hypoplasia of the pituitary gland and "ectopic" enhancing pituitary tissue (*arrow*) at the level of the infundibulum.

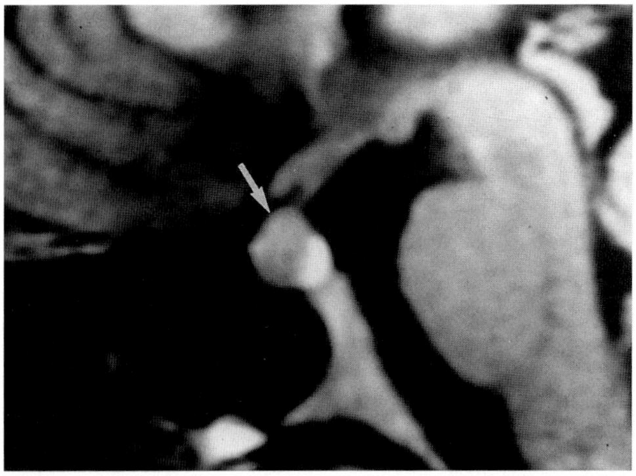

Figure 3-9A: Pituitary gland hyperplasia during pregnancy. Unenhanced sagittal T1-weighted MR image in a pregnant patient showing pituitary hyperplasia (*arrow*), especially involving the anterior lobe.

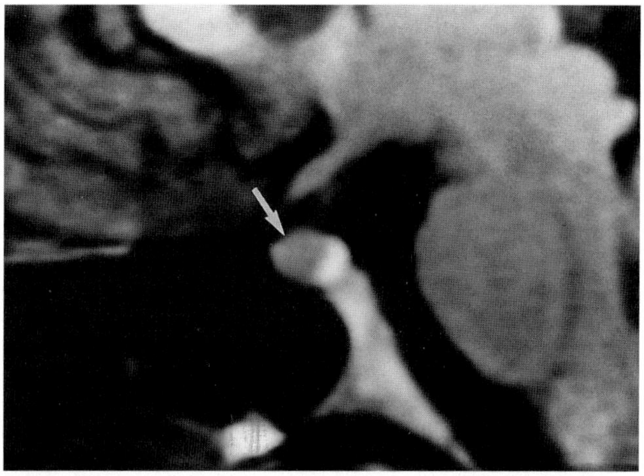

Figure 3-9B: Unenhanced sagittal T1-weighted MR image in the postpartum period in the same case as that in Figure 3-9A, showing that the pituitary gland (*arrow*) has returned to normal size (compare with Figure 3-9A).

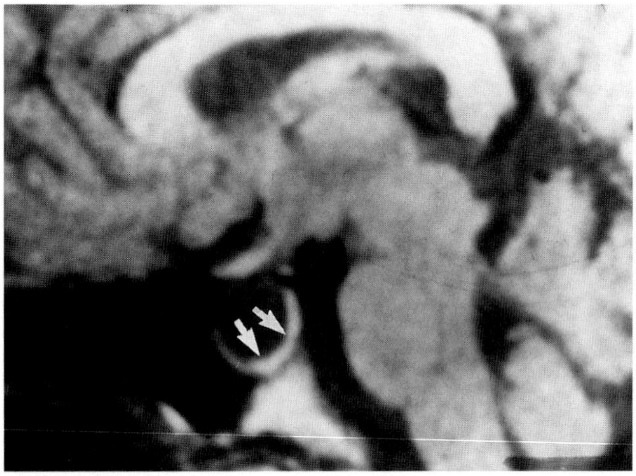

Figure 3-10A: Partially empty, enlarged sella turcica. Sagittal midline T1-weighted MR image showing an enlarged sella turcica that is filled with relatively hypointense cerebrospinal fluid. The pituitary tissue is compressed posteroinferiorly into a thin crescent (*arrows*).

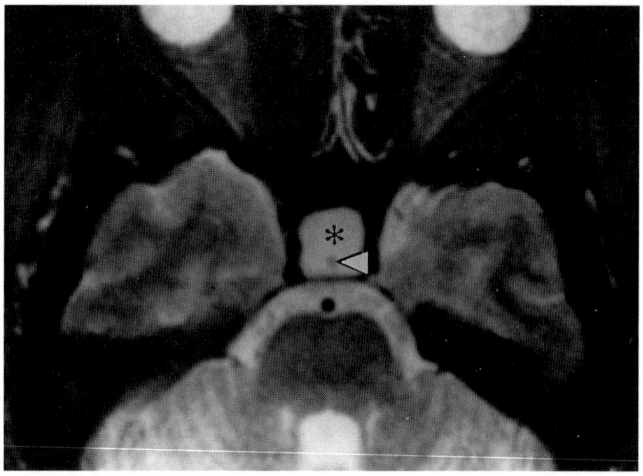

Figure 3-10B: Axial T2-weighted MR image showing hyperintense cerebrospinal fluid (*asterisk*) within the partially empty sella turcica, and the descending pituitary infundibulum (*arrowhead*).

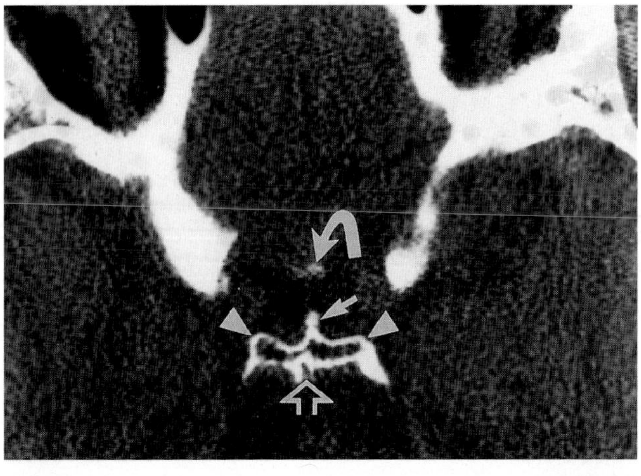

Figure 3-11: Duplicated sella turcica/intrasellar bony spike. Axial CT showing a midline bony spur (*solid arrow*) extending from the dorsum sellae (*open arrow*). In such a case the lateral posterior clinoid processes (*arrowheads*) are seen on either side of what might be termed the *median posterior clinoid process* (Jinkins) (*solid arrow*) . This may represent a duplicated sella turcica or a congenital intrasellar bony spike. The patient exhibited no evidence of pituitary dysfunction. The dorsum sellae (*curved arrow*) is also noted.

Pituitary Infundibulum Variants

Deviation of the pituitary infundibulum on coronal magnetic resonance images has generally been used to support the presence of a microadenoma. However, in one study 46% of normal patients had a more or less pronounced tilt of the pituitary infundibulum. This tilt was due to a developmental lateral eccentricity of the pituitary gland in relationship to the midline of the brain in 34% and to developmental eccentric insertion of the pituitary infundibulum of the midline of the gland in another 12%. This high frequency of infundibulum deviation in patients without pituitary disease suggests that such displacement should not be used by itself to support the presence of pituitary microadenoma.

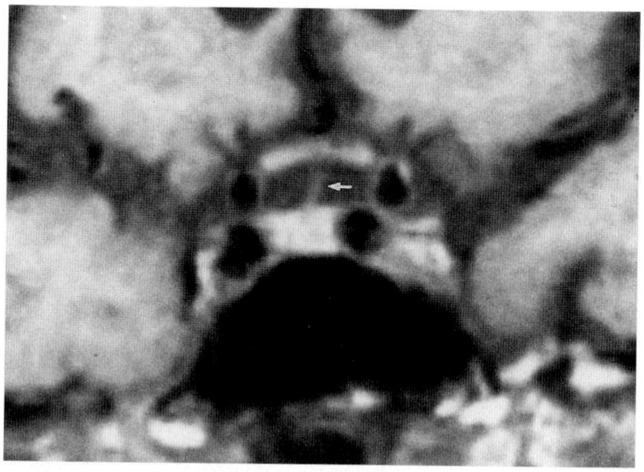

Figure 3-12: Constitutional deviation of the pituitary infundibulum. Unenhanced coronal T1-weighted MR image in a normal subject showing the eccentric position of the pituitary gland with respect to the cerebral interhemispheric fissure. There is also asymmetry of the carotid flow voids with respect to the cerebral midline and the midline of the sphenoid sinus. This results in a normal (nonpathologic) pituitary infundibular tilt (*arrow*) toward the right.

Vascular Supply to the Pituitary Gland

1. The arterial supply of the pituitary gland and hypothalamus is primarily via the superior and inferior hypophyseal arteries, which are small branches of the cavernous segment of the internal carotid artery.
2. Branches of the superior hypophyseal arteries enter the basal portion of the medial eminence of the posterior lobe of the pituitary gland where they form a dense plexus of capillary loops. The blood in this capillary bed picks up hypothalamic hormones and carries them to the venous sinusoids of the anterior lobe of the pituitary gland (adenohypophysis); this network of capillaries, venous channels, and venous sinusoids constitutes the hypothalamic-hypophyseal portal system.
3. The venous system of the anterior lobe of the pituitary gland drains into the cavernous venous sinuses.
4. The arterial supply of the pars nervosa of the pituitary gland is via the inferior hypophyseal arteries. The infundibulum is supplied by branches of the superior hypophyseal arteries.
5. The venous system of the posterior lobe of the pituitary gland drains into the cavernous venous sinuses.

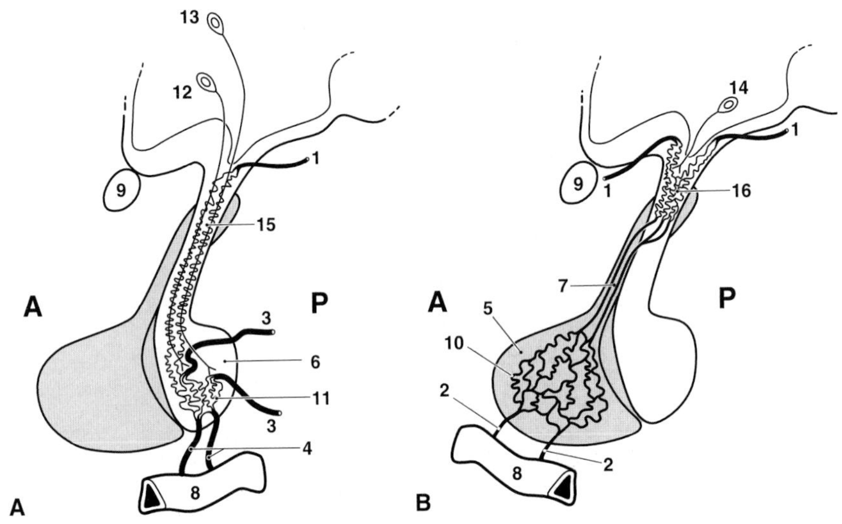

Figure 3-13: Lateral schematic of the normal vascular anatomy of the pituitary gland. **A:** Vascular supply to the pars nervosa of the neurohypophysis. **B:** Hypothalamic-hypophyseal portal system.

1 Superior hypophyseal artery branches
2 Inferior–anterior pituitary veins to cavernous venous sinus
3 Inferior hypophyseal artery branches
4 Inferior–posterior pituitary veins to cavernous venous sinus
5 Pars distalis of the adenohypophysis
6 Pars nervosa of the neurohypophysis
7 Long portal vessels of the hypothalamic-hypophyseal portal system
8 Cavernous venous sinus
9 Optic chiasm
10 Venous sinusoids of the anterior lobe of the pituitary gland
11 Capillary vascular system of the posterior lobe of the pituitary gland
12, 13 Supraoptic and paraventricular nuclei of hypothalamus that produce oxytocin and antidiuretic hormone (vasopressin)
14 Hypothalamic (infundibular) nucleus that releases factors to inhibit or stimulate the hormone release of the adenohypophysis
15 Arteries of the infundibulum (trabecular arteries)
16 Capillary network of the medial eminence

THE CAVERNOUS VENOUS SINUSES

Anatomy

1. The paired lateral cavernous venous sinuses are irregular, trabeculated venous plexuses, rather than single lumen cavernous venous structures, that normally drain from front to back and superiorly to inferiorly. However, because these venous sinuses are valveless, the direction of flow is reversible.
2. The major veins that drain into the cavernous venous sinus include (a) the superior and inferior ophthalmic veins, (b) the sphenoparietal venous sinus, (c) the superficial middle cerebral (sylvian) vein, (d) the inferior cerebral veins, (e) the veins draining the pituitary gland, and, occasionally, (f) the frontal meningeal veins.
3. In the midline, the two lateral cavernous venous sinuses are interconnected via (a) the anterior and posterior intercavernous venous sinuses running in the floor of the pituitary fossa, and (b) the basilar venous plexus on the posterior surface of the clivus.
4. The venous drainage of the cavernous venous sinus on each side includes (a) the superior and inferior petrosal sinuses directly, and (b) the pterygoid venous plexus beneath the skull base via cranial emissary veins.
5. The internal carotid artery together with its accompanying sympathetic neural plexus passes through the cavernous venous sinus.
6. The neural structures that pass through the cavernous venous sinus include the third, fourth, and sixth cranial nerves (CN-III, IV, and VI) and the first (oculomotor) and second (maxillary) divisions of the fifth cranial nerve (CN-V1, CN-V2). The first and second divisions of the fifth cranial nerves pass partly or completely within the dural wall of the cavernous venous sinus; in the former case medially they are covered primarily by venous endothelium.
7. The dura mater of the cavernous venous sinuses reflect medially over the superior surface of the pituitary gland to form the diaphragma sellae; this structure is pierced centrally by an aperture that transmits the pituitary infundibulum.

See also Chapter 2U, The Paired Cavernous Venous Sinuses.

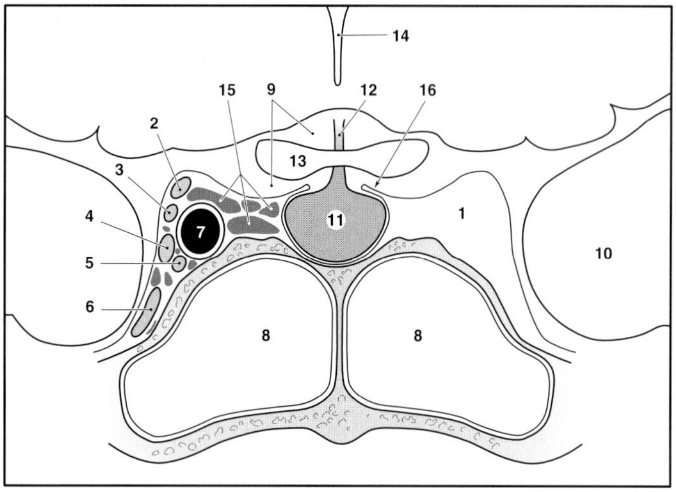

Figure 3-14: Coronal schematic of the contents of the cavernous venous sinuses and surrounding structures.
1 Cavernous venous sinus on the left side
2 Cranial nerve III (oculomotor) (CN III)
3 Cranial nerve IV (trochlear) (CN IV)
4 Cranial nerve V1 (ophthalmic) (CN V1)
5 Cranial nerve VI (abducens) (CN VI)
6 Cranial nerve V2 (maxillary division) (CN V2)
7 Internal carotid artery
8 Sphenoid sinus
9 Suprasellar cistern
10 Temporal lobe
11 Pituitary gland
12 Pituitary infundibulum
13 Optic chiasm
14 Third ventricle
15 Venous sinusoids of cavernous venous sinus on the right side
16 Diaphragma sellae

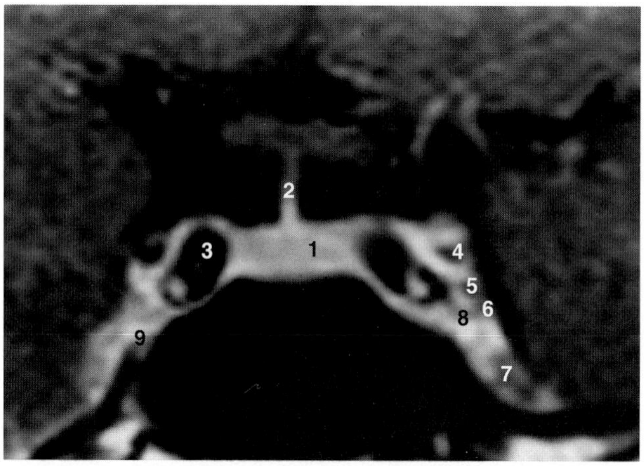

Figure 3-15: Cavernous venous sinuses. Enhanced coronal T1-weighted MR image showing the anatomic detail of the left cavernous venous sinus and surrounding structures.
1 Pituitary gland
2 Pituitary infundibulum
3 Internal carotid artery (flow void)
4 Oculomotor (CN III) nerve
5 Trochlear (CN IV) nerve
6 Trigeminal (CN V) nerve, first division (CN V1: ophthalmic nerve)
7 Trigeminal (CN V) nerve, second division (CN V2: maxillary nerve)
8 Abducens (CN VI) nerve
9 Cavernous venous sinus sinusoids

CHAPTER 4

The Orbit

OVERVIEW

1. The shape of the orbit is conical with its apex directed posteriorly.
2. The orbital roof is formed by the frontal bone anteriorly and the lesser wing of the sphenoid bone posteriorly.
3. The orbital floor is formed by the maxillary bone, the zygomatic bone, and the orbital process of the palatine bone.
4. The medial orbital wall is formed by the frontal process of the maxillary bone, the lacrimal bone, the lamina papyracea, and the sphenoid bone.
5. The lateral orbital wall is formed by the orbital process of the zygomatic bone and the greater wing of the sphenoid bone.
6. The periosteal layer that lines the bony orbit is termed the periorbita.
7. The superior orbital fissure transmits
   a. The third, fourth, ophthalmic (first) division of the fifth (e.g., supraorbital nerve) and sixth cranial nerves (CN III, IV, V1, VI)
   b. Branches of the lacrimal/middle meningeal arteries
   c. The superior ophthalmic vein connecting with the cavernous venous sinus posteriorly, and
   d. sympathetic and parasympathetic (e.g., lacrimal nerve) neural fibers
8. The inferior orbital fissure transmits
   a. The infraorbital nerve (branch of the maxillary [second] division of the fifth cranial nerve: CN-V2) and the zygomatic nerve
   b. The infraorbital artery and inferior ophthalmic vein, and
   c. Neural branches from the pterygopalatine ganglion
9. The optic foramen/canal transmits
   a. the optic nerve (CN II), and
   b. the ophthalmic artery
10. The nasolacrimal duct foramen in the medial wall of the orbit transmits the nasolacrimal duct, which conducts tears that ultimately drain into the inferior nasal meatus of the nasal passageway.
11. The supraorbital notch/foramen transmits
    a. the supraorbital artery
    b. the supraorbital vein, and
    c. the supraorbital nerve (branch of the ophthalmic [first] division of the fifth cranial nerve: CN-V1)
12. The infraorbital groove, canal, and foramen transmit
    a. The infraorbital nerve (branch of the maxillary [second] division of the fifth cranial nerve: CN-V2)
    b. The inferior ophthalmic vein

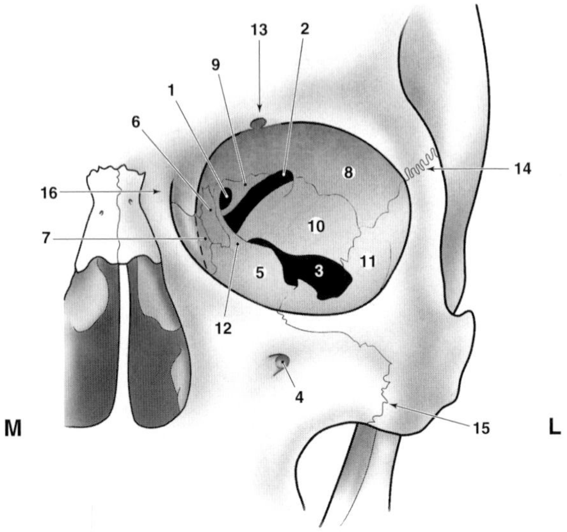

Figure 4-1A: Frontal schematic of the bony orbit on the left side. *M,* medial; *L,* lateral.

1 Optic canal
2 Superior orbital fissure
3 Inferior orbital fissure
4 Infraorbital foramen
5 Orbital process of the maxillary bone
6 Ethmoid bone
7 Lacrimal bone
8 Orbital plate of the frontal bone
9 Sphenoid bone (lesser wing)
10 Sphenoid bone (greater wing)
11 Zygomatic bone
12 Orbital process of the palatine bone
13 Supraorbital notch
14 Zygomaticofrontal suture
15 Zygomaticomaxillary suture
16 Frontomaxillary suture

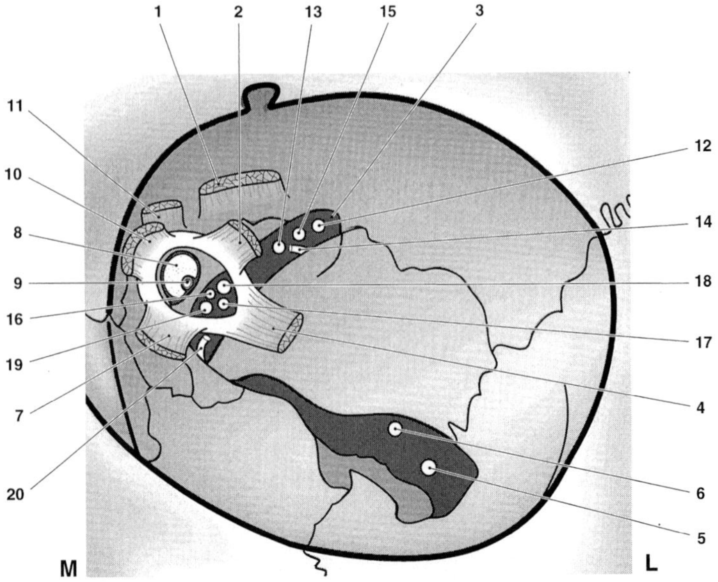

Figure 4-1B: Schematic showing the relationship of the structures at the apex of the orbit on the left side. *M*, medial; *L*, lateral.

1 Levator palpebrae superioris muscle
2 Superior rectus muscle
3 Superior orbital fissure
4 Lateral rectus muscle
5,6 Zygomatic and infraorbital nerves passing through the inferior orbital fissure
7 Inferior rectus muscle
8,9 Optic nerve (CN II) and ophthalmic artery emerging through the optic canal
10 Medial rectus muscle
11 Superior oblique muscle
12 Lacrimal nerve
13 Ophthalmic nerve CN V1
14 Superior ophthalmic vein
15 Trochlear nerve (CN IV)
16 Nasociliary nerve
17 Abducens nerve (CN VI)
18 Superior division of oculomotor nerve (CN III)
19 Inferior division of oculomotor nerve (CN III)
20 Inferior ophthalmic vein

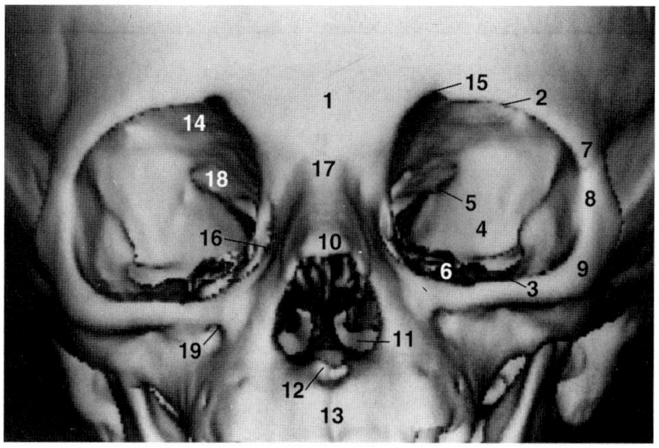

Figure 4-2: The bony orbit. Three-dimensional CT image in the frontal projection showing the orbits and surrounding bony structures.

1 Glabella of frontal bone
2 Supraorbital margin
3 Infraorbital margin
4 Greater wing of sphenoid bone
5 Superior orbital fissure
6 Inferior orbital fissure
7 Zygomatic process of frontal bone
8 Frontal process of zygomatic bone
9 Zygomatic bone
10 Nasal bones
11 Inferior nasal concha
12 Anterior nasal spine
13 Intermaxillary suture
14 Orbital plate of frontal bone
15 Supraorbital notch
16 Nasolacrimal groove in lacrimal bone
17 Nasion
18 Lesser wing of sphenoid bone
19 Infraorbital foramen

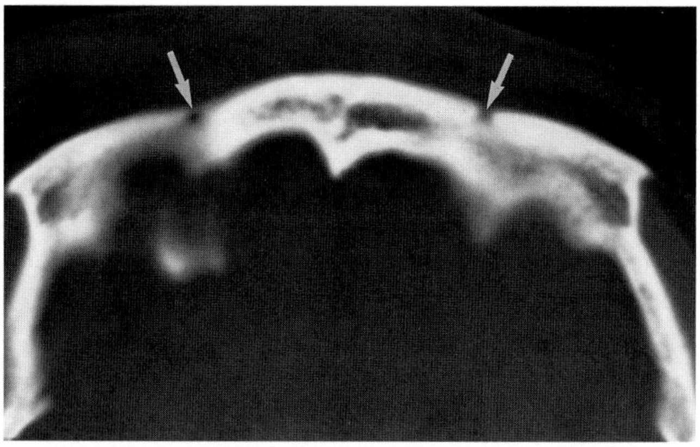

Figure 4-3A: The supraorbital foramina/notches. Axial CT image showing the supraorbital notches (*arrows*) bilaterally.

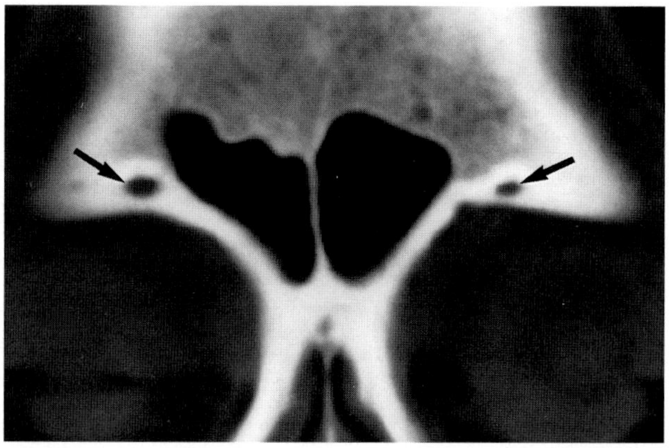

Figure 4-3B: Supraorbital foramina/canals. Coronal CT image showing complete supraorbital bony canals/foramina (*arrows*) bilaterally.

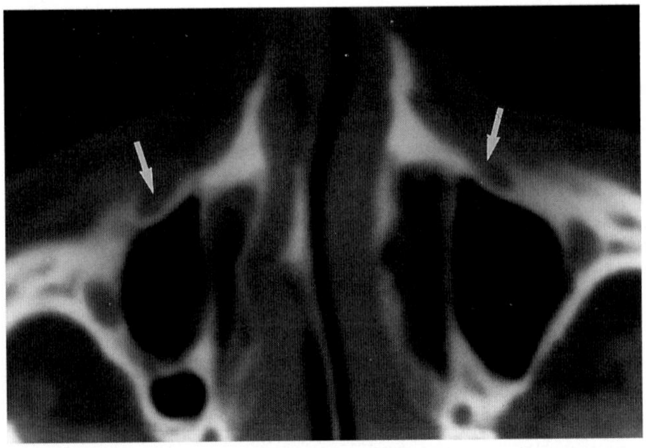

Figure 4-4A: The infraorbital foramina and canals. Axial CT image showing the infraorbital foramina (*arrows*).

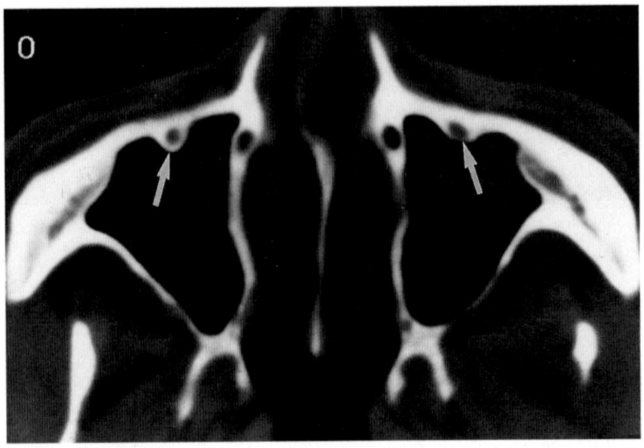

Figure 4-4B: The infraorbital canals. Axial CT image showing the infraorbital canals (*arrows*) bilaterally.

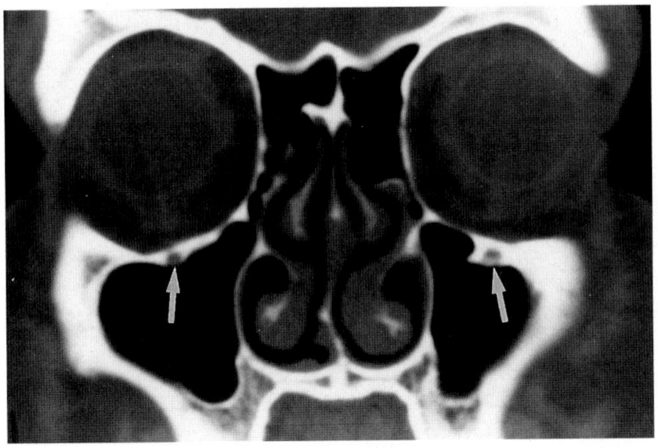

Figure 4-4C: Coronal CT image again showing the infraorbital canals (*arrows*).

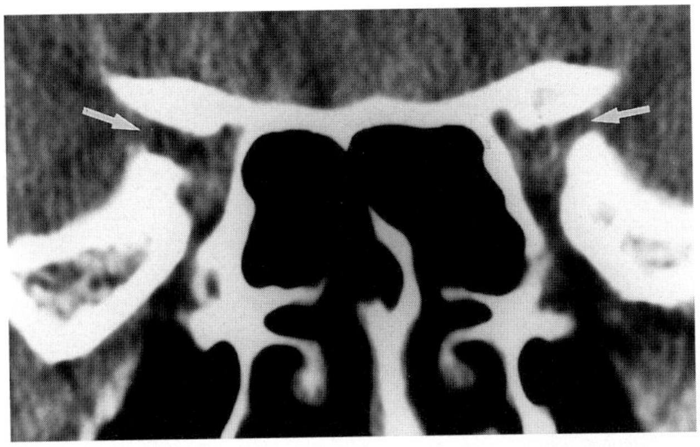

Figure 4-5: The superior orbital fissure. Coronal CT image showing the superior orbital fissures (*arrows*) bilaterally.

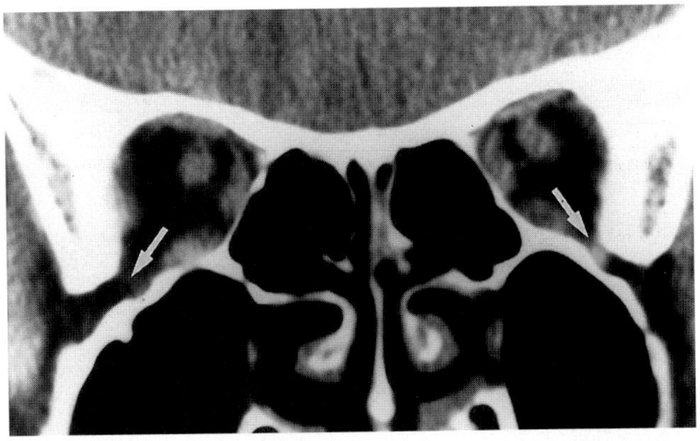

Figure 4-6: The inferior orbital fissure. Coronal CT image showing the inferior orbital fissures (*arrows*) bilaterally.

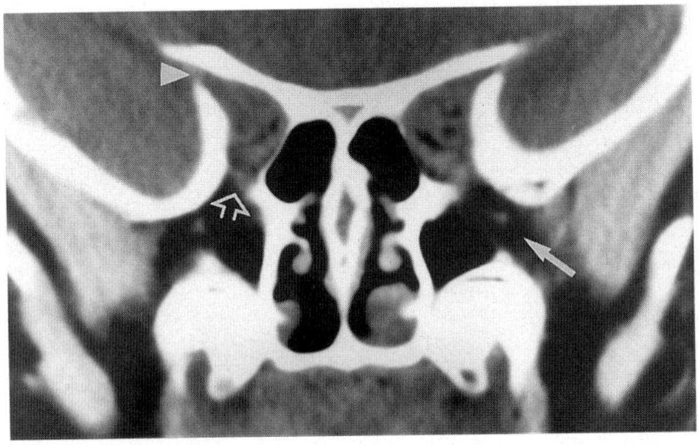

Figure 4-7: Superior and inferior orbital fissures, and connection with the pterygopalatine fossae. Coronal CT image showing the superior (*arrowhead*) and inferior (*open arrow*) orbital fissures and the pterygopalatine fossa (*solid arrow*).

THE GLOBE AND OPTIC NERVE/SHEATH COMPLEX

1. The globe is a round or oval structure that has five layers in its wall, described from inward to outward: (a) the retina, (b) Bruch's membrane, (c) the choroid, (d) the sclera, and (e) Tenon's capsule.
2. The transparent cornea is continuous with the sclera at the limbus (i.e., corneoscleral junction). The limbus is circumscribed by the sinus venosus sclerae or the canal of Schlemm. The venous sinus is separated from the anterior chamber by loose trabecular tissue, the trabecular meshwork. Aqueous fluid from the aqueous humor filters through the trabecular meshwork and into the sinus venosus sclerae which subsequently drains into the episcleral venous plexus which in turn drains into the anterior ciliary veins.
3. The uvea (uveal tract) is the pigmented tissue beneath the sclera. The three components of the uvea are: (a) the choroid, (b) the ciliary body, and (c) the iris.
   a. The choroid is a pigmented vascular layer of the globe. It extends from the optic nerve head to the ciliary body. The blood supply and drainage of the choroid is as follows:
      i. The posterior part of the choroid is supplied from the short posterior ciliary arteries that in turn arise from the ophthalmic artery.
      ii. The anterior part of the choroid is supplied from the long posterior ciliary arteries which in turn arise from a common origin, with the short posterior ciliary arteries from the ophthalmic artery, and from the recurrent ciliary arteries which in turn arise from the arterial circle of the iris, an anastomotic arc between the long posterior ciliary and the anterior ciliary arteries. The anterior ciliary arteries in turn arise from muscular arterial branches of the anterior orbit.
      iii. The venous drainage of the choroid is into four or more vortex veins. The two superior vortex veins drain into the superior ophthalmic vein; the two inferior vortex veins drain into the inferior ophthalmic vein.
   b. The ciliary body secretes the aqueous humor. The ciliary body also contains muscles that attach to the periphery of the lens and control the lens shape. The ciliary muscle is innervated by parasympathetic fibers from the oculomotor nerve (CN-III) via the short ciliary nerves.
   c. The iris is a disc-shaped structure that is attached peripherally to the ciliary body and is perforated centrally by the round pupil. It contains smooth muscle: the dilator pupillae and sphincter pupillae muscles. This muscle allows dilatation and constriction of the pupil. The dilator pupillae muscle is innervated by sympathetic fibers from the long ciliary nerves. The sphincter pupillae muscle is innervated by parasympathetic fibers from the oculomotor nerve (CN-III). Less melanin pigment in the iris results in a blue coloration; greater degrees of melanin result in a mottled and eventually a brown coloration.
4. The zonule of the lens is a suspensory ligament running between the lens and the ciliary body. When the ciliary body relaxes, the zonule tenses and flattens the lens (for focusing). Contraction of the ciliary body causes the zonule to relax, thereby resulting in a bulging of the anterior convexity of the lens (near focusing).
5. The anterior segment of the globe consists of an anterior and posterior chamber. The anterior and posterior chambers are subdivided by the iris and communicate with one another via the pupil. The anterior segment lies between the rear surface of the cornea and the front surface of the lens. Clear, fluid aqueous humor circulates within the anterior segment.
6. The posterior segment of the globe is located posterior to the lens and its supporting ligament, the zonule. It contains a clear, jelly-like material termed the vitreous humor.
7. The lens lies posterior to the iris and is separated from it by the posterior chamber. The posterior surface of the lens is separated from the anterior aspect of the vitreous humor by the fluid-filled retrolenticular space. The lens is a biconvex transparent structure having a central nucleus and a peripheral cortex. The lens has a gelatinous consistency that is firmer in the nucleus than in the cortex. The posterior surface has a more con-

vex curvature than the anterior surface. The suspensory ligament, or zonule, connects the lens to the ciliary body and suspends the lens in place.

8. The retina is the thin, transparent, inner, light-sensitive coat of the globe. It extends from posteriorly to its serrated margin, the ora serrata, situated approximately halfway from the midplane of the globe in the vertical direction to the limbus. The retina is attached at the ora serrata to both the choroid and to the vitreous body. The retina histologically has 10 layers. The photoreceptor cells are located in the outer areas of the retina and the neural fibers are found in the inner layer. No photoreceptors are found at the optic disc. The fovea centralis is the thinnest part of the retina and is the most light-sensitive.
9. The optic disc (optic nerve head, optic papilla) is the site where the nerve enters the retina. The central retinal artery and vein enter and drain via the optic disc. The optic disc is not light-sensitive (i.e., "blind spot").
10. The macula lutea is located several millimeters lateral to the optic disc. It is a depression in globe approximately the size of the optic disc. At its center is found the fovea centralis.
11. The fovea centralis is a capillary-free zone located in the center of the macula lutea. The absence of vessels allows light to pass without obstruction directly to the fovea. The fovea centralis is the most light-sensitive area of the retina and is composed almost entirely of cones, the color-sensitive photoreceptors.
12. Bruch's membrane is an acellular, amorphous, sheet-like structure lying between the retina and the choroid of the globe.
13. The sclera is a fibrous covering of the globe that is opaque and relatively avascular. It extends from the limbus (i.e., junction of cornea and sclera) to the back of the globe. When the sclera is perforated by numerous neural bundles of the optic nerve, the region is called the lamina cribrosa. The extraocular muscles insert into the external aspect of the sclera.
14. The hyaloid canal runs from the posterior surface of the lens to the optic nerve head. During embryogenesis of the globe, it transmits the hyaloid artery; this artery normally involutes at approximately 30 weeks gestation. In the fully developed globe, the hyaloid canal persists as a thin fibrous structure that may be filled with a relatively more watery fluid as compared to the surrounding vitreous humor.
15. The conjunctiva is a transparent mucous membrane that forms the conjunction between the cornea and the sclera. It covers the internal palpebral (lid) surfaces and extends onto the external aspect of the cornea and sclera.
16. Tenon's capsule (fascia bulbi) is a thin fibrous capsule that covers the majority of the globe and extends from the periphery of the cornea anteriorly to the insertion of the optic nerve posteriorly. The inner surface of Tenon's capsule is incompletely separated from the sclera by a fluid-filled space, the episcleral space. Fibrous strands traverse the episcleral space to attach Tenon's capsule to the underlying sclera. Tenon's capsule supports the globe and allows for its movement in all directions.
17. Tenon's capsule and the extraocular muscle sheaths project to adjacent orbital structures to form check ligaments. These check ligaments limit the actions of the extraocular muscles. The check ligaments include the medial check ligament from Tenon's capsule to the lacrimal bone, the lateral check ligament from the lateral rectus muscle sheath to the zygomatic bone, the check ligament from the superior rectus muscle sheath to the levator palpebrae superioris muscle, the check ligament from the inferior rectus muscle sheath to the lower eyelid, the check ligament from the superior oblique muscle sheath to the trochlea, and the check ligament from the inferior oblique muscle to the lateral aspect of the orbital floor.
18. The orbital septum is a fibrous membrane arising circumferentially from the periosteum of the orbital rim. The septum extends inward to join the tarsal plates of the upper and lower eyelids. The orbital septum is pierced by the levator palpebrae superioris, the check ligament of the inferior rectus muscle, and the lacrimal, supratrochlear, infratrochlear, and supraorbital vessels and nerves.
19. The upper and lower tarsal plates have free borders peripherally, the ciliary border, and

are attached centrally to the orbital septum and medial and lateral palpebral ligaments at the orbital border. The levator palpebrae superioris inserts into the upper tarsal plate. A band of muscle passes from the inferior rectus muscle to the lower tarsal plate. Tarsal (meibomian) glands are modified sebaceous glands found in the tarsal plates that secrete an oily secretion via ducts at the free margin of the eyelids that lubricates and retards tear evaporation on the surface of the globe.

20. The central retinal artery divides at the optic disc into superior and inferior branches that give rise to medial (nasal) and lateral (temporal) branches (four branches total). The terminal branches of the retinal artery are end arteries, not anastomosing with other terminal branches. The branches of the central retinal artery give nutrient supply to the inner area of the retina comprising the neural fibers. The outer area of the retina, composed of photoreceptors, receives its nutrient supply by diffusion from the overlying choroidal vessels. Retinal veins accompany the retinal artery and its branches. The central retinal vein drains the main superior and inferior retinal veins at the optic disc.
21. The upper and lower eyelids cover the anterior surface of the globe. The opening between the two lids is termed the palpebral fissure. The external surface of the eyelid is covered by skin, whereas the internal surface is covered by conjunctiva. The chief muscle of the eyelids is the orbicularis oculi muscle. The upper and lower lids meet medially and laterally at the medial (inner) and lateral (outer) canthi. Internally the lids have a structure composed of the tarsal plates along the border of the lids and the orbital septum into which the tarsal plates insert. The lacrimal papillae and tarsal gland ducts empty onto the anterior surface of the globe at the lid margins. The eyelashes arise from the ciliary portion of the eyelids, that part of each eyelid lateral to the medially placed lacrimal papilla(e).
22. The optic nerve sheath is continuous anteriorly with the sclera and Tenon's capsule on the posterior surface of the globe, and posteriorly with the intracranial dura mater.
23. The optic subarachnoid space contained within the optic nerve sheath and surrounding the optic nerve is continuous with the intracranial subarachnoid space.

TABLE 4-1: The Five Layers of the Wall of the Globe

1. Retina: the neural/sensory stratum of the globe
2. Bruch's membrane: an acellular, amorphous, sheet-like structure
3. Uvea (uveal tract): a richly vascular/pigmented tissue consisting of three components:
   a. Iris
   b. Ciliary body
   c. Choroid of the globe
4. Sclera: the fibrous tunic of the globe
5. Tenon's capsule: a fibroelastic membrane that covers the sclera of the globe

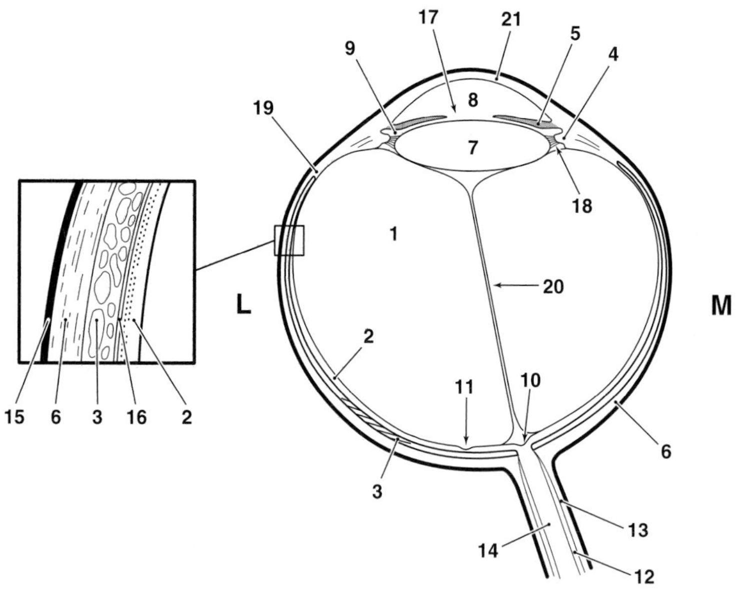

Figure 4-8: Axial schematic section showing the anatomy of the globe and the ocular layers on the right side. *M,* medial; *L,* lateral.

1 Posterior segment (vitreous humor)
2 Retina
3 Choroid
4 Ciliary body (uvea)
5 Iris
6 Sclera
7 Lens
8 Anterior chamber } anterior segment (aqueous
9 Posterior chamber } humor)
10 Optic disc (optic nerve head)
11 Fovea
12 Optic subarachnoid space
13 Optic nerve sheath
14 Optic nerve
15 Tenon's capsule
16 Bruch's membrane
17 Pupil
18 Zonule
19 Limbus (corneoscleral junction)
20 Remnant of hyaloid canal
21 Cornea

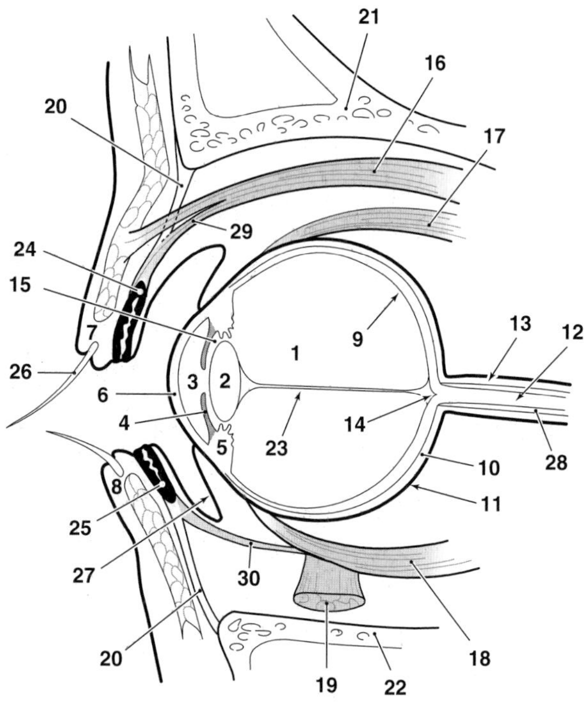

Figure 4-9: Sagittal schematic section of the anterior orbit showing the globe and related structures of the orbit (globe not to scale).

1 Vitreous humor
2 Lens
3 Anterior chamber
4 Iris
5 Ciliary body
6 Cornea
7 Upper eyelid
8 Lower eyelid
9 Retina
10 Choroid
11 Sclera
12 Optic nerve
13 Optic nerve sheath
14 Optic disc (optic nerve head)
15 Posterior chamber
16 Levator palpebrae superioris muscle
17 Superior rectus muscle
18 Inferior rectus muscle
19 Inferior oblique muscle
20 Orbital septum (upper and lower aspects)
21 Bony orbital roof
22 Bony orbital floor
23 Remnant of hyaloid canal
24 Superior tarsal plate
25 Inferior tarsal plate
26 Eyelash
27 Bulbar conjunctiva
28 Optic subarachnoid space
29 Check ligament to inferior tarsal plate
30 Check ligament to superior tarsal plate

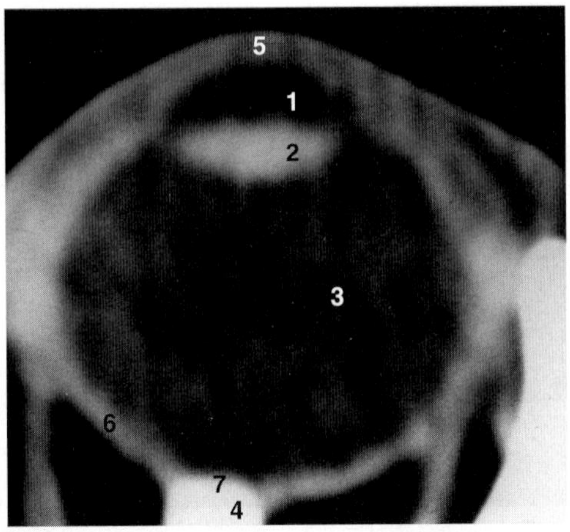

Figure 4-10A: The globe. Axial CT image of the left globe following intrathecal contrast administration showing the normal appearance of the left globe.
1 Anterior chamber of the anterior segment
2 Lens
3 Posterior segment
4 Contrast media within the subarachnoid space of the optic nerve sheath
5 Cornea
6 Wall of globe
7 Optic disc (optic nerve head/papilla)

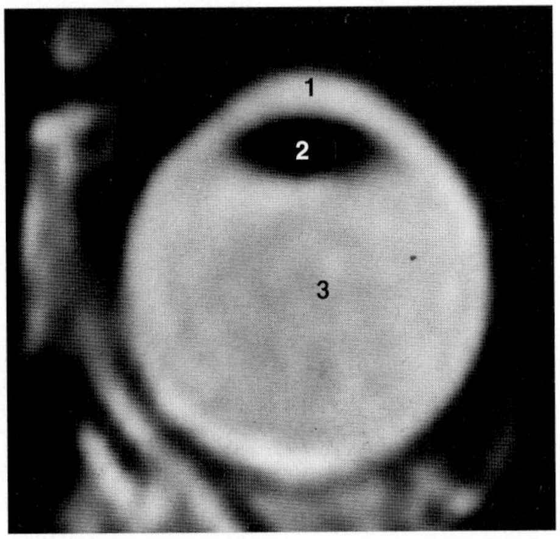

Figure 4-10B: Axial T2-weighted MR image showing the normal appearance of the left globe.
1 Cornea and anterior chamber of the anterior segment
2 Lens
3 Posterior segment

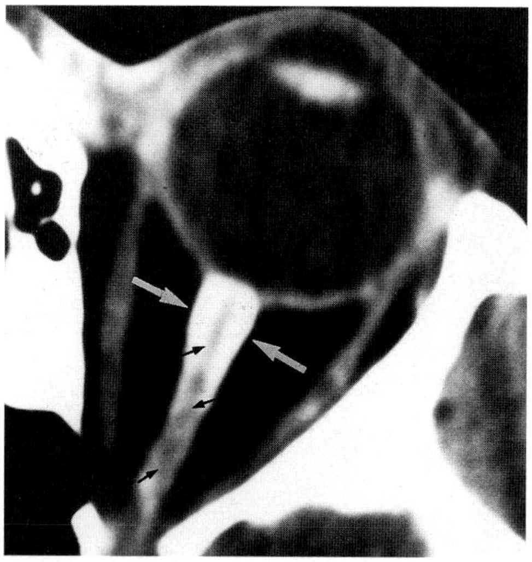

Figure 4-11A: Optic nerve/sheath complex. Axial CT of the left orbit obtained after water-soluble intrathecal water-soluble contrast administration showing opacification of the subarachnoid space of the optic nerve sheath (*white arrows*). The optic nerve can be seen as a linear filling defect (*black arrows*) within the contrast column.

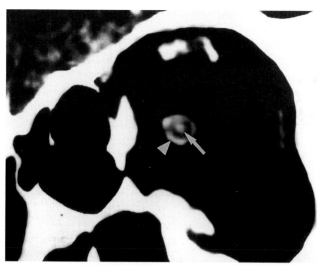

Figure 4-11B: Coronal CT image of the left orbit following intravenous iodinated contrast administration showing the optic nerve sheath (*arrowhead*), the circumferential hypodense optic subarachnoid space, and the centrally placed optic nerve (*arrow*) of the left eye.

Figure 4-11C: Coronal T2-weighted MR image of the left eye showing the retrobulbar orbital structures.

1 Superior rectus muscle and levator palpebrae superioris muscle
2 Medial rectus muscle
3 Inferior rectus muscle
4 Lateral rectus muscle
5 Cerebrospinal fluid in perioptic subarachnoid space
6 Optic nerve
7 Retroorbital fat
8 Optic nerve sheath
9 Orbital blood vessel

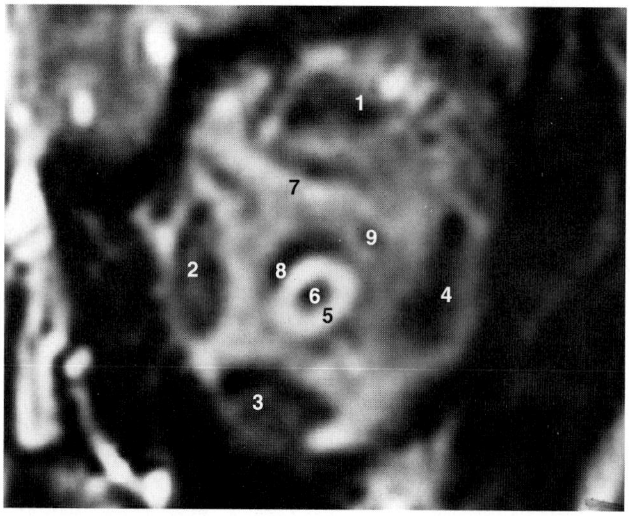

THE OPTIC PATHWAY

Overview

1. From peripherally to centrally the optic pathway consists of
   a. The retina
   b. The optic nerves
   c. The optic chiasm
   d. The optic tracts
   e. The lateral geniculate bodies
   f. The optic radiations (hemispheric white matter transmitting the optic association fibers), and
   g. The visual (calcarine, striate) cortices
2. The optic nerve inserts into the back of the globe at the optic nerve head (optic disc, optic papilla) to ramify within the retina.
3. The optic nerve fibers partially decussate in the optic chiasm.
4. The lateral geniculate body is a thalamic sensory relay nucleus.
5. The visual (calcarine, striate) cortex is located in the medial aspect of the inferior occipital lobes on each side.

The Visual Pathway

1. The primary visual or striate cortex (Brodmann cortical area 17) is located in the gyri surrounding and in the walls of the posterior aspect of the calcarine sulcus. It is referred to as the striate cortex because of the morphologically prominent visual stria it contains.
2. The striate cortex is nearly surrounded (except anteriorly) by the parastriate cortex (Brodmann cortical area 18), which in turn is largely surrounded by the peristriate cortex (Brodmann area 19).
3. Primary visual signals reach the striate cortex from the lateral geniculate body. Secondary visual signals reach the parastriate and peristriate areas from the striate cortex and the pulvinar; to a lesser degree, primary visual signals also directly project to the parastriate and peristriate cortices.
4. Optic area commissural fibers interconnect the parastriate and peristriate cortices via the posterior aspect of the corpus callosum; the striate cortices proper have few callosal interconnections.
5. Projections from the striate, parastriate, and peristriate cortices to the superior colliculi and pretectal area of the brain stem control the visual reflexes of fixation and accommodation. Projections to the frontal eye fields influence the voluntary turning of the eyes toward visual stimuli.
6. Other secondary visual areas are located in the middle and inferior temporal gyri.
7. Retinal (retinotopic) neural projections within the primary visual (calcarine striate) cortex come from the ipsilateral halves of each retina. The upper portions of the retina (lower visual field) project to the visual cortex above the calcarine sulcus; the lower portions of the retina (upper visual field) project to the visual cortex below the calcarine sulcus. For this reason the "visual field" maps of the striate cortex are essentially upside down. A disproportionately large cortical area is devoted to central (macular) vision (central 6 ° of vision).

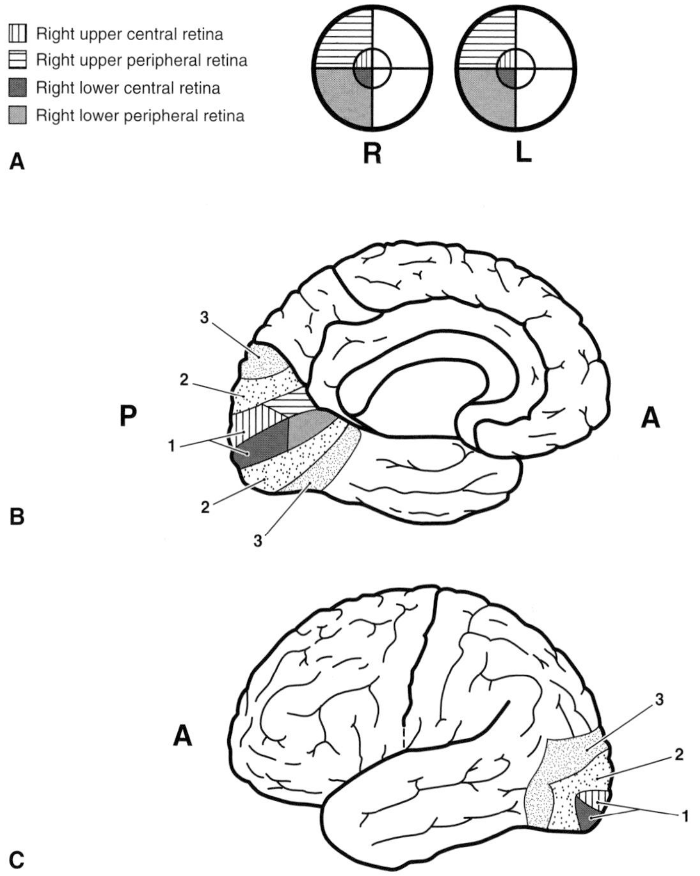

Figure 4-12: A: Schematics of the retinotopic projections within the visual (striate) cortex. **B:** Medial aspect of left hemisphere. **C:** Lateral aspect of left hemisphere. *A*, anterior; *P*, posterior; *R*, right globe retina; *L*, left globe retina (as seen on fundrescopic examination).

1 Primary visual (striate) cortex
2 Parastriate cortex
3 Peristriate cortex

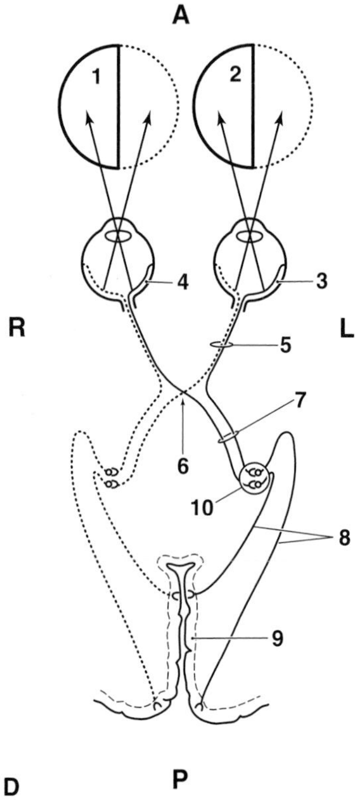

Figure 4-12D: Schematic of the visual pathway (CN II) viewed from above. *L*, left; *R*, right; *A*, anterior; *P*, posterior.

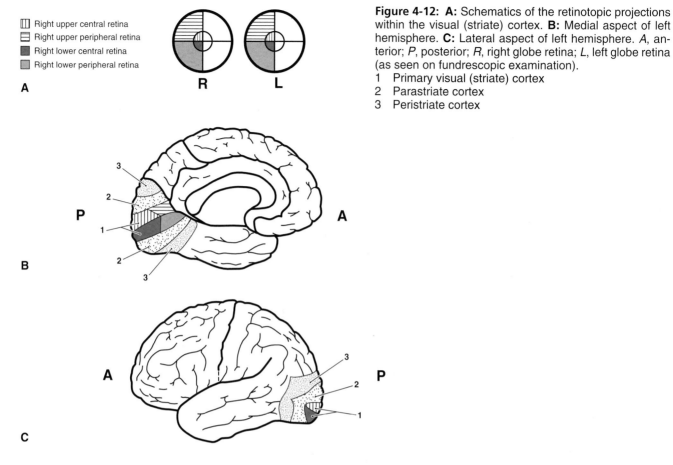

1 Temporal visual field of the left hemispheric visual (calcarine) cortex
2 Nasal visual field of the left hemispheric visual (calcarine) cortex
3 Temporal retina
4 Nasal retina
5 Optic nerve
6 Optic chiasm
7 Optic tract
8 Optic radiation
9 Visual (calcarine) cortex of the left hemisphere
10 Lateral geniculate body of the left side

THE EXTRAOCULAR MUSCLES OF THE ORBIT

1. The extraocular muscles are seven in number and include (a) the medial rectus, (b) superior rectus, (c) inferior rectus, (d) lateral rectus, (e) superior oblique, (f) inferior oblique, and (g) levator palpebrae superioris muscles.
2. The superior, inferior, lateral, and medial rectus muscles originate in the annulus of Zinn at the optic foramen in the orbital apex and insert onto the outer surface of the globe.
3. The superior oblique muscle originates from the orbital roof, superomedial to the optic foramen, and inserts into the superior-outer surface of the globe. The anterior tendon of the superior oblique muscle passes through a fibrocartilaginous ring, the trochlea, that is in turn attached to the trochlear fovea of the frontal bone. The tendon moves within the trochlea in a similar fashion to a rope within a pulley. The trochlea may occasionally be calcified.
4. The inferior oblique muscle originates from the orbital floor at the orbital plate of the maxillary bone and inserts into the inferior-outer surface of the globe.
5. The levator palpebrae superioris muscle originates from the orbital roof, near the origin of the superior rectus muscle, and inserts into the upper eyelid.

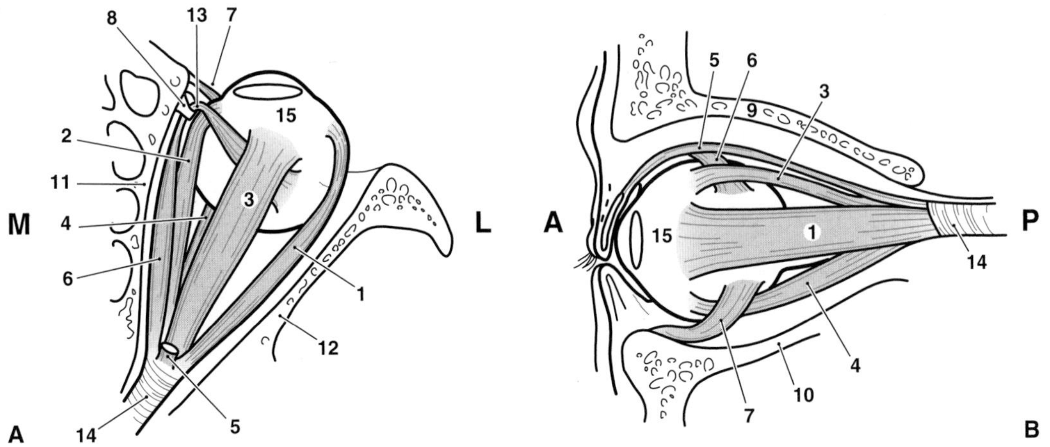

Figure 4-13: Superior and lateral schematics of the extraocular muscles of the left eye with the tissues above and lateral to the muscle cone removed, respectively. In the superior view the levator palpebrae superioris muscle has also been removed. **A:** Superior schematic of the extraocular muscles, *M*, medial; *L*, lateral. **B:** Lateral schematic of the extraocular muscles. *A*, anterior; *P*, posterior.

1 Lateral rectus muscle
2 Medial rectus muscle
3 Superior rectus muscle
4 Inferior rectus muscle
5 Levator palpebrae superioris muscle (resected in **A**)
6 Superior oblique muscle
7 Inferior oblique muscle
8 Trochlea
9 Orbital roof
10 Orbital floor
11 Medial orbital wall
12 Lateral orbital wall
13 Anterior tendon of the superior oblique muscle
14 Annulus of Zinn
15 Globe (outer surface)

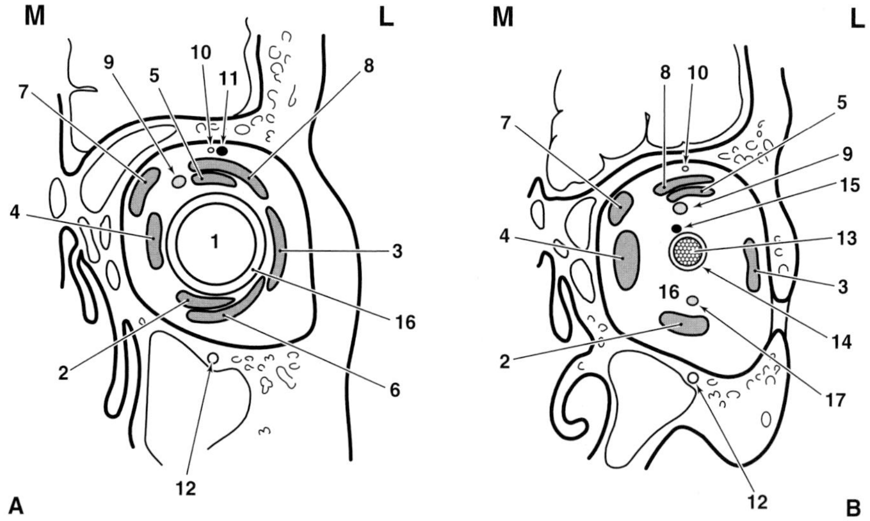

Figure 4-14: Coronal cross-section schematic of the orbital structures on the left side. **A:** Anterior orbit. **B:** Posterior orbit. *M,* medial; *L,* lateral.

1 Posterior aspect of the globe
2 Inferior rectus muscle
3 Lateral rectus muscle
4 Medial rectus muscle
5 Superior rectus muscle
6 Inferior oblique muscle
7 Superior oblique muscle
8 Levator palpebrae muscle
9 Superior ophthalmic vein
10 Supraorbital nerve (V1)
11 Supraorbital artery
12 Infraorbital nerve (V2)
13 Optic nerve
14 Optic nerve sheath
15 Ophthalmic artery
16 Wall of globe
17 Inferior ophthalmic vein

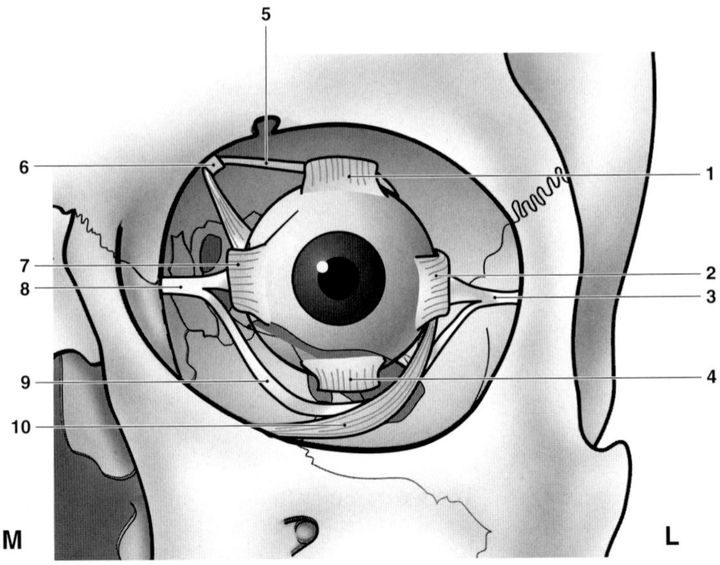

Figure 4-15: Schematic of the ligaments and extraocular muscles of the eye (anterior view). *M,* medial; *L,* lateral.

1 Superior rectus muscle
2 Lateral rectus muscle
3 Lateral check ligaments
4 Inferior rectus muscle
5 Superior oblique muscle
6 Trochlea
7 Medial rectus muscle
8 Medial check ligament
9 Suspensory ligament
10 Inferior oblique muscle

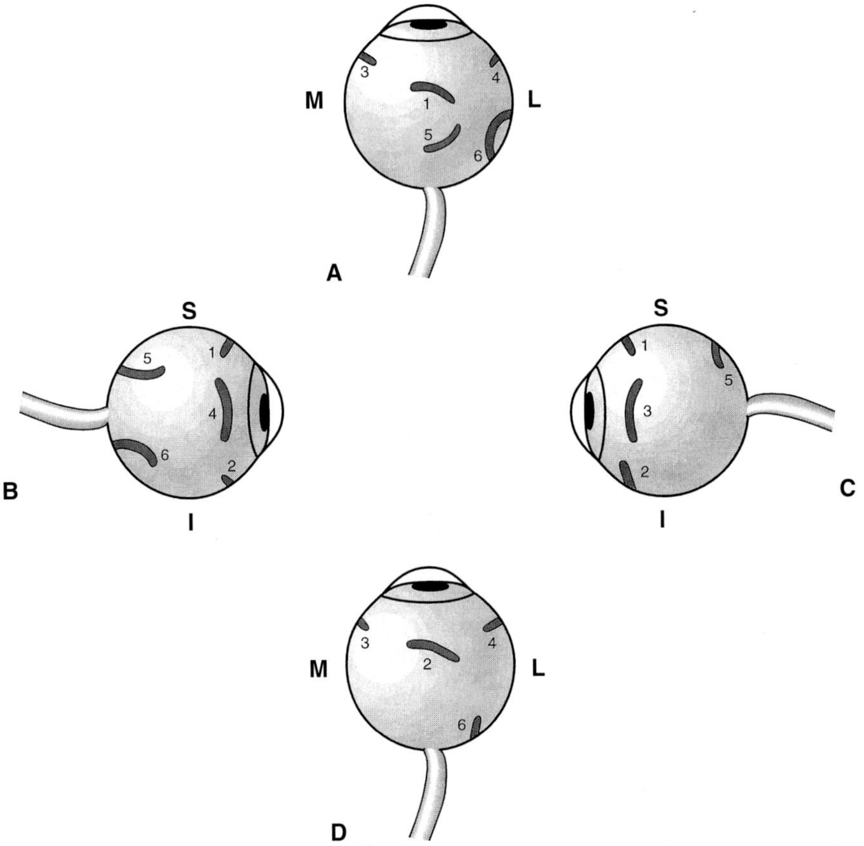

Figure 4-16: Schematic of the surfaces of the left eye showing the sites of attachment of the extraocular muscles. **A:** Superior aspect. **B:** Lateral aspect. **C:** Medial aspect. **D:** Inferior aspect. *M,* medial; *L,* lateral; *S,* superior; *I,* inferior.

1 Superior rectus
2 Inferior rectus
3 Medial rectus
4 Lateral rectus
5 Superior oblique
6 Inferior oblique

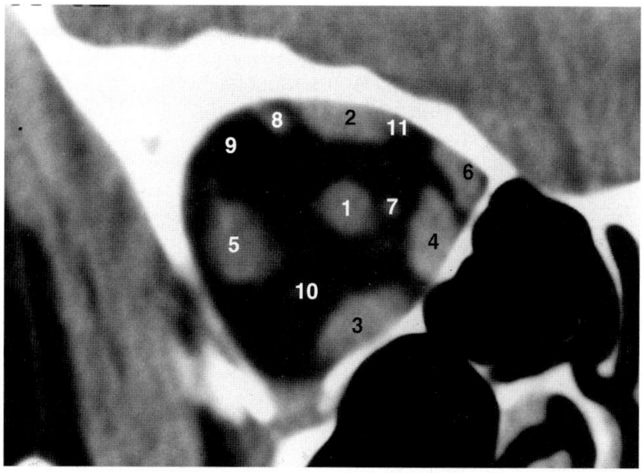

Figure 4-17A: The extraocular muscles and related orbital structures. Coronal CT image on the right side showing:
1 Optic nerve/sheath complex
2 Superior rectus
3 Inferior rectus muscle
4 Medial rectus muscle
5 Lateral rectus muscle
6 Superior oblique muscle
7 Ophthalmic artery
8 Superior ophthalmic vein
9 Retrobulbar fat
10 Inferior ophthalmic vein
11 Levator palpebrae superioris muscle

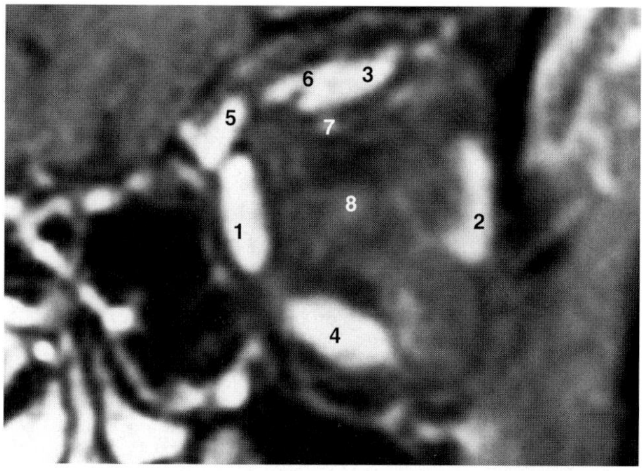

Figure 4-17B: The extraocular muscles and related orbital structures. Coronal contrast-enhanced T1-weighted MR image with fat suppression on the left side showing:
1 Medial rectus muscle
2 Lateral rectus muscle
3 Superior rectus muscle
4 Inferior rectus muscle
5 Superior oblique muscle
6 Levator palpebrae superioris muscle
7 Superior ophthalmic vein
8 Nonenhancing optic nerve/sheath complex.

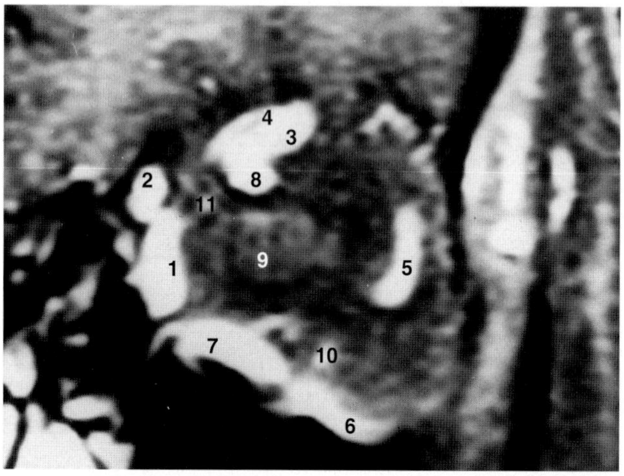

Figure 4-17C: The extraocular muscles and related orbital structures. Coronal enhanced T1-weighted MR image with fat suppression acquired at a more anterior level than that of Figure 4-17B on the left side showing:
1 Medial rectus muscle
2 Superior oblique muscle
3 Superior rectus muscle
4 Levator palpebrae superioris muscle
5 Lateral rectus muscle
6 Inferior rectus muscle
7 Origin of inferior oblique muscle
8 Superior ophthalmic vein
9 Nonenhancing optic nerve/sheath complex
10 Inferior ophthalmic vein
11 Branch of ophthalmic artery

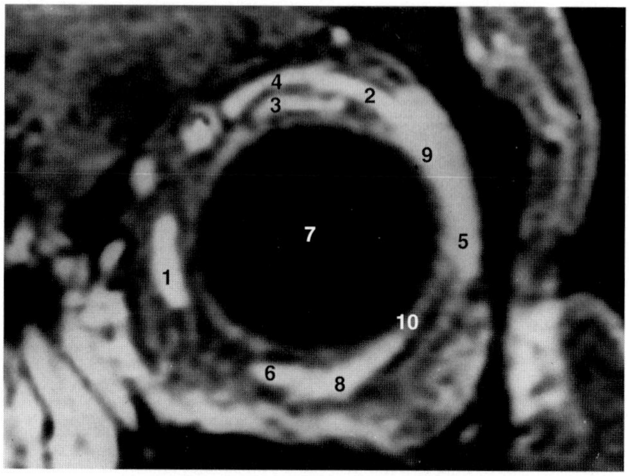

Figure 4-17D: The extraocular muscles and related orbital structures. Coronal enhanced T1-weighted MR image with fat suppression acquired at a more anterior level than that of Figure 4-17A on the left side showing:
1 Medial rectus muscle
2 Terminal superior oblique muscle
3 Superior rectus muscle
4 Levator palpebrae superioris muscle
5 Lateral rectus muscle
6 Inferior rectus muscle
7 Globe—vitreous humor
8 Terminal inferior oblique muscle
9 Point of attachment of superior oblique muscle
10 Point of attachment of inferior oblique muscle

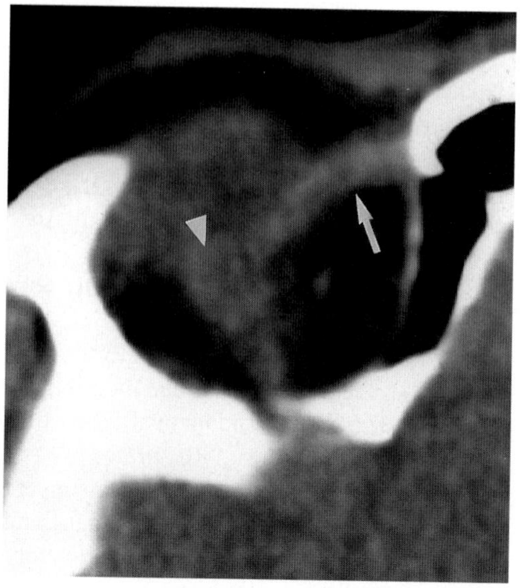

Figure 4-17E: The extraocular muscles and related orbital structures. Axial CT image showing the anterior extent of the superior oblique muscle (*arrow*) on the right side at the level of its insertion into the globe (*arrowhead*).

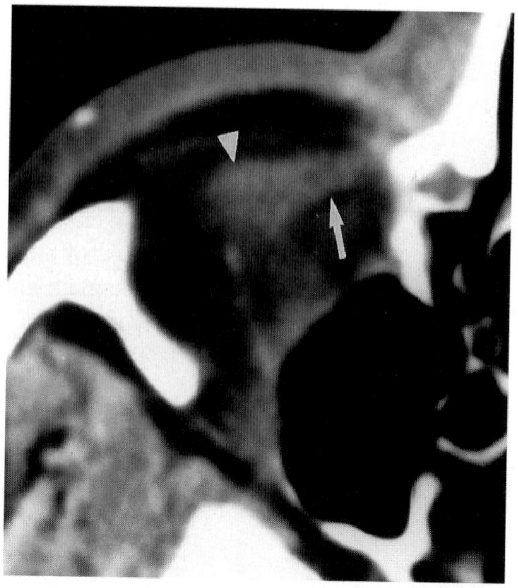

Figure 4-17F: The extraocular muscles and related orbital structures. Axial CT image showing the anterior extent of the inferior oblique muscle (*arrows*) on the right side at the level of its insertion into the globe (*arrowhead*).

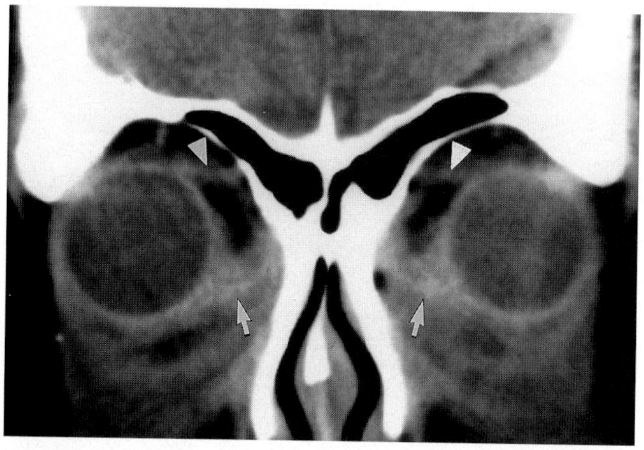

Figure 4-17G: The extraocular muscles and related orbital structures. Coronal CT image showing the anterior extent of the superior (*arrowheads*) and inferior (*arrows*) oblique extraocular muscles at the levels of their insertion into the globes.

THE LACRIMAL APPARATUS

1. The lacrimal apparatus on each side consists of the lacrimal gland, the lacrimal canaliculi, the lacrimal sac, and the nasolacrimal duct.
2. The lacrimal gland lies in the lacrimal fossa of the zygomatic process of the frontal bone located superolaterally in the anterior aspect of the orbit.
3. The lacrimal gland is tubuloacinar in form; its secretory units (acini) grossly resemble those of the salivary glands.
4. The main innervation of the lacrimal gland is from the parasympathetic nervous system.
5. The lacrimal gland produces tears that drain via the lacrimal excretory ducts (approximately six in number) onto the anterior surface of the globe and the eyelids.
6. Many small accessory lacrimal glands at or near the conjunctival fornix of the upper and lower eyelids drain independently onto the anterior globe surface.
7. Drainage of tears from the eye surface progresses into the lacrimal sac (upper extent of the nasolacrimal duct) via the medially located superior and inferior canaliculi.
8. Drainage of the lacrimal sac is via the nasolacrimal duct proper and ultimately through the valve of Hasner into the inferior meatus of the nasal cavity.

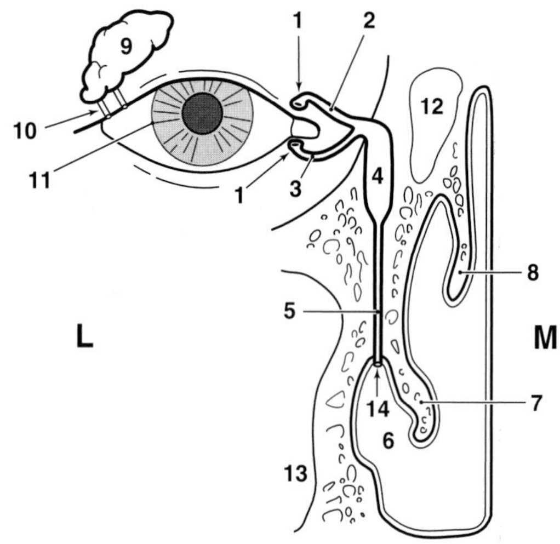

Figure 4-18A: Coronal schematic of the lacrimal apparatus on the right side. *M*, medial; *L*, lateral.
1 Lacrimal papillae
2 Superior lacrimal canaliculus
3 Inferior lacrimal canaliculus
4 Lacrimal sac
5 Nasolacrimal duct
6 Inferior nasal meatus
7 Inferior concha
8 Middle concha
9 Lacrimal gland
10 Lacrimal gland excretory ducts
11 Globe
12 Ethmoid air cells
13 Maxillary sinus
14 Valve of Hasner (nasolacrimal duct foramen)

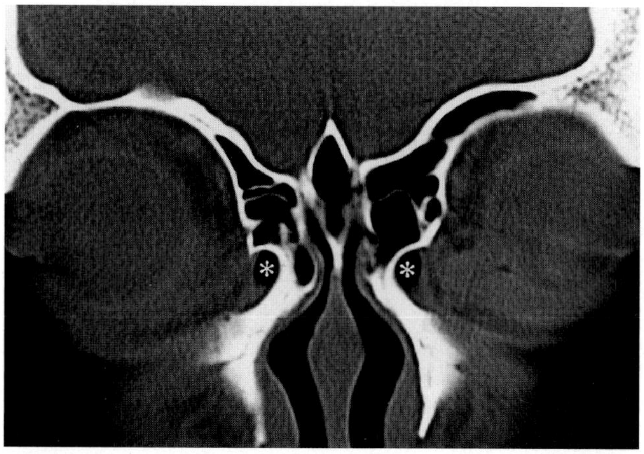

Figure 4-18B: The lacrimal sacs. Coronal CT image showing air within the lacrimal sacs (*asterisks*) bilaterally.

THE ARTERIAL SUPPLY AND VENOUS DRAINAGE OF THE ORBIT

1. The main arterial supply to the orbit is via the ophthalmic artery which originates from the internal carotid artery.
2. The central retinal artery is usually the first branch originating from the ophthalmic artery. It penetrates the optic nerve sheath distally and enters the optic nerve proper approximately 1.25 cm behind the optic nerve head. Subsequently, it divides into four branches, each supplying a quadrant of the retina (superior, inferior, medial, lateral retinal arterial branches).
3. The ciliary arteries include the long and short posterior ciliary arteries and the anterior ciliary arteries. The short posterior ciliary arteries penetrate the globe at the level of the optic nerve; the long posterior ciliary arteries pierce the globe along the periphery of the optic nerve head; the anterior ciliary arteries pierce the globe at the sclerocorneal junction. These vessels supply the choroid, ciliary processes, conjunctiva, and iris.
4. Normally the arterial flow in the orbit is in the frontal (anterior) direction.
5. The main collateral arterial flow to the orbit is from the lacrimal artery, a branch of the middle meningeal artery, via the superior orbital fissure. This artery is sometimes referred to as the "meningolacrimal" artery.
6. The main venous drainage of the orbit is via the superior and inferior ophthalmic veins.
7. The ophthalmic veins anastomose posteriorly with the cavernous venous sinus, and anteriorly with the angular frontal vein and anterior facial vein. The drainage of the venous system of the orbit can be either in the anterior direction into the anterior facial vein(s), or in the posterior direction into the cavernous venous sinus. Preferentially, the venous flow is from anterior to posterior, although because the orbital veins are valveless the venous flow may be the reverse of this, i.e., posterior to anterior.
8. The central retinal vein initially accompanies the optic nerve. It then leaves the nerve to undertake a variable course in the subarachnoid space and subsequently pierces the optic nerve sheath to drain into the superior ophthalmic vein or directly into the cavernous venous sinus.

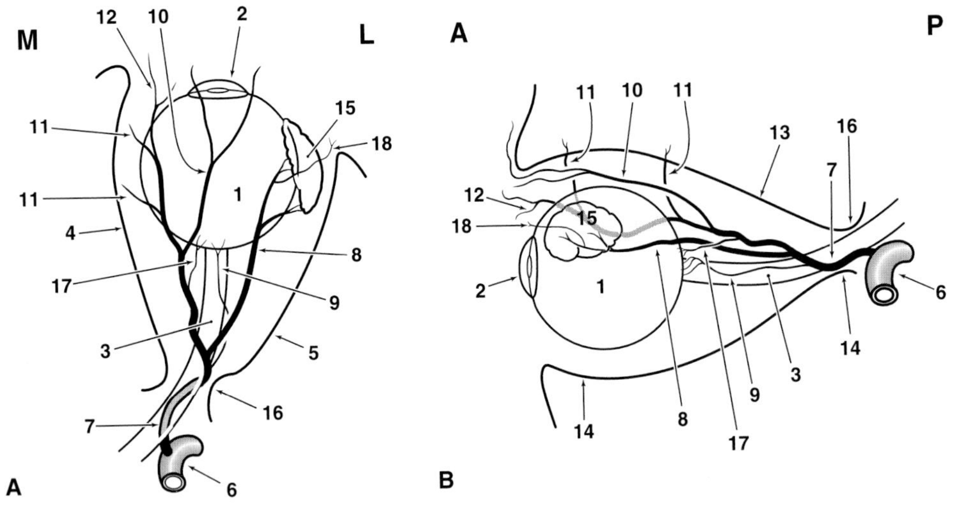

Figure 4-19: Schematics of the normal ophthalmic artery and its main branches on the left side. **A:** Superior schemiatic of the ophthalmic artery. **B:** Lateral schematic of the ophthalmic artery. *M,* medial; *L,* lateral; *A,* anterior; *P,* posterior.

1 Globe
2 Cornea
3 Optic nerve/sheath complex
4 Medial orbital wall
5 Lateral orbital wall
6 Internal carotid artery
7 Ophthalmic artery trunk
8 Lacrimal artery
9 Central retinal artery
10 Supraorbital artery
11 Anterior and posterior ethmoidal branches of the ophthalmic artery
12 Medial palpebral branches of ophthalmic artery
13 Orbital roof
14 Orbital floor
15 Lacrimal gland
16 Optic canal
17 Short posterior ciliary artery
18 Lateral palpebral branch of lacrimal artery

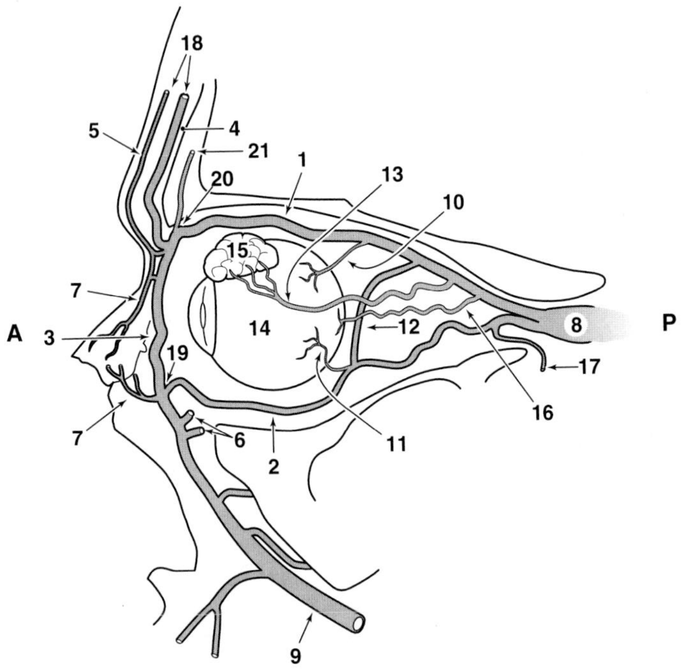

Figure 4-20: Lateral schematic of the venous system of the orbit on the left side. *A,* anterior; *P,* posterior.

1 Superior ophthalmic vein
2 Inferior ophthalmic vein
3 Angular vein (proximal extent of facial vein)
4 Supraorbital vein
5 Supratrochlear vein
6 Inferior palpebral veins
7 External nasal vein(s)
8 Cavernous venous sinus
9 Facial vein proper
10 Superior vortical vein(s)
11 Inferior vortical vein(s)
12 Apsidal vein
13 Lacrimal vein
14 Globe
15 Lacrimal gland
16 Central retinal vein
17 Anastomosis with pterygoid venous plexus
18 Anastomosis with frontal tributaries of the superficial temporal vein
19 Anastomosis of inferior ophthalmic vein with angular (facial) vein (variable)
20 Anastomosis with frontal diploic vein (variable)
21 Frontal diploic vein

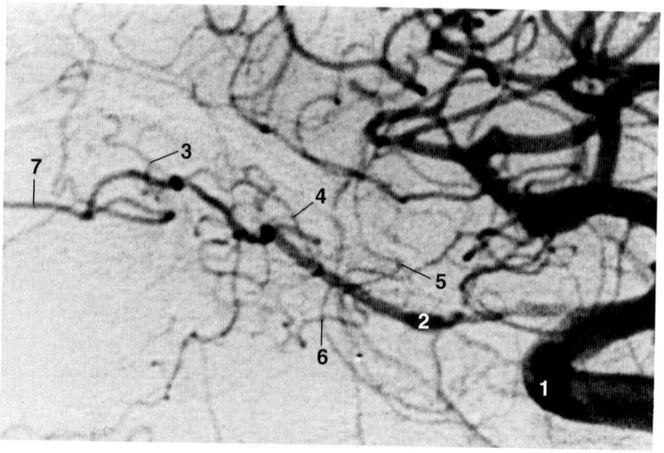

Figure 4-21A: The ophthalmic artery. Internal carotid angiogram in the lateral projection showing some of the major branches of the ophthalmic artery.
1 Internal carotid artery
2 Ophthalmic artery trunk
3 Anterior ethmoidal arterial branch(es)
4 Middle ethmoidal arterial branch(es)
5 Posterior ethmoidal arterial branch(es)
6 Branch to central retinal artery
7 Supratrochlear artery

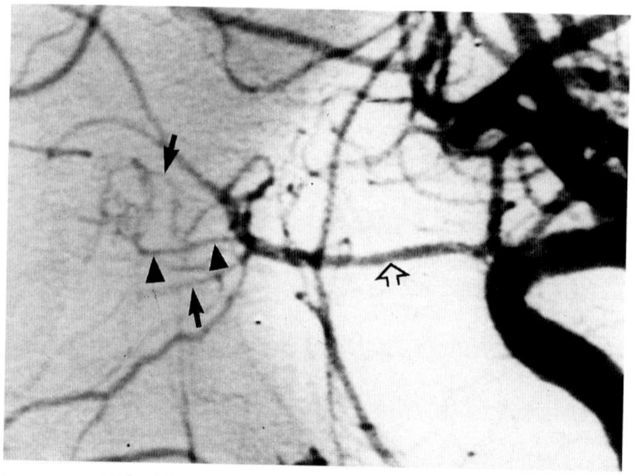

Figure 4-21B: The central retinal/short ciliary arteries. Carotid arteriogram in the lateral projection showing the ophthalmic artery proper (*open arrow*), the central retinal artery (*arrowheads*), and short ciliary arteries (*solid arrows*).

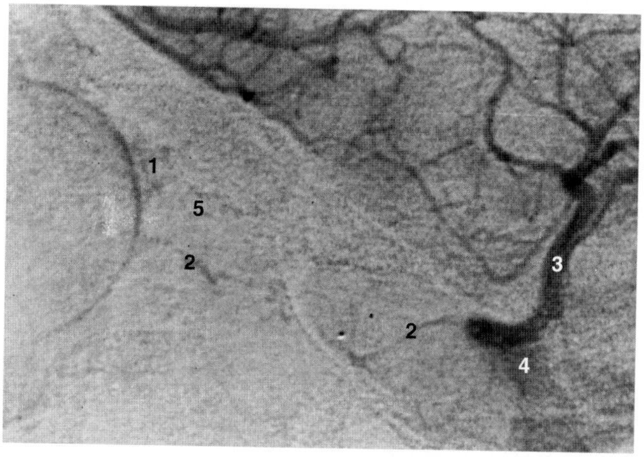

Figure 4-22: Central retinal/vortical veins. Venous phase of internal carotid arteriogram in the lateral projection showing the choroidal blush and central retinal vortical vein(s) draining posteriorly into the cavernous venous sinus.
1 Choroidal blush in the posterior globe
2 Central retinal vein
3 Superficial middle cerebral (Sylvian) vein
4 Cavernous venous sinus
5 Vortical veins

ORBIT VARIANTS

Bony Orbit Variants

- Hypoplasia of the orbit
- Hyperplasia of the orbit secondary to underlying orbital contents (mass forming malformation)
- Malformation of the shape of the orbit secondary to abnormal coronal/metopic suture closure

Globe Variants

Varying Shape of Globe

- Round globe
- Oval globe
- Staphyloma
- Coloboma

Calcifications of Globe

- Drusen of the optic nerve head
- Limbus calcifications

Lens Abnormalities

- Absence of the lens (aplasia: aphakia)
- Calcification of the lens
- Dislocation of the lens

Extraocular Muscles/Adnexia Variants

- Trochlea calcification/ossification
- Hypertrophy
- Atrophy

Optic Nerve/Sheath Complex Variants

- Patulous optic nerve sheath
- Incomplete patency of the optic subarachnoid space from the optic nerve head through the cranial subarachnoid space
- Benign meningeal calcifications in the optic nerve sheath

Orbital Vasculature Variants

- Hypoplasia (atresia) of the ophthalmic artery with compensatory enlargement of the meningolacrimal artery
- Ophthalmic artery originating from the middle meningeal artery
- Middle meningeal artery originating from the ophthalmic artery
- Optic nerve varix
- Unnamed variations in size of the ophthalmic veins and their drainage patterns

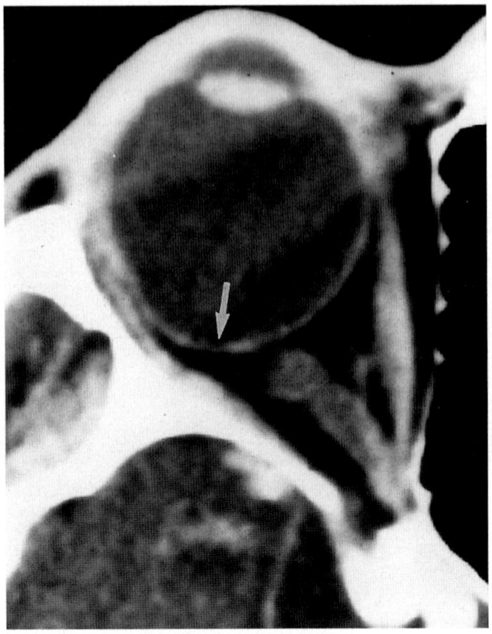

Figure 4-23A: Ocular staphyloma. Axial CT image showing a staphyloma (*arrow*: focal outward bulge of wall of globe) of the right globe.

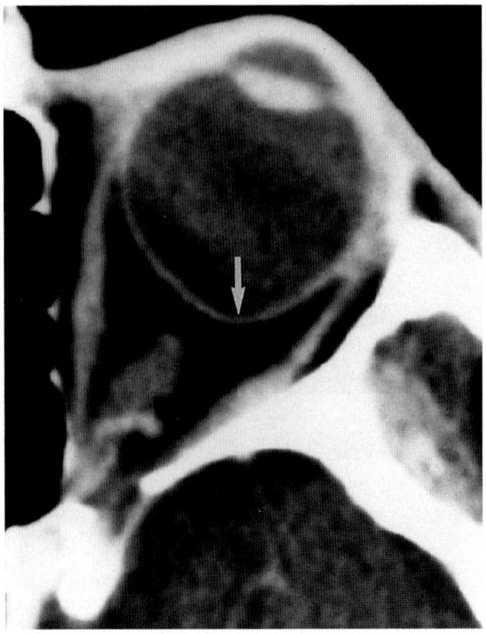

Figure 4-23B: Axial CT image showing a similar although smaller staphyloma (*arrow*) of the left globe in the same patient.

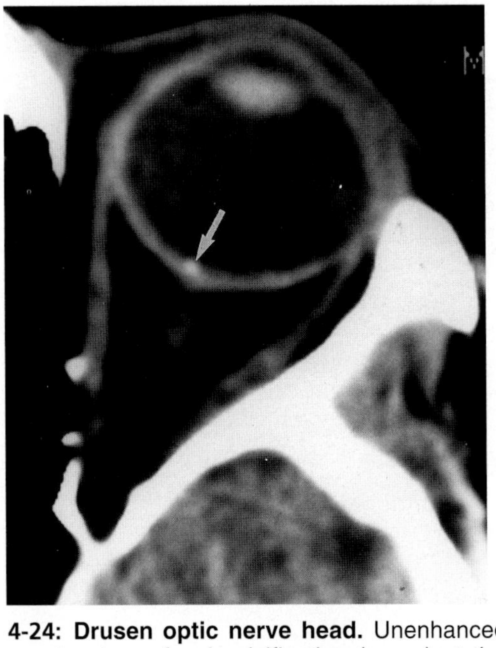

Figure 4-24: Drusen optic nerve head. Unenhanced axial CT image showing a focal calcification (*arrow*) at the optic nerve head (disc) representing a drusen (benign idiopathic accumulations of calcified, proteinaceous material beneath the surface of the optic nerve head).

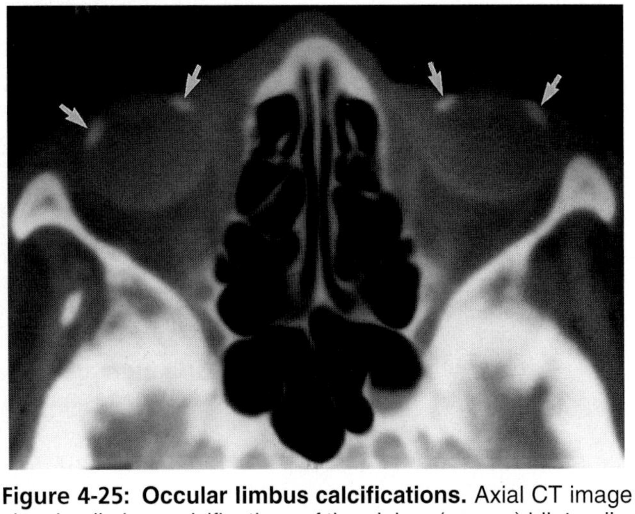

Figure 4-25: Occular limbus calcifications. Axial CT image showing limbus calcifications of the globes (*arrows*) bilaterally.

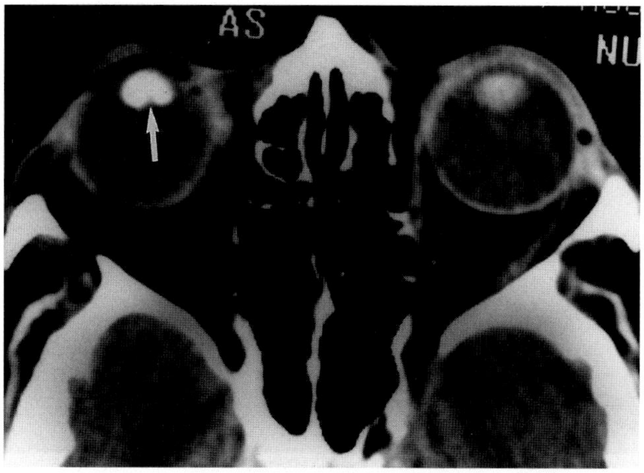

Figure 4-26: Calcified ocular lens. Axial CT showing calcification of the ocular lens (*arrow*) on the right side.

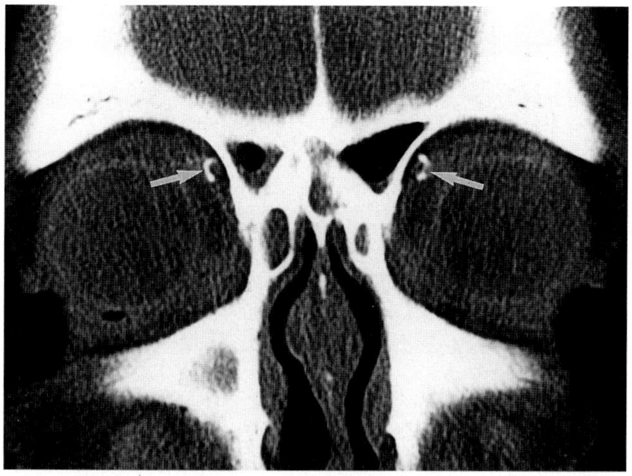

Figure 4-27: Trochlea calcification/ossification. Coronal unenhanced CT image showing calcification/ossification (*arrows*) of the trochlea of the superior oblique extraocular muscles on each side.

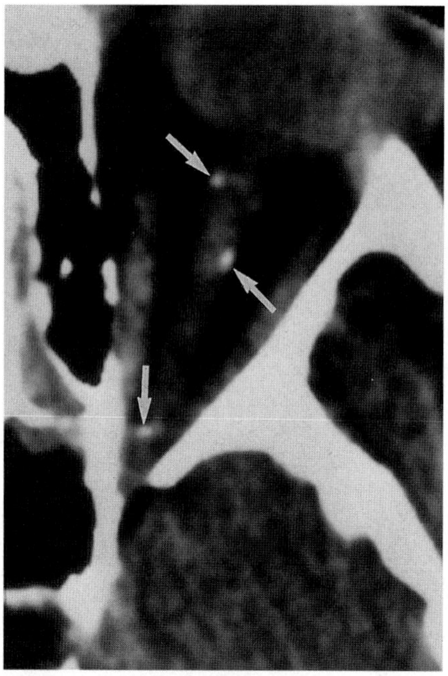

Figure 4-28: Benign calcification of the optic nerve sheath. Axial CT image showing several benign calcifications (*arrows*) in the optic nerve sheath.

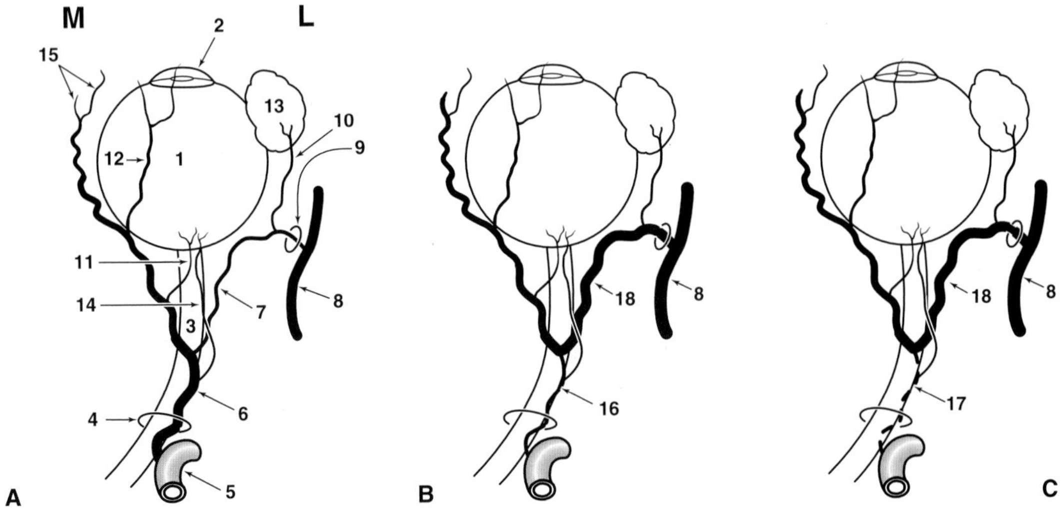

Figure 4-29: Superior schematic of the main variations of the ophthalmic artery on the left side. **A:** Dominant configuration. **B:** Configuration in ophthalmic artery hypoplasia. **C:** Configuration in ophthalmic artery atresia (*dashed line*). *M,* medial; *L,* lateral.

1 Globe
2 Cornea
3 Optic nerve/sheath complex
4 Optic canal
5 Internal carotid artery
6 Ophthalmic artery trunk originating from the internal carotid artery
7 Normally small ophthalmic artery anastomosis with branch of middle meningeal artery (normal “meningolacrimal” artery)
8 Middle meningeal artery
9 Lateral aspect of superior orbital fissure
10 Lacrimal artery
11 Short posterior ciliary arteries
12 Supraorbital artery
13 Lacrimal gland
14 Central retinal artery
15 Medial palpebral and supratrochlear branches of the ophthalmic artery
16 Developmentally hypoplastic proximal ophthalmic artery
17 Developmentally atretic proximal ophthalmic artery (dashed line)
18 Developmentally enlarged ophthalmic artery anastomosis with middle meningeal artery (hypertrophied “meningolacrimal” artery)

CHAPTER 5

Facial Structures

SUPERFICIAL ANATOMIC FEATURES OF THE FACE AND EXTERNAL EAR

1. The nose is pyramidal in shape and is pierced inferiorly by the external nares or nostrils. The nares are separated in the midline by the nasal septum. The tip of the nose is termed the apex. The lateral surfaces end inferiorly in the alae nasi (nasal alae). The point at the junction of the upper nose with the frontal bone in the midline is termed the nasion. The median frontal elevation just above the nasion is called the glabella.
2. The lips are represented by two soft tissue folds that surround the oral orifice. The skin of the lips is continuous with the mucosa of the oral cavity at the transitional or vermilion border. Laterally the upper and lower lips are delimited at the right and left oral fissures. Externally in the midline, the upper lip exhibits a shallow vertical groove, the philtrum, demarcated by paired lateral ridges. Internally the upper and lower lips are connected to the upper and lower gums, respectively, by a medial labial frenulum.
3. The cheeks are continuous with the lips anteriorly and are demarcated by the bilateral nasolabial sulci. The cheek tends to be outwardly convex due to underlying skeletal muscle and a biconvex buccal fat pad.
4. The external ear consists of the auricle (pinna) and the external auditory meatus. The auricle superficially consists of several eminences and depressions, including the helix, or external rim; the auricular tubercle, lying along the posterosuperior rim of the helix; the antihelix, an internal curved ridge paralleling the helix that divides into two crura superiorly; the triangular fossa, situated between these latter two crura; the scaphoid fossa, representing the depression between the helix and antihelix; the concha, or the space of the auricle partly encircled by the antihelix and partly divided by the crus of the helix; the cymba concha, or the area of the concha lying above the crus of the helix; the tragus, a small flap of soft tissue projecting from the anterior margin of the auricle and partially overlying the external auditory meatus; the antitragus, a similar small soft-tissue flap projecting upward and separated from the tragus by the intertragic incisure; and the lobule, a soft tissue projection extending from the inferior aspect of the auricle.

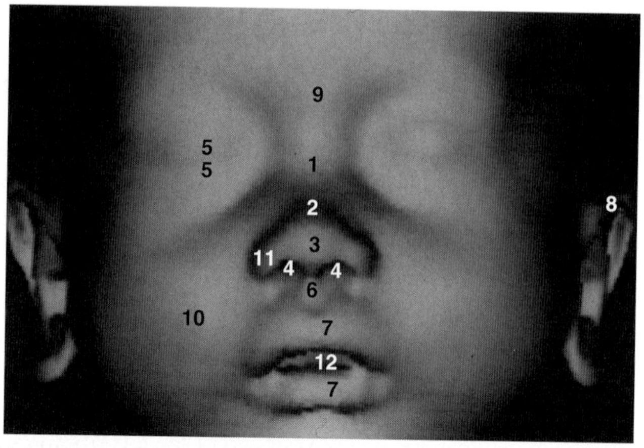

Figure 5-1: Surface anatomy of the face. Three-dimensional image in an infant showing the surface anatomy of the face.

1 Root of nose
2 Bridge of nose
3 Apex of nose
4 External nares
5 Upper and lower lids of the eyes
6 Philtrum
7 Upper and lower lips
8 Auricle
9 Glabella
10 Cheek
11 Nasal ala
12 Oral orifice

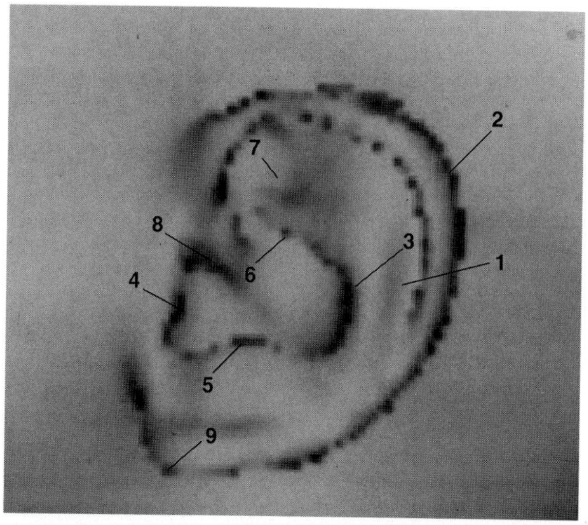

Figure 5-2A: Surface anatomy of the external ear (auricle [pinna] and external auditory meatus). Three-dimensional CT image showing surface anatomy of the left external ear.

1 Scaphoid fossa
2 Helix
3 Antihelix
4 Tragus
5 Antitragus
6 Concha
7 Triangular fossa
8 External auditory canal (meatus)
9 Lobule

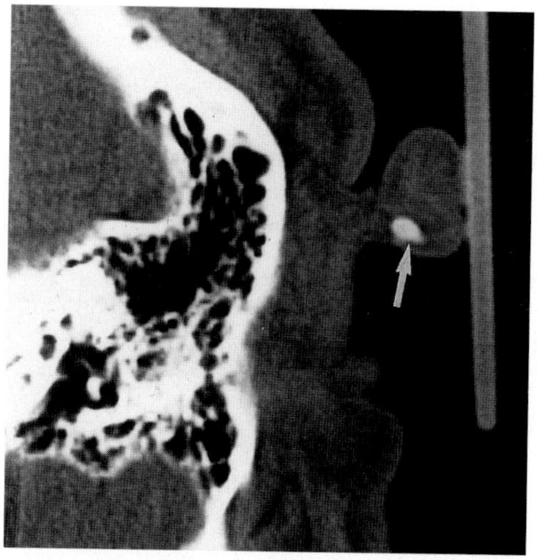

Figure 5-2B: Ossification of pinna cartilage of external ear. Axial CT scan showing ossification (*arrow*) of the pinna cartilage of the external ear on the right side.

FACIAL BONY ANATOMY

1. The facial skeleton is composed of bones of the face that may attach to form a part of the cranium.
2. All together, the facial skeleton consists of 14 bones, including the paired maxillae, the paired palatine bones, the paired zygomatic bones, the paired inferior nasal conchae, the paired lacrimal bones, the paired nasal bones, and the unpaired vomer and mandible.
3. The two maxillae join at the intermaxillary suture to form the upper jaw. The four paired processes of the maxilla include frontal, zygomatic, alveolar, and palatine.
4. The palatine processes of the two maxillae join in the midline to form the anterior portion of the hard palate. The horizontal plates of the two palatine bones join in the midline to form the posterior portion of the hard palate.
5. The two zygomatic bones form part of the lateral aspect and floor of the orbit, and the anterior aspect of the zygomatic arch. Each zygomatic bone has four processes: frontal, orbital, maxillary, and temporal.
6. The two inferior nasal conchae are curved bones emanating from the lateral walls of the nasal cavities. They form the bony core of the inferior nasal turbinates.
7. The two lacrimal bones form a small portion of the medial walls of the orbits.
8. The two nasal bones are joined in the midline at the internasal suture. They form the upper part of the nose.
9. The single midline vomer forms the posterior aspect of the bony nasal septum.
10. The mandible consists of a single body crossing the midline in a U shape, two rami, two coronoid processes, and two condyles. The condyles articulate with the temporal bones at the glenoid fossae to form the temporomandibular joints.

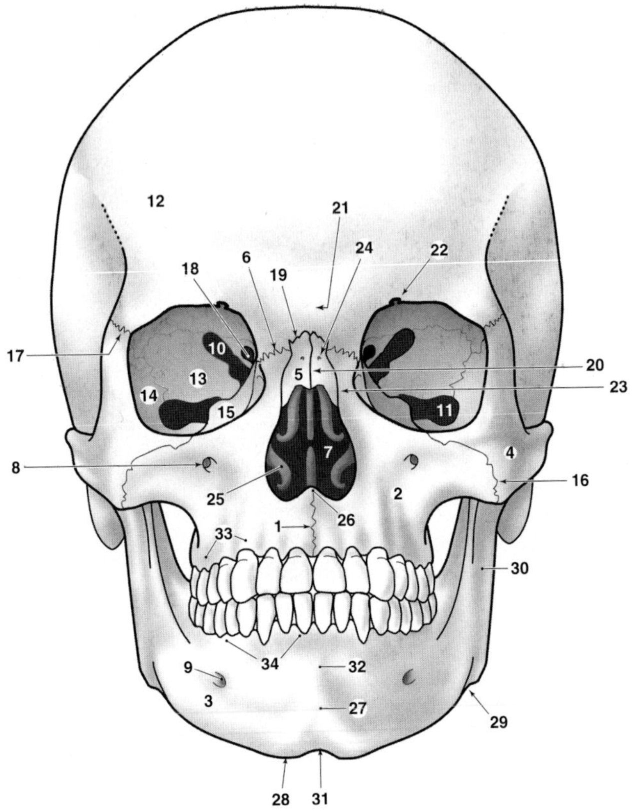

Figure 5-3: Frontal schematic of the facial bones.
1 Intermaxillary suture
2 Maxilla
3 Body of mandible
4 Zygomatic bone
5 Nasal bone
6 Frontomaxillary suture
7 Piriform aperture (anterior nasal aperture)
8 Infraorbital foramen
9 Mental foramen
10 Superior orbital fissure
11 Inferior orbital fissure
12 Frontal bone
13 Greater wing of sphenoid bone
14 Orbital process of zygomatic bone
15 Orbital process of maxillary bone
16 Zygomaticomaxillary suture
17 Zygomaticofrontal suture
18 Optic foramen
19 Frontonasal suture
20 Internasal suture
21 Glabella
22 Supraorbital notch
23 Nasomaxillary suture
24 Nasal vascular foramen
25 Inferior nasal concha
26 Anterior nasal spine
27 Mental protuberance
28 Mental tubercle
29 Angle of mandible
30 Ramus of mandible
31 Mental symphysis (fused)
32 Median external ridge of mandible
33 Alveolar process of maxilla
34 Alveolar process of mandible

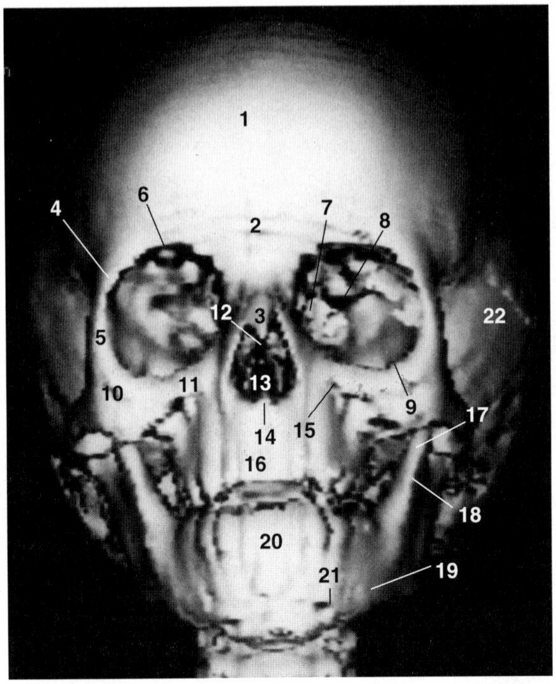

Figure 5-4A: Surface anatomy of the face. Three-dimensional CT image of skull in the frontal projection showing the surface anatomy.
1 Frontal bone
2 Glabella
3 Nasal bones
4 Zygomatic process of frontal bone
5 Frontal process of zygomatic bone
6 Supraorbital margin
7 Optic canal
8 Superior orbital fissure
9 Infraorbital margin
10 Zygomatic bone
11 Zygomatic process of maxillary bone
12 Middle nasal concha
13 Nasal apertures
14 Anterior nasal spine
15 Infraorbital foramen
16 Alveolar process of maxillary bone
17 Condyle of mandible
18 Ramus of mandible
19 Angle of mandible
20 Alveolar process of mandible
21 Mental foramen
22 Temporal squamosa

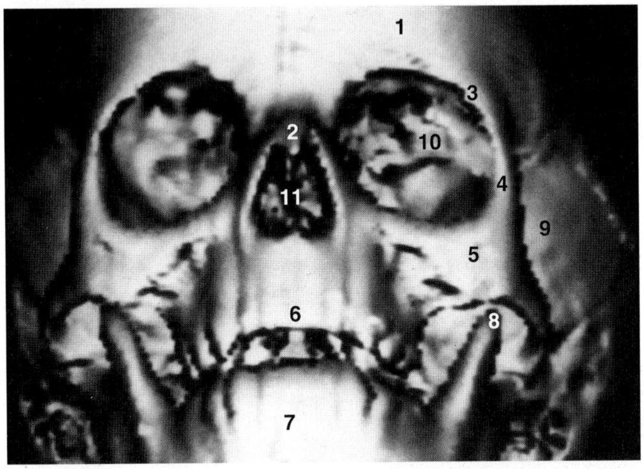

Figure 5-4B: Three-dimensional CT image in a 20 degree inclined anteroposterior projection showing the surface features of the facial bones.
1 Frontal bone
2 Nasal bones
3 Zygomatic process of frontal bone
4 Frontal process of zygomatic bone
5 Zygomatic bone
6 Alveolar process of maxilla
7 Alveolar process of mandible
8 Coronoid process of mandible
9 Temporal bone squama
10 Orbit
11 Nasal passageways

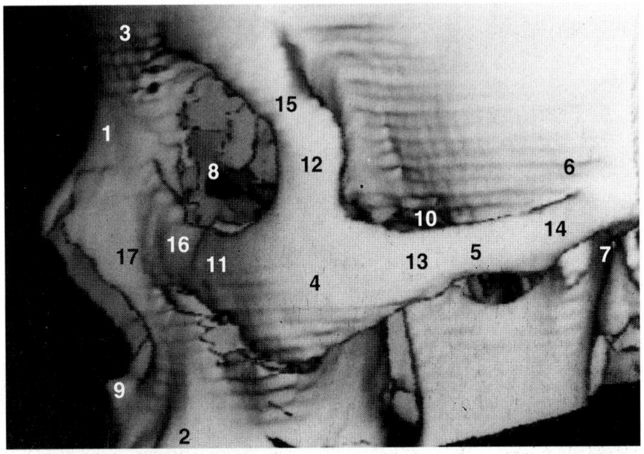

Figure 5-4C: Facial bones. Three-dimensional CT image in the lateral projection showing the facial bones on the left side.
1 Nasal bone(s)
2 Alveolar process of maxilla
3 Frontal bone
4 Zygoma
5 Zygomatic arch
6 Squamous portion of temporal bone
7 Condyloid process of mandible
8 Orbit
9 Anterior nasal spine
10 Deep temporal fossa
11 Maxillary process of zygoma
12 Frontal process of zygoma
13 Temporal process of zygoma
14 Zygomatic process of temporal bone
15 Zygomatic process of frontal bone
16 Zygomatic process of maxilla
17 Nasal process of maxilla

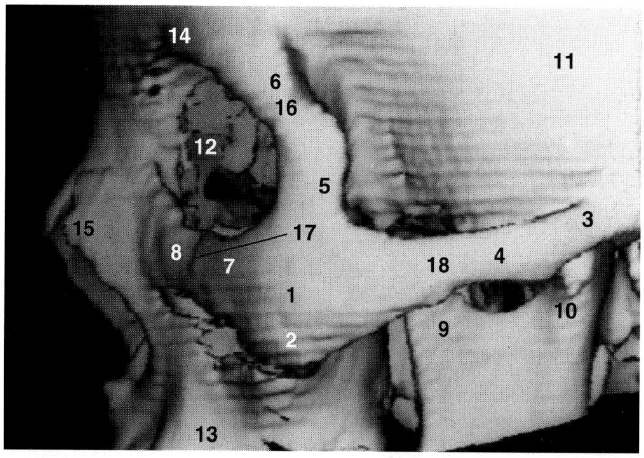

Figure 5-5A: Zygomatic arch. Three-dimensional CT image in the lateral projection showing the normal anatomy of the zygomatic arch on the left side.
1 Zygoma (zygomatic bone)
2 Malar emminance of zygomatic bone
3 Zygomatic process of the temporal bone
4 Zygomatic arch at site of zygomaticotemporal suture
5 Frontal process of the zygoma
6 Zygomatic process of the frontal bone
7 Maxillary process of the zygoma
8 Zygomatic process of the maxilla
9 Coronoid process of mandible
10 Condylar process of mandible
11 Squamous portion of the temporal bone
12 Orbit
13 Maxilla
14 Frontal bone
15 Nasal bone
16 Site of zygomaticofrontal suture
17 Site of zygomaticomaxillary suture
18 Temporal process of zygoma

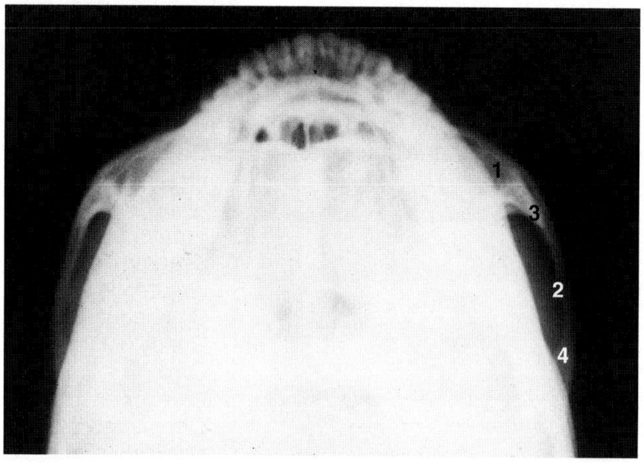

Figure 5-5B: Zygomatic arch. Submentovertex projection of the skull showing the zygomatic arches.
1 Zygoma (zygomatic bone)
2 Zygomatic arch
3 Temporal process of zygoma
4 Zygomatic process of temporal bone

THE NASAL BONES

1. The nasal bones are paired structures, joined at the midline by the longitudinal sagittal internasal suture.
2. The superior border of the nasal bone on each side joins the frontal bone at the frontonasal suture; the inferior border of each nasal bone is continuous with the paired lateral nasal cartilages; the lateral borders of the nasal bones join the frontal processes of the maxillae at the paired nasomaxillary sutures; medially and posteriorly, the two nasal bones project backward as a midline vertical (nasal) crest becoming a part of the nasal septum. The vertical (nasal) crest articulates with the nasal septal cartilage, the perpendicular plate of the ethmoid bone, and the nasal spine of the frontal bone.
3. The external surface of each nasal bone may be pierced by a vascular nasal (venous) foramen.

THE NASAL SEPTUM

1. The unpaired midline nasal septum forms the medial wall of each nasal passageway.
2. The nasal septum is composed anterosuperiorly of the vertical (nasal) crest of the nasal bones and the nasal spine of the frontal bone; anteriorly, the nasal septal cartilage; superiorly, the perpendicular plate of the ethmoid bones; inferiorly, the vomer (bone), and the maxillary and palatine nasal crests; and posterosuperiorly, the sphenoid rostrum below and the sphenoid nasal crest above.

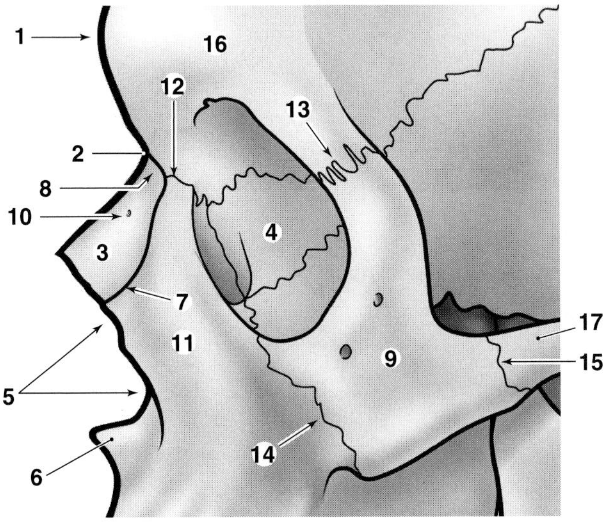

Figure 5-6: Lateral schematic of the facial bones in and surrounding the nasal region.

1 Glabella (median, inferior external elevation of the frontal bone)
2 Nasion (depression at the root of the nose)
3 Nasal bone
4 Lacrimal bone
5 Piriform aperture (anterior nasal aperture)
6 Anterior nasal spine
7 Nasomaxillary suture
8 Frontonasal suture
9 Zygomatic bone
10 Nasal bone vascular foramen
11 Maxillary bone
12 Frontomaxillary suture
13 Zygomaticofrontal suture
14 Zygomaticomaxillary suture
15 Zygomaticotemporal suture
16 Frontal bone
17 Zygomatic process of temporal bone

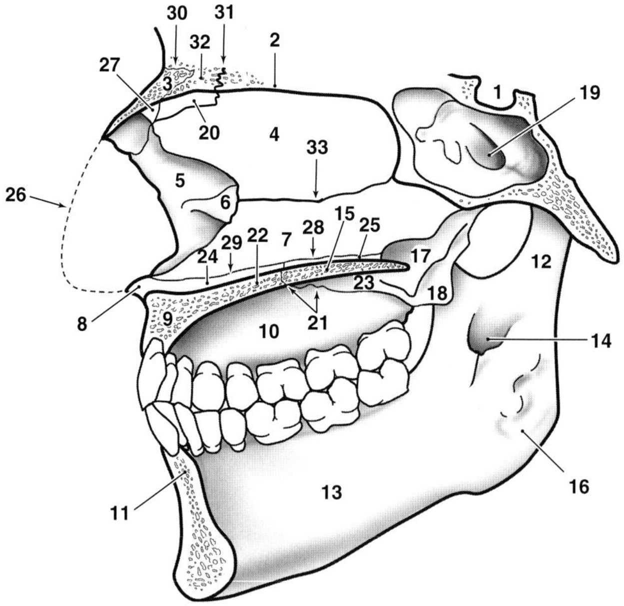

Figure 5-7: Midline sagittal schematic of the nasal septum. (The left half of the bony facial structure has been removed.)

1 Sella turcica
2 Cribriform plate of ethmoid bone
3 Nasal bone(s)
4 Perpendicular plate of ethmoid bone
5 Maxillary bone
6 Inferior nasal concha
7 Vomer
8 Anterior nasal spine
9 Alveolar process of maxillary bone
10 Palatine process of maxillary bone laterally
11 Alveolar process of mandible
12 Neck of mandible
13 Body of mandible
14 Mandibular foramen
15 Horizontal plate of the palatine bones at the midline interpalatine suture
16 Angle of mandible
17 Medial lamina (ala) of pterygoid process
18 Lateral lamina (ala) of pterygoid process
19 Sphenoid sinus
20 Nasal crest of frontal bone
21 Palatomaxillary suture
22 Palatine process of the maxillary bone at the midline intermaxillary suture
23 Palatine bone
24 Nasal crest of the maxilla
25 Nasal crest of palatine bone(s)
26 Outline of margin of nasal septal cartilage
27 Vertical crest of nasal bones
28 *Palatovomeral suture* (Jinkins)
29 *Maxillovomeral suture* (Jinkins)
30 Frontonasal suture
31 Fronto-ethmoidal suture
32 Frontal bone
33 Vomero-ethmoidal suture

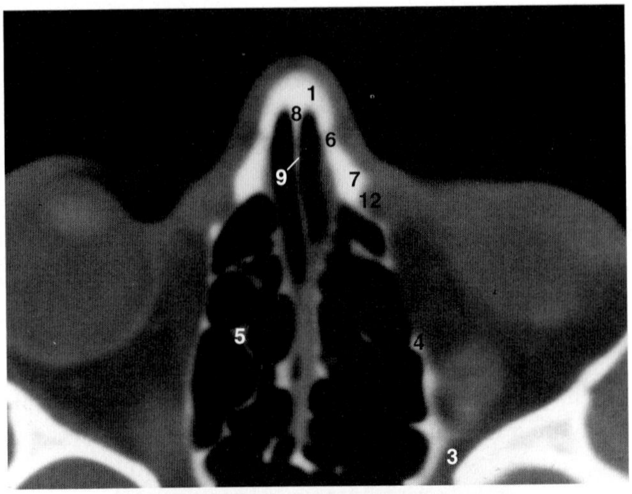

Figure 5-8A: The nasal bones. Axial CT scan showing the nasal bones.

1 Nasal bone
2 Nasolacrimal sulcus (groove) of lacrimal bone
3 Inferior orbital fissure
4 Lamina papyracea
5 Ethmoid air cells
6 Nasomaxillary suture
7 Nasal process of maxillary bone
8 Vertical crest of nasal bones
9 Perpendicular plate of ethmoid bone

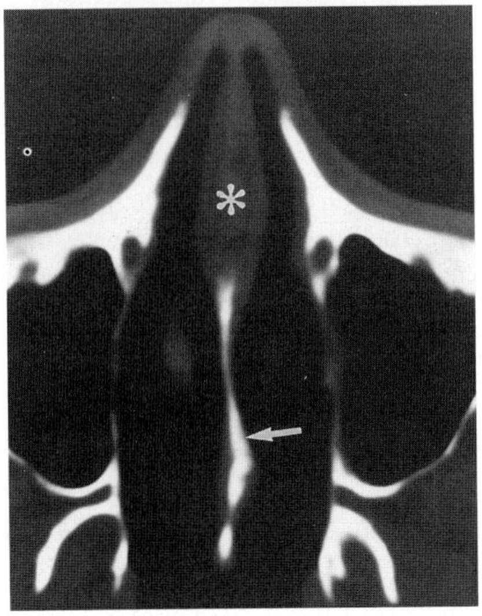

Figure 5-8B: Axial CT image showing the vomer (*arrow*) and the anterior nasal septal cartilage (*asterisk*).

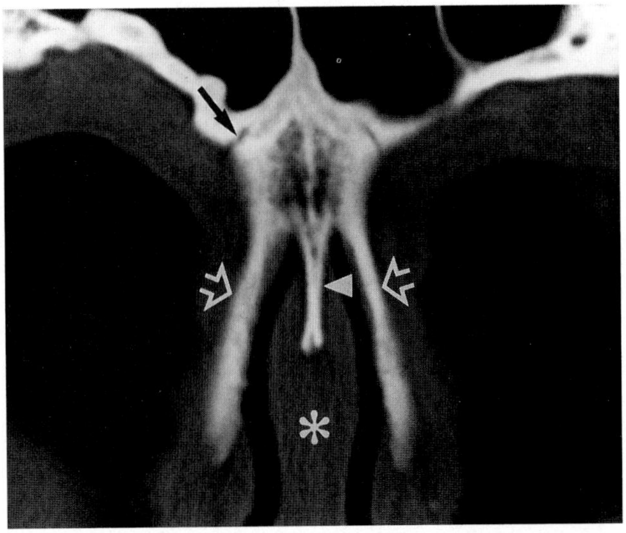

Figure 5-8C: CT image in the coronal plane showing the frontonasal sutures (*arrows*), the vertical crest of the nasal bones (*arrowhead*), the anterior nasal septal cartilage (*asterisk*), and the nasal bones (*open arrows*) fused in the midline.

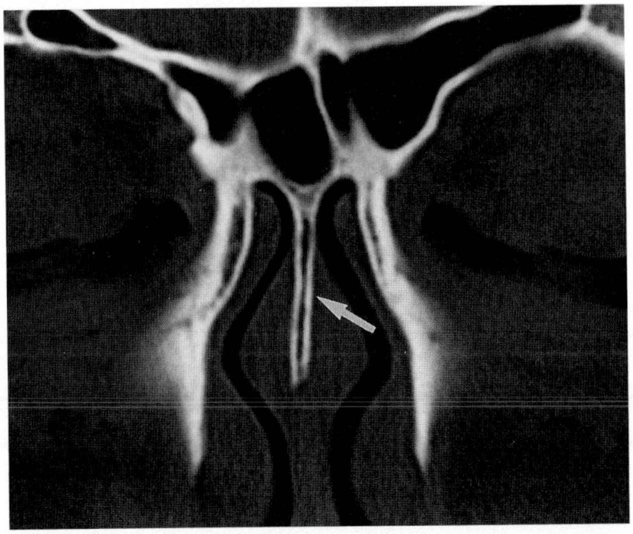

Figure 5-8D: CT image in the coronal plane showing the perpendicular plate of ethmoid bone (*arrow*).

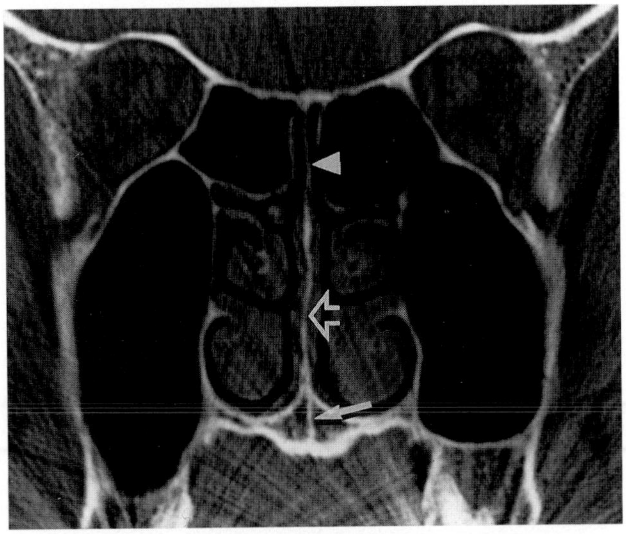

Figure 5-8E: Coronal CT image showing the intermaxillary suture (*solid arrow*), the vomer (*open arrow*), and the perpendicular plate of the ethmoid bone (*arrowhead*).

THE MANDIBLE

1. The mandible has a horizontally curved body and two posteriorly directed mandibular rami.
2. The U-shaped (axial plane) alveolar part or process of the mandible contains 16 alveoli or tooth sockets for the roots of the mandibular teeth.
3. Anteriorly in the midline, the point of fusion of the embryologic mandibular symphysis menti may reveal a small external median mental ridge. Inferiorly, there may be a midline external mental protuberance and paired mental tubercles immediately lateral to the midline. Internally in the anterior midline, upper and lower mental spines may be present.
4. The mandibular ramus runs upward and backward from the body of the mandible, thereby yielding the angle of the mandible at the junction of the two. The coronoid process extends anterosuperiorly from the rami and the condylar processes extend posterosuperiorly. The condylar process terminates as the head or condyle of the mandible, articulating with the glenoid fossa of the temporal bone on each side.
5. The mandibular ramus is pierced medially by the mandibular foramen. The paired mandibular canals (one on each side) run anteriorly from the mandibular foramina. The mandibular canals contain the inferior alveolar (dental) nerve [branch of the mandibular (third) division of the fifth cranial nerve: CN-V3)] and inferior alveolar (dental) vessels (artery and vein). At the level of the first and second premolar teeth, the inferior alveolar nerve divides into two parts: (a) an incisive branch that travels within the incisive canal and (b) a mental branch. The incisive nerve innervates the first premolar, canine, and incisor teeth as well as the regional gingivae. The paired mental foramina on the anterior, outer surface of the mandible at the level of the apexes of the premolar teeth transmit the mental vessels and nerves. The mental nerves supply the regional gingivae and skin of the lower lip and chin.
6. There are many unnamed accessory mandibular foramina.
7. The muscles providing mandibular movement include the paired lateral and medial pterygoid, temporalis, masseter, digastric, and geniohyoid muscles.
8. A longitudinal (hyperostotic) ridge may form along the inner aspect of the alveolar process of the mandible, the mandibular torus (torus mandibularis).

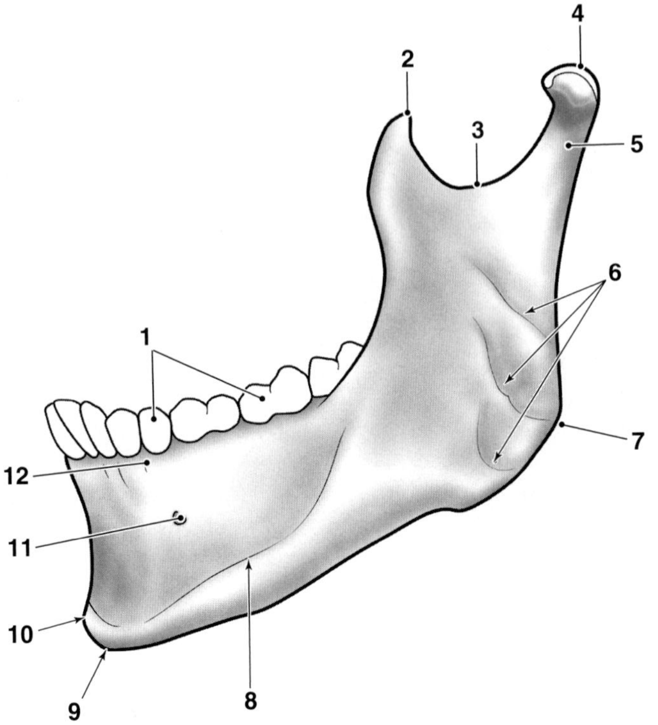

Figure 5-9: Lateral schematic of the mandible showing its external surface.

1 Mandibular teeth
2 Coronoid process
3 Mandibular notch
4 Head of mandible
5 Neck of mandible
6 Irregularities in area of insertion of the masseter muscle
7 Angle of mandible
8 Oblique line
9 Mental tubercle
10 Mental protuberance
11 Mental foramen
12 Alveolar process

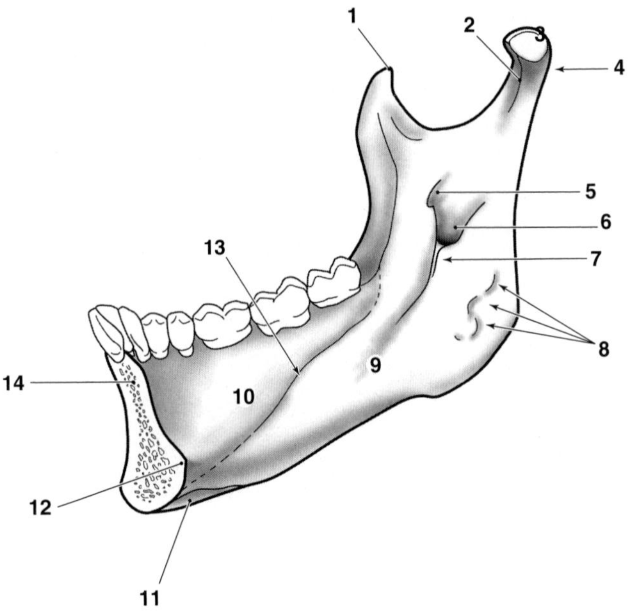

Figure 5-10: Medial schematic of the mandible showing its internal surface.

1 Coronoid process
2 Fossa for lateral pterygoid muscle insertion
3 Head of mandible
4 Neck of mandible
5 Lingula
6 Mandibular foramen
7 Mylohyoid groove
8 Surface irregularities in area of the medial pterygoid muscle insertion
9 Submandibular fossa
10 Sublingual fossa
11 Digastric fossa
12 Internal mental spine (protuberance)
13 Mylohyoid line
14 Alveolar process

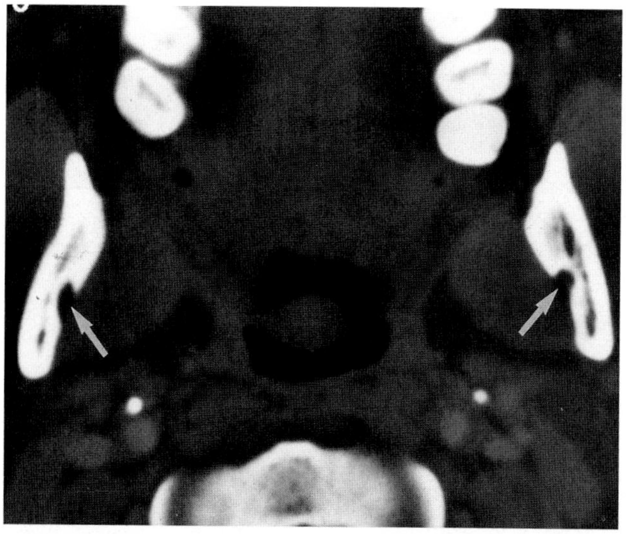

Figure 5-11A: Mandibular and mental foramina and canals. Axial CT image showing mandibular foramina (*arrows*).

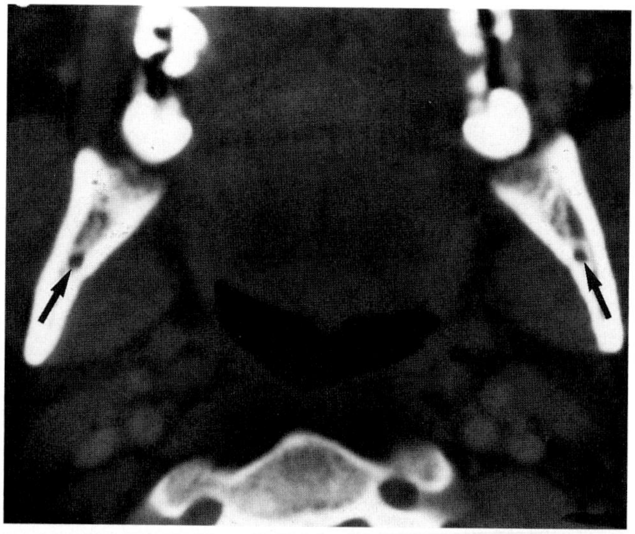

Figure 5-11B: Axial CT image showing the mandibular canals (*arrows*).

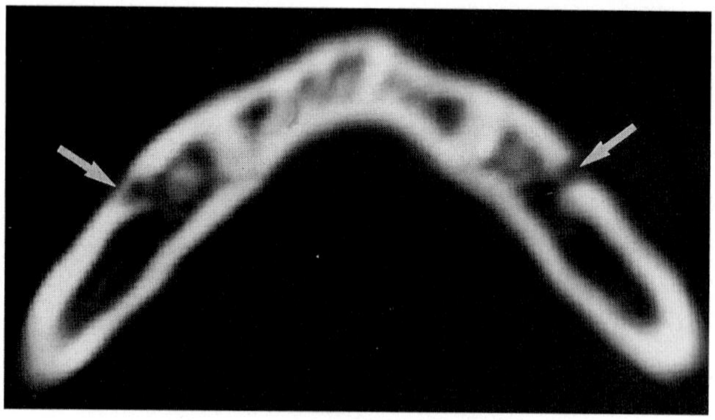

Figure 5-11C: Axial CT image through the anterior mandible showing the mental foramina (*arrows*).

MANDIBULAR VARIANTS

- Mandibular hypoplasia
- Mandibular hyperplasia (prognathism)
- Accessory mandibular neurovascular foramina
- Torus mandibularis

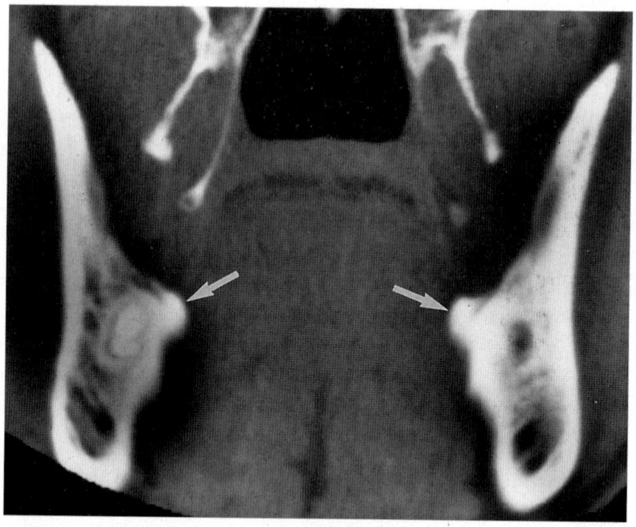

Figure 5-12: Torus mandibularis. Coronal CT image showing torus mandibularis bilaterally (*arrows*).

THE TEMPOROMANDIBULAR JOINT

1. The osseous portion of the temporomandibular joint (TMJ) is composed of the mandibular condyle, glenoid fossa, and the articular tubercle of the temporal bone.
2. The articulating surfaces of the TMJ are covered with a thin layer of dense fibrous tissue.
3. The TMJ articular disc is a biconcave fibrous structure located between the articular surfaces of the mandibular condyle and the glenoid fossa of the temporal bone. The anterior and posterior portions of the articular disc are referred to as the anterior and posterior bands, respectively.
4. The TMJ is surrounded by a joint capsule, with the articular disc interposed between the superior and inferior articular TMJ spaces.
5. During opening of the jaw, the articular disc normally partially dislocates together with the mandibular condyle in the anterior direction. Following closing of the jaw, the articular disc and mandibular condyle return to their resting position within the glenoid fossa.
6. The capsule and ligaments of the TMJ are as follows:
   a. The TMJ capsule arises from the neck of the mandibular condyle and inserts into the margin of the glenoid fossa. Synovial membrane lines the joint capsule internally.
   b. The ligaments of the TMJ are three in number: the temporomandibular, the stylomandibular, and the sphenomandibular (pterygomandibular) ligaments. They are named for their origin and insertion points.
7. The TMJ innervation is primarily via the auriculotemporal branch of the mandibular division of the trigeminal nerve (CN-V3). Some neural fibers also arise from the masseteric branch of the mandibular nerve (CN-V3).
8. The arterial supply to the TMJ is from the superficial temporal and internal maxillary arteries.

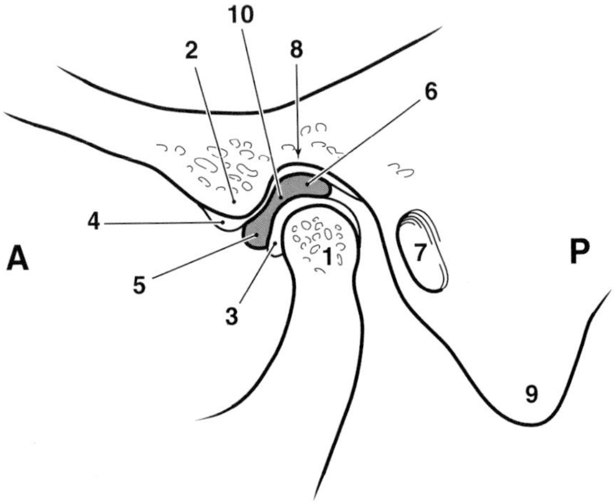

Figure 5-13: Sagittal cross-sectional schematic of the left temporomandibular joint in the closed-mouth position. *A*, anterior; *P*, posterior.
1 Mandibular condyle
2 Articular tubercle of temporal bone
3 Inferior joint space
4 Superior joint space
5 Anterior band of the articular disc
6 Posterior band of the articular disc
7 External auditory canal
8 Glenoid fossa
9 Mastoid process of temporal bone
10 Intermediate zone of the articular disc

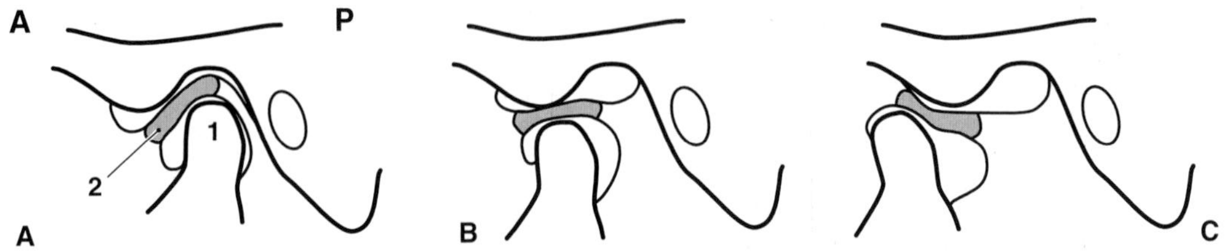

Figure 5-14: Lateral schematics of the left temporomandibular joint in various degrees of opening. Note the normal partial anterior dislocation of the mandibular condyle *(1)* and articular disc *(2)* upon opening of the jaw. **A:** Jaw closed. **B:** Jaw partially opened. **C:** Jaw fully opened. *A,* anterior; *P,* posterior.

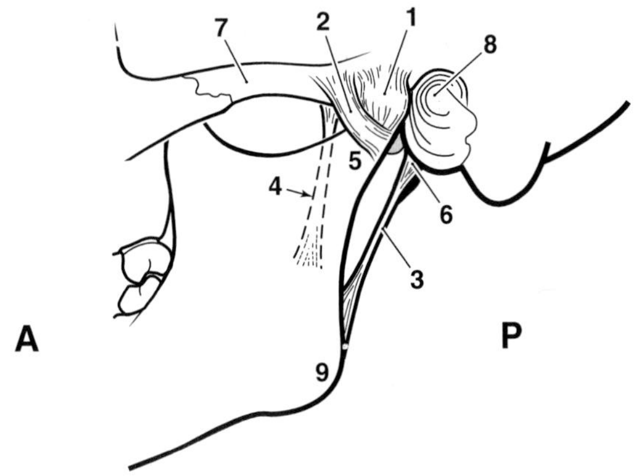

Figure 5-15: Lateral schematic of the temporomandibular capsule and ligaments. *A,* anterior; *P,* posterior.
1 Temporomandibular joint capsule
2 Temporomandibular ligament
3 Stylomandibular ligament
4 Sphenomandibular ligament
5 Neck of mandible
6 Styloid process of temporal bone
7 Zygomatic process of temporal bone
8 External auditory meatus
9 Angle of mandible

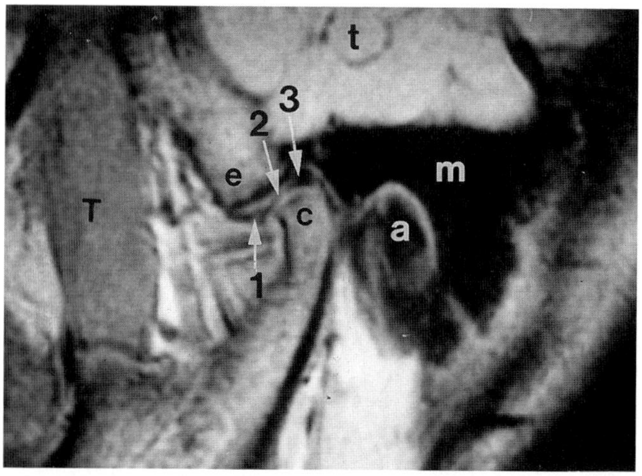

Figure 5-16A: The temporomandibular joint. Sagittal T1-weighted MR image in the closed-mouth position of the temporomandibular joint (anterior to reader's left). Note the articular disc [*(arrows)*: *(1)* anterior band, *(2)* intermediate zone, *(3)* posterior band] superior to the mandibular condyle *(c)*, the articular tubercle (*e*, eminence), the temporalis muscle *(T)*, the external auditory meatus *(a)*, the temporal lobe *(t)*, and the mastoid air cells *(m)*.

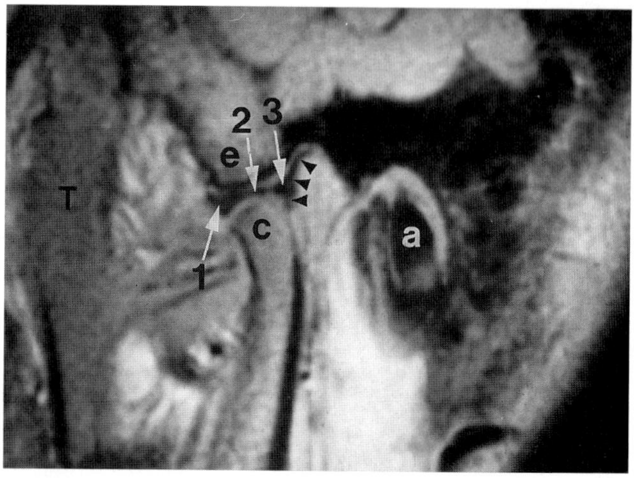

Figure 5-16B: Sagittal T1-weighted MR image in the open-mouth position. Note the anterior condylar *(c)* translation to the level of the apex of the articular tubercle (*e*, eminence) and its relationship to the articular disc [(*arrows*): *(1)* anterior band, *(2)* intermediate zone, *(3)* posterior band], the limit of posterior band and posterior attachment (*arrowheads*), the temporalis muscle *(T)*, the external auditory meatus *(a)*.

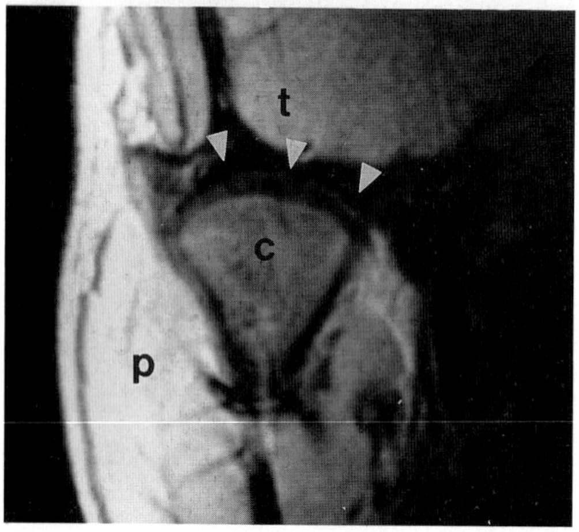

Figure 5-16C: Coronal T1-weighted MR image in the closed-mouth position. Note that there is no sideways (i.e., lateral or medial) articular disc (*arrowheads*) displacement. Also note the mandibular condyle *(c)*, the parotid gland *(p)*, and the temporal lobe *(t)*.

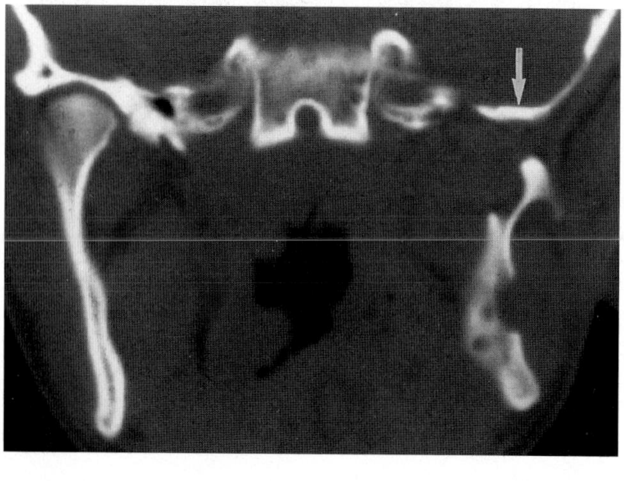

Figure 5-17: Dysplastic temporomandibular joint. Coronal CT shows hypoplasia and deformity of the mandibular neck, condyle, and head on the left side and related nonformation of the glenoid fossa (*arrow*).

THE BONY (HARD) PALATE

1. The bony (i.e., "hard") palate is composed of the paired palatine processes of the maxillary bones and the paired horizontal plates of the palatine bones. A third, temporarily separate bone, the incisive bone (premaxillary bone), usually fuses with the maxilla during development.
2. The bones of the hard palate are joined at the posterior cruciform suture of the palate formed by the intermaxillary (anteriorly) and interpalatine (posteriorly) sutures in the midline running longitudinally, and the palatomaxillary suture running transversely. A temporary second transverse suture runs anteriorly between the incisive bone and the maxilla and might be termed the *maxilloincisive suture* (Jinkins); the two temporary incisive bones will form the *interincisive suture* (Jinkins). This will in turn form the *anterior cruciform suture of the palate* (Jinkins).
3. The posterior border of the hard palate projects backward in the midline to form the posterior nasal spine. Anteriorly the maxillae project forward to form the anterior nasal, spine.
4. The U-shaped maxillary alveolar arch has 16 alveoli or tooth sockets for the roots of the maxillary teeth.
5. The midline incisive foramen in the incisive bone splits superiorly or remains joined to form the paired incisive canals. This foramen communicates with the nasal cavity, and transmits the terminal rami of the greater palatine vessels and the nasopalatine nerve. The nasopalatine nerve descends through the incisive canal to supply the mucosa overlying the anterior part of the hard palate.
6. The greater palatine foramina and paired lateral canals are located near the lateral palatine border, posterior to the palatomaxillary suture. These canals transmit the left and right greater palatine vessels and nerves. The greater palatine nerves descend through the greater palatine canals and exit the foramina to supply the gums, mucosa, and glands overlying the posterior aspect of the hard palate.
7. The lesser palatine foramina and canals, usually numbering two on each side, are located posterior to the greater palatine foramina and pierce the pyramidal processes of the palatine bones. Accessory lesser foramina may be present in 30% to 70% of anatomic specimens. These canals transmit the lesser palatine vessels and nerves. The lesser palatine nerves descend through the lesser palatine canals and exit the foramina to supply the uvula, tonsil, and soft palate.
8. In addition to sensory impulses, the palatine nerve [branch of the maxillary (second) division of the fifth cranial nerve: CN-V2] conveys regional taste related impulses to the pterygopalatine ganglion.
9. The margins of the intermaxillary and interpalatine sutures are elevated in some individuals to form an irregular longitudinal (hyperostotic) ridge, the palatine torus (torus palatinus). Similarly, a longitudinal (hyperostotic) maxillary ridge, the maxillary torus (torus maxillarus), may form along the inner aspect of the alveolar process of the maxillae palatal to the upper molar teeth.

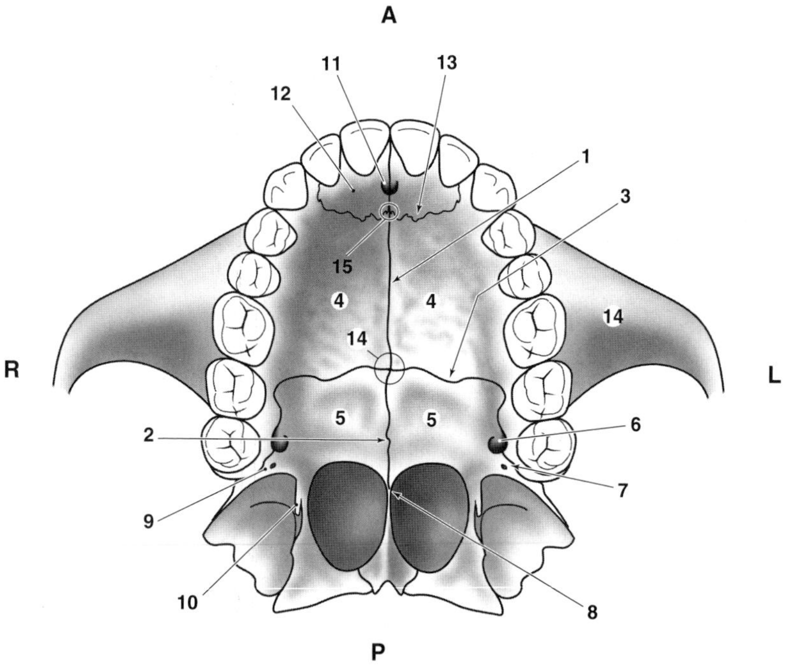

Figure 5-18: Schematic of the hard palate from below. *A,* anterior; *P,* posterior; *L,* left; *R,* right.

1 Intermaxillary suture
2 Interpalatine suture
3 Palatomaxillary suture
4 Left and right palatine processes of the maxillary bone
5 Left and right horizontal plates of the palatine bones
6 Greater palatine foramen
7 Lesser palatine foramen
8 Posterior nasal spine
9 (Tubercle) pyramidal process of the palatine bone
10 Hamulus of the medial pterygoid plate
11 Incisive foramen
12 Incisive bone
13 Maxilloincisive suture
14 Posterior cruciform (cross-shaped) suture
15 Anterior cruciform (cross-shaped) suture

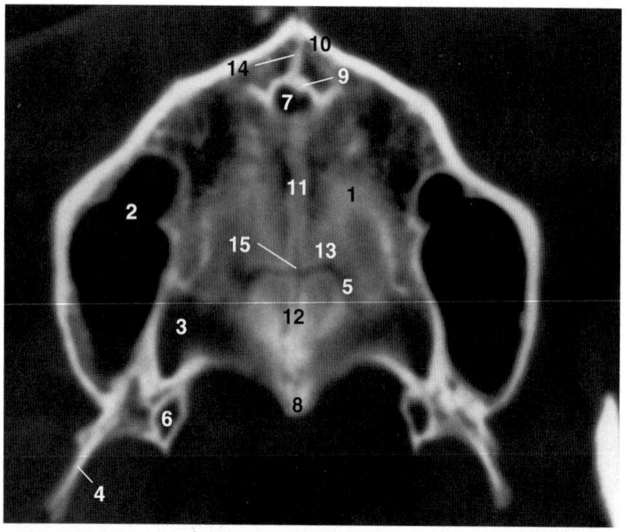

Figure 5-19A: The hard palate. Axial CT image showing the hard palate.

1 Palatine process of maxillary bone
2 Maxillary sinus
3 Greater palatine canal/foramen
4 Lateral pterygoid plate
5 Pallatomaxillary suture
6 Lesser palatine canal/foramen
7 Incisive canal/foramen
8 Posterior nasal spine
9 Remnant of maxillo-incisive suture (anterior cruciform suture)
10 Primitive remnant of incisive bone
11 Intermaxillary suture
12 Interpalatine suture
13 Horizontal plate of palatine bone
14 Interincisive suture
15 Posterior cruciform suture

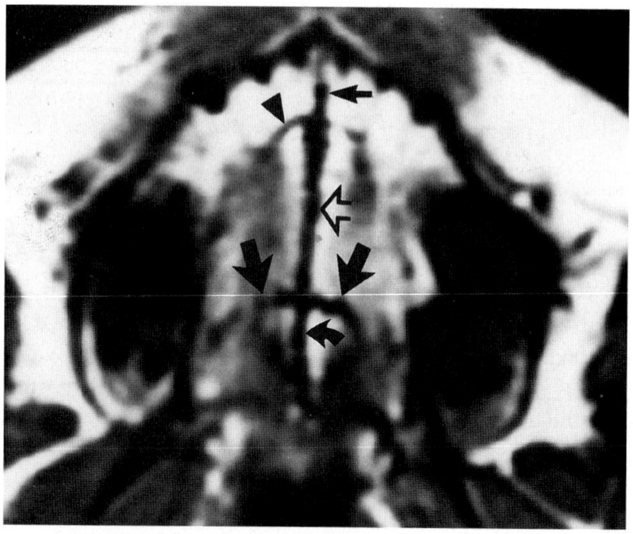

Figure 5-19B: Cruciform sutures of the hard palate. Axial T1-weighted MR image showing the incisive suture (*arrowhead*), the palatomaxillary suture (*large solid arrows*), the intermaxillary suture (*open arrow*), the interpalatine suture (*curved arrow*), and the interincisive suture (*small solid arrow*). These intersecting sutures thereby create anterior and posterior cruciform (i.e., cross-shaped) sutures.

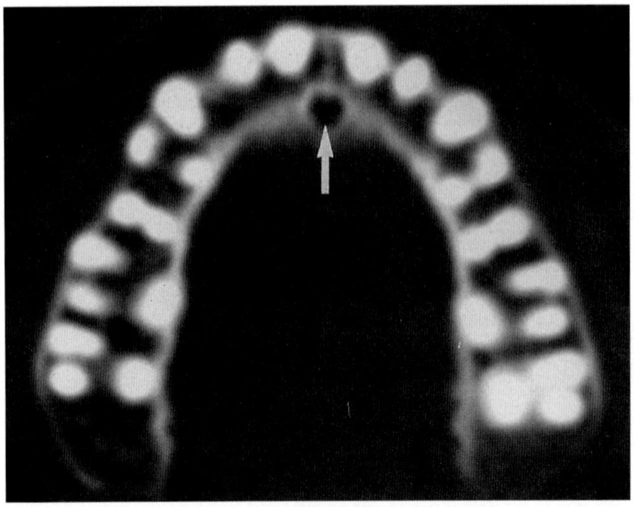

Figure 5-20A: The incisive foramen and canal(s). Axial CT image showing the joined inferior aspect of the incisive canal(s)/foramen (*arrow*).

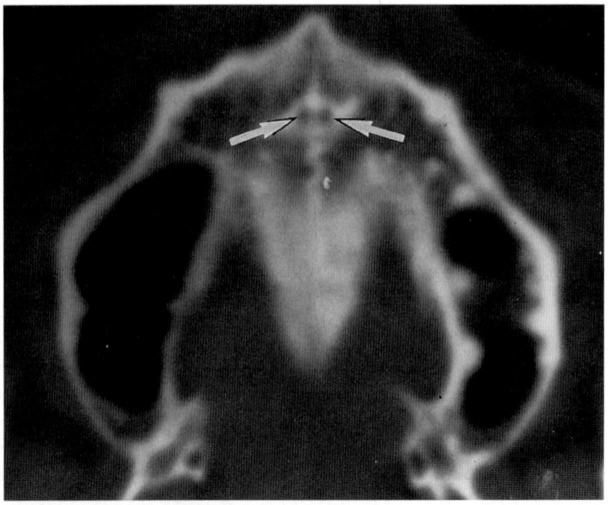

Figure 5-20B: Axial CT image showing the separated superior aspect of the incisive canals (*arrows*) within the anterior hard palate.

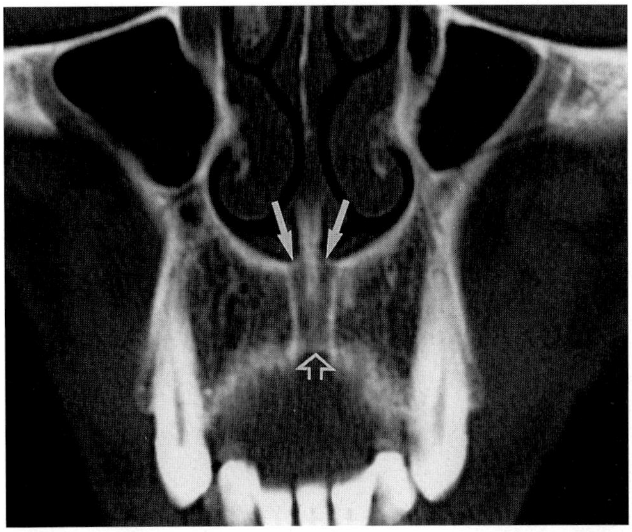

Figure 5-20C: Coronal CT image showing the paired incisive canals within the anterior hard palate. Note that they are separated superiorly (*solid arrows*) and joined inferiorly at the level of the incisive foramen (*open arrow*).

MAXILLAE AND HARD PALATE VARIANTS

- Hypoplasia of maxilla
- Partial/complete cleft palate
- Accessory neurovascular foraminae
- Torus palatinus
- Torus maxillarus

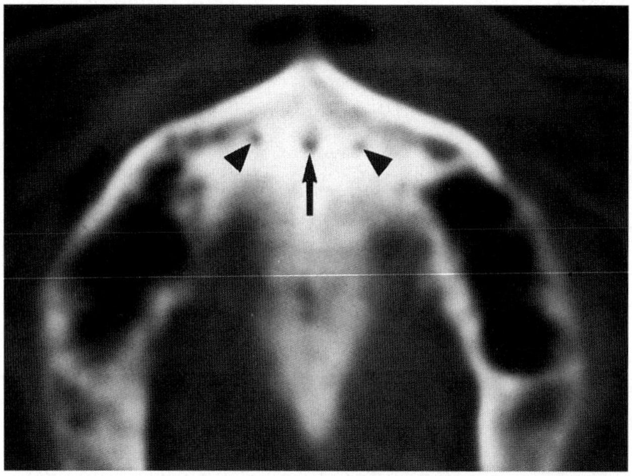

Figure 5-21: Accessory incisive canals. Axial CT image showing the primary incisive canal in the midline (*arrow*), flanked by accessory incisive canals laterally (*arrowheads*).

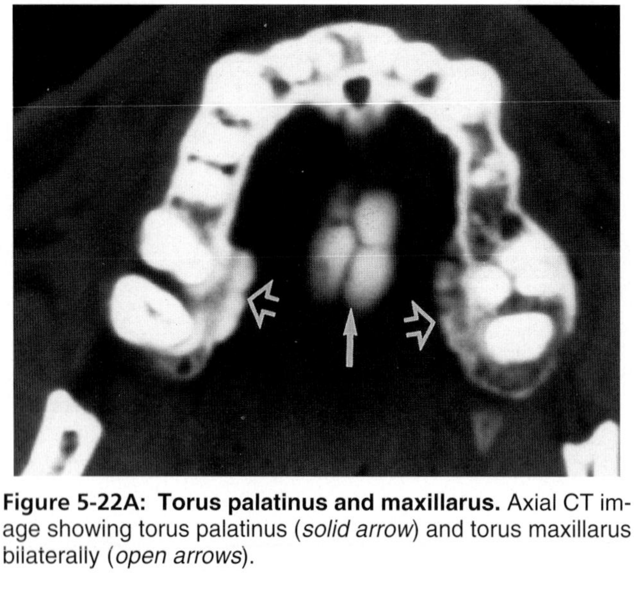

Figure 5-22A: Torus palatinus and maxillarus. Axial CT image showing torus palatinus (*solid arrow*) and torus maxillarus bilaterally (*open arrows*).

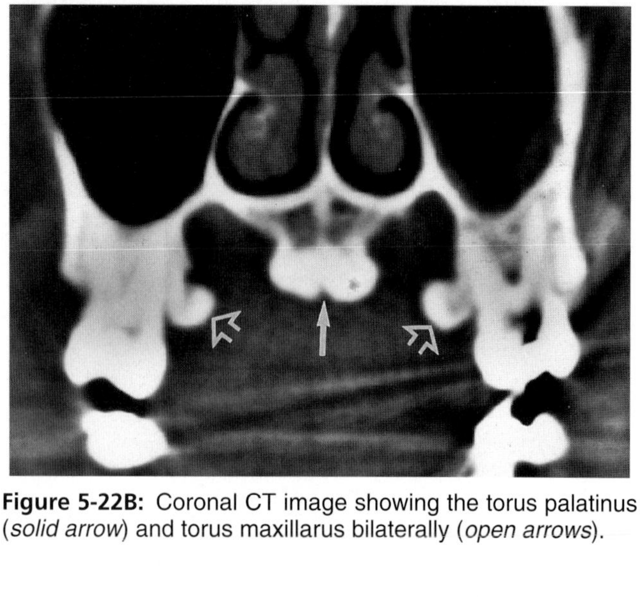

Figure 5-22B: Coronal CT image showing the torus palatinus (*solid arrow*) and torus maxillarus bilaterally (*open arrows*).

ANATOMY, ENUMERATION, AND VARIATIONS OF THE PERMANENT TEETH

1. The four basic types of teeth include incisors, canines, premolars, and molars.
2. There are typically 4 incisors, 2 canines, 4 premolars, and 6 molars for a total of 16 teeth in each of the upper (maxilla) and lower (mandible) jaws (i.e., 32 teeth in all).
3. Variations in the number and form of the permanent teeth is not uncommon.
   a. Hypodontia refers to a developmental absence of one or more teeth. The third molar is the most frequently absent tooth. In decreasing order of frequency, other missing teeth include the maxillary lateral incisors, the maxillary or mandibular second premolars, the mandibular central incisors, and the maxillary first premolars.
   b. Hyperdontia refers to developmentally additional or supernumerary teeth. This occurs with much greater frequency in the maxilla than in the mandible. Most commonly the supernumerary teeth occur on the palatal aspect of the incisors or distal to the molars. Rarely, supernumerary premolars develop.
   c. Macrodontia refers to a developmentally overlarge tooth or teeth and microdontia overly small tooth or teeth.
   d. Hyperodontia tends to be associated with macrodontia; hypodontia tends to be associated with microdontia.

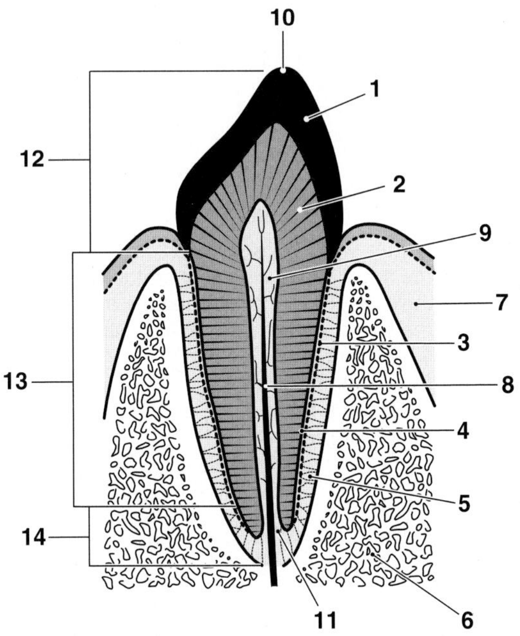

Figure 5-23: Longitudinal section schematic of a permanent tooth after eruption.
1 Enamel
2 Dentine
3 Cementoblasts
4 Cementum
5 Periodontal ligament
6 Bone of tooth socket (maxillary or mandibular alveolar process)
7 Gingivae
8 Dental neurovascular plexus (artery, vein, sensory nerves, sympathetic plexus)
9 Pulp chamber
10 Buccal cusp
11 Apical foramen
12 Crown
13 Root
14 Apex

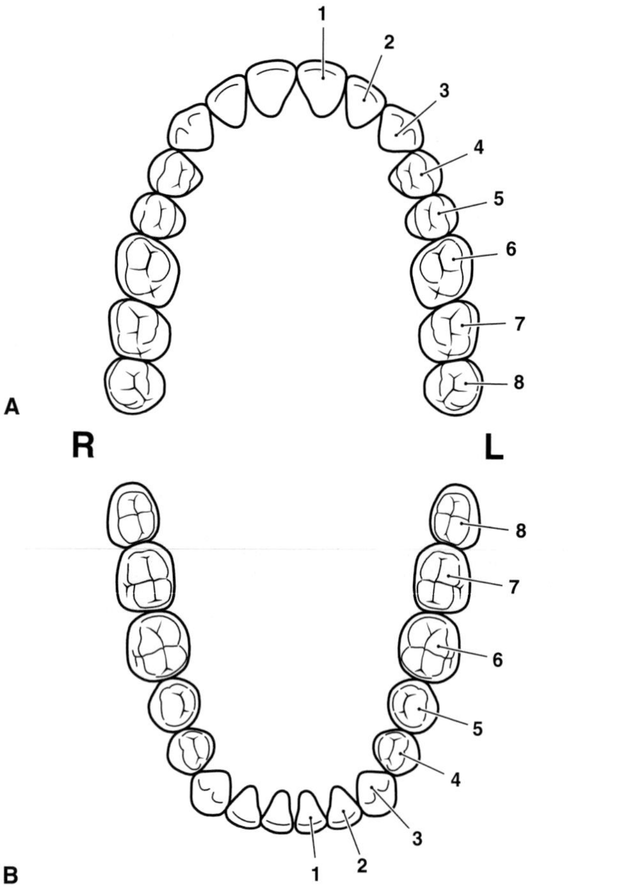

Figure 5-24: Schematics of the spatial relationship of the maxillary and mandibular teeth. **A:** Maxillary teeth. **B:** Mandibular teeth. *R*, right; *L*, left.

1 First incisor
2 Second incisor
3 Canine
4 First premolar
5 Second premolar
6 First molar
7 Second molar
8 Third molar

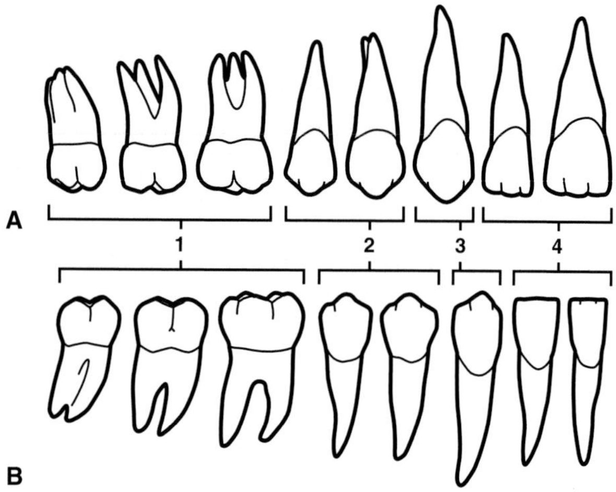

Figure 5-25: External lateral schematic of the permanent teeth of the maxilla and mandible on the right side. The teeth are shown removed from their respective alveolar processes. **A:** Maxillary teeth on the right side. **B:** Mandibular teeth on the right side.

1 Molar teeth
2 Premolar teeth
3 Canine teeth
4 Incisor teeth

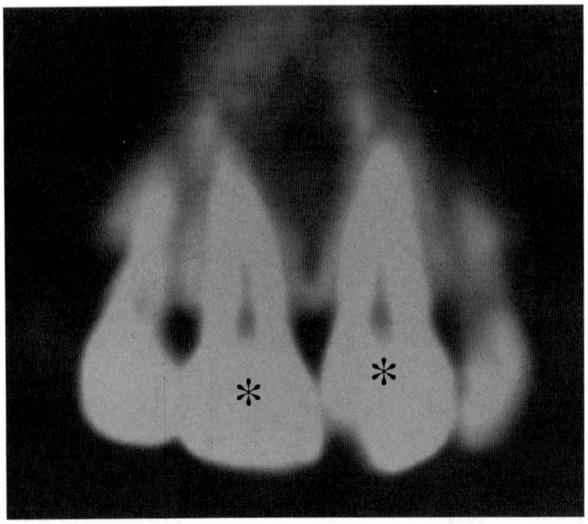

Figure 5-26: The maxillary incisors. Magnified coronal CT image showing the maxillary incisors (*asterisks*).

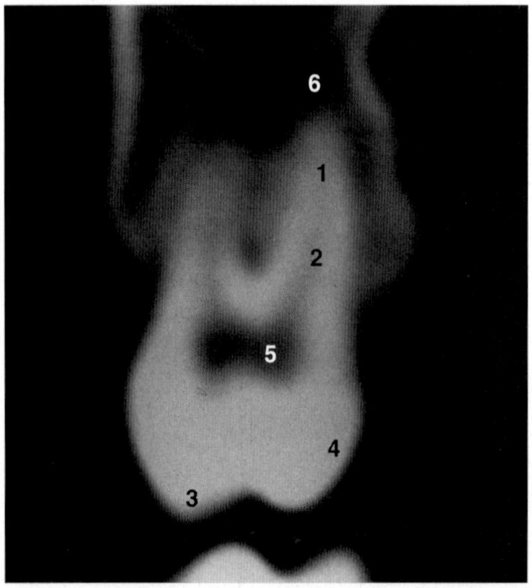

Figure 5-27: A molar tooth. Magnified coronal CT image showing the normal anatomy of a maxillary molar tooth.
1 Root
2 Neck
3 Crown
4 Enamel
5 Pulp
6 Alveolar process of maxilla

CHAPTER 6

Paranasal Sinuses and Nasal Passageways

THE PARANASAL SINUSES

1. The paranasal sinuses are paired, mucosally lined air spaces within the facial bones and skull base.
2. The paranasal sinuses are divided into four groups: frontal, maxillary, ethmoid, and sphenoid. These sinuses are primarily housed in the bones for which they are named.
3. The paranasal sinus mucosa is continuous with that of the nasal passageways via paranasal sinus apertures (ostia) in the lateral wall of the nasal cavity.
4. Mucus is secreted by glands in the mucosa and is moved toward the paranasal sinus ostia by cilia on the mucosal surface.
5. The functions of the paranasal sinuses are uncertain; speculations on their evolutionarily derived function include voice resonance modification, facial strengthening, and facial group contour determination (e.g., gender, sexual maturity, group identity).

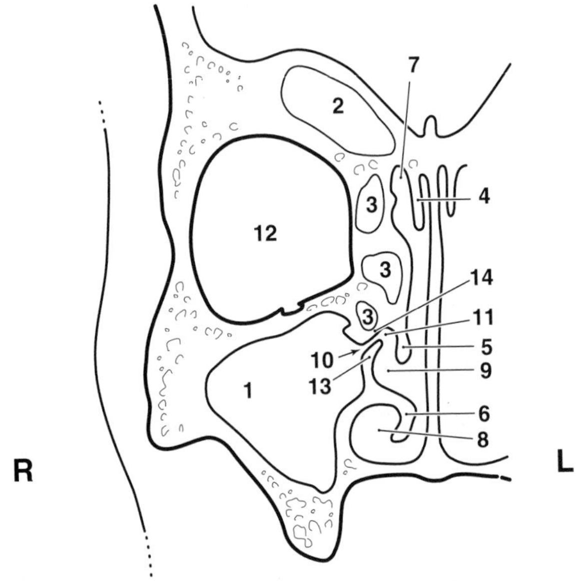

Figure 6-1: Coronal schematic of the frontal, maxillary, and ethmoid sinuses on the right side. *R*, right; *L*, left.
1 Maxillary sinus
2 Frontal sinus
3 Ethmoid air cells
4 Superior turbinate (concha)
5 Middle turbinate (concha)
6 Inferior turbinate (concha)
7 Superior meatus
8 Inferior meatus
9 Middle meatus
10 Maxillary sinus ostium } Osteomeatal complex
11 Semilunar hiatus } Osteomeatal complex
12 Orbit
13 Uncinate process
14 Ethmoid infundibulum

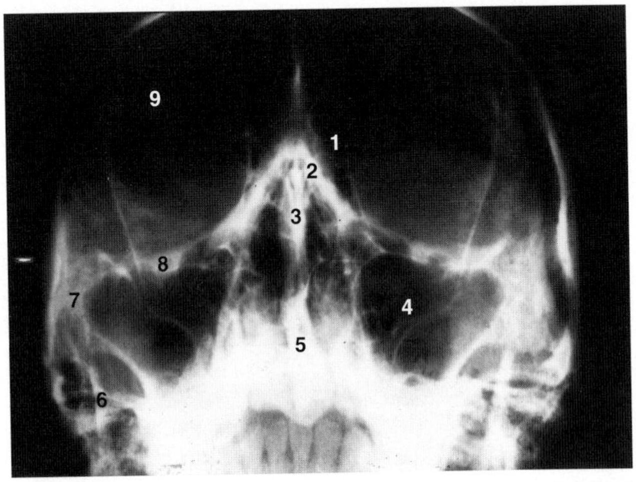

Figure 6-2: The paranasal sinuses. Conventional radiograph of the skull in the Waters projection showing the paranasal sinuses.
1 Ethmoid air cells
2 Nasal bone
3 Bony nasal septum
4 Maxillary sinus
5 Alveolar (dental) arch/ridge
6 Mastoid air cells
7 Zygomatic bone
8 Floor of orbit
9 Orbit

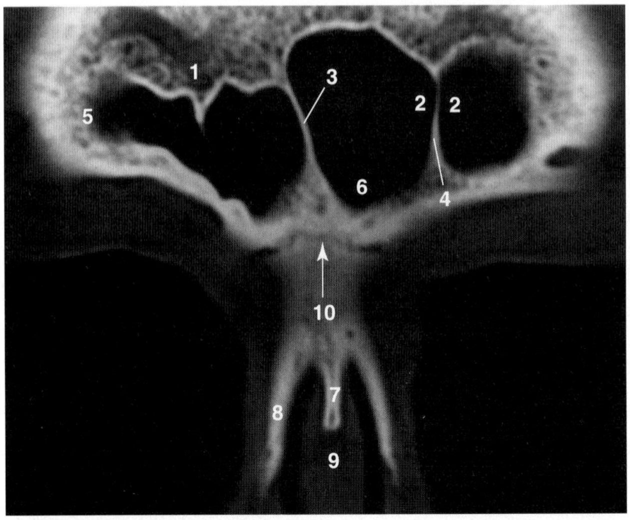

Figure 6-3: Nasal bones and frontal sinuses. Coronal CT scan showing the nasal bones and frontal sinuses.

1 Frontal bone
2 Frontal sinuses
3 Median septum
4 Lateral septum
5 Lateral recess
6 Nasal recess
7 Vertical crest of nasal bones
8 Nasal bone
9 Cartilaginous portion of nasal septum
10 Frontonasal suture

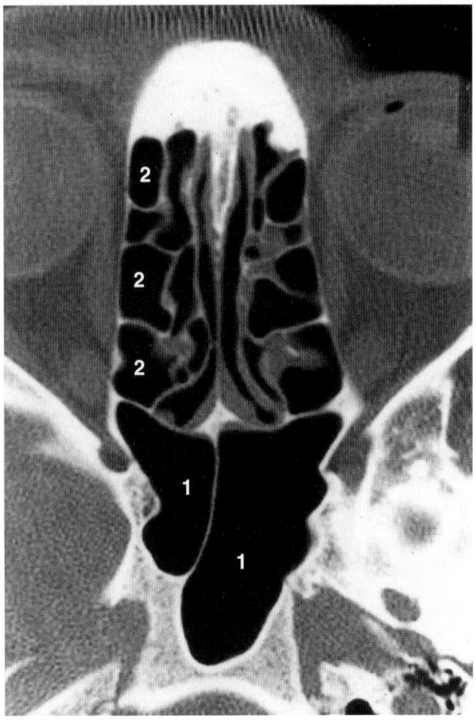

Figure 6-4: The ethmoid and sphenoid sinuses. Axial CT image showing the ethmoid and sphenoid sinuses.

1 Sphenoid sinus
2 Ethmoid air cells

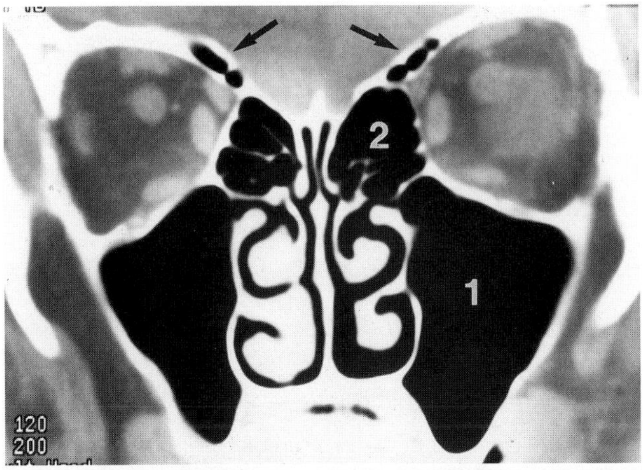

Figure 6-5: The maxillary and ethmoid sinuses. Coronal CT image showing the normal appearance of maxillary (1) and ethmoid (2) sinuses. There is some extension of the ethmoid air cells into the bony roofs of the orbits (*arrows*).

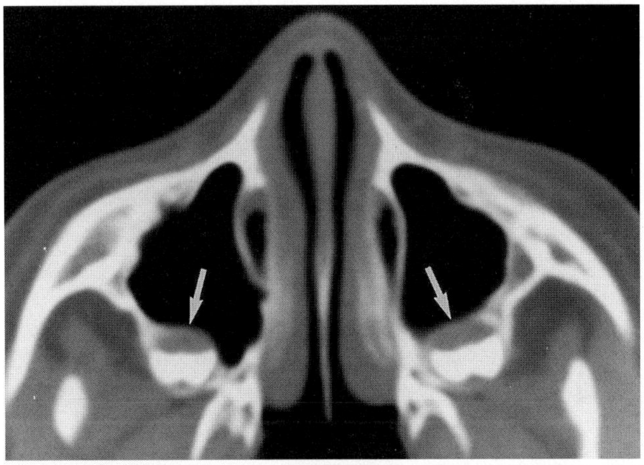

Figure 6-6: Unerupted molar teeth protruding into the maxillary sinuses. Axial CT image showing the normal appearance of the maxillary sinuses in an adolescent. Note the unerupted molar teeth (*arrows*) protruding into the posteroinferior aspect of the maxillary sinuses.

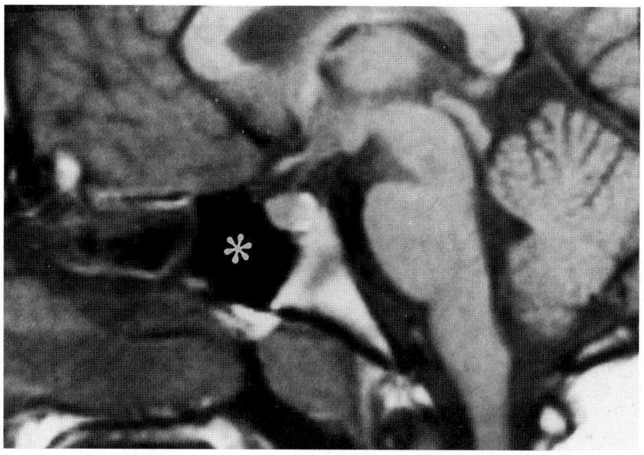

Figure 6-7: The sphenoid sinus. Unenhanced sagittal T1-weighted MR image showing the normal appearance of the aerated sphenoid sinus (*asterisk*).

THE NASAL PASSAGEWAYS

1. The nasal passageways are paired, air-filled cavities, lined by mucosa and separated by the nasal septum.
2. The external openings anteriorly are the piriform or anterior nasal apertures; the internal openings posteriorly are the paired choanae (posterior nasal apertures).
3. The nasal floor is made up of the hard palate (palatine processes of the maxillae and horizontal plates of the palatine bones).
4. The lateral wall has three mucosally lined bony projections called turbinates (conchae). The superior and middle turbinates are part of the ethmoid bone. The inferior turbinate is an independent bone. There may be a fourth small turbinate, supreme turbinate (60%), located above the superior turbinate.
5. The portion of the nasal passageway lateral and inferior to each turbinate is called a nasal meatus and is named for the suprajacent turbinate (e.g., inferior meatus, middle meatus, superior meatus, supreme meatus).
6. The medial wall is composed of the septal cartilage anteriorly, the vertical plate of the ethmoid bone superiorly, and the vomer (bone) inferiorly.
7. The nasal roof is formed by portions of the nasal, frontal, ethmoid, and sphenoid bones.
8. The olfactory area is located in the superior nasal tarbinate, the opposed portion of the nasal septum, and the intervening nasal roof. These areas contain the sensory terminations of the olfactory nerve (CN-I).

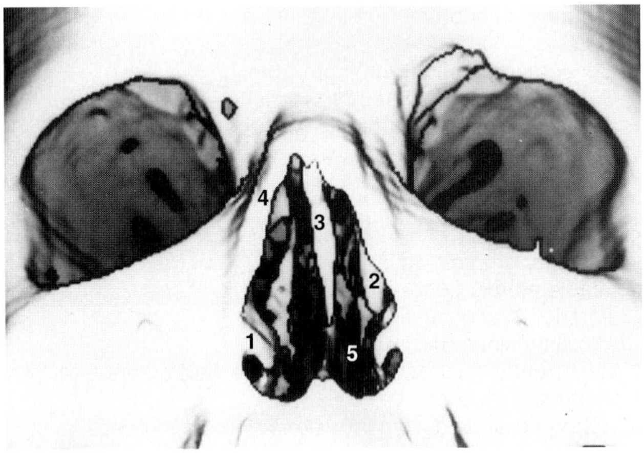

Figure 6-8: The nasal passageways. Three-dimensional CT image showing the bony nasal passageway anatomy.
1 Inferior concha
2 Middle concha
3 Nasal septum
4 Nasal bone
5 Nasal passageway

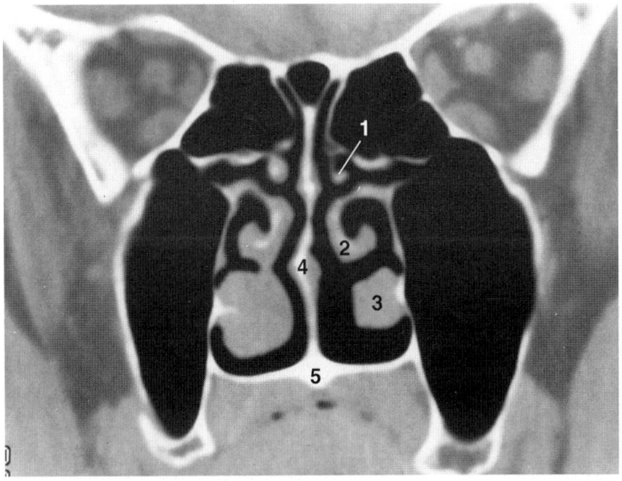

Figure 6-9: The nasal turbinates. Coronal CT image showing the nasal turbinates bilaterally together with the corresponding meati.
1 Superior nasal turbinate
2 Middle nasal turbinate
3 Inferior nasal turbinate
4 Bony nasal septum
5 Hard (bony) palate

DRAINAGE OF THE PARANASAL SINUSES

1. The frontal sinus drains (a) into the frontoethmoid recess via an independent frontal paranasal sinus ostium, or (b) into the middle meatus via the nasofrontal duct. From there the drainage is into the middle meatus of the nasal passageway.
2. The anterior ethmoid air cells drain either directly into the middle meatus via an independent ethmoid paranasal sinus ostium(ia), or into the frontoethmoidal recess via the nasofrontal duct and thereafter into the middle meatus. Frequently present in the ethmoidal air cells is the ethmoid bulla, representing the outwardly convex wall of the largest ethmoid cell; the ethmoid bulla is found at the level of the maxillary sinus infundibulum. The drainage of the middle ethmoid cells is via an ostium(ia) in the ethmoid bulla into the middle meatus. The posterior ethmoid air cells drain into the superior or supreme meati via an independent ostium(ia).
3. The maxillary sinus primarily drains via the *osteomeatal complex* consisting of (a) the maxillary sinus ostium, (b) the hiatus semilunaris, and (c) the middle meatus. An assessory maxillary sinus ostium frequently is present inferoposterior to the hiatus semilunaris.
4. The sphenoid sinus drains via the sphenoid ostia directly into the sphenoethmoidal recess just posterior to the superior meatus.

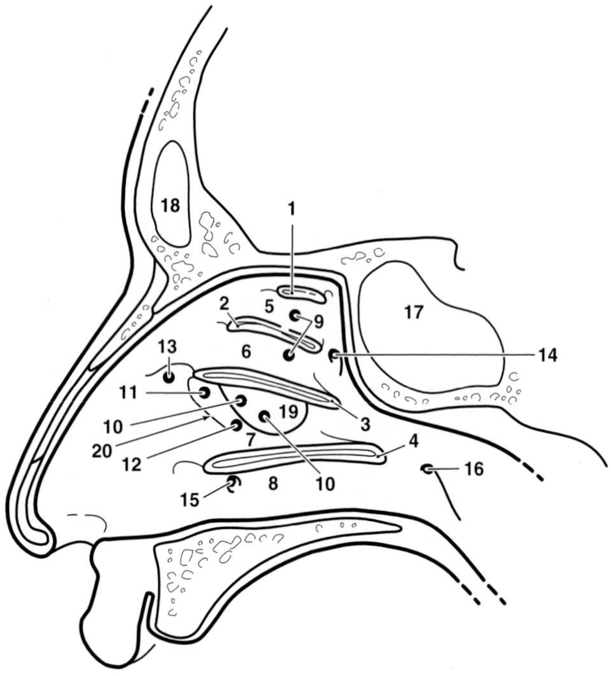

Figure 6-10: Lateral schematic of the lateral wall of the nasal passageway with the nasal septum and conchae removed showing the drainage ostia of the paranasal sinuses, the nasolacrimal duct, and the eustachian (auditory) tube.

1 Cut edge of supreme turbinate (concha) (present in 60% of patients)
2 Cut edge of superior turbinate (concha)
3 Cut edge of middle turbinate (concha)
4 Cut edge of inferior turbinate (concha)
5 Supreme meatus
6 Superior meatus
7 Middle meatus
8 Inferior meatus
9 Posterior ethmoid ostia
10 Middle ethmoid ostia
11 Anterior ethmoid ostium(ia)
12 Maxillary sinus ostium(ia)
13 Nasofrontal duct ostium (drains the frontal sinus in frontoethmoid recess)
14 Sphenoid sinus ostium in sphenoethmoidal recess
15 Ostium of the nasolacrimal duct
16 Orifice of the eustachian tube
17 Sphenoid sinus
18 Frontal sinus
19 Ethmoid bulla
20 Hiatus semilunaris

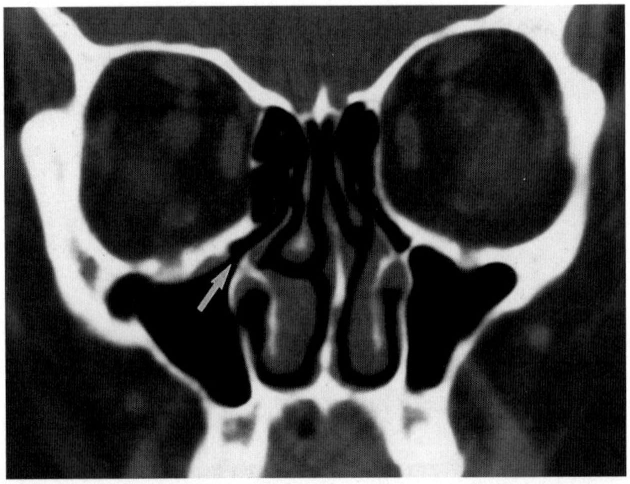

Figure 6-11: The osteomeatal complex. Coronal CT image showing the normal appearance of the osteomeatal complex (*arrow*) on the right side.

MAXILLARY SINUS VARIANTS

- Laterally asymmetric maxillary sinuses
- Aplastic or hypoplastic maxillary sinus(es)
- Hyperplastic maxillary sinus(es)
- Accessory maxillary sinus air cells
- Aerated recesses of maxillary sinus
    - Palatine recess
    - Alveolar recess
    - Infraorbital recess

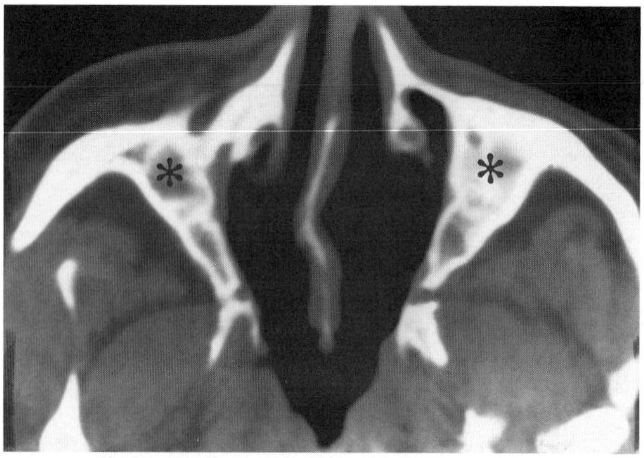

Figure 6-12A: Aplasia of maxillary sinuses. Axial CT image in an adult showing aplasia of both maxillary sinuses (*asterisks*).

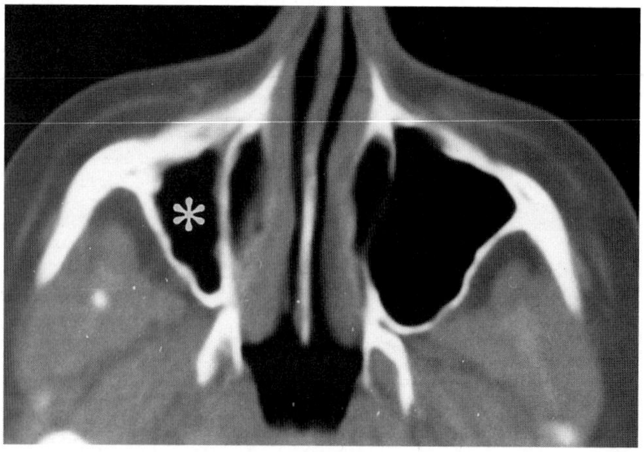

Figure 6-12B: Hypoplastic maxillary sinus. Axial CT image showing a hypoplastic maxillary sinus (*asterisk*) on the right side.

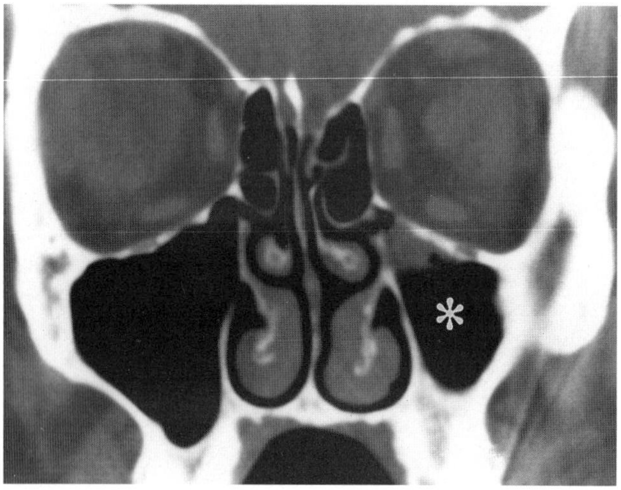

Figure 6-12C: Asymmetric paranasal sinuses and cribriform plates. Coronal CT image showing hypoplasia of the maxillary sinus (*asterisk*) on the left side. Mild mucosal thickening in the roof of the left maxillary sinus is also noted. Note the compensatory enlargement of the nasal passageway, the ethmoid air cells, and the cribriform plate on the left side.

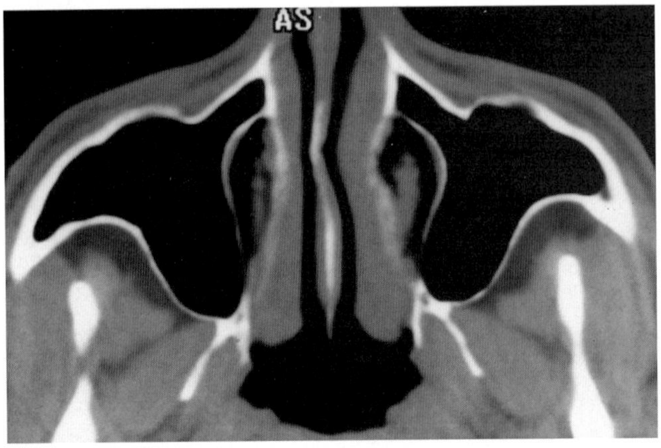

Figure 6-13A: Bilateral hyperplastic maxillary sinuses. Axial CT image showing mildly hyperplastic maxillary sinuses.

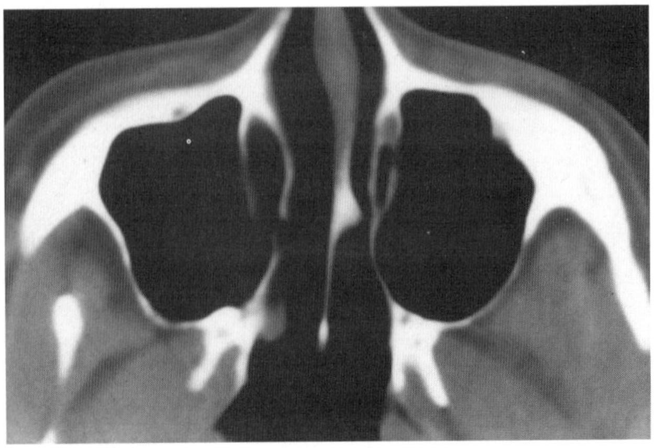

Figure 6-13B: Axial CT image in a different patient showing ballooned maxillary sinuses.

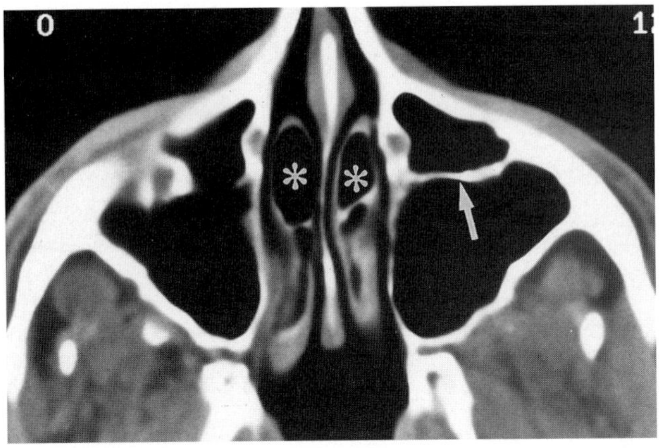

Figure 6-14A: Accessory maxillary sinus. Axial CT image showing an accessory maxillary sinus (*arrow*) on the left side anteriorly. Note also the concha bullosae bilaterally (*asterisks*).

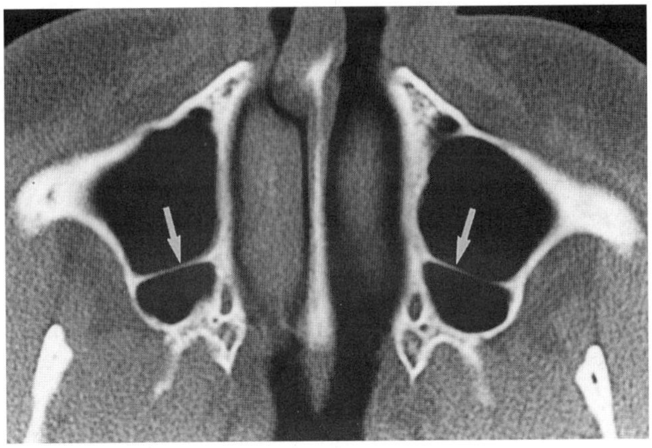

Figure 6-14B: Axial CT image showing accessory maxillary sinuses (*arrows*) bilaterally, posteriorly.

ETHMOID AIR CELL VARIANTS

- Hypoplastic ethmoid air cells
- Laterally asymmetric ethmoid air cells
- Hyperplastic ethmoid air cells, with extension into:
- The bony orbital roof
- The sphenoid bone
- Haller air cells (air cell extension into floor of the orbit: the orbital plate of the maxillary bone)
- Agger nasi air cells (anteriormost ethmoid air cells)
- Ethmoid bullae

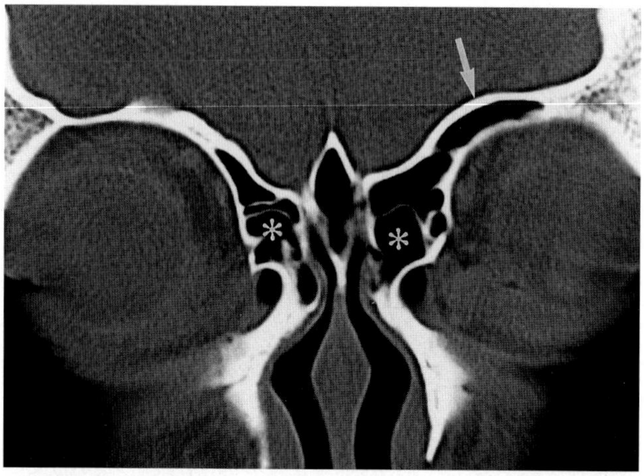

Figure 6-15: Agger nasi air cells. Coronal CT image showing Agger nasi air cells (asterisks: anteriormost ethmoid air cells) and ethmoid air cell extension into the bony roof of the left orbit (*arrow*).

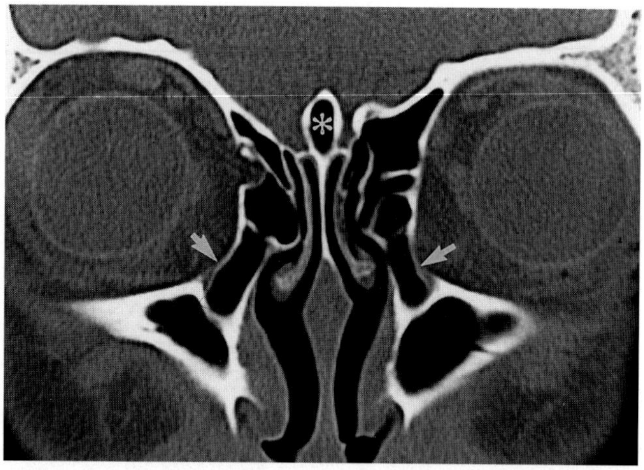

Figure 6-16: Haller cells and crista galli aeration. Coronal CT image showing aeration of the crista galli (*asterisk*) and Haller cells (*arrows*) extending into the bony floor of the orbit.

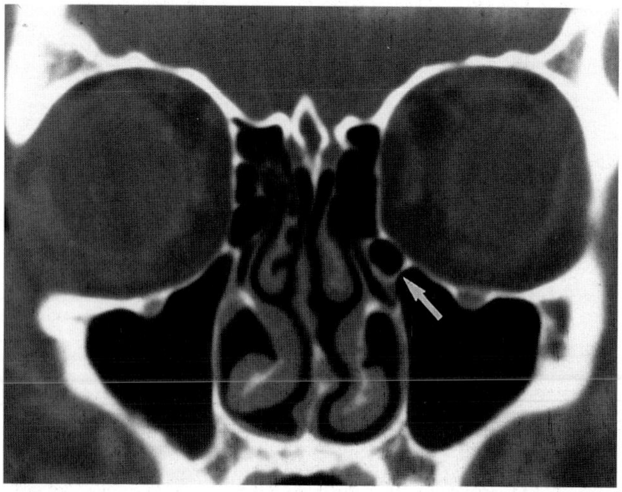

Figure 6-17: Haller paranasal sinus air cell. Coronal CT image showing a Haller air cell (*arrow*) of the ethmoid paranasal sinuses extending into the floor of the bony orbit on the left side.

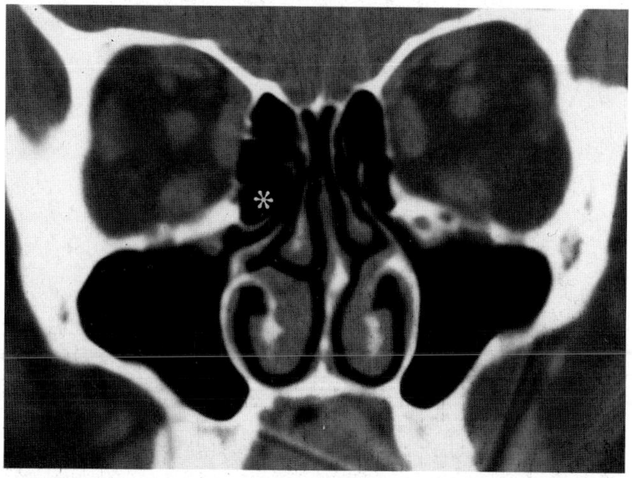

Figure 6-18: Asymmetric ethmoid air cells. Coronal CT image showing an ethmoid bulla (*asterisk*) and mild lateral asymmetry in size of the ethmoid air cells. Note also mild leftward deviation of the nasal septum.

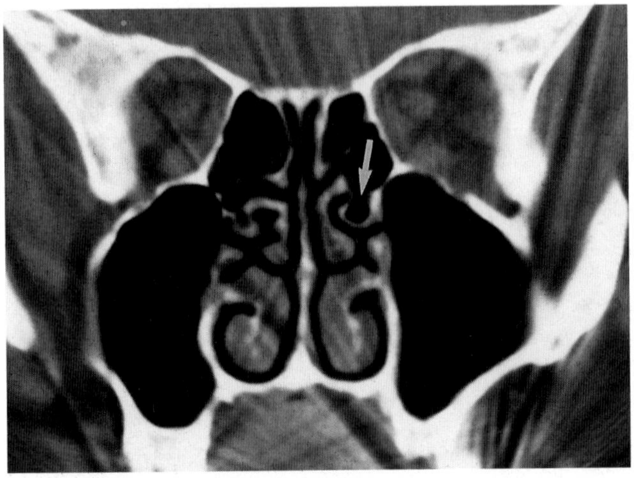

Figure 6-19: The ethmoid bulla. Coronal CT image showing the ethmoid bulla (*arrow*) on the left side.

FRONTAL SINUS VARIANTS

- Aplastic or hypoplastic frontal sinus (unilateral, bilateral)
- Hyperplastic frontal sinus
- Frontal air cell bulla
- Pneumatization of the crista galli
- Pneumatization of the bony orbital roof
- Pneumatization of the base of the nasal bones

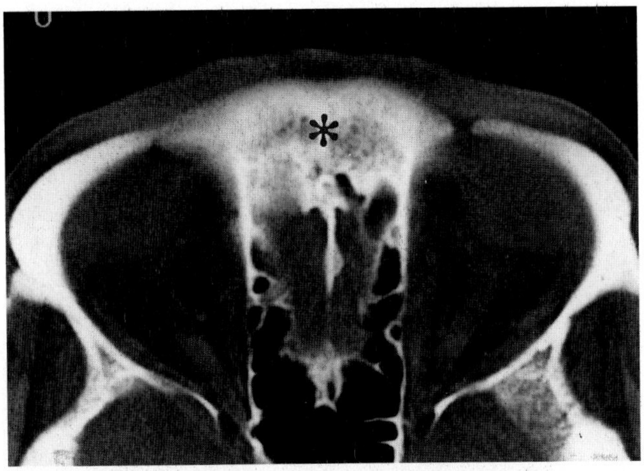

Figure 6-20A: Aplasia of frontal sinus. Axial CT image showing aplasia of the frontal sinus (*asterisk*).

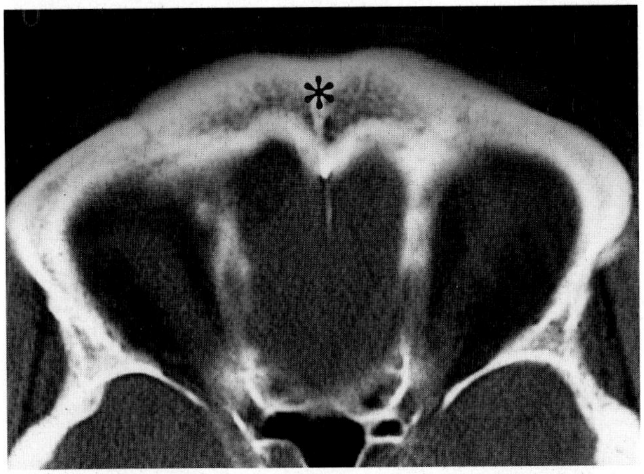

Figure 6-20B: Axial CT image at a higher level than that of Figure 6-20A showing aplasia of the frontal sinus (*asterisk*).

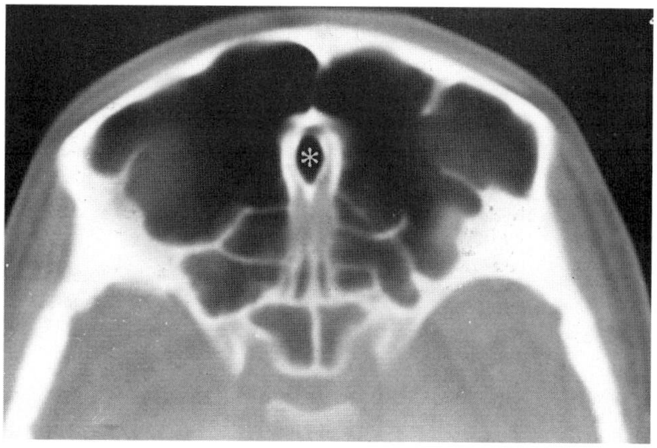

Figure 6-21A: Hyperplastic frontal sinus and aeration of the crista galli. Axial CT image showing the hyperplastic frontal sinuses extending onto the bony orbital roofs. The ethmoid air cells are similarly extending laterally. Note also the aeration of the crista galli (*asterisk*).

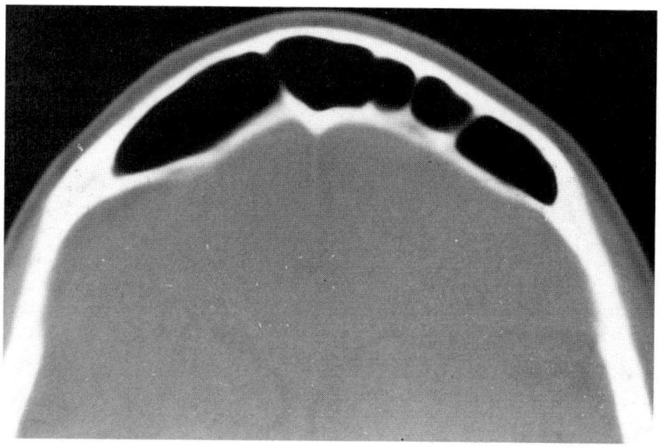

Figure 6-21B: Axial CT image showing mildly hyperplastic frontal sinuses extending upward and laterally into the frontal bone.

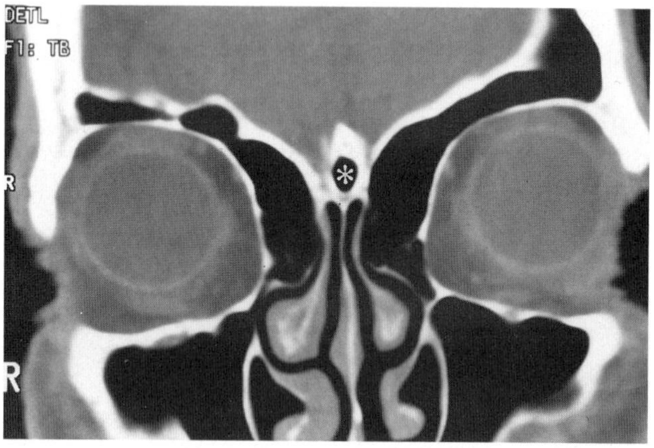

Figure 6-21C: Coronal CT image again showing extension of the frontal sinus into the bony roof of the orbits bilaterally. Note also the aeration of the crista galli (*asterisk*).

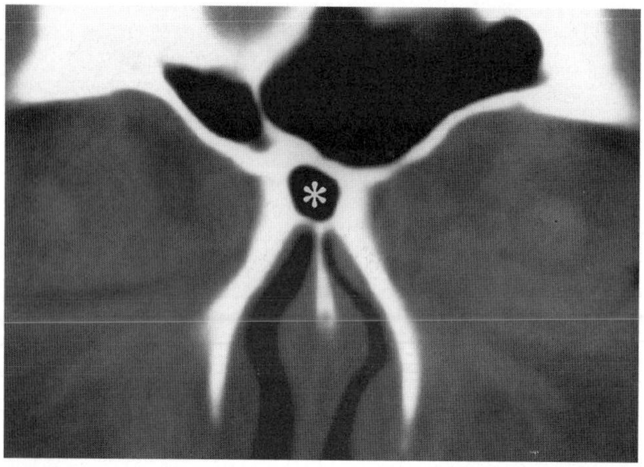

Figure 6-22A: Aeration of base (bridge) of nose from paranasal sinuses. Coronal CT image showing aeration of the bridge of the nose (*asterisk*).

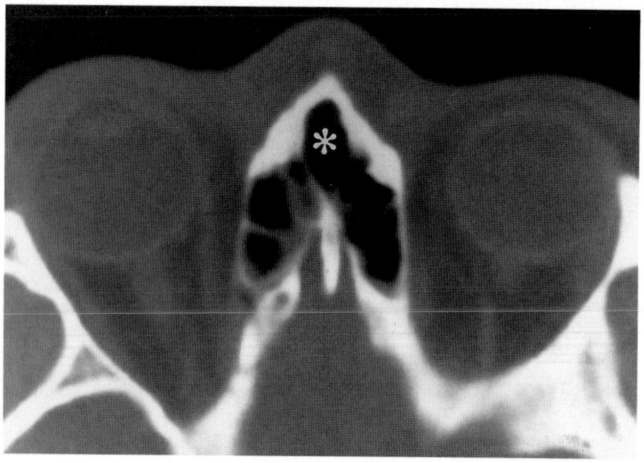

Figure 6-22B: Axial CT again showing aeration of the bridge of the nose (*asterisk*), likely extending from the ethmoid air cells.

SPHENOID SINUS VARIANTS

- Aplastic or hypoplastic sphenoid sinus
- Generally hyperplastic sphenoid sinus
- Aerated recesses of the sphenoid sinus
  - Lateral recess in lesser wing of sphenoid bone
  - Inferolateral recess in greater wing of sphenoid bone
  - Pterygoid recess
  - Septal recess (nasal septum)
  - Vomeral recess
- Air cell extension into the anterior clinoid process(es) of the sella turcica
- Air cell extension into the dorsum sellae and the posterior clinoid processes of the sella turcica
- Air cell extension into the region of the bony pterygoid plates and fossa

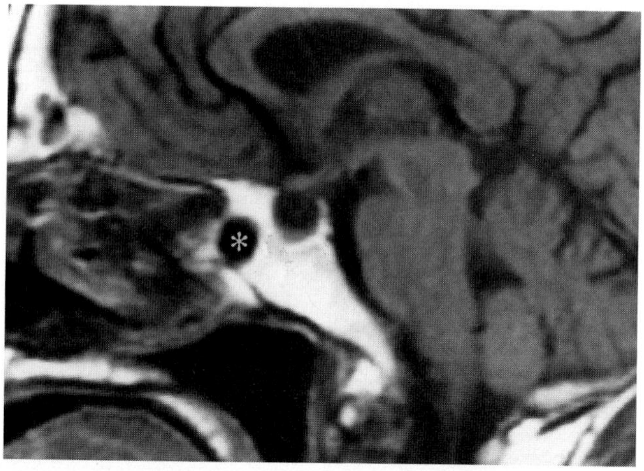

Figure 6-23: Hypoplastic sphenoid sinus. Unenhanced sagittal T1-weighted MR image showing a hypoplastic sphenoid sinus (*asterisk*).

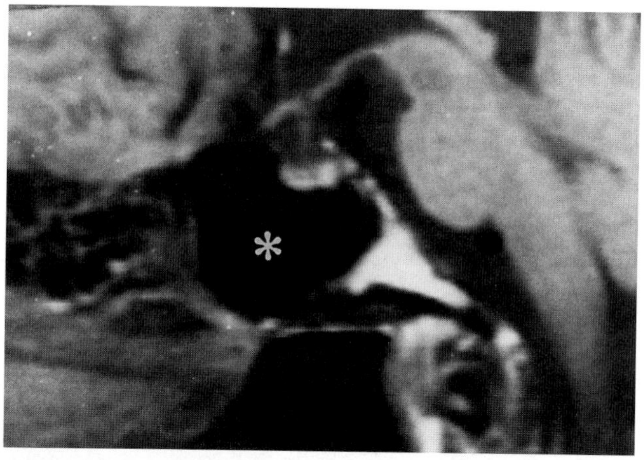

Figure 6-24: Hyperplastic sphenoid sinus. Unenhanced sagittal T1-weighted MR image showing mild hyperplasia of the sphenoid sinus (*asterisk*).

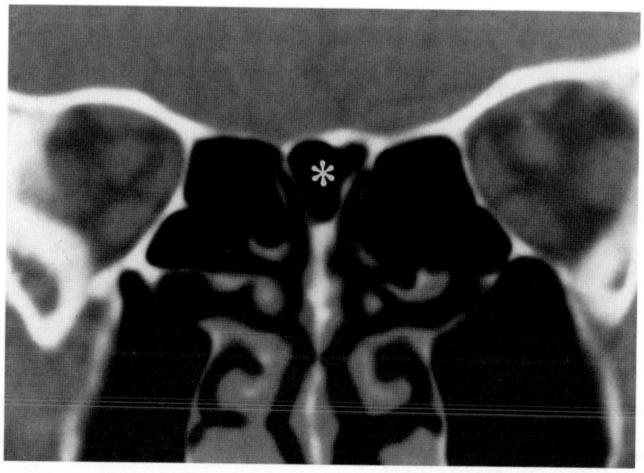

Figure 6-25: Vomeral recess of the sphenoid sinus. Coronal CT image showing a rostral recess (*asterisk*) of the sphenoid sinus originating from the rostrum of the sphenoid bone in the midline and extending into the superior–posterior aspect of the vomer in the nasal septum.

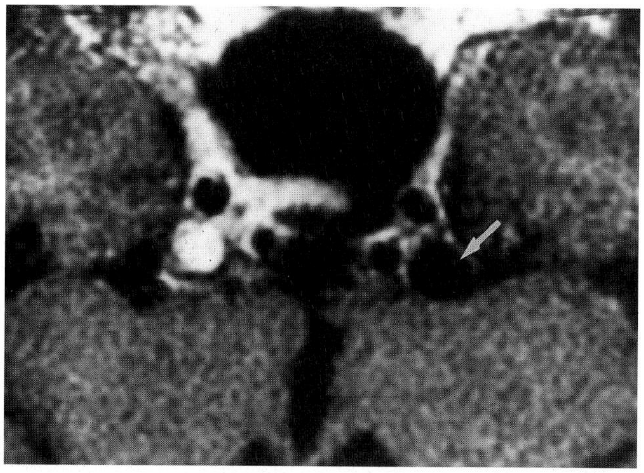

Figure 6-26A: Aerated clinoid processes. Magnified axial T1-weighted MR image showing aeration of the anterior clinoid process (*arrow*) on the left side.

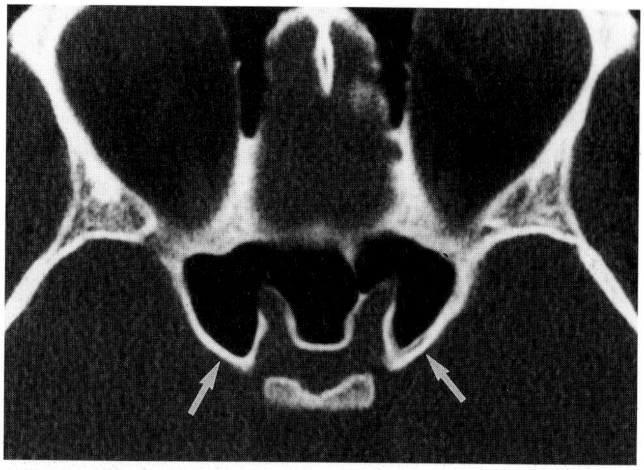

Figure 6-26B: Axial CT image showing aerated anterior clinoid processes (*arrows*) bilaterally.

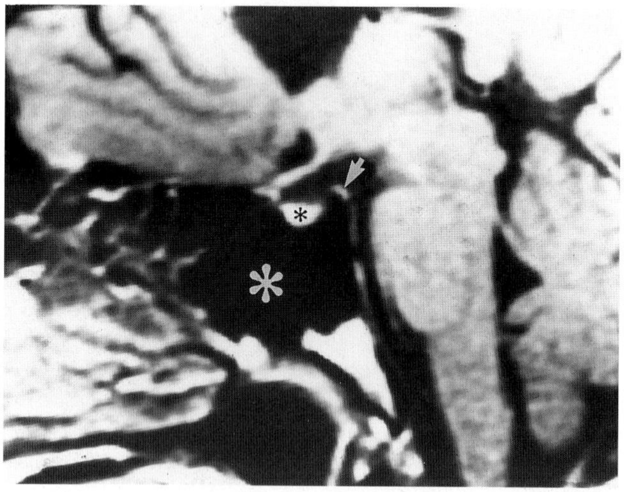

Figure 6-26C: Sagittal T1-weighted MR image showing aeration of the posterior clinoid process (*arrow*). Note the marked aeration of the sphenoid sinus (*white asterisk*) completely surrounding the pituitary gland (*black asterisk*).

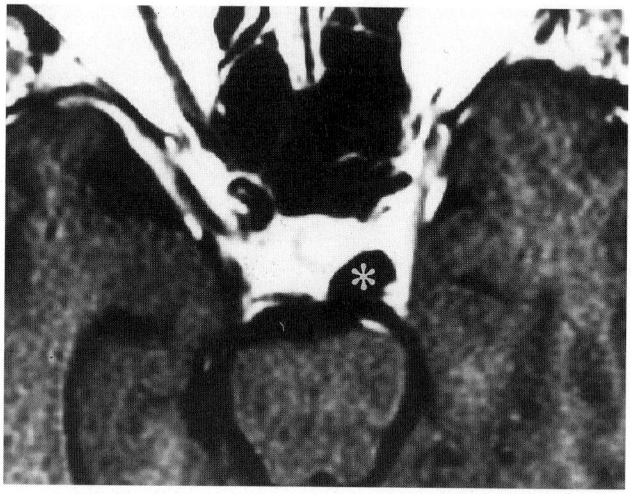

Figure 6-26D: Axial T1-weighted MR image again showing aeration of the posterior clinoid process (*asterisk*) on the left side.

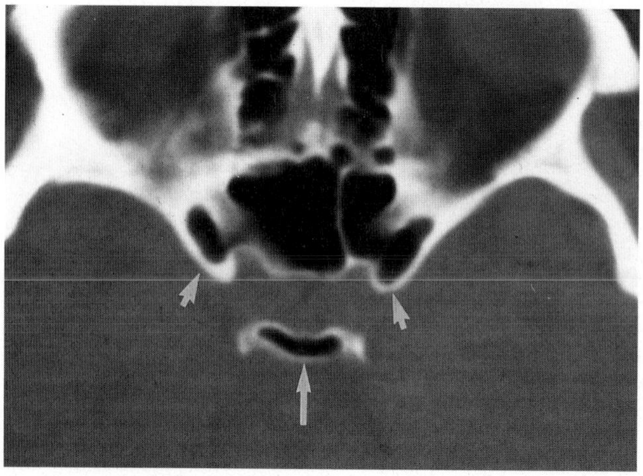

Figure 6-26E: Axial CT image showing pneumatization of anterior clinoid processes (*small arrows*) and the dorsum sella (*large arrow*), both extensions of the sphenoid sinuses.

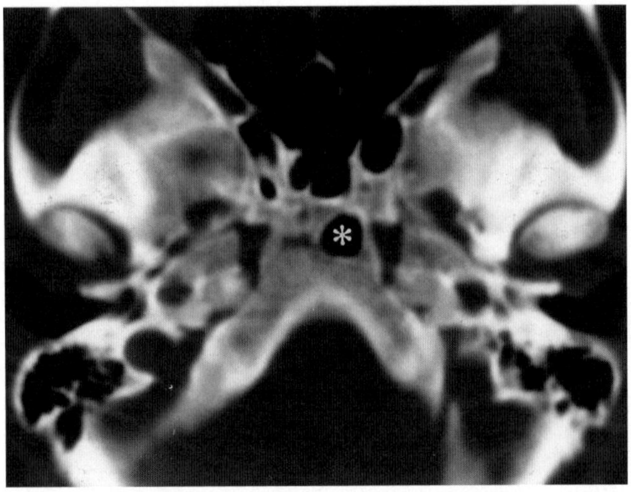

Figure 6-27: Hyperpneumatization of the clivus. Axial CT image showing mild hyperpneumatization of the clivus (*asterisk*) from the sphenoid sinus.

NASAL PASSAGEWAY VARIANTS

- Nasal septum deviation
- Asymmetric nasal passageways
- Septal spur or ridge
- Supreme turbinate
- Unilateral/bilateral hypoplasia of the superior, middle, or inferior turbinates
- Paradoxical (i.e., reversed) curve of the middle/inferior turbinate(s)
- Concha bullosa (pneumatization) of the middle turbinate (most common), the superior turbinate, or the inferior turbinate
- Aerated supreme turbinate
- Deviation of the uncinate process
- Uncinate process bullus formation
- Asymmetric cribriform plate

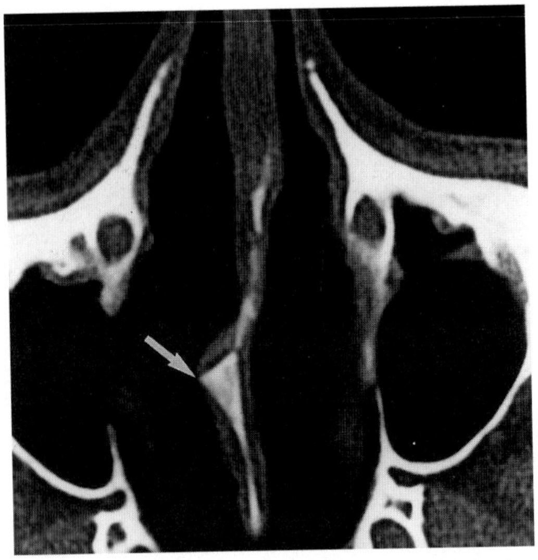

Figure 6-28A: Nasal septal spur. Axial CT image showing a nasal septal spur (*arrow*) on the right side. Note the nasal septal deviation in the direction of the side of the spur.

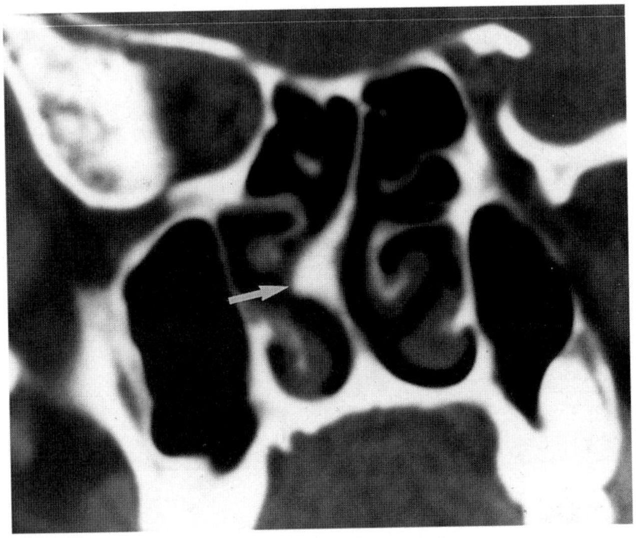

Figure 6-28B: Coronal CT image in a different patient again showing a nasal spur (*arrow*) on the right side. Note the nasal septal deviation in the direction of the side of the spur.

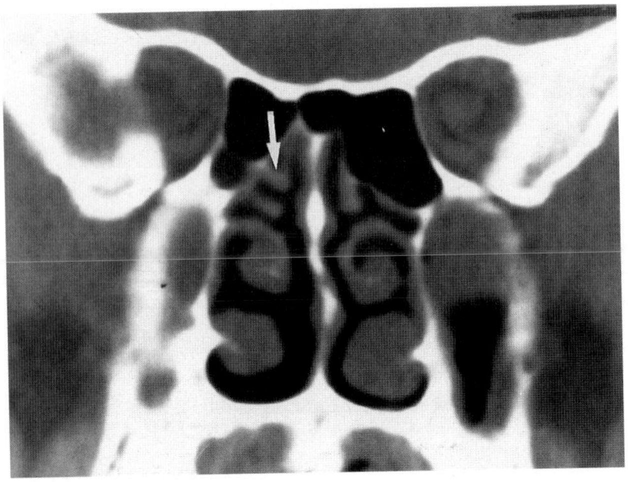

Figure 6-29: Supreme turbinate. Coronal CT image showing a supreme turbinate (*arrow*) on the right side.

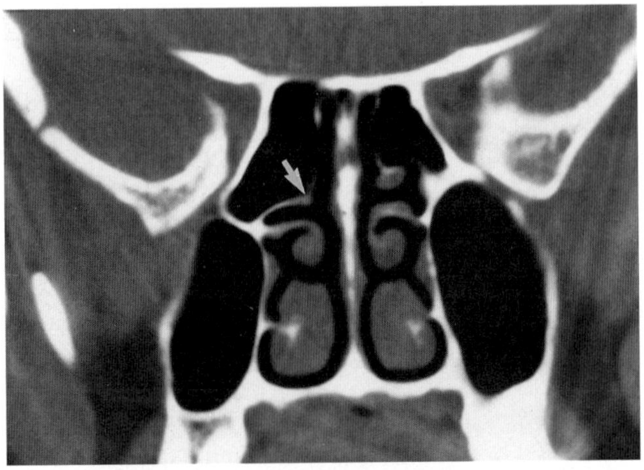

Figure 6-30: Hypoplasia of superior turbinate. Coronal CT image showing a unilateral hypoplastic superior turbinate (*arrow*) on the right side.

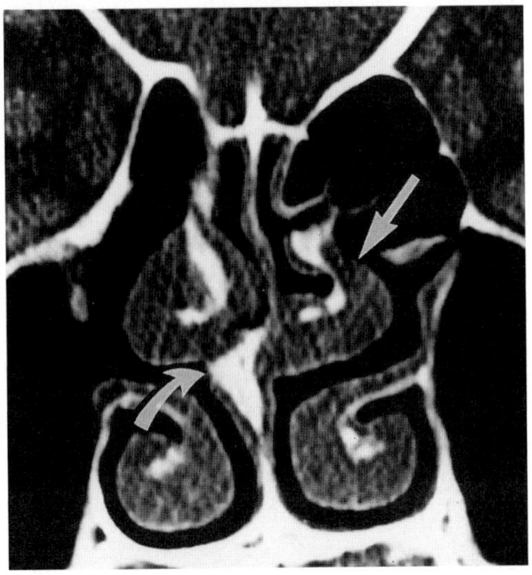

Figure 6-31A: Paradoxic (reversed curve) turbinates. Coronal CT image showing paradoxical middle turbinate (*straight arrow*) on the left side and nasal septal spur (*curved arrow*) on the right side. Compare with the direction of curve of the other conchae.

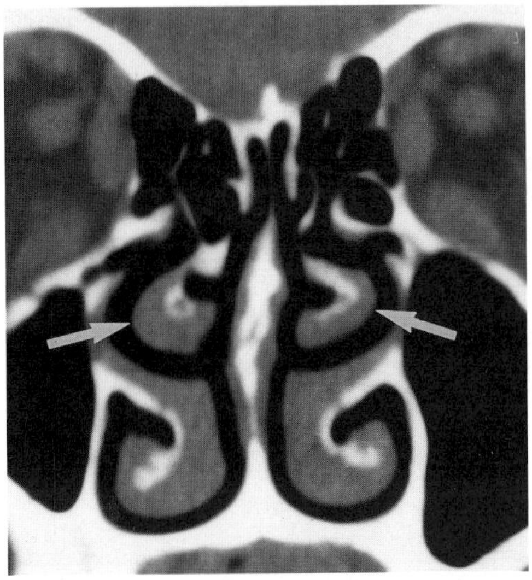

Figure 6-31B: Coronal CT image showing paradoxical (reverse curve) middle conchae (*arrows*) bilaterally.

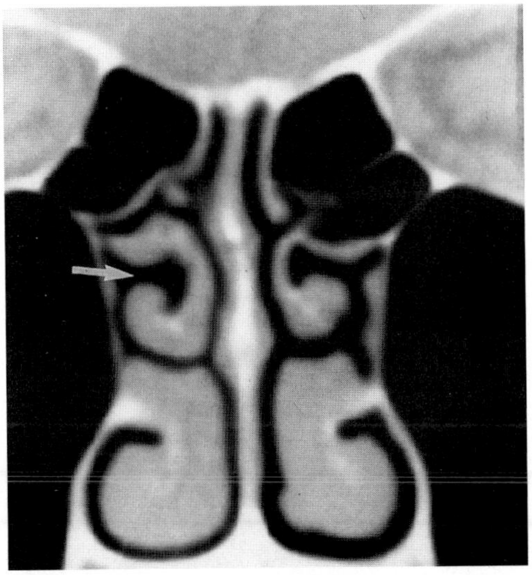

Figure 6-31C: Coronal CT image showing the normal outward curve of the middle turbinate posteriorly (*arrow*).

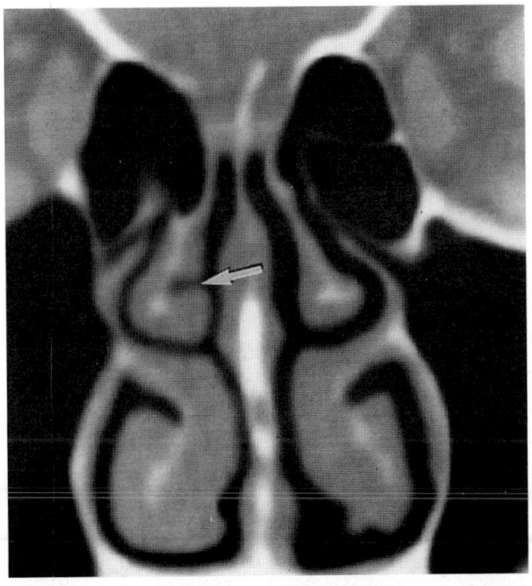

Figure 6-31D: Coronal CT image anterior to that of Figure 6-31C showing that the curve of the right middle turbinate is reversed inwardly (*arrow*). This is typical of the reverse curve of the middle turbinate: the curve begins normally posteriorly but then "warps" into a reverse curve as it progresses anteriorly.

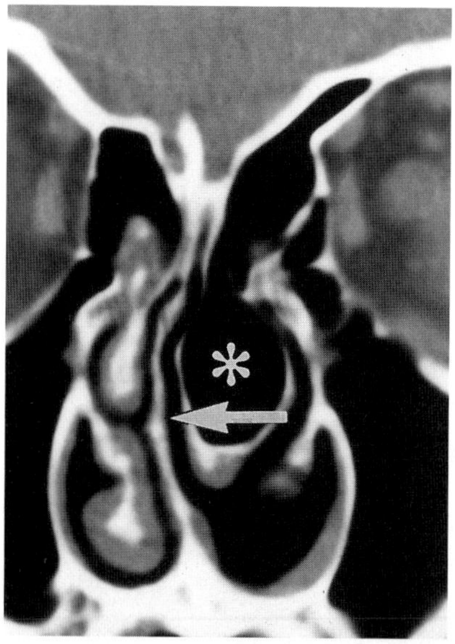

Figure 6-32A: Concha bullosa and contralateral nasal septal deviation. Coronal CT image showing a concha bullosa (*asterisk*), involving the middle turbinate, associated contralateral nasal septal deviation (*arrow*), hypoplasia/atrophy of the left inferior turbinate, and enlargement of the nasal passageways on the left side.

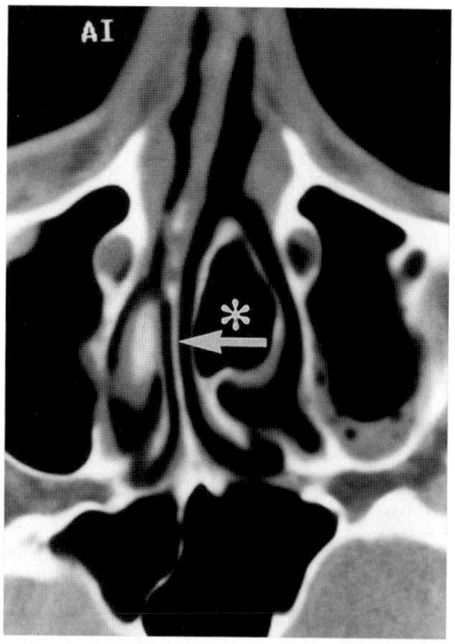

Figure 6-32B: Axial CT image in the same case as that in Figure 6-32A, again showing the concha bullosa (*asterisk*) and associated nasal septal deviation (*arrow*).

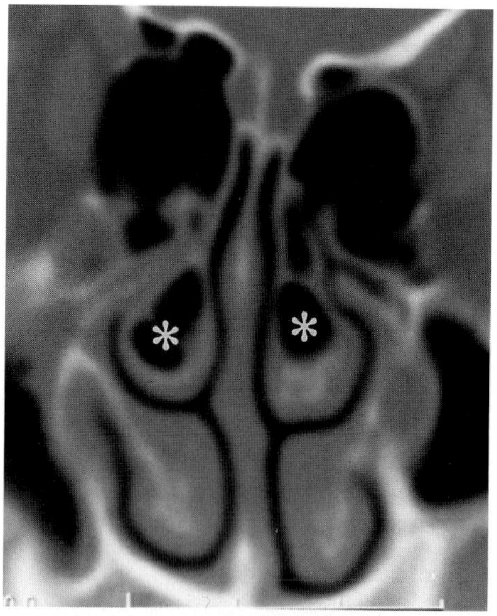

Figure 6-32C: Bilateral concha bullosae with balanced nasal septum. Coronal CT image showing bilateral conchae bullosae involving the middle nasal turbinates and a relatively balanced (midline) nasal septum (*asterisks*).

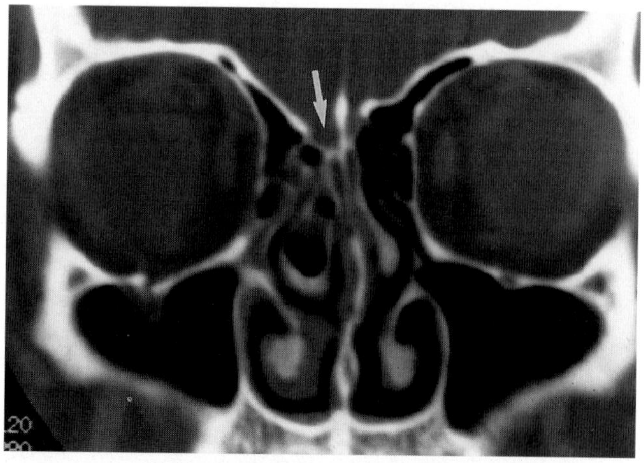

Figure 6-33: Asymmetric cribriform plate. Coronal CT image showing a broader and deeper cribriform plate (*arrow*) on the right side and lesser aeration of the right-sided ethmoid air cells. Also note the middle turbinate conchae bullosa on the right side and septal deviation toward the left side.

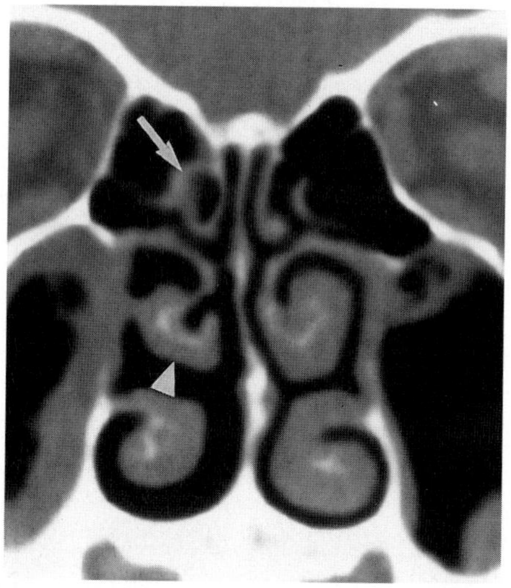

Figure 6-34: Concha bullosa involving a superior turbinate. Coronal CT showing a concha bullosa (*arrow*) involving the superior turbinate on the right side. A paradoxical (reverse) curve is also seen to involve the right middle turbinate (*arrowhead*).

CHAPTER 7

The Spine

7A Spinal Column

OVERVIEW

1. The spinal column is composed of 5 subdivisions totaling 33 individual segments. These include 3 unfused subdivisions: cervical (7 segments), thoracic (12 segments), and lumbar (5 segments); and 2 partially or completely fused subdivisions: the sacrum (5 segments) and coccyx (4 segments).
2. While the overall total number of vertebrae remains more or less constant, the numbers of vertebrae designated to each subdivision may alter slightly. These designations are somewhat artificial and are often based on whether or not the vertebra is rib bearing (e.g., thoracic subdivision), or whether or not the vertebra is fused to the adjacent fused segment, e.g., "sacralized" L-5 vertebra (fused) or "lumbarized" S-1 vertebra (unfused). Counting downward from C-1 and taking into account segmental anomalies (e.g., C-7 cervical ribs, absence of ribs on T-12, rudimentary ribs on L1-2, "sacralization" of L-5 or "lumbarization" of S-1) correctly attributed to the numbered vertebral segment is the most accurate method of vertebral enumeration.
3. Each unfused vertebra is composed of an anterior vertebral body and a posterior bony "neural" arch.
4. The posterior bony neural arch is formed by two pedicles and two laminae.
5. The laminae have seven processes: four articular (two pair: superior and inferior), two transverse, and one spinous.
6. Below C-2, the unfused vertebrae are joined by the intervertebral disc, the posterior spinal facet (zygapophyseal) joints, and various spinal ligaments.

SPECIAL FEATURES OF THE C-1 AND C-2 VERTEBRAE

C-1 Vertebra (Atlas)

1. The atlas, C-1, articulates with the occipital condyles of the skull superiorly and the lateral masses of C-2 inferiorly.
2. C-1 lacks a true body and therefore is ring-like, consisting of an anterior and posterior bony arch and two lateral masses.
3. The posterior border of the anterior arch of C-1 has an articulation surface for the anterior aspect of the odontoid process of C-2.
4. The transverse processes of C-1 are perforated by the foramina transversaria which transmit the vertebral arteries, veins, and nerves.
5. The paired superior laminar grooves are sometimes completely encircled by bone, thereby forming true bony foramina (arcuate foramina: approximately 14% incidence). When incomplete, the margins of this groove may give rise to bony partially bridging spurs. The grooves transmit the vertebral artery and the first cervical spinal nerve (C-1) on each side.
6. The longus colli muscles attach to the anterior tubercle of C-1.
7. The rectus capitus minor muscles attach to the posterior tubercle of C-1.
8. Many cases show unnamed paired tubercles off of the medial surface of the lateral masses of C-2 for the insertion of the transverse atlantal ligament. These might be termed the *transverse atlantal tubercles* (Jinkins).
9. There frequently is an unnamed vascular foramen on the medial surface of the lateral mass posterosuperior to the transverse atlantal tubercle. This foramen might be termed the *paratubercular vascular foramen of C-1* (Jinkins).

C-2 Vertebra (Axis)

1. The most distinctive feature of the C-2 vertebra, or axis, is the vertically directed odontoid process or dens (i.e., "tooth-like").
2. The odontoid process has two synovial articular surfaces: one directed anteriorly with

the posterior surface of the anterior arch of C-1, and the other posteriorly directed with the transverse atlantal ligament.

3. The transverse processes of C-2 are perforated by the foramina transversaria which transmit the vertebral arteries, veins, and nerves.
4. There often is an unnamed vascular (nutrient) foramen/channel on one or both sides of the odontoid process entering the superior surface of the body of C-2. This foramen might be termed the *paraodontal vascular foramen channel of C-2* (Jinkins).

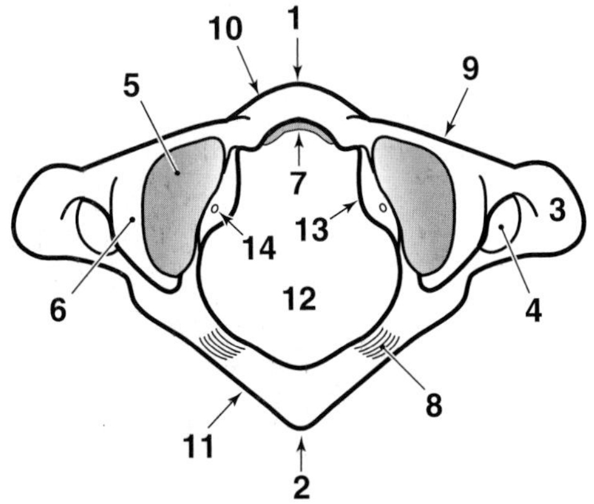

Figure 7A-1: Superior schematic of the C-1 vertebra (atlas).
1 Anterior tubercle (longus colli and anterior longitudinal ligament insertion)
2 Posterior tubercle (rectus capitus minor insertion)
3 Transverse process
4 Foramen transversarium for vertebral artery/veins
5 Superior articular surface for articulation with occipital condyle (atlantooccipital joint)
6 Lateral mass on the right
7 Articular surface for odontoid process of C-2
8 Superior groove for vertebral artery and C-1 spinal nerve (when a complete bony foramen is present it is termed *arcurate foramen*)
9 Lateral mass on the left
10 Anterior bony arch
11 Posterior bony neural arch (lamina)
12 Central spinal canal
13 Transverse atlantal tubercle (point of transverse atlantal ligament insertion)
14 Paratubercular vascular foramen of C-1

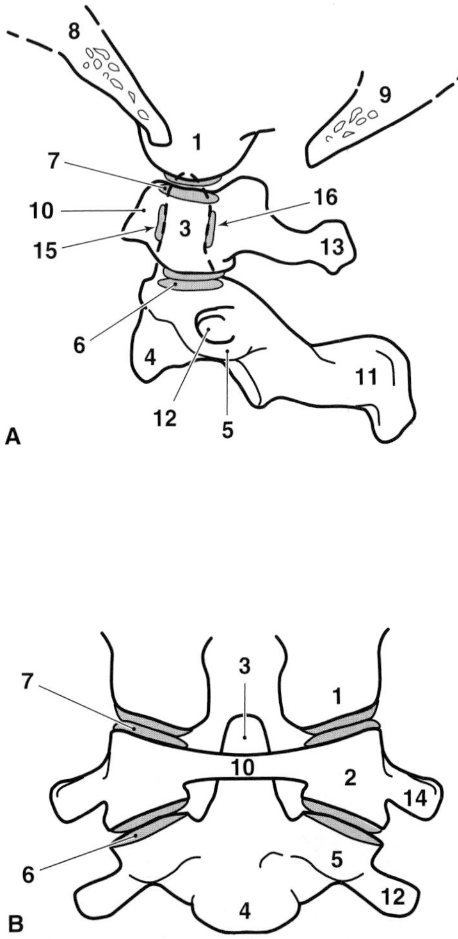

Figure 7A-2: Schematics of the articulations between the C-1 vertebra (atlas) and the C-2 vertebra (axis). **A:** Lateral schematic. **B:** Frontal schematic.
1 Occipital condyle
2 Lateral mass of C-1
3 Odontoid process (dens)
4 Body of C-2
5 Lateral mass of C-2
6 Atlantoaxial joint
7 Atlantooccipital joint
8 Clivus
9 Occipital bone
10 Anterior bony arch of C-1
11 Spinous process of C-2
12 Transverse process of C-2
13 Posterior bony arch of C-1
14 Transverse process of C-1
15 Articulation between the odontoid process and the anterior arch of C-1 (median anterior odontoarcal joint)
16 Articulation between the odontoid process and the transverse atlantal ligament (median posterior odontoatlantal joint)

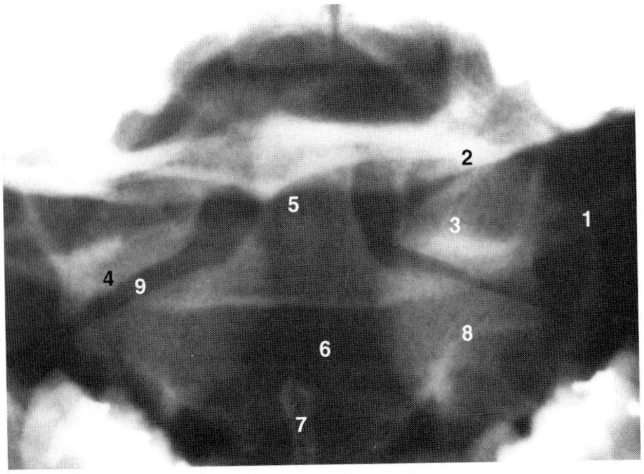

Figure 7A-3A: The craniocervical junction, C-1 and C-2. Conventional radiograph in the "open-mouth" frontal projection showing the atlas (C-1) and the axis (C-2).
1 Transverse process of C-1
2 Atlantooccipital joint
3 Lateral mass of C-1
4 Inferior articular process of C-1
5 Odontoid process of C-2
6 Body of C-2
7 Spinous process of C-2
8 Superior articular process of C-2
9 Atlantoaxial joint (C1-2)

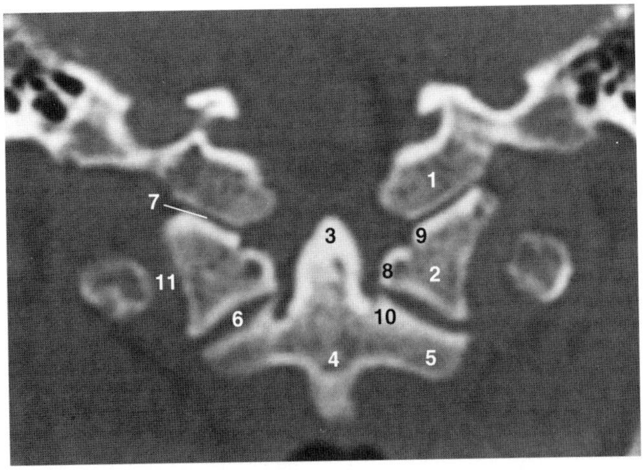

Figure 7A-3B: Coronal CT image showing the normal appearance of craniocervical junction.
1 Occipital condyle
2 Lateral mass of C-1 (atlas)
3 Odontoid process (dens)
4 Body of C-2 (axis)
5 Lateral mass of C-2 (axis)
6 Atlantoaxial joint (C1-2)
7 Atlantooccipital joint
8 Transverse atlantal tubercle on left side
9 Paratubercular vascular foramen of C-1
10 Paraodontal vascular foramen of C-2
11 Foramen transversarium of C-1 on right side

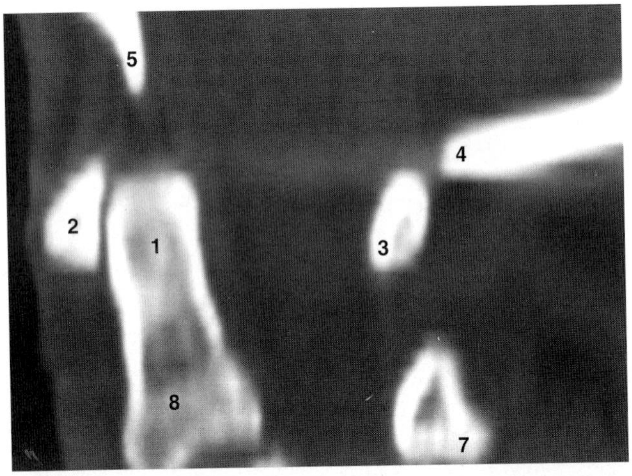

Figure 7A-3C: Craniovertebral junction. Midline sagital CT reconstruction showing the craniovertebral junction.
1 Odontoid process
2 Anterior arch of C-1
3 Posterior arch of C-1
4 Opisthion arch of C-1
5 Basion
6 Foramen magnum
7 Posterior arch of C-2
8 Body of C-2

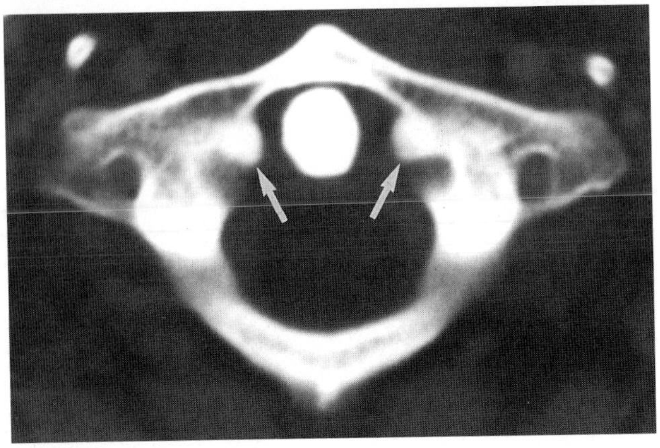

Figure 7A-4: The transverse atlantal tubercles. Axial CT image showing the transverse atlantal tubercles (*arrows*) for insertion of the transverse atlantal ligament.

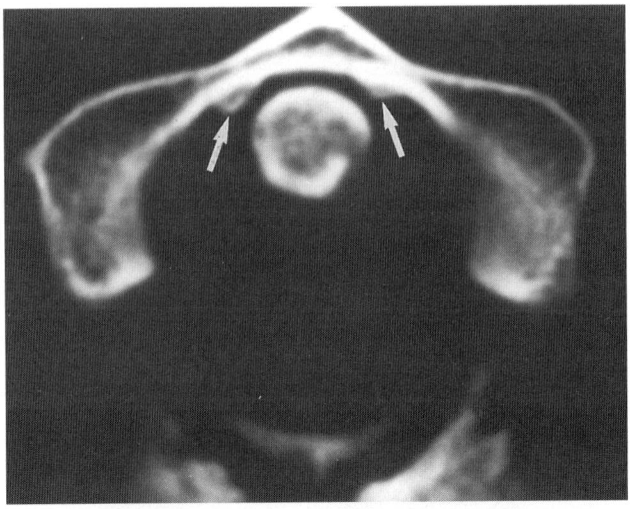

Figure 7A-5: Median anterior odontoarcal joint tubercles. Axial CT in a young patient showing the anterior atlantodental joint tubercles (*arrows,* Jinkins) on both sides.

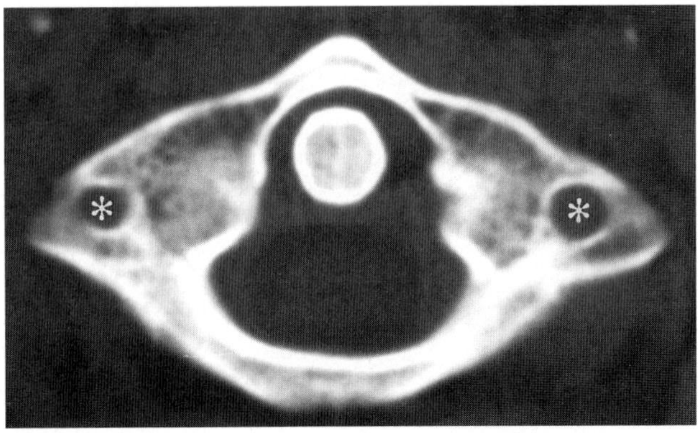

Figure 7A-6: The foramina transversaria of C-1. Axial CT image showing the foramina transversaria bilaterally (*asterisks*). Note the asymmetric foraminal calibre.

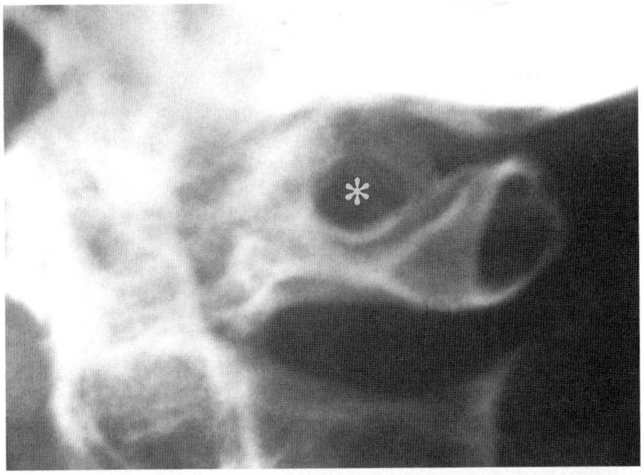

Figure 7A-7A: The arcuate foramen of C-1. Conventional radiograph in the lateral projection showing the arcuate foramen at C-1 transmitting the vertebral artery (*asterisk*), the C-1 spinal nerve, and the vertebral veins on each side.

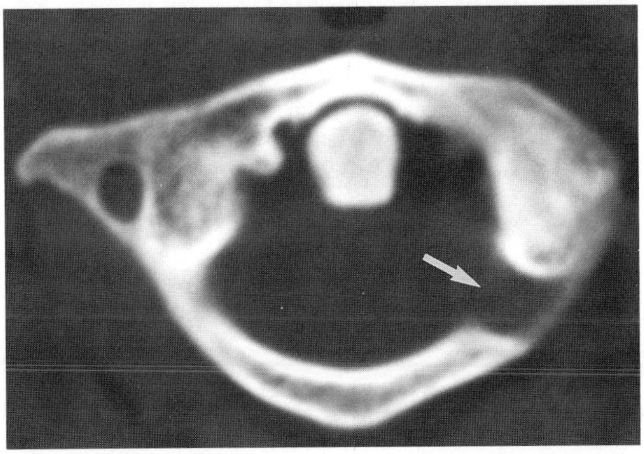

Figure 7A-7B: Asymmetric arcuate grooves/foramen(ina). Axial CT image showing a unilateral arcuate groove/foramen (*arrow*) for the vertebral artery, C-1 spinal nerve, and vertebral veins on the left.

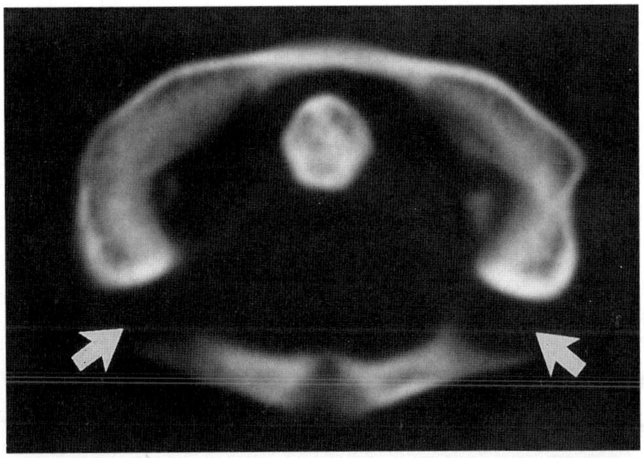

Figure 7A-7C: Axial CT image in a different patient showing bilateral vertebral artery arcuate grooves/foramina (*arrows*). Note also the spina bifida occulta involving the posterior bony neural arch of C-1.

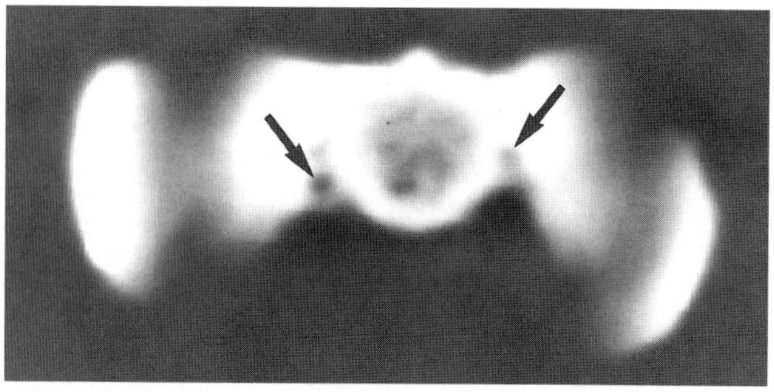

Figure 7A-8A: Paraodontal vascular foramina channel(s) of C-2. Axial CT image showing paraodontal vascular nutrient channels bilaterally (*arrows*) extending into the body of C-2.

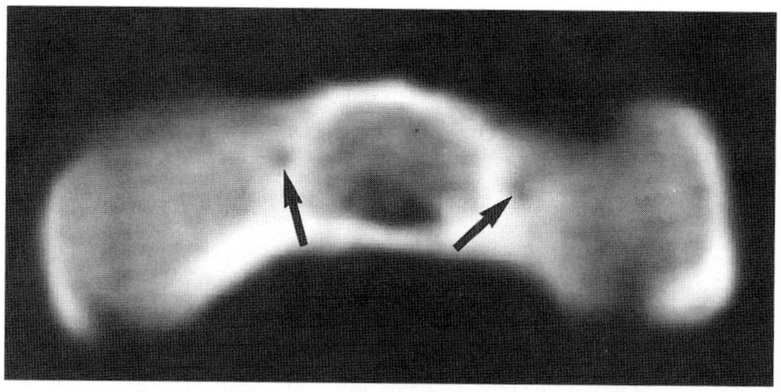

Figure 7A-8B: Axial CT image again showing the paraodontal vascular channels (*arrows*) of C-2.

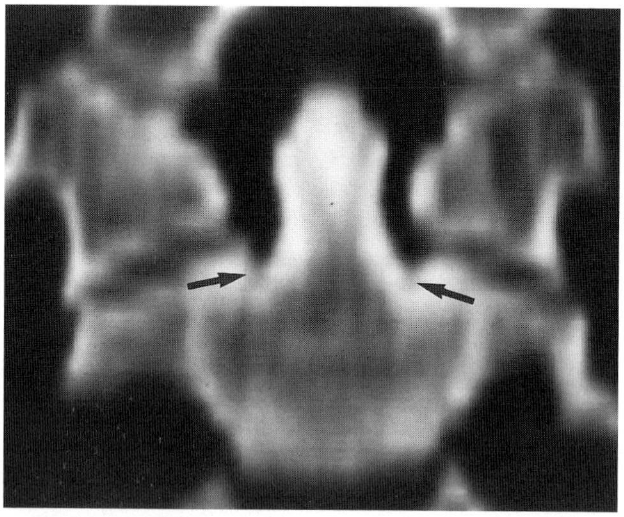

Figure 7A-8C: Reformatted CT image in the coronal plane showing the proximal extent of the paradontal vascular channels of C-2 bilaterally (*arrows*).

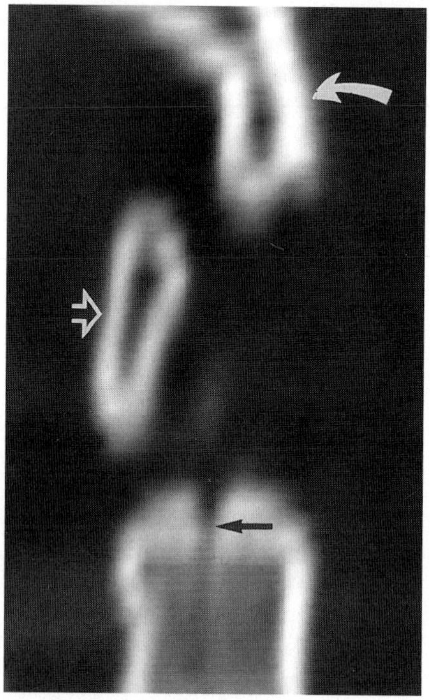

Figure 7A-8D: Reformatted sagittal CT image showing the paradontal vascular channel (*straight solid arrow*) within the lateral mass of C-2 on the right side. Anterior is to the reader's left. Also note the anterior arch of C-1 (*open arrow*) and the clivus (*curved arrow*).

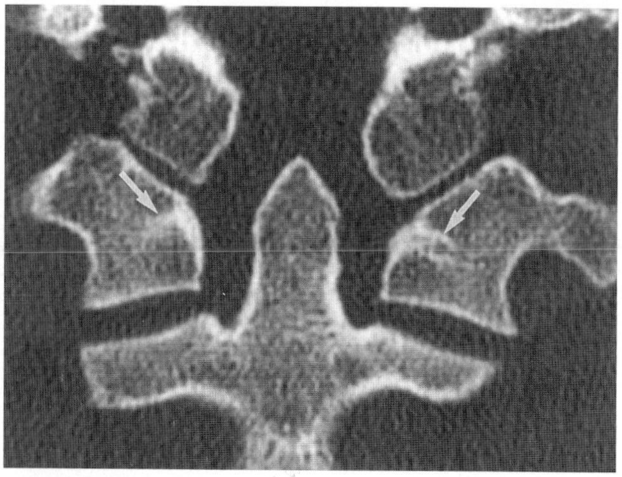

Figure 7A-9: The paratubercular vascular nutrient channels. Coronal CT image showing sclerosis surrounding paratubercular vascular channels (*arrows*) in the lateral masses of C-1 bilaterally.

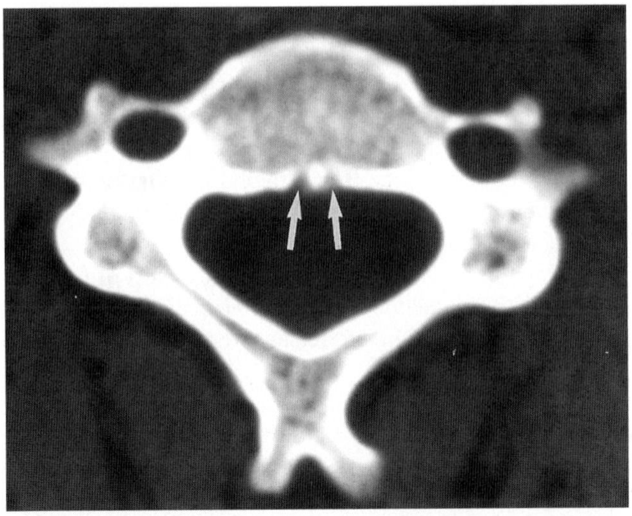

Figure 7A-10A: Cervical basivertebral venous channels. Axial CT image showing the nutrient foramen(ina) in the cervical spine in the region of the basivertebral vein (*arrows*).

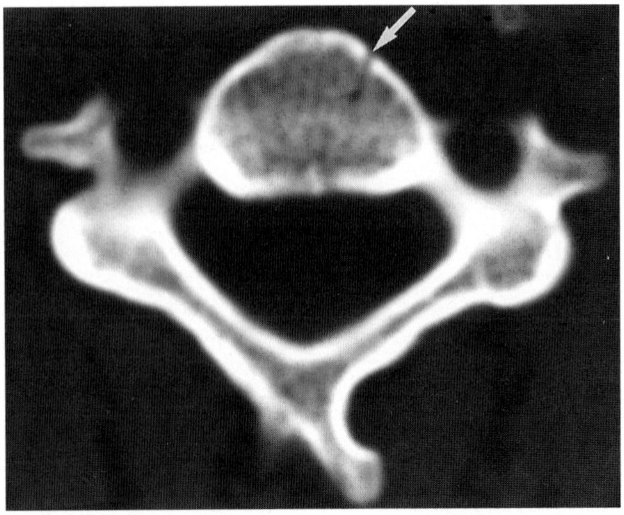

Figure 7A-10B: Axial CT image showing an anterior vertebral body nutrient canal (*arrow*).

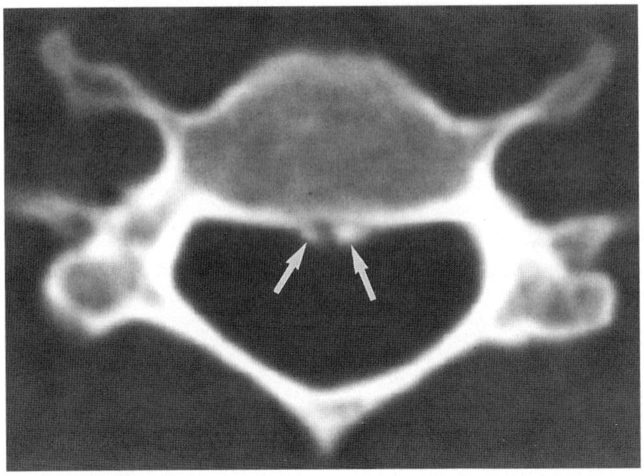

Figure 7A-10C: Basivertebral vascular foramen operculum. Axial CT image showing a typical bony cap on the basivertebral vein foramen (*arrows*) in the midcervical spine, the basivertebral vascular foramen operculum.

OTHER SPECIAL FEATURES OF THE CERVICAL SPINE

1. The cervical vertebrae are the smallest unfused segments of the vertebral column. All may contain foramina transversaria varying in size from individual to individual; the vertebral arteries only traverse these foramina from the C-1 through the C-4, C-5, C-6, or C-7 (most common lowest level: C-6) vertebrae. The vertebral veins and nerves may also pass through the foramina transversaria. Not infrequently partial or complete accessory foramina transversaria accompany the main foramina.
2. The uncinate processes, projecting lips extending from the lateral aspect of the superior surface of the vertebral bodies, are unique to the cervical spine. These processes in part restrict lateral gliding motion. They are often referred to as the uncovertebral joints or joints of Luschka.
3. The spinous processes of the middle and upper cervical vertebrae are frequently bifid.
4. The spinal canal in the cervical region tends to be oval in shape in the axial plane.
5. The basivertebral vascular foramina enter the posterior surface of the vertebral bodies in the midline, roughly midway between the top and bottom of the corpus. These foramina transmit the basivertebral veins and arteries. These vascular foraminal channels are often paired. In the cervical spine, these foramina may be partially covered by a cap of bone joined to the posterior surface of the vertebral body. This bony cap might be termed the *basivertebral vascular foramen operculum* (Jinkins).
6. The normal sagittal curvature of the cervical spine is lordotic.

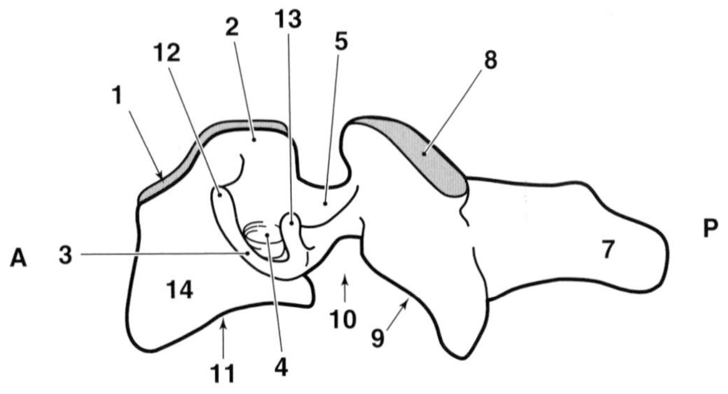

A

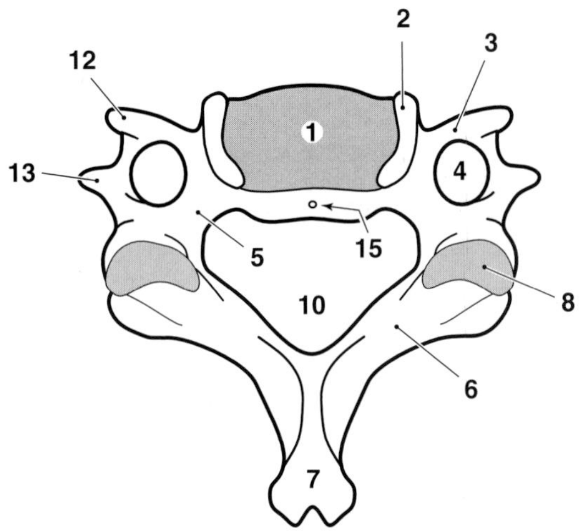

B

Figure 7A-11: Schematics of a midcervical vertebra. **A:** Lateral schematic. **B:** Superior schematic. *A*, anterior; *P*, posterior.

1 Superior vertebral end plate
2 Uncinate process
3 Transverse process
4 Foramen transversarium
5 Pedicle
6 Lamina
7 Spinous process (partially bifid)
8 Superior posterior articular facet joint surface
9 Inferior posterior articular facet joint surface
10 Central spinal canal
11 Inferior vertebral end plate
12 Anterior tubercle of transverse process
13 Posterior tubercle of transverse process
14 Vertebral body
15 Basivertebral vascular foramen

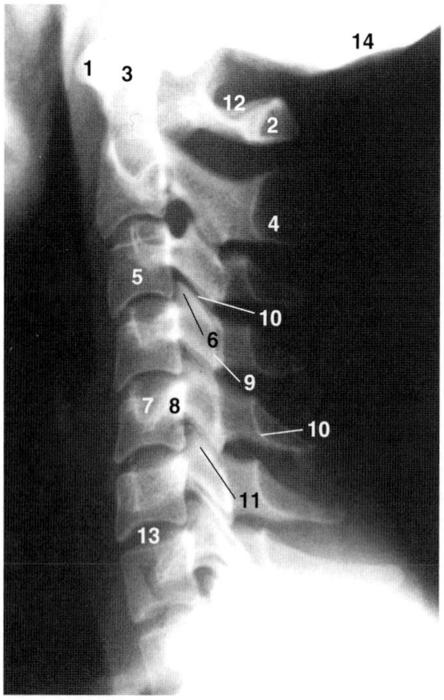

Figure 7A-12A: Conventional radiographic anatomy of cervical spine. Conventional radiograph in the lateral projection showing the normal anatomy of the cervical spine.

1 Anterior arch of C-1
2 Spinous process of C-1
3 Odontoid process (dens) of C-2
4 Spinous process of C-2
5 Vertebral body (C-3)
6 Superior articular process of posterior spinal facet (zygapophyseal) joint
7 Anterior tubercle of transverse process overlying vertebral body
8 Posterior tubercle of transverse process
9 Inferior articular process of posterior spinal facet (zygapophyseal) joint
10 Spinous process of C-5
11 Posterior spinal facet (zygapophyseal) joint
12 Groove(s) in posterior bony arch of C-1 for the vertebral artery(ies)
13 Intervertebral disc space
14 Occipital bone

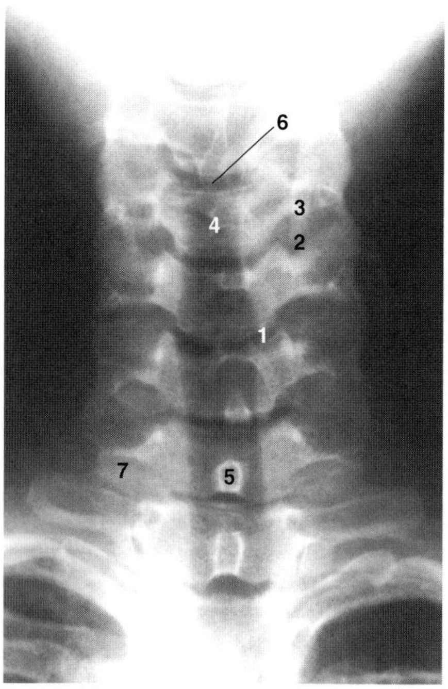

Figure 7A-12B: Conventional radiograph in the anteroposterior projection showing the normal anatomy of the cervical spine.

1 Uncovertebral joint
2 Inferior articular process (posterior spinal facet joint)
3 Superior articular process (posterior spinal facet joint)
4 Vertebral body
5 Spinous process
6 Intervertebral disc space
7 Transverse process

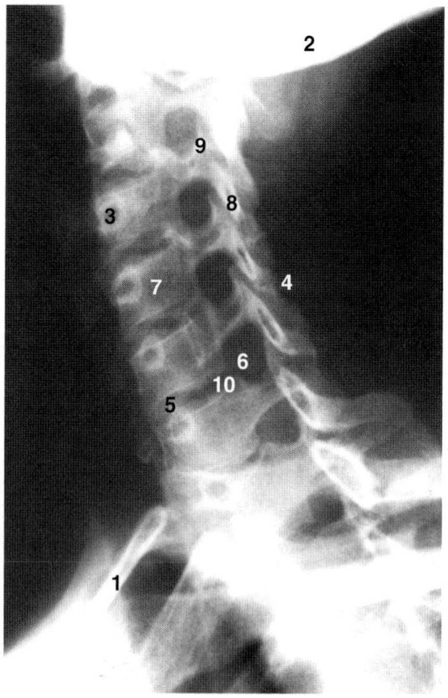

Figure 7A-12C: Conventional radiograph in the oblique projection showing the normal anatomy of the cervical spine.

1 First rib
2 Occipital bone
3 Transverse process
4 Spinous process
5 Intervertebral disc space
6 Intervertebral neural foramen
7 Vertebral body
8 Inferior articular process
9 Superior articular process
10 Uncovertebral joint

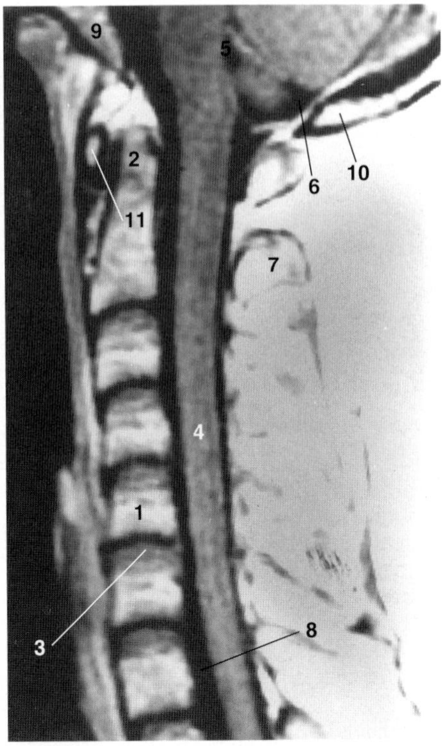

Figure 7A-13A: Magnetic resonance anatomy of the cervical spine. Sagittal T1-weighted MR image showing the normal anatomy of the cervical spine.

1 Vertebral body
2 Odontoid process (dens)
3 Intervertebral disc
4 Spinal cord
5 Medulla oblongata
6 Cisterna magna
7 Spinous process
8 Spinal subarachnoid space
9 Clivus
10 Occipital bone
11 Anterior arch of C-1

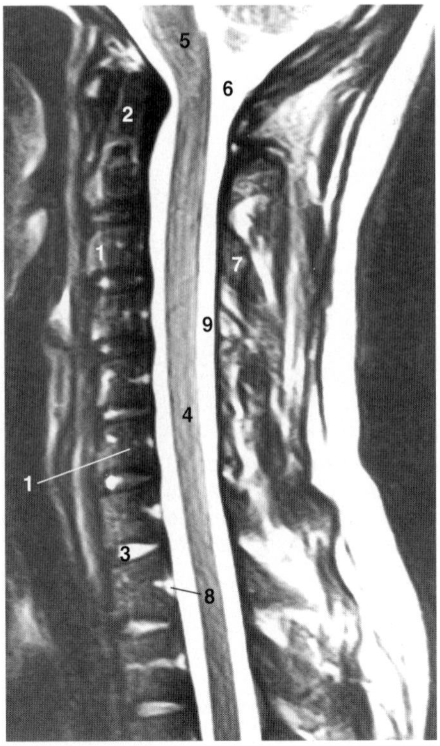

Figure 7A-13B: Sagittal T2-weighted MR image again showing the normal anatomy of the cervical spine.

1 Vertebral body
2 Odontoid process (dens)
3 Intervertebral disc
4 Cervical spinal cord
5 Medulla oblongata
6 Cisterna magna
7 Spinous process
8 Basivertebral vein (posterior aspect)
9 Spinal subarachnoid space

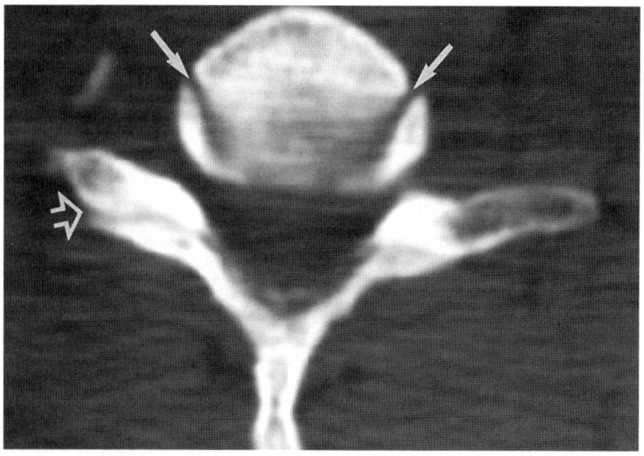

Figure 7A-14A: The uncovertebral joints and mid-cervical articulations. Axial CT image showing the uncovertebral joints (joints of Luschka) in the midcervical spine (*solid arrows*) as well as the posterior spinal facet (zygapophyseal) joints (*open arrow*).

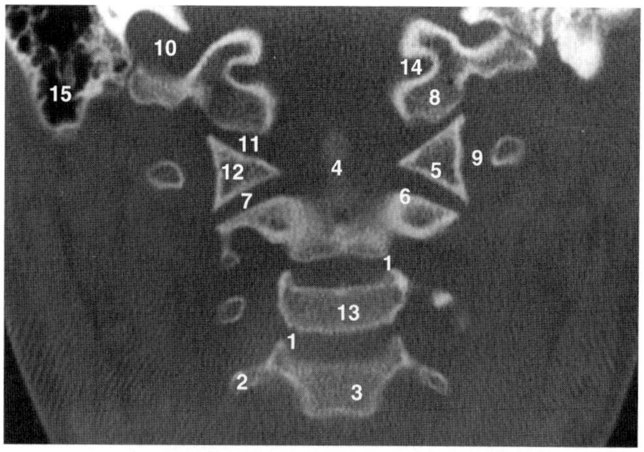

Figure 7A-14B: The upper cervical vertebrae and craniovertebral junction. Coronal CT image showing the upper cervical vertebrae, and craniovertebral junction.

1 Uncovertebral joints
2 Transverse process of C-4 vertebra
3 C-4 vertebral body
4 Odontoid process (dens) of C-2
5 Inferior articular surface of lateral mass of C-1 on left side
6 Superior articular surface of lateral mass of C-2 on left side
7 Atlantoaxial joint on right side
8 Occipital condyle on right side
9 Foramen transversarium of C-1 on left side
10 Jugular foramen (sigmoid venous sinus bony canal) on right side
11 Atlantooccipital joint on right side
12 Lateral mass of C-1 on right side
13 C-3 vertebral body
14 Hypoglossal canal (CN XII)
15 Mastoid process on right side

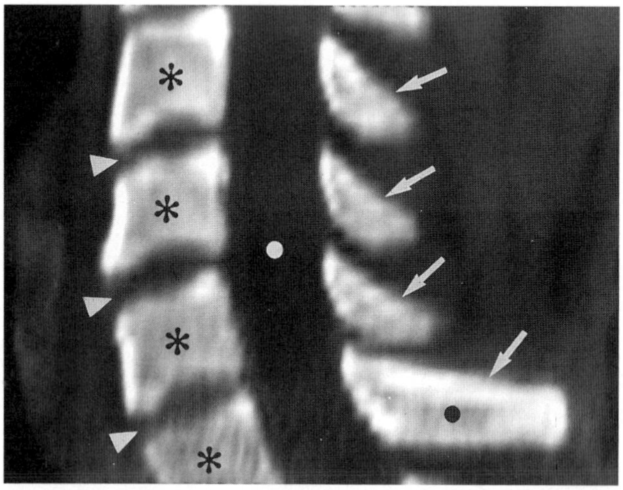

Figure 7A-14C: The lower cervical spine (C-4 to C-7). Midline sagittal CT reconstruction showing the spinous processes (*arrows*), the vertebral bodies (*asterisks*), and the intervetebral discs (*arrowheads*). Note the typically elongated C-7 spinous process (*black dot*), and the central spinal canal (*white dot*).

SPECIAL FEATURES OF THE THORACIC SPINE

1. The thoracic vertebrae increase in size in a craniocaudal direction.
2. The superoinferior dimension of the thoracic vertebral bodies is smaller anteriorly than posteriorly (i.e., normal anterior wedge shape).
3. The bodies of the thoracic vertebrae have a synovial joint surface that posterolaterally articulates with the heads of the ribs. These *costocorpal facet joints* may be shared with their neighbor (*costocorpal demifacet joint*: T-1 to T8-9) or they may be complete and not shared (*complete costocorpal facets*: T9-10 to T-12).
4. Some of the transverse processes of the thoracic vertebrae have one or more synovial joint surfaces for articulation with a tubercle of a rib (*costotransverse facet joint* (Jinkins)).
5. The normal sagittal curvature of the thoracic spine is kyphotic.

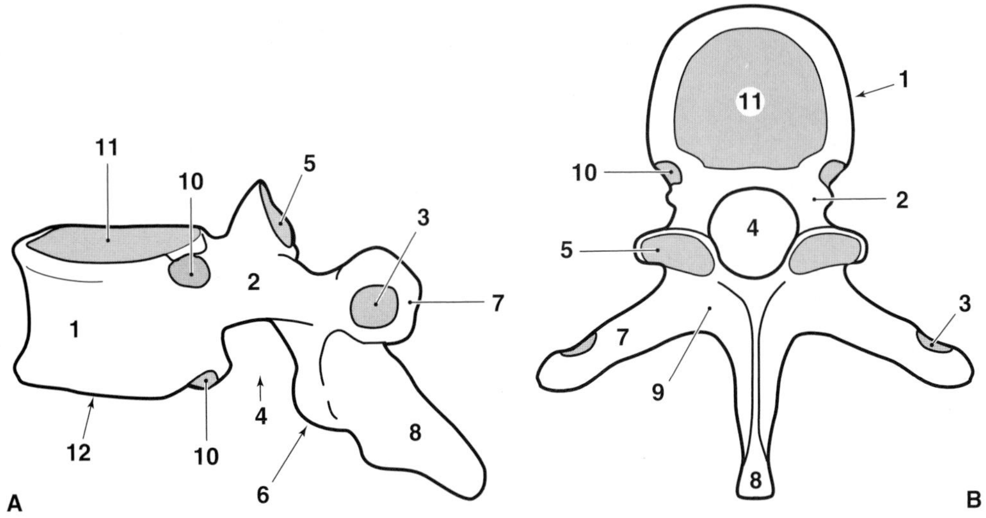

Figure 7A-15: Schematics of a thoracic vertebra. **A:** Lateral schematic. **B:** Superior schematic.

1 Vertebral body
2 Pedicle
3 Costotransverse facet joint surface on transverse process
4 Central spinal canal
5 Superior articular surface of posterior spinal facet (zygapophyseal) joint
6 Inferior articular surface of posterior spinal facet (zygapophyseal) joint
7 Transverse process
8 Spinous process
9 Lamina
10 Upper and lower costocorpal demifacet joint surfaces for articulation with head of rib (T-1 to T8-9)
11 Superior vertebral end plate
12 Inferior vertebral end plate

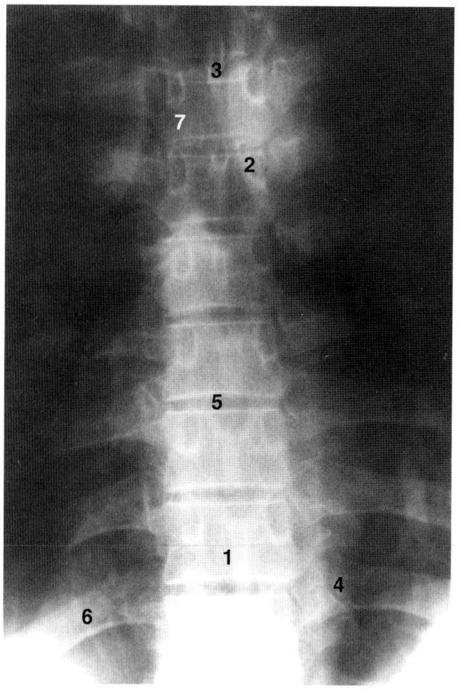

Figure 7A-16A: Conventional radiographic and CT anatomy of the thoracic spine. Conventional radiograph in the frontal projection showing the normal anatomy of the thoracic spine.
1 Vertebral body
2 Pedicle
3 Spinous process
4 Transverse process
5 Intervertebral disc space
6 Rib
7 Trachea

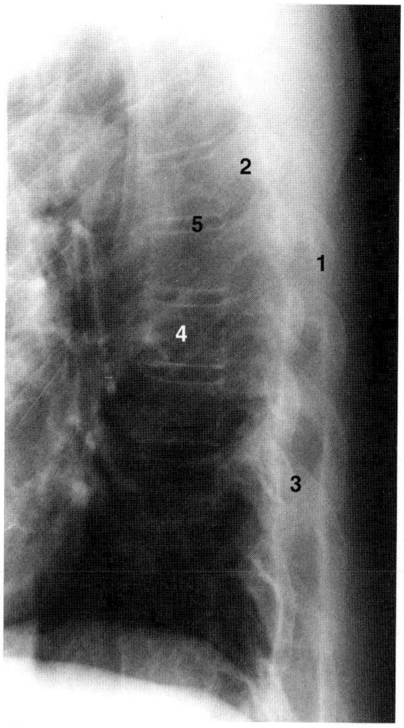

Figure 7A-16B: Conventional radiograph in the lateral projection showing the normal anatomy of the thoracic spine.
1 Rib
2 Pedicle
3 Spinous process
4 Vertebral body
5 Intervertebral disc space

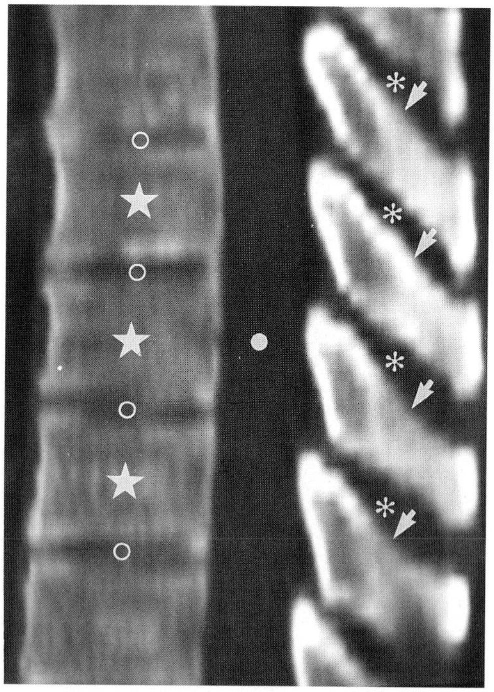

Figure 7A-16C: Midline sagittal CT reconstruction showing the spinous processes (*arrows*), the interspinous space (*asterisk*), the vertebral bodies (*stars*),the intervertebral discs (*circles*), and the central spinal canal (*dot*).

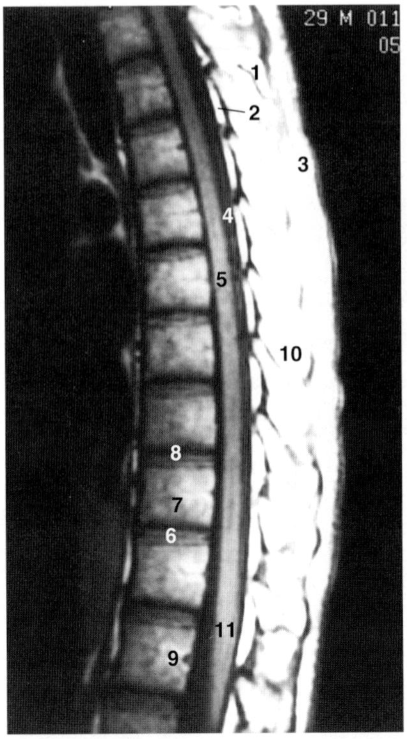

Figure 7A-17A: Magnetic resonance anatomy of thoracic spine. Sagittal T1-weighted MR image showing the normal anatomy of the thoracic spine.

1 Interspinous fat
2 Posterior epidural fat pad
3 Subcutaneous fat
4 Spinal subarachnoid space
5 Thoracic spinal cord
6 Intervertebral disc
7 Vertebral body
8 Inferior vertebral end plate (with superimposed chemical chemical shift artifact)
9 Basivertebral vein foramen/channel
10 Spinous process
11 Conus medullaris

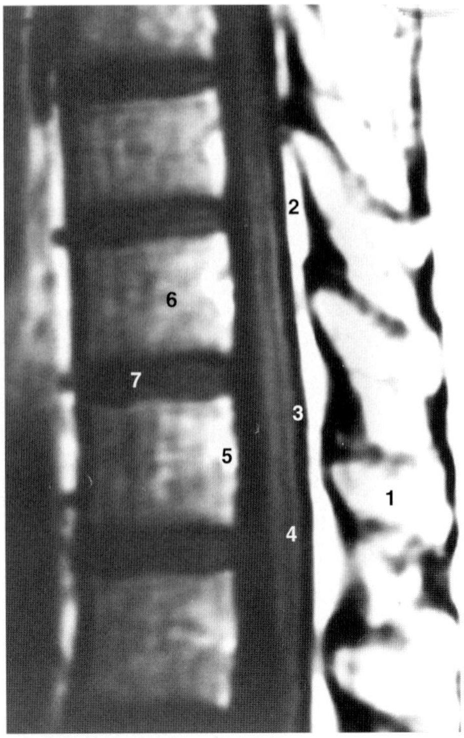

Figure 7A-17B: Magnified intravenous gadolinium-enhanced T1-weighted image showing the normal anatomy of the lower thoracic spine.

1 Spinous process
2 Posterior epidural fat pad
3 Spinal subarachnoid space
4 Conus medullaris
5 Enhancing basivertebral vein
6 Vertebral body
7 Intervertebral disk

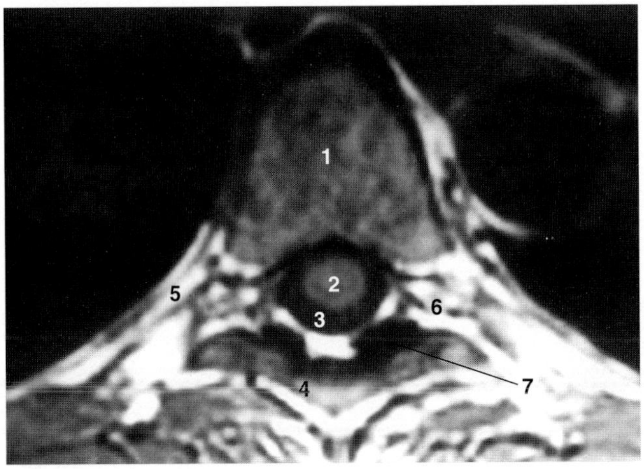

Figure 7A-17C: Axial T1-weighted MR image at T-5 showing normal anatomy at this thoracic level.

1 Vertebral body
2 Thoracic spinal cord
3 Spinal subarachnoid space
4 Lamina
5 Rib
6 Spinal neural foramen
7 Posterior spinal facet (zygapophyseal) joint

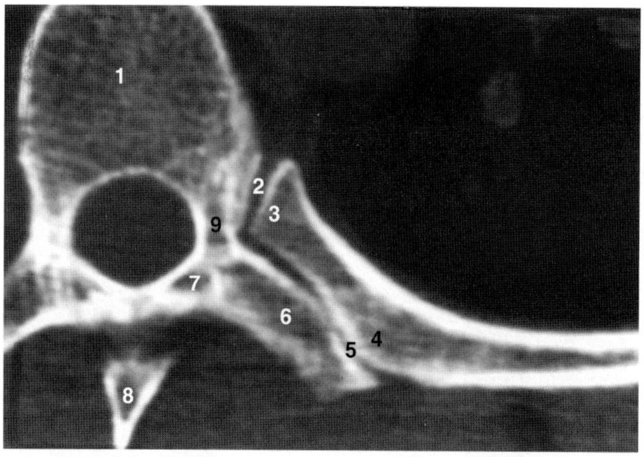

Figure 7A-18: Costal articulations with spinal column. Axial CT image showing the rib articulations in the midthoracic region.

1 Vertebral body
2 Costocorpal facet joint
3 Head of rib
4 Tubercle of rib
5 Costotransverse facet joint
6 Transverse process
7 Lamina
8 Spinous process
9 Pedicle

SPECIAL FEATURES OF THE LUMBAR SPINE

1. The lumbar vertebrae are the largest segments of the nonfused spinal column.
2. Generally, the superoinferior dimension of L-2 to L-5 is greater anteriorly than posteriorly (i.e., posterior wedge shape). The L2-3 through the L5-S1 intervertebral discs have a similar posterior wedge configuration. The L-1 vertebral body is shaped more like the thoracic vertebrae (i.e., anterior wedge shape). There is much individual variation among these findings.
3. The transverse processes in the lumbar spine are actually homologs of the ribs. The accessory process, a small tubercle projecting from the posterior surface of the transverse process medially, is actually the rudimentary true transverse process.
4. The structure of the fifth lumbar vertebra will alter depending on whether it is completely unfused or if it is partially fused to the sacrum (i.e., sacralized).
5. The L-5 spinous process is normally somewhat hypoplastic. The lumbar spinal canal tends to be oval to triangular in shape in the axial plane.
6. The normal sagittal curvature of the lumbar spine is lordotic.

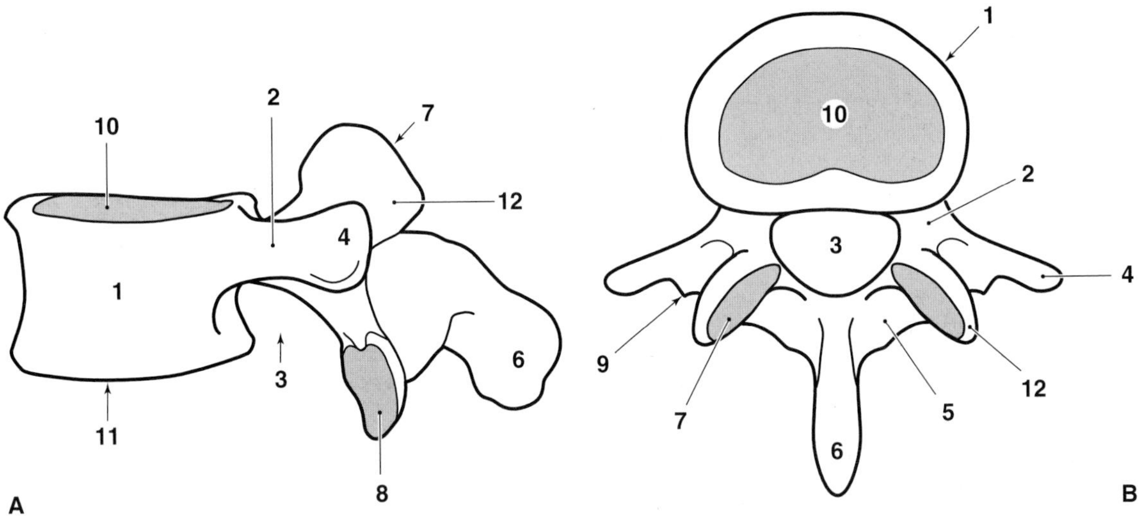

Figure 7A-19: Schematics of a lumbar vertebra. **A:** Lateral schematic. **B:** Superior schematic.
1 Vertebral body
2 Pedicle
3 Central spinal canal
4 Lumbar transverse process (homolog of rib)
5 Lamina
6 Spinous process
7 Superior-posterior spinal facet (zygapophyseal) joint surface
8 Inferior-posterior spinal facet (zygapophyseal) joint surface
9 Accessory process (rudimentary true transverse process)
10 Superior vertebral end plate
11 Inferior vertebral end plate
12 Mamillary process

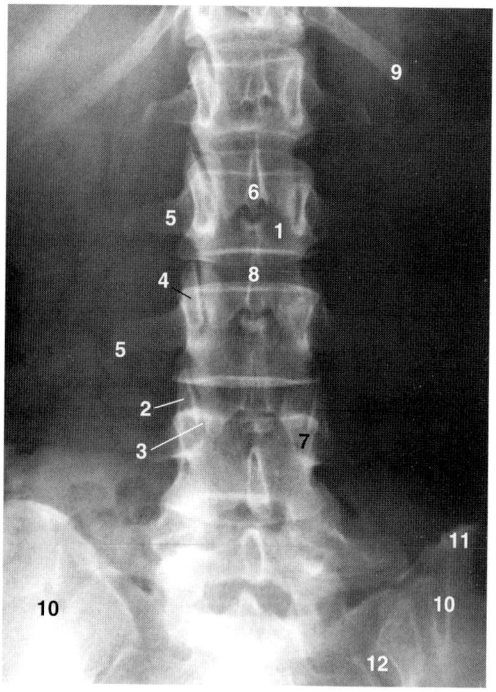

Figure 7A-20A: Conventional radiographic anatomy of the lumbar spine. Conventional radiograph in the anteroposterior projection showing the normal anatomy of the lumbar spine.

1 Vertebral body
2 Superior articular process of posterior spinal facet (zygapophyseal) joint
3 Inferior articular process of posterior spinal facet (zygapophyseal) joint
4 Posterior spinal facet joint
5 Transverse process
6 Spinous process
7 Pedicle
8 Intervertebral disc space
9 Twelfth rib
10 Iliac wing
11 Iliac crest
12 Sacroiliac joint

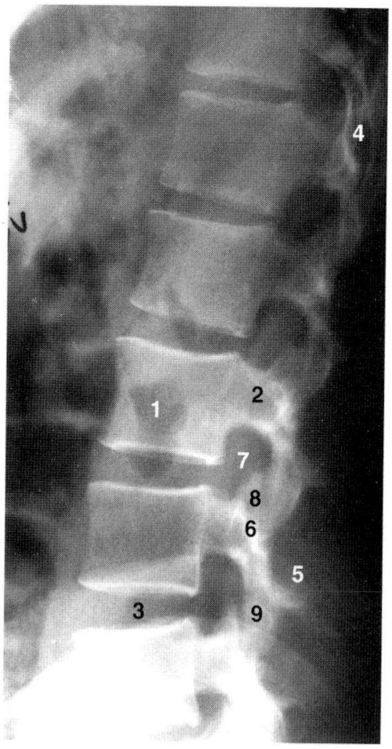

Figure 7A-20B: Conventional radiograph in the lateral projection showing the normal anatomy of the lumbar spine.

1 Vertebral body
2 Pedicle
3 Intervertebral disc space
4 Twelfth rib
5 Spinous process
6 Pars interarticularis
7 Intervertebral (neural) foramen
8 Superior articular process of posterior spinal facet (zygapophyseal) joint
9 Inferior articular process of posterior spinal facet (zygapophyseal) joint

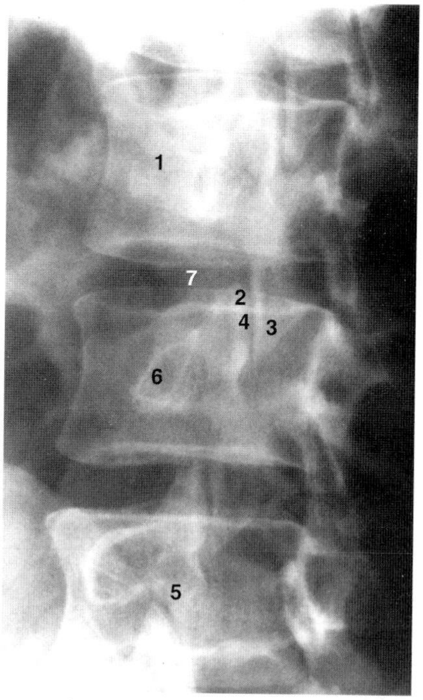

Figure 7A-20C: Conventional radiograph in the oblique projection showing the anatomy of the lumbar spine.

1 Pedicle
2 Superior articular process
3 Inferior articular process
4 Facet joint
5 Pars interarticularis
6 Transverse process
7 Intervertebral disc space

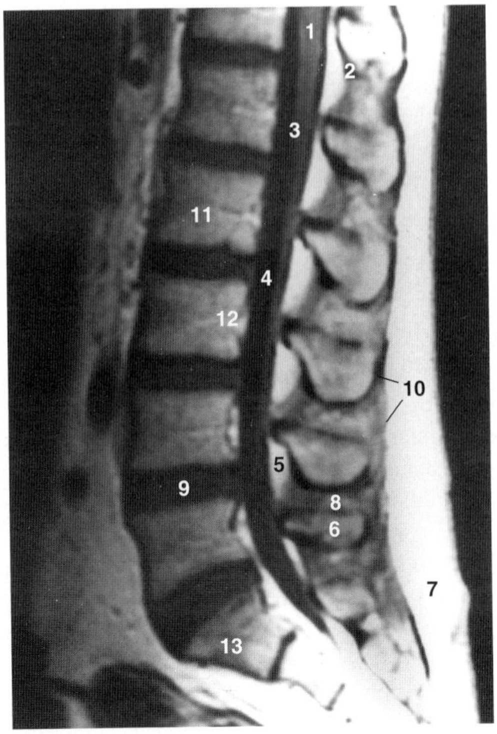

Figure 7A-21A: Magnetic resonance anatomy of the lumbar spine. Sagittal T1-weighted MR image showing the normal anatomy of the lumbar spine.

1 Distal thoracic spinal cord (conus medullaris)
2 Ligamentum flavum
3 Cauda equina
4 Spinal subarachnoid space
5 Retrothecal fat pad
6 Spinous process
7 Subcutaneous fat
8 Interspinous ligament
9 Intervertebral disc
10 Supraspinous ligament
11 Body of L-2 vertebra
12 Basivertebral venous channel
13 Body of S-1 vertebra

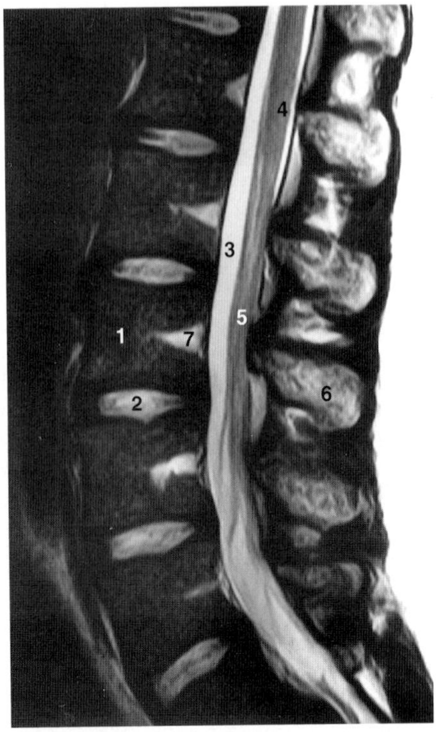

Figure 7A-21B: Sagittal T2-weighted MR image showing the normal anatomy of the lumbar spine.

1 Vertebral body
2 Intervertebral disc
3 Spinal subarachnoid space
4 Conus medullaris
5 Nerve roots of cauda equina
6 Spinous process
7 Basivertebral vein/channel

SPECIAL FEATURES OF THE SACRUM

1. The sacrum is composed of five partially or completely fused segments.
2. Laterally the sacrum articulates with the iliac bones to form the sacroiliac joints. The lateral sacral ala that articulate with the ilia are the fused transverse (anterior quarter) and costal (posterior three quarters) processes of the sacral vertebrae.
3. The fused sacral segments articulate with the fifth lumbar vertebra cranially and the coccygeal segments caudally.
4. At the junctions of the sacral vertebral segments there are four ventral sacral neural foramina. These foramina transmit the ventral divisions of the upper sacral spinal nerves (S-1 to S-4) and the lateral sacral arteries.
5. There are also four dorsal sacral neural foramina that transmit the dorsal divisions of the upper sacral spinal nerves (S-1 to S-4).
6. The rudimentary nonarticulating articular processes of the fifth sacral segment form the nonfused sacral cornua. They are connected by a ligamentous structure to the coccygeal cornua. This might be termed the *intercornual sacrococcygeal ligament* (Jinkins).
7. The laminae of the fifth sacral vertebral segment are not fused in the midline posteriorly, resulting in an aperture into the sacral spinal canal, the sacral hiatus. The fifth sacral spinal nerves (S-5) exit from the sacral hiatus and traverse laterally beneath the sacral cornua.
8. The middle or median sacral crests are formed by fusion of rudimentary sacral spinous processes.
9. The fused posterior articular facet processes form a series of posterior sacral tubercles that together constitute the intermediate sacral crests.
10. The fused rudimentary sacral transverse processes combine to form the lateral crests of the sacrum.
11. The sacral spinal canal tends to be triangular or oval in shape in the axial plane.
12. The normal sagittal shape of the sacrum is kyphotic.

SPECIAL FEATURES OF THE COCCYX

1. The coccyx typically consists of four fused or partially fused rudimentary vertebral segments; however, the total number of segments present may vary from three to five.
2. The upper surface of the first coccygeal segment articulates with the inferior surface of the fifth sacral segment. This sacrococcygeal articulation usually fuses with age.
3. The intercoccygeal joints are symphyses, consisting of discs of fibrocartilage. Occasionally there is a synovial joint between the first and second coccygeal segments. With age the intercoccygeal joints usually become fused.
4. There is no coccygeal central spinal canal. The pedicles, laminae, and spinous processes are absent.
5. The coccygeal segments diminish in size in a craniocaudal direction; the last segment is usually a simple rounded ossicle.
6. The rudimentary articular processes of the first coccygeal segment form the paired coccygeal cornua.
7. The fifth sacral spinal nerves exit below the sacral cornua and above the coccygeal cornua.
8. There may be a single coccygeal spinal nerve (Cx1) exiting on each side of the coccyx.
9. The normal sagittal curvature of the coccyx is a continuation of the kyphotic curve of the sacrum.

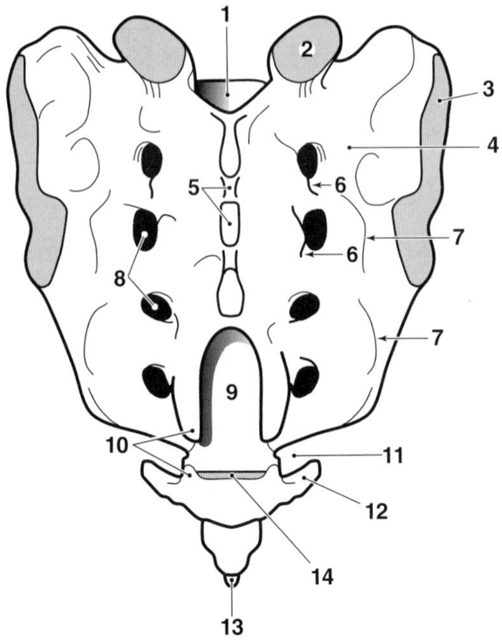

Figure 7A-22: Schematic of the dorsal (posterior) surface of the sacrum and coccyx.
1 Sacral central spinal canal
2 Superior articular (posterior) facet of S-1 articulating with L-5
3 Sacral auricular surface of sacroiliac joint
4 Sacral tuberosity
5 Median sacral crest
6 Intermediate sacral crest
7 Lateral sacral crest
8 Dorsal sacral neural foramina
9 Sacral hiatus
10 Cornua of sacrum and coccyx
11 Sacrococcygeal notch
12 Transverse process of coccyx
13 Apex of coccyx

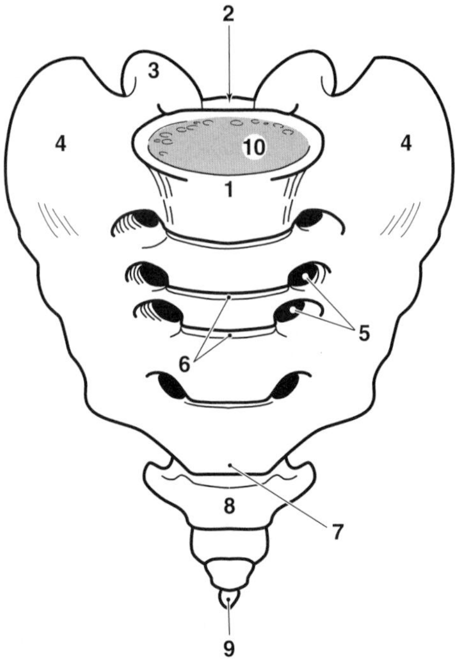

Figure 7A-23: Schematic of the ventral (anterior) surface of the sacrum and coccyx.
1 Sacral promontory
2 Sacral central spinal canal
3 S-1 articular posteriorspinal facet process
4 Sacral ala
5 Ventral sacral neural foramina
6 Rudimentary sacral intervertebral discs
7 Apex of sacrum
8 Base of coccyx
9 Apex of coccyx
10 Superior vertebral end plate of S-1 vertebral body

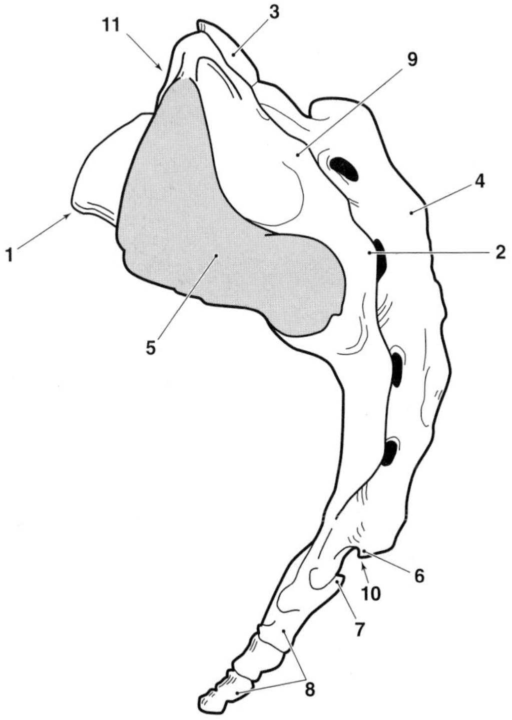

Figure 7A-24: Lateral schematic of the sacrum and coccyx.
1 Sacral promontory
2 Intermediate sacral crest
3 S-1 articular process
4 Median sacral crest
5 Sacral articular surface of sacroiliac joint
6 Cornu of sacrum
7 Cornu of coccyx
8 Coccyx
9 Sacral tuberosity
10 Sacral hiatus
11 Sacral central spinal canal

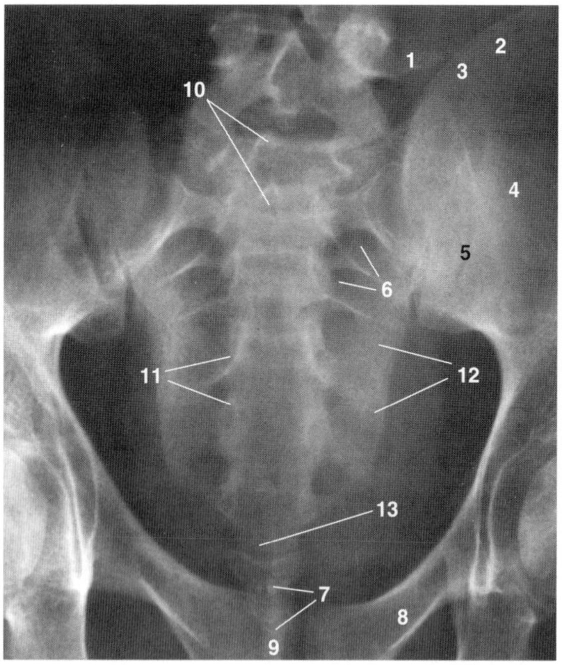

Figure 7A-25A: Conventional radiographic anatomy of the sacrum and coccyx. Conventional radiograph in the anteroposterior projection showing the normal anatomy of the sacrum and coccyx.

1 Transverse process, L-5
2 Iliac crest
3 Iliac wing
4 Ala of sacrum
5 Sacroiliac joint
6 Sacral foramina
7 Coccyx
8 Ramus of pubis
9 Symphysis pubis
10 Median sacral crest and spinous tubercles
11 Intermediate sacral crest and articular tubercles
12 Lateral sacral crest and transverse tubercles
13 Sacrococcygeal junction

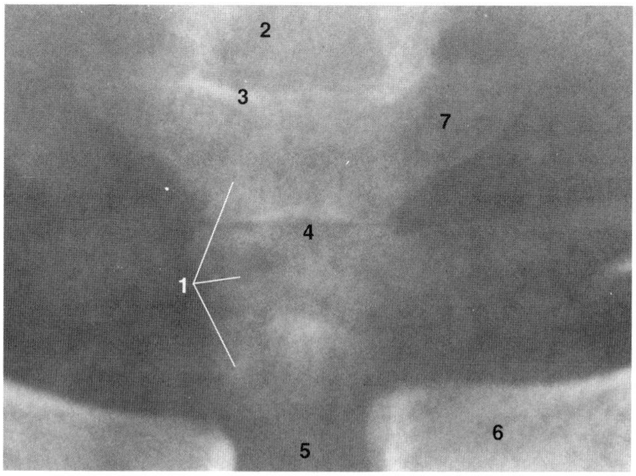

Figure 7A-25B: Conventional radiograph in the frontal projection showing the normal anatomy of the coccyx.

1 Coccyx
2 Terminal sacrum
3 Fused sacrococcygeal junction
4 Unfused coccygeal segments
5 Symphysis pubis
6 Superior ramus of pubis
7 Cornu of first coccygeal segment on the left side

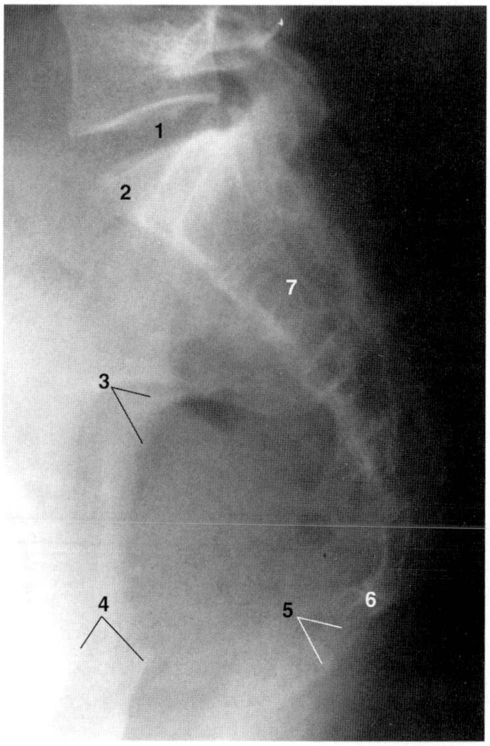

Figure 7A-25C: Conventional radiograph in the lateral projection showing the normal anatomy of the sacrum and coccyx.

1 Intervertebral disc space at L-5 to S-1
2 Sacral promontory
3 Greater sciatic notches
4 Ischial spines
5 Coccyx
6 Sacrococcygeal junction
7 Sacral canal

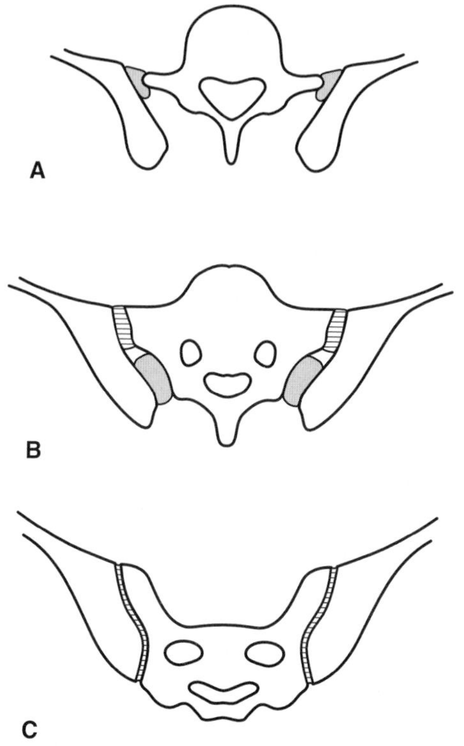

Figure 7A-26: Schematics showing the normal anatomy of the sacroiliac joint at the upper **(A)**, middle **(B)**, and lower **(C)** levels.

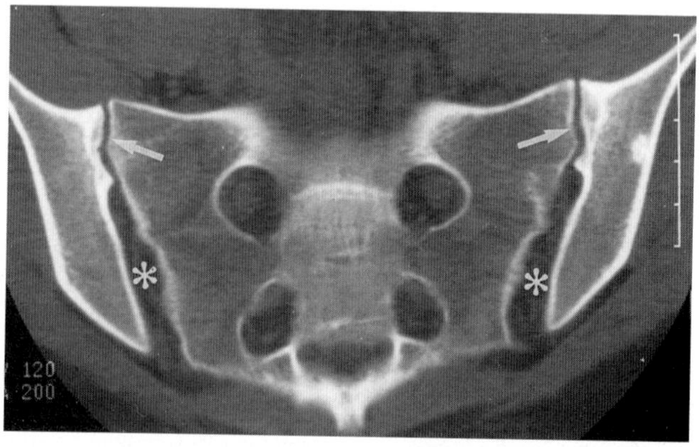

Figure 7A-27: Midsacroiliac joint semicoronal CT showing the articular portion of the midsacroiliac joint anterosuperiorly (*arrows*) and the ligamentous (fibrous) portion posteroinferiorly (*asterisks*).

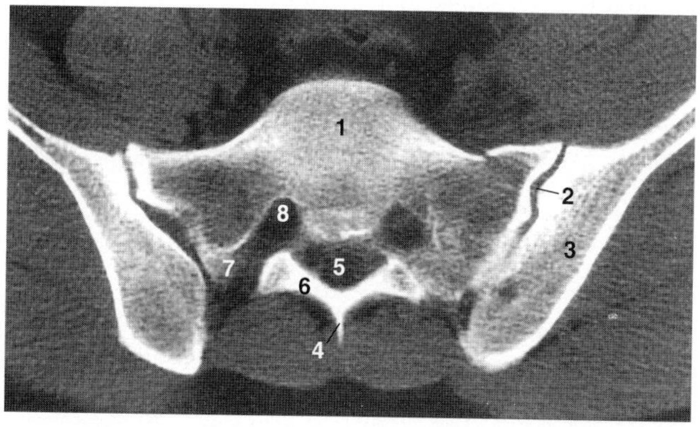

Figure 7A-28A: Axial CT anatomy of the lower sacrum. Normal anatomy.
1 Sacral body
2 Sacroiliac joint
3 Iliac bone
4 Sacral spinous process
5 Central sacral spinal canal
6 Lamina
7 Dorsal sacral neural foramen
8 Ventral sacral neural foramen

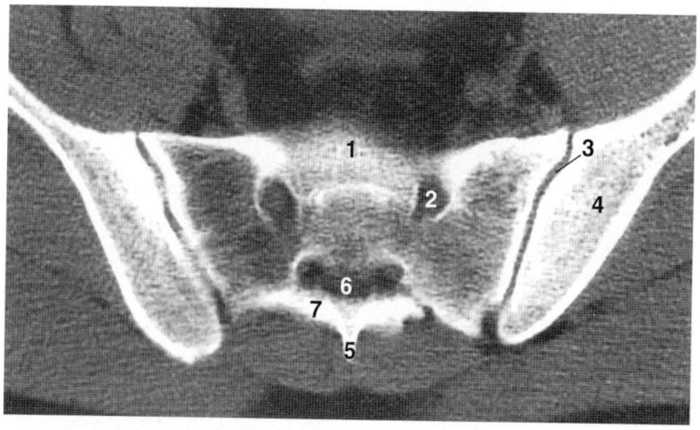

Figure 7A-28B: Axial CT image showing the normal anatomy of the lower sacrum below that of Figure 7A-28A.
1 Body of sacrum
2 Ventral sacral neural foramen
3 Sacroiliac joint
4 Iliac bone
5 Sacral spinous process
6 Sacral central spinal canal
7 Lamina

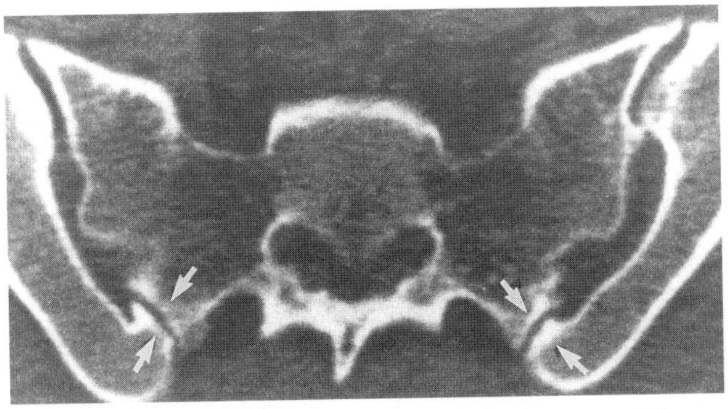

Figure 7A-29A: Sacroiliac joint variations. Axial CT scan showing bilateral accessory sacroiliac joints (*arrows*) posteriorly.

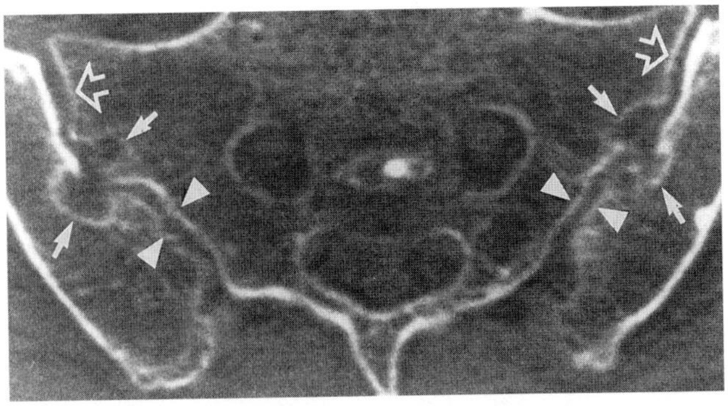

Figure 7A-29B: Axial CT scan showing bilateral semicircular pseudodefects (*arrows*) between the primary sacroiliac joints (*open arrows*) and accessory sacroiliac joints (*arrowheads*).

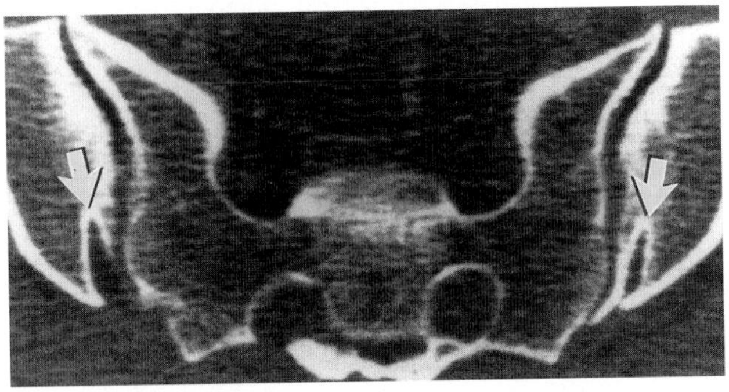

Figure 7A-29C: Axial CT image showing a bipartite appearance (*arrows*) of the iliac bony plate at the inferoposterior aspect of the sacroiliac joint.

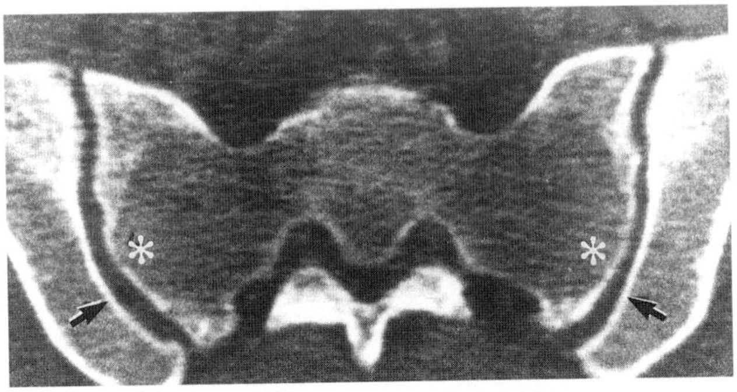

Figure 7A-29D: Axial CT image showing bilateral crescent-shaped iliac bony plates (*arrows*) surrounding the prominent sacrum (*asterisks*) bilaterally posterosuperiorly.

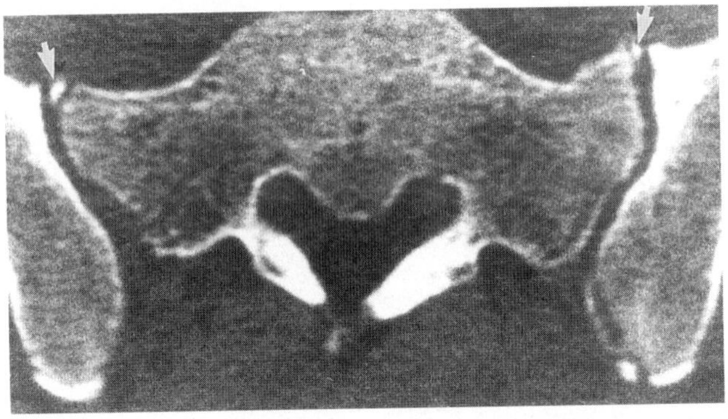

Figure 7A-29E: Axial CT scan showing bilateral accessory ossification centers (*arrowheads*) of the sacral wings. (Courtesy of P.K. Prassopoulos, M.D., N. Gourtsoyiannis, M.D., C.P. Faflia, M.D., and A.E. Voloudaki, M.D.)

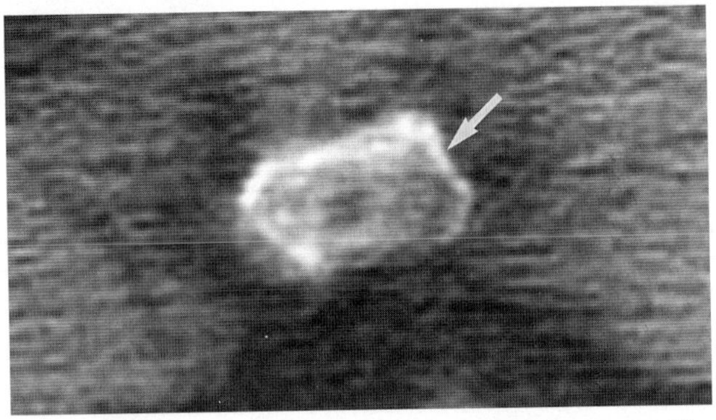

Figure 7A-30: CT anatomy of the coccyx. Axial magnified CT image showing the normal anatomy of one of the coccygeal elements coccyx (*arrow*).

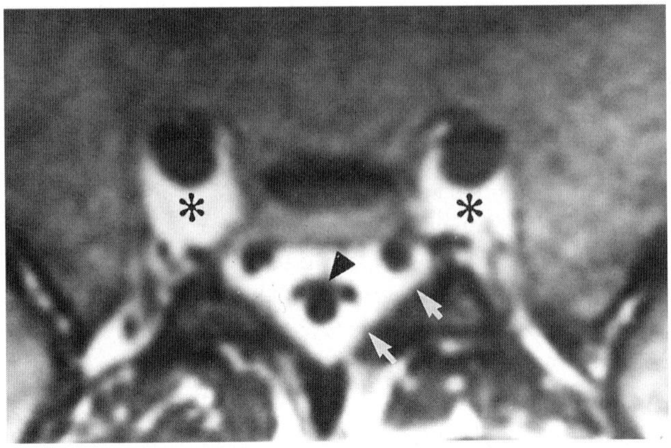

Figure 7A-31A: Magnetic resonance image of sacrum. Axial T1-weighted MR image acquired at the level of S-3 shows the sacral spinal canal (*arrows*), the terminal thecal sac (*arrowhead*), and the dorsal sacral neural foramina (*asterisks*).

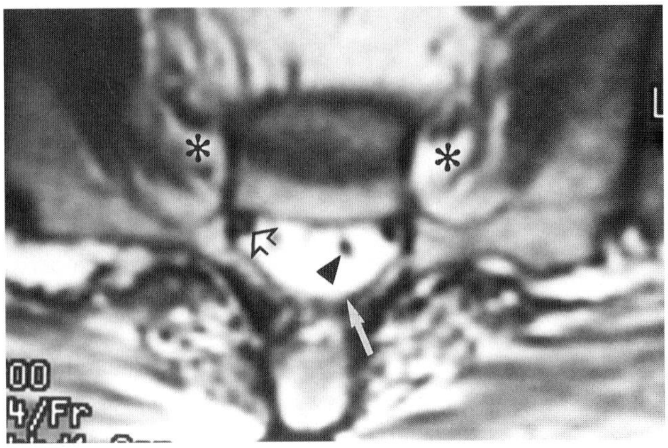

Figure 7A-31B: Axial T1-weighted MR image acquired at the S4-5 level shows the ventral sacral neural formaina (*asterisks*) and the terminal sacral canal (*solid arrow*) below the termination of the thecal sac. The S-5 (*open arrow*) and Cx1 (*arrowhead,* first coccygeal nerve) nerve root/sheath complexes are visualized.

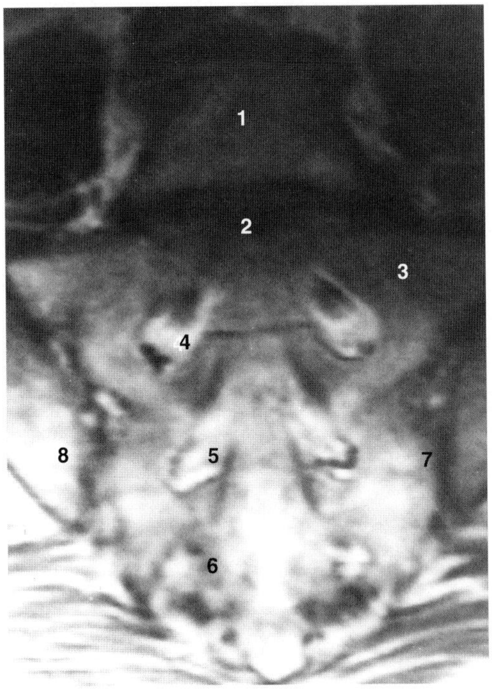

Figure 7A-31C: Magnetic resonance anatomy of the sacrum. Unenhanced coronal T1-weighted MR image showing the normal appearance of the sacrum and ventral sacral neural foramina.

1 L-5 vertebral body
2 S-1 vertebral body
3 Ala of the sacrum
4 Left S-1 ventral sacral neural foramen
5 Left S-2 ventral sacral neural foramen
6 Left S-3 ventral sacral neural foramen
7 Sacroiliac joint
8 Iliac bone

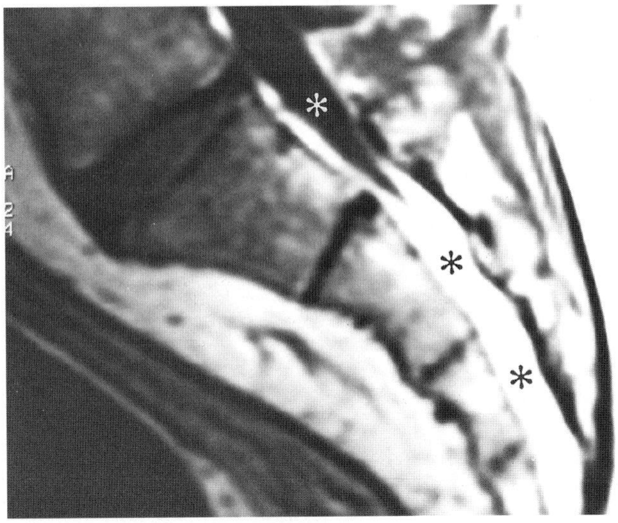

Figure 7A-31D: The sacrum. Sagittal T1-weighted image showing the sacrum. Note the fat (*black asterisks*) within the central sacral canal and the terminal thecal sac (*white asterisk*).

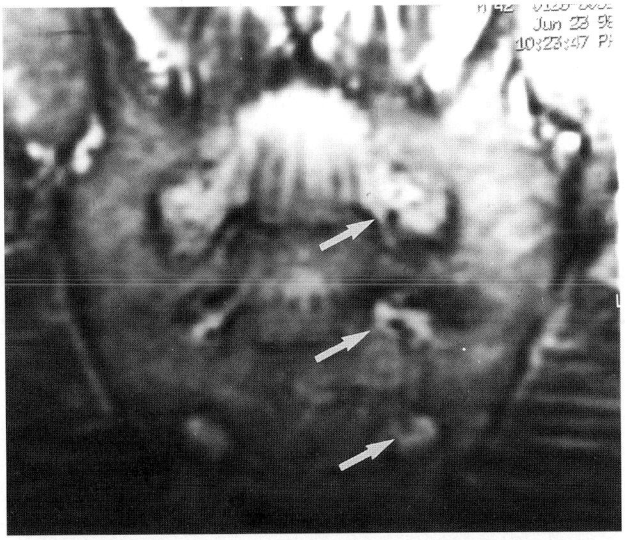

Figure 7A-31E: Coronal T1-weighted MR image acquired posterior to that of Figure 7A-31C showing the dorsal sacral neural foramina (*arrows*).

THE INTERVERTEBRAL SPINAL NEURAL FORAMINA

1. The intervertebral or spinal neural foramina are the main lateral pathways to and from the central spinal canal. Cranially, the foramen magnum is the main longitudinal aperture, and the sacral hiatus is the caudal longitudinal orifice.
2. The boundaries of the spinal neural foramina are (a) anteriorly, the inferior posterolateral aspect of the craniad vertebral body, the posterolateral aspect of the intervertebral disc, and the superior posterolateral aspect of the caudal vertebral body; (b) superiorly, the inferior margin of the pedicle of the craniad vertebral body; (c) inferiorly, the superior margin of the pedicle of the caudal vertebral body; and (d) posteriorly, the ventral surface of the posterior spinal facet (zygapophyseal) joint.
3. The walls of the neural foramina are covered by fibrous tissue, which may be periosteal (vertebral), perichondrial (posterior facet joint margin), anular (intervertebral disc), or capsular (posterior facet joint synovium) in origin.
4. The longitudinal axis of the cervical neural foramina is directed obliquely anterolaterally, whereas the longitudinal axes of the thoracic and lumbar neural foramina are directed laterally.
5. The spinal neural foramina contain the segmental spinal nerve/sheath complexes, one or more recurrent meningeal (sinu-vertebral) nerves, a spinal (radiculomeningeal) artery, a simple or plexiform venous structure, and varying amounts of fat.
6. Although individually segmentally variable, the position of the nerves and vessels in the neural foramina generally progressively changes with the level in the spine: cervical, inferior recess of neural foramen; thoracic, midforamen; lumbar, superior recess of neural foramen.

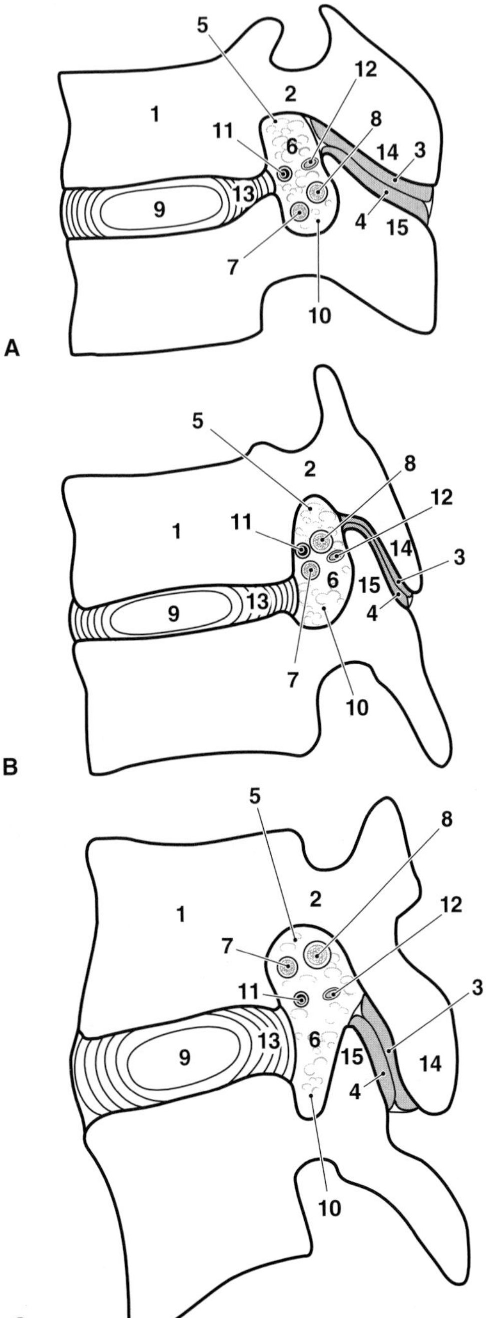

Figure 7A-32: Parasagittal cross-section schematics of the contents of the neural foramina at the cervical, thoracic, and lumbar levels. **A:** Cervical level. **B:** Thoracic level. **C:** Lumbar level.

1 Vertebral body
2 Pedicle
3 Inferior surface of posterior articular facet joint
4 Superior surface of posterior articular facet joint
5 Superior recess of neural foramen
6 Fat in neural foramen
7 Ventral nerve root
8 Dorsal nerve root/ganglion
9 Nucleus pulposus of intervertebral disc
10 Inferior recess of neural foramen
11 Radiculomedullary artery
12 Radiculomedullary vein
13 Anulus fibrosus of intervertebral disc
14 Inferior articular process of posterior facet (zygapophyseal) joint
15 Superior articular process of posterior facet (zygapophyseal) joint

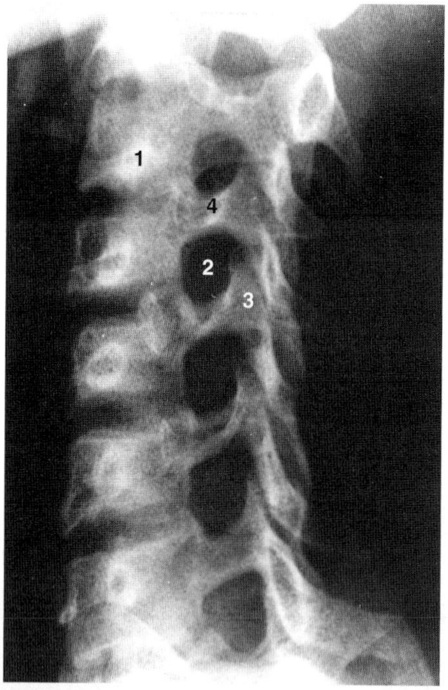

Figure 7A-33A: The intervertebral/neural foramina. Conventional radiograph in the oblique projection showing the normal configuration of the cervical intervertebral foramina.
1 Vertebral body of C-3
2 C-3/C-4 intervertebral foramen
3 C-3/C-4 posterior spinal/zygapophyseal facet joint
4 C-4 pedicle

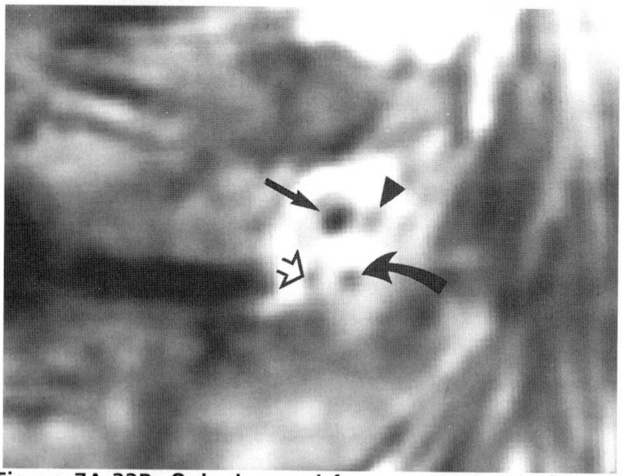

Figure 7A-33B: Spinal neural foramen anatomy. Sagittal T1-weighted MR image showing hyperintense fat surrounding the dorsal nerve root/ganglia (*straight solid arrow*), the ventral nerve root (*curved arrow*), and possibly an exiting radiculomedullary vein (*arrowhead*) and an entering radiculomedullary artery (*open arrow*).

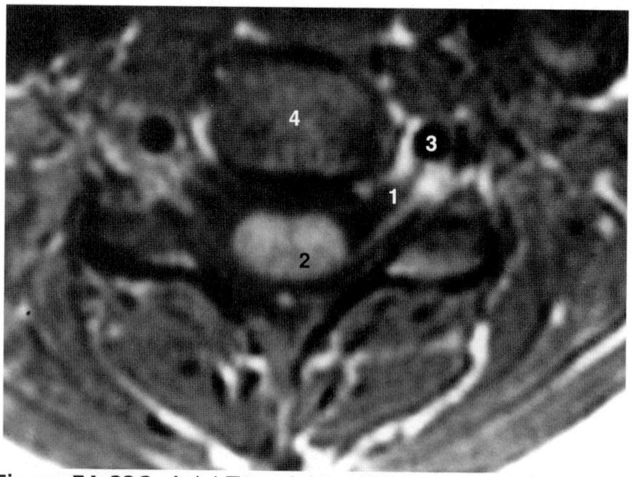

Figure 7A-33C: Axial T1-weighted MR image acquired at the C-5 level showing the poor visualization of the cervical spinal neural foramina on this acquisition.
1 Spinal neural foramen
2 Spinal cord
3 Vertebral artery
4 Vertebral body

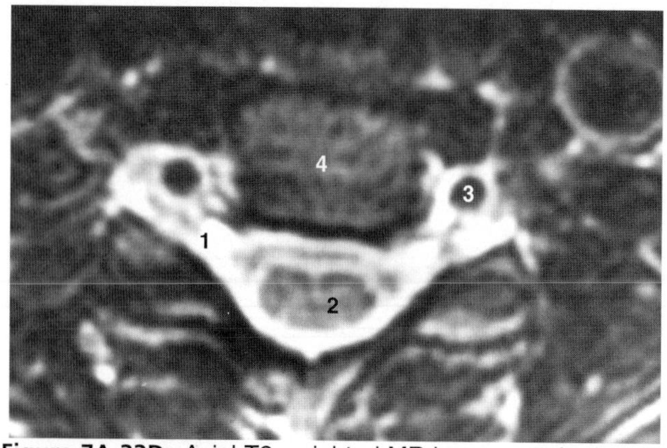

Figure 7A-33D: Axial T2-weighted MR image acquired at the C-5 level showing the normal appearance of the cervical spinal neural foramina.
1 Spinal neural foramen
2 Spinal cord
3 Vertebral artery
4 Vertebral body

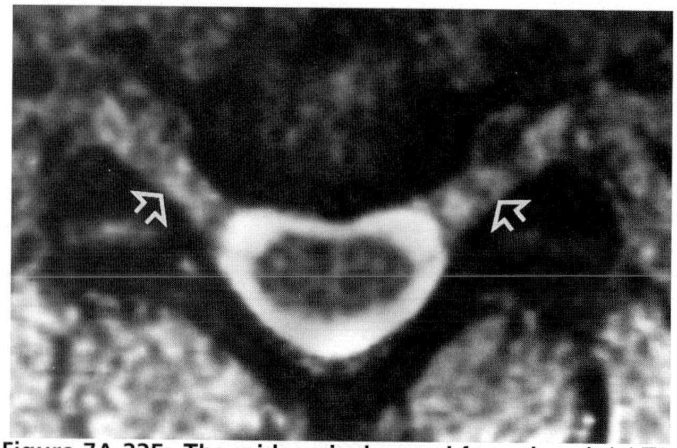

Figure 7A-33E: The midcervical neural foramina. Axial T2-weighted MR image shows the cervical spinal neural foramina (*arrows*).

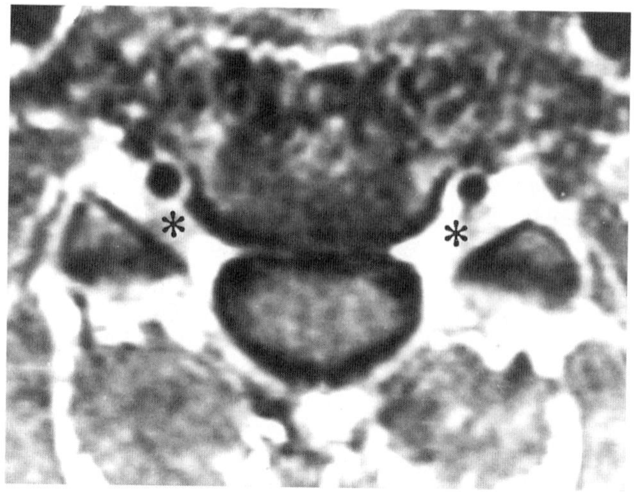

Figure 7A-33F: Axial intravenous contrast-enhanced T1-weighted MR image shows enhancement of the venous structures within the cervical spinal neural foramina (*asterisks*).

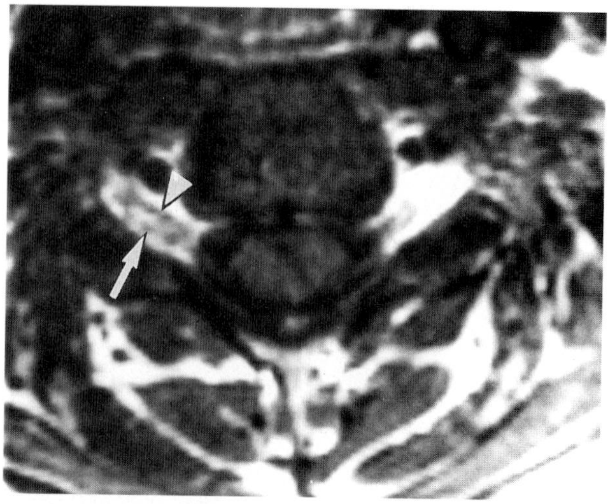

Figure 7A-33G: Cervical nerve roots. Intravenous contrast-enhanced axial T1-weighted MR image showing the exiting ventral (*arrowhead*) and dorsal (*arrow*) nerve roots in the mid-cervical region.

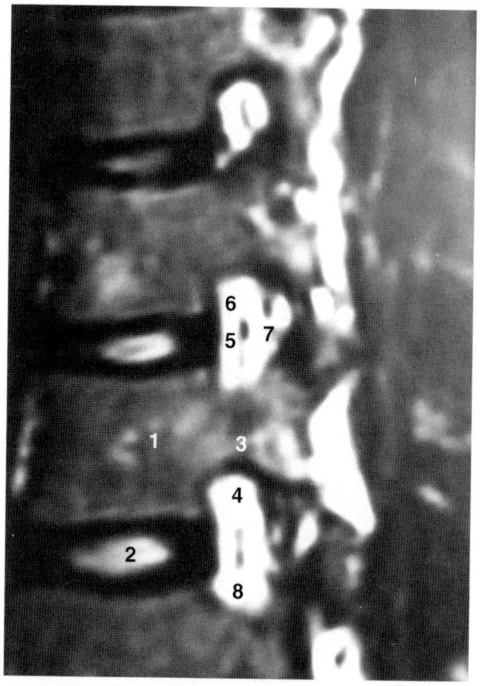

Figure 7A-33H: Thoracic spinal neural foramina. Sagittal T2-weighted MR image showing the normal appearance of the thoracic spinal neural foramina.

1 Vertebral body
2 Intervertebral disc
3 Pedicle
4 Superior recess of neural foramen
5 Ventral spinal nerve root
6 Dorsal spinal nerve root
7 Spinal radiculomedullary artery or vein
8 Inferior recess of spinal neural foramen

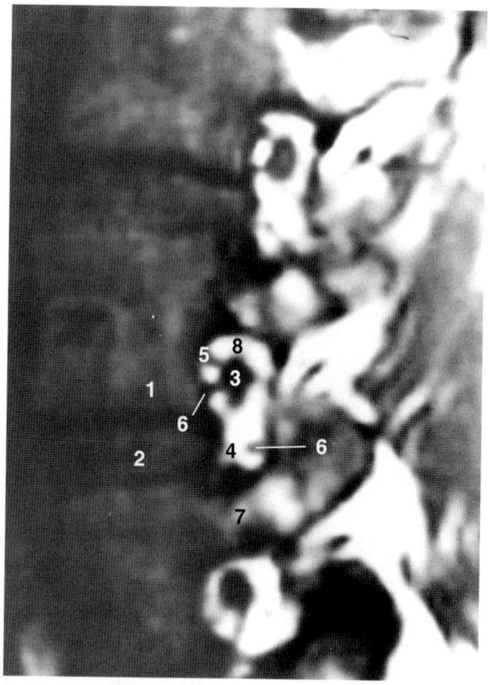

Figure 7A-33I: Lumbar spinal neural foramina. Sagittal T1-weighted MR image showing the normal appearance of the lumbar spinal neural foramina.

1 Lumbar vertebral body
2 Lumbar intervertebral disc
3 Dorsal nerve root ganglion
4 Inferior recess of neural foramen
5 Ventral nerve root
6 Radiculomedullary blood vessels
7 Pedicle
8 Superior recess of spinal neural foramen

THE POSTERIOR SPINAL FACET (ZYGAPOPHYSEAL) JOINTS

1. The paired superior and inferior vertebral articular processes are also known as the zygapophyses; therefore the posterior spinal facet joints are also known as the zygapophyseal joints.
2. The posterior spinal facet (zygapophyseal) joints are of the synovial variety, i.e., hyaline-covered articular cartilage enclosed within an articular capsule.
3. The posterior spinal facet joints vary in shape, size, and spatial orientation according to the vertebral level. The posterior spinal facet joint angulation in the axial plane may be unequal in degree from one side to the other, a phenomenon referred to as *zygapophyseal joint tropism*. This tropism is most prominent in the mid and lower lumbar region (L3-4, L4-5), and at the lumbosacral junction (L5-S1).
4. The minisci (or, more properly, miniscoids) of the lumbar posterior spinal facet (zygapophyseal) joints.
   a. There are two groups of miniscoids extending into the posterior spinal facet joints: ventral and dorsal, and superior and inferior.
   b. The ventral and dorsal miniscoids are only rudimentary fibrous structures that in humans apparently represent no more than capsular invaginations into the posterior spinal facet joints.
   c. The superior and inferior polar miniscoids contain varying proportions of fat, connective tissue, blood vessels, and synovium. Some may contain neurons. These meniscoids are believed to represent synovial reflections. Some are fibroadipose miniscoids while others are simply fat pads.
   d. The proportionally differing components of the polar miniscoids in the young reflect individual embryonically determined differences. In adults these meniscoidal components progressively alter with repetitive stresses on the posterior spinal facet joints.

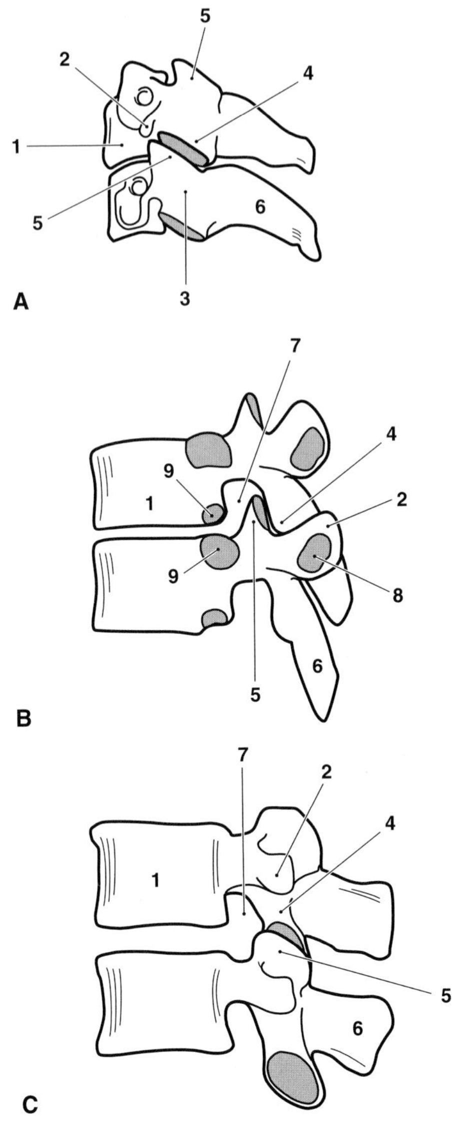

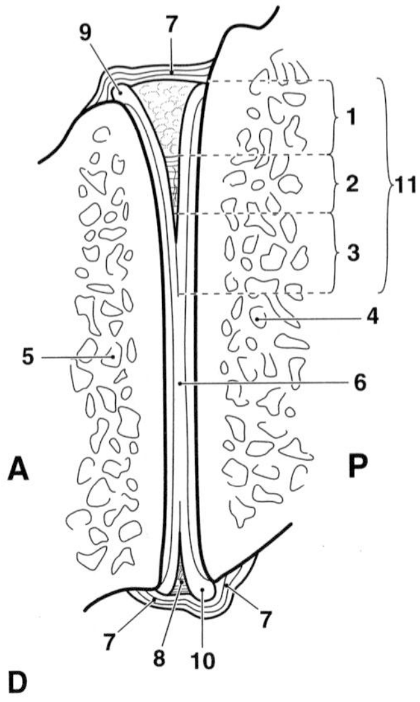

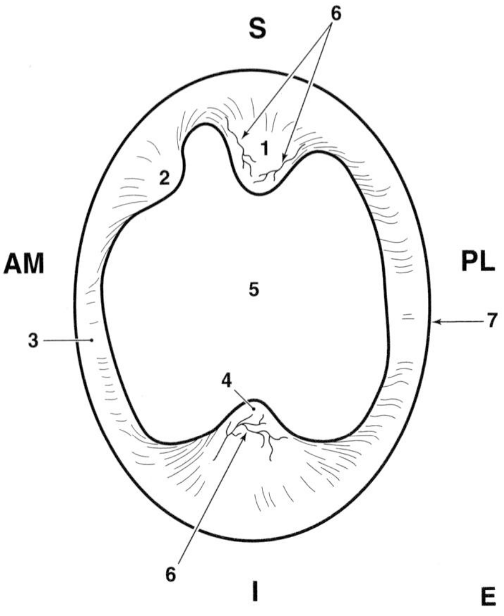

Figure 7A-34A: Schematic of the cervical, thoracic, and lumbar posterior spinal facet (zygapophyseal) joints. **A:** Cervical level. **B:** Thoracic level. **C:** Lumbar level.

1 Vertebral body
2 Transverse process
3 Articular column/lateral mass (cervical spine only)
4 Inferior posterior articular facet/process
5 Superior posterior articular facet/process
6 Spinous process
7 Intervertebral foramen
8 Transverse process articulation for rib (costotransverse facet joint)
9 Superior and inferior demifacets for articulation with head of rib (T-1 to T8-9) (costocorpal facet joint)

Figure 7A-34D: Schematics of the lumbar miniscoids of the posterior spinal facet (zygapophyseal) joints. Sagittal oblique schematic of a lumbar posterior spinal facet (zygapophyseal) joint showing the polar miniscoids. *A,* anterior; *P,* posterior.

1 Loose connective and adipose (fat) tissue within superior polar miniscoid
2 Synovial tissue and blood vessels (also possibly neural tissue)
3 Dense connective tissue
4 Inferior articular process of suprajacent posterior spinal facet (zygapophyseal) joint
5 Superior articular process of subajacent posterior spinal facet (zygapophyseal) joint
6 Joint space
7 Synovial membrane
8 Inferior polar miniscoid (synovial tissue and blood vessels and possibly neural tissue)
9 Superior articular recess
10 Inferior articular recess
11 Superior polar miniscoid

Figure 7A-34E: *En face* schematic of miniscoid of lumbar posterior spinal facet (zygapophyseal) joint. *AM,* anteromedial; *PL,* posterolateral; *S,* superior; *I,* inferior.

1 Superior polar fibradipose miniscoid
2 Adipose tissue pad
3 Synovial membrane
4 Inferior polar fibroadipose miniscoid
5 Joint space
6 Blood vessels and possible neural radicles
7 Joint capsule

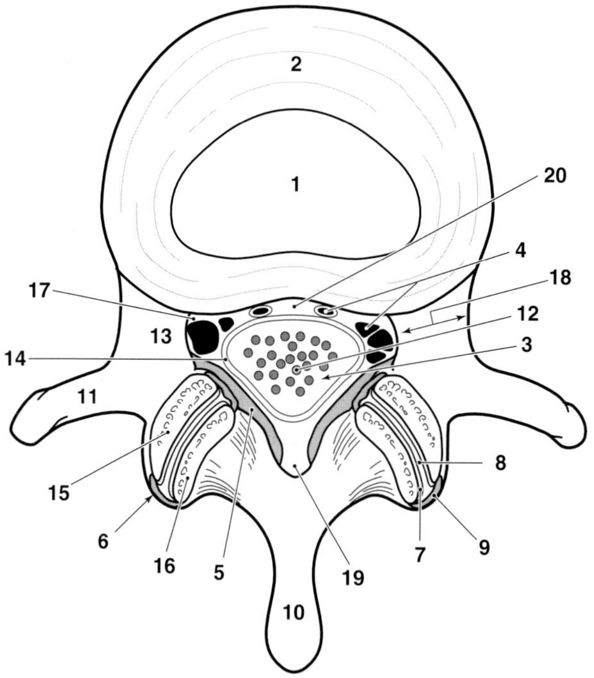

Figure 7A-35: Axial cross section schematic of the intervertebral disc, posterior spinal facet (zygapophyseal) joints, and central spinal canal in the lumbar area.
1 Nucleus pulposus
2 Anulus fibrosus
3 Spinal subarachnoid space with nerve roots of cauda equina and filum terminale
4 Anterior epidural arteries and veins
5 Ligamentum flavum
6 Posterior spinal facet (zygapophyseal) joint
7 Articular cartilage of posterior spinal facet (zygapophyseal) joint
8 Posterior spinal facet (zygapophyseal) joint space
9 Synovial membrane and capsular ligament of posterior spinal facet joint
10 Spinous process
11 Transverse process
12 Filum terminale
13 Pedicle
14 Parietal spinal meninges (dura and arachnoid maters)
15 Cut surface of superior articular facet (zygapophyseal) process
16 Cut surface of inferior articular facet (zygapophyseal) process
17 Lateral recess of central spinal canal
18 Lateral extent of intervertebral (neural) foramen (above pedicle)
19 Median retrothecal fat pad
20 Anterior epidural space (fat)

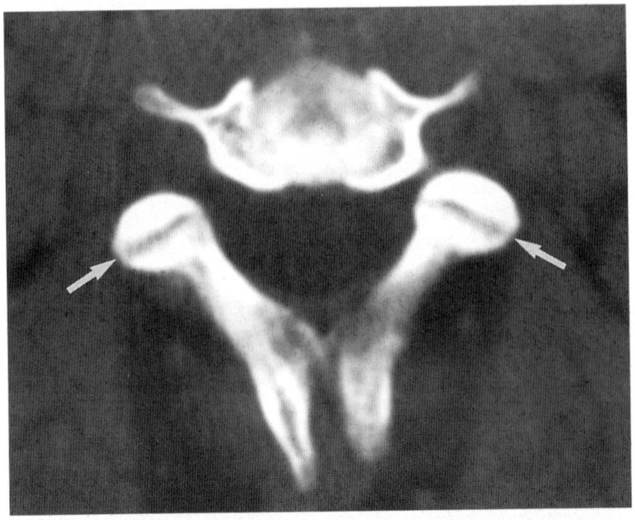

Figure 7A-36A: The cervical posterior spinal facet (zygapophyseal) joints. Axial CT image at C2-3 showing the oblique orientation of the posterior spinal facet joints (*arrows*) at this level.

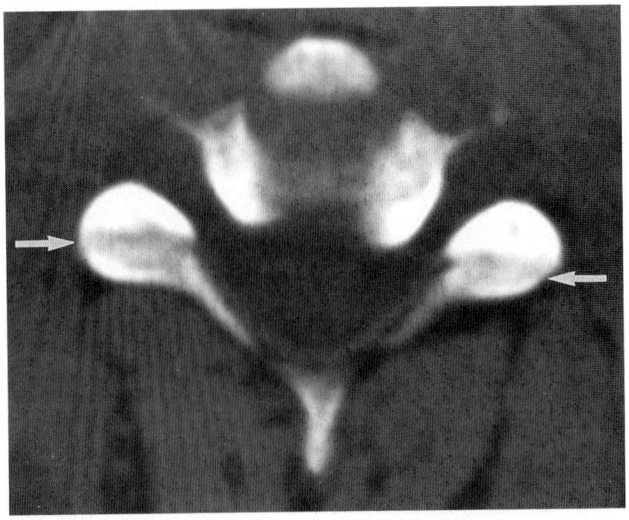

Figure 7A-36B: Axial CT image at C4-5 showing the coronal orientation of the posterior spinal facet joints (*arrows*) at this level.

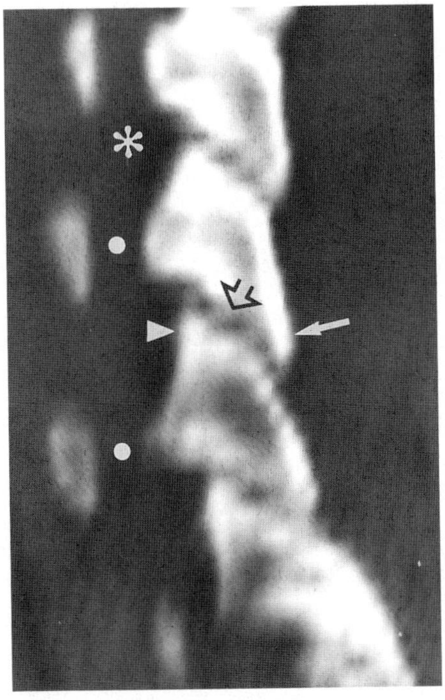

Figure 7A-36C: Parasagittal CT reconstruction through the mid-lower cervical spine showing a superior articular facet process (*arrowhead*), an inferior articular facet process (*solid arrow*), posterior spinal facet joints (*open arrow*), the lateral aspect of a neural foramen (*asterisk*), and the foramina transversaria (*dots*).

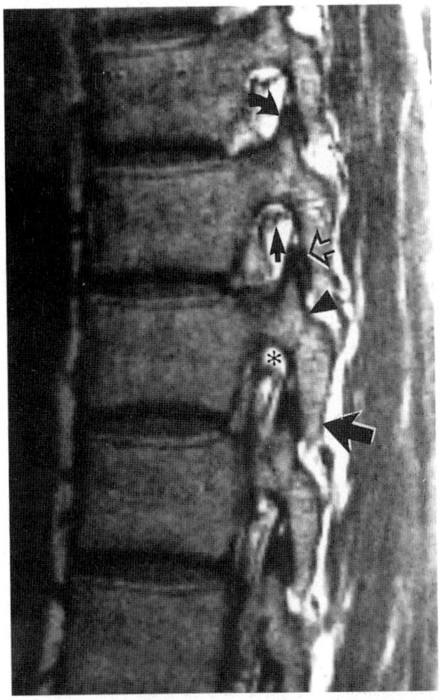

Figure 7A-36D: Thoracic posterior spinal facet joints. Parasagittal T1-weighted MR image showing an inferior facet process (*large straight arrow*), a superior facet process (*curved arrow*), the pars interarticularis (*arrowhead*), a facet joint (*open arrow*), fat in a neural foramen (*asterisk*), and an exiting spinal nerve roots and vessels (*small straight arrow*).

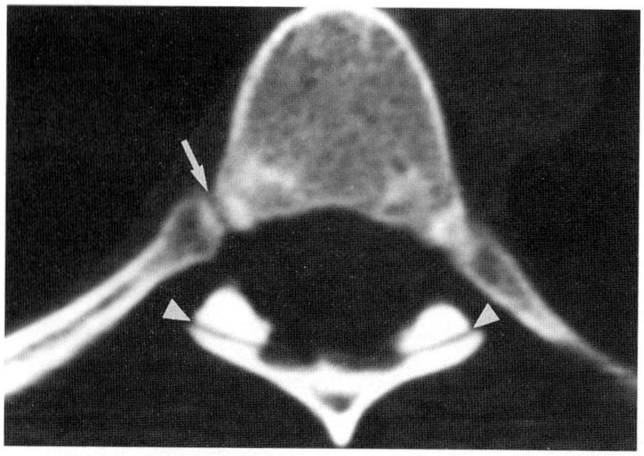

Figure 7A-36E: Thoracic posterior spinal facet (zygapophyseal) joints and costovertebral facet. Axial CT image showing the posterior spinal facet joints (*arrowheads*) bilaterally and the costovertebral facet (*arrow*) on the right side. Note the near coronal orientation of the posterior spinal facet joints.

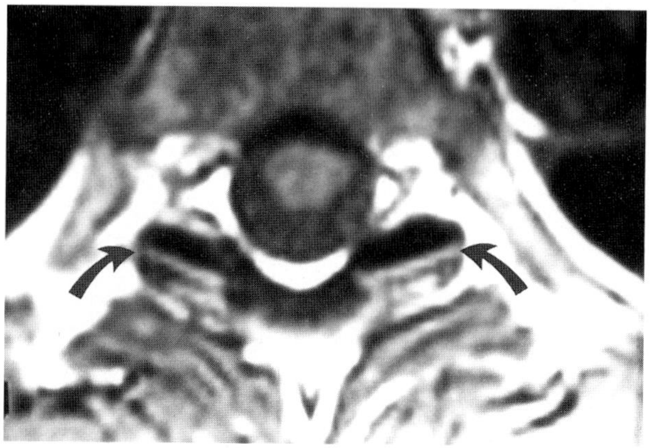

Figure 7A-36F: Axial T1-weighted MR image showing the facet joints (*arrows*) in the midthoracic level.

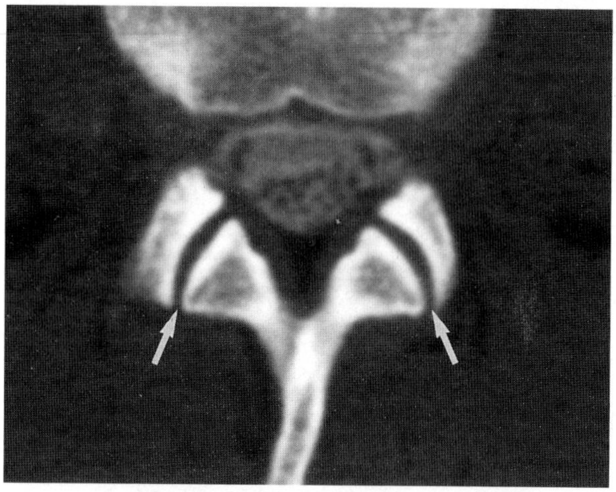

Figure 7A-36G: Upper lumbar posterior spinal facet (zygapophyseal) joints. Axial CT myelogram at L2-3 showing the steep oblique orientation of the posterior spinal facet joints (*arrows*) at this level.

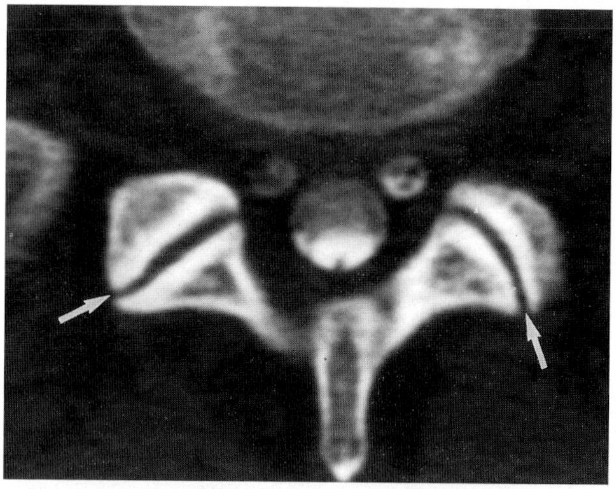

Figure 7A-36H: Lumbosacral junction posterior spinal facet (zygapophyseal) joints with tropism. Axial CT myelogram at L-5 to S-1, showing the oblique angle of the posterior spinal facet joints (*arrows*) at this level. Note the lateral asymmetry in the facet joint angulation (zygapophyseal joint tropism).

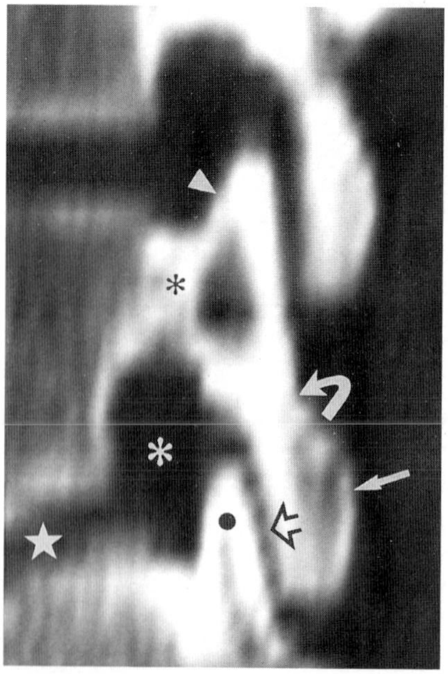

Figure 7A-36I: Parasagittal CT reconstruction at the lumbosacral junction showing the L-5 inferior facet process (*solid arrow*), the L-5 superior facet process (*arrowhead*), the L-5 pars interarticularis (*curved arrow*), the L-5 to S-1 facet joint (*open arrow*), the L-5 to S-1 intervertebral (neural) foramen (*white asterisk*), the L-5 pedicle (*black asterisk*), the L-5 to S-1 intervertebral disk (*star*), and the superior facet process of S-1 (*dot*).

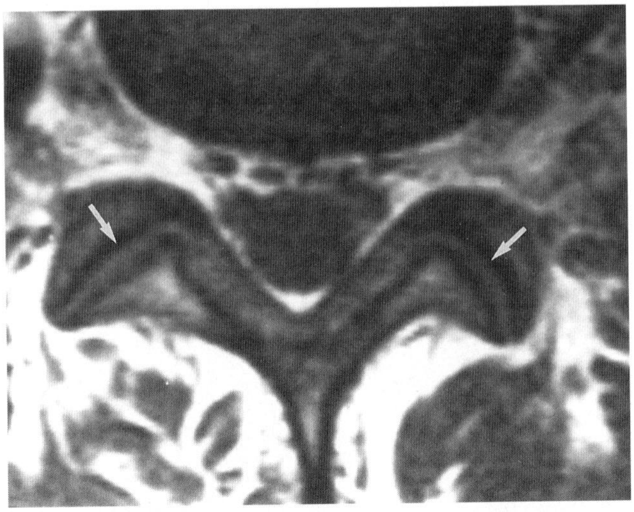

Figure 7A-36J: Normal lumbar posterior spinal facet joint enhancement. Unenhanced axial T1-weighted MR image showing normal lumbar posterior facet joints (*arrows*).

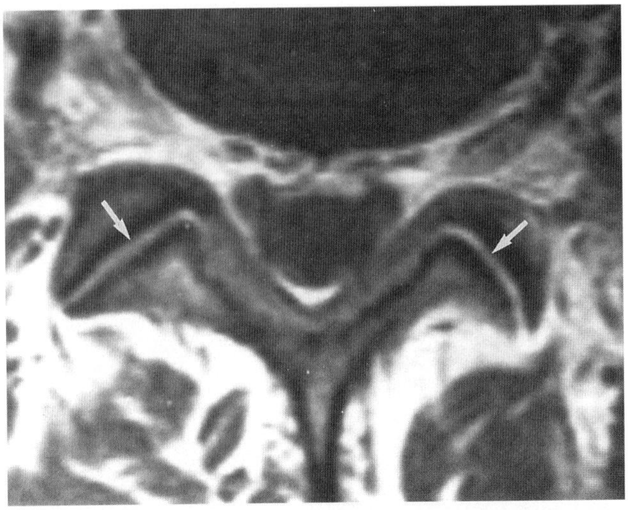

Figure 7A-36K: Axial "triple-dose" (0.3 mmol/kg) intravenous gadolinium-enhanced MR image in same case as Figure 7A-36J, showing normal enhancement of the posterior facet joints (*arrows*) (compare with Figure 7A-36J).

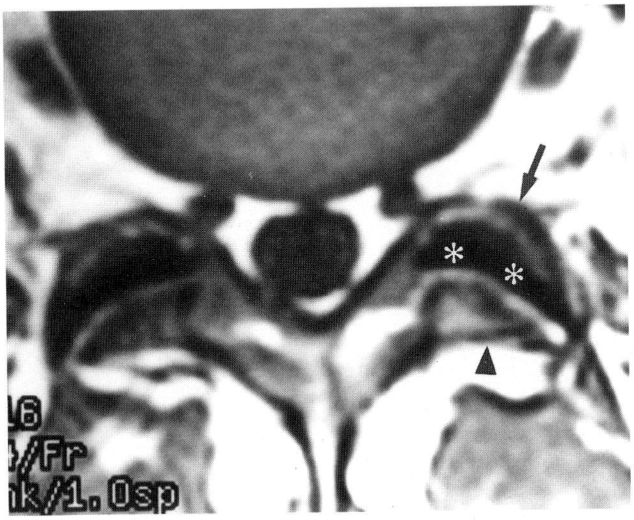

Figure 7A-36L: Lumbar posterior spinal facet (zygapophyseal) joints. Axial T1-weighted MR image showing the superior facet process of S-1 (*arrow*), the inferior facet process of L-5 (*arrowhead*), and the posterior spinal facet joint (*asterisks*).

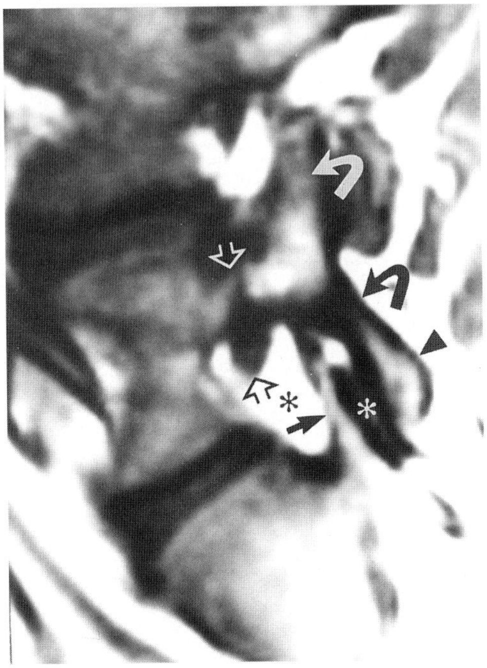

Figure 7A-36M: Parasagittal T1-weighted MR image showing again the superior facet process of S-1 (*solid arrow*), the inferior facet process of L-5, and the posterior spinal facet joint (*white asterisk*). Also note fat within the L-5 to S-1 neural foramen (*black asterisk*), the L-5 spinal nerve/dorsal root ganglion (*black open arrow*), the pars interarticularis of L-5 (*black curved arrow*), the superior articularis process of L-5 (*white curved arrow*), and the pedicle of L-5 (*white open arrow*).

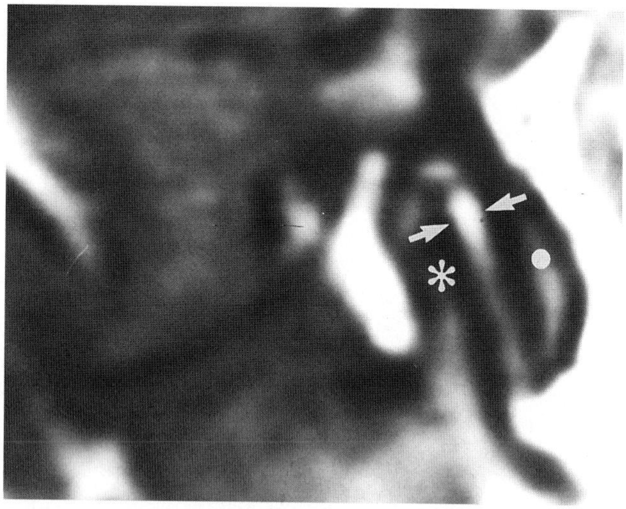

Figure 7A-36N: Lumbar posterior spinal facet (zygapophyseal) joint polar miniscoids. Parasagittal T1-weighted MR image shows the superior articular process of S-1 (*asterisk*), the inferior articular process of L-5 (*dot*), and hyperintense fat (*arrows*) within the superior polar miniscoid/fat pad.

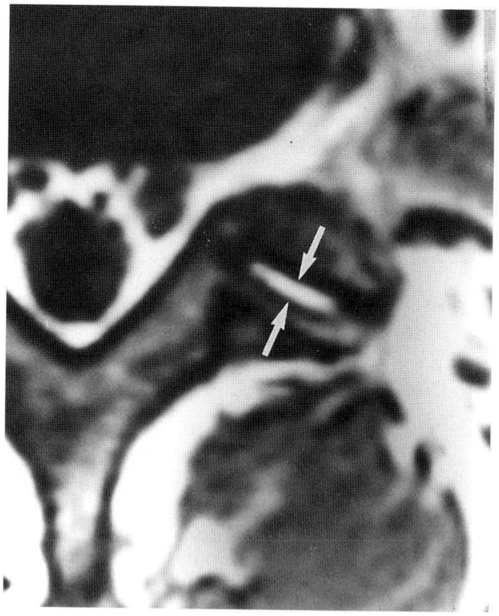

Figure 7A-36O: Axial T1-weighted MR image in same case as that in Figure 7A-36N again shows the hyperintense fat (*arrows*) within the superior polar miniscoid/fat pad.

THE CRANIOCERVICAL LIGAMENTS

1. The membrana tectoria is the craniad extension of the posterior longitudinal ligament from the posterior surfaces of the bodies of C-1 to C-2 to the posteroinferior surface of the clivus.
2. The anterior atlantooccipital membrane joins the anterior arch of C-1 to the anterior margin of the foramen magnum.
3. The posterior atlantooccipital membrane interconnects the posterior arch of C-1 with the posterior and lateral margins of the foramen magnum.
4. The cruciform ligament is composed of the transverse atlantal ligament, and the superior and inferior longitudinal bands. The transverse atlantal ligament connects the lateral masses of C-1 (at the transverse atlantal tubercles) with the posterior surface of the odontoid process, at which point it is covered by articular cartilage. The superior longitudinal band inserts onto the posteroinferior surface of the clivus and the inferior longitudinal band inserts onto the posterior surface of the body of C-2.
5. The apical (dental) ligament of the odontoid process interconnects the tip (apex) of the odontoid with the anterior margin of the foramen magnum (basion).
6. The anterior longitudinal ligament extends from the anterior surface of C-1 and C-2 to the anteroinferior surface of the clivus.
7. The alar ligaments obliquely interconnect the posterolateral surface of the odontoid process to the medial surfaces of the occipital condyles.

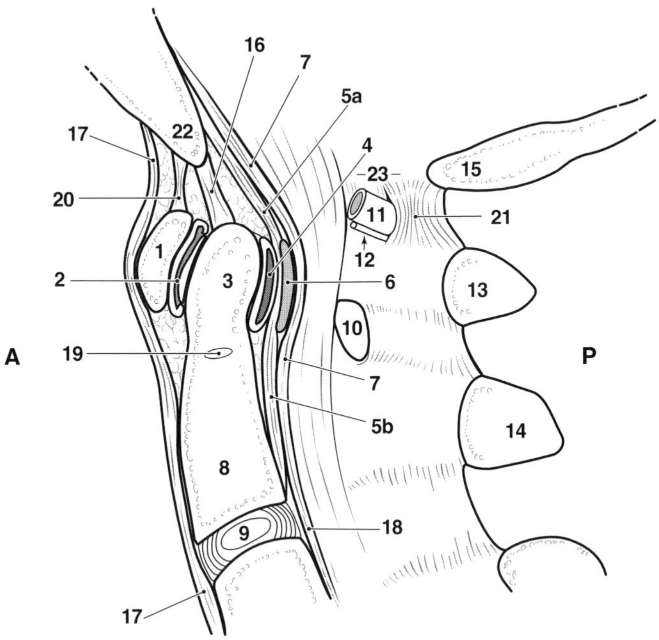

Figure 7A-37: Midline sagittal section schematic of the craniocervical ligaments. The left half of the spine, cranium, and all of the spinal cord have been removed. *A*, anterior; *P*, posterior.

1 Anterior bony arch of C-1
2 Synovial joint between the posterior surface of the anterior arch of C-1 and the anterior surface of the odontoid process
3 Odontoid process (dens) of C-2
4 Synovial joint between the anterior surface of the transverse atlantal ligament and the posterior surface of the odontoid process
5 Longitudinal components of the cruciate ligament:
  a. Superior longitudinal band of cruciate ligament
  b. Inferior longitudinal band of cruciate ligament
6 Transverse component of the cruciate ligament: transverse atlantal ligament
7 Membrana tectoria (superior extension of posterior longitudinal ligament)
8 Body of C-2
9 Intervertebral disc (C2-3)
10 C1-2 intervertebral (neural) foramen (for C-2 neurovascular structures)
11 Vertebral artery on right side
12 C-1 spinal nerve on right side
13 Posterior bony arch of C-1
14 Spinous process of C-2
15 Opisthion (occipital bone) (posterior margin of foramen magnum)
16 Apical odontoid (dental) ligament
17 Anterior longitudinal ligament
18 Posterior longitudinal ligament
19 Disc remnant at junction of base of the odontoid process and the centrum of C-2 (remnant of C1-2 intervertebral disc: variably present)
20 Anterior atlantooccipital membrane
21 Posterior atlantooccipital membrane
22 Basion (basiocciput) (anterior margin of foramen magnum)
23 Foramen magnum

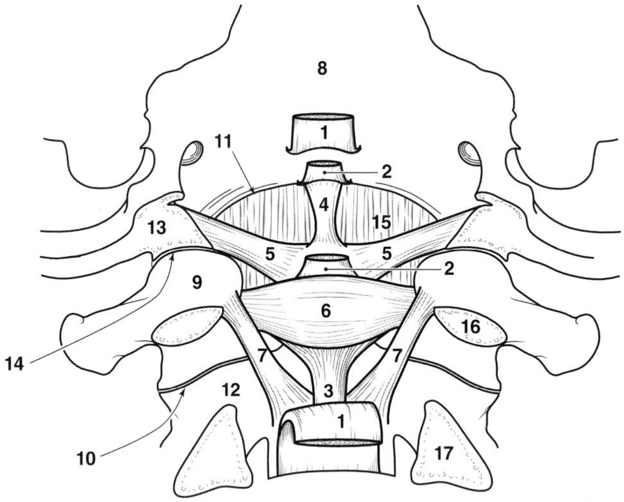

Figure 7A-38: Posterior schematic of the craniocervical ligaments. The posterior spinal elements, posterior aspect of the occipital bone, and spinal cord/brain stem have been removed, and the membrana tectoria and superior band of the cruciform ligament have been cut and partially resected.

1 Cut ends of membrana tectoria (superior extension of posterior longitudinal ligament)
2 Cut ends of partially resected superior longitudinal band of cruciform ligament
3 Inferior longitudinal band of cruciform ligament
4 Apical odontoid (dental) ligament
5 Alar ligaments
6 Transverse atlantal ligament
7 Accessory atlantoaxial ligaments
8 Basiocciput (clivus)
9 Lateral mass of C-1
10 Lateral atlantoaxial articulation
11 Anterolateral margin of foramen magnum
12 Lateral mass of C-2
13 Occipital condyle
14 Atlantooccipital articulation
15 Anterior atlantooccipital membrane
16 Cut surface of C-1 pedicle
17 Cut surface of C-2 pedicle

LIGAMENTS AND INTERVERTEBRAL DISCS OF THE SPINAL COLUMN BELOW C-2

1. The anterior longitudinal ligament extends along the length of the anterior aspect of the spinal column. It is attached superiorly to the clivus and extends caudally to insert into the sacrum. It is thickest in the lumbar spine and thinnest in the cervical spine. The longitudinal fibers of the anterior longitudinal ligament blend with the underlying outermost anulus fibrosus of the intervertebral discs, and the vertebral periosteum and perichondrium.
2. The posterior longitudinal ligament lies over the posterior aspect of the spinal column and forms the anterior surface of the central spinal canal. Superiorly it is contiguous with the membrana tectoria that in turn attaches to the posteroinferior surface of the clivus. Inferiorly the posterior longitudinal ligament inserts into the sacrum. In between it is attached with variable degrees of firmness to the vertebral periosteum, the outermost fibers of the posterior anulus fibrosus of the intervertebral discs, and the peripheral posterior margins of the hyaline cartilage of the vertebral end plates, where they reach sufficiently posteriorly to make contact.
3. The intervertebral discs are formed of a central semiliquid nucleus pulposus and an outer fibrous laminated anulus fibrosus. Intervertebral discs are present between the bodies of the vertebrae from C-2/3 to the sacrum; synovial joints are present at the atlantooccipital and the atlantoaxial articulations. The intervertebral discs are thickest in craniocaudal diameter in the lumbar region and thinnest in the upper thoracic area. The disc is continuous above and below with the vertebral endplate, a thin, vascularized layer of hyaline cartilage lining the superior and inferior surfaces of the vertebral bodies. While blood vessels supply the periphery of the intervertebral discs, the central areas are normally avascular in the adult; nutrition of the disc is primarily supplied by diffusion of fluids and solutes from the adjacent vascularized vertebrae and vertebral end plates.
4. The anulus fibrosus is composed of a narrow outer collagenous rim and a broader inner fibrocartilaginous sector. The laminae of the anulus fibrosus consist of overlapping layers of obliquely oriented fibrous bands running in a criss-cross fashion between adjacent vertebral bodies. Across the posterior portion of the intervertebral disc, the fibers of the anulus fibrosus run more vertically than obliquely. The anular fibers insert superiorly and inferiorly into the periphery of the articular surfaces (i.e., vertebral end plates) and surrounding bone of the adjacent vertebral bodies.
5. The center of the nucleus pulposus is nearer to the posterior than the anterior surface of the intervertebral disc. At birth the nucleus pulposus is large and is composed of gelatinous mucoid material containing scattered notochordal cells. By the end of the first decade the notochordal cells disappear. Over time the mucoid material of the nucleus pulposus is progressively replaced by fibrocartilage from the surrounding hyaline cartilage plates of the adjacent vertebral bodies and from the anulus fibrosus. At the same time, the margins of the nucleus pulposus gradually become less distinct from the anulus fibrosus.
6. The paired ligamenta flava originate and insert into the laminae of the adjacent vertebral bodies. The fibers of the medial aspect of the ligamenta flava may blend with or give rise to the anteriormost fibers of the interspinous ligament.
7. The interspinous ligaments interconnect the spinous processes of the vertebrae. They are heaviest in the lumbar area, thinner in the thoracic region, and poorly developed in the cervical spine. They are generally directed in an oblique posterior-cranial direction. From ventral to dorsal: anteriorly (ventrally) the interspinous ligament arises from the medial extents of the two ligamenta flava and inserts into the suprajacent spinous process; midway it originates in the subjacent spinous process and inserts into the suprajacent spinous process; and posteriorly (dorsally) it originates in the subjacent spinous process and inserts into the supraspinous ligament at levels where it exists (i.e., C-1 to L-5). Caudally (i.e., L-5 to S-1) the posterior aspect of the interspinous ligament(s) inserts into the overlying tendons of the erector spinae muscles.

8. The supraspinous ligament interconnects the posterior midline bony arch of C-1 and the tips of the spinous processes from C-2 to L-5 (variation of termination of supraspinous ligament: L-3 to L-5). It extends craniad from the posterior midline bony arch of C-1 to insert into the external occipital protuberance as the ligamentum nuchae. At the termination of the supraspinous ligament, the supraspinous ligament fibrous tissue blends with the erector spinae muscle tendons in the midline, which in turn insert into the midline (median) sacral spinous tubercles.
9. The intertransverse ligaments either are minor independent connections between the transverse processes of the vertebrae or are blended with adjacent intertransverse muscles attaching to the spine.
10. The iliolumbar ligament originates from the tip and anteroinferior aspect of the transverse process of the fifth lumbar vertebra. The inferior portion, the lumbosacral ligament, arises from the fifth transverse process on each side and terminates in the lateral surface of the sacrum anterosuperiorly; the superior portion partially arises from the quadratus lumborum and transverse process of L-5 on each side and terminates in the iliac crest and thoracolumbar fascia.
11. In the sacrococcygeal area, the anterior sacrococcygeal ligament is an extension of the anterior longitudinal ligament and inserts onto the anterior surface of the sacrum and coccyx. The deep dorsal sacrococcygeal ligament extends similarly from the posterior longitudinal ligament to the posterior surface of the sacrum. The superior posterior sacrococcygeal ligament roofs the dorsal aspect of the sacral spinal canal. The paired intercornual sacrococcygeal ligaments connect the sacral cornua to the coccygeal cornua on each side.
12. At the caudal end of the spine, the anococcygeal ligament connects the coccyx with the anorectum. Included in this ligament are the presacral fascia, the tendinous plate of the pubococcygeus muscle, the muscular raphe of the iliococcygeus muscle, the posterior attachments of the puborectalis muscle, and the sphincter ani externus muscle. The terminal segment is attached to the overlying skin by an unnamed grouping of fibrous tissue.

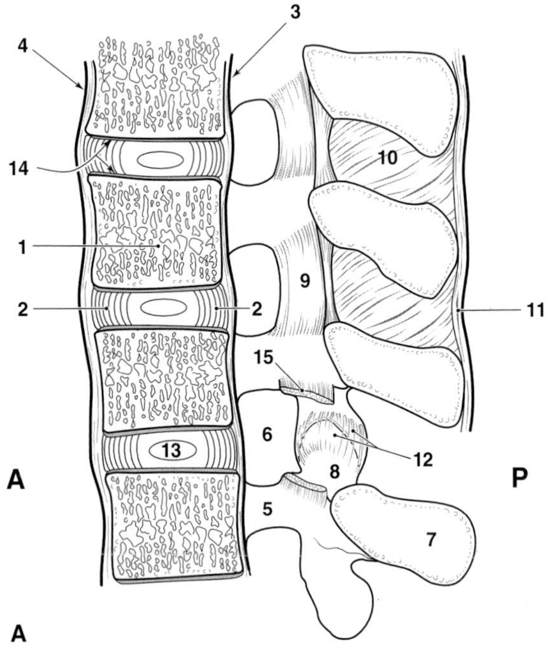

A

Figure 7A-39A: Sagittal section schematic of the spinal ligaments and intervertebral discs. The left half of the spine, as well as the neurovascular elements and meninges, has been removed. *A,* anterior; *P,* posterior.

1 Vertebral body
2 Anterior and posterior aspect of anulus fibrosus
3 Posterior longitudinal ligament
4 Anterior longitudinal ligament
5 Pedicle
6 Neural (intervertebral) foramen
7 Spinous process
8 Superior articular process of the posterior spinal facet joint on the right side
9 Ligamentum flavum
10 Interspinous ligament (note posterocranial orientation of fibers)
11 Supraspinous ligament
12 Capsular ligament of the posterior spinal facet (zygapophyseal) joint
13 Nucleus pulposus
14 Hyaline cartilage of superior and inferior vertebral end plates
15 Cut surface of excised ligamentum flavum

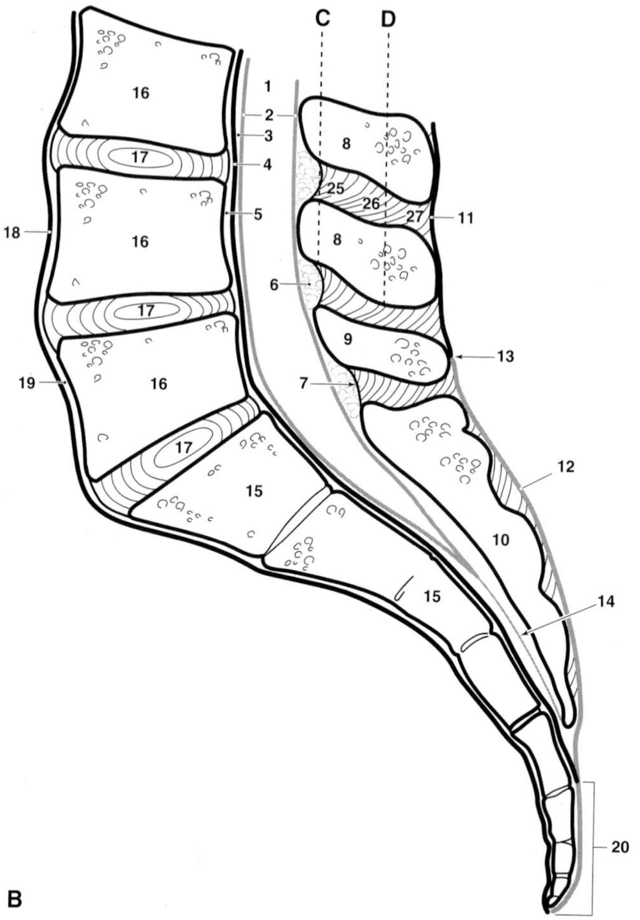

B

Figure 7A-39B: Midline sagittal schematic of the lumbosacral spinal ligaments and related spaces.

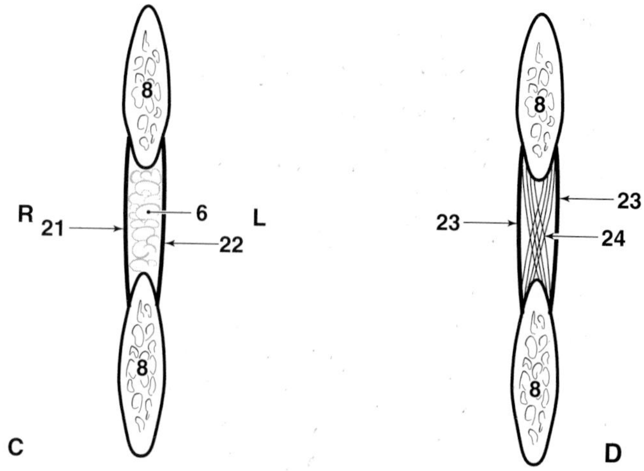

C

D

Figure 7A-39C: Coronal schematic through anterior aspect of interspinous ligament and adjacent spinous processes.
Figure 7A-39D: Coronal schematic through mid-aspect of interspinous ligament and adjacent spinous processes. *R*, right; *L*, left

1 Spinal subarachnoid space
2 Thecal sac
3 Anterior epidural space
4 Posterior longitudinal ligamemt
5 Retrovertebral subligamentous space
6 Retrothecal fat pad (posterior epidural space)
7 Junction of halves of interspinous ligament with the ligamenta flava
8 Normal spinous processes of L-3 and L-4
9 Normally hypoplastic spinous process of L-5
10 Midline sacral spinous tubercles
11 Supraspinous ligament
12 Erector spinae muscle tendons and deep fibers of the lumbosacral fascia
13 Variation in termination of supraspinous ligament (L-3 to L-5)
14 Filum terminale
15 Sacral spinal segments
16 Lumbar vertebral bodies
17 Lumbar intervertebral discs
18 Anterior longitudinal ligament
19 Prevertebral subligamentous space
20 Coccyx
21 Right half of interspinous ligament anteriorly
22 Left half of interspinous ligament anteriorly
23 Combined right and left halves of the interspinous ligament in its middle and posterior extent
24 Fibers of interspinous ligament shown crossing the midline
25 Anterior (ventral) segment of interspinous ligament originating in ligamenta flava on each side and terminating in inferior margin of the suprajacent craniad spinous process*
26 Middle segment of interspinous ligament originating in superior margin of the subajacent spinous process and terminating in the inferior margin of the suprajacent spinal process*
27 Posterior (dorsal) segment of interspinous segment originating in the superior margin of the subjacent spinous process and terminating in the supraspinous ligament (at levels where it exists: C-1 to L-5) or the erector spinae muscle tendons (below the level of the termination supraspinous ligament)*

*Note the posterocranial orientation of the fibers of the interspinous ligament. *C*, level of section in Figure 7A-39C; *D*, level of section in Figure 7A-39D.

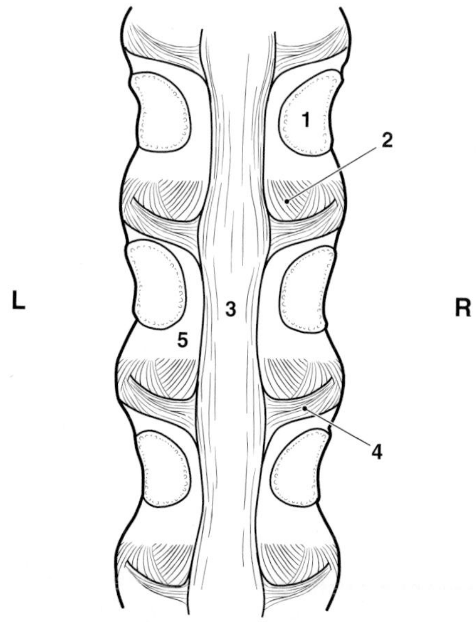

E

Figure 7A-39E: Posterior schematic of the spinal ligaments. The posterior vertebral elements, thecal sac, and neural elements have been removed. *R*, right; *L*, left.
1 Cut edge of pedicle
2 Outer fibers of the anulus fibrosus of the intervertebral disc
3 Posterior longitudinal ligament
4 Lateral extension of the posterior longitudinal ligament
5 Vertebral body

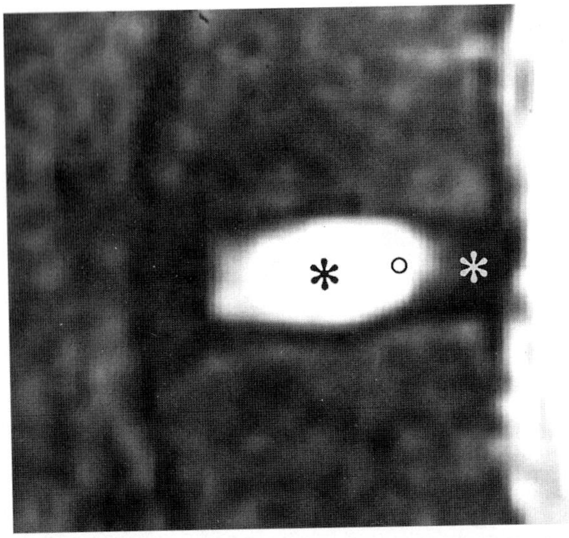

Figure 7A-40A: The intervertebral disc. Sagittal T2-weighted MR image of a lumbar intervertebral disc showing a hyperintense nucleus pulposus (*black asterisk*) centrally and hypointense peripheral annulus fibrosus fibers (*white asterisk*). Note the lack of definition between the border of the nucleus pulposus and the central anular fibers (*circle*).

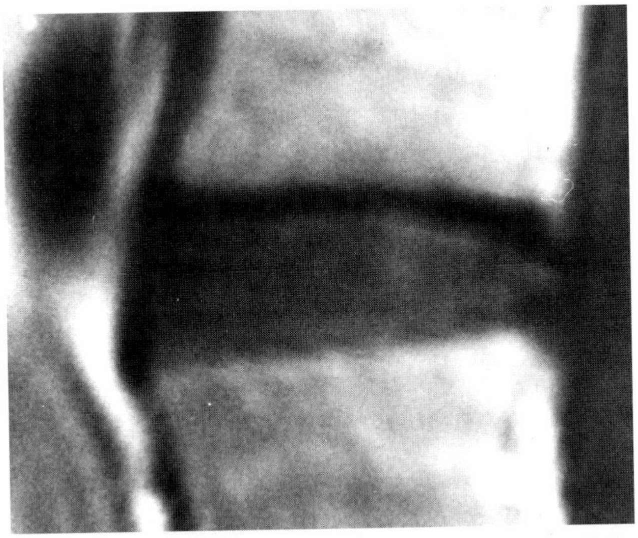

Figure 7A-40B: Normal intervertebral disc enhancement. Sagittal T1-weighted MR image showing a normal L4-5 intervertebral disc. Note the typical wedge configuration, narrower posteriorly than anteriorly.

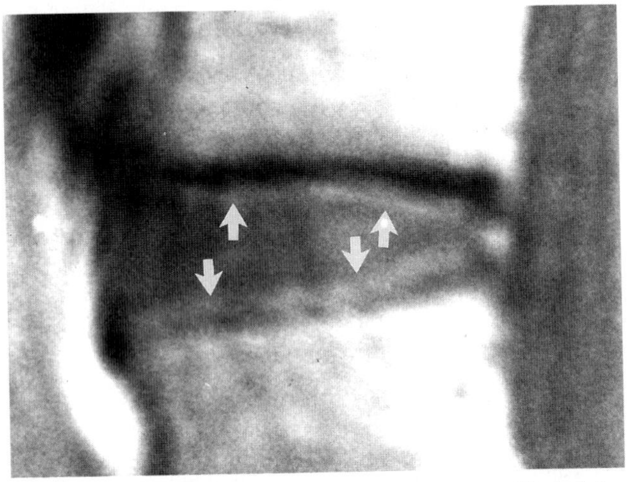

Figure 7A-40C: Sagittal "triple-dose" (0.3 mmol/kg), intravenous gadolinium-enhanced, time-delayed (45-minute) MR image in same case as that in Figure 7A-40B, showing intravertebral disc enhancement (*arrows*) paralleling the vertebral end plates. This represents normal diffusion of contrast medium into the disc from the vascularized vertebral end plates. Compare with Figure 7A-40B.

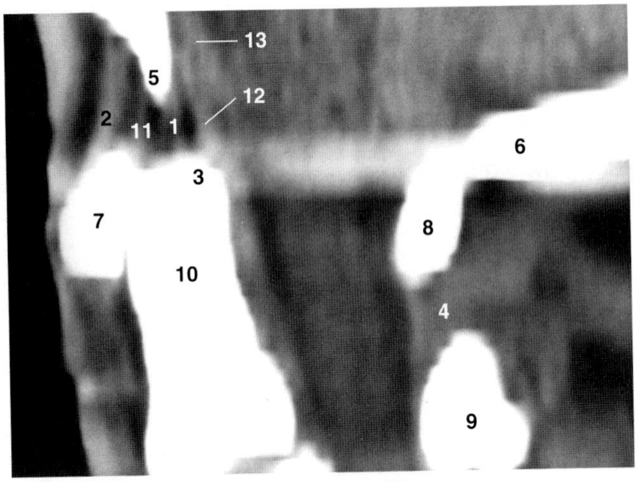

Figure 7A-40D: Craniovertebral ligaments. Sagittal CT reconstruction at the craniovertebral junction showing the ligamentous and bony structures.

1 Apical ligament
2 Anterior longitudinal ligament
3 Posterior longitudinal ligament, cruciate ligament
4 Interspinous ligament at C2-3
5 Basion
6 Opisthion
7 Anterior arch of C-1
8 Posterior arch of C-1
9 Posterior arch of C-2
10 Odontoid process (dens)
11 Anterior atlantooccipital membrane
12 Superior longitudinal band of cruciate ligament
13 Membrane tectoria

SPINAL LIGAMENT VARIANTS

- Hypoplastic/aplastic spinal ligaments (theoretical)
- Calcification/ossification of the spinal ligaments (pathologic)
- Hypertrophy/redundancy of the spinal ligaments (aging; degenerative–pathologic)

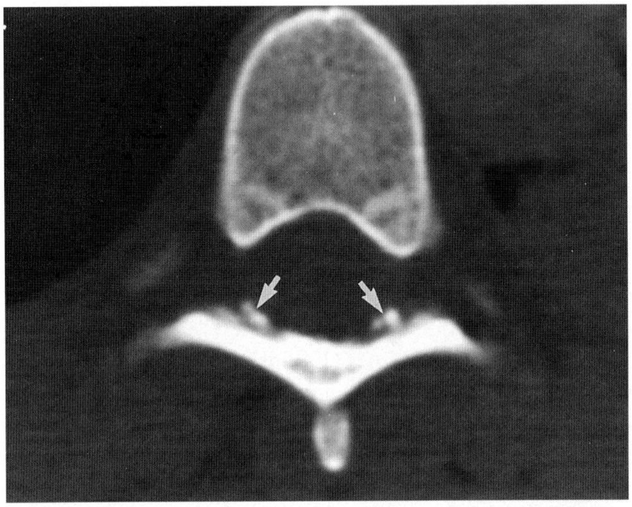

A

Figure 7A-41A: Ligamentum flavum insertion ossification. Axial CT in the thoracic region showing normal ossifications (*arrows*) at the insertions of the ligamenta flava.

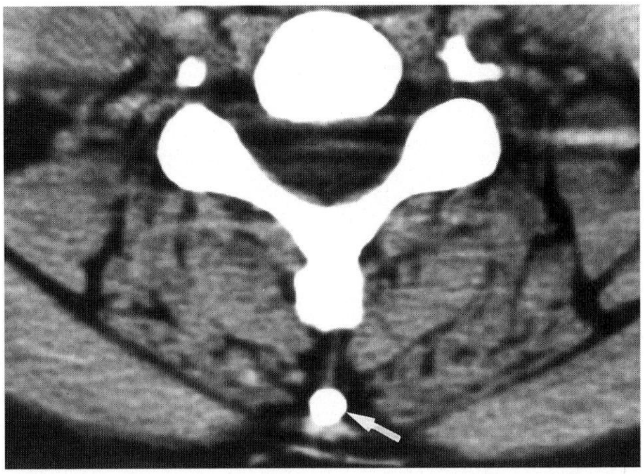

B

Figure 7A-41B: Ossification of the ligamentum nuchae. Axial CT showing ossification of the ligamentum nuchae (*arrow*).

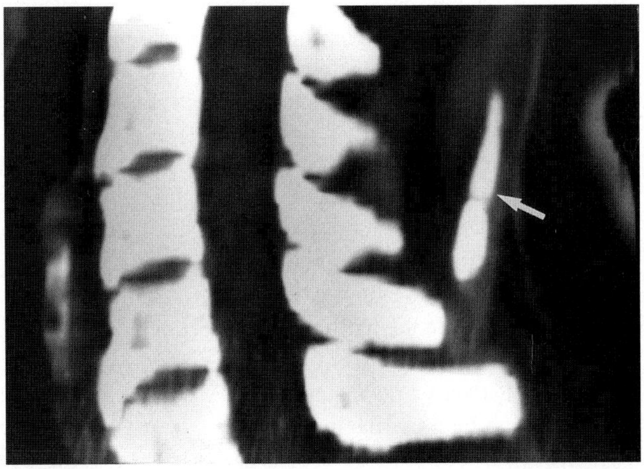

C

Figure 7A-41C: Sagittal CT reconstruction of same case as that in 7A-41B, showing the ligamentum nuchae ossification (*arrow*).

OSSIFICATION OF THE VERTEBRAL COLUMN

Ossification of the C-1 (Atlas) Vertebrae

1. The first cervical vertebrae has three primary ossification centers: one for the anterior arch and one each for the two regions consisting of the lateral masses and halves of the posterior vertebral neural arch.
2. Synchondroses form anteriorly and between the anterior arch and the paired posterior neural arches [*arconeural synchondrosis* (Jinkins)], and posteriorly between the two ossification centers of the bony neural arch [*intraneural synchondrosis* (Jinkins)].
3. The first cervical vertebra has no secondary ossification centers.

Ossification of the C-2 (Axis) Vertebra

1. The second cervical vertebra has five primary ossification centers: one in the centrum, one in each half of the posterior vertebral neural arch, and one in each half of the shaft or stem of the odontoid process.
2. Secondary ossification centers are two in number and occur at the apex of the odontoid process and at the anular epiphysis inferior to the centrum of C2. The apical ossification center, the cuneiform cartilage, appears late, usually at 5 to 8 years of life. It usually fuses with the main mass of the odontoid process by age 12 years.
3. Synchondroses form between the ossification centers of the shaft of the odontoid process and the centrum [*odontocentral synchondrosis* (Jinkins)]; the shaft of the odontoid and the ossification centers of the posterior neural arches (odontoneural synchondrosis), the posterior neural arches and the centrum (neurocentral synchondrosis); between the posterior neural arch in the midline posteriorly (intraneural synchondrosis); between the paired primary ossification centers of the odontoid shaft [*longitudinal intraodontoid shaft synchondrosis* (Jinkins)], and between the paired ossification centers of the odontoid shaft and the secondary ossification center of the odontoid tip/apex (the cuneiform cartilage) [*apical intraodontoid synchondrosis* (Jinkins)].
4. The base of the odontoid process at its junction with the body of C-2 is separated during development by a cartilaginous disc. This disc may represent an embryologic remnant of the C1-2 intervertebral disc; there may be contained rudiments of the adjacent epiphyses of the atlas and axis. The disc may remain cartilaginous until old age.

The Ossification of C-3 to C-6 and T-1 to T-12 Vertebrae

1. The typical vertebra (C-3 to L-5) ossifies from three primary vertebral ossification centers: one in the centrum and one in each half of the posterior vertebral (neural) arch. For the centrum, the earliest ossification occurs in the lower thoracic and upper lumbar regions in the ninth to tenth week of gestation and progresses thereafter craniocaudally.
2. During the first postnatal years, the centrum is connected to the posterior vertebral neural arch by a cartilaginous synchondrosis, the neurocentral synchondrosis. A similar cartilagineous synchondrosis exists at the junction of the two halves of the neural arch in the midline posteriorly, which might be called the *intraneural synchondrosis* (Jinkins). These synchondroses normally unite sometime between birth and age 6 years.
3. It should be noted that the centrum is not synonymous with the vertebral body. The posterolateral portions of the vertebral body are formed from the anterior extents of the posterior neural arch ossification centers. Thus, the centrum during development constitutes less than the volume of the adult vertebral body, and the posterior neural arch ossification center makes up more than the posterior bony neural arch proper.

4. Around the time of puberty, five secondary vertebral ossification centers appear: one at the apex of the spinous and each transverse process, and one at each anular epiphysis abutting the intervertebral disc on the upper and lower surfaces of the vertebral body. Bifid spinous processes will naturally have two secondary ossification centers.

Ossification of the C-7 Vertebra

1. Paired primary ossification centers are present in the C-7 vertebra for the costal processes.
2. These ossification centers usually appear at 6 months of age and fuse with the transverse processes and vertebral body between the fifth and sixth years.
3. Occasionally, these coastal processes remain separate to form cervical ribs associated with C-7. Very rarely cervical ribs form on the C-4, C-5, and/or C-6 vertebrae.

Ossification of the L-1 to L-5 Vertebrae

In addition to the typical primary and secondary vertebral ossification centers, two additional secondary centers are present at the base of the mamillary processes on each side, representing vestiges of the costal elements at this level in the spine. These secondary ossification centers or epiphyses fuse with the primary ossification centers at approximately 25 years of age. Other secondary or accessory or ossification centers peculiar to this level of the spine include the apices of the articular processes of the zygapophyseal joints and the accessory processes.

Ossification of the Sacrum

Typical primary ossification centers include one for the centrum and two for the posterior neural arch. Two additional primary centers appear for the costal element remnants.

Ossification of the Coccyx

1. The first coccygeal segment has a single primary ossification center for its centrum and two additional primary centers for the coccygeal cornua.
2. The remaining coccygeal segments have a single ossification center.
3. There are no secondary coccygeal ossification centers.
4. While the first coccygeal segment begins to ossify shortly after birth, the remaining segments ossify at different times up to the twentieth year of life.
5. The various coccygeal segments fuse irregularly between segments over a period of 30 years or more; in later life the coccyx may unite with the sacrum.

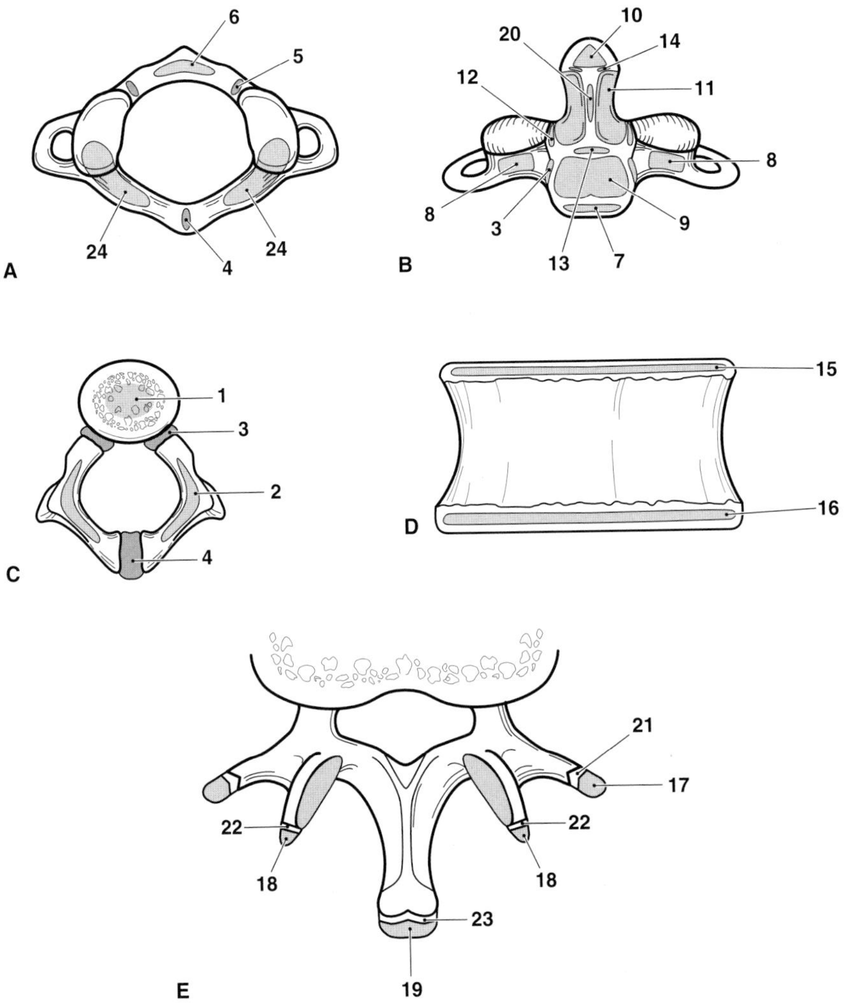

Figure 7A-42: Schematics of the ossification centers and synchondroses of the vertebral column. **A:** Primary ossification centers of C-1 at 8 weeks. **B:** Primary and secondary ossification centers of C-2. **C:** Primary ossification centers of typical midcervical vertebra at 8 weeks. **D:** Secondary ossification centers of epiphyseal plates of vertebral body at puberty. **E:** Secondary ossification centers of lumbar vertebrae.

1 Primary ossification center of centrum of C-3 (eighth week)
2 Primary ossification centers of neural arch of C-3 (eighth week)
3 Neurocentral synchondrosis(es)
4 Posterior median intraneural synchondrosis
5 Arconeural synchondrosis(es)
6 Primary ossification center of anterior arch of C-1(first year)
7 Secondary ossification center of the vertebral body of C-2 (puberty)
8 Primary ossification centers of the neural arch of C-2 (7 to 8 weeks)
9 Primary ossification center of the centrum of C-2 (vertebral body) (fourth month)
10 Secondary ossification center of apex of odontoid process (cuneiform cartilage) (5 to 8 years)
11 Bilateral primary ossification centers for the stem of the odontoid process (sixth month)
12 Odontoneural synchondrosis
13 Odontocentral synchondrosis
14 Apical intraodontoid synchondrosis
15 Secondary ossification center of epiphyseal plate of upper surface of centrum (vertebral body) (puberty)
16 Secondary ossification center of epiphyseal plate of lower surface of centrum (vertebral body) (puberty)
17 Secondary ossification center of the transverse process(es) (puberty)
18 Secondary ossification center of the mamillary process(es) (puberty) (lumbar vertebrae)
19 Secondary ossification center of the spinous process(es)
20 Longitudinal intraodontoid synchondrosis (secondary)
21 Intratransverse synchondrosis (secondary)
22 Mammillozygapophyseal synchondrosis (secondary)
23 Intraspinous synchondrosis (secondary)
24 Primary ossification center(s) of neural arch of C-1

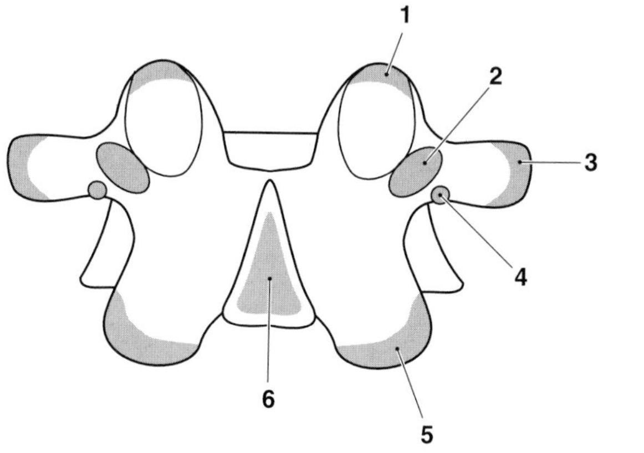

Figure 7A-43: Schematic of posterior aspect of accessory ossification centers of the lumbar vertebrae.

1 Accessory ossification center of apex of superior articular process of posterior spinal facet (zygapophyseal) joint
2 Accessory ossification center of mamillary process
3 Accessory ossification center of apex of transverse process
4 Accessory ossification center of accessory process
5 Accessory ossification center of apex of inferior articular process of posterior facet (zygapophyseal) joint
6 Accessory ossification center of apex of spinous process

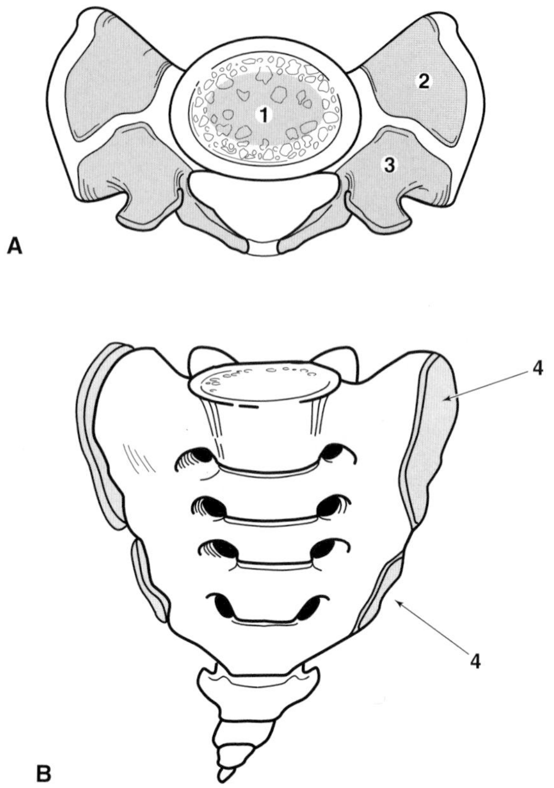

Figure 7A-44: Schematics of ossification centers of the sacrum. **A:** Primary ossification centers (4 years of age). **B:** Secondary ossification centers at sacroiliac joints (25 years of age.)

1 Primary ossification center for body (corpus)
2 Primary ossification center for costal element analog
3 Primary ossification center for vertebral arch analog
4 Secondary sacral ossification centers of epiphyseal plates for sacroiliac joints

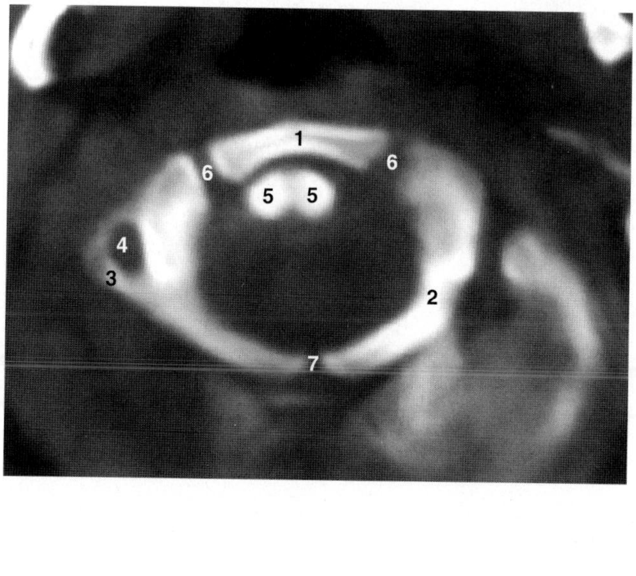

Figure 7A-45: Ossification centers and synchondroses of C-1. Axial CT image showing the developing atlas (C-1) in an infant.

1 Primary ossification center of the anterior bony arch of C-1
2 Primary ossification centers of the posterior bony neural arch of C-1
3 Transverse process of atlas (C-1)
4 Foramen transversarium
5 Paired primary ossification centers of the shaft of the odontoid process (dens) of C-2
6 Arcocentral synchondroses between the primary ossification centers of the anterior bony arch and the paired lateral centers of the lateral mass/posterior bony neural arch of C-1
7 Posterior-median intraneural synchondrosis between the paired primary centers of ossification in the posterior bony neural arch of C-1

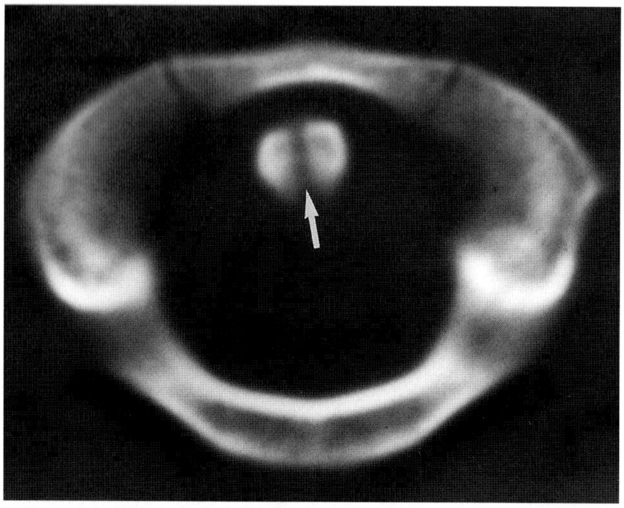

Figure 7A-46A: Ossification centers and synchondroses of C-2. Axial CT image showing the developing odontoid process. The paired primary ossification centers of the odontoid shaft are ossified but have not yet fused in the midline at the longitudinal intraodontoid synchondrosis (*arrow*).

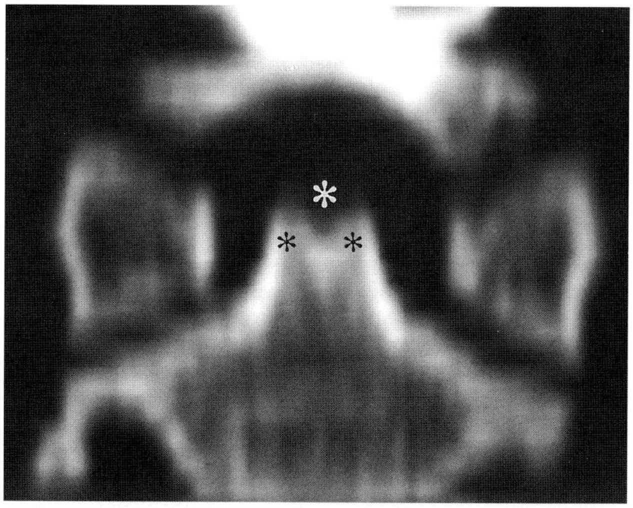

Figure 7A-46B: Reformatted CT image in the coronal plane showing the developing odontoid process. The primary ossification centers of the lateral masses of the odontoid shaft are ossified (*black asterisks*); however, the secondary ossification center of the odontoid tip apex (*white asterisk*) is not yet ossified. This secondary ossification center (cuneiform cartilage) lies in and just superior to the cleft in the upper aspect of the odontoid stem located beneath the *white asterisk*.

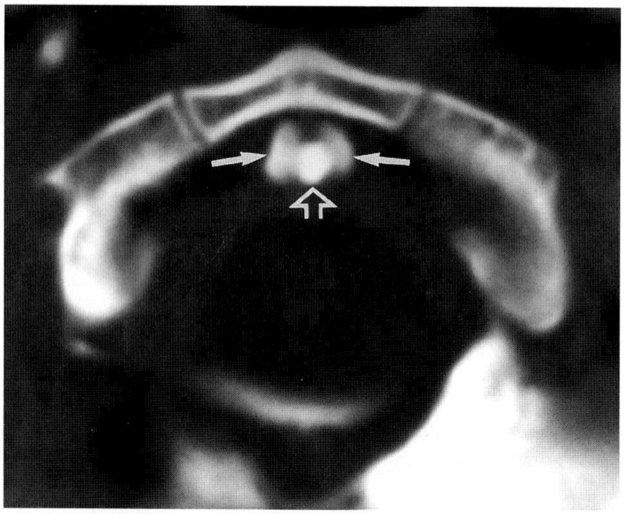

Figure 7A-46C: Axial CT images showing ossification of the paired lateral primary ossification centers of the shaft of the odontoid process (*closed arrows*) and the single midline secondary ossification center of the odontoid tip/apex (*open arrow*, cuneiform cartilage).

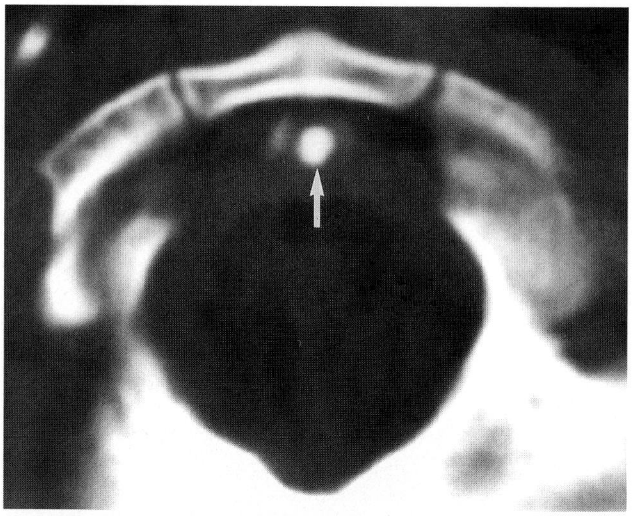

Figure 7A-46D: Axial CT image at a section above that of Figure 7A-46C showing the secondary ossification center of the tip/apex of the odontoid process (*arrow*, cuneiform cartilage).

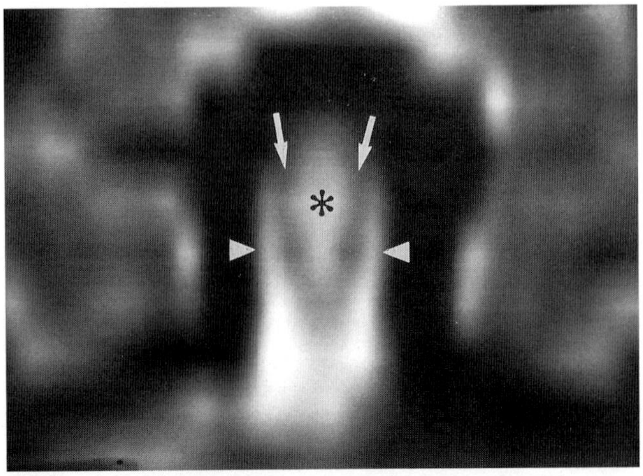

Figure 7A-46E: Odontoid ossification centers. Coronal CT reconstruction image in an adolescent showing the fusion of the single secondary ossification center of the odontoid apex (*asterisk:* cuneiform cartilage) with the paired fused primary ossification center (*arrowheads*) of the odontoid shaft. Note the apical intraodontoid synchondrosis (*arrows*).

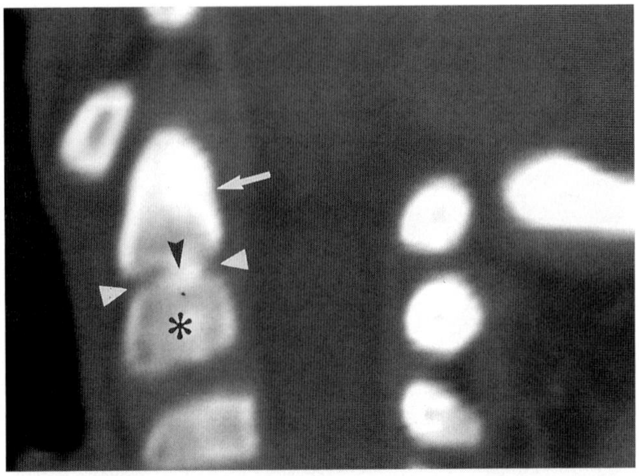

Figure 7A-46F: Sagittal CT reconstruction showing the odontocentral synchondrosis (*white arrowheads*) between the odontoid stem (*arrow*) and the ossification of the centrum of C-2 (*asterisk*). Some ossification of the odontocentral synchondrosis is taking place in the middle of the synchondrosis (*black arrowhead*).

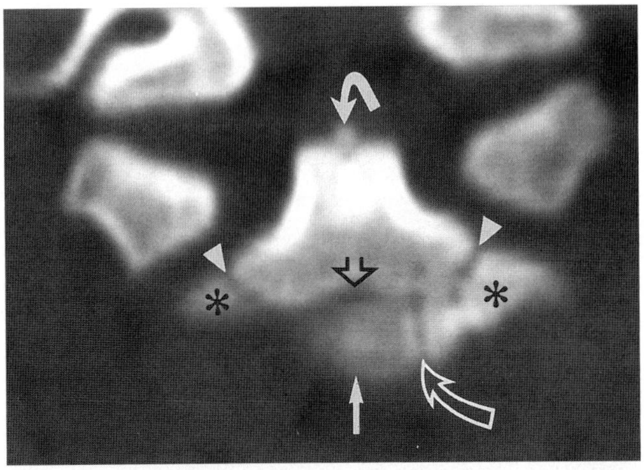

Figure 7A-46G: Coronal reconstruction showing the odontocentral synchondrosis (*open straight arrow*), the odontoneural synchondrosis (*arrowheads*), the centrum C-2 (*solid arrow*), the posterior bony neural arches of C-2 (*asterisks*), the unfused secondary ossification center of the odontoid tip/apex (*solid curved arrow,* cuneiform cartilage), and the neurocentral synchondrosis on the left (*open curved arrow*).

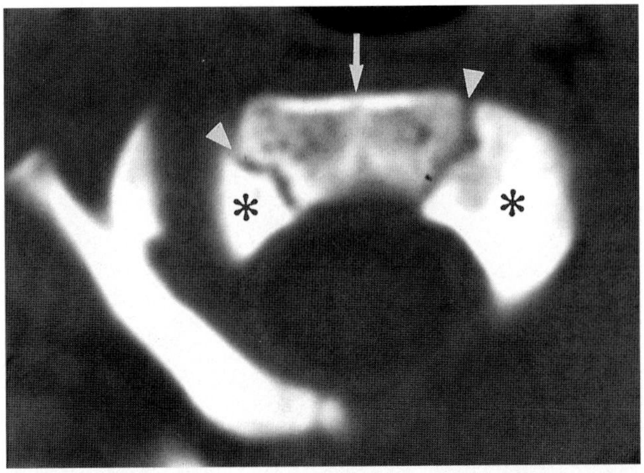

Figure 7A-46H: Axial CT image showing the odontoneural synchondroses (*arrowheads*) between the primary ossification centers of the base of the odontoid process (*arrow*) and the paired primary ossification centers (*asterisk*) of the posterior bony neural arch. The paired lateral ossification centers of the odontoid stem have already fused.

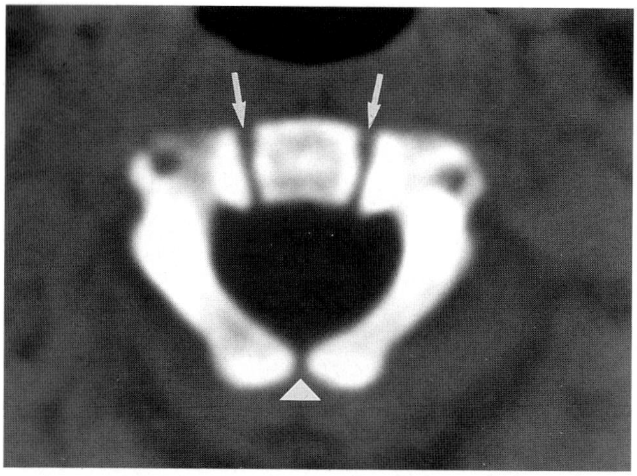

Figure 7A-46I: Axial CT image at a lower level than that of Figure 7A-46C showing the paired neurocentral synchondroses (*arrows*) and the single posterior intraneural synchondrosis (*arrowhead*).

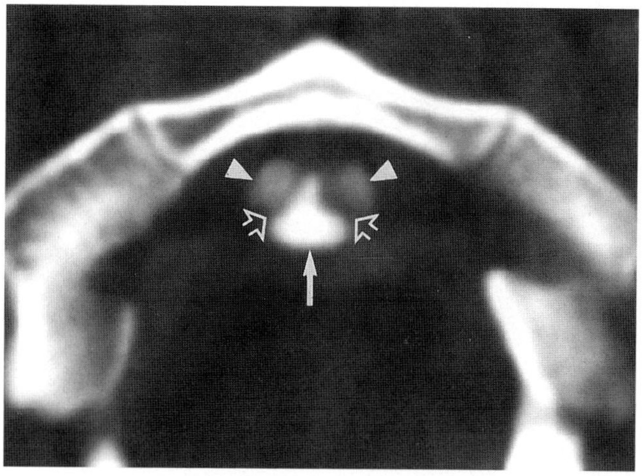

Figure 7A-46J: Axial CT image in an older child showing the developing odontoid process of C-2. The paired primary ossification centers of the lateral masses of the odontoid shaft are indicated (*arrowheads*), as is the unfused but ossifying secondary ossification center of the odontoid tip/apex (*solid arrow*, cuneiform cartilage). The apical intraodontoid synchondroses (*open arrows*) are also noted.

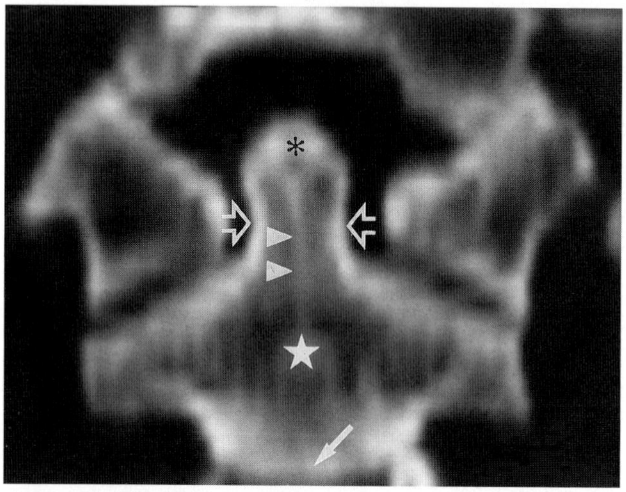

Figure 7A-46K: Reformatted CT image in the coronal plane in an adult showing C-2 ossification and fusion. The secondary ossification centers of the tip/apex of the odontoid (*asterisk*) and the epiphyseal plate (*straight arrow*), the paired primary ossification centers of the odontoid shaft (*open arrows*), and the centrum of C-2 (*star*) have fused across the various synchondroses. Sclerosis along the line of fusion (*arrowheads*) between the primary ossification centers of the odontoid shaft is also noted.

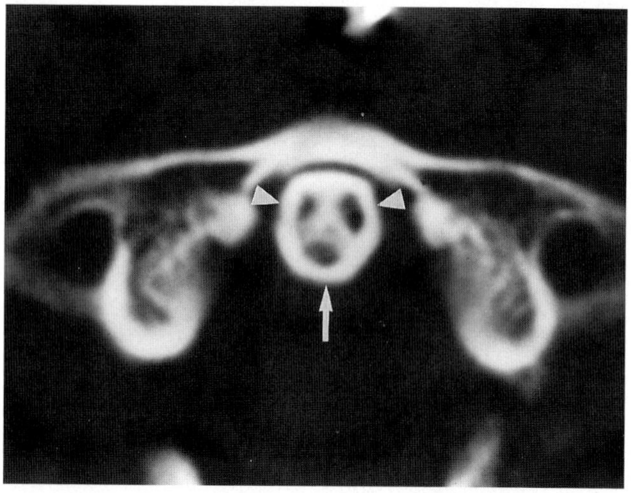

Figure 7A-46L: Axial CT image in an adult showing sclerosis at the sites of fusion of the junctions (synchondroses) between the two primary (*arrowheads*) and secondary (*arrow*) ossification centers of the odontoid process yielding an appearance of a three-spoked wheel ("Mercedes Benz") in the axial plane.

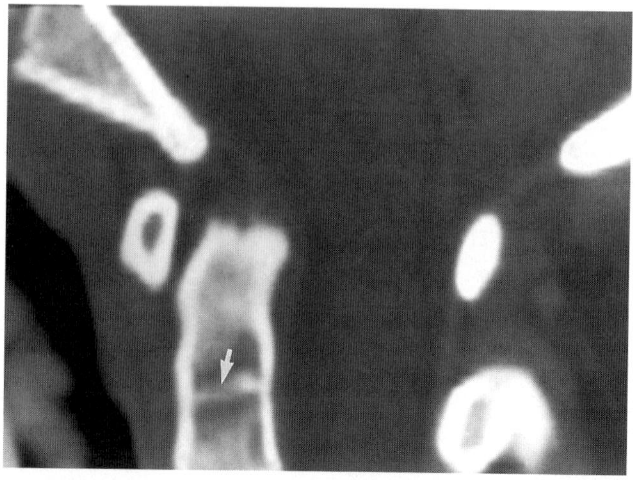

Figure 7A-47A: Odontocentral synchondrosis. Sagittal CT reconstruction in a child (7 years of age) showing a remnant of the odontocentral synchondrosis (*arrow*) representing the embryonic vestige of the C1-2 intervertebral disc.

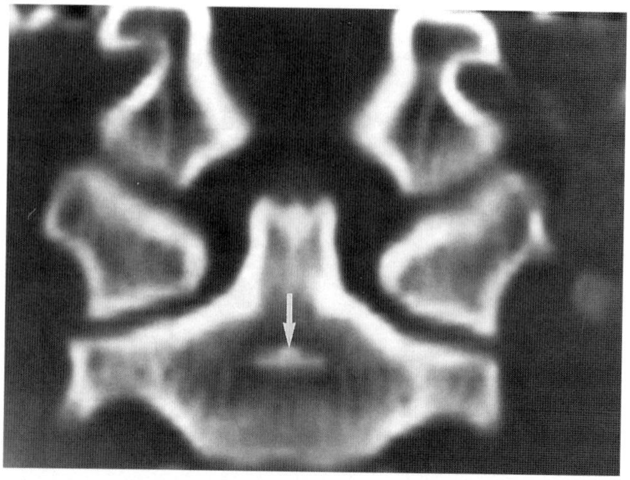

Figure 7A-47B: Odontocentral synchondrosis. Coronal CT reconstruction showing the vestige of the odontocentral synchondrosis (*arrow*).

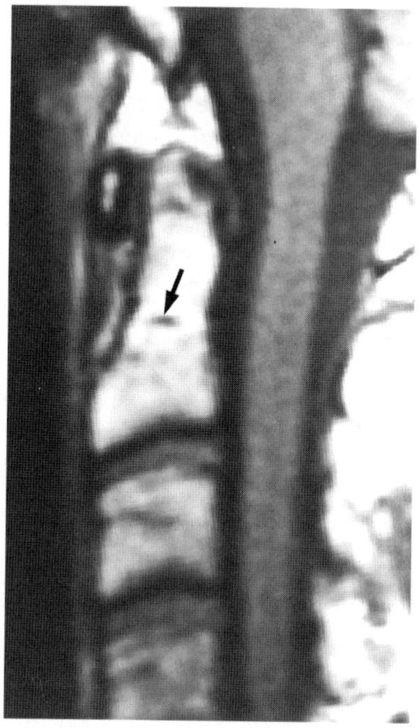

Figure 7A-48: Odontocentral synchondrosis. Magnified sagittal T1-weighted MR image shows the vestige of cartilaginous disc material (*arrow,* vestigal C1-2 intervertebral disc) at the junction of the base of the odontoid process and the body of C-2 (odontocentral synchondrosis).

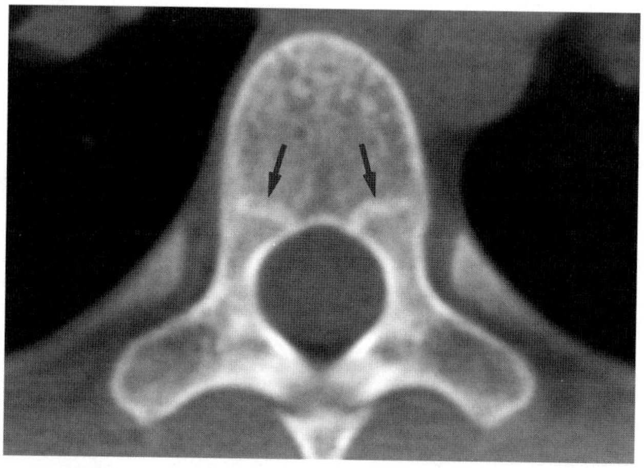

Figure 7A-49: Neurocentral synchondrosis. Axial CT image in an adolescent in the thoracic region showing sclerosis along the neurocentral synchondrosis between the paired posterior bony arch ossification centers and the unpaired ossification of the vertebral centrum (*arrows,* neurocentral synchondrosis).

7B Spinal Cord

OVERVIEW

1. The spinal cord gray matter is located deep with respect to the more superficially positioned spinal cord white matter.
2. The gray matter has a butterfly or "H" configuration in the axial plane. The two "wings" are connected by the anterior and posterior transverse gray commissures.
3. The gray matter of the spinal cord consists primarily of neurons, neurites, and neuroglia.
4. The gray matter is arranged into anterior (ventral) gray columns and posterior (dorsal) gray columns. A lateral gray column is also present at some levels (T-2 to L-1).
5. In the thoracic region, the volume of gray matter is relatively small; the volume of gray matter in the cervical and lumbar areas is greater because of the large number of neurons innervating the upper and lower extremities, respectively. This produces the characteristic cervical and lumbar spinal cord enlargements.
6. The central canal of the spinal cord longitudinally traverses the anterior and posterior transverse gray commissures and is normally only a potential space. It is composed primarily of ependymal cells encircled by a zone of neuroglia, neurons, and nerve fibers, known as the substantia gelantinosa centralis. The central canal runs the entire length of the spinal cord, broadens into the fourth ventricle cranially, at the obex and extends for 5 to 6 mm into the filum terminale caudally.
7. The white matter of the spinal cord consists largely, although not solely, of neural fibers that are arranged in longitudinal white columns or funiculi. The general groups of columns or funiculi are designated dorsal, lateral, and ventral.

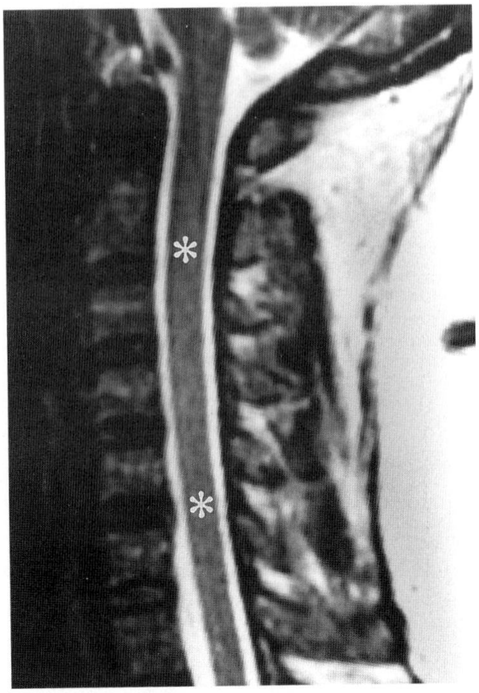

Figure 7B-1A: Cervical spinal cord. Sagittal T2-weighted MR image showing the cervical spinal cord (*asterisks*).

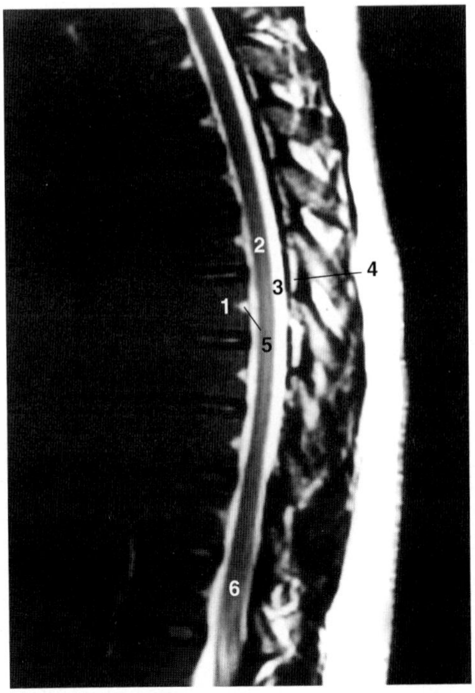

Figure 7B-1B: Thoracic spinal cord. Sagittal T2-weighted MR image showing the normal anatomy of the thoracic spinal cord.
1 Vertebral body
2 Midthoracic spinal cord
3 Spinal subarachnoid space
4 Retrothecal fat pad
5 Basivertebral vein/foramen
6 Conus medullaris

Figure 7B-1C: Conus medullaris. Sagittal T2-weighted MR image showing in detail the conus medullaris (*asterisks*) and upper cauda equina (*arrowheads*).

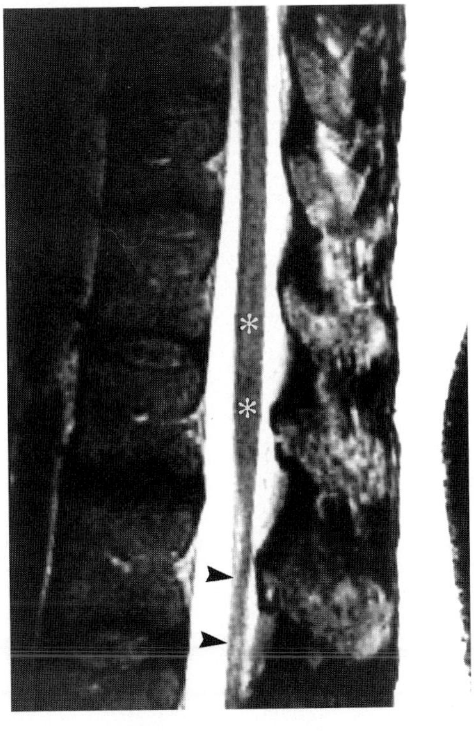

GRAY MATTER NUCLEI AND COLUMNS OF THE SPINAL CORD

1. The gray matter of the spinal cord is divided into longitudinally oriented columns and laminae.
2. The dorsal (posterior) gray column (horn) is primarily the site of termination of sensory fibers. The dorsal column (a) integrates and modulates sensory data, (b) acts as a relay area to pass on data to higher centers in the brainstem, cerebellum, and thalamus, and (c) serves as an integral part of reflex arcs.
3. The paired dorsal column nuclei (neuronal groups) include the posteromarginal nucleus (zone), the substantia gelatinosa, and the principal sensory nucleus (nucleus proprius); the dorsal nucleus of Clarke (nucleus dorsalis) extends solely from C-8 to L-3 or L-4.
4. The ventral (anterior) gray column (horn) consists primarily of lower motor neurons that innervate striated muscle.
5. The paired ventral columns (neuronal groups) include the medial motor column that innervates the axial musculature; the central motor column consisting of the phrenic nucleus (innervation of diaphragm musculature) and the lumbosacral nucleus (unknown function); and the lateral motor column present in the cervical and lumbar spinal cord enlargements that innervate the musculature of the extremities.
6. The intermediolateral (lateral or intermediate) cell column consists primarily of preganglionic sympathetic neurons; it is found only in the thoracic and lumbar levels. The intermediolateral cell column is involved in visceral functions and reflexes.
7. The laminae of Rexed basically represent a cytoarchitectonic map of the spinal cord gray matter. These laminae are based on the histologic size, shape, cytologic features, and density of neurons in the spinal cord gray matter. Nine or ten such laminae have been described; these laminae run the length of the spinal cord.

TABLE 7B-1: Major Spinal Cord Gray Matter Nuclei and Columns

Nucleus or column	Spinal levels	Function
Dorsal Columns/Nuclei		
Posteromarginal nucleus	All levels	All three nuclei receive primary sensory information; the first two appear to modulate this information, whereas the principal sensory nucleus is associated more with transmission to higher centers and with reflex connections
Substantia gelatinosa	All levels	
Principal sensory nucleus (nucleus proprius)	All levels	
Dorsal nucleus of Clarke (nucleus dorsalis)	C-8 to L3-4	Nucleus of origin of the dorsal spinocerebellar tract
Posteromarginal nucleus		
Substantia gelatinosa		
Principal sensory nucleus (nucleus proprius)		
Lateral Column		
Intermediolateral nucleus (column)	C-8, to T1-2 to L1-3	Centers for autonomic reflexes; nuclei of origin of sympathetic and parasympathetic preganglionic fibers
Intermediomedial nucleus (column)	T1-2 to L1-3	
Sacral parasympathetic gray column	S-2 to S-4	
Ventral Columns		
Medial motor column	All levels	Lower motor neurons innervating axial musculature
Central motor column		
Phrenic nucleus	C-3 to C-7	Lower motor neurons innervating diaphragm
Lumbosacral nucleus	L-2 to S-1	Unknown
Lateral motor column	C-5 to T-1 and 1 to S-3	Lower motor neurons innervating muscles of the upper extremity Lower motor neurons innervating muscles of the lower extremity

Modified from Burt AM. Major spinal cord nuclei and columns. In: *Textbook of neuroanatomy*. Philadelphia: WB Saunders, 1993:128.

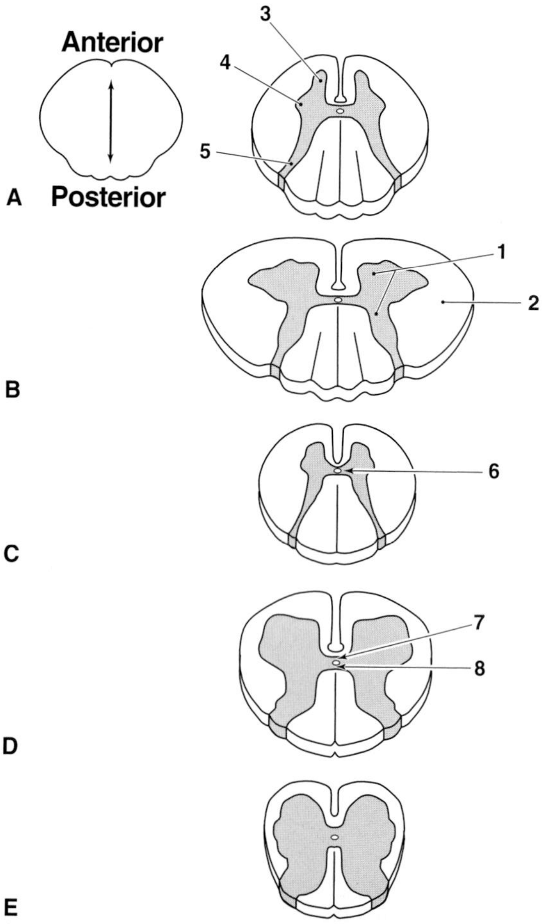

Figure 7B-2 Top: Axial schematics of the configuration of the gray/white matter at different segments of the spinal cord. **A:** Upper cervical segment. **B:** Lower cervical segment. **C:** Thoracic segment. **D:** Lumbar segment. **E:** Sacral segment.

1 Deep gray matter
2 Superficial white matter
3 Anterior gray column (ventral horn)
4 Lateral gray column (intermediolateral column)
5 Posterior gray column (dorsal horn)
6 Central canal of spinal cord (potential space)
7 Anterior transverse gray commissure
8 Posterior transverse gray commissure

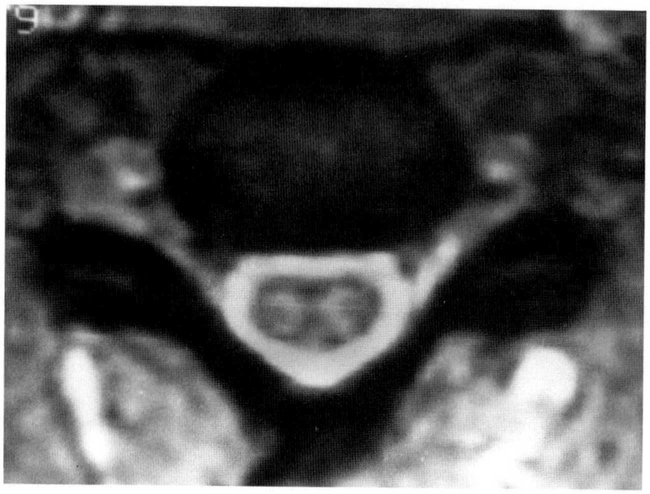

Figure 7B-2 Bottom: Magnetic resonance image of the gray/white matter of the spinal cord. Axial T2-weighted image showing the normal appearance of the gray and white matter in the spinal cord.

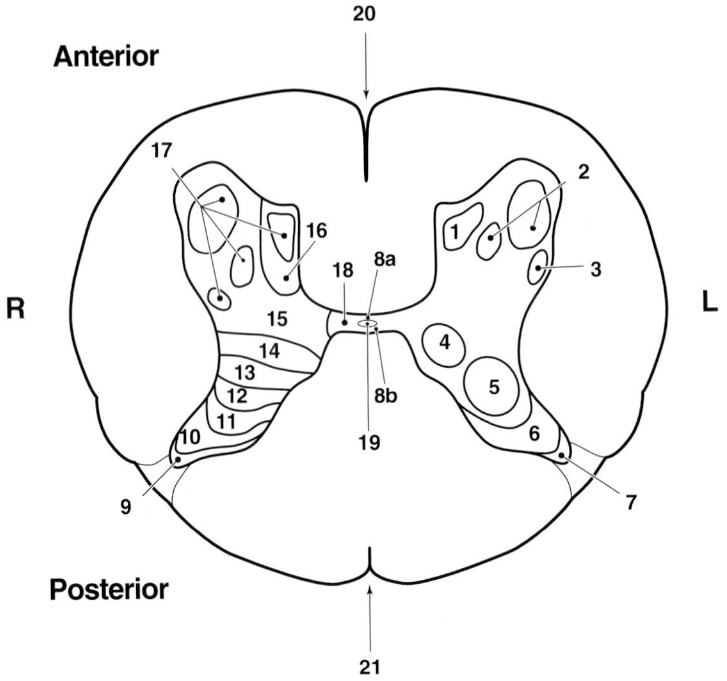

Figure 7B-3: Axial schematic of the spinal cord showing a composite of the gray matter columnar and nuclear organization (1–8), and Rexed's laminae (9–18). *R,* right; *L,* left.

1 Medial motor column
2 Lateral motor column
3 Intermediolateral cell column
4 Nucleus dorsalis (dorsal nucleus of Clarke)
5 Principal sensory nucleus (nucleus proprius)
6 Substantia gelatinosa
7 Posteromarginal nucleus
8 Anterior (a) and posterior (b) transverse central gray commissure
9 Lamina I
10 Lamina II
11 Lamina III
12 Lamina IV
13 Lamina V
14 Lamina VI
15 Lamina VII
16 Lamina VIII
17 Lamina IX
18 Lamina X
19 Central canal of spinal cord (potential space)
20 Anterior median fissure
21 Posterior median fissure

ASCENDING AND DESCENDING TRACTS OF THE SPINAL CORD

Ascending or descending neural fibers of the spinal cord are grouped into tracts or fasciculi according to function. These tracts are generally named according to origin and termination.

Ascending Spinal Tracts

1. Ascending tracts transmit somatosensory data. These ascending tracts run in three columns of the white matter: the dorsal, lateral, and ventral columns.
2. The functions of the ascending pathways include (a) conscious sensation (somatic, visceral), (b) reflex mediation (somatic, visceral), and (c) motor center guidance (cerebellum, brain stem, diencephalon, basal ganglia, cerebrum).
3. Ascending pathways mediating conscious sensation include the lateral spinothalamic tract (pain, temperature), anterior (ventral) spinothalamic tract (touch), and the dorsal columns (fasciculus gracilis and cuneatus: touch, form, texture, position sense).
4. Ascending pathways mediating unconscious sensation include the dorsal and ventral spinocerebellar tracts (coordination) and the spinoreticular/spinotectal tracts (somatic and visceral reflexes). The viscerosensory autonomic tracts, controlling breathing, elimination, blood pressure, pulse, sweating, other glandular secretions, and gastrointestinal/colonic motility, are found primarily in the ventrolateral quadrant of the spinal cord and travel with the ventral and lateral spinothalamic tracts.

Descending Spinal Tracts

1. The sources of descending tracts are either in the spinal cord/dorsal nerve roots or in the cerebral cortex and brain stem. No descending spinal tracts originate in the cerebellum, diencephalon, or basal ganglia.
2. The largest descending spinal tracts are the corticospinal tracts: the lateral corticospinal tract (crossed innervation of motor neurons: major) and the ventral (anterior) corticospinal tract (uncrossed innervation of motor neurons: minor). The corticospinal tracts mediate voluntary contraction of skeletal muscles.
3. The descending tracts from the brain stem include the tectospinal tract (in response to reflex movements in head and neck), rubrospinal tract (precise, well-controlled movements), coeruleospinal tract (modulation of sensory input, control of autonomic and somatic motor neuron activity), vestibulospinal tract (modulation of lower motor neuron activity in response to vestibular sensory information), reticulospinal tracts (affects somatic and visceral motor functions), and raphe spinal tract (inhibits the transmission of sensory signals entering the spinal cord). As noted above, the autonomic visceromotor tracts (together with the viscerosensory tracts) occupy the ventrolateral quadrant of the spinal cord, travel principally with the ventral and lateral spinothalamic tracts, and influence respiratory, gastrointestinal bladder, cardiovascular, and glandular activity.

Intersegmental and Intrasegmental Neural Fibers of the Spinal Cord

1. Intersegmental and intrasegmental neural fibers of the spinal cord relay information between different spinal segments and between the two sides of the spinal cord, respectively. These fibers either ascend and descend to different levels in the spinal cord (intersegmental) or cross the midline to the opposite side of the spinal cord (intrasegmental).
2. The largest number of intersegmental fibers ascend and descend within the fasciculus proprius to terminate on neurons at other levels of the spinal cord on the same side.
3. Intersegmental primary somatosensory fibers entering the spinal cord in the dorsal

nerve root bifurcate and ascend/descend in the dorsolateral fasciculus of Lissauer before terminating in the dorsal horn.

4. Intrasegmental spinal neural fibers cross the midline in the ventral (anterior) white commissure. These fibers originate and terminate on neurons in opposite sides of the spinal cord.

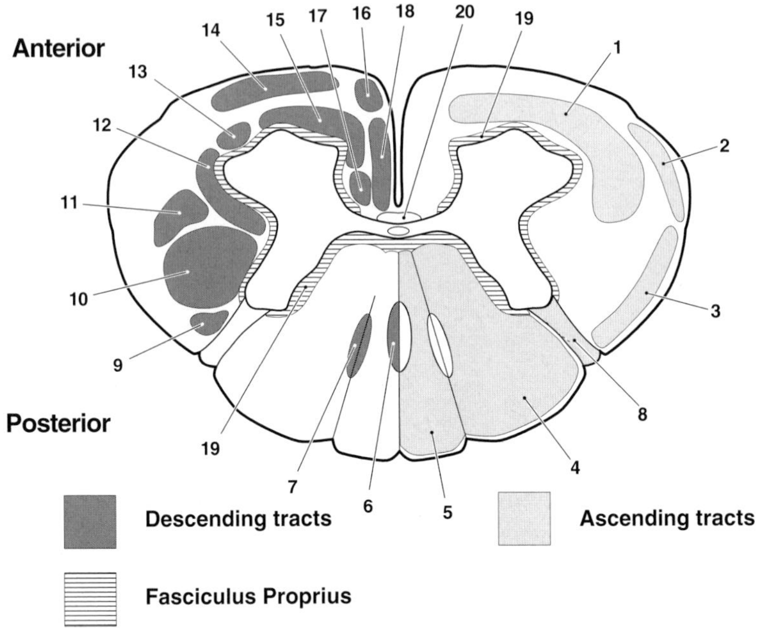

Figure 7B-4: Axial schematic of the spinal cord showing the ascending and descending tracts and the fasciculus proprius.

1 Anterolateral system [anterior (ventral) and lateral spinothalamic, spinotectal, spinoreticular tracts]
2 Ventral spinocerebellar tract
3 Dorsal spinocerebellar tract
4 Fasciculus cuneatus (dorsal column)
5 Fasciculus gracilis (dorsal column)
6 Septomarginal fasciculus
7 Interfascicular fasciculus
8 Dorsolateral fasciculus of Lissauer
9 Raphe spinal tract
10 Lateral corticospinal tract
11 Rubrospinal tract
12 Lateral reticulospinal tract
13 Lateral tectospinal tract
14 Vestibulospinal tract
15 Medial reticulospinal tract
16 Medial tectospinal tract
17 Medial longitudinal fasciculus
18 Ventral corticospinal tract
19 Fasciculus proprius
20 Ventral (anterior) white commissure

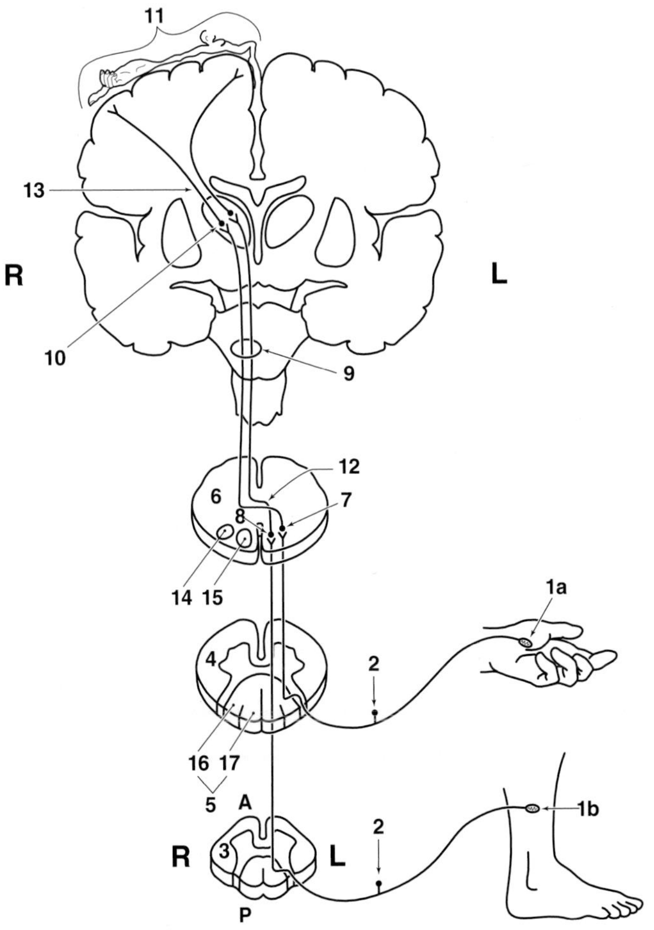

Figure 7B-5: Longitudinal schematic of the dorsal column (funiculus) showing the ascending somatosensory pathway for proprioception, touch-pressure, and vibratory sensation. *A,* anterior; *P,* posterior; *L,* left; *R,* right.

1 Receptors for proprioception (position sense), touch-pressure, and vibratory sensation in the upper (a) and lower (b) extremities
2 Primary sensory neuron in the dorsal root ganglion of the spinal nerve
3 Conus medullaris
4 Cervical spinal cord
5 Dorsal column
6 Medulla oblongata
7 Secondary sensory neuron in nucleus cuneatus
8 Secondary neuron in nucleus gracilis
9 Medial lemniscus
10 Ventral posterolateral nucleus of the thalamus (tertiary sensory neurons)
11 Postcentral gyrus (somatosensory cortex) with overlying somatotopic homunculus
12 Lemniscal decussation
13 Internal capsule
14 Nucleus cuneatus
15 Nucleus gracilis
16 Fasciculus cuneatus
17 Fasciculus gracilis

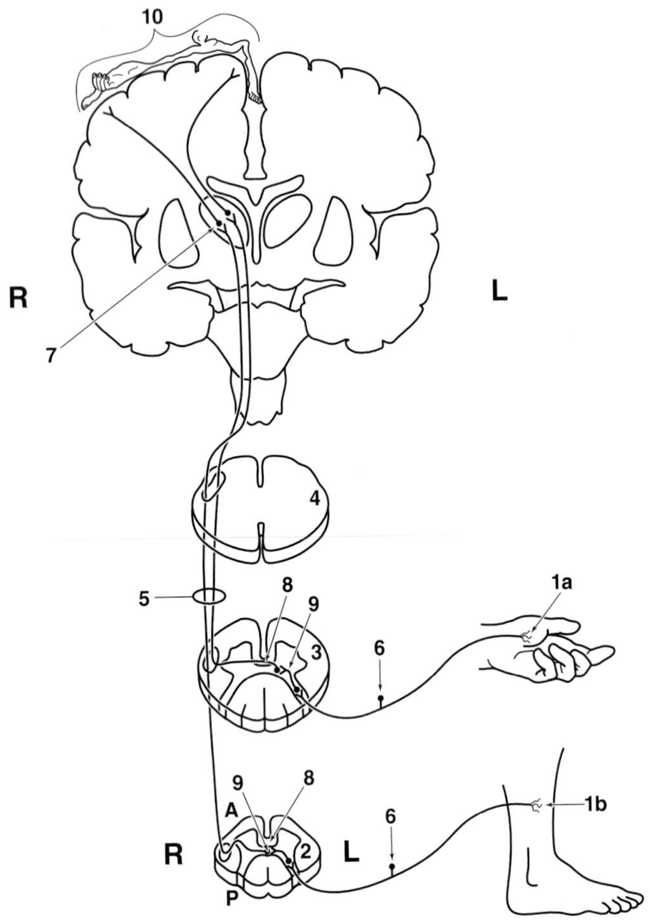

Figure 7B-6A: Longitudinal schematic of the lateral spinothalmic tract showing the ascending somatosensory pathway for pain and temperature. *A,* anterior; *P,* posterior; *R,* right; *L,* left.

1 Receptors for pain and temperature in the upper (a) and lower (b) extremities
2 Conus medullaris
3 Cervical spinal cord
4 Medulla oblongata
5 Lateral spinothalamic tract
6 Primary sensory neuron in the dorsal root ganglion of the spinal nerve
7 Ventral posterolateral nucleus of thalamus
8 Anterior white commissure of spinal cord
9 Spinal cord interneuron
10 Postcentral gyrus (somatosensory cortex) with overlying somatotopic homunculus

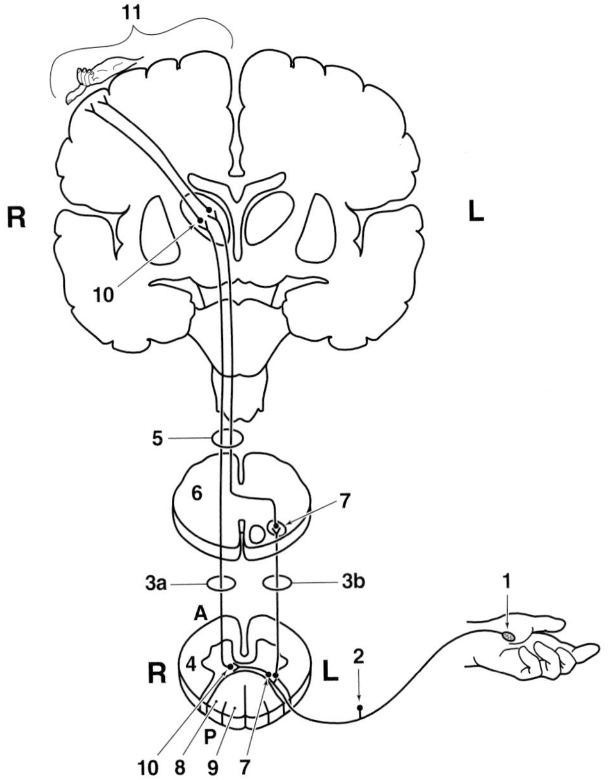

Figure 7B-6B: Longitudinal schematic of the anterior spinothalamic tract showing the ascending somatosensory pathway for light touch. *A,* anterior; *P,* posterior; *R,* right; *L,* left.

1 Receptor for light touch
2 Primary sensory neuron in the dorsal root ganglion of the spinal nerve
3a Crossed axons of ascending fibers in contralateral anterior spinothalamic tract
3b Uncrossed axons of ascending fibers in ipsilateral anterior spinothalamic tract
4 Lumbar spinal cord
5 Anterior spinothalamic tract
6 Lower medulla oblongata
7 Spinal cord interneuron
8 Nucleus cuneatus
9 Nucleus gracilis
10 Ventral posterolateral nucleus of thalamus
11 Postcentral gyrus (somatosensory cortex) with overlying somatotopic homunculus

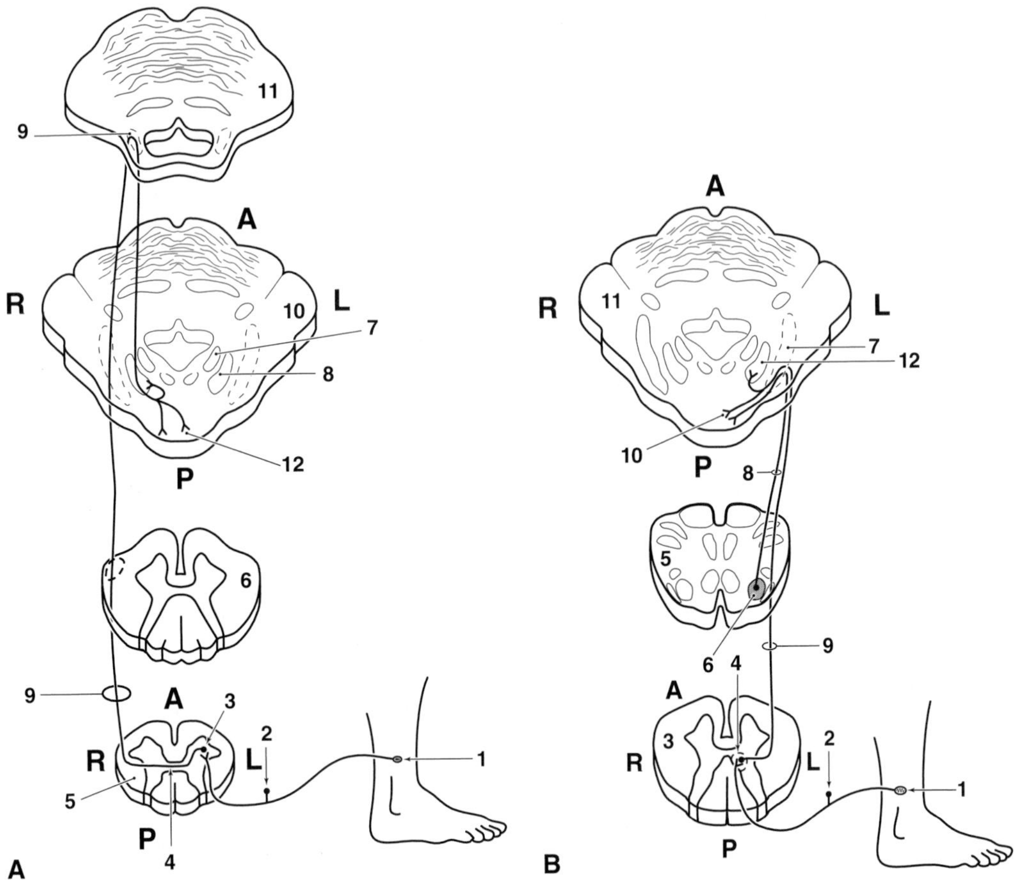

Figure 7B-7: Longitudinal schematic showing the spinocerebellar pathways that convey proprioceptive sensory impulses to the cerebellum. *A,* anterior; *P,* posterior; *R,* right; *L,* left.

A: Anterior (ventral) crossed spinocerebellar tract

1 Receptors in the golgi tendon organs
2 Sensory neuron in dorsal root ganglion
3 Nucleus in the anterior spinocerebellar tract
4 Axons crossing the gray matter commissure to contralateral side
5 Conus medullaris
6 Cervical spinal cord
7 Superior cerebellar peduncle
8 Dentate nucleus
9 Rostral loop of anterior (ventral) spinocerebellar tract
10 Lower pons
11 Upper pons
12 Cortex of cerebellar vermis

B: Posterior (dorsal) uncrossed spinocerebellar tract

1 Receptors in the golgi tendon organs, muscle spindles and pressure receptors
2 Sensory neuron in dorsal root ganglion
3 Conus medullaris
4 Nucleus dorsalis of Clarke (secondary neuron)
5 Caudal medulla oblongata
6 Accessory cuneate nucleus
7 Inferior cerebellar peduncle
8 Cuneocerebellar tract
9 Posterior spinocerebellar tract
10 Cortex of cerebellar vermis
11 Lower pons
12 Dentate nucleus

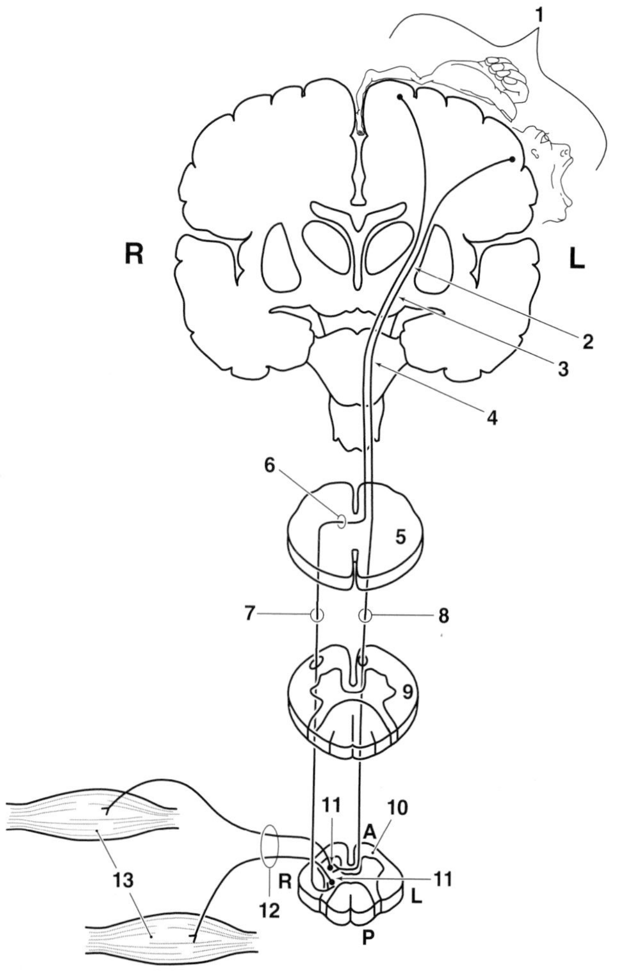

Figure 7B-8A: Longitudinal schematic of the uncrossed anterior (uncrossed motor function) and crossed lateral (crossed motor function) corticospinal (pyramidal) tracts. *A,* anterior; *P,* posterior; *R,* right; *L,* left.

1 Precentral gyrus (somatomotor cortex) with overlying somatotopic homunculus
2 Corticospinal tract in internal capsule
3 Corticospinal tract in cerebral peduncle/cruz cerebri
4 Corticospinal tract in upper brain stem
5 Medulla oblongata
6 Pyramidal decussation (corticospinal tract fibers)
7 Crossed lateral corticospinal tract
8 Uncrossed anterior (ventral) corticospinal tract
9 Cervical spinal cord
10 Conus medullaris
11 Lower motor neuron
12 Ventral root of spinal nerve
13 Skeletal muscle

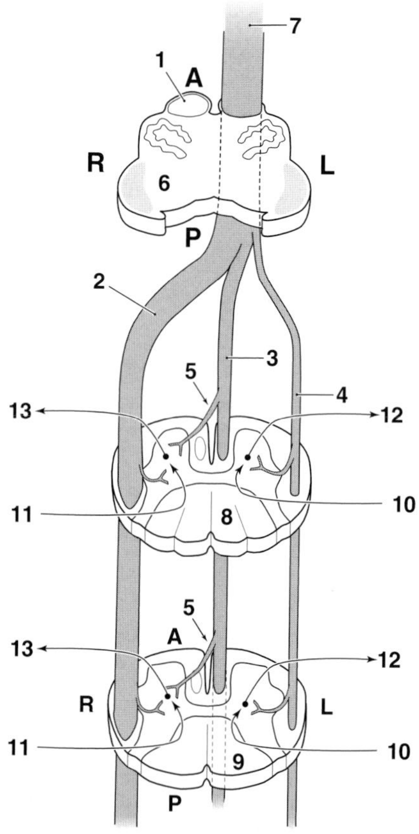

Figure 7B-8B: Detailed schematic of the corticospinal tracts. Ninety percent of fibers cross in lower medulla to descend in the contralateral lateral corticospinal tract. Eight percent of fibers do not cross in the medulla, but descend in the ipsilateral anterior corticospinal tract and cross at the level of the respective spinal segments at or near the exit from the spinal cord. Only 2% remain uncrossed in the ipsilateral corticospinal tract. *A,* anterior; *P,* posterior; *R,* right; *L,* left.

1 Medullary pyramid
2 Crossed (contralateral) lateral corticospinal tract (90%)
3 Uncrossed (ipsilateral) anterior (ventral) corticospinal tract (8%)
4 Uncrossed (ipsilateral) lateral corticospinal tract (2%)
5 Spinal segmental crossing of fibers of ipsilateral anterior (ventral) corticospinal tract
6 Medulla oblongata
7 Combined unilateral pyramidal tract above medulla oblongata
8 Cervical spinal cord
9 Lumbar spinal cord
10 Ipsilateral lower motor neuron
11 Contralateral lower motor neuron
12 To ipsilateral skeletal muscle
13 To contralateral skeletal muscle

SOMATOTOPIC REPRESENTATION OF THE SPINAL CORD

1. A general somatotopic organization can be found for motor function (e.g., flexors, extensors) and body regions in the anterior gray columns of the spinal cord.
2. A more precisely localized laminar somatotopic arrangement can be found in the dorsal funiculi (columns), the corticospinal tract, and the anterolateral columns (spinothalamic tracts). These laminae are organized largely by level of origin of the neural fibers and progress by sublaminae from the sacral through the lumbar and thoracic to the cervical levels.

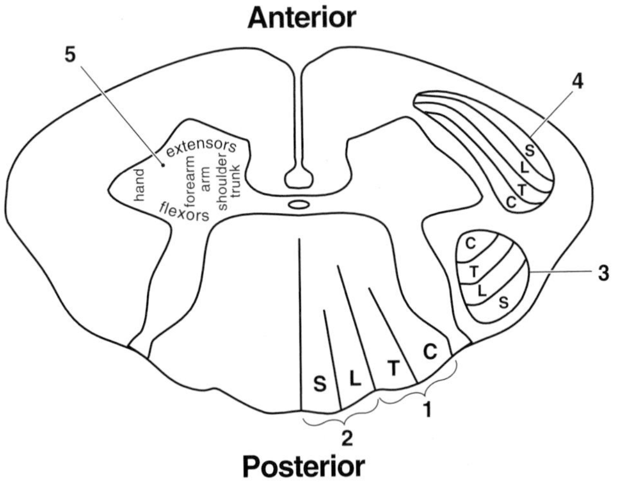

Figure 7B-9: Axial schematic showing the general somatotopic organization of the high cervical spinal cord. *C,* cervical somatotopic area; *T,* thoracic somatotopic area; *L,* lumbar somatotopic area; *S,* sacral somatotopic area.
1 Fasciculus cuneatus (dorsal column) (sensory)
2 Fasciculus gracilis (dorsal column) (sensory)
3 Lateral corticospinal tract (motor)
4 Anterior and lateral spinothalamic tracts (sensory)
5 Deep gray matter motor neurons (flexors, extensors)

7C SPINAL VASCULATURE

ARTERIAL SUPPLY TO THE SPINAL CORD AND SPINAL COLUMN

1. The arterial supply to the spinal cord is via a series of radiculomedullary arteries.
2. Because of the relatively greater longitudinal growth of the spinal column as compared to the spinal cord and nerve roots during embryogenesis, there is an effective developmental "stretching" of some of the lumbosacral radiculomedullary arteries, resulting in a craniad vascular diversion. This is especially marked in the lower thoracic region. One of the major radiculomedullary arteries to manifest this craniad arterial diversion is termed the artery of Adamkiewicz (arteria radicularis magna) supplying the lower thoracic cord to include the conus medullaris and nerve roots of the cauda equina.
3. The radiculomedullary arteries enter the spine with the spinal nerves via the intervertebral (neural) foramina and terminate in the spinal cord.
4. The major radiculomedullary arteries vary between individuals and differ irregularly among side of spinal entry, level of spinal entry, number, size, and artery of origin.
5. Radiculomedullary arteries may originate from the vertebral arteries, the ascending cervical artery (from the thyrocervical trunk), the deep cervical artery (from the costocervical trunk), the intercostal arteries, the lumbar and sacral paraspinal arteries, and the iliac arteries.

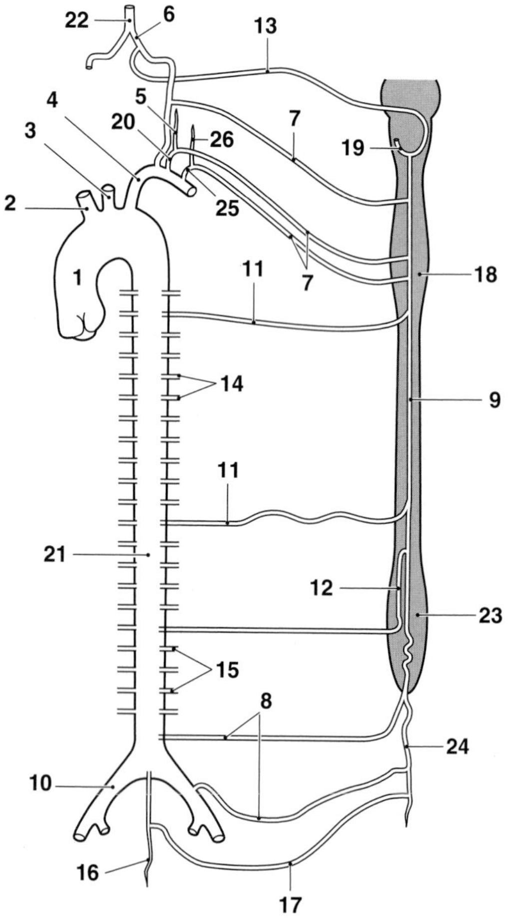

Figure 7C-1: Frontal schematic of the various potential major arterial routes to the spinal cord via the anterior spinal artery.

1 Aortic arch
2 Innominate artery
3 Left common carotid artery
4 Left subclavian artery
5 Ascending cervical artery
6 Left vertebral artery
7 Cervical anterior radiculomedullary arteries
8 Upper sacral anterior radiculomedullary arteries
9 Anterior spinal artery to spinal cord
10 Common iliac artery
11 Thoracic anterior radiculomedullary arteries
12 Artery of Adamkiewicz
13 Anterior radiculomedullary artery from left vertebral artery
14 Intercostal arteries
15 Lumbar paraspinal arteries
16 Median sacral artery
17 Lower sacral anterior radiculomedullary artery
18 Cervical spinal cord
19 Anterior radiculomedullary artery from right vertebral artery (resected)
20 Thyrocervical trunk
21 Descending aorta
22 Basilar artery
23 Conus medullaris
24 Major ascending/descending arterial radicle to cauda equina and filum terminale
25 Costocervical trunk
26 Deep cervical artery

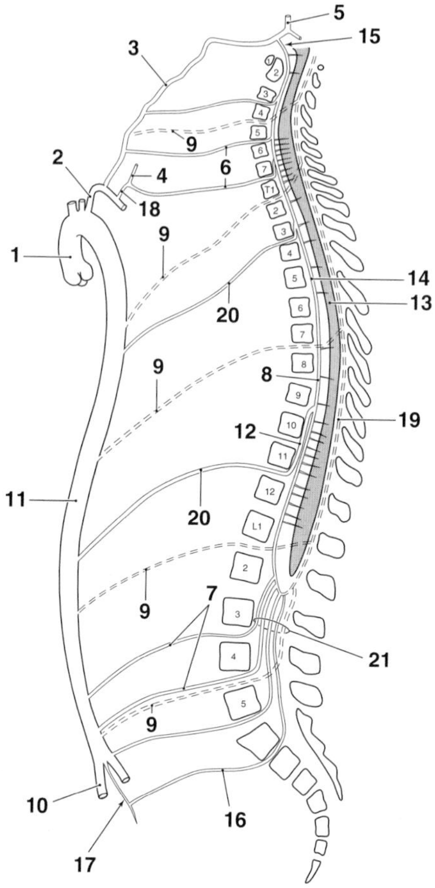

Figure 7C-2: Lateral schematic of the various potential major arterial supply routes to the spinal cord via the anterior and posterior spinal arteries. *Solid vascular wall,* feeding radiculomedullary arteries, anterior spinal artery(ies); *dashed vascular wall,* feeding radiculomedullary arteries, posterior spinal artery(ies). Vertebrae are individually numbered.

1 Aortic arch
2 Left subclavian artery
3 Left vertebral artery
4 Ascending cervical or deep cervical artery
5 Basilar artery
6 Cervical anterior radiculomedullary arteries
7 Lumbar anterior radiculomedullary arteries
8 Anterior spinal artery
9 Cervical, thoracic, lumbar, and sacral posterior radiculomedullary arteries
10 Common iliac artery
11 Descending aorta
12 Artery of Adamkiewicz
13 Spinal cord
14 Anterior spinal artery to spinal cord
15 Anterior radiculomedullary artery from vertebral artery
16 Sacral anterior radiculomedullary artery(ies).
17 Median sacral artery
18 Thyrocervical trunk or costocervical trunk
19 Posterior spinal artery(ies)
20 Thoracic anterior radiculomedullary arteries
21 Ascending/descending vascular supply to cauda equina

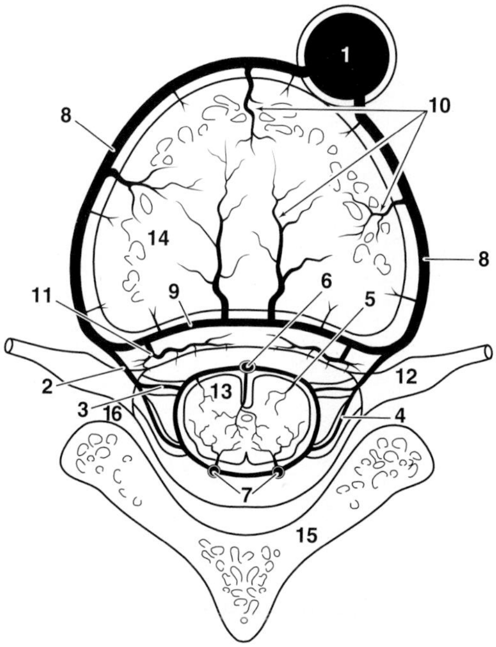

Figure 7C-3: Axial schematic of the arterial supply to the spine.

1 Aorta
2 Primary radiculomedullary artery
3 Anterior radiculomedullary artery
4 Posterior radiculomedullary artery
5 Penetrating medullary artery branch
6 Anterior spinal artery
7 Posterior spinal arteries
8 Segmental spinal artery(ies) (e.g., intercostal, lumbar, and sacral paraspinal arteries)
9 Posterior central spinal artery
10 Penetrating nutrient arteries to vertebral body
11 Anterior meningeal artery
12 Spinal nerve with dorsal root ganglion
13 Spinal cord
14 Vertebral body
15 Spinal lamina
16 Intervertebral (neural) foramen

Note: At any one level, numbers 3 and 4 may alternatively be atretic resulting in the majority or all of the blood supply at that level running within either the anterior or the posterior radiculomedullary arteries.

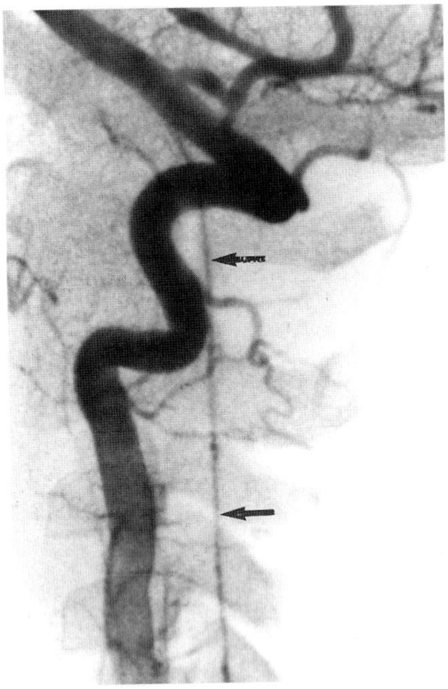

Figure 7C-4A: Spinal cord radiculomedullary arteries. Digital subtraction film from a left vertebral angiogram in the lateral projection showing the anterior spinal artery (*arrows*) originating from the distal vertebral artery.

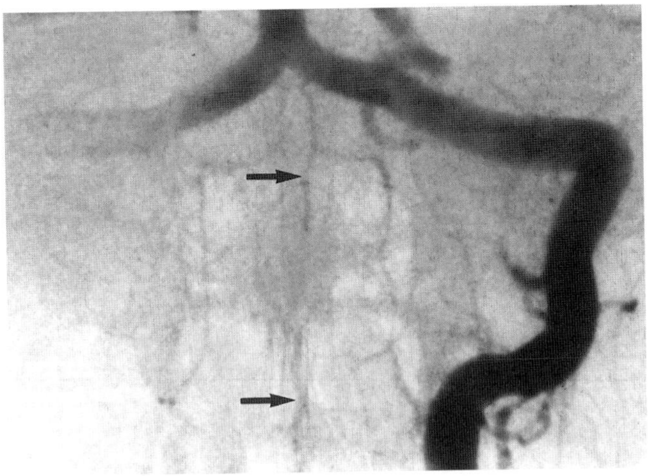

Figure 7C-4B: Digital subtraction film from a left vertebral angiogram in the anteroposterior projection showing the anterior spinal artery (*arrows*) originating from the left vertebral artery.

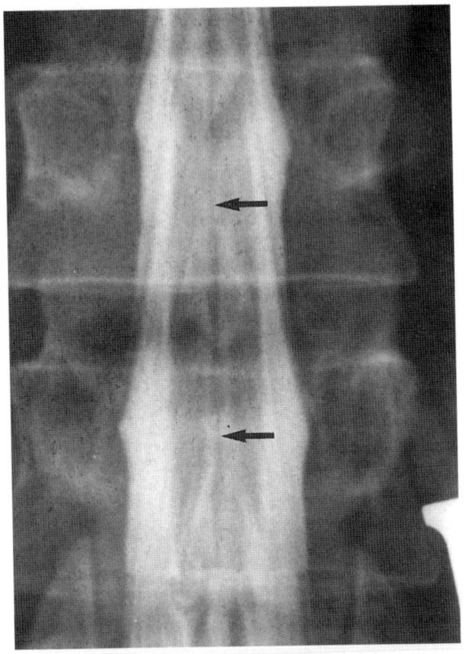

Figure 7C-5: Anterior spinal artery. Conventional myelogram in the frontal projection showing the filling defect corresponding to the anterior spinal artery (*arrows*) on the anterior surface of the spinal cord.

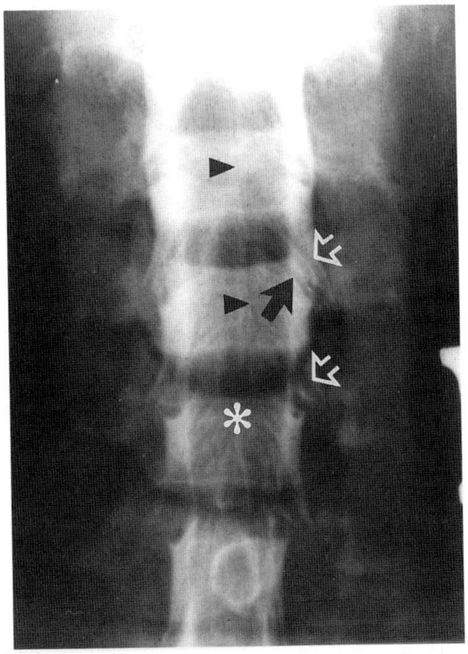

Figure 7C-6: Anterior spinal artery. Cervical myelogram in the frontal projection showing the spinal cord (*asterisk*), spinal nerve roots (*open arrows*), anterior spinal artery (*arrowheads*), and a major cervical radiculomedullary artery (*solid straight arrow*).

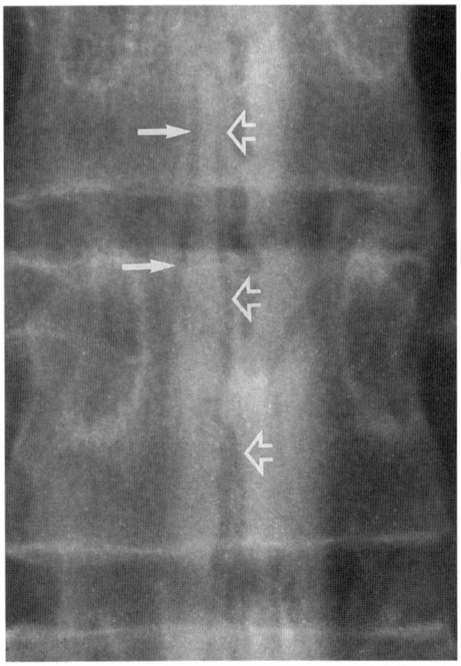

Figure 7C-7A: Artery of Adamkiewicz. Conventional water-soluble contrast myelogram in the posteroanterior projection showing filling defects corresponding to the artery of Adamkiewicz (*solid arrows*) and the anterior spinal artery (*open arrows*).

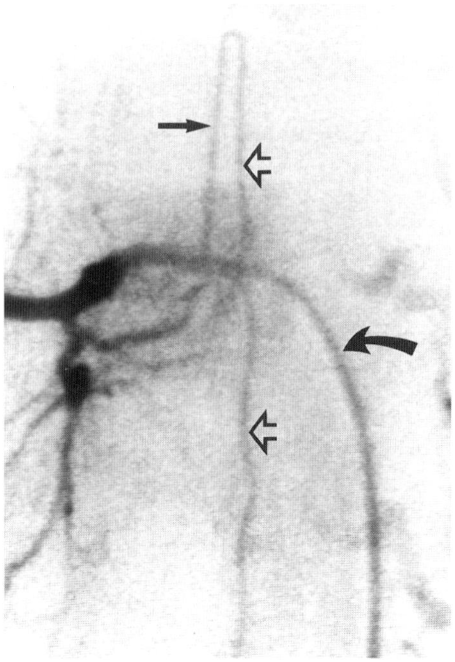

Figure 7C-7B: Digital subtraction film from an angiogram of a lower thoracic intercostal artery in the anteroposterior projection shows the artery of Adamkiewicz (*solid arrow*) and the anterior spinal artery (*open arrows*) (*curved arrow,* catheter).

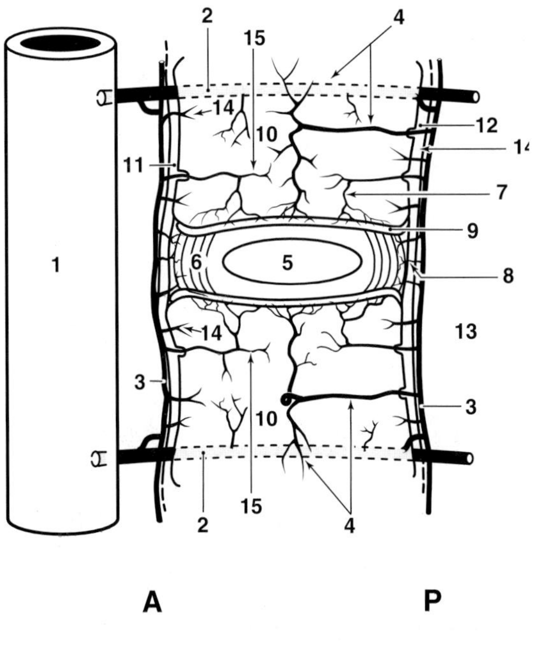

Figure 7C-8A: Midsagittal schematic of the arterial vascular supply of the vertebral bodies and intervertebral discs in the adult (lumbar region). The posterior bony elements of the spine are not shown. *A,* anterior; *P,* posterior.

1 Descending aorta
2 Segmental spinal arteries over vertebral surface (*dashed vascular wall*)
3 Intersegmental anastomosing spinal arteries on vertebral surface
4 Penetrating intraosseous nutrient arteries (*shading*)
5 Nucleus pulposus
6 Anulus fibrosus
7 Arterioles/capillaries supplying vertebral end plate
8 Arterioles/capillaries supplying the peripheral lamellae of the anulus fibrosus
9 Vertebral end plate
10 Vertebral bodies
11 Anterior longitudinal ligament
12 Posterior longitudinal ligament
13 Central canal of spinal column
14 Vessels supplying the longitudinal ligaments and periosteum of the vertebrae

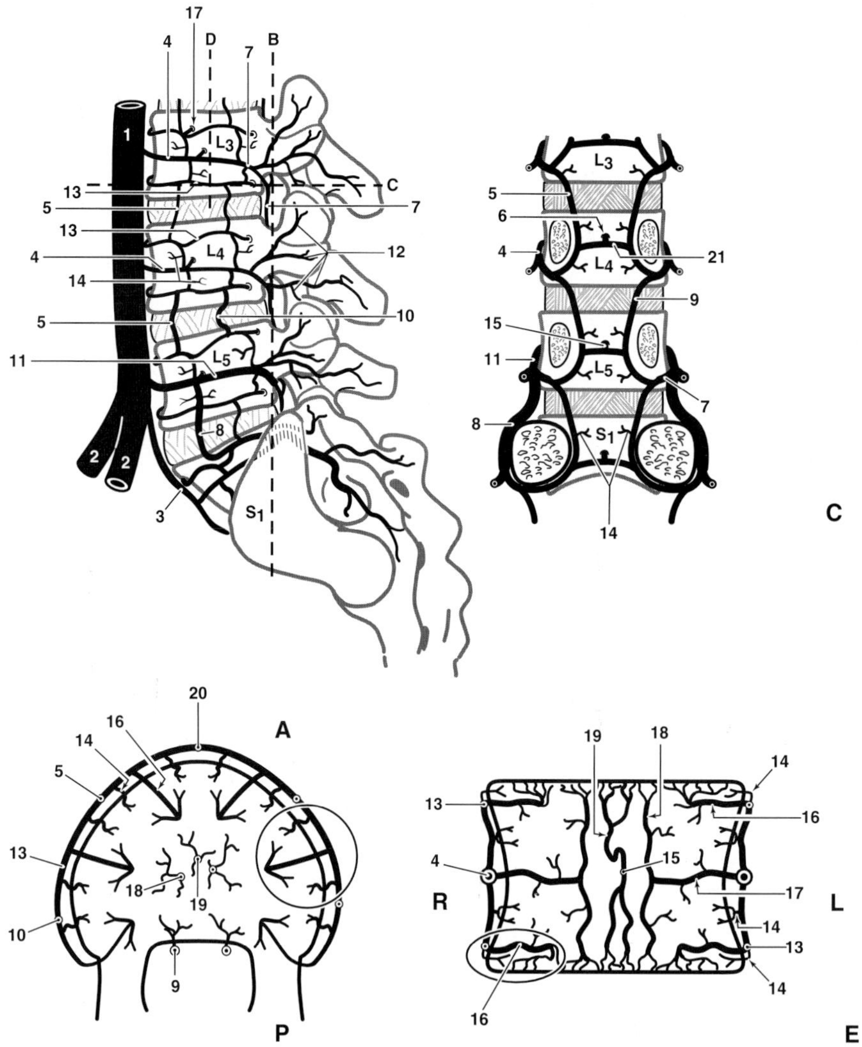

Figure 7C-8B–E: Schematics of the arterial supply to the lumbar spine and lumbosacral junction. **B:** Lateral aspect. **C:** Posterior aspect with posterior bony neural arch and thecal sac removed. **D:** Axial section through the vertebral metaphysis (see **B** for plane of section) **E:** Coronal section (see **B** for plane of section). (Modified from Ratcliffe JF. The arterial anatomy of the adult human lumbar vertebral body: a microarteriographic study. *J Anat* 1980;131:57–79.)

1 Aorta
2 Common iliac arteries
3 Median sacral artery
4 Lumbar paraspinal arteries
5 Anterolateral intervertebral longitudinal arterial anastomoses (Jinkins)
6 Posterior basivertebral vascular foramen
7 Radiculomedullary artery entering spinal neural foramen
8 Lateral intervertebral longitudinal arterial anastomosis at the lumbosacral junction
9 Posterior intraspinal intervertebral longitudinal arterial anastomosis
10 Posterolateral intraspinal intervertebral longitudinal arterial anastomosis
11 Paraspinal artery at the lumbosacral junction (larger caliber than at levels above)
12 Arterial branches to posterior spinal elements (spinous process, transverse processes, posterior articular facet processes, pars interarticulares, laminae, posterior spinal ligaments and muscles)
13 Anterolateral metaphyseal transverse vertebral arterial anastomoses (superior and inferior)
14 Periosteal/cortical arteries
15 Basivertebral corpal artery
16 Metaphyseal artery
17 Anterolateral corpal artery(ies)
18 Branch of lateral corpal artery(ies)
19 Branch of basivertebral corpal artery
20 Anterior intervertebral longitudinal arterial anastomosis
21 Posterior transverse vertebral arterial anastomosis

ARTERIAL SUPPLY TO THE PARENCHYMA OF THE SPINAL CORD

1. The arterial supply to the spinal cord parenchyma is via radiculomedullary arteries arising from the vertebral, ascending cervical deep cervical, intercostal, lumbar, iliac, and sacral paraspinal arteries.
2. The plexus of arterial vessels formed by the single longitudinal anterior spinal artery and the two longitudinal posterior spinal arteries on the pial surface of the spinal cord is called the arterial vasocorona.
3. The surface arterial anastomoses are present both circumferentially and longitudinally.
4. The anterior spinal artery gives off a branch that penetrates the anterior median sulcus (the artery of the anterior median sulcus), thereafter ramifying within the deep gray matter of the spinal cord on each side. Lateralizing branch arteries may be bilaterally asymmetric in distribution.
5. Elsewhere branch arteries from the arterial vasocorona of varying size penetrate the spinal cord directly, creating an irregular overlapping watershed in the axial plane with the terminal vessels from the artery of the anterior median sulcus.
6. Parenchymal arterial overlapping watersheds also occur in the longitudinal plane between the various terminal branches of the aforementioned penetrating arteries supplying the spinal cord.

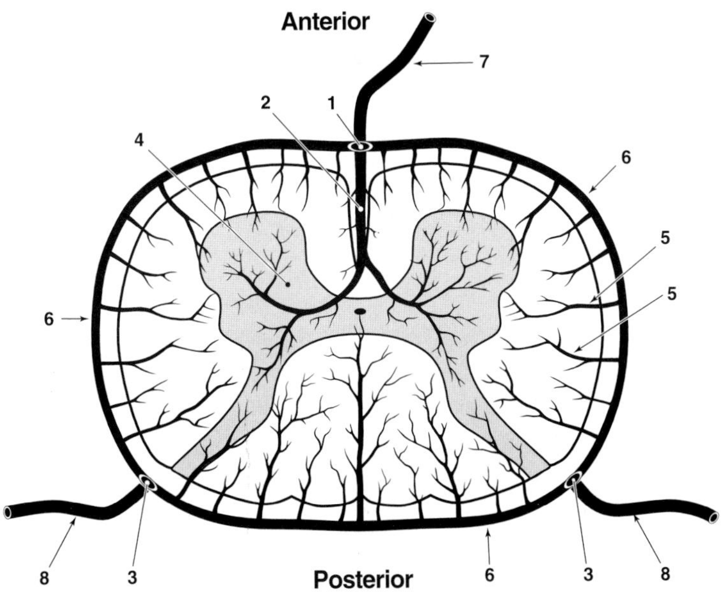

Figure 7C-9: Axial schematic of the circumferential anastomotic pattern of the arterial supply to the spinal cord.
1 Longitudinal anterior spinal artery
2 Artery of the anterior median sulcus
3 Longitudinal posterior spinal arteries
4 Deep gray matter of spinal cord
5 Penetrating spinal cord arteries
6 Superficial circumferential arterial anastomoses (arterial vasocorona)
7 Anterior radiculomedullary artery
8 Posterior radiculomedullary arteries

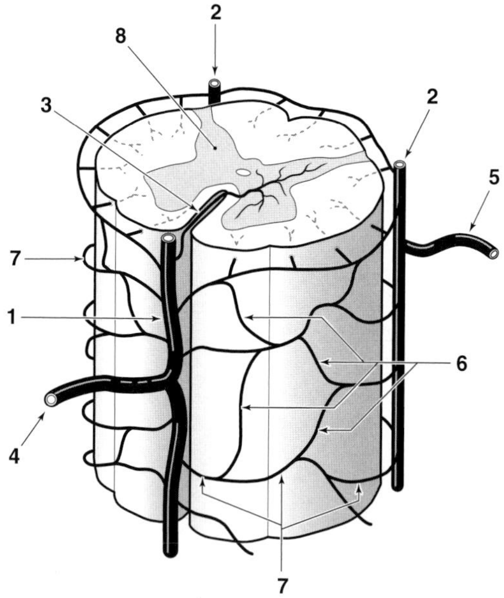

Figure 7C-10: Oblique schematic of the superficial longitudinal and circumferential arterial anastomoses of the spinal cord: the arterial vasocorona.

1 Anterior spinal artery
2 Posterior spinal arteries
3 Artery of the anterior median sulcus
4 Anterior radiculomedullary artery
5 Posterior radiculomedullary artery
6 Longitudinal arterial anastomoses
7 Circumferential arterial anastomoses
8 Deep gray matter of spinal cord

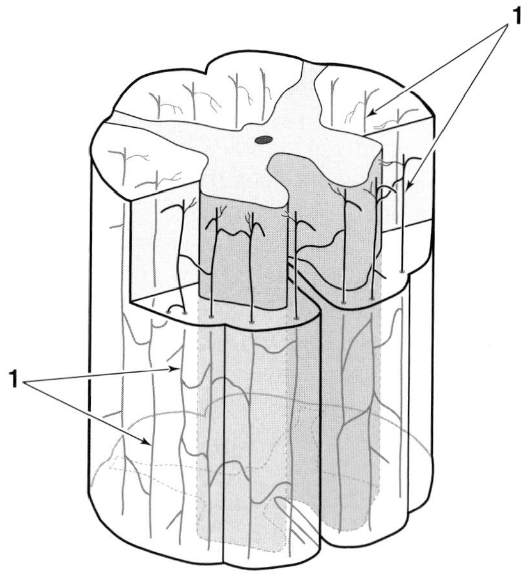

Figure 7C-11: Cutaway three-dimensional schematic of the deep longitudinal arterial anastomosis of the spinal cord. *1,* Deep longitudinal arterial anastomoses of the spinal cord.

VENOUS DRAINAGE OF THE SPINE

1. The main venous drainage of the structures within the central canal of the spinal column is via the anterior and posterior internal vertebral veins. This epidural venous plexus lies between the dura of the thecal sac and the periosteum of the vertebrae. Anastomoses occur between the anterior internal vertebral veins and the posterior internal vertebral veins (spinal epidural venous plexus). These veins contain no valves.
2. The supra- and infrapediculate veins connect the anterior internal vertebral veins and the ascending external vertebral veins running longitudinally lateral to the bases of the pedicles.
3. The ascending longitudinal veins drain into the lumbar segmental veins, which in turn run transversely to drain into the inferior vena cava.
4. The basivertebral vein, which drains the vertebral body, potentially flows in both directions: posteriorly into the anterior internal vertebral veins, and anteriorly and laterally into the external segmental spinal veins.
5. The intervertebral veins accompany the segmental spinal nerves through the intervertebral (neural) foramina. These veins drain the anterior and posterior radiculomedullary veins of the spinal cord, and the internal and external vertebral venous plexi.
6. The intervertebral discs drain into veins serving the vascularized vertebral end plates and the peripheral anulus fibrosus. From there the venous drainage is into larger tributaries such as the basivertebral venous plexus, the anterior internal vertebral veins, or the external segmental spinal veins.

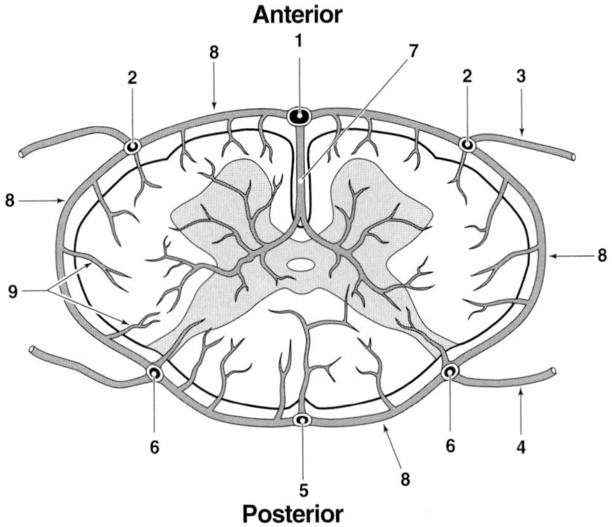

Figure 7C-12: Axial schematic of the spinal cord venous drainage.
1 Longitudinal anteromedian vein
2 Longitudinal anterolateral vein
3 Anterior radiculomedullary vein
4 Posterior radiculomedullary vein
5 Longitudinal posteromedian vein
6 Longitudinal posterolateral veins
7 Vein(s) of the anteromedian sulcus
8 Venous vasocorona of spinal cord
9 Penetrating spinal cord veins

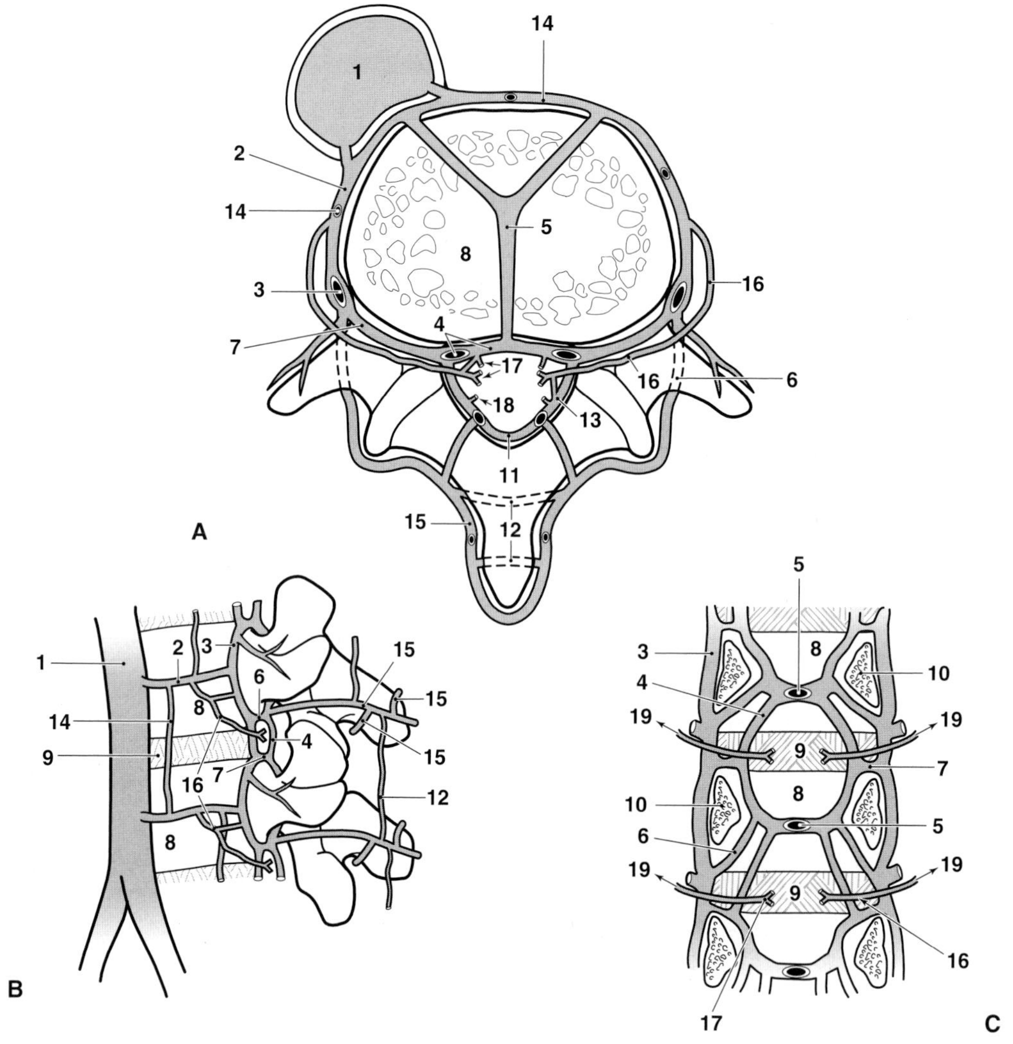

Figure 7C-13: Schematic of the venous system of the lumbar spine. The venous drainage at other spinal levels follows a similar if varying pattern. **A:** Axial schematic section through midvertebral body; the spinal cord has been removed. **B:** Lateral schematic. **C:** Posterior schematic with thecal sac and posterior bony elements removed.

1 Inferior vena cava
2 Spinal (lumbar paraspinal) segmental veins
3 Ascending vertebral veins
4 Anterior internal vertebral veins (venous plexus)
5 Basivertebral vein
6 Infrapediculate veins
7 Suprapediculate veins
8 Vertebral body
9 Intervertebral disc
10 Cut edge of pedicle
11 Posterior internal vertebral veins (venous plexus)
12 Interspinous anastomosis
13 Lateral transverse venous plexus
14 Anterior external venous plexus
15 Posterior external venous plexus
16 Intervertebral veins (cut ends of radiculomedullary veins; spinal cord removed)
17 Anterior medullary vein draining spinal cord
18 Posterior medullary vein draining spinal cord
19 To the spinal (lumbar paraspinal) segmental vein(s).

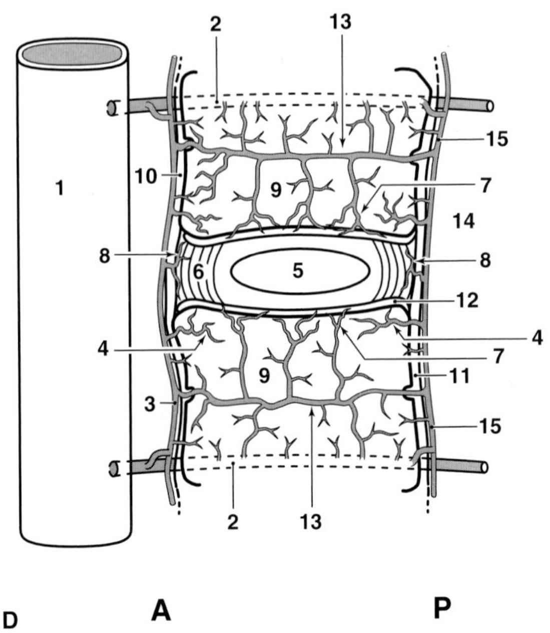

Figure 7C-13D: Midsagittal schematic of the venous drainage of the vertebral bodies and intervertebral discs in the adult (lumbar region). The posterior bony elements of the spine are not shown. *A*, anterior; *P*, posterior.

1 Inferior vena cava
2 Spinal segmental veins on vertebral surface (dashed vascular wall)
3 Anterior external vertebral venous plexus on vertebral surface
4 Penetrating intraosseous veins (*shading*)
5 Nucleus pulposus
6 Anulus fibrosus
7 Venules draining vertebral end plate
8 Venules draining the peripheral lamellae of the anulus fibrosus
9 Vertebral bodies
10 Anterior longitudinal ligament
11 Posterior longitudinal ligament
12 Vertebral end plate
13 Basivertebral venous plexus (*shading*)
14 Central canal of spinal column
15 Anterior internal vertebral veins (venous plexus)

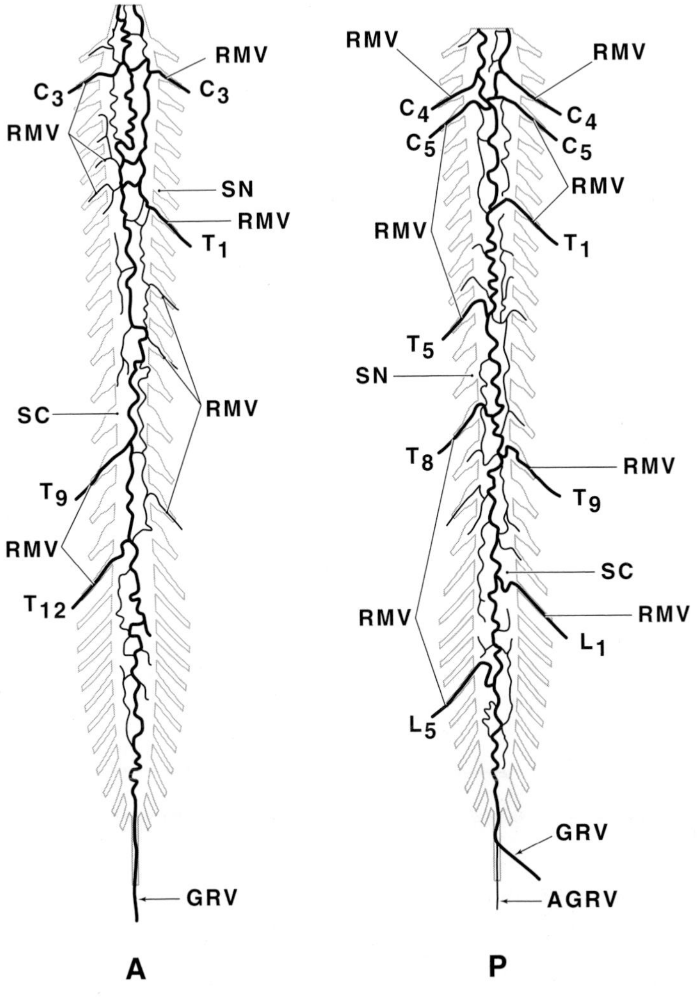

Figure 7C-14: Schematic of the anterior and posterior spinal cord veins and radiculomedullary veins. The irregular anastomotic vascular network is typical of the venous system draining the spinal cord. The schematics should only serve as a general conceptual overview that will vary greatly from patient to patient. *A*, anterior aspect; *P*, posterior aspect; *SC*, spinal cord; *SN*, spinal nerve; *GRV*, great radicular vein of cauda equina; *AGRV*, accessory great radicular vein of cauda equina; *RMV*, radiculomedullary vein(s); *C, T, L*, cervical, thoracic, lumbar radiculomedullary veins.

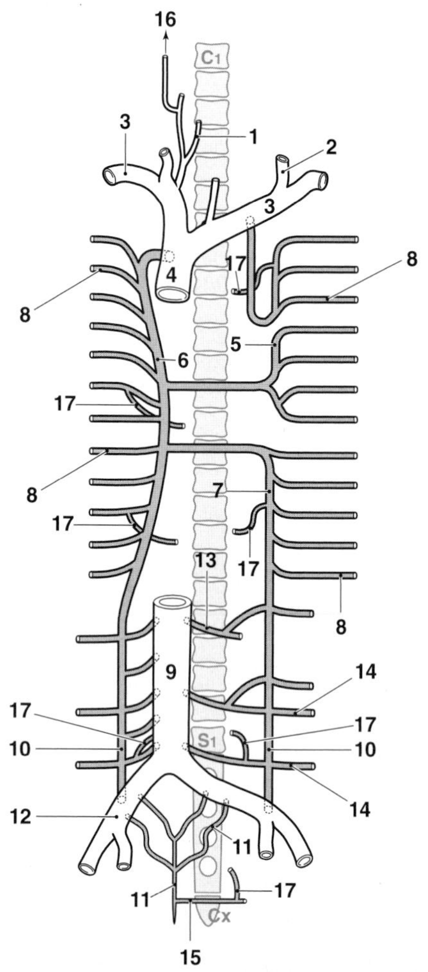

Figure 7C-15: Schematic of the major venous drainage of the spine.

1 Posterior jugular vein (drains cervical vertebral venous plexus)
2 Internal jugular vein (drains cervical vertebral venous plexus)
3 Right and left brachiocephalic veins
4 Superior vena cava
5 Superior hemiazygos vein
6 Azygos vein
7 Inferior hemiazygos vein
8 Posterior intercostal veins (segmental veins draining spinal column)
9 Inferior vena cava
10 Ascending lumbar veins
11 Median and lateral sacral veins
12 Common iliac vein
13 Renal vein
14 Lumbar segmental veins (segmental veins draining spinal column)
15 Sacral segmental vein (segmental veins draining spinal column)
16 Cervical vertebral venous plexus
17 Intervertebral veins (draining radiculomedullary veins)

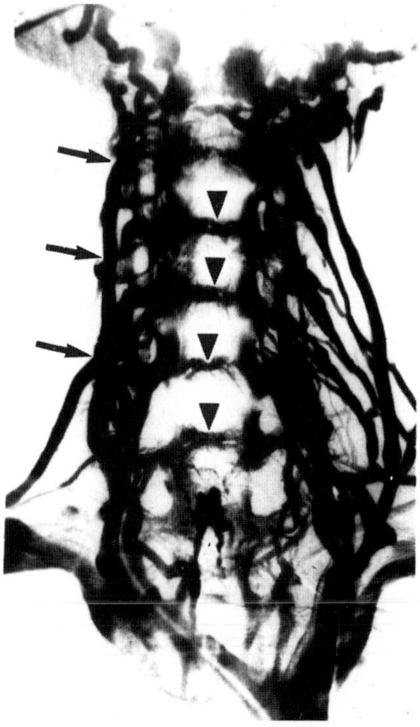

Figure 7C-16A: Cervical and lumbar epidural veins. Cervical epidural venogram in the frontal projection showing the internal epidural spinal venous plexus (*arrowheads*) as well as the external perivertebral spinal venous plexus (*arrows*). (Courtesy of J. Theron, M.D.)

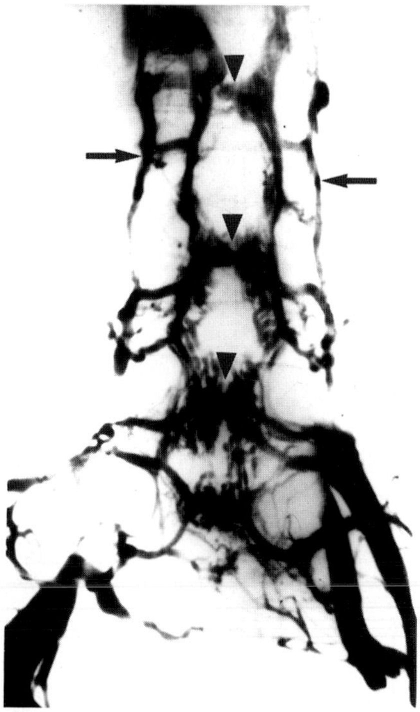

Figure 7C-16B: Lumbar epidural venogram in the frontal projection showing the internal epidural spinal venous plexus (*arrowheads*) as well as external perivertebral spinal venous plexus (*arrows*). (Courtesy of J. Theron, M.D.)

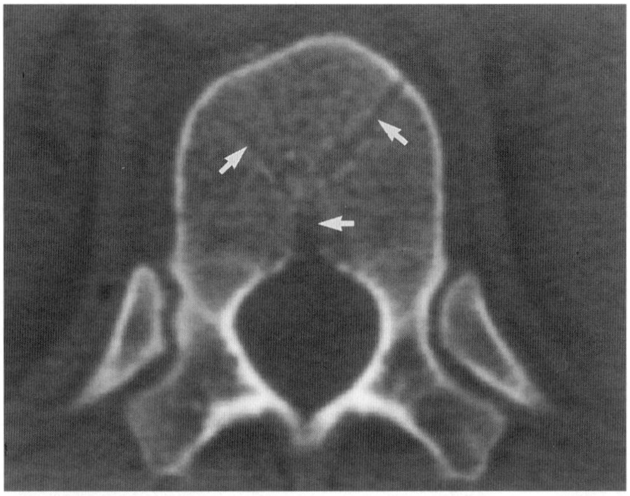

Figure 7C-17: Basivertebral venous channels. Axial image showing the typical "Y"-shaped basivertebral venous channels in a thoracic vertebra (*arrows*).

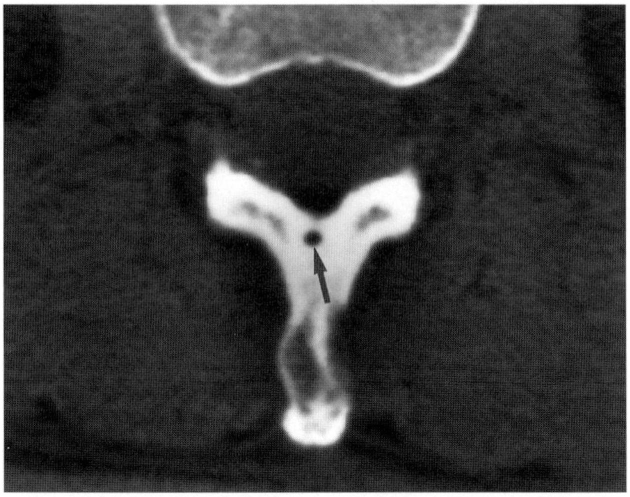

Figure 7C-18A: Spinous process vascular nutrient channel. Axial CT images showing a transverse spinous process vascular nutrient canal (*arrow*).

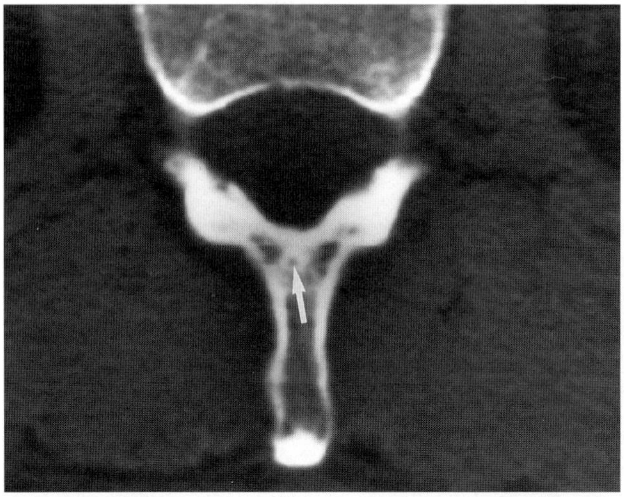

Figure 7C-18B: Axial CT image showing a continuation of the transverse spinous process vascular nutrient canal (*arrow*).

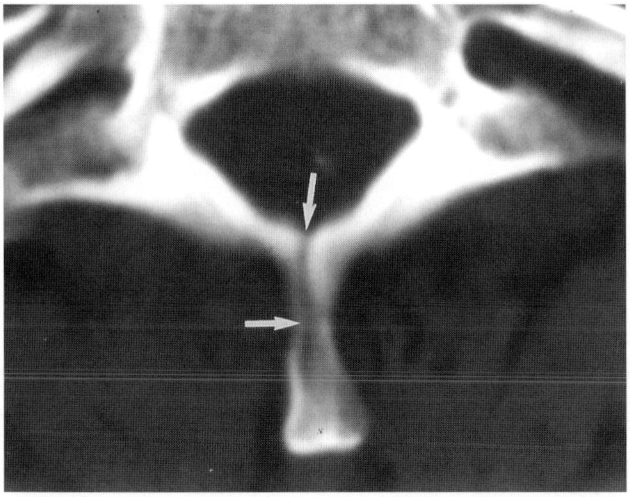

Figure 7C-18C: Axial CT image in another patient showing a longitudinal spinous process vascular nutrient groove/channel (*arrows*).

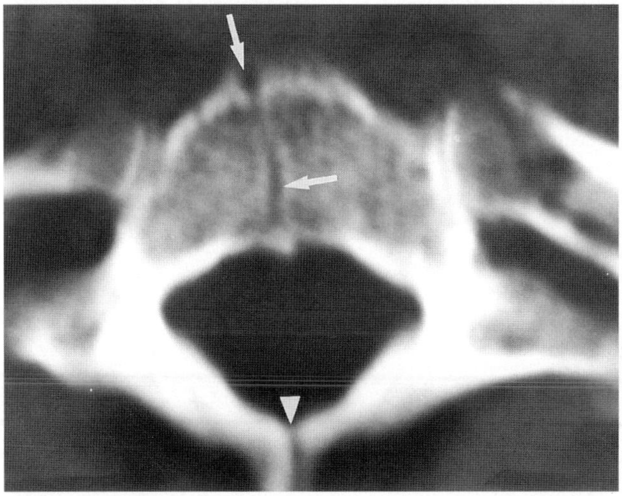

Figure 7C-18D: Axial CT image in the upper thoracic region showing a vertebral body vascular nutrient channel (*arrows*) and spinous process vascular channel/cleft (*arrowhead*).

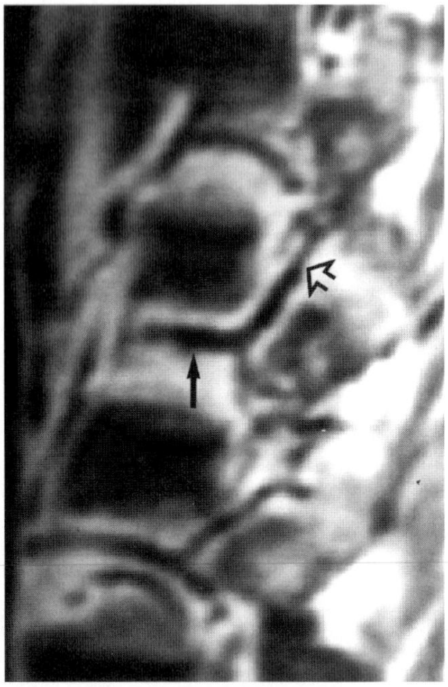

Figure 7C-19A: Spinal veins. Parasagittal T1-weighted MR image shows a lumbar segmental vein (*solid arrow*) and an ascending vertebral vein (*open arrow*).

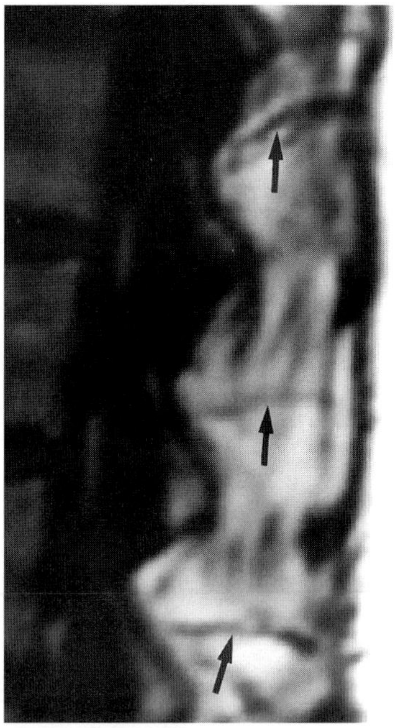

Figure 7C-19B: Parasagittal T1-weighted MR image shows a part of the posterior external venous plexus (i) (*arrows*).

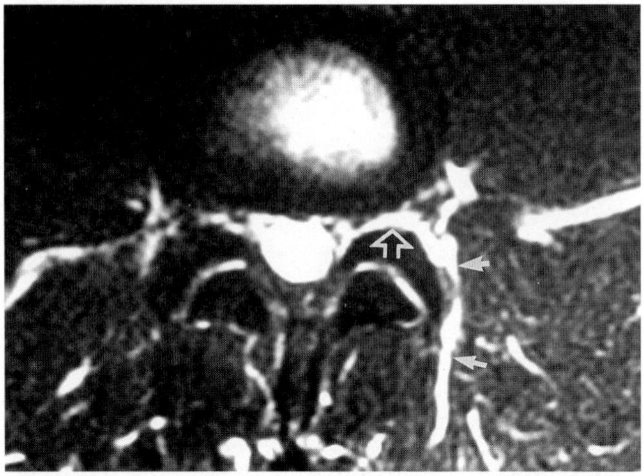

Figure 7C-19C: Axial T2-weighted fat-suppressed MR image showing the intrapediculate vein (*open arrow*) and the posterior external venous plexus (*solid arrows*).

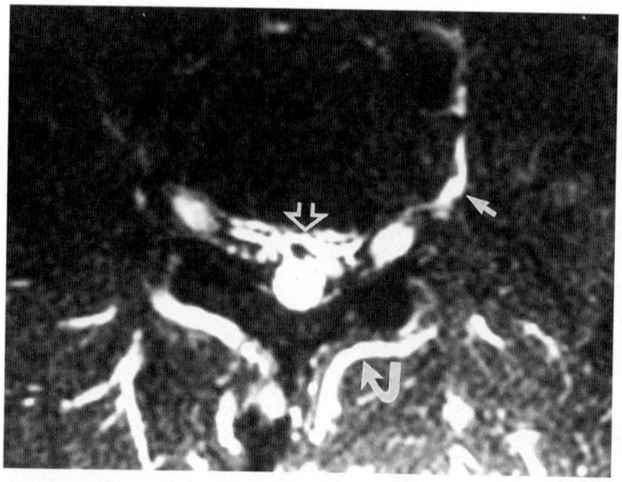

Figure 7C-19D: Axial T2-weighted fat suppressed MR image shows the anterior internal vertebral veins (*open arrow,* epidural venous plexus), the anterior external venous plexus (*solid straight arrow*), and the posterior external venous plexus (*curved arrow*).

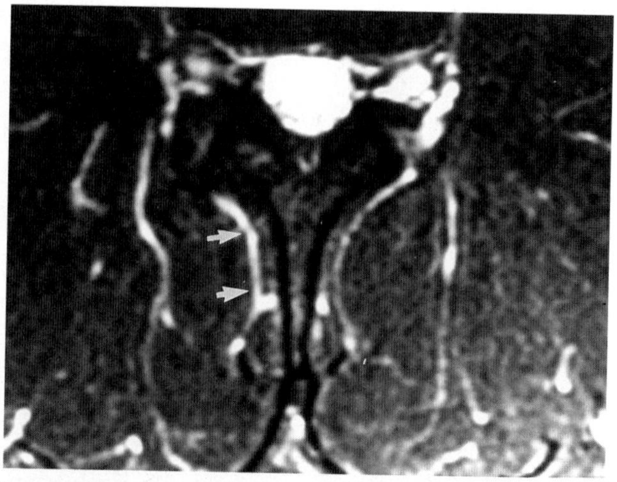

Figure 7C-19E: Axial T2-weighted, fat-suppressed image shows the posterior external venous plexus (*arrows*).

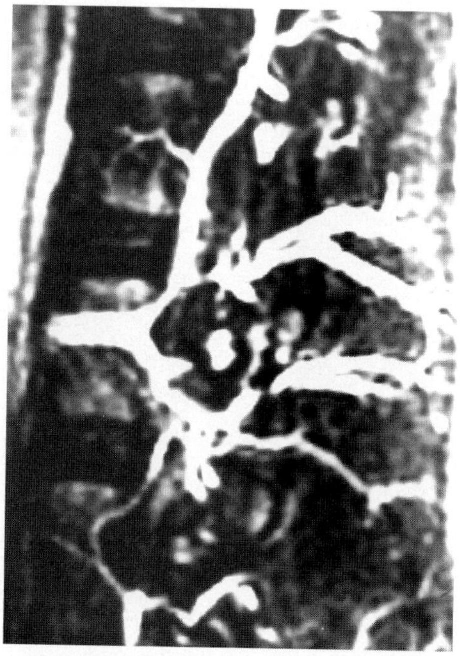

Figure 7C-20: Paravertebral venous plexus. Sagittal T2-weighted fat suppressed MR image showing the paravertebral external venous plexus.

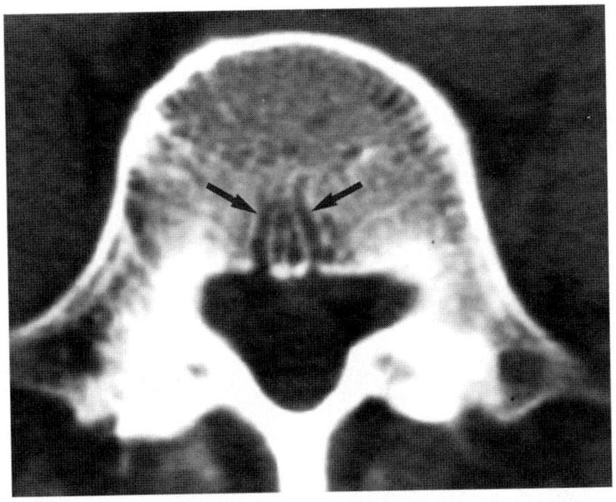

Figure 7C-21: Basivertebral vein/arterial channels. Axial CT showing dual basivertebral venous/arterial channels (*arrows*) communicating with the anterior epidural space of the central spinal canal.

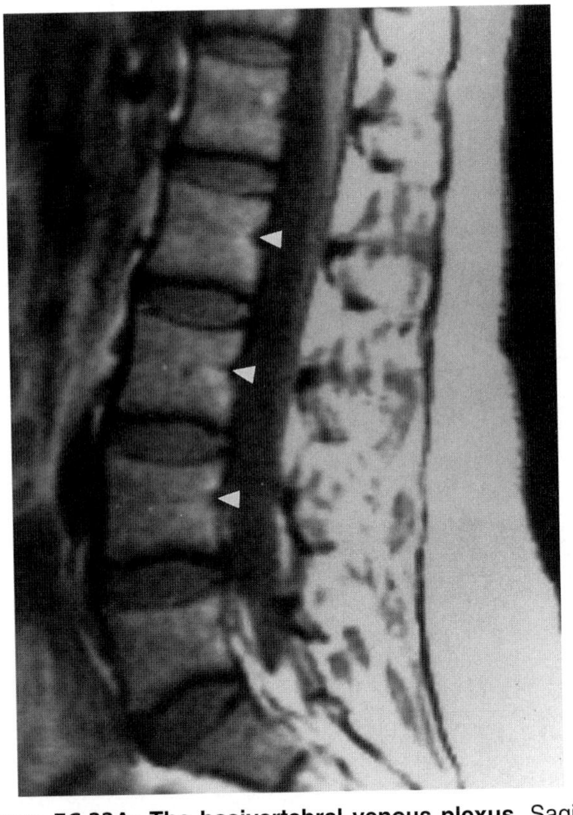

Figure 7C-22A: The basivertebral venous plexus. Sagittal T1-weighted MR image showing the basivertebral venous plexus foramina (*arrowheads*).

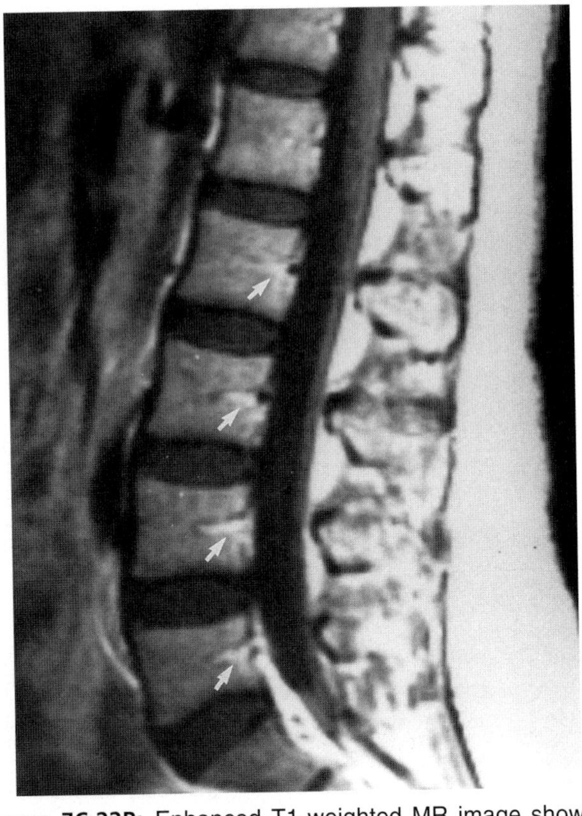

Figure 7C-22B: Enhanced T1-weighted MR image showing enhancement of the basivertebral venous plexi at every level (*arrows*).

VASCULAR SUPPLY TO THE CAUDA EQUINA

1. Craniad arterial and venous vascular radicles normally accompany the nerve roots at their origin from the conus medullaris. This may in part represent major or minor tributaries from the artery of Adamkiewicz.
2. There is also caudal arterial inflow and venous outflow from distal radiculomedullary arterial or venous radicles that accompany each nerve root as it exits the intervertebral neural foramen. The craniad and caudal arterial systems anastomose freely; similarly, the craniad and caudal venous systems anastomose freely.
3. Ordinarily there is no intervening vascular supply to the lumbosacral nerve roots of the cauda equina along their longitudinal course.
4. The vascular watershed of the cauda equina normally is found at the junction of the proximal and middle thirds of the longitudinal extent of the intrathecal segments of the nerve roots.

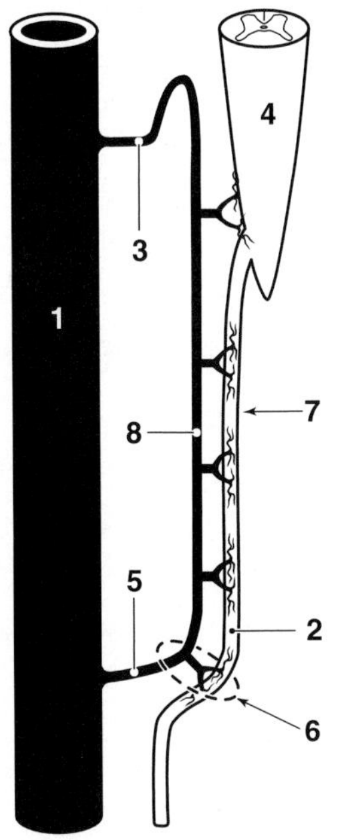

Figure 7C-23: Schematic of normal dual arterial supply to lumbosacral neural radicles of cauda equina and anastomotic arcade. The venous drainage of the cauda equina follows a similar pattern.

1 Abdominal aorta
2 Lumbosacral nerve root of the cauda equina
3 Craniad radiculomedullary artery
4 Conus medullaris
5 Caudal radiculomedullary artery
6 Level of spinal intervertebral neural foramen
7 Vascular watershed at the junction of proximal and middle thirds of the cauda equina
8 Anastomotic arcade of cauda equina

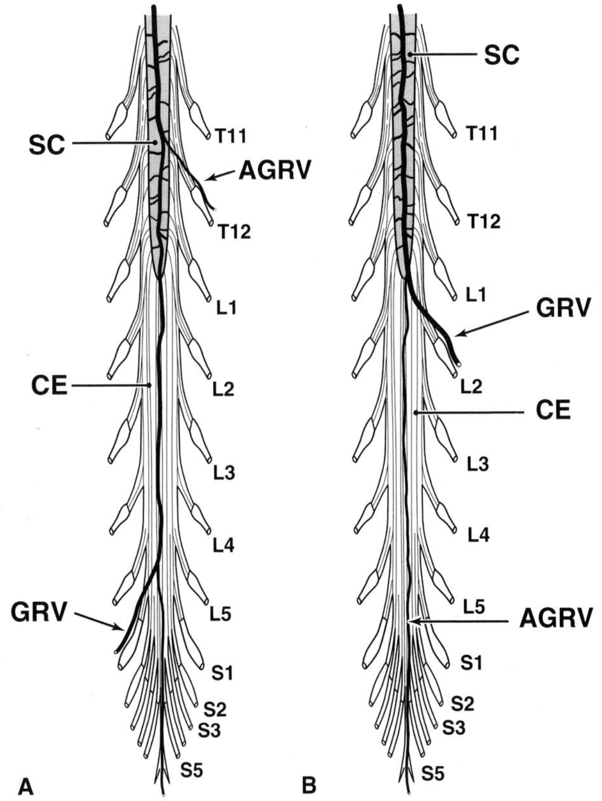

Figure 7C-24: Schematic of the superficial veins of the ventral surface of the conus medullaris and cauda equina. **A:** General example of the major venous anatomy present in one quarter of cadaveric specimens. Note the great radicular vein (GRV) accompanying an exiting sacral nerve root, and the accessory great radicular vein (AGRV) exiting with a thoracic nerve root. **B:** General example of the major venous anatomy present in three quarters of cadaveric specimens. Note the GRVs exiting the spine with a lumbar nerve root on the left. A small AGRV accompanies the filum terminale distally. *SC,* spinal cord; *CE,* cauda equina; *T, L, S,* numbered thoracic/lumbar/sacral spinal nerves.

VASCULAR SUPPLY TO THE SPINAL NERVE ROOTS AND PROXIMAL SPINAL NERVES

1. Radiculomedullary arteries and veins supply and drain the spinal nerve roots.
2. Transverse and longitudinal arterial and venous arterial coils compensate for limited degrees of stretch and axial deformation that may occur with normal somatic movements.

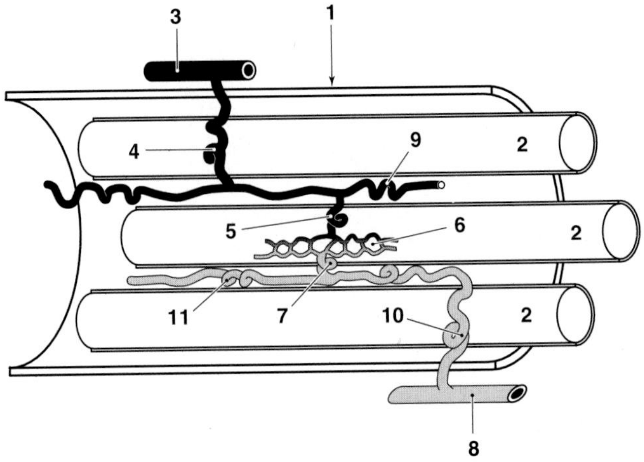

Figure 7C-25: Schematic of the spinal nerve root arterial vascular supply and venous drainage
1 Nerve root pia or dural sheath
2 Neural axons
3 Superficial nerve root artery (arterial vasa nervorum) arising from segmental radiculomedullary artery
4 Penetrating branch artery with compensating transverse arterial coils
5 Arteriole with compensating transverse coil
6 Neural capillary network
7 Venule with compensating transverse coil
8 Superficial nerve root vein (venous vasa nervorum) draining into radiculomedullary vein
9 Compensating longitudinal arterial coils
10 Draining branch vein with compensating transverse venous coils
11 Compensating longitudinal venous coils

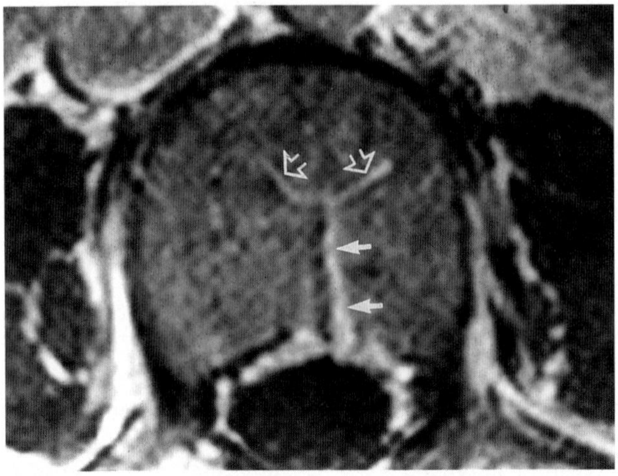

Figure 7C-26A: Basivertebral vein channels. Contrast-enhanced axial T1-weighted MR image showing the trunk of the basivertebral vein channel (*closed arrows*), communicating with the anterior intraspinal epidural venous plexus, and its main branches (*open arrows*).

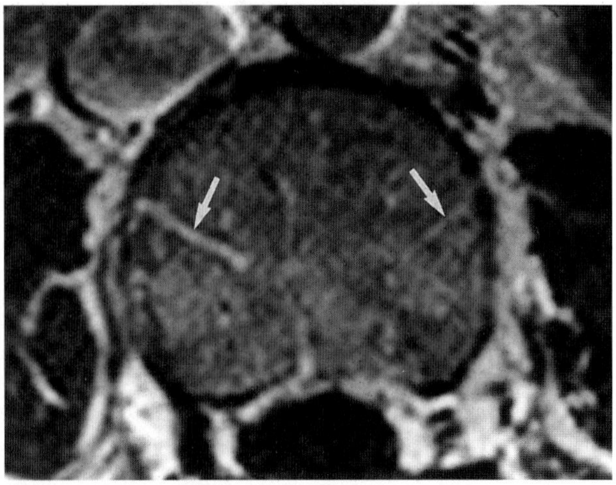

Figure 7C-26B: Subjacent contrast-enhanced axial T1-weighted MR image showing the exiting anterior venous branches (*arrows*) of the basivertebral vein.

7D Anatomy of Spinal Nerve Roots, Spinal Nerves, and Spinal Nerve Plexi

SPINAL NERVE EXIT PATTERNS

1. The cervical pairs of spinal nerves exit above the corresponding vertebral body with the exception of the C-8 spinal cord segment that gives rise to a pair of spinal nerves (C-8) that exit between C-7 and T-1.
2. Below this, the thoracic, lumbar, sacral, and coccygeal pairs of spinal nerves exit below the corresponding numbered vertebral column segments.
3. Lateral to the dorsal root ganglion (consisting of bipolar sensory neurons), the dorsal and ventral roots join to form the spinal nerve proper. Immediately distal to this joinder, the spinal nerve splits into ventral and dorsal rami. Depending on the spinal level, the ventral ramus then gives off and/or receives the gray and white rami of the paraspinal sympathetic chain.

SPINAL NERVE PLEXI

Overview

1. Anastomoses between two or more portions of spinal nerve roots (e.g., dorsal and ventral roots) form the spinal nerves.
2. The spinal neural plexi consist of groups of anastomosing spinal nerves.
3. The paired spinal neural plexi include the cervical plexus, the brachial plexus, the lumbar plexus, the sacral plexus, and the coccygeal plexus.

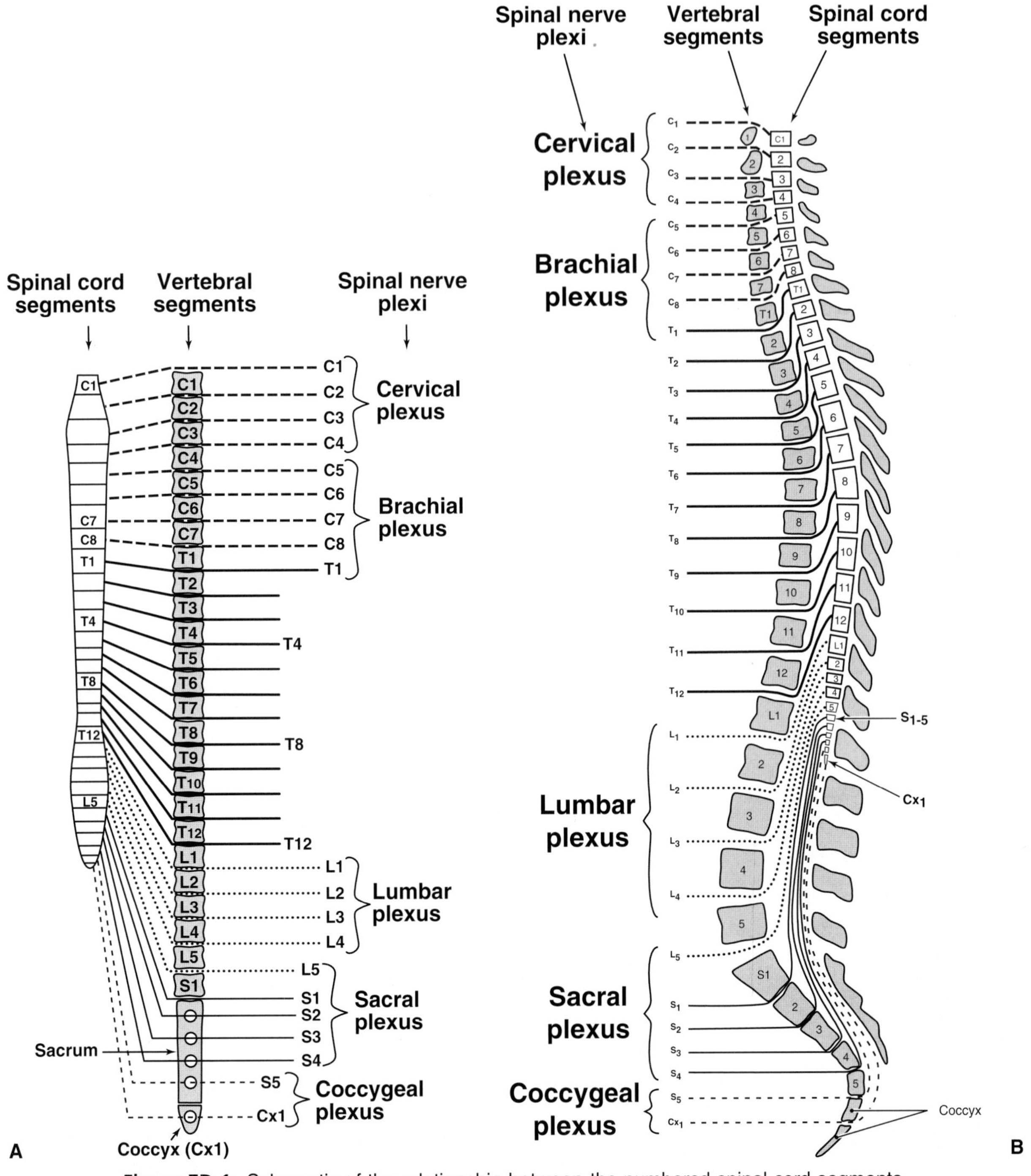

Figure 7D-1: Schematic of the relationship between the numbered spinal cord segments, spinal nerves, and vertebral bodies in the adult. **A:** Frontal view. **B:** Sagittal view. *C,* cervical; *T,* thoracic; *L,* lumbar; *S,* sacral; *Cx,* coccygeal.

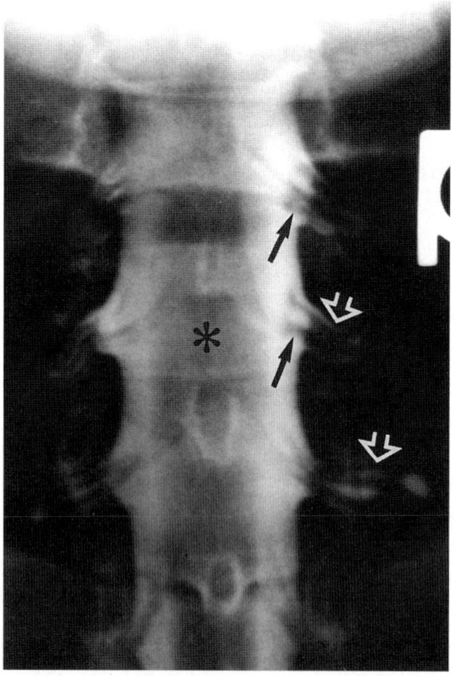

Figure 7D-2: Spinal cord nerve roots. Cervical myelogram in the frontal projection showing the spinal cord (*asterisk*), dorsal and ventral nerve roots (*closed arrows*), and nerve root sleeves (*open arrows*).

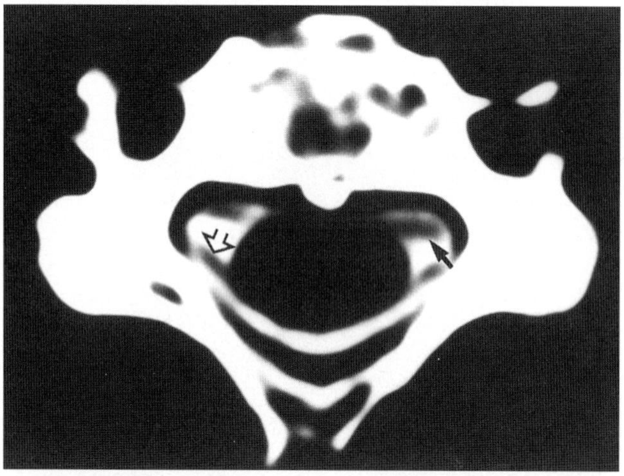

A

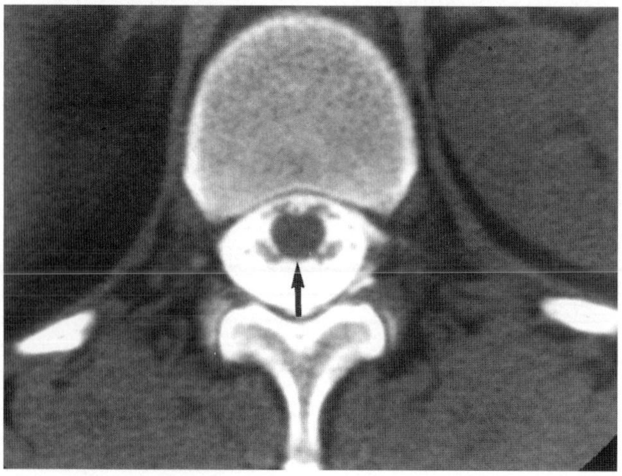

B

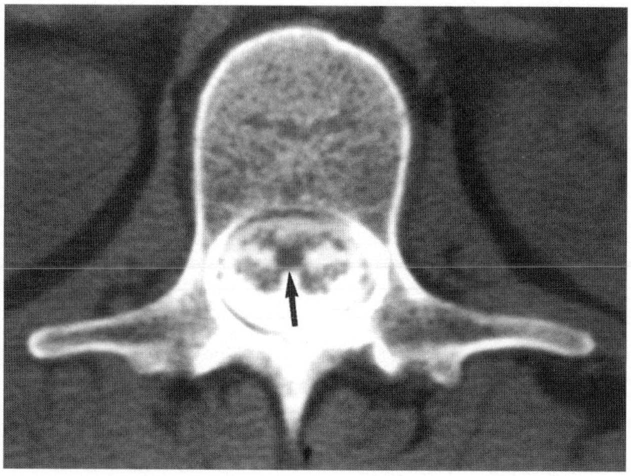

C

Figure 7D-3: Spinal cord and nerve roots. Axial CT myelogram at different levels showing the normal appearance of the spinal cord and nerve roots. **A:** The C-4 vertebral level (*open arrow,* dorsal root; *solid arrow*, ventral root). **B:** The T-12 to L-1 vertebral level (*arrow,* conus medullaris). **C:** The L1-2 vertebral level (*arrow,* tip of spinal cord). (*continued*)

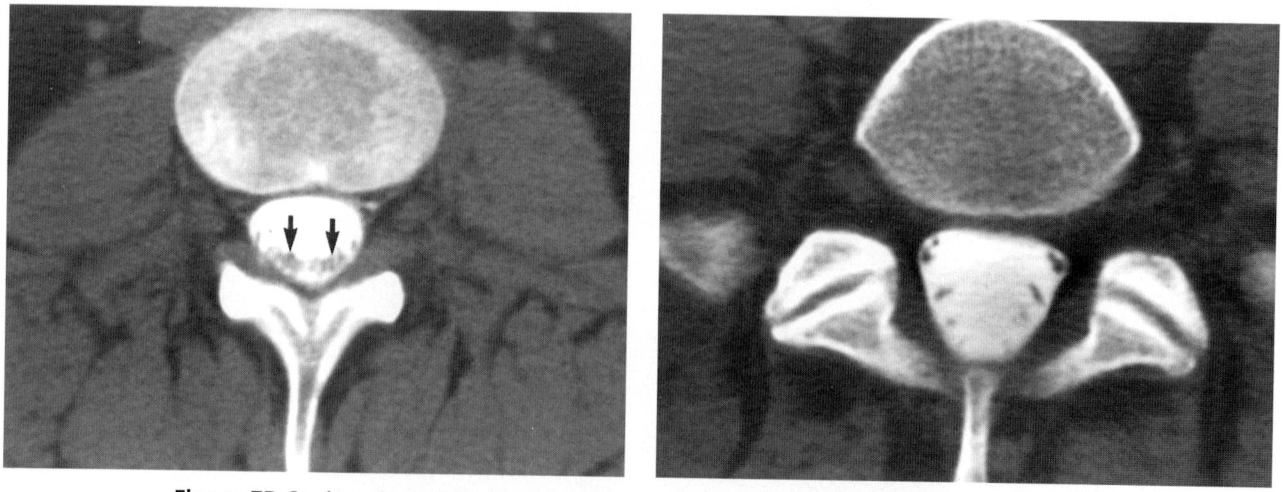

Figure 7D-3: ***(continued)*** **D:** The L4-5 vertebral level (*arrows,* cauda equina). **E:** The L-5 to S-1 vertebral level (note general peripheral location of intrathecal nerve roots at this level).

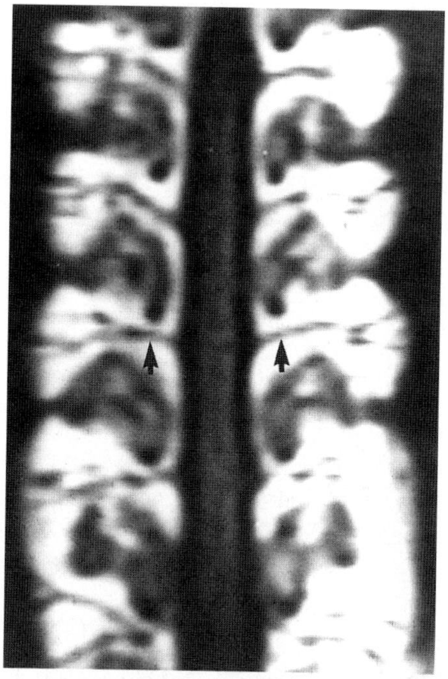

Figure 7D-4: Spinal nerves. Coronal T1-weighted MR image at the midthoracic level showing the exiting and branching thoracic spinal nerves (*arrows*) at multiple levels bilaterally.

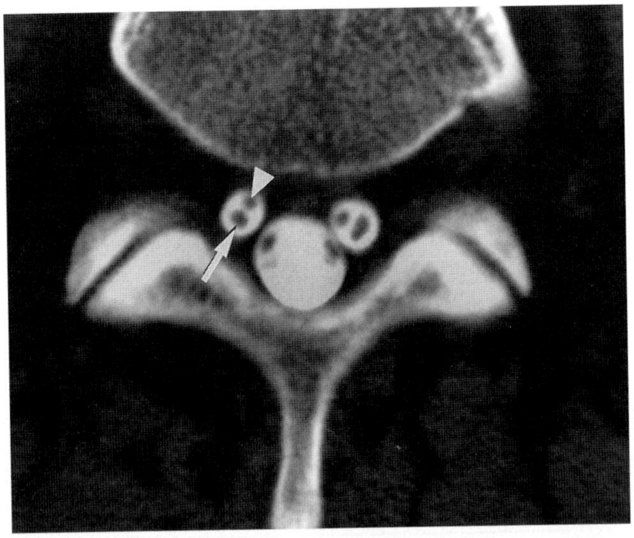

Figure 7D-5: Dorsal and ventral spinal nerve roots. Axial CT myelogram showing the dorsal (*arrow*) and ventral (*arrowhead*) nerve roots bilaterally within the exiting spinal nerve root sheath.

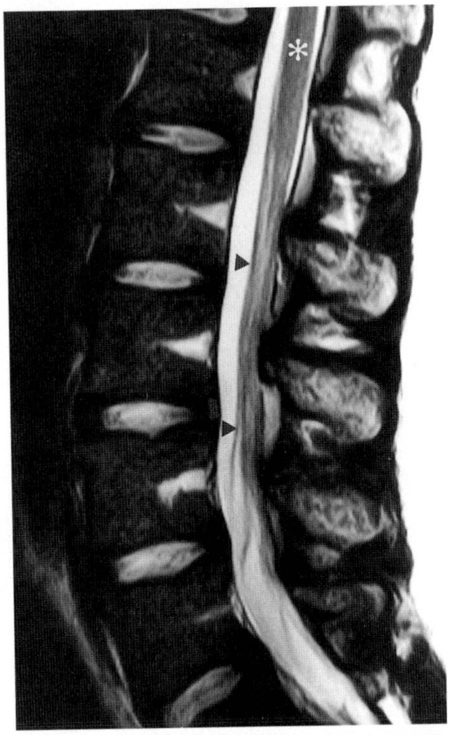

Figure 7D-6: The cauda equina. Sagittal T2-weighted MR image showing the normal appearance of the conus medullaris (*asterisk*) and the nerve roots of the cauda equina (*arrowheads*).

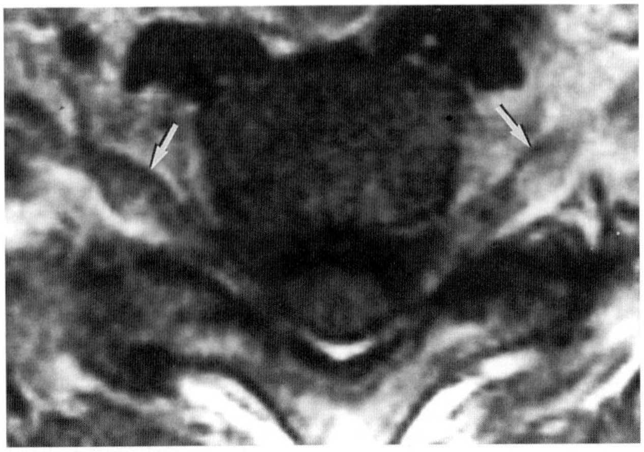

Figure 7D-7A: Dorsal root ganglia: cervical spine. Axial T1-weighted MR image showing the extraforaminal location of the dorsal root ganglia (*arrows*) at this level.

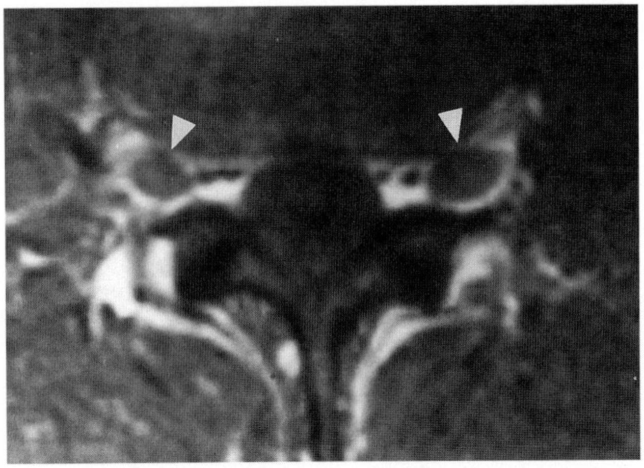

Figure 7D-7B: The dorsal root ganglia. Unenhanced axial T1-weighted MR image at L-5 level showing the normal appearance of the dorsal root ganglia (*arrowheads*).

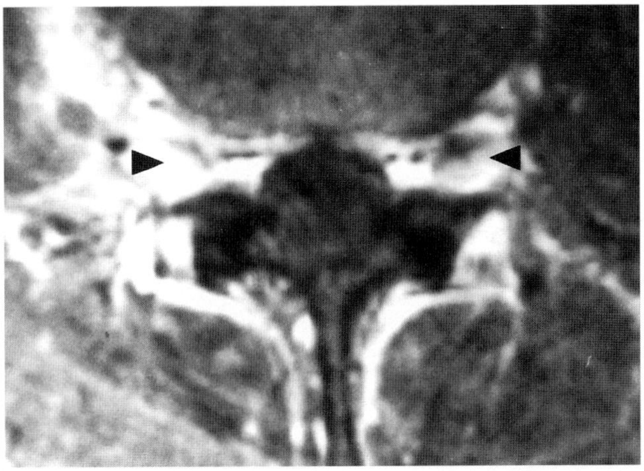

Figure 7D-7C: Contrast-enhanced axial T1-weighted MR image of the same case as that of Figure 7D-7B, showing normal enhancement of the dorsal root ganglia (*arrowheads*). Note the absence of intrathecal enhancement.

The Cervical Neural Plexus

1. The cervical neural plexus is composed of the ventral rami of the first four spinal nerves (C-1 to C-4). Minor parts of the C-5 spinal nerve may also be incorporated.
2. The distribution of the cervical neural plexus is to the nuchal muscles, the diaphragm, and the cutaneous tissues of the head, neck, and chest.
3. The three general groups of nerves comprising the cervical neural plexus are: the ascending superficial branches, the descending superficial branches, and the deep branches.
4. The ascending superficial branches of the cervical neural plexus include: the lesser occipital nerve (C-2), the great auricular nerve (C-2, C-3), and the transverse cutaneous nerve of the neck (C-2, C-3). The ascending superficial branches provide regional cutaneous innervation.
5. The descending superficial branches of the cervical neural plexus include the supraclavicular nerves (medial, intermediate, and lateral: C-3, C-4). The descending superficial branches provide regional cutaneous innervation
6. The deep medial branches of the cervical neural plexus include the ansa ("loop") cervicalis (C-1, C-2, C-3) innervating all of the infrahyoid muscles excluding the thyrohyoid; the phrenic nerve (C-3, C-4, C-5), the sole motor supply to the diaphragm; and muscular neural branches to the rectus capitis lateralis (C-1), rectus capitis anterior (C-1, C-2), longus capitis (C-1, C-2, C-3), and longus colli (C-4) muscles.
7. The deep lateral branches of the cervical neural plexus include muscular branches to the sternocleidomastoid (C-2), trapezius (C-3, C-4), levator scapulae (C-3), and scalenus medius (C-4) muscles.

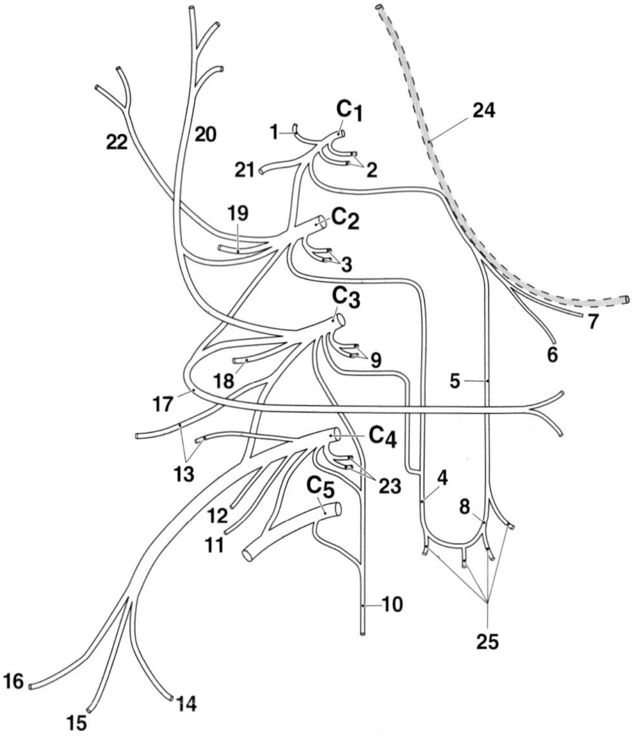

Figure 7D-8: Schematic of the cervical neural plexus on the right side. (*C-1* to *C-5*, cervical spinal nerves).

1 To rectus capitis lateralis muscle
2 To rectus capitis anterior and longus capitis muscles
3 To longus capitis and longus cervicalis muscles
4 Inferior root of ansa ("loop") cervicalis
5 Superior root of ansa ("loop") cervicalis
6 To thyrohyoid muscle
7 To geniohyoid muscle
8 Ansa ("loop") cervicalis
9 To longus capitis, longus colli, and scalenus medius muscles
10 Phrenic nerve
11 To scalenus medius muscle
12 To levator scapulae muscle
13 To trapezius muscle
14 Medial supraclavicular nerve
15 Intermediate supraclavicular nerve
16 Lateral supraclavicular nerve
17 Transverse cutaneous nerve of neck
18 To levator scapulae muscle
19 To sternocleidomastoid muscle
20 Great auricular nerve
21 To vagus nerve
22 Lesser occipital nerve
23 To longus colli muscle
24 Hypoglossal nerve
25 To all infrahyoid muscles except the thyrohyoid

The Brachial Neural Plexus

1. The brachial neural plexus is composed of the ventral rami of the lower four cervical spinal nerves (C-5 to C-8) and a part of the ventral ramus of the first thoracic spinal nerve (T-1). The ventral rami of the C-4 and T-2 spinal nerves may also variably make small contributions to the brachial plexus.
2. Before the anastomosis to form the brachial plexus, neural branches originating directly from the ventral roots of the cervical spinal nerves include nerves to scaleni and longus colli muscles (C-5 to C-8), a neural branch to the phrenic nerve (C-5), the dorsal scapular nerve (C-5), and the long thoracic nerve (C-5 to C-7).
3. The first order proximal neural anastomosis of the brachial plexus are the neural trunks, which include the upper cervical neural trunk (C-5 and C-6), the middle cervical neural trunk (C-7), and the lower cervical neural trunk (C-8 and T-1).
4. Nerves arising directly from the neural trunks of the brachial plexus include the nerve to the subclavius muscle (C-5 and C-6) and the suprascapular nerve (C-5 and C-6).
5. The second-order intermediate neural anastomoses of the brachial plexus are the neural cords, which include the lateral cervical neural cord (anterior divisions of the upper and middle trunks), the medial cervical neural cord (anterior division of the lower trunk), and the posterior cervical neural cord (posterior divisions of the anterior, middle, and lower trunks).
6. Nerves arising from the lateral cervical neural cord of the brachial plexus include the lateral pectoral (C-5 to C-7), musculocutaneous (C-5 to C-7), and the lateral root of the median (C-6 and C-7) nerves.
7. Nerves arising from the medial cervical neural cord of the brachial plexus include the medial pectoral nerve (C-8 and T-1), the medial cutaneous nerve of the forearm (C-8 and T-1), the medial cutaneous nerve of the arm (C-8 and T-1), the ulnar nerve (C-8 and T-1), and the medial root of the median (C-8 and T-1) nerves.
8. Nerves arising from the posterior cervical neural cord of the brachial plexus include the upper subscapular (C-6 and C-7), the thoracodorsal (C-6 to C-8), the lower subscapular (C-5 and C-6), the axillary (C-5 and C-6), and the radial (C-5, C-6, C-7, and T-1) nerves.

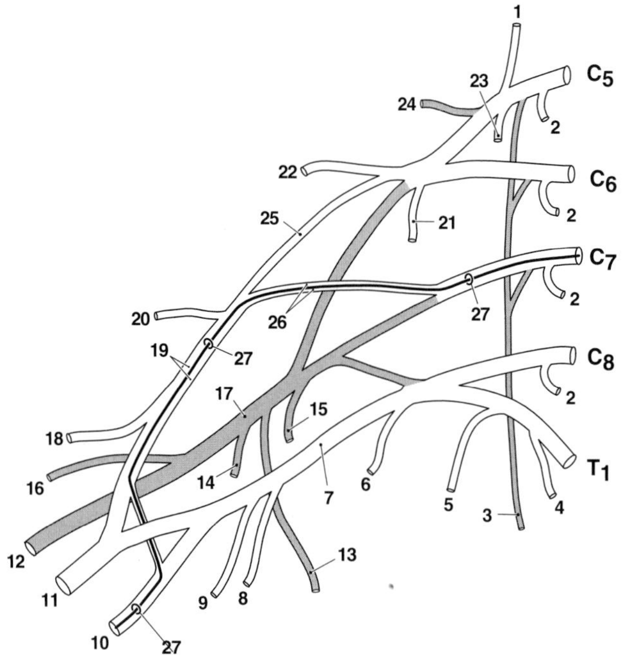

Figure 7D-9: Schematic of the brachial neural plexus on the right side. The posterior divisions and their counterparts are shaded. The fibers from C-7 joining the ulnar nerve are shown as a black line. *C-5* to *T-1,* cervical and thoracic spinal nerves.

1 Contributing neural branches to brachial plexus from C-4 spinal nerve (variable)
2 Neural branches to scaleni muscles
3 Long thoracic nerve to serratus anterior muscle
4 Contributing neural branch to brachial plexus from T-2 spinal nerve (variable)
5 First intercostal nerve
6 Medial pectoral nerve
7 Medial cord
8 Medial cutaneous nerve of arm
9 Medial cutaneous nerve of forearm
10 Ulnar nerve
11 Median nerve
12 Radial nerve
13 Thoracodorsal nerve
14 Lower subscapular nerve (to subscapularis and teres major muscles)
15 Upper subscapular nerve (to subscapularis and teres major muscles)
16 Axillary nerve
17 Posterior cord
18 Musculocutaneous nerve
19 Lateral cord
20 Lateral pectoral nerve
21 Nerve to subclavius muscle
22 Suprascapular nerve to supraspinatus and infraspinatus muscles
23 Neural branch to phrenic nerve
24 Dorsal scapular nerve to rhomboid muscles
25 Anterior division of upper trunk
26 Anterior division of middle trunk
27 Fibers from C-7 joining the ulnar nerve

The Lumbar Neural Plexus

1. The lumbar neural plexus is composed of the ventral rami of the first three lumbar spinal nerves (L-1 to L-3), most of the fourth lumbar spinal nerve (L-4), and a branch of the last thoracic (T-12) spinal nerve.
2. The neural branches of the lumbar plexus include muscular (T-12, L-1, L-2, L-3, L-4), iliohypogastric (L-1), ilioinguinal (L-1), genitofemoral (L-1, L-2), lateral femoral cutaneous (L-2, L-3), femoral (L-2 to L-4), obturator (L-2 to L-4), and accessory obturator (L-3 and L-4) nerves.
3. The muscular neural branches supply the quadratus lumborum (T-12, L-1 to L-4), psoas minor (L-1), psoas major (L-2 to L-4), and iliacus (L-2 and L-3) muscles.

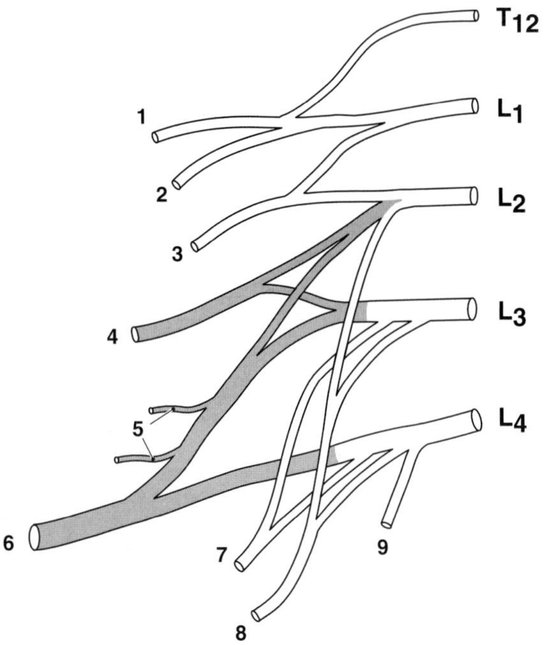

Figure 7D-10: Schematic of the lumbar neural plexus. The anterior divisions of ventral primary rami are *unshaded*; the posterior divisions of ventral primary rami are *shaded*. *T-12* to *L-4*, thoracic and lumbar spinal nerves.
1 Iliohypogastric nerve
2 Ilioinguinal nerve
3 Genitofemoral nerve
4 Lateral femoral cutaneous nerve
5 Nerve to iliopsoas muscle
6 Femoral nerve
7 Accessory obturator nerve
8 Obturator nerve
9 Branch of L-4 to lumbosacral trunk (sacral neural plexus)

The Sacral Neural Plexus

1. The sacral neural plexus is composed of the ventral rami of the lumbosacral trunk, the ventral rami of the first three sacral spinal nerves (S-1 to S-3), and part of the fourth sacral spinal nerve (S-4).
2. The lumbosacral trunk is composed of part of the ventral ramus of the L-4 spinal nerve and all of the ventral ramus of the L-5 spinal nerve.
3. The named sacral ventral rami together with the lumbosacral trunk converge at the greater sciatic foramen to form the upper and lower sacral neural bands.
4. The upper sacral neural band is composed of the lumbosacral trunk (L-4 to L-5) combined with the first, second, and the majority of the third sacral ventral rami (S-1 to S-3). It becomes a part of the sciatic nerve.
5. The lower sacral neural band is composed of portions of the ventral rami of the third and fourth sacral spinal nerves (S-3 to S-4). It becomes the pudendal nerve. The pudendal nerve proper subsequently receives a small branch from the ventral ramus of the second sacral spinal nerve (S-2).

The Coccygeal Neural Plexus

1. The coccygeal neural plexus is composed of a portion of the ventral ramus of the fourth sacral (S-4) spinal nerve, all of the ventral ramus of the fifth sacral (S-5) spinal nerve, and the ventral ramus of the sole coccygeal (Cx1) spinal nerve.
2. The coccygeal plexus gives rise to the anococcygeal nerves and cutaneous neural branches supplying the overlying skin.

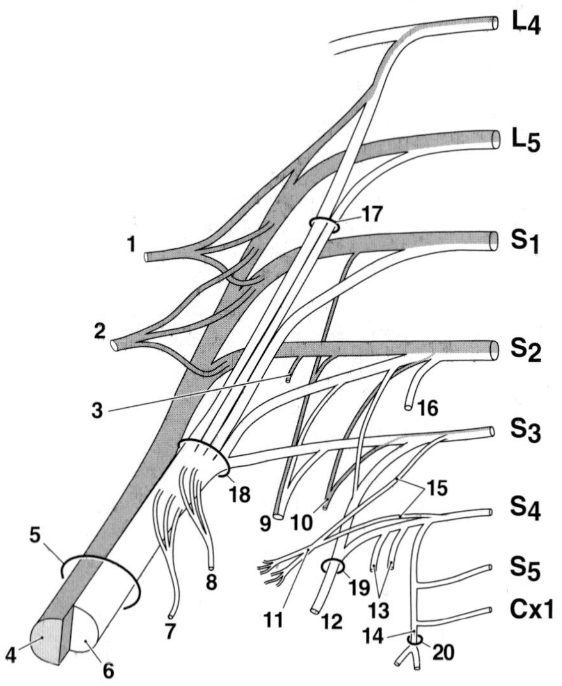

Figure 7D-11: Schematic of the sacral and coccygeal neural plexi on the right side. The ventral neural rami are *unshaded*; the dorsal neural rami and the nerves derived from them are *shaded*. *L-4, L-5, S-1 to S-5, Cx1,* lumbar, sacral, and coccygeal spinal nerves.

1 Superior gluteal nerve
2 Inferior gluteal nerve
3 Neural branch to piriformis muscle
4 Common peroneal nerve
5 Sciatic nerve
6 Tibial nerve
7 To quadratus femoris and inferior gemellus muscle
8 To obturator internus and superior gemellus muscle
9 Posterior femoral cutaneous nerve
10 Perforating cutaneous nerve
11 Pelvic splanchnic nerve
12 Pudendal nerve
13 Neural branches to levator ani, coccygeus, and sphincter ani externus muscles
14 Anococcygeal nerves
15 Visceral neural branches
16 Visceral neural branch
17 Lumbosacral trunk
18 Upper sacral neural band
19 Lower sacral neural band
20 Coccygeal neural plexus

THE SEGMENTAL PATTERN OF SOMATIC SENSORY INNERVATION

1. Somites are mesodermal segments that develop on each side of the embryonic neural tube.
2. The somites differentiate into dermatomes (skin), myotomes (skeletal muscle), and sclerotomes (skeleton and related connective tissue, such as joints and ligaments).
3. Each somite is innervated by one somatic spinal nerve that consists of somatic and autonomic fibers. The innervation to the dermis is directed to the somite's dermatome, that to the skeletal muscles is directed to the somite's myotome, and that to the bone, joints, and ligaments is directed to the somite's sclerotome.
4. Because of this innervation pattern, dermatomal, myotomal, and sclerotomal innervation charts may be generated based on clinically gathered sensory information from large numbers of patients.
5. However, these dermatome, myotome, and sclerotome demarcations are variable in part because of (a) overlapping innervation between somites, (b) intraindividual lateral asymmetry, and (c) interindividual somatic innervation variations, and (d) the complex peripheral and central somatic and autonomic innervation pathways.

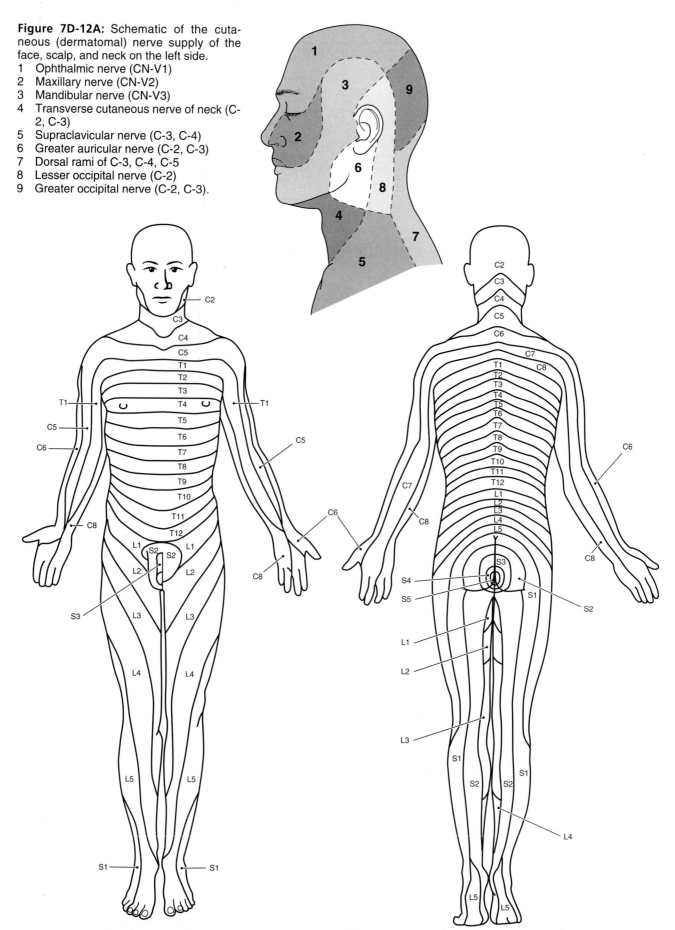

Figure 7D-12A: Schematic of the cutaneous (dermatomal) nerve supply of the face, scalp, and neck on the left side.

1 Ophthalmic nerve (CN-V1)
2 Maxillary nerve (CN-V2)
3 Mandibular nerve (CN-V3)
4 Transverse cutaneous nerve of neck (C-2, C-3)
5 Supraclavicular nerve (C-3, C-4)
6 Greater auricular nerve (C-2, C-3)
7 Dorsal rami of C-3, C-4, C-5
8 Lesser occipital nerve (C-2)
9 Greater occipital nerve (C-2, C-3).

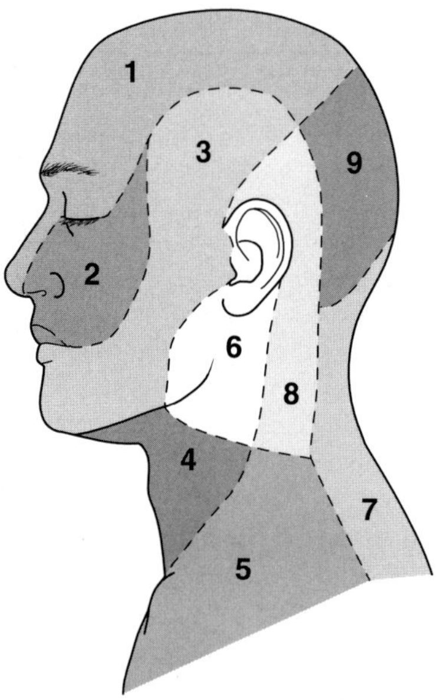

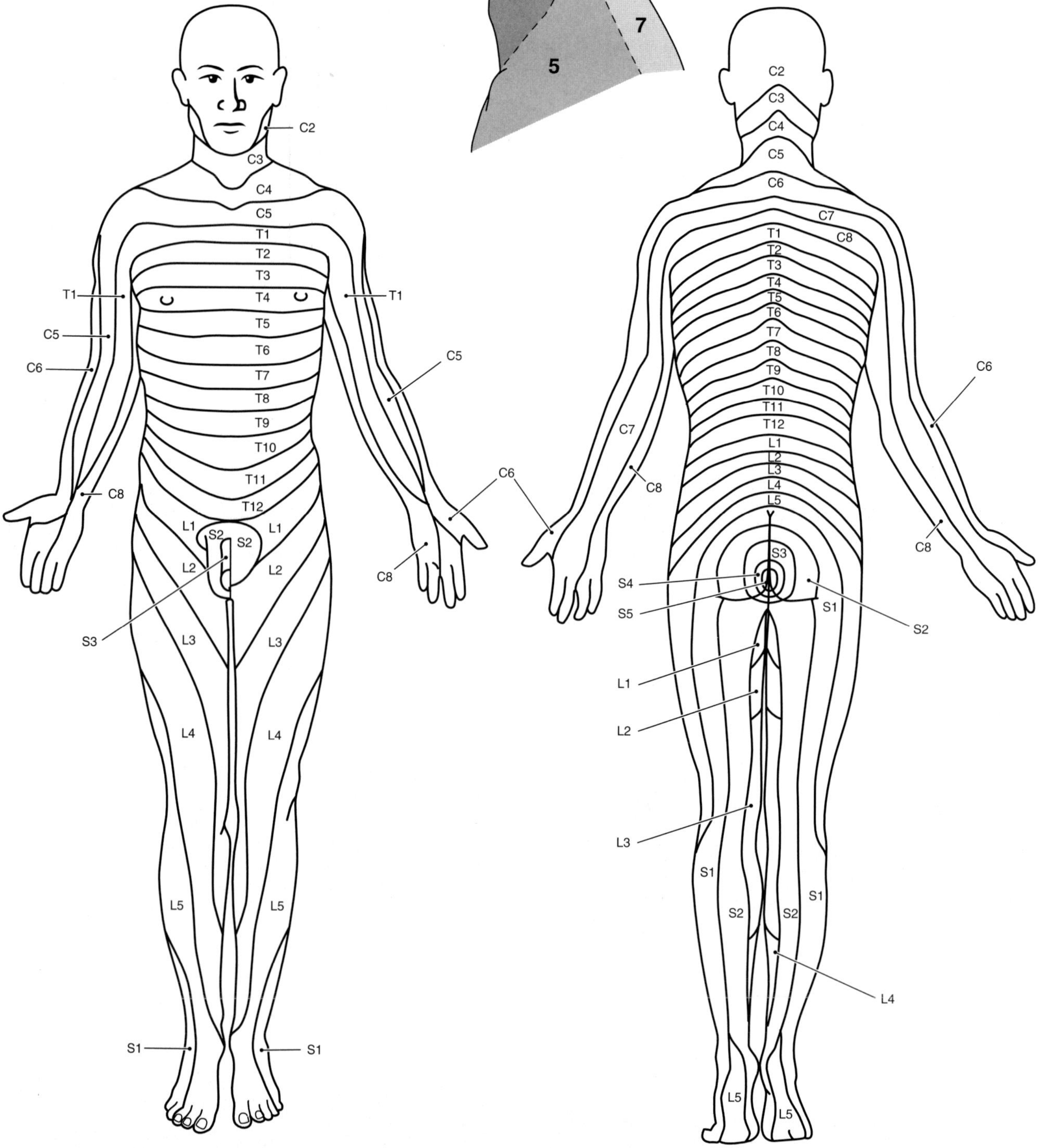

Figure 7D-12B: Schematic showing the anterior and posterior dermatomal maps below the head. **Left:** Anterior aspect. **Right:** Posterior aspect. *C, T, L, S,* cervical, thoracic, lumbar, and sacral spinal nerve innervation.

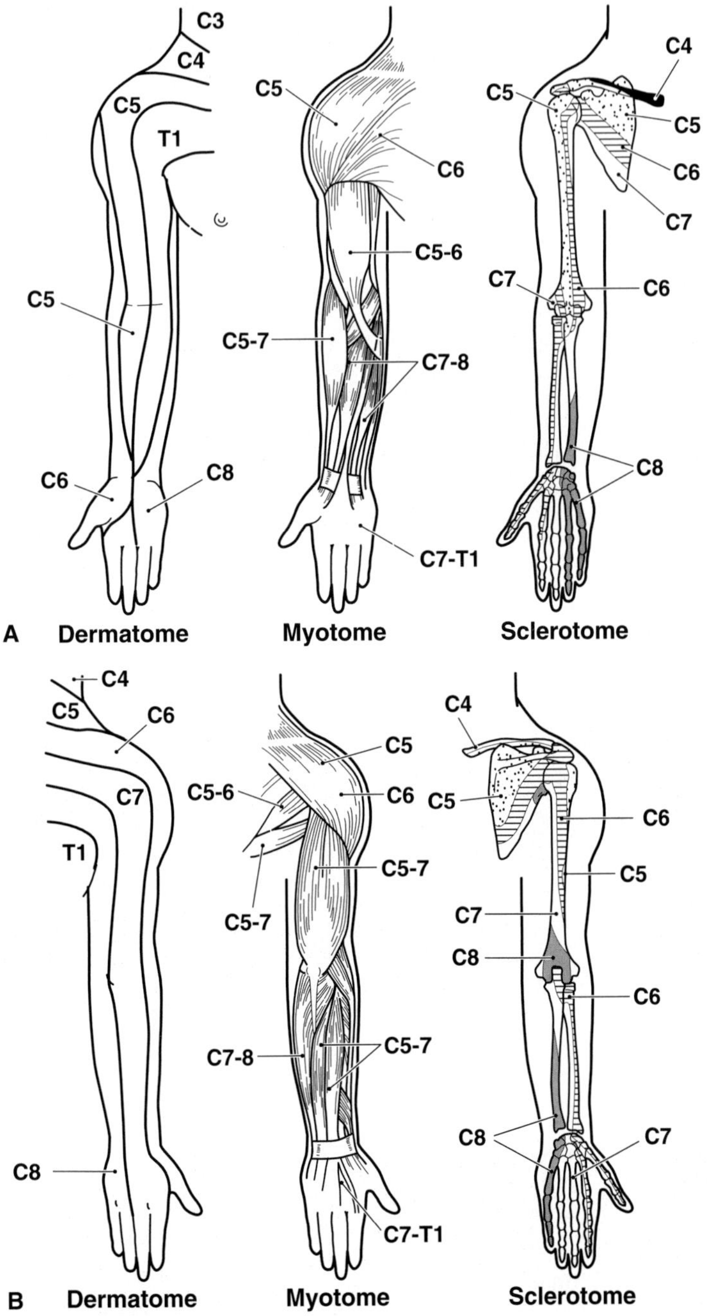

Figure 7D-13: Schematic of the anterior and posterior maps of the dermatomes, myotomes, and sclerotomes of the upper extremities. (For specific innervation of the muscles of the extremities, see Appendix, pp. 695–696.) **A:** Anterior aspect. **B:** Posterior aspect. (Modified from Inman VT, Saunders JB. The clinicoanatomical aspects of the lumbosacral region. *Radiology* 1942;38:669–678.)

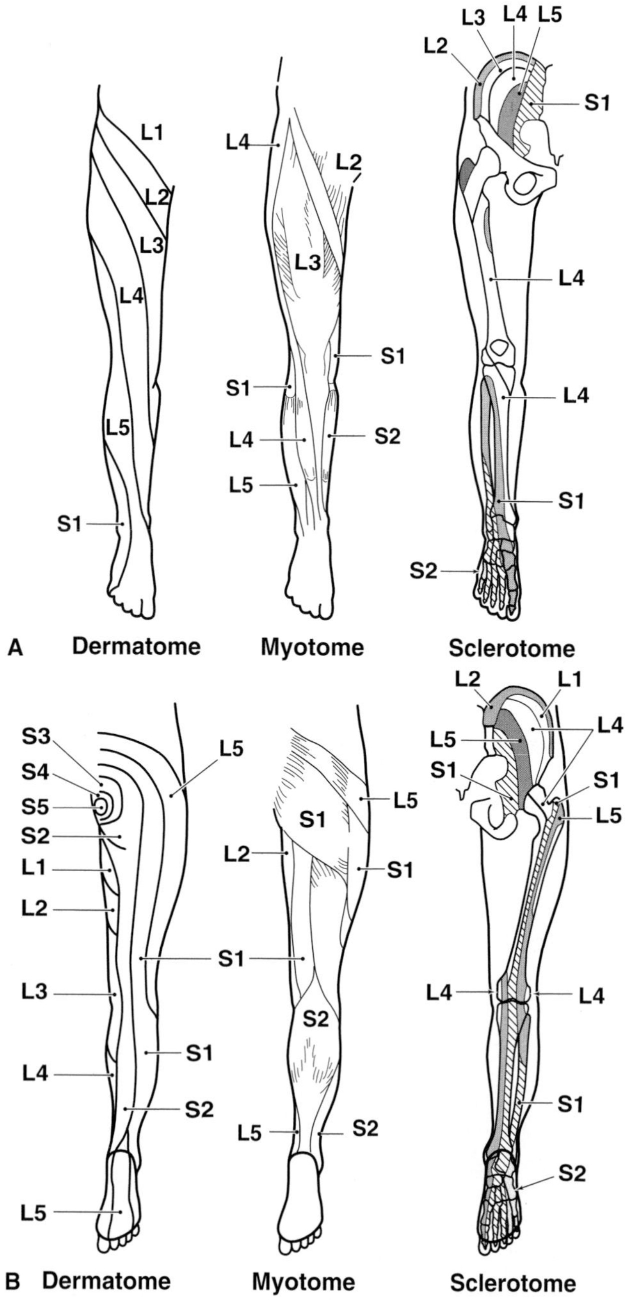

Figure 7D-14: Schematic of the anterior and posterior maps of the dermatomes, myotomes, and sclerotomes of the lower extremities. (For specific innervation of the muscles of the extremities, see Appendix, pp. 695–696.) **A:** Anterior aspect. **B:** Posterior aspect. (Modified from Inman VT, Saunders JB. The clinicoanatomical aspects of the lumbosacral region. *Radiology* 1942;38:669–678.)

SPINAL REFLEX ARCS

1. Skin, muscle, and joint receptors have sensory afferent axons that reach the spinal cord via the dorsal root of the spinal nerve. In the spinal cord they synapse with interneurons that in turn synapse with a somatic motor efferent neuron situated in the ventral horn of the gray matter of the spinal cord. Their motor efferent axons leave the spinal cord via the ventral root of the spinal nerve and innervate skeletal muscle. These afferent and efferent axons and neurons constitute a reflex arc and are part of the somatic nervous system.
2. Visceral afferent sensory axons proceed from the periphery toward the spinal cord via the dorsal root of the spinal nerve root. In the spinal cord they synapse via interneurons that in turn synapse with a visceral efferent neuron. The efferent visceral motor axon exits the spinal cord via the ventral spinal nerve root en route to a visceral motor neuron. The visceral motor neurons are grouped outside the central nervous system (CNS) in clusters forming the visceral motor ganglia. The visceral motor neuron axons subsequently innervate target organs (e.g., visceral smooth muscle, secretory glands, smooth muscle in the walls of blood vessels). These visceral afferent and visceral efferent axons and neurons constitute a reflex arc and are part of the autonomic nervous system.
3. Similar somatic and autonomic reflex arcs are believed to exist at the level of the cranial nerves and brain stem.

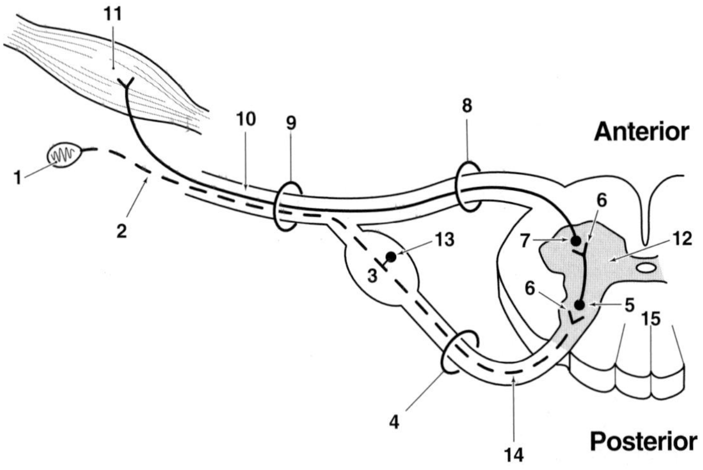

Figure 7D-15: Schematic of a segmental somatic reflex arc on the right side.
1 Somatic sensory receptor
2 Distal limb of somatic sensory afferent axon
3 Dorsal root ganglion
4 Dorsal root of spinal nerve
5 Spinal cord interneuron
6 Synapse(s)
7 Somatic motor neuron in ventral horn of spinal cord gray matter
8 Ventral root of spinal nerve
9 Combined spinal nerve
10 Somatic motor efferent axon
11 Skeletal muscle
12 Gray matter of spinal cord
13 Somatic afferent sensory neuron cell body
14 Proximal limb of somatic sensory afferent axon
15 Spinal cord

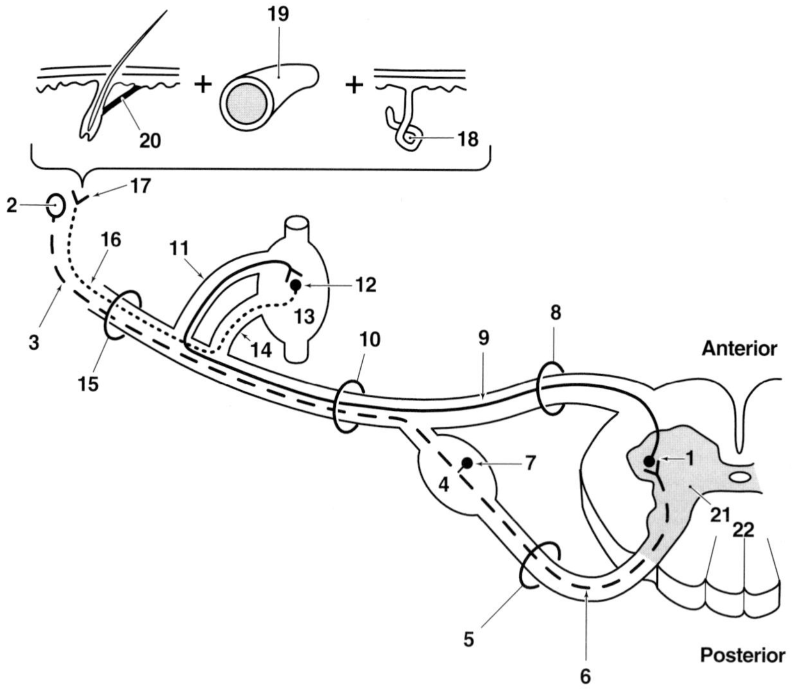

Figure 7D-16: Schematic of a theoretical sympathetic reflex arc with synapse in the paraspinal sympathetic chain on the right side.

1 Sympathetic preganglionic efferent neuron in spinal cord with synapse
2 Sympathetic afferent (sensory) receptor
3 Distal limb of afferent sympathetic axon
4 Dorsal root ganglion
5 Dorsal nerve root
6 Proximal limb of afferent sympathetic axon
7 Sympathetic afferent (sensory) neuron cell body
8 Ventral nerve root
9 Efferent preganglionic sympathetic axon
10 Combined spinal nerve
11 White ramus communicans
12 Sympathetic ganglionic efferent neuron (in paraspinal sympathetic ganglion with synapse)
13 Paraspinal sympathetic chain/ganglion
14 Gray ramus communicans
15 Peripheral nerve
16 Efferent postganglionic sympathetic axon
17 Visceral efferent nerve ending in 18–20 (see below)
18 Smooth muscle in sebaceous gland
19 Smooth muscle in blood vessel
20 Erector pili smooth muscle
21 Gray matter of spinal cord
22 Spinal cord

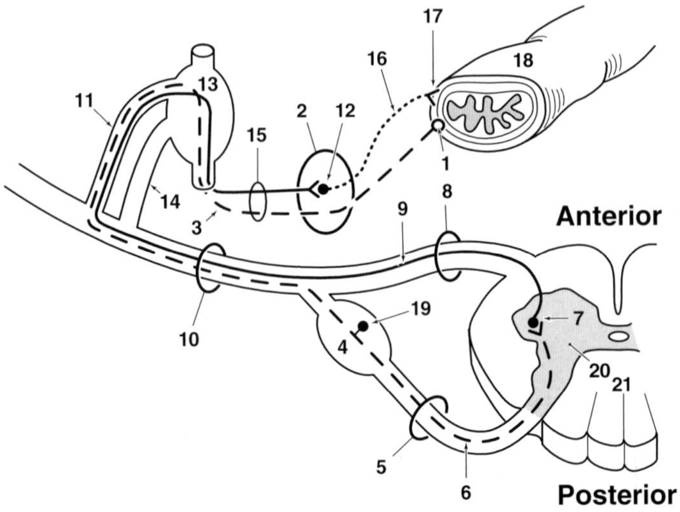

Figure 7D-17: Schematic of a theoretical parasympathetic reflex arc with synapse in intermediate ganglia (ciliary, pterygopalatine, submandibular, and otic ganglia) on the right side.

1 Parasympathetic afferent (sensory) receptor
2 Parasympathetic (effector) ganglion (e.g. ciliary, pterygopalatine, submandibular, and otic ganglia; abdominal visceral parasympathetic synapses in/near target organs)
3 Distal limb of parasympathetic afferent axon
4 Dorsal root ganglion
5 Dorsal nerve root
6 Proximal limb of afferent parasympathetic axon
7 Parasympathetic efferent neuron cell body in spinal cord with synapse
8 Ventral nerve root
9 Efferent preganglionic parasympathetic axon
10 Combined spinal nerve
11 White ramus communicans
12 Visceral sympathetic motor neuron cell body
13 Paraspinal sympathetic ganglion/chain
14 Gray ramus communicans
15 Visceral splanchnic nerve
16 Postganglionic efferent parasympathetic motor axon
17 Visceral efferent nerve ending
18 Intestine (or other parasympathetically innervated organ)
19 Parasympathetic afferent (sensory) neuron cell body
20 Gray matter of spinal cord
21 Spinal cord

SPINAL INNERVATION

The anatomic basis for the origin and mediation of clinical signs and symptoms related to the spine rests with (a) afferent and efferent somatic neural branches emanating from the ventral and dorsal rami of the spinal nerve, (b) neural rami projecting directly to and originating from the paravertebral autonomic (sympathetic) neural plexus, and (c) the dorsal and ventral spinal nerve roots and spinal nerves themselves. These fibers originate and terminate in the spinal column and related nonneural perispinal and intraspinal tissues, in the spinal nerves and their ramifications in regional neural tissue intimately related to the spinal elements, and in the peripheral neural and nonneural tissues.

Somatic Innervation of Ventral Spinal Elements

The anatomic basis for discogenic and vertebrogenic pain rests partially with afferent somatic fibers originating from the recurrent meningeal nerve (sinuvertebral nerve of Luschka) supplying the posterior longitudinal ligament, the meninges, the blood vessels, the posterior extent of the outermost fibers of the anulus fibrosus, and a portion of the periosteum of the vertebral body and related issues over an inconstant range. Irregular, unnamed afferent branches directly emanating from the rami of the somatic spinal nerves themselves also contribute to direct anterior spinal and perispinal soft tissue innervation.

Somatic Innervation of Dorsal Spinal Elements

The posterior spinal facet (zygapophyseal) joints (laminae, transverse and spinous processes) as well as the surrounding bone and posterior spinal muscular and ligamentous tissues receive their innervation primarily from the dorsal rami of the spinal nerves. There may also be innervation to the dorsal spinal elements from neural fibers arising directly from the ventral ramus and from the combined spinal nerve itself before its bifurcation into the dorsal and ventral rami.

Additional Theoretical Innervations of Spinal Elements

In addition to the local somatic spinal afferent nerves innervating the spinal column, there are nerve fibers innervating the nerves themselves, the *nervi nervorum*. These nervi nervorum are theoretically of three types. First, there are afferent sensory fibers to the nerve radicles traversing the spinal column. These are responsible for local neural sensation and even localized pain when the nerve itself is injured. Second, there are regional sympathetic afferent fibers which enter the paraspinal sympathetic chain via the gray rami communicantes and return to the CNS via the white rami communicantes. These fibers relay afferent information from the spinal roots, nerves, and surrounding spinal and perispinal tissues to the sympathetic nervous system. Third, there are regional sympathetic efferent fibers that carry out sympathetic actions (e.g., vasoactive functions) upon the spinal roots, nerves, and surrounding tissues.

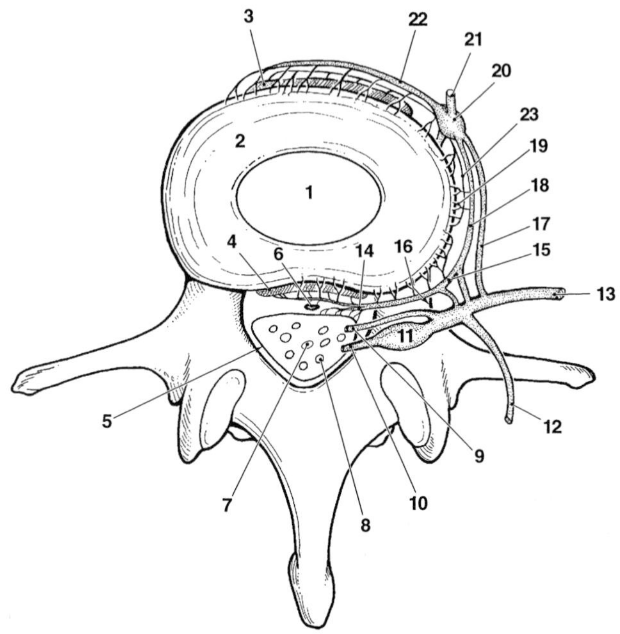

Figure 7D-18 Schematic of somatic and autonomic innervation of ventral spinal canal and structures of ventral aspect of spinal column.

1 Nucleus pulposus
2 Anulus fibrosus
3 Anterior longitudinal ligament/vertebral periosteum
4 Posterior longitudinal ligament/vertebral periosteum
5 Meninges of thecal sac
6 Epidural vasculature
7 Filum terminale
8 Intrathecal lumbosacral nerve root
9 Ventral nerve root
10 Dorsal nerve root
11 Dorsal root ganglion
12 Dorsal ramus of spinal nerve
13 Ventral ramus of spinal nerve
14 Recurrent meningeal nerve (sinuvertebral nerve of Luschka)
15 Autonomic (sympathetic) branch to recurrent meningeal nerve
16 Direct somatic branch from ventral ramus of spinal nerve to lateral disc surface
17 White ramus communicans (multilevel irregular lumbosacral distribution, often missing from L-2 to S-2 inclusive)
18 Gray ramus communicans (multilevel irregular lumbosacral distribution)
19 Lateral sympathetic branches projecting from gray ramus communicans
20 Paraspinal sympathetic ganglion (PSG)
21 Craniocaudal extension of paraspinal sympathetic chain
22 Anterior paraspinal sympathetic ramus(i) projecting to PSG
23 Lateral paraspinal sympathetic ramus(i) projecting to PSG

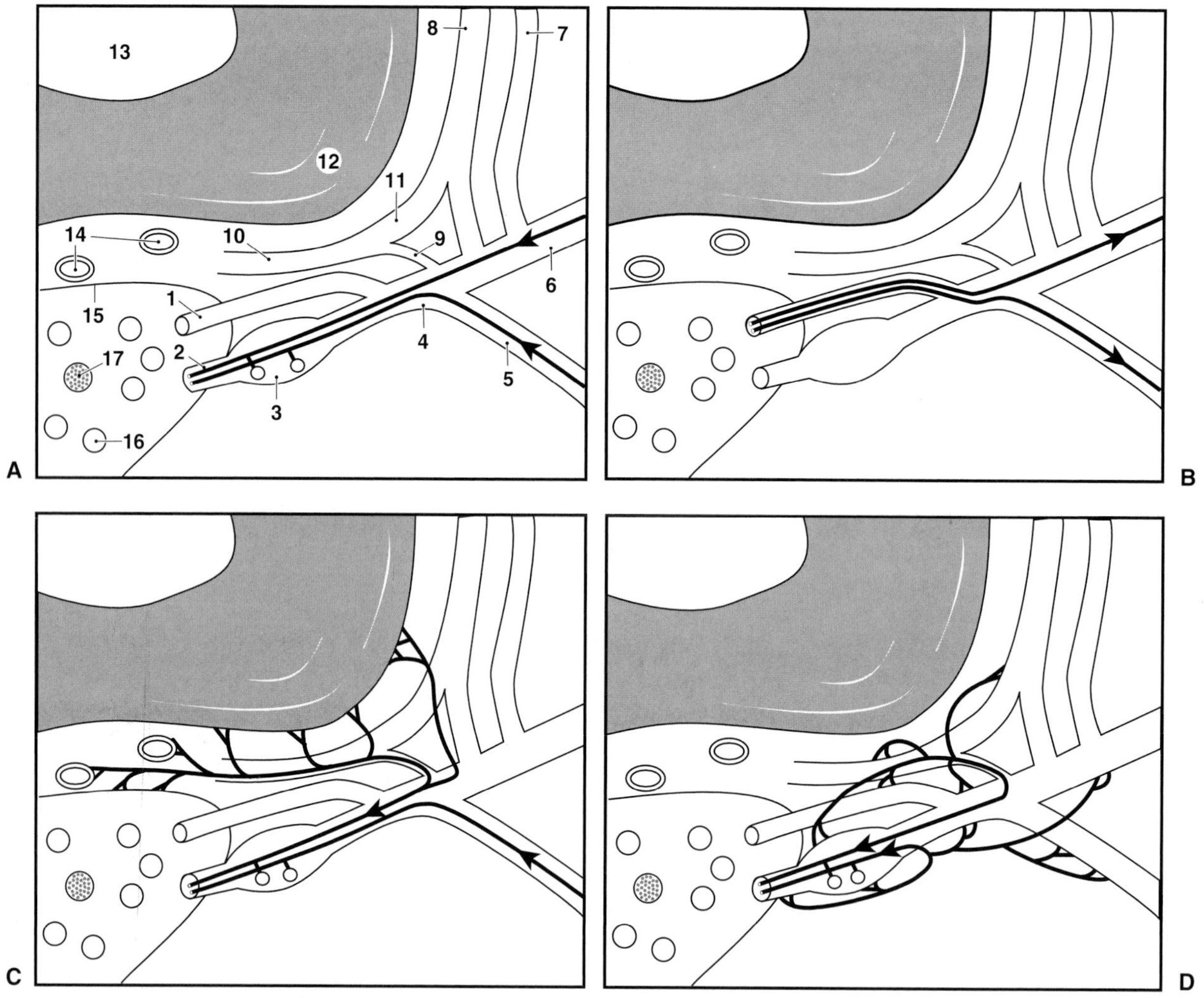

Figure 7D-19: Schematic of local and peripheral somatic innervation of spinal column and related structures. **A:** Somatic afferent sensory neural fibers from *peripheral* ventral and dorsal tissues. **B:** Somatic efferent motor neural fibers to *peripheral* ventral and dorsal tissues. **C:** *Local* somatic afferent sensory neural fibers from ventral (e.g., peripheral disc, epidural tissues, dura mater vertebral periosteum), and dorsal tissues (e.g., facet joints, posterior spinal ligaments, periosteum). **D:** *Local* radicular afferent *nervi nervorum*.

1 Ventral nerve root
2 Dorsal nerve root
3 Dorsal root ganglion
4 Combined spinal nerve
5 Dorsal ramus of spinal nerve
6 Ventral ramus of spinal nerve
7 White ramus communicans (not found or irregularly found caudal to L-2)
8 Gray ramus communicans (multilevel irregular lumbosacral distribution)
9 Branch to recurrent meningeal nerve from spinal nerve
10 Recurrent meningeal nerve (sinuvertebral nerve of Luschka)
11 Autonomic (sympathetic) branch to recurrent meningeal nerve from gray ramus communicans
12 Anulus fibrous
13 Nucleus pulposus
14 Epidural vasculature
15 Meninges of thecal sac
16 Intrathecal lumbosacral nerve root
17 Filum terminale

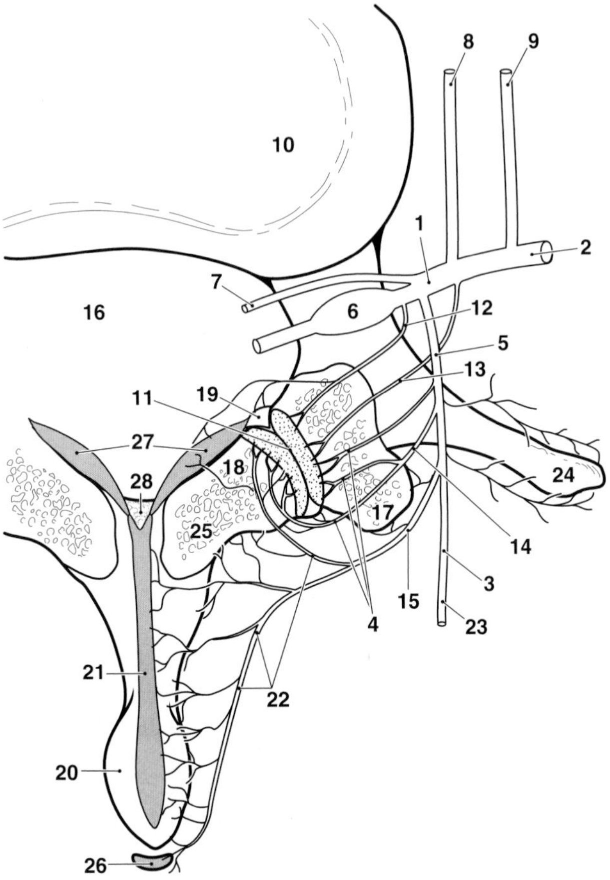

Figure 7D-20: Schematic diagrams outlining innervation of the structures of the dorsal (posterior) aspect of the spinal column.

1 Main trunk of spinal nerve
2 Ventral ramus of spinal nerve
3 Lateral branch of dorsal ramus of spinal nerve
4 Neural fibers to posterior dorsal ramus of spinal nerve
5 Dorsal ramus of spinal nerve
6 Dorsal nerve root and ganglion
7 Ventral nerve root
8 Gray ramus communicans
9 White ramus communicans
10 Intervertebral disc
11 Articular cartilage of posterior spinal facet (zygapophyseal) joint
12 Neural fibers from main trunk of spinal nerve
13 Neural fibers to posterior facet joint from ventral ramus of spinal nerve
14 Neural fibers to posterior facet joint from dorsal ramus
15 Medial branch of dorsal ramus
16 Central spinal canal
17 Superior articular facet process
18 Inferior articular facet process
19 Zygapophyseal joint space and capsule
20 Spinous process
21 Interspinous ligament
22 Medial neural branches ramifying within posterior spinal facet joint, the lamina, spinous process, interspinous ligament, and supraspinous ligament
23 Branch of dorsal ramus ramifying within posterior perispinous tissues
24 Transverse process
25 Lamina
26 Supraspinous ligament
27 Ligamenta flavum
28 Median retrothecal fat pad

THE AUTONOMIC NERVOUS SYSTEM

Overview

1. The autonomic nervous system innervates the viscera, glands, blood vessels, and other nonstriated (smooth) muscle–containing tissues.
2. There are three parts of the autonomic nervous system: sympathetic, parasympathetic, and enteric.
3. Autonomic efferent pathways are interrupted by peripheral synapses; at least two neurons are interposed between the spinal cord and the autonomic peripheral effectors.
4. The nerve cell bodies of the primary efferent neurons (preganglionic neurons) are found in the autonomic nuclei of the cranial nerves and in the lateral gray columns of the spinal cord.
5. Efferent axons traverse the cranial and spinal nerves to arrive at peripheral autonomic ganglia where synapses occur.
6. The secondary effector efferent autonomic neurons (postganglionic neurons) supply, via their axon processes, smooth muscle or glandular cells.
7. One preganglionic neuron may synapse with 15 to 20 postganglionic neurons. This multisynaptic phenomenon is greater in the sympathetic than in the parasympathetic nervous system.
8. Autonomic afferent fibers are similar to somatic afferent ones. The origin of autonomic afferent fibers are bipolar neurons found in the cranial nerve ganglia and spinal nerve dorsal root ganglia.
9. The peripheral afferent autonomic neural processes (axons) traverse from the periphery without synaptic interruption.
10. The central autonomic neural processes (axons) of the afferent autonomic neurons project from the cranial nerve ganglia and spinal nerve dorsal root ganglia to the CNS (brain stem, spinal cord).

The Sympathetic Nervous System

1. The sympathetic nervous system consists of the paired paraspinal sympathetic trunks (chains) together with their branches, plexi, and subsidiary ganglia.
2. The sympathetic nervous system innervates the sweat glands, piloerector muscles, the muscular wall of the blood vessels, the heart, lungs, abdominal viscera, pelvic viscera, esophagus, iris musculature, and urogenital tract.
3. The efferent preganglionic sympathetic fibers exit the CNS via the ventral nerve roots. They enter the paraspinal sympathetic chain via white rami communicantes. These white rami exist primarily in the thoracolumbar region (T-1 to L-3) and midsacral region (S-2,3 to Cx1).
4. Efferent preganglionic sympathetic fibers may then (a) immediately synapse with the postganglionic neuron(s), (b) ascend or descend to a different paraspinal sympathetic ganglion before synapsing, or (c) exit the paraspinal sympathetic chain and travel to one of the peripheral sympathetic ganglia or plexi before synapsing with the postganglionic neuron(s).
5. After synapsing, the peripheral neural process (axon) of the postganglionic sympathetic neuron may (a) exit immediately back to the spinal nerve via a gray ramus communicans, or (b) ascend or descend within the paraspinal sympathetic chain to a different level before exiting via a gray ramus communicans, to ramify within the peripheral tissues.

The Parasympathetic Nervous System

1. The preganglionic parasympathetic fibers run within the third, seventh, ninth, tenth, and eleventh cranial nerves, and within the second to fourth sacral spinal nerves.

2. The cell bodies of the postganglionic neurons are located peripherally in either discrete intermediate ganglia or scattered within the walls of the viscera.
3. Four peripheral intermediate ganglia are found in the cranial portion of the parasympathetic system: the ciliary, pterygopalatine, submandibular, and otic ganglia. These ganglia are the site of the cranial postganglionic parasympathetic neuron cell bodies; afferent fibers and postganglionic sympathetic efferent fibers also traverse the parasympathetic ganglia, without synapsing, from peripheral and more central sources, respectively.
4. In the sacral region, the preganglionic parasympathetic fibers exit the CNS via ventral rami of the second to fourth sacral spinal nerves to join the pelvic splanchnic nerves.
5. The splanchnic parasympathetic nerves serve the pelvic viscera. The peripheral processes of these nerves synapse with the postganglionic parasympathetic neurons in small ganglia within the walls of the pelvic viscera. Therefore, the postganglionic parasympathetic pelvic efferent fibers are quite short.
6. The cranial innervation of the parasympathetic nervous system includes branches of the: occulomotor nerve (CN-III: to ciliary muscle, sphincter pupillae muscle), facial nerve (CN-VII: to submandibular gland, sublingual gland, lacrimal gland, nasal/palatal mucosal glands), glossopharyngeal nerve (CN-IX: to parotid gland, oral mucosal glands), and vagus nerve (CN-X: to heart, bronchi/bronchioles, stomach, intestines).
7. The pelvic innervation of the parasympathetic nervous system includes branches to the urinary bladder, to penile and clitoral erectile tissue, and to blood vessels of the testes, ovaries, uterus, and colon distal to the terminal transverse segment.

Descending Cerebral Autonomic Pathways

1. The cerebral nuclear regions giving rise to descending autonomic fibers include
   a. Hypothalamic nuclei: paraventricular nucleus, nuclei in the lateral and posterior hypothalamic areas, supramamillary nuclei, and dorsomedial nucleus.
   b. Visceral nuclei of the oculomotor complex.
   c. Locus ceruleus
   d. Nucleus of the solitary tract (nucleus solitarius)
   e. Neurons in the reticular formation of the brain stem
2. These descending autonomic fibers terminate upon visceral cell (neurons) groups in the spinal cord (e.g., intermediolateral cell column, sacral preganglionic cell groups) that in turn innervate visceral and peripheral smooth muscle, cardiac muscle, and the viscera.

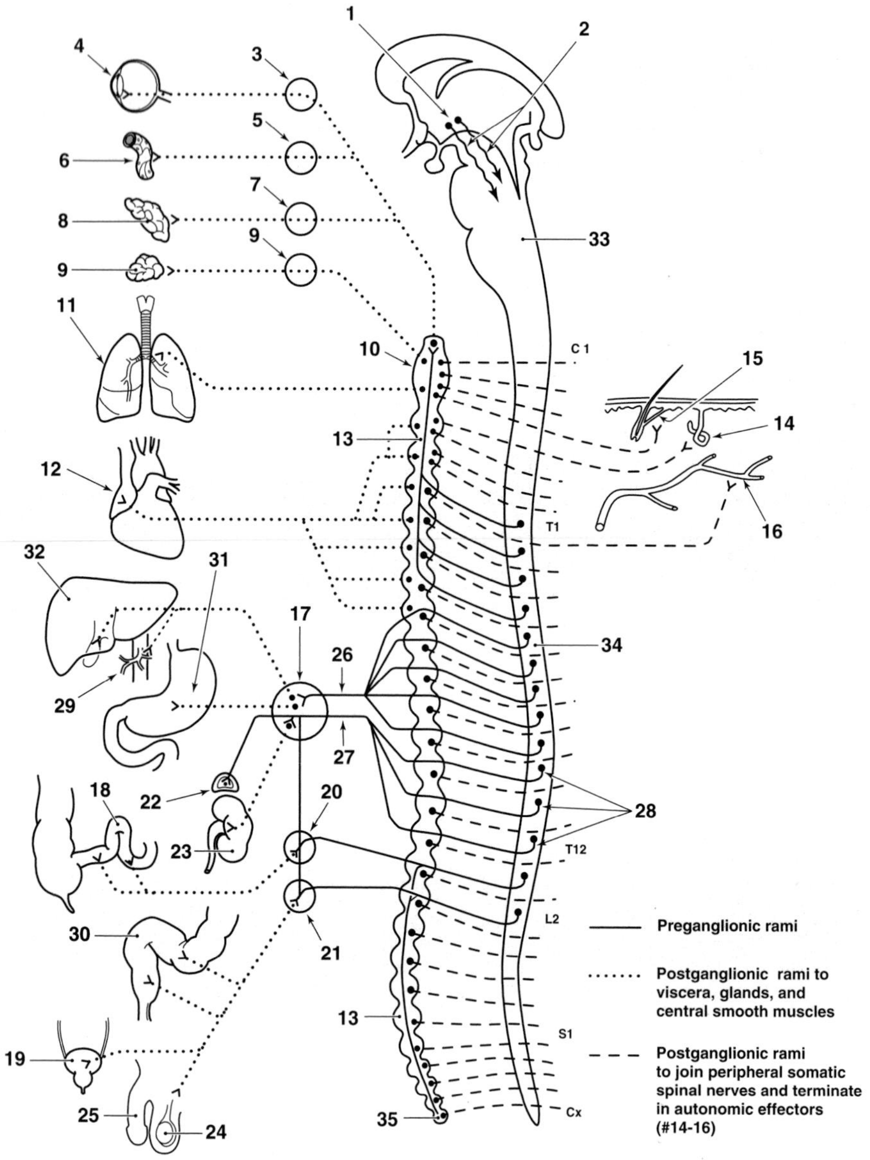

Figure 7D-21: Schematic of the sympathetic division of the autonomic nervous system. *C, T, L, S, Cx,* cervical, thoracic, lumbar, sacral, and coccygeal spinal cord segments.

1 Inflow into sympathetic nervous system from the hypothalamus
2 Descending autonomic pathways
3 Ciliary ganglion (traversing sympathetic fibers without synapse)
4 Globe
5 Pterygopalatine ganglion (traversing sympathetic fibers without synapse)
6 Blood vessels and mucous membranes of extracranial head and neck
7 Otic ganglion (traversing sympathetic fibers without synapse)
8 Glands associated with eye, (lacrimal gland) nasal cavity, and oral cavity
9 Submandibular gland and ganglion (traversing sympathetic fibers without synapse)
10 Superior cervical sympathetic ganglion
11 Respiratory system
12 Central circulatory system
13 Paraspinal sympathetic chain
14 Sweat glands
15 Hair follicle muscle
16 Peripheral blood vessel (smooth muscle)
17 Celiac ganglion
18 Small intestine
19 Urinary bladder
20 Superior mesenteric ganglion
21 Inferior mesenteric ganglion
22 Adrenal gland
23 Kidney
24 Reproductive system (testes)
25 External genitalia
26 Greater splanchnic nerve
27 Lesser splanchnic nerve
28 Gray rami communicantes
29 Abdominal vessels
30 Large intestine
31 Stomach
32 Liver and biliary ducts
33 Brain stem
34 Spinal cord
35 Terminal coccygeal sympathetic ganglion

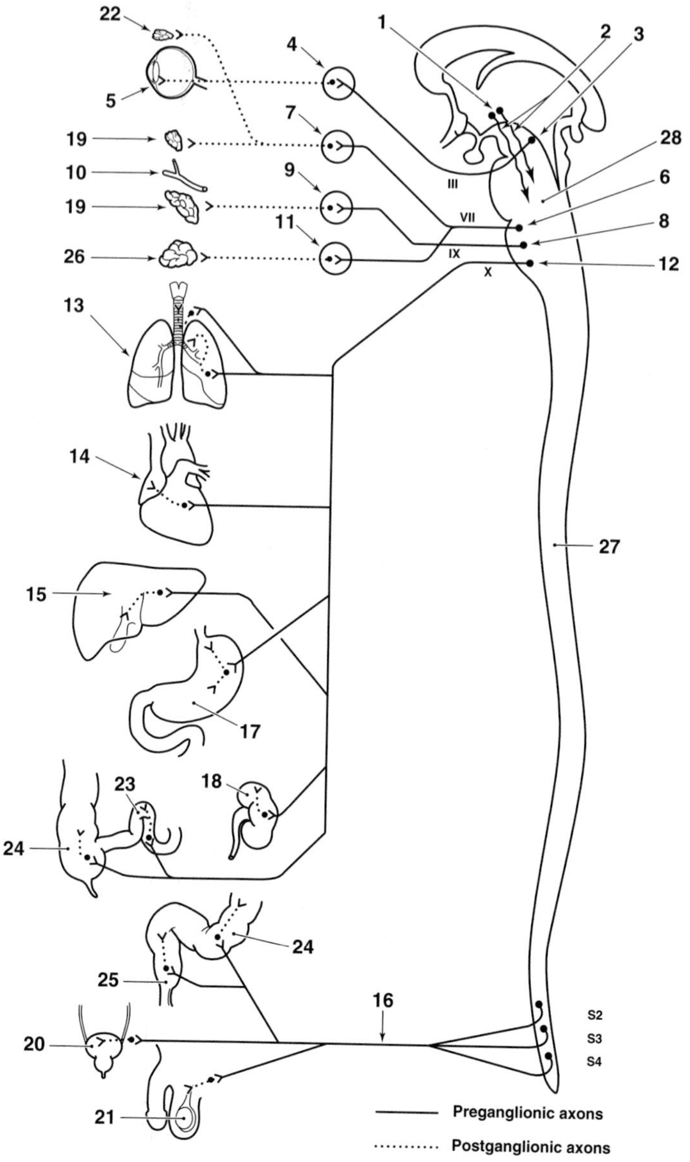

Figure 7D-22: Schematic of the parasympathetic division of the autonomic nervous system. *III, VII, IX, X,* oculomotor, facial, glossopharyngeal, vagus cranial nerves; *S-2 to S-4,* sacral spinal cord segments.

1 Inflow into parasympathetic nervous system from hypothalamus
2 Descending autonomic pathways
3 Edinger-Westphal nucleus
4 Ciliary ganglion (with parasympathetic synapse)
5 Ciliary muscle
6 Superior salivatory nucleus
7 Pterygopalatine ganglion (with parasympathetic synapse)
8 Inferior salivatory nucleus
9 Otic ganglion (with parasympathetic synapse)
10 Blood vessels of head and neck region
11 Submandibular ganglion (with parasympathetic synapse)
12 Dorsal vagal nucleus
13 Respiratory system
14 Central circulatory system
15 Liver
16 Pelvic splanchnic nerves
17 Stomach
18 Kidney
19 Salivary glands
20 Urinary bladder
21 Reproductive system
22 Lacrimal gland
23 Small intestine
24 Colon
25 Rectum
26 Submandibular gland
27 Spinal cord
28 Brain stem

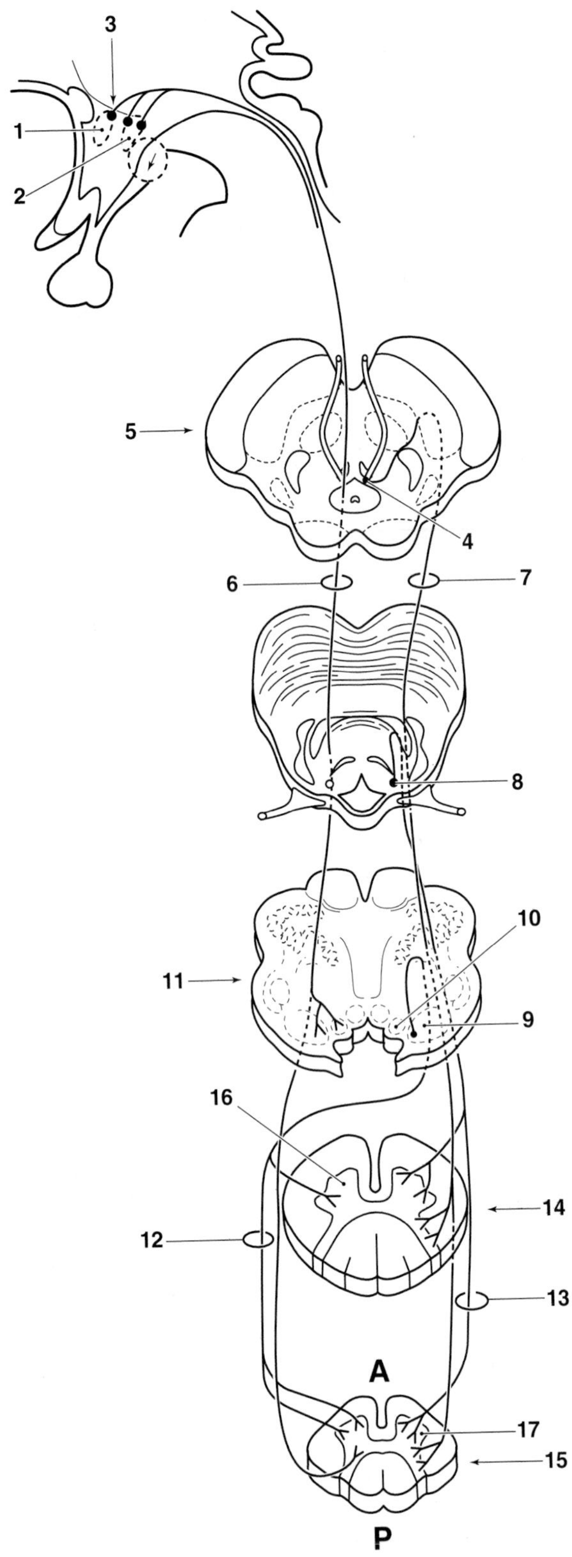

Figure 7D-23: Schematic of the descending autonomic projections to the spinal cord. *A*, anterior; *P*, posterior.

1 Paraventricular nucleus
2 Posterior hypothalamus
3 Hypothalamus
4 Oculomotor visceral nuclei
5 Midbrain
6 Hypothalamic spinal projections
7 Oculomotor spinal projections
8 Locus ceruleus
9 Nucleus solitarius (solitary nucleus)
10 Dorsal motor nucleus of the vagus nerve (CN-X)
11 Medulla
12 Spinal projections of the nucleus solitarius
13 Spinal projections of the locus ceruleus
14 Cervical spinal cord
15 Thoracic spinal cord
16 Phrenic nerve nucleus
17 Anterior horn and intermediate gray matter

SPINAL NERVE ROOT, SPINAL NERVE, SPINAL ROOT SLEEVE, AND NERVE PLEXUS VARIANTS

- Conjoined nerve roots/sleeve
- Fibrolipoma of filum terminale
- Variations in the grouping and branching of the spinal neural plexi

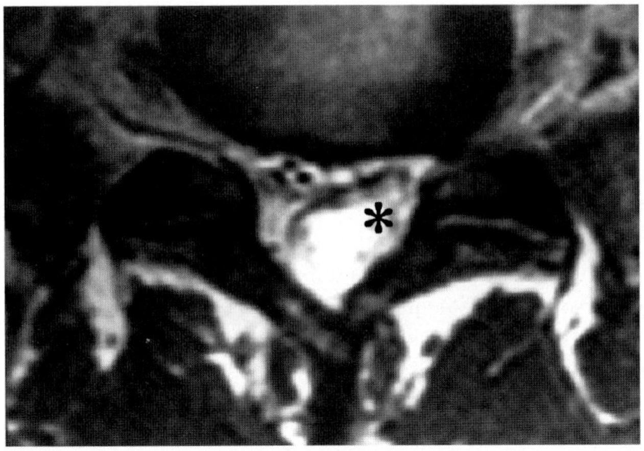

Figure 7D-24: Conjoined root/sleeve. Axial T2-weighted MR image showing that the contents of the conjoined nerve root sleeve (*asterisk*) contains multiple exiting nerve roots and that otherwise the root sleeve contents follows cerebrospinal fluid intensity.

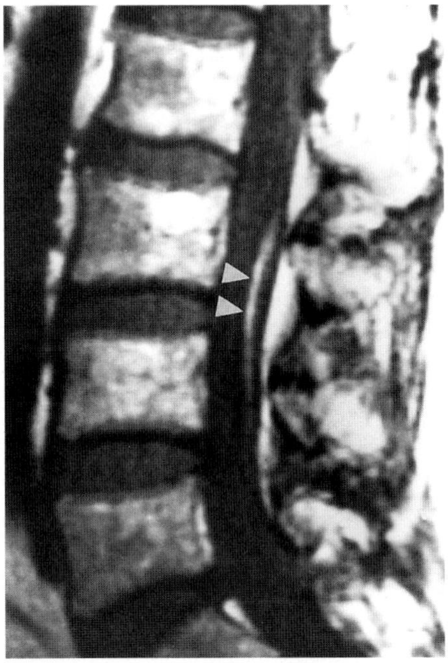

Figure 7D-25A: Fibrolipoma of the filum terminale. Sagittal T1-weighted MR images showing curvilinear hyperintense intratracheal material (*arrowheads*) representing a fibrolipoma of the filum terminale.

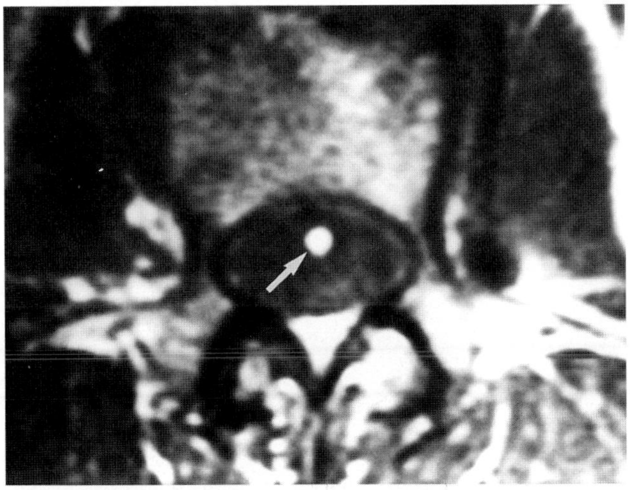

Figure 7D-25B: Axial T1-weighted MR image showing the hyperintense fibrolipoma (*arrow*).

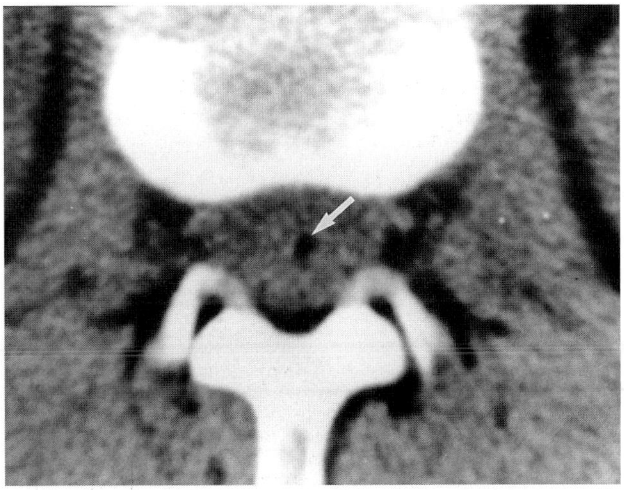

Figure 7D-25C: Axial CT showing the hypodense fibrolipoma (*arrow*).

7E Spinal Meninges

OVERVIEW

1. The meninges of the spine are continuous with those of the cranium.
2. The spinal meninges, much like the cranial meninges, consist of the spinal pachymeninges (dura mater) and the spinal leptomeninges (arachnoid mater and pia mater), with the exception that the dura mater has only one layer in the spine, and there are intermediate and outer layers of the arachnoid mater in the spine. From the spinal cord outward, the spinal meningeal layers include pia mater on the surface of the spinal cord, intermediate layer of arachnoid matter associated with the pia mater, outer layer of arachnoid mater associated with the dura mater, and, finally, the dura mater.
3. Exiting or entering vessels and nerves have a thin covering of leptomeningeal cells throughout their course within the subarachnoid space. The leptomeninges of the spinal nerve fuses with the perineurium of the peripheral spinal nerve as the spinal nerve exits the thecal sac; in turn, the dura mater of the spinal nerve root sheath fuses with the epineurium of the peripheral spinal nerve.
4. The pia mater on the surface of the spinal cord is continuous with the denticulate (dentate) ligaments. These ligaments are fibrous structures that originate in the pial/subpial connective tissue of the spinal cord laterally between the ventral and dorsal nerve roots and insert into the dura mater laterally. There are approximately 21 ligaments on each side extending from the foramen magnum to the T-12 to L-1 spinal segmental level.
5. Similar spinal cord ligaments include the dorsal, dorsolateral, and ventral ligaments of the spinal cord. Such "ligaments" are irregular, fenestrated structures that attach the pial surface of the spinal cord to the parietal arachnoid mater. These arachnoid trabeculae are found throughout the spine in segments traversed by the spinal cord.
6. Caudal to the conus medullaris, the filum terminale is invested in pia mater, but no distinct spinal ligaments are found.

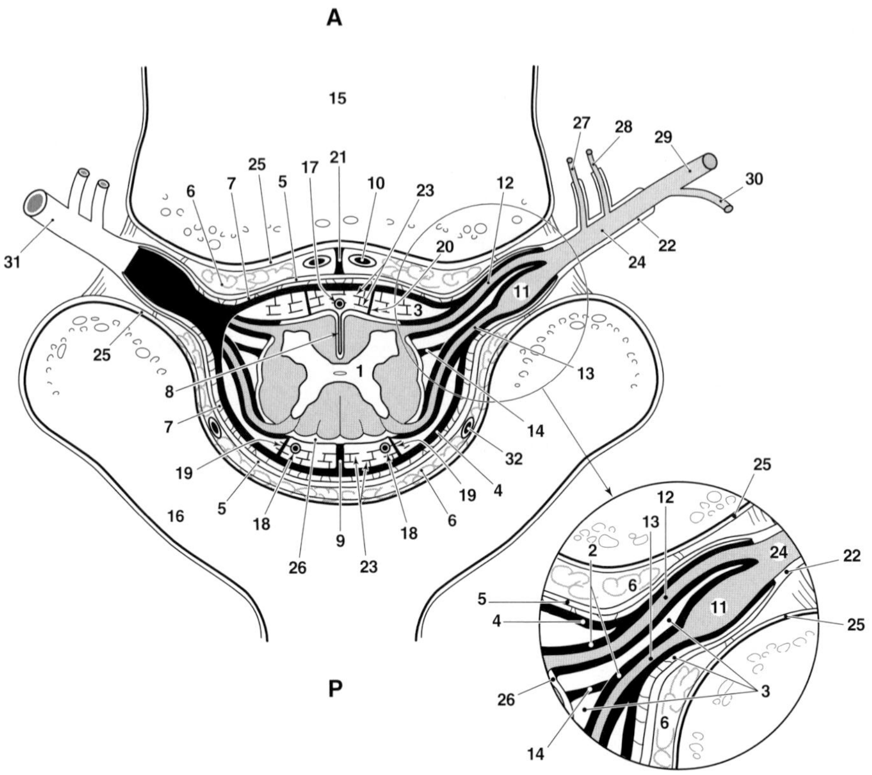

Figure 7E-1: Axial schematic of the spinal canal showing the spinal meninges and related tissues. *A*, anterior; *P*, posterior.

1 Deep gray matter of spinal cord
2 Pia mater on surface of spinal nerve roots
3 Subarachnoid space
4 Outer layer of arachnoid mater
5 Dura mater
6 Epidural space
7 Subdural space
8 Anterior median fissure of spinal cord
9 Dorsal ligament
10 Anterior epidural venous plexus
11 Dorsal root ganglion
12 Ventral nerve root
13 Dorsal nerve root
14 Denticulate (dentate) ligaments of spinal cord
15 Vertebral body
16 Vertebral lamina
17 Anterior spinal artery
18 Posterior spinal arteries
19 Dorsolateral ligaments of spinal cord
20 Ventral ligaments
21 Anterior median septum (attaches outer aspect of dura mater to posterior vertebral periosteum)
22 Peri- and epineurium of spinal nerve
23 Intermediate layers of arachnoid mater
24 Spinal nerve proper
25 Vertebral periosteum
26 Pia mater on surface of spinal cord
27 Gray ramus communicans
28 White ramus communicans
29 Ventral ramus of spinal nerve
30 Dorsal ramus of spinal nerve
31 Perineurium of spinal nerve
32 Posterior epidural venous plexus

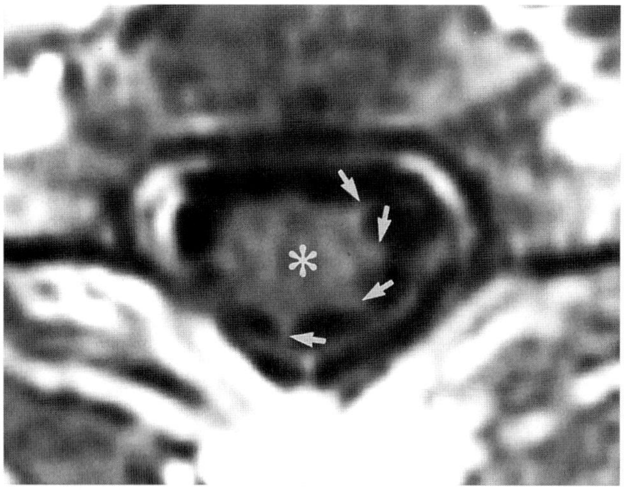

Figure 7E-2A: The dentate ligaments and arachnoid trabeculae. Axial T1-weighted MR image of the mid-cervical spinal cord (*asterisk*) showing some of the spinal dentate ligaments/arachnoid trabeculae (*arrows*).

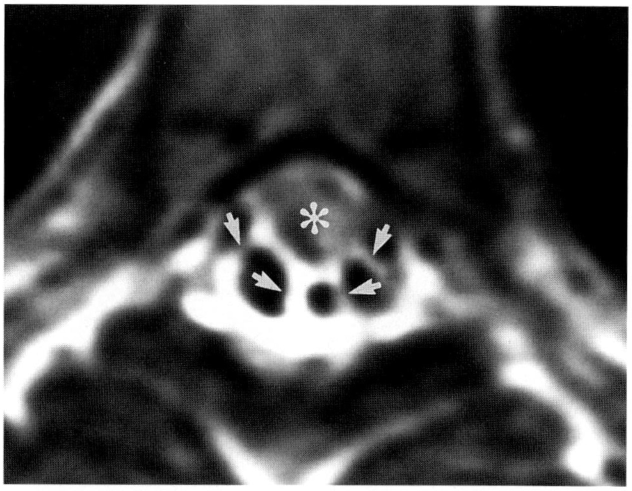

Figure 7E-2B: Axial T2-weighted MR image showing voids within the cerebrospinal fluid between the arachnoid trabeculae (*arrows*) surrounding the spinal cord (*asterisk*).

TABLE 7E-1: The Structures, Coverings, and Spaces of the Spine from Outward to Inward

Structure	Space	Contents of space
Bone (vertebrae)	Intraosseous	Bone, blood vessels, lymphatics, nerves
	Subperiosteal space (potential space)	Bridging blood vessels
Periosteum		
	Epidural space (potential space)	Fat, vessels, nerves
Dura mater		
	Subdural space (potential space)	Bridging blood vessels
Outer layer of arachnoid mater		
	Subarachnoid space	Inner layer of arachnoid mater, cerebrospinal fluid, blood vessels, spinal cord ligaments
Pia mater		Subpial and bridging blood vessels
	Subpial space (potential space)	
Spinal cord/nerve root	Intramedullary/intraneural space	Neural tissue, blood vessels

SPINAL MENINGES VARIANTS

- Conjoined nerve root sleeve
- Perineural root sleeve (Tarlov) cyst
- Lateral spinal meningocele
- Patulous thecal space
- Low termination of thecal sac
- High termination of thecal sac

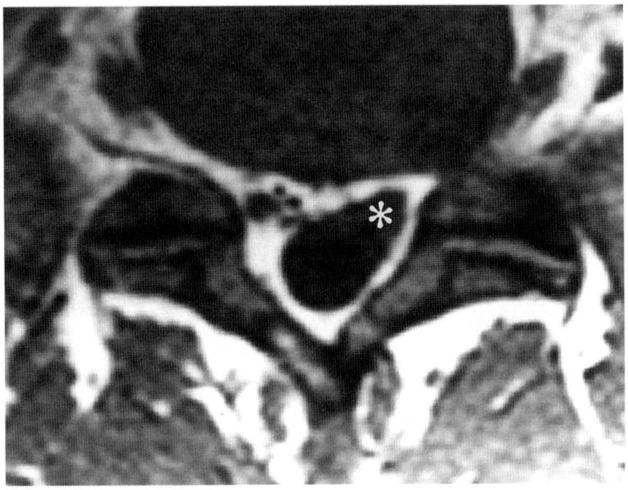

Figure 7E-3: Conjoined spinal nerve root sleeve. Axial T1-weighted MR image sharing an enlarged, conjoined spinal nerve root sleeve (*asterisk*) originating on the left side.

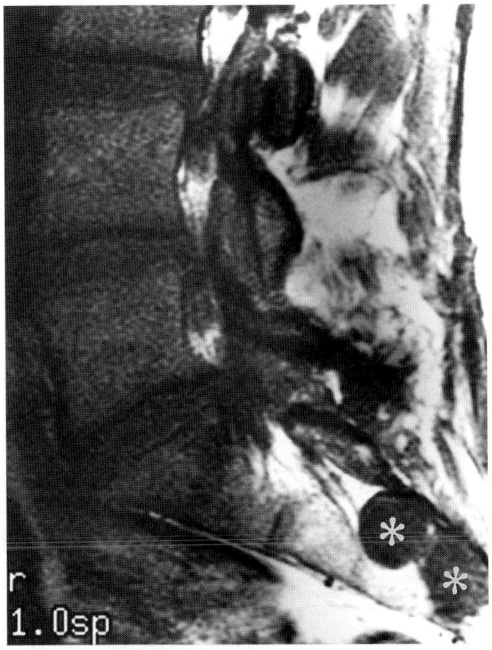

Figure 7E-4A: Perineural root sleeve (Tarlov) cysts. Sagittal T1-weighted MR image showing two perineural root sleeve cysts (*asterisks*) in the sacral region.

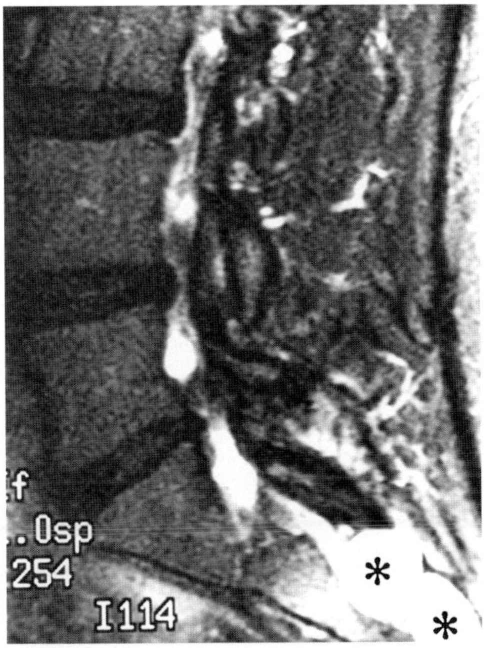

Figure 7E-4B: Sagittal T2-weighted MR image showing the root sleeve cysts (*asterisks*). Note that the intensity of the cysts follows closely that of cerebrospinal fluid.

7F Paraspinal Muscles

THE INTRINSIC MUSCLES OF THE SPINE

1. The intrinsic muscles of the spine extend from the skull to the pelvis and collectively control the motion and posture of the spinal column.
2. The intrinsic muscles of the spine include the extensors and rotators of the head and neck (splenius capitis, splenius cervicis muscles), the extensors and rotators of the spine (erector spinae, transversospinalis and rotatores muscles), and the short segmental spinal muscles (interspinales, intertransversarii).
3. The individual components of the extensors and rotators of the spine include (a) the erector spinae, divided into three columns—the iliocostalis muscles (iliocostalis lumborum, thoracis, cervicis), longissimus muscles (longissimus thoracis, cervicis, capitis), and spinalis muscles (thoracis, cervicis, capitis); and (b) the transversospinalis consisting of the semispinalis muscles (semispinalis thoracis, cervicis, capitis), the multifidus muscles, and the rotatores muscles (rotatores thoracis, cervicis, lumborum).
4. The individual components of the short segmental spinal muscles include (a) the interspinales muscles extending between the apexes and bodies of the spinous processes of contiguous vertebrae, and (b) the intertransversarii muscles extending between the transverse processes of the vertebrae.

TABLE 7F-1: The Intrinsic Muscles of the Back

Muscles	Origin	Insertion
A. Extensors and Rotators of the Head and Neck		
Splenius capitis	Lower half of ligamentum nuchae, spinous processes and supraspinous ligaments of C-7 and upper 3–4 thoracic vertebrae	Mastoid process, occipital bone
Splenius cervicis	Spinous processes of T-3 to T-6	Transverse processes of upper 2–3 cervical vertebrae
B. Extensors and Rotators of the Spine		
1. Erector spinae muscles		
a. Iliocostalis group		
Iliocostalis cervicis	Angles of 3rd to 6th ribs	Transverse processes of C-4, C-5, and C-6
Iliocostalis thoracis	Angles of lower 6 ribs	Angles of upper 6 ribs, transverse process of C-7
Iliocostalis lumborum	Iliac crest	Inferior borders of angles of lower 6 or 7 ribs
b. Longissimus group		
Longissimus capitis	Transverse processes of upper 4 or 5 thoracic vertebrae, articular processes of lower 3 or 4 cervical vertebrae	Posterior margin of mastoid process
Longissimus cervicis	Transverse processes of upper 4 or 5 thoracic vertebrae	Transverse processes of C-2 to C-6
Longissimus thoracis	Transverse processes of lumbar vertebrae	Transverse processes of all thoracic and upper lumbar vertebrae and 9th and 10th ribs
c. Spinalis group		
Spinalis capitis	Medial part of semispinalis capitis	Insert with semispinalis capitis in occipital bone
Spinalis cervicis	Lower part of ligamentum nuchae and related spinous processes	Spinous process of axis and occasionally spinal processes of vertebrae below
Spinalis thoracis	Spinous processes of T-11 to L-2 vertebrae	Spinous processes of upper thoracic vertebrae
2. Transversospinalis muscles		
Semispinalis capitis	Tips of the transverse processes of upper 6th or 7th thoracic and C-7 vertebrae; articular processes of C-4, C-5, and C-6; occasionally spinous processes of C-7 and T-1	Occipital bone
Semispinalis cervicis	Transverse processes of upper 5 or 6 thoracic vertebrae	Spinous processes of C-2 to C-5
Semispinalis thoracis	Transverse processes of T-6 to T-10	Spinous processes of C-6, C-7, and T-1 to T-4 vertebrae
Multifidus	Sacrum, ilium, mamillary processes and posterior facet (zygapophyseal) joint capsule of lumbar, thoracic, and lower 4 cervical vertebrae	Spinous processes of all vertebrae 1–3 segments superior to the one of origin
Rotatores cervicis, thoracis and lumborum	Transverse processes of all vertebrae	Lower border and lateral surface of the lamina of all vertebrae superior to the one of origin
3. Short segmental spinal muscles		
Interspinales	Superior surface of all spinous processes	Inferior surface of spinous processes of all vertebrae superior to the one of origin
Intertransversarii	Transverse processes of all vertebrae	Transverse processes of all vertebrae superior to the one of origin

Modified from Smoker WRK, Harnsbuger HR. Differential diagnosis of head and neck lesions based on their spore of origin, 2. The infrahyoid portion of the neck, *AJR* 1991; 157: 155–159.

THE NECK MUSCLES

Anterior and Lateral Muscles of the Neck

1. These muscle groups include the superficial and lateral cervical muscles, the suprahyoid muscles, and the infrahyoid muscles.
2. The anterior superficial and lateral cervical group includes the platysma, trapezius, and sternocleidomastoid muscles.
3. The suprahyoid group includes the digastric, stylohyoid, mylohyoid, and geniohyoid muscles.
4. The infrahyoid group includes the sternohyoid, sternothyroid, thyrohyoid, and omohyoid muscles.

Anterior and Lateral Vertebral Muscles

1. The anterior vertebral group includes the longus colli, longus capitis, rectus capitis anterior, and rectus capitis lateralis muscles.
2. The lateral vertebral group includes the scalenus anterior, scalenus medius, scalenus posterior, and scalenus minimus muscles.

The Suboccipital Muscles

The suboccipital muscles include the rectus capitis posterior major, rectus capitis posterior minor, obliquus capitis superior, and obliquus capitis inferior muscles.

THE ANTERIOR SPINAL MUSCLES BELOW THE NECK

1. Anterior spinal muscles below the neck include the muscles of the iliac and pelvic regions.
2. The muscles of the iliac region that involve the spine are the psoas major, psoas minor and the iliacus muscles. The psoas major and iliacus combined are known as the iliopsoas.
3. Muscles in the pelvic region that involve the sacrum or coccyx include the piriformis, coccygeus and levator ani muscles.
4. In addition, the left and right crura of the diaphragm insert into the anterior aspect of the lumbar spine.

SUPERFICIAL MUSCLES OF THE BACK AND TRUNK ATTACHING TO THE EXTREMITIES

Muscles Connecting the Upper Limbs with the Spinal Column

The muscles that connect the upper limbs with the spinal column include the trapezius, rhomboid major, rhomboid minor, levator scapulae, and latissimus dorsi muscles.

Muscles Connecting the Lower Limbs with the Spinal Column

The muscles that connect the lower extremities to the spinal column include the gluteus maximus, psoas major, psoas minor, and iliacus muscles.

TABLE 7F-2: The Neck Muscles

Muscles	Origin	Insertion
A. Anterior Superficial and Lateral Muscles of the Neck		
1. Superficial and lateral cervical muscles		
Platysma	Fascia of pectoralis major and deltoid muscles	Mandibular body, lower lip, skin of lower face
Trapezius	Occiput, external occipital protuberance ligamentum nuchae, spinous processes, and supraspinous ligaments from C-7 to T-12	Lateral third of clavicle, acromion processes, scapular spine
Sternocleidomastoid	Mastoid process of temporal bone, occipital bone	Manubrium of the sternum, medial third of clavicle
2. Suprahyoid muscles		
Digastric	Anterior belly: mandible Posterior belly: mastoid notch of temporal bone	Greater cornu of hyoid bone
Stylohyoid	Styloid process	Body of hyoid bone
Mylohyoid	Mandible	Median fibrous raphe, symphysis menti, hyoid bone
Geniohyoid	Inferior mental spine of mandible	Body of hyoid bone
3. Infrahyoid muscles		
Sternohyoid	Medial aspect of clavicle, posterior sternoclavicular ligament, posterior aspect of manubrium sterni	Body of hyoid bone
Sternothyroid	Manubrium sterni, cartilage of 1st rib	Thyroid cartilage
Thyrohyoid	Thyroid cartilage	Greater conu and body of hyoid bone
Omohyoid	Inferior belly: upper border of scapula Superior belly: intermediate tendon of omohyoid muscle	Intermediate tendon of omohyoid muscle Body of hyoid bone
B. Suboccipital Muscles		
Obliquus capitis superior	Upper surface of the transverse process of atlas	Occipital bone
Obliquus capitis inferior	Lateral surface of the the spinous process and adjacent lamina of axis	Inferior aspect of the transverse process of atlas
Rectus capitis posterior major	Spinous process of axis	Lateral part of inferior nuchal line and occipital bone
Rectus capitis posterior minor	Tubercle on the posterior arch of atlas	Medial part of nuchal line and occipital bone
C. Anterior and Lateral Vertebral Muscles		
1. Anterior vertebral muscles		
Longus coli	Inferior oblique part: anterior bodies of T-1 to T-3 Superior oblique part: anterior tubercles of transverse processes of C-3 to C-5 Vertical intermediate part: anterior bodies of C-5 to T-3	Anterior tubercles of transverse processes of C-5 to C-6 Anterior tubercle of anterior arch of C-1 Anterior bodies of C-2 to C-4
Longus capitus	Inferior surface of basilar part of occipital bone	Anterior tubercles of the transverse processes of C-3 to C-6
Rectus capitus anterior	Anterior surface of lateral mass of C-1 and base of C-1 transverse processes	Occipital bone anterior to occipital condyle
Rectus capitus lateralis	Transverse process of C-1	Interior surface of jugular process of the occipital bone
2. Lateral vertebral muscles		
Scalenus anterior	Anterior tubercles of the the transverse processes of C-3 to C-6	First rib
Scalenus medius	Transverse processes of C-2 to C-7	First rib
Scalenus posterior	Transverse processes of C-4 to C-6	Second rib
Scalenus minimus	Transverse process of C-7	First rib

TABLE 7F-3: The Superficial Muscles of the Back and Trunk

Muscles	Origin	Insertion
Trapezius	Occipital bone, ligamentum nuchae, spinous process of C-7 and all thoracic vertebrae	Lateral third of clavicle, acromion process and scapular spine
Latissimus dorsi	Spinous processes of lower 6 thoracic vertebrae, thoracolumbar fascia, iliac crest, lower 3 or 4 ribs	Floor of bicipital groove
Rhomboid minor	Lower ligamentum nuchae, spinous processes of C-7 and T-1 vertebrae	Medial end of scapular spine
Rhomboid major	Spinous processes and supraspinous ligaments of T-2 to T-5 vertebrae	Medial scapular border between root of spine and inferior angle
Levator scapulae	Transverse process of C-1 to C-4 vertebrae	Superior medial border of scapula
Gluteus maximus	Posterior gluteal line of ilium, dorsal surface of lower part of sacrum, lateral margin of coccyx, sacrotuberous ligament	Iliotibial tract of fascia lata, greater tuberosity of femur

Modified from Asur AMR, Lee MJ. Grant's atlas of anatomy. Baltimore: Williams & Wilkins 1881: 239.

TABLE 7F-4: The Muscles of the Pelvic Floor Attaching to the Spine

Muscle	Origin	Insertion
Levator ani (a broad muscular sheet that is divisible into two parts: the pubococcygeus and iliococcygeus muscles)		
Pubococcygeus	Pubic bone	Coccyx, urethra, prostrate (males), vagina (females), rectum, central tendon of perineum, anococcygeal raphe
Iliococcygeus	Obturator fasciae between the obturator canal and the ischial spine	Coccyx, anococcygeal raphe

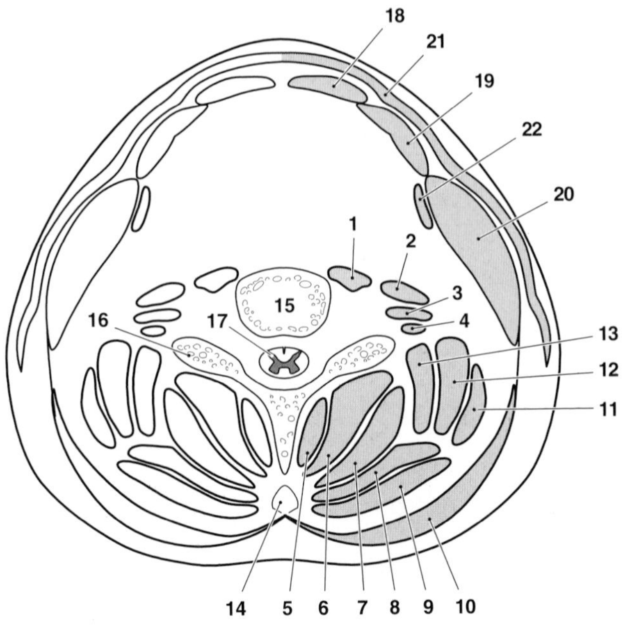

Figure 7F-1: Axial schematic of the muscles of the infrahyoid neck.

1 Longus colli muscle
2 Anterior scalene muscle
3 Middle scalene muscle
4 Posterior scalene muscle
5 Greater multifidus muscle
6 Lesser multifidus muscle
7 Semispinalis capitis muscle
8 Semispinalis cervicis muscle
9 Splenius muscle
10 Trapezius muscle
11 Levator scapulae muscle
12 Longus capitis muscle
13 Longus cervicis muscle
14 Ligamentum nuchae
15 Vertebral body
16 Posterior vertebral bony arch
17 Spinal cord
18 Sternohyoid muscle
19 Sternothyroid muscle
20 Sternocleidomastoid muscle
21 Platysma muscle
22 Omohyoid muscle

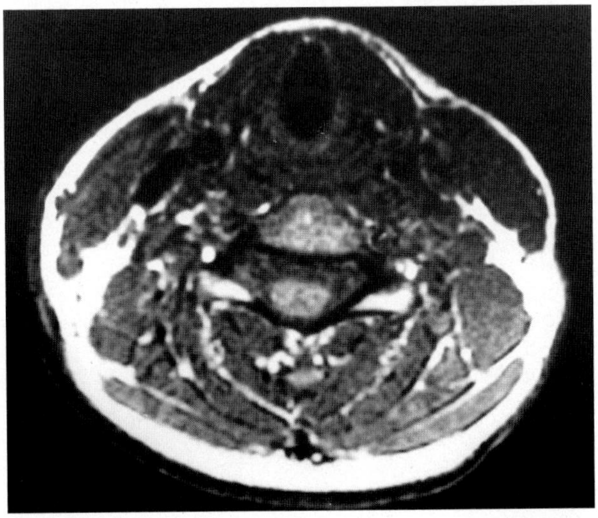

Figure 7F-2: Muscles of the infrahyoid neck. Axial T1-weighted MR image showing the muscles of the infrahyoid neck.

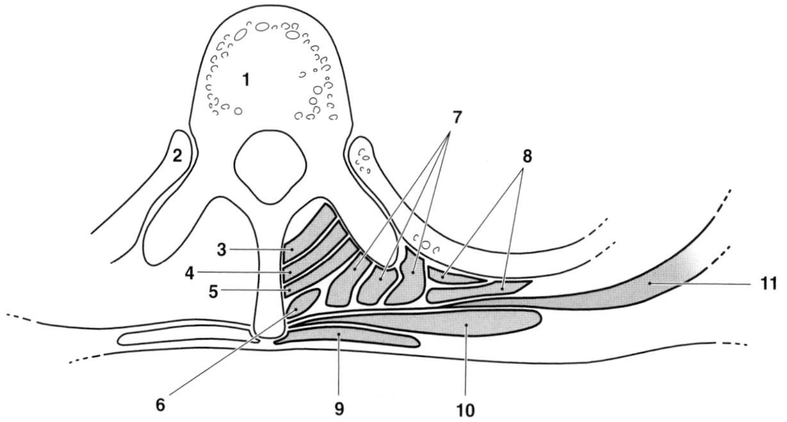

Figure 7F-3: Axial schematic of the paraspinal muscles in the thoracic region on the left side.

1 Thoracic vertebra
2 Rib
3 Rotatores muscle
4 Multifidus muscle
5 Semispinalis muscle
6 Spinalis muscle
7 Longissimus (cervicis, thoracis) muscle
8 Iliocostalis (cervicis, thoracic, lumborum) muscle
9 Trapezius muscle
10 Latissimus dorsi muscle
11 Serratus posterior muscle

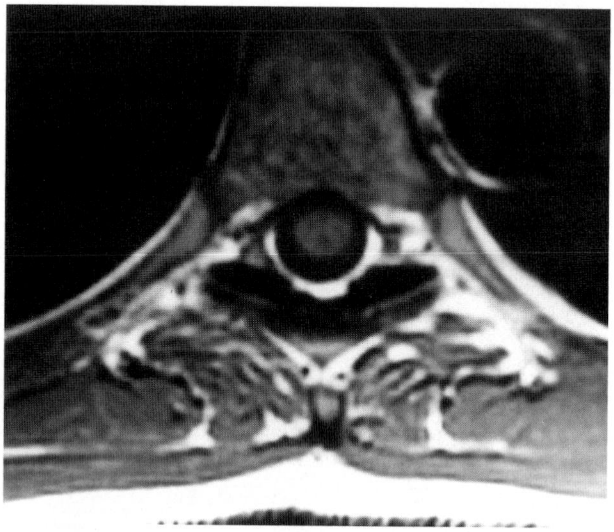

Figure 7F-4: Paraspinal muscles of the thoracic region. Axial T1-weighted MR image showing the paraspinal muscles in the thoracic region.

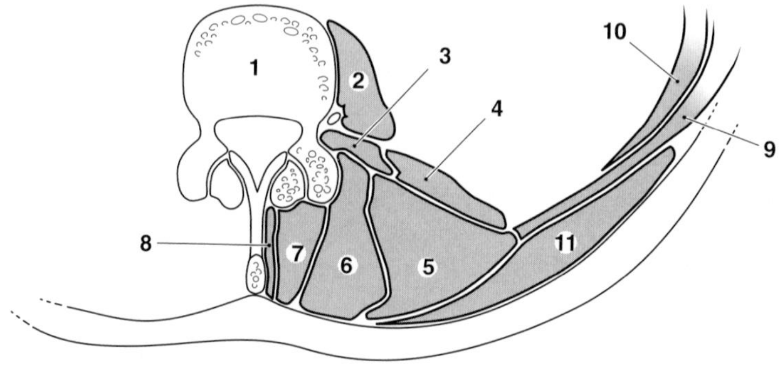

Figure 7F-5: Axial schematic of the paraspinal muscles in the lumbar region on the left.
1 Lumbar vertebra
2 Psoas muscle
3 Intertransversarii muscle
4 Quadratus lumborum muscle
5 Thoracocosstalis muscle
6 Longissimus muscle
7 Multifidus muscle
8 Interspinalis muscle
9 External oblique muscle
10 Internal oblique muscle
11 Latissimus dorsi muscle

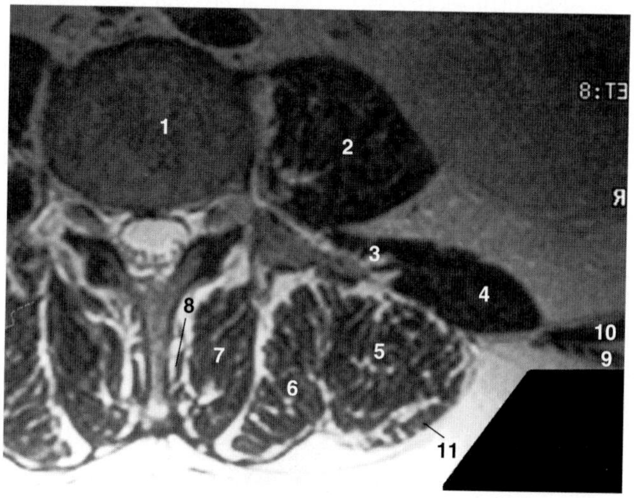

Figure 7F-6: Axial T1-weighted MR image showing the paraspinal muscles of the lumbar region.
1 Lumbar vertebra
2 Psoas muscle
3 Intertransversarii muscle
4 Quadratus lumborum muscle
5 Thoracocosstalis muscle
6 Longissimus muscle
7 Multifidus muscle
8 Interspinalis muscle
9 External oblique muscle
10 Internal oblique muscle
11 Latissimus dorsi muscle

7G Variants of the Spinal Column

FORMATION OF THE SPINAL OSSIFICATION CENTERS VARIANTS

Aplasia/Hypoplasia of Spinal/Costal Ossification Center(s)

- Absent neural arch: complete, unilateral
- Absent pedicle
- Unilateral absence of bifid spinous process
- Incomplete/absent cervical foramen transversarium/transverse process
- Asymmetric/accessory foramina transversaria
- Abnormalities of centrum formation: hemivertebra, butterfly vertebra, wedge vertebrae (lateral and dorsal)
- Absent rib(s) [e.g., aplastic twelfth rib(s)]

Accessory Supernumerary Spinal/Costal Ossification Center(s)

- Accessory primary supernumerary spinal/costal ossification center(s)
- Accessory secondary/supernumerary spinal/costal ossification center(s)
- Accessory ossification center in anterior arch of C-1
- Accessory ossification center in posterior neural arch (C-1 to S-5)
- Bifid/trifid spinous process
- Cervical ribs (supernumerary)
- Lumbar ribs (supernumerary)
- Arcuate process of C-1

FUSION OF SPINAL SYNCHONDROSIS VARIANTS

- Posterior spina bifida (nonfusion of posterior intraneural synchondrosis)
- Anterior spina bifida at C-1 (nonfusion of accessory ossification centers of anterior arch of C-1: interarchal synchondrosis)
- Retrosomatic cleft (nonfusion of neurocentral synchondrosis)
- Paraspinous cleft (nonfusion of accessory ossification centers of posterior neural arch)
- Os odontoideum (nonfusion of odontocentral synchondrosis)
- Occipital vertebra(e)/sclerotome(s) formation [nonfusion of primitive occipital sclerotome intervertebral synchondrosis(es)]
- Accessory ossicle of spinous process (nonfusion of neurospinous synchondrosis)
- Accessory ossicle of transverse process (nonfusion of neurotransverse synchondrosis)
- Accessory ossicle of mamillary process (nonunion of neuromamillary synchondrosis)
- Persistence of the odontocentral synchondrosis (remnant of primitive C1-2 intervertebral disc)

SPINAL MARROW CONTENT VARIANTS

- Variations in ratio and distribution of hematopoietic and fatty spinal marrow by region (e.g., odontoid process) and by age (e.g., increasing marrow fat with age).
- Focal variations in bone/fat content of marrow
  - Bone island
  - "Fat" island

SPINAL VASCULAR FORAMINA/CHANNELS VARIANTS

- Asymmetric cervical foramina transversaria
- Accessory cervical foramina transversaria
- Accessory vertebral vascular nutrient foramina/channels

SPINAL CANAL SIZE VARIANTS

- Central spinal canal stenosis: hypoplasia of posterior bony neural arch primary ossification centers
- Central spinal canal enlargement: hyperplasia of posterior bony neural arch primary ossification centers

SPINAL COLUMN CONTOUR VARIANTS

- Scoliosis
- Kyphosis

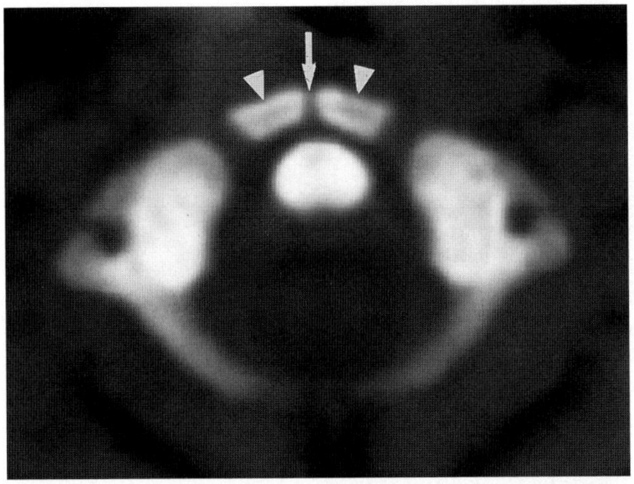

Figure 7G-1: Split primary ossification center of anterior arch of C-1. Axial CT image showing the midline secondary intraarchal synchondrosis (*arrow*) splitting the anterior arch of C-1 into two equal primary ossification centers (*arrowheads*), i.e., bipartite primary ossification center of anterior arch of C-1.

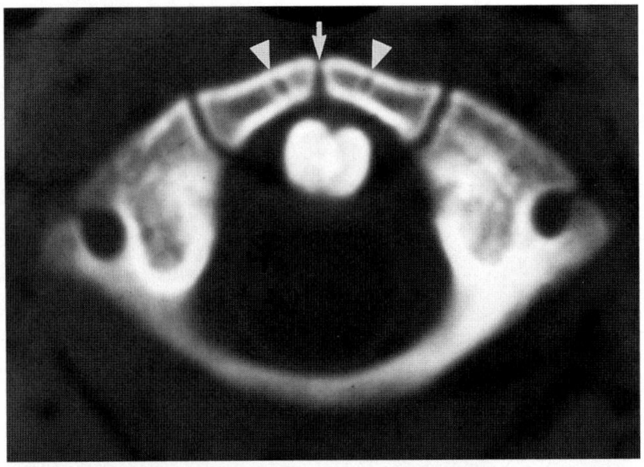

Figure 7G-2: Symmetric, split (quadripartite), primary accessory ossification center of the anterior arch of C-1. Axial CT image in an infant showing the midline intraarchal accessory synchondrosis (*arrow*) splitting the primary ossification center of the anterior arch of C-1 into two equal halves. Also note the partially fused, paired lateral intraarchal accessory synchondroses (*arrowheads*) on either side of the midline accessory synchondrosis. This effectively splits the primary anterior arch ossification center into four equal accessory parts (i.e., quadripartite primary ossification center of anterior arch of C-1).

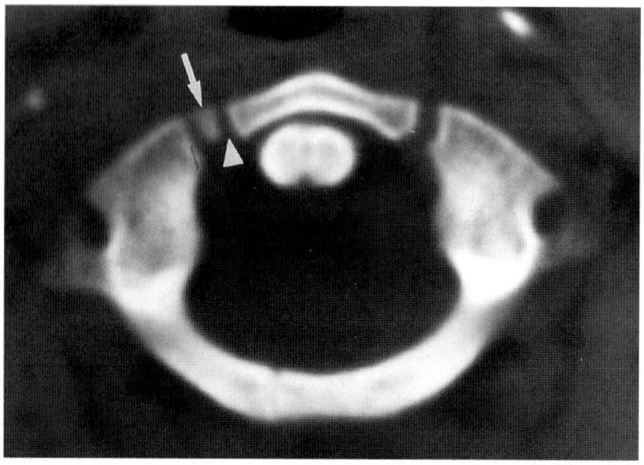

Figure 7G-3: Asymmetric, unilateral split (bipartite) primary ossification center of anterior arch of C-1. Asymmetric, unilateral split (bipartite) primary ossification center of anterior arch of C-1. Axial CT scan in a child showing a unilateral split (bipartite) primary ossification center of the anterior arch of C-1 resulting in a unilateral accessory primary ossification center (*arrow*) and a single lateral intraarchal accessory synchondrosis (*arrowhead*) (i.e., bipartite primary ossification center of anterior arch of C-1).

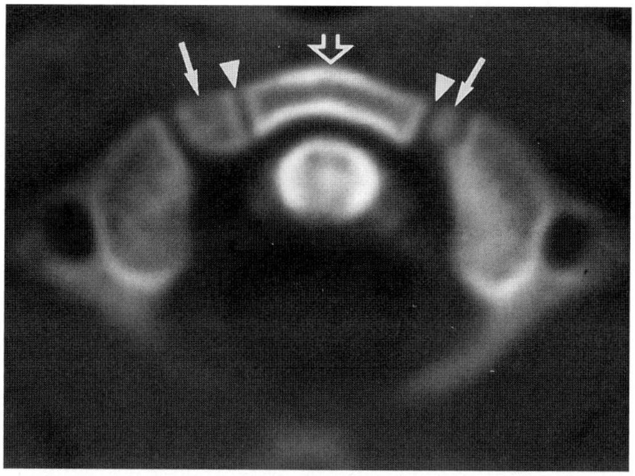

Figure 7G-4: Asymmetric bilateral split (tripartite) primary ossification center of the anterior arch of C-1. Axial CT image in a child showing lateral intraarchal accessory synchondroses (*arrowheads*) splitting of the primary ossification center of the anterior arch of C-1 into three unequal parts. Note the two accessory primary ossification centers (*solid arrows*) on either side of the main primary ossification center (*open arrow*) of the anterior arch of C-1 (i.e., tripartite primary ossification center of the anterior arch of C-1).

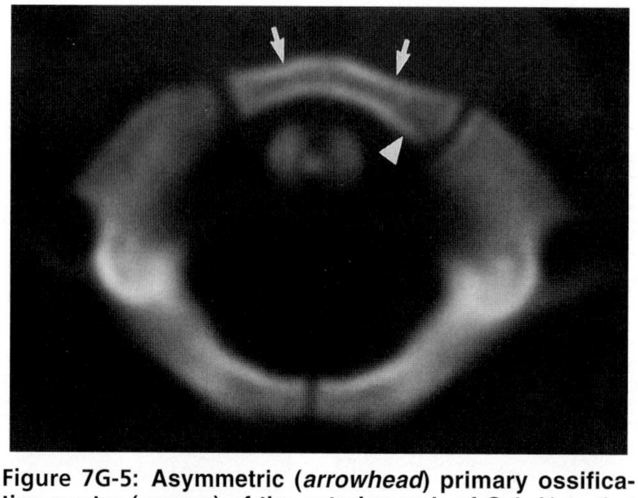

Figure 7G-5: Asymmetric (*arrowhead*) primary ossification center (*arrows*) of the anterior arch of C-1. Note that the neuroarchal synchondrosis is placed further laterally on the left side than the right.

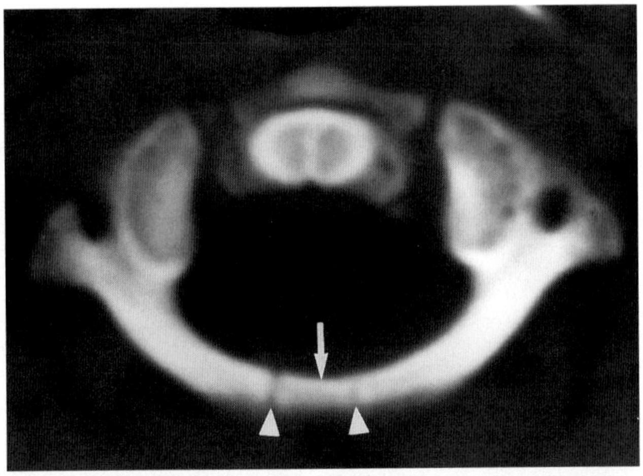

Figure 7G-6: Accessory intraneural primary ossification center of the posterior arch of C-1. Axial CT scan in a child showing an accessory median intraneural primary ossification center of the posterior arch of C-1 (*arrow*), and bilateral accessory intraneural synchondroses (*arrowheads*: Jinkins).

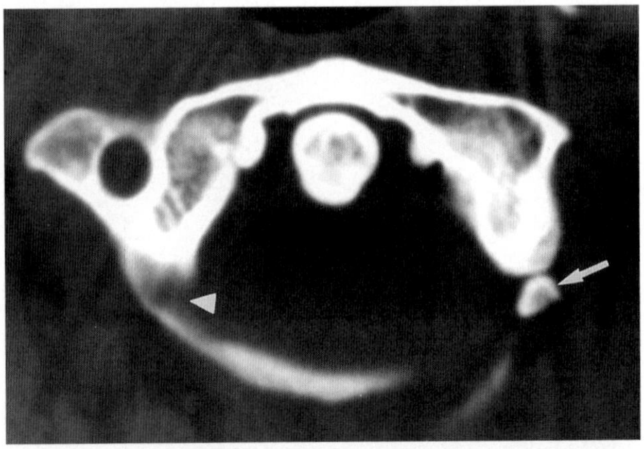

Figure 7G-7: Accessory, unfused ossicle within the arcuate ligament (arch) of C-1. Axial CT image showing a unilateral accessory, unfused ossicle (*arrow,* arcuate ossicle) within the arcuate ligament of C-1 on the left side. This likely arose from an accessory ossification center within the arcuate ligament. The arcuate groove (*arrowhead*) on the right side is also identified.

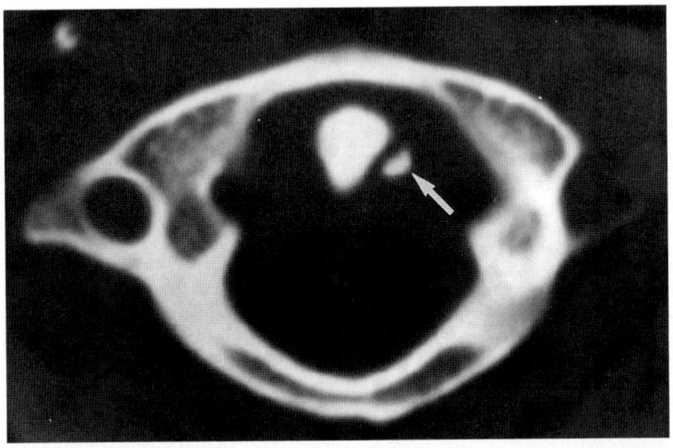

Figure 7G-8A: Accessory odontoid ossicle. Axial CT image in a 12-year-old showing an accessory odontoid ossicle (*arrow*) likely arising from an unfused secondary accessory ossification center of the apex of the odontoid process.

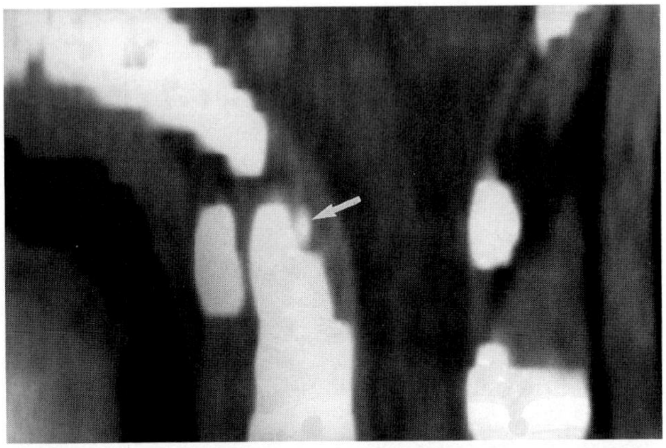

Figure 7G-8B: Accessory odontoid ossicle. Sagittal reconstruction showing the accessory odontoid ossicle (*arrow*).

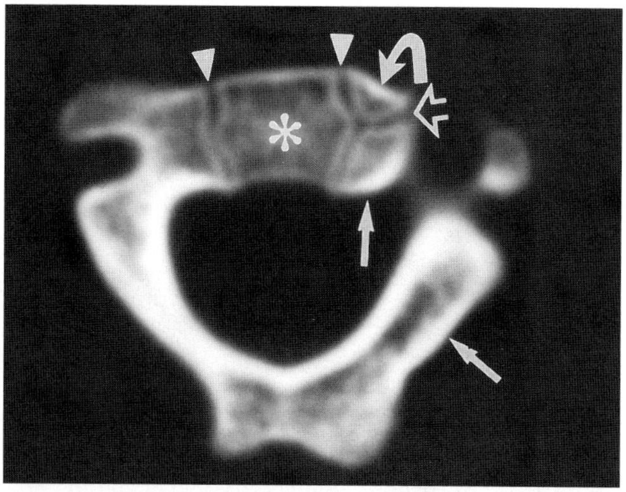

Figure 7G-9: Accessory vertebral ossification center of C-2. Axial CT image showing a split or accessory ossification center of the posterior bony neural arch of C-2 on the left side in a child. The primary ossification center of the centrum (body) of C-2 (*asterisk*), the neurocentral synchondroses (*arrowheads*), and the aberrant anterior intraneural synchondrosis (*open arrow*) splitting the anterior accessory ossification center (*curved arrow*) of the posterior neural arch on the left from the main primary ossification center (*solid arrows*) are also noted.

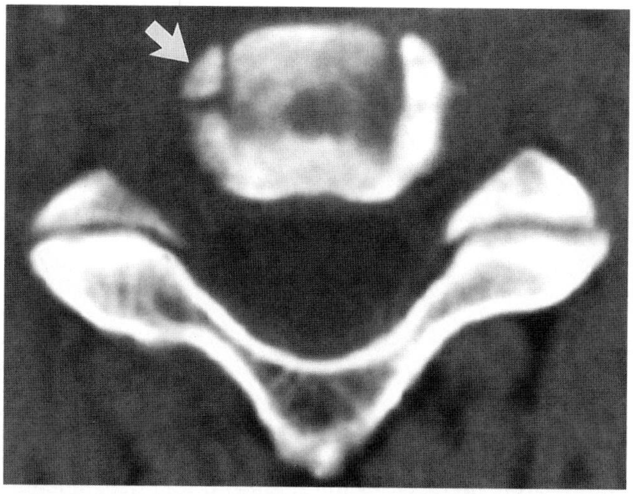

Figure 7G-10: Accessory ossification center within the uncinate process. Axial CT image acquired at the C-3 level showing an accessory ossification center (*arrow*) on the right side anteriorly. Note the relatively smooth margins and the absence of displacement, thereby distinguishing the accessory ossification center from a fracture fragment.

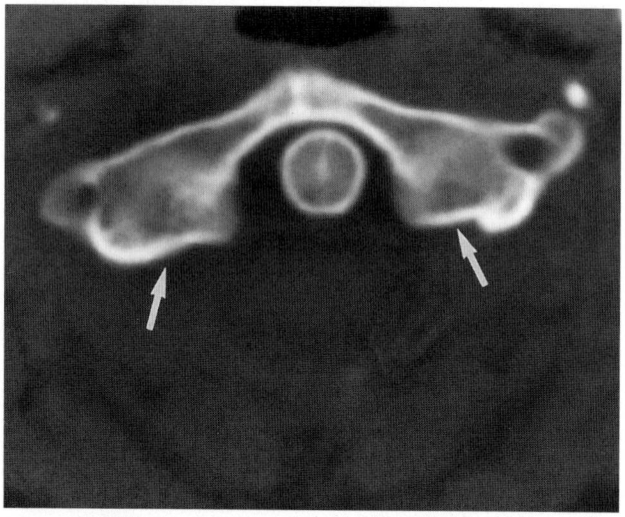

Figure 7G-11A: Aplasia of the posterior bony neural arch. Axial CT image showing aplasia of the posterior bony neural arch of C-1, with cortical bone forming the posterior margins of the lateral masses (*arrows*).

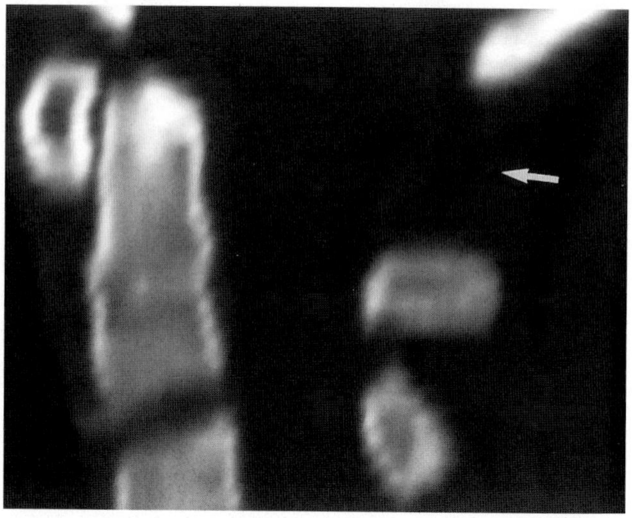

Figure 7G-11B: Sagittally reformatted CT image showing aplasia of the posterior bony neural arch of C-1 (*arrow*).

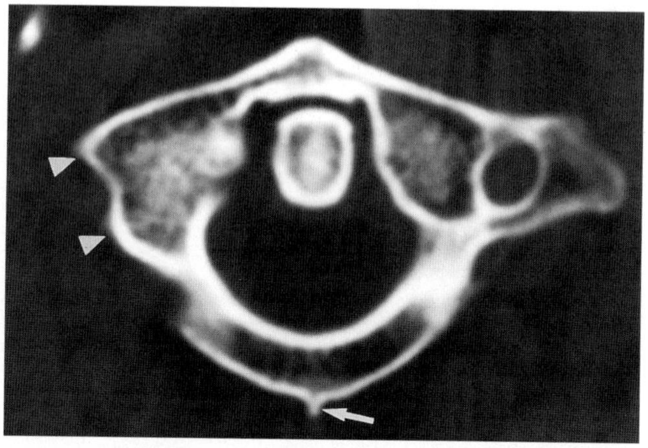

Figure 7G-12: Absent transverse process. Axial CT image showing vestigial right C-1 spinous process (*arrow*) and an incomplete bony foramen transversarium (*arrowheads*) resulting from an absent transverse process on the right side.

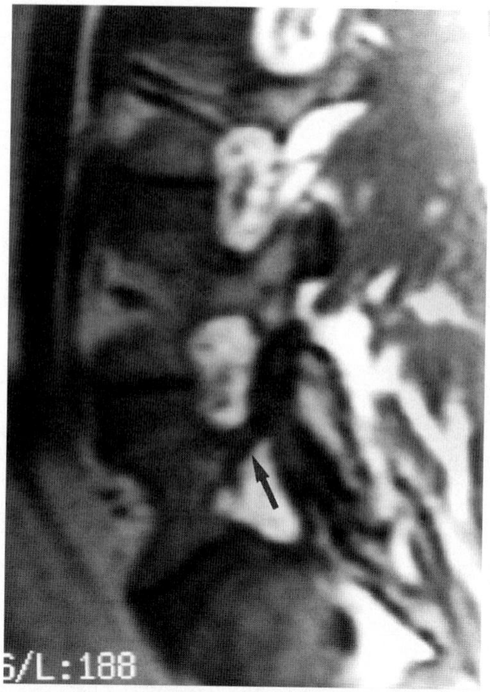

Figure 7G-13: Hypoplastic lumbar pedicle. Sagittal T1-weighted MR image showing a hypoplastic pedicle (*arrow*) at the L-5 level on the right.

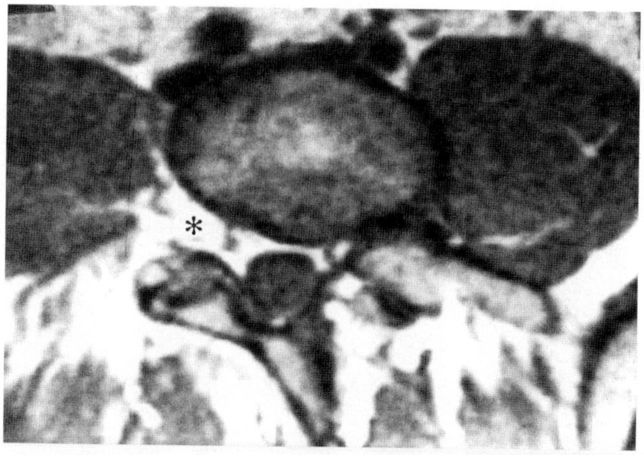

Figure 7G-14A: Agenesis of a lumbar vertebral pedicle and articular process. Unenhanced axial T1-weighted image showing the absence (*asterisk*) of the right L-5 pedicle. Note the shortening of the left L-5 pedicle.

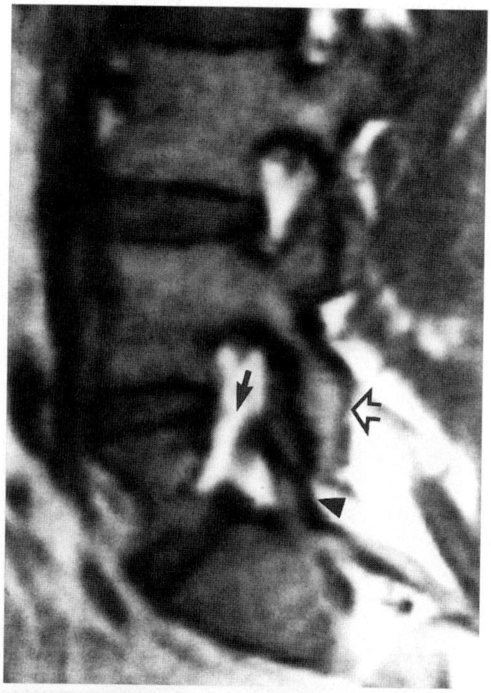

Figure 7G-14B: Sagittal T1-weighted MR image showing absence (solid arrow) of the right L-5 pedicle and facet. Note the articulation of the inferior articular facet of L-4 (*open arrow*) with the superior articular facet of S-1 (*arrowhead*).

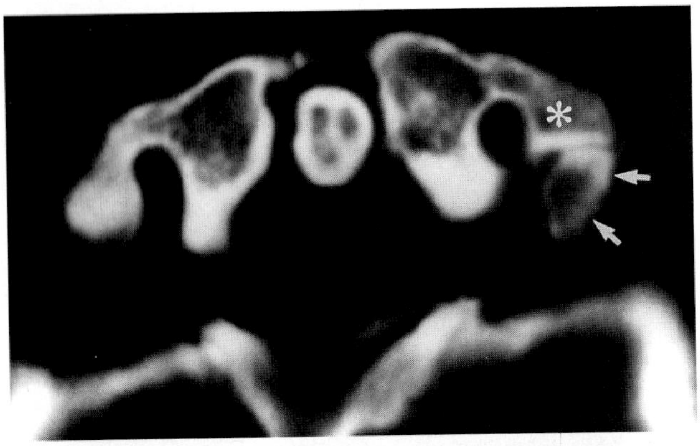

Figure 7G-15: Cervical transverse process accessory ossicle. Axial CT image showing an unfused accessory ossicle (*arrows*) comprising the posterior aspect of the transverse process extending posteriorly from the anterior aspect of the transverse process (*asterisk*) on the left side.

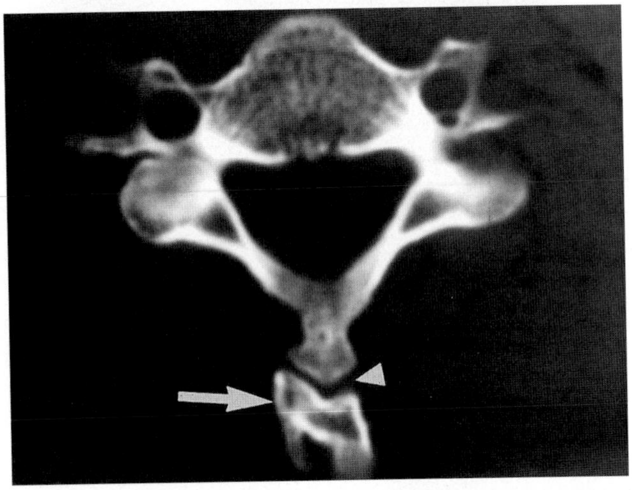

Figure 7-16A: Unfused secondary ossification center of vertebral spinous process at the C-6 level. Axial CT image showing an unfused secondary ossification center (*arrow*) of the spinous process. Note the apparent pseudoarthrosis formation at the level of the unfused synchondrosis (*arrowhead*).

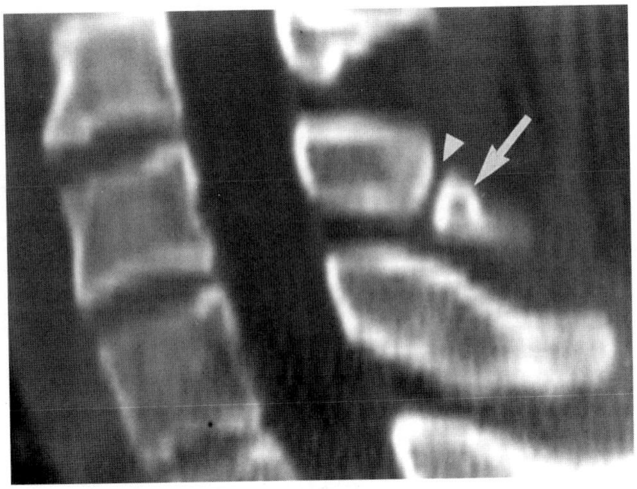

Figure 7-16B: Sagittal reconstruction again showing the unfused secondary ossification center (*arrow*) and the synchondrosis/ pseudoarthrosis (*arrowhead*).

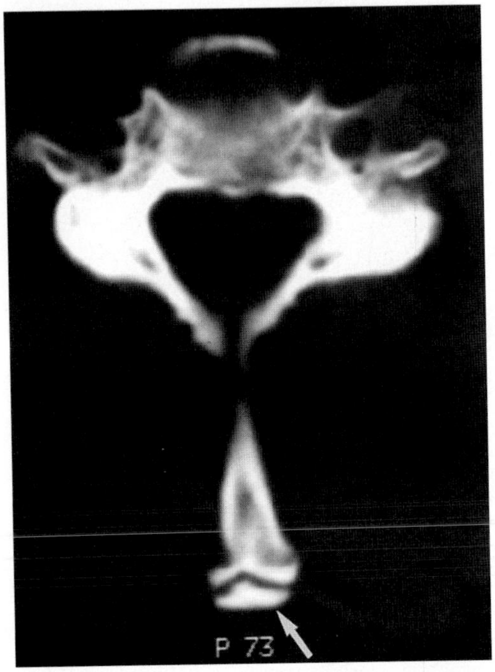

Figure 7G-17A: Unfused spinous process accessory ossicle at the C-7 level. Axial CT image showing the unfused spinous process accessory ossicle (*arrow*) (i.e., unfused secondary ossification center).

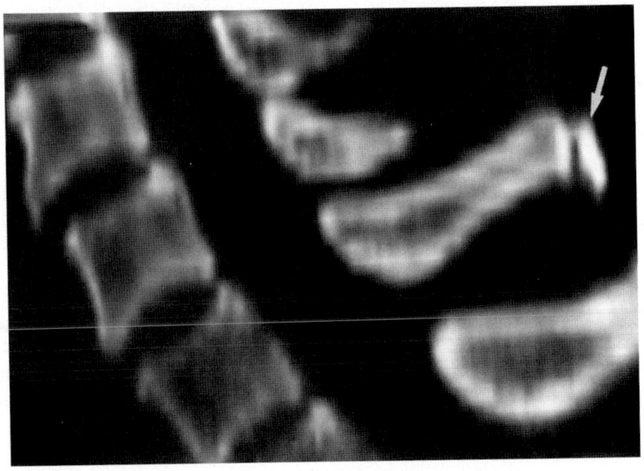

Figure 7G-17B: Sagittally reformatted CT image showing an unfused spinous process accessory ossicle (*arrow*).

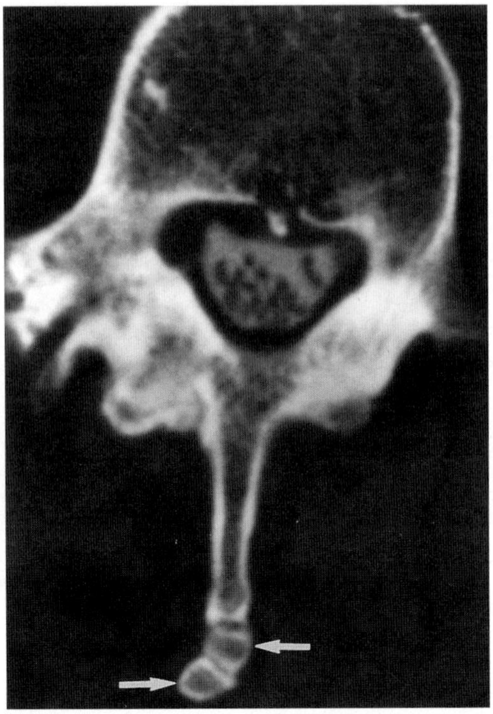

Figure 7G-18: Accessory spinous process ossicles at the L-4 level. Axial CT showing double accessory ossicles (*arrows*) off of the tip of the L-4 spinous process.

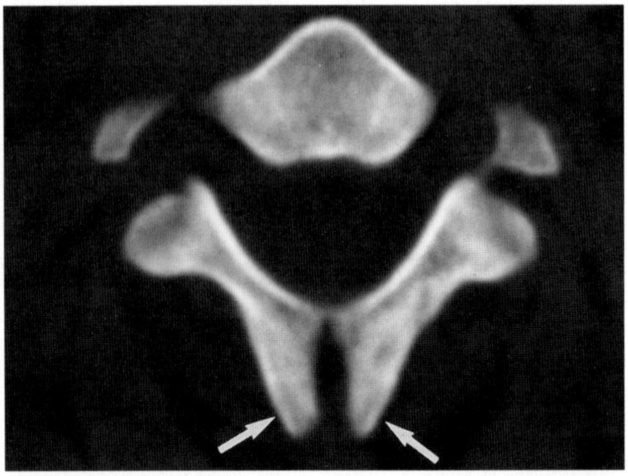

Figure 7G-19: Laterally bifid spinous process at the C-3 level. Axial CT image showing a laterally bifid (*arrows*) spinous process of the C-3 vertebra.

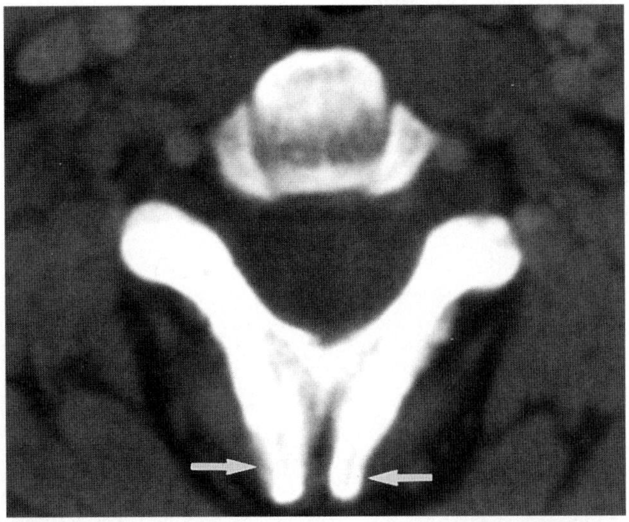

Figure 7G-20: Laterally bifid spinous process at the C-4 level. Axial CT image showing a laterally bifid spinous process of the C-4 vertebra (*arrows*).

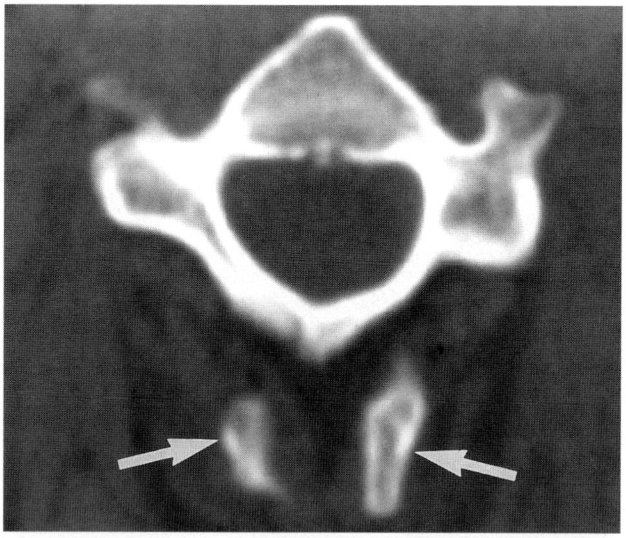

Figure 7G-21A: Inferior fusion of bifid spinous processes in the midcervical region. Axial CT image showing bifid spinous processes (*arrows*) of an upper cervical vertebrae.

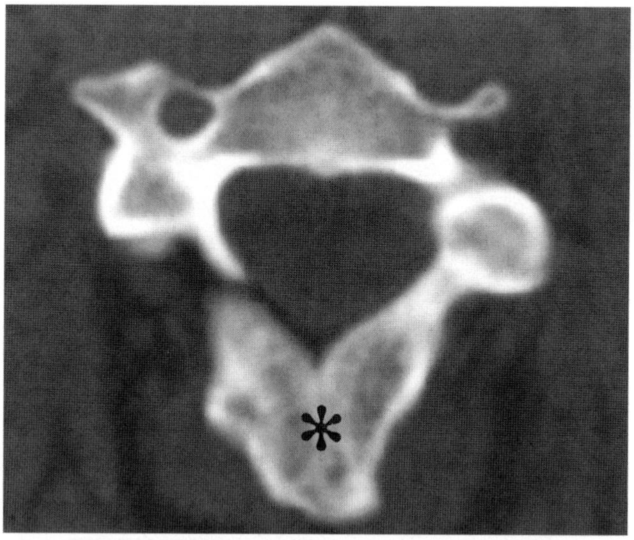

Figure 7G-21B: Axial CT image acquired at a lower level than that of Figure 7G-22A showing midline fusion (*asterisk*) of the bifid spinous process.

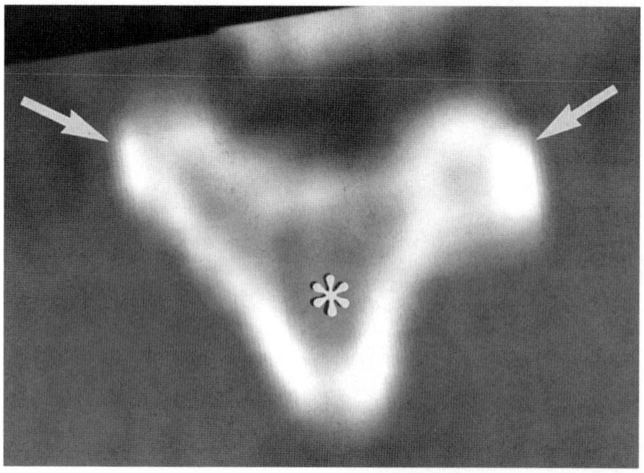

Figure 7G-21C: Coronal CT reconstruction showing the bifid spinous processes superiorly (*arrows*) and the midline inferior fusion (*asterisk*).

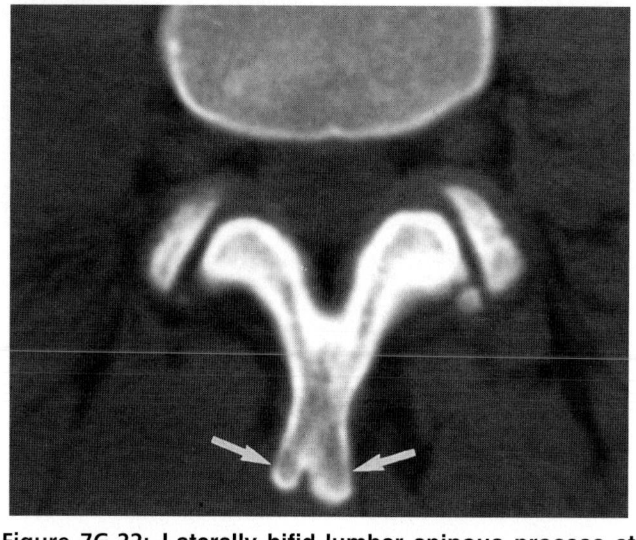

Figure 7G-22: Laterally bifid lumbar spinous process at the L-2 level. Axial CT image showing a bifid spinous process (*arrows*) extending from the L-2 vertebrae.

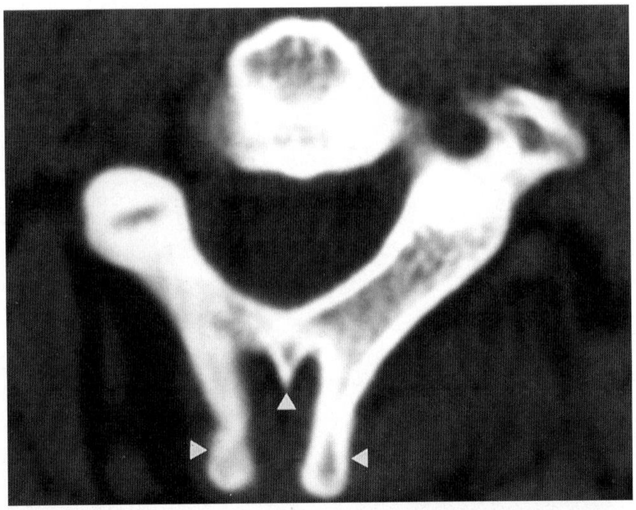

Figure 7G-23: Trifid cervical spinous process. Axial CT image showing a trifid (three in number) spinous process (*arrowheads*) of C-3.

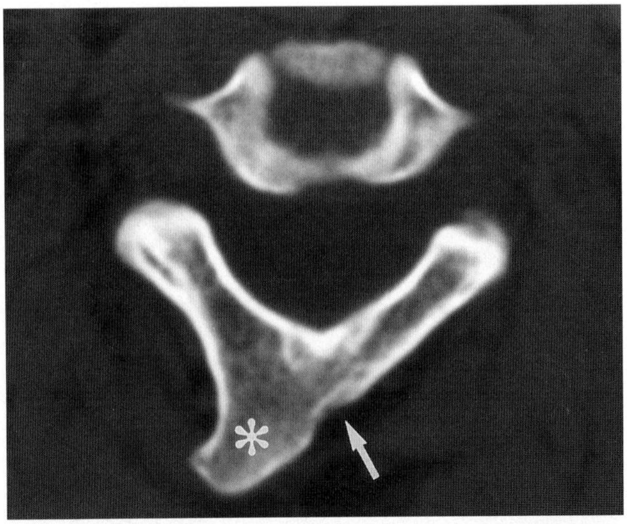

Figure 7G-24: Unilateral hypoplasia of otherwise bifid cervical spinous process. Axial CT image showing the right side of a bifid spinous process (*asterisk*) at C-2 but absence of the bifid spinous process on the left (*arrow*).

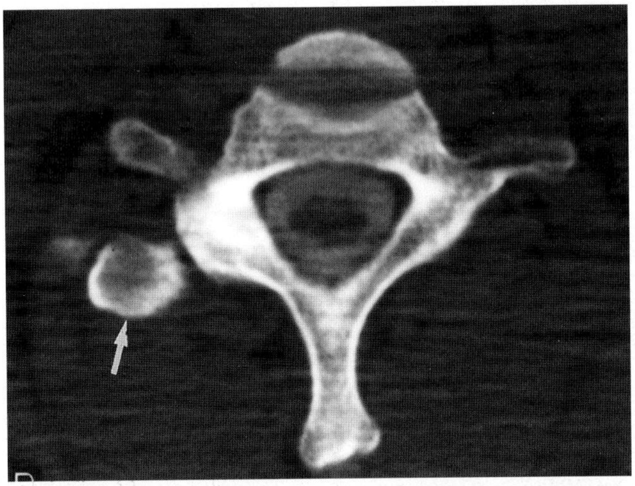

Figure 7G-25A: Unilateral elevation of right T-1 transverse process. Axial CT image showing an elevated T-1 transverse process (*arrow*) and rib on the right side.

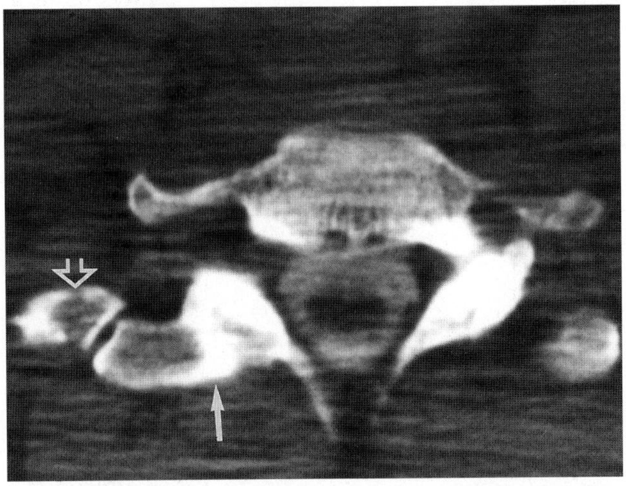

Figure 7G-25B: Axial CT image acquired at a lower level than that of Figure 7G-26A showing the base of the transverse process of T1 (*solid arrow*) and the right first rib (*open arrow*).

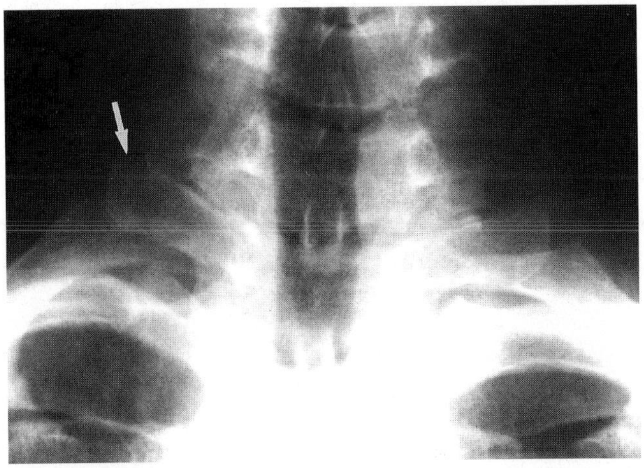

Figure 7G-25C: Anteroposterior conventional radiograph showing the elevated transverse process of T1 (*arrow*) and medial aspect of the first rib on the right side.

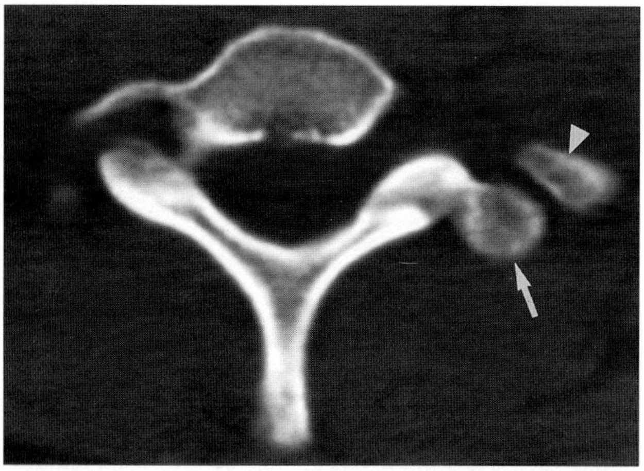

Figure 7G-26: Unilateral elevation of the left T1 transverse process. Axial CT showing unilateral elevation of the transverse process (*arrow*) and first rib (*arrowhead*) on the left side.

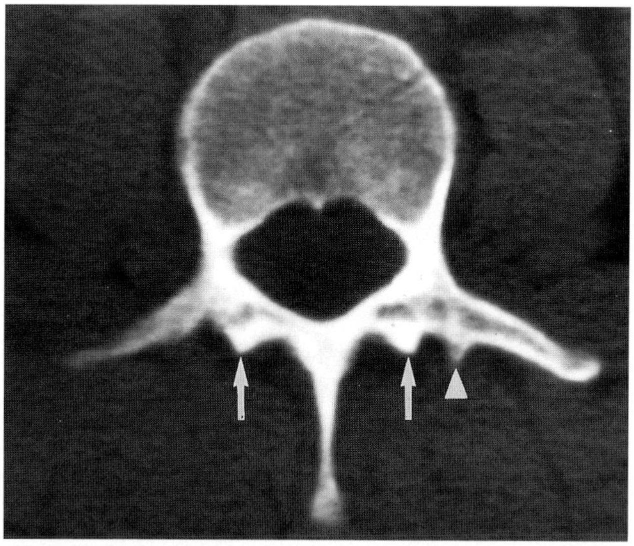

Figure 7G-27: Vertebral mamillary and accessory (mamillary) processes. Axial CT image showing vertebral mamillary processes bilaterally (*arrows*) and an accessory (mamillary) process (*arrowhead*) on the left side.

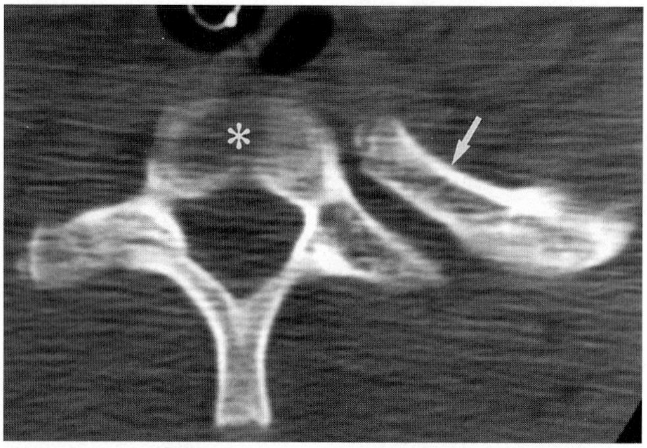

Figure 7G-28: Unilateral C-7 cervical rib. Axial CT image showing a unilateral cervical rib (*arrow*) on the left side articulating with the C-7 vertebral body (*asterisk*).

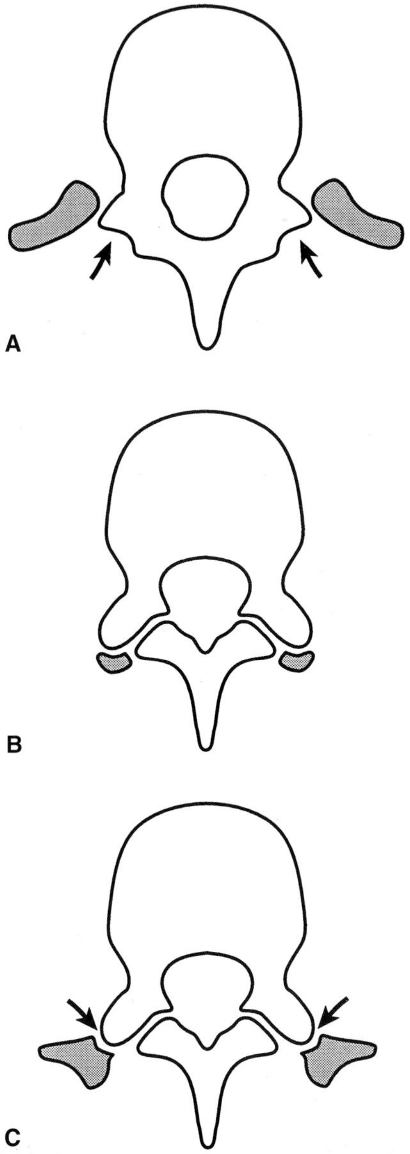

Figure 7G-29: Schematics of accessory ossification centers of supernumerary ribs of the craniad lumbar vertebrae. A: Accessory ossification centers (*shading*) of supernumerary ribs of a lumbar vertebra anterior to hypoplastic transverse processes (*arrows*). **B:** Accessory ossification centers (*shading*) of ununited ossicles (hypoplastic supernumerary "ribs") of the mamillary processes of a lumbar vertebra. **C:** Accessory ossification centers (*shading*) of supernumerary ribs forming from the mamillary processes of a lumbar vertebra. Note that the accessory ribs may either articulate with (*arrow*) or be separate from the posterior spinal facet (zygapophyseal) joints.

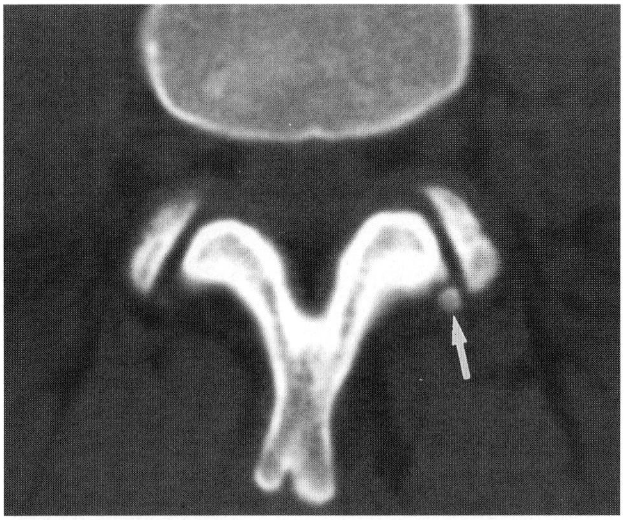

Figure 7G-30: Unilateral vestigial rudimentary rib extending from the posterior aspect of L-2 vertebra. Axial CT image in a young adult showing a vestigial rudimentary rib (*arrow*) extending from the posterior aspect (? mamillary process) of the L-2 vertebra on the left side.

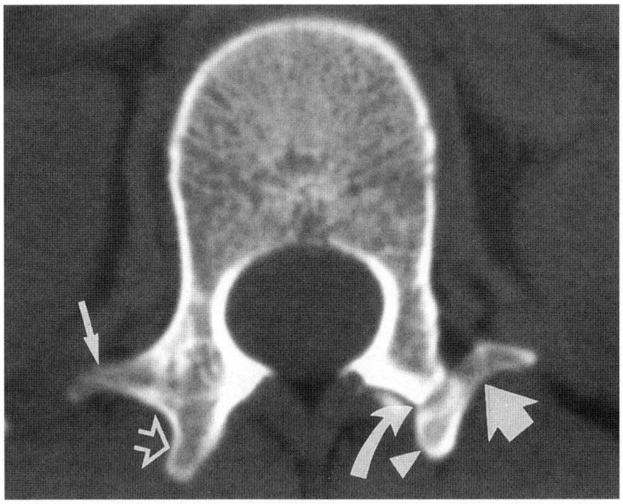

Figure 7G-31: Unilateral vestigial rudimentary rib extending from articulation with L-1 vertebra. Axial CT image in a young adult showing the transverse process on the right side (*small closed straight arrow*), the mamillary process on the right side (*open arrow*), and a rudimentary accessory rib (no. 13) on the left side (*large closed straight arrow*) articulating (*curved arrow*) with the L-1 vertebra. Also note the analogous portions of the accessory rib on the left side: the head of the rib (*arrowhead*) corresponding to the mamillary process and the rib itself (*large closed straight arrow*) corresponding to the transverse process (compare with the right side).

SPINAL COLUMN DEVELOPMENTAL VERTEBRAL CLEFT VARIANTS

- Neurocentral cleft (theoretical) (1)
- Pedicular (retrosomatic) cleft (2)
- Isthmic (pars interarticularis) cleft (3)
- Retroisthmic cleft (4)
- Paraspinous cleft (5)
- Spina bifida (anterior: median intracorpal, posterior: median intraspinous) (6)
- Transverse process cleft (transverse process accessory ossicle) (7)
- Spinous process cleft with duplicated spinous process (8)
- Mammillary process cleft (mammillary process accessory ossicle) (9)
- Spinous process groove(s) (superior, inferior)
- Paraspinous (intralaminar) groove(s)

(1–9 refer to numbers in Figure 7G-32.)

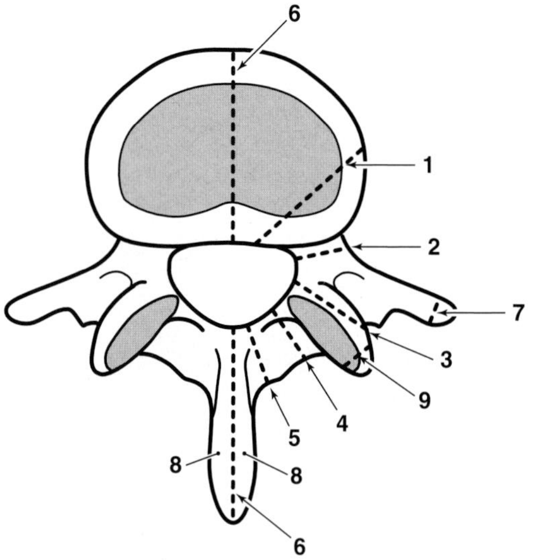

Figure 7G-32: Spinal column develpomental vertebral cleft variants
1 Neurocentral cleft (theoretical)
2 Pedicular (retrosomatic) cleft
3 Isthmic (pars interarticularis) cleft
4 Retroisthmic cleft
5 Paraspinous cleft
6 Spina bifida (anterior: median intracorpal, posterior: median intraspinous)
7 Transverse process cleft (transverse process accessory ossicle)
8 Spinous process cleft with duplicated spinous process
9 Mammillary process cleft (mammillary process accessory ossicle)

TABLE 7G-1: Disorders of Formation and Segmentation of the Spinal Column

Disorders of vertebral formation	Disorders of vertebral segmentation
▸ Lateral hemivertebra ▸ Lateral wedge vertebra "Butterfly" vertebra Dorsal wedge vertebra ▸ Spina bifida (hypoplasia of midline posterior bony vertebral arch) ▸ Hypoplasia/aplasia of a pedicle/articular process ▸ Posterior bony arch hypoplasia resulting in developmental spinal stenosis (central spinal canal stenosis, lateral recess stenosis of central spinal canal, neural foramen stenosis) ▸ Notochord remnant	▸ Complete intervertebral failure of segmentation (e.g., "block" vertebrae, Klippel-Feil syndrome) ▸ Unilateral intervertebral failure of segmentation ▸ Anterior or posterior intervertebral failure of segmentation ▸ Failure of segmentation of adjacent articular processes/spinous processes ▸ Supplemental spinal segments (e.g., "lumbarized" first sacral segment) ▸ Assimilated spinal segments (e.g., atlantooccipital assimilation, "sacralization" of the fifth lumbar segment) ▸ Pedicle fusion bars

Modified from Jinkins JR, da Costa Leite C. *Neurodiagnostic imaging: pattern analysis and differential diagnosis*. Philadelphia: Lippincott-Raven Publishers, 1998:73.

TABLE 7G-2: Classification of Spinal Scoliosis

Idiopathic

Infantile
Juvenile
Adolescent
Adult

Congenital

Vertebral formation anomalies
Vertebral segmentation anomalies
Mixed formation-segmentation anomalies

Acquired

Neuromuscular
1. Neuropathic
   a. Upper motor neuron abnormalities (e.g., cerebral palsy, spinocerebellar degeneration, syringohydromyelia, diastematomyelia spinal cord trauma, spinal cord tumor)
   b. Lower motor neuron abnormalities (e.g., poliomyelitis, nerve root trauma, paraspinal muscle atrophy, myelocele/lipomyelocele, lipomyelocele/lipomyelomeningocele)
   c. Dysautonomia
2. Myopathic
   a. Arthrogryposis
   b. Muscular dystrophy

Neurofibromatosis
Mesenchymal dysplasia
1. Marfan's syndrome
2. Ehlers-Danlos syndrome
3. Homocystinuria

Posttraumatic
1. Spinal fracture or dislocation
2. Sequela of spinal irradiation

Contracture-related, following external burn
Osteochondrodystrophies
1. Achondroplasia
2. Spondyloepiphyseal dysplasia

Neoplastic
1. Benign neoplasms of spinal column, paraspinal soft tissues, spinal cord, or nerve roots
2. Malignant neoplasms of spinal column, paraspinal soft tissues, spinal cord, or nerve roots

Metabolic
1. Rickets
2. Juvenile osteoporosis
3. Osteogenesis imperfecta

Functional
1. Postural
2. Compensatory: short lower extremity
3. Secondary to muscular spasm or unilateral pain (lateral bending, not true scoliosis)

Modified from Jinkins JR, da Costa Leite C. *Neurodiagnostic imaging: pattern analysis and differential diagnosis*. Philadelphia: Lippincott-Raven Publishers, 1998:73.

TABLE 7G-3: Classification of Spinal Kyphosis

Congenital (e.g., spinal dislocation, dorsal wedge vertebra)
Scheuermann's disease
Paralytic
Posttraumatic
Postinflammatory (e.g., tuberculosis, ankylosing spondylitis)
Postsurgical
Postirradiation
Metabolic (i.e., osteoporosis, osteogenesis imperfecta)
Neoplastic
Spondyloepiphyseal dysplasia
Mucopolysaccharidosis
Postural

Modified from Jinkins JR, da Costa Leite C. *Neurodiagnostic imaging: pattern analysis and differential diagnosis*. Philadelphia: Lippincott-Raven Publishers, 1998:73.

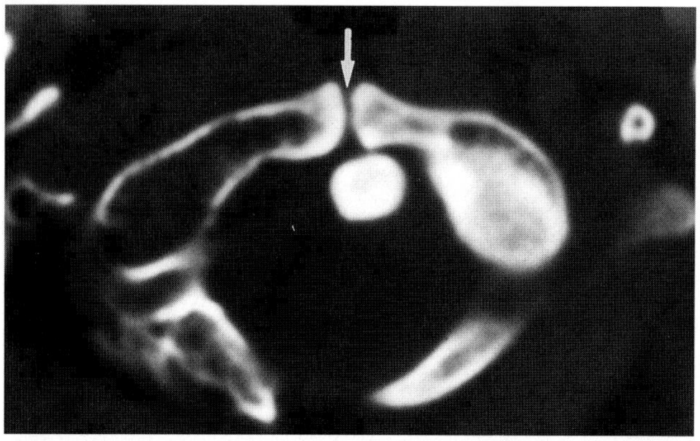

Figure 7G-33A: Anterior spina bifida at C-1. Magnified axial CT image shows an anterior spina bifida (*arrow*) involving the anterior arch of C-1.

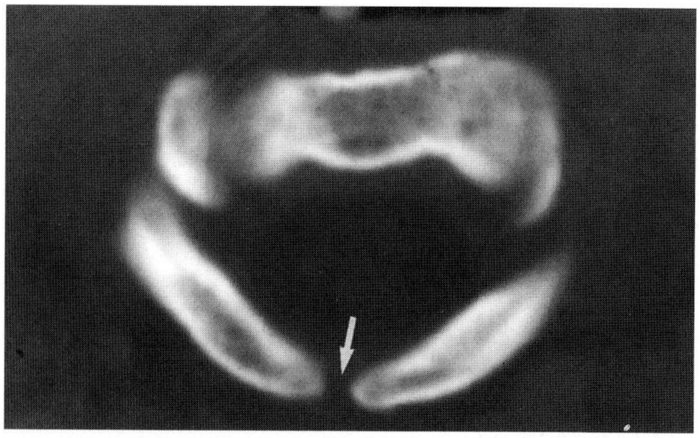

Figure 7G-33B: Complete posterior spina bifida at C-1. Axial CT image showing a posterior spina bifida at C-1 (*arrow*).

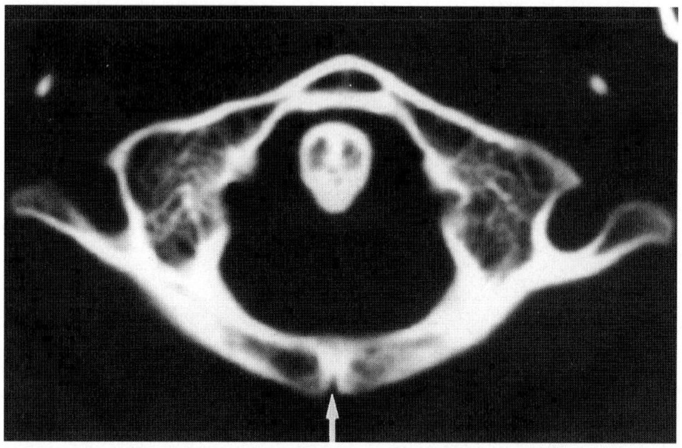

Figure 7G-33C: Incomplete posterior spina bifida at C-1. Axial CT image showing an incomplete spina bifida involving the posterior bony arch (*arrow*) of C-1.

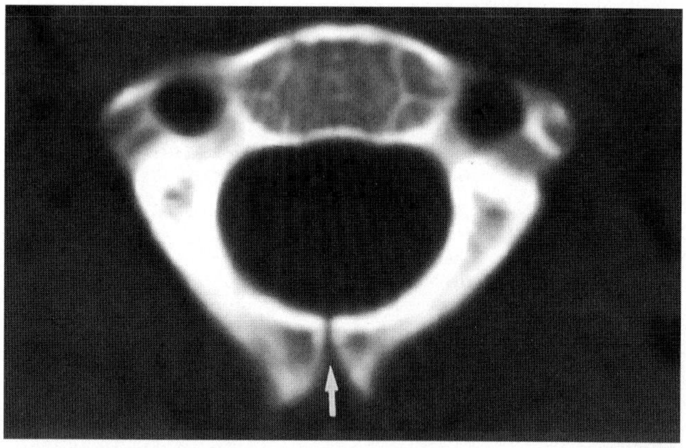

Figure 7G-33D: Posterior spina bifida at C-2. Axial CT image showing a posterior spina bifida involving the posterior bony arch of C-2 (*arrow*).

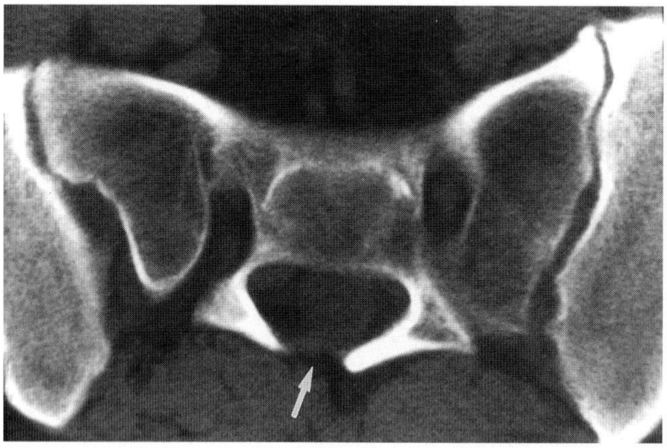

Figure 7G-33E: Sacral posterior spina bifida. Axial CT showing a posterior spina bifida (*arrow*) of the second sacral segment.

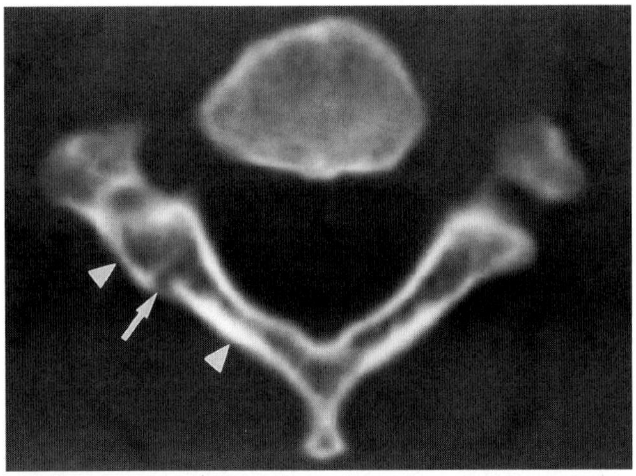

Figure 7G-34: Fused cervical retroisthmic cleft: accessory synchondrosis of spinal lamina. Axial CT image in an adult showing a fused synchondrosis (*arrow*) on the right side between two accessory primary ossification centers (*arrowheads*) of the bony neural arch. This would be consistent with a fused retroisthmic cleft.

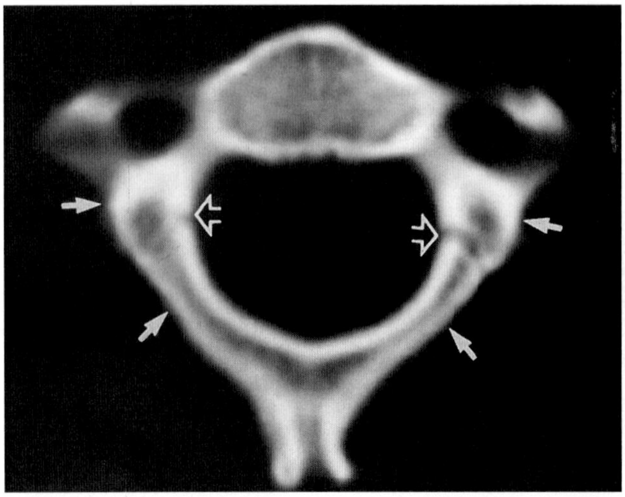

Figure 7G-35: Incomplete cervical retroisthmic clefts. Magnified axial CT image showing incomplete retroisthmic clefts bilaterally (*arrows*). This represents fused synchondroses (*open arrows*) between two accessory primary ossification centers (*arrows*) on each side.

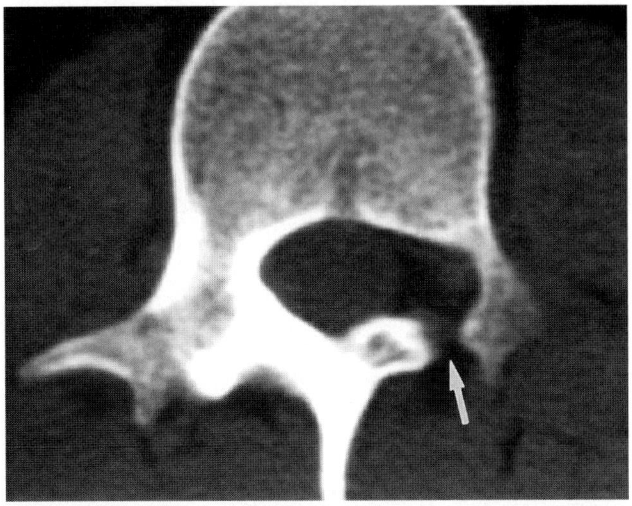

Figure 7G-36: Lumbar retroisthmic cleft. Axial CT image showing a retroisthmic cleft in the L-2 vertebra on the left side (*arrow*). Also noted are the hypoplastic left pedicle, transverse process, and pars interarticularis.

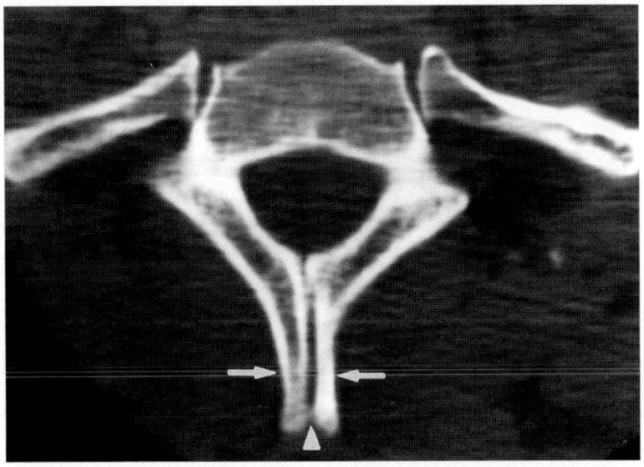

Figure 7G-37A: Laterally duplicated thoracic spinous processes with midline intraspinous process cleft (posterior spina bifida). Axial CT showing two spinous processes (*arrows*) at the T-1 and a midline spinous process cleft (*arrowhead*).

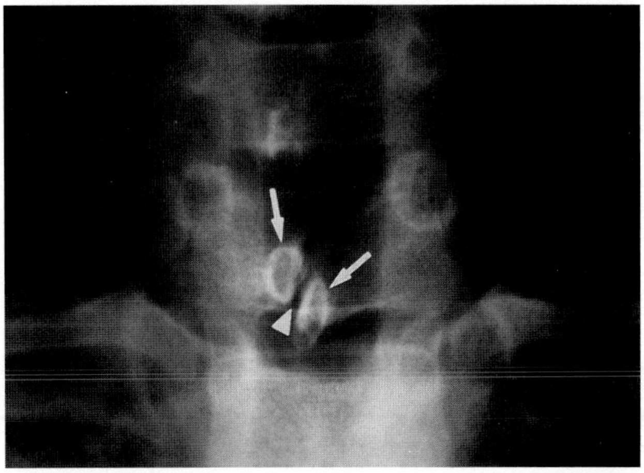

Figure 7G-37B: Conventional radiograph in the anteroposterior projection in the same case as that shown in Figure 7G-37A, again showing the duplicated spinous processes of T-1 (*arrows*) and the midline cleft (*arrowhead*).

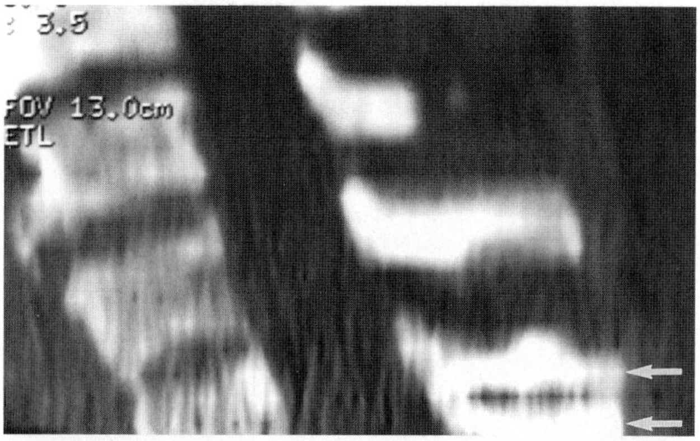

Figure 7G-38A: Sagittally bifid spinous processes and paraspinous clefts with duplicated posterior bony neural arches. Sagittally reformatted CT image showing sagittally duplicated spinous processes (*arrows*).

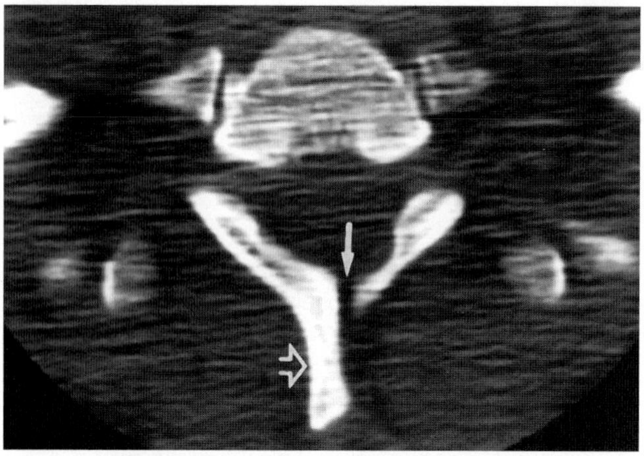

Figure 7G-38B: Axial CT image showing the superior duplicated spinous process (*open arrow*) and the adjacent paraspinous cleft (*closed arrow*) on the left side. The bony neural arch is also duplicated.

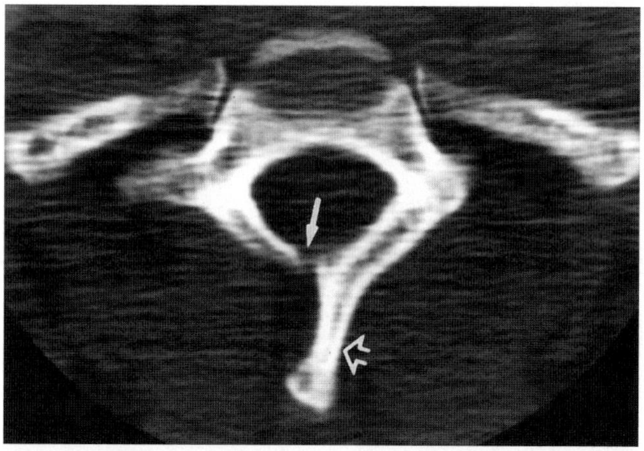

Figure 7G-38C: Axial CT image in bone window showing the inferior duplicated spinous process (*open arrow*) and the paraspinous cleft (*closed arrow*) on the right side. The bony neural arch is also duplicated.

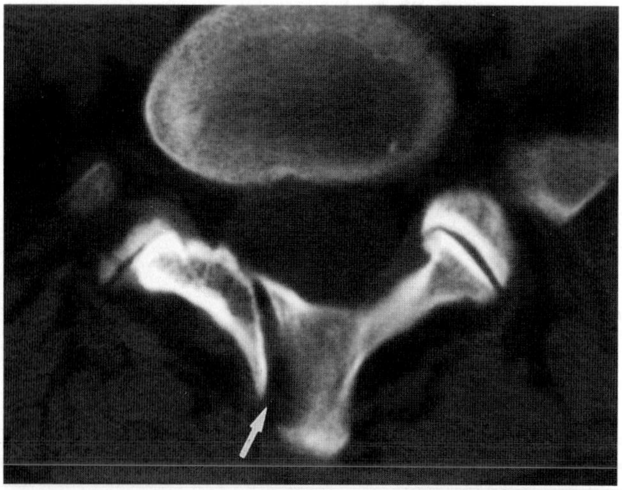

Figure 7G-39: Lumbar paraspinous cleft. Axial CT image showing a paraspinous cleft (*arrow*) in the lamina of L-5 on the right side.

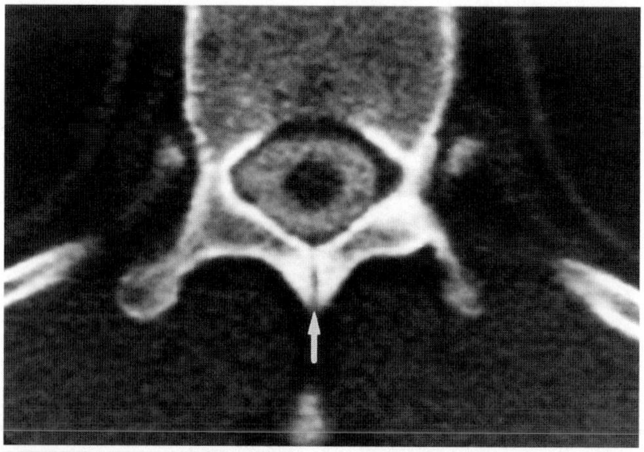

Figure 7G-40: Superior spinous groove. Axial CT myelogram showing a superior spinous process groove (*arrow*).

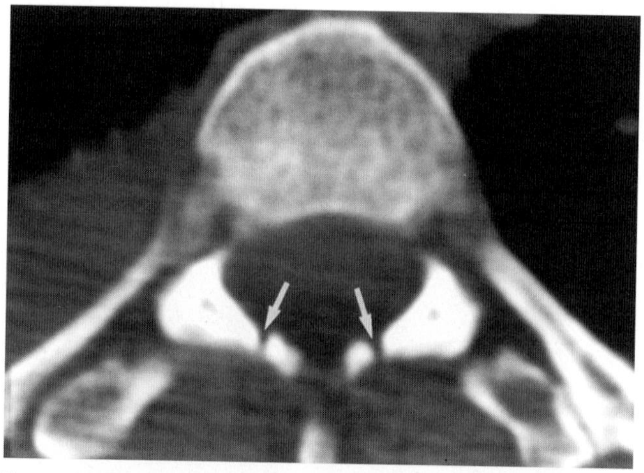

Figure 7G-41A: Paraspinous (intralaminar) grooves/clefts. Axial CT image showing the upper extent of the paraspinous (intralaminar) grooves bilaterally (*arrows*).

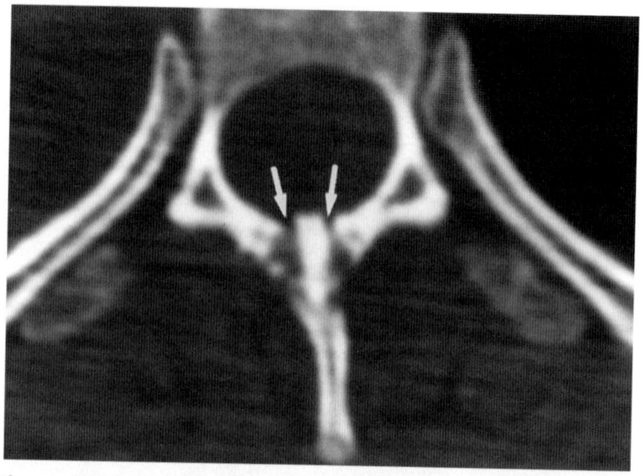

Figure 7G-41B: Axial CT image showing the midextent of the paraspinous grooves/clefts (*arrows*).

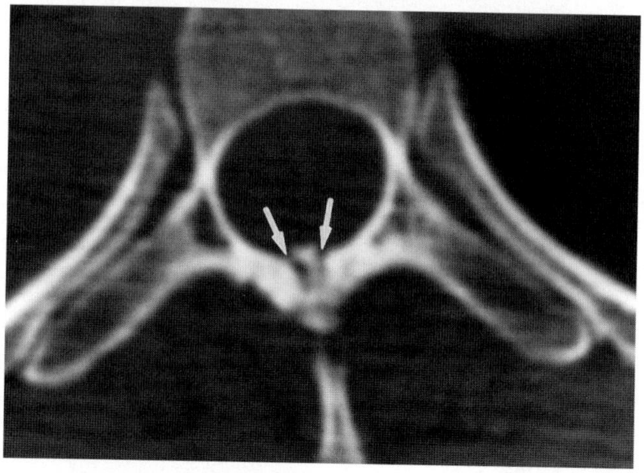

Figure 7G-41C: Axial CT image showing the terminal/inferior extent of the paraspinous grooves/clefts (*arrows*). Note that the lamina are completely fused posteriorly.

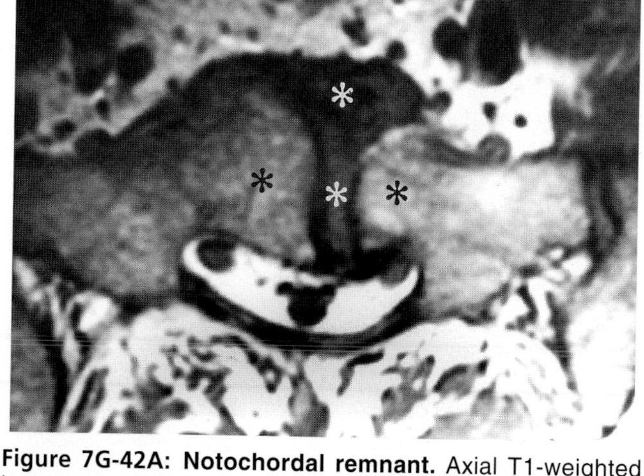

Figure 7G-42A: Notochordal remnant. Axial T1-weighted image at the S-1 level showing a notochordal remnant (*white asterisks*) resulting in a split vertebral body (*black asterisks*, "butterfly" vertebra).

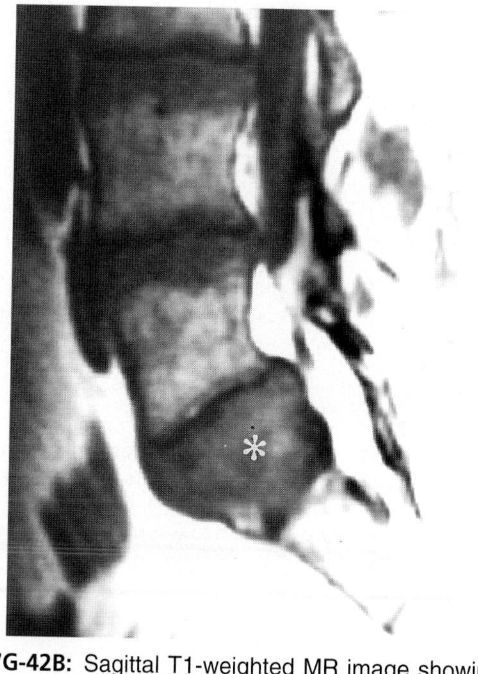

Figure 7G-42B: Sagittal T1-weighted MR image showing the notochord remnant (*asterisk*) in the midline. Note that the intensity of the remnant is approximately the same as that of intervertebral disc material elsewhere in the lumbar spine.

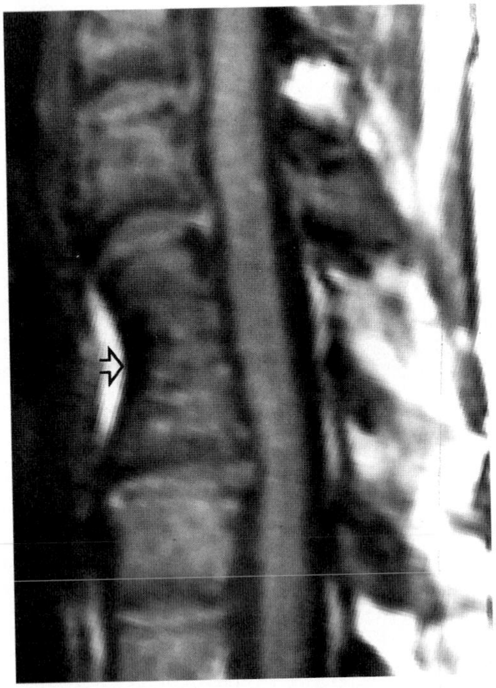

Figure 7G-43A: Segmentation anomaly: congenital C-spine block vertebra (abnormal segmentation) with associated adjacent degeneration. Sagittal T1-weighted MR image shows the typical waist configuration (*arrow*) of the C-5 to C-6 junction compatible with a congenital block vertebrae.

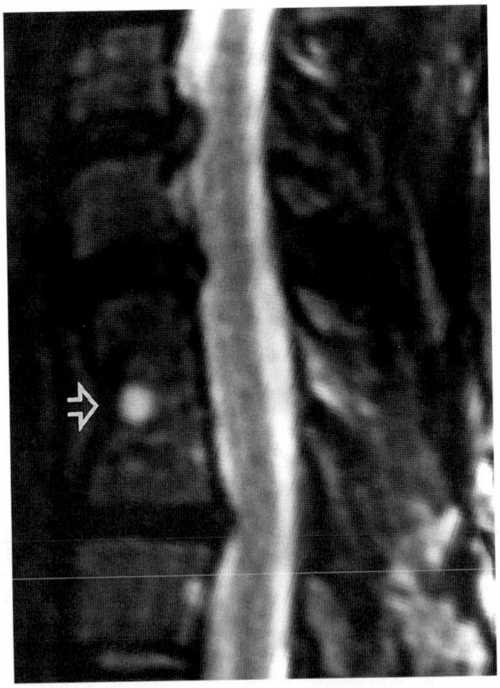

Figure 7G-43B: Sagittal T2-weighted MR image showing the hypoplastic (i.e., waist shape) of the failure of segmentation (*arrow*) of C-5 to C-6. Note the degenerative change above and below this level.

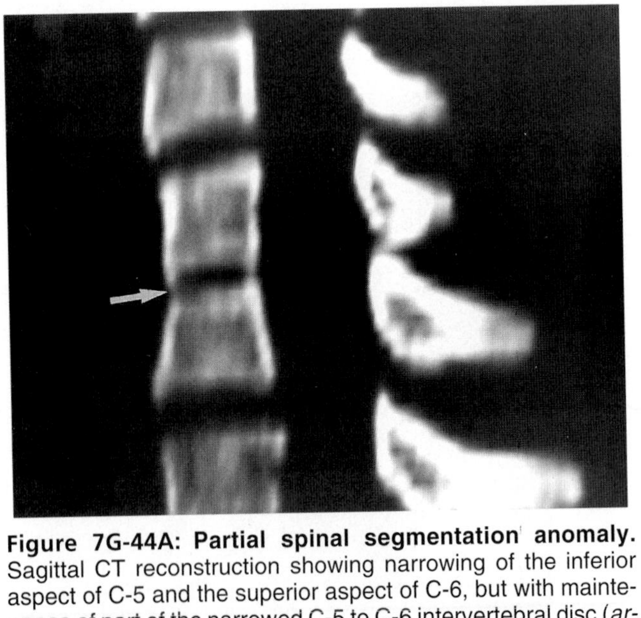

Figure 7G-44A: Partial spinal segmentation anomaly. Sagittal CT reconstruction showing narrowing of the inferior aspect of C-5 and the superior aspect of C-6, but with maintenance of part of the narrowed C-5 to C-6 intervertebral disc (*arrow*). Note that the spinous processes are not fused.

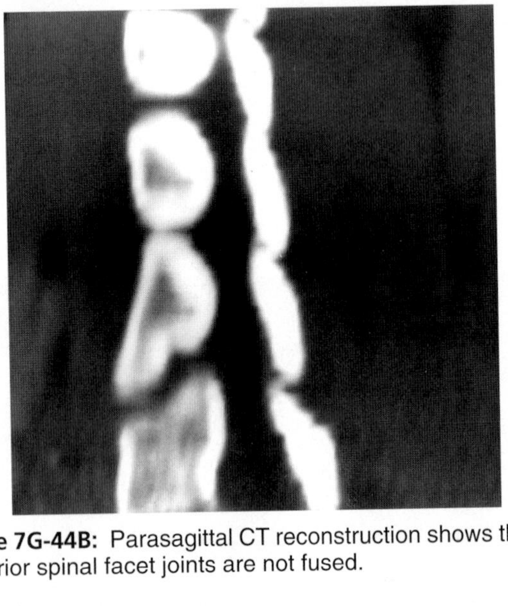

Figure 7G-44B: Parasagittal CT reconstruction shows that the posterior spinal facet joints are not fused.

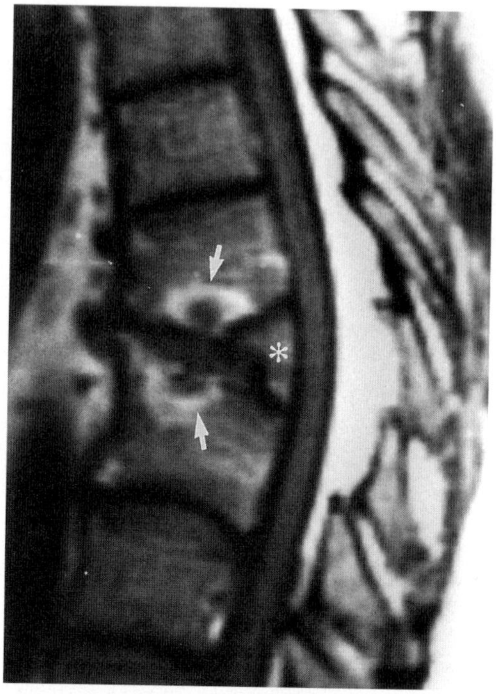

Figure 7G-45: Congenital kyphosis associated with dorsal wedge vertebrae and Schmorl nodes. Sagittal T1-weighted MR image showing a mild thoracic kyphosis due to a dorsal wedge-shaped T-8 vertebral body (*asterisk*). Note also the focal central hypointensity representing Schmorl nodes with surrounding marrow hyperintensity (*arrows*) involving the inferior end plate of T-7 and the superior end plate of T-9.

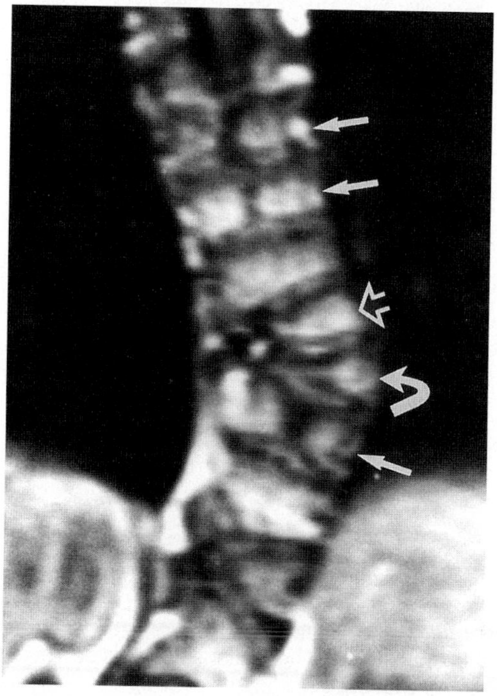

Figure 7G-46A: Congenital scoliosis associated with multiple anomalies of vertebral formation. Coronal T1-weighted MR image of the thoracic pine showing multiple anomalies of vertebral formation (*curved arrow,* lateral hemivertebra; *open arrow,* lateral wedge vertebra; *closed arrows,* butterfly vertebra).

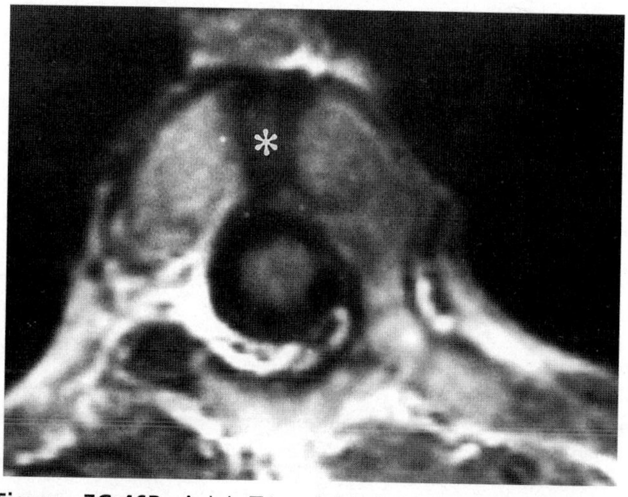

Figure 7G-46B: Axial T1-weighted MR image acquired through the midthoracic region showing a midline cleft (*asterisk*) in the T-5 vertebral body compatible with a butterfly vertebrae.

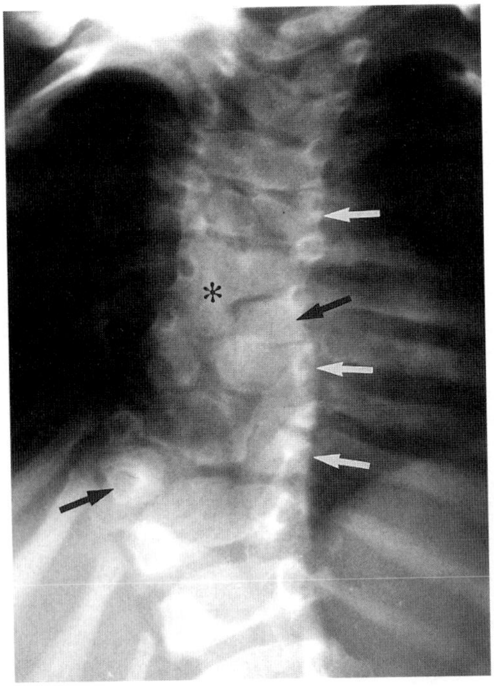

Figure 7G-47: Congenital scoliosis associated with multiple anomalies of vertebral segmentation and formation. Conventional radiograph in the frontal projection showing multiple segmentation and fusion anomalies of the thoracic spine. A complex combination of lateral hemivertebra (*black arrows*), butterfly vertebra (*white arrows*), and fused segments (*asterisk*) is identified, together with multisegment widening of the spinal canal.

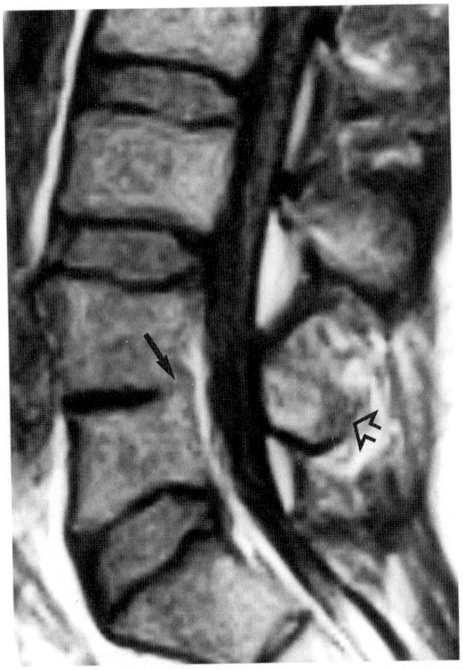

Figure 7G-48A: Lumbar spinal segmentation anomaly involving the vertebral body, posterior spinal facet joints, and spinous processes. Unenhanced sagittal T1-weighted MR image showing partial fusion (*solid arrow*) of L-4 to L-5 vertebral bodies posteriorly. Note also the narrowing of the anteroposterior diameter of the vertebral bodies at the L-4 to L-5 level and the single fused spinous process (*open arrow*).

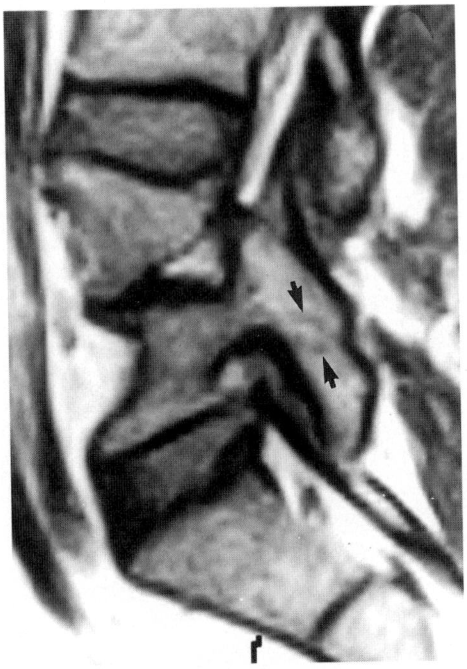

Figure 7G-48B: Sagittal T1-weighted MR image acquired on the patient's left side showing fusion of the L-4 to L-5 facet joint (*arrows*) indicated by the continuity of fatty marrow signal across the articulation. The patient's right side revealed the same findings (not shown).

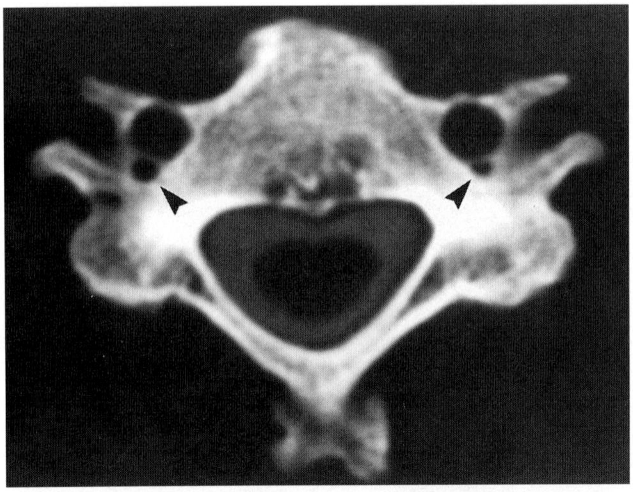

Figure 7G-49: Accessory posterior foramina transversaria. Axial CT image filmed on bone window settings shows accessory vertebral foramina transversaria laterally bifid (*arrowheads*) spinous process of the C-3 vertebra.

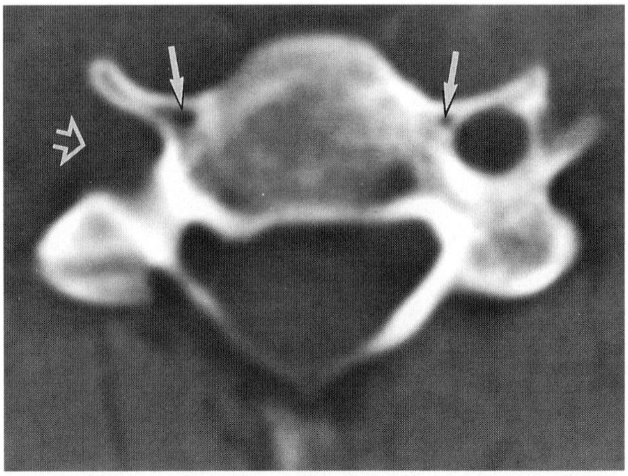

Figure 7G-50: Anterior accessory foramina transversaria: hypoplastic cervical transverse process. Axial CT image showing an anterior accessory transverse foramina bilaterally (*solid arrows*). Also note that the bony ring of the foramen transversarium is incomplete on the right side (*open arrow*).

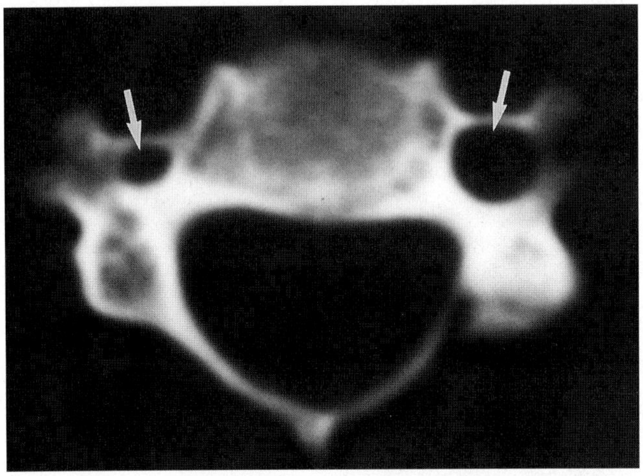

Figure 7G-51: Asymmetric cervical foramen transversarium. Axial CT image showing asymmetry in foramina transversaria of the cervical spine (*arrows*).

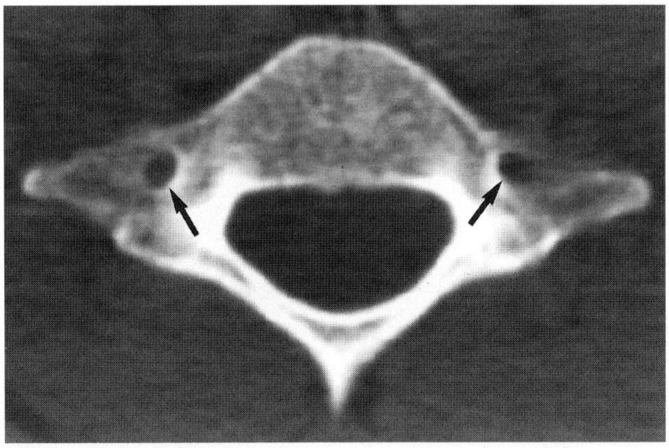

Figure 7G-52: Cervical foramina transversaria below level of traverse of vertebral arteries. Axial CT image showing small size of the foramina transversaria at the level of C-7 in the cervical spine (*arrows*). The vertebral arteries do not traverse the foramina at this level.

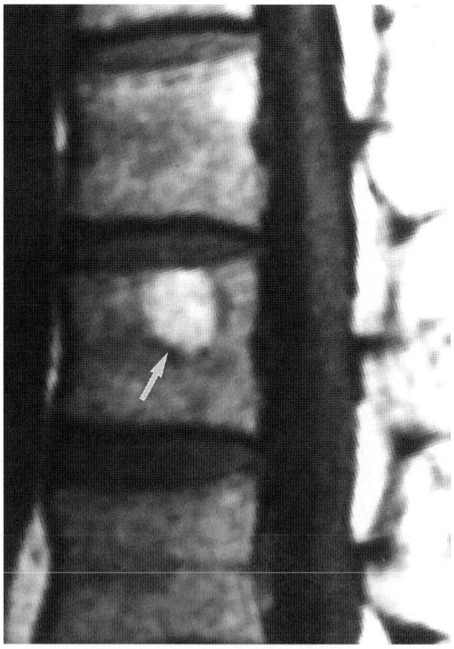

Figure 7G-53A: Vertebral bone marrow "fat" island. Unenhanced sagittal T1-weighted MR image showing a well-defined, round, hyperintense area (*arrow*) at L-5 vertebral body.

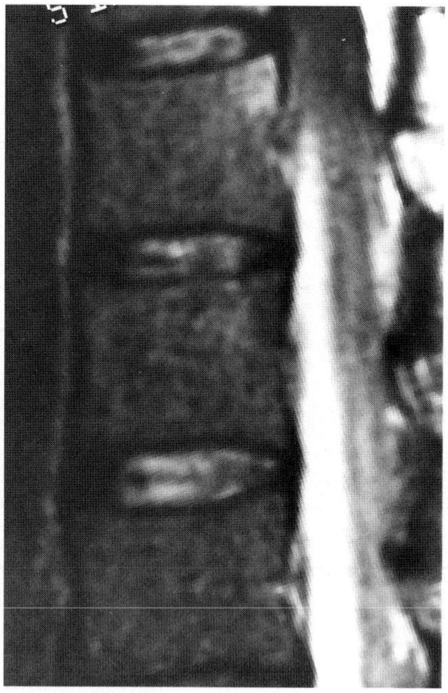

Figure 7G-53B: Sagittal T1-weighted MR image with fat suppression shows the signal of the L-5 area identified in Figure 7G-53A to be suppressed to isointensity with surrounding vertebral marrow, indicating it to be a "fat island" or a benign focal area of increased bone marrow fat.

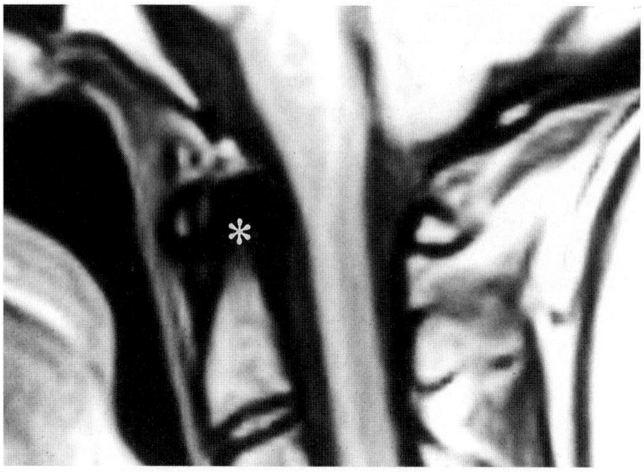

Figure 7G-54: Odontoid marrow MR signal. Sagittal T1-weighted MR image showing poor marrow fat content with the upper odontoid process (*asterisk*).

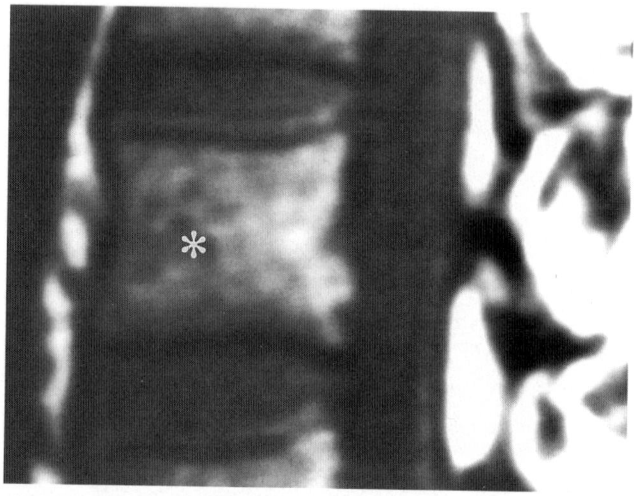

Figure 7G-55A: Age-related variation in vertebral marrow composition. Sagittal T1-weighted MR image in an adolescent showing predominantly hypointense vertebral marrow (*asterisk*) indicating a predominance of hematopoietic marrow.

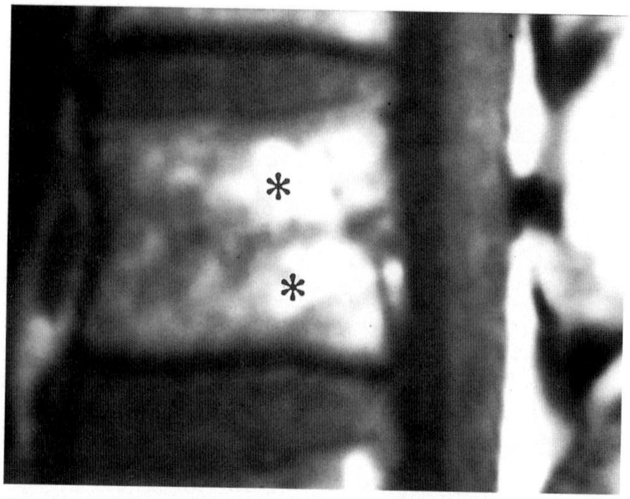

Figure 7G-55B: Sagittal T1-weighted MR image in a young adult showing a moderate degree of hyperintense vertebral marrow (*asterisks*) indicating an increase in fatty marrow and a decrease in hematopoietic marrow.

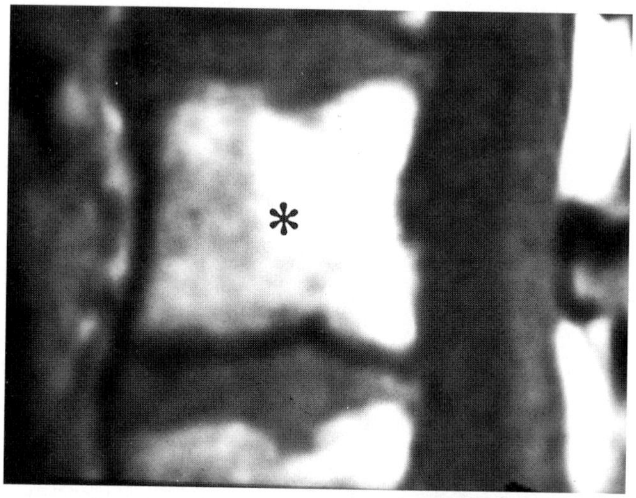

Figure 7G-55C: Sagittal T1-weighted MR image in an elderly adult showing predominantly hyperintense vertebral marrow (*asterisk*) indicating a predominance of fatty marrow.

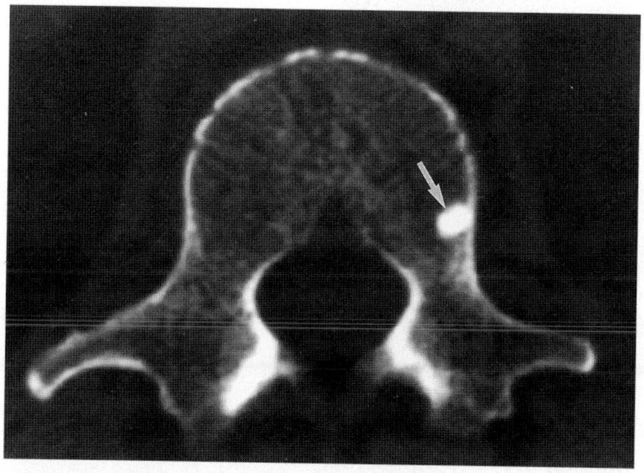

Figure 7G-56A: Vertebral bone "island." Axial CT image showing a bone island (*arrow*) in a lumbar vertebral body.

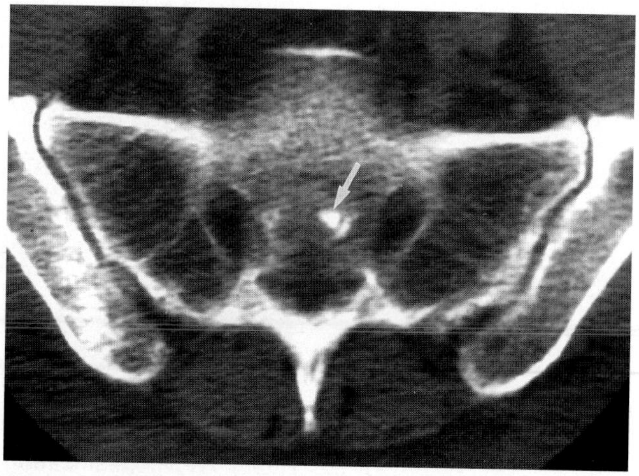

Figure 7G-56B: Axial CT image showing a similar bone island in the sacrum (*arrow*).

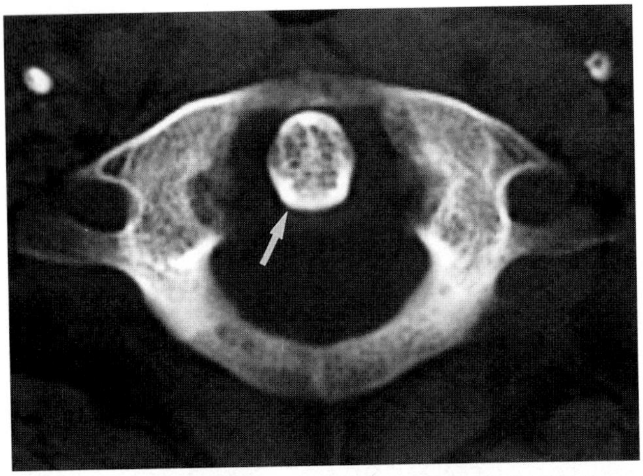

Figure 7G-57A: Ossified apical ligament. Axial CT image showing the normal odontoid apex (*arrow*).

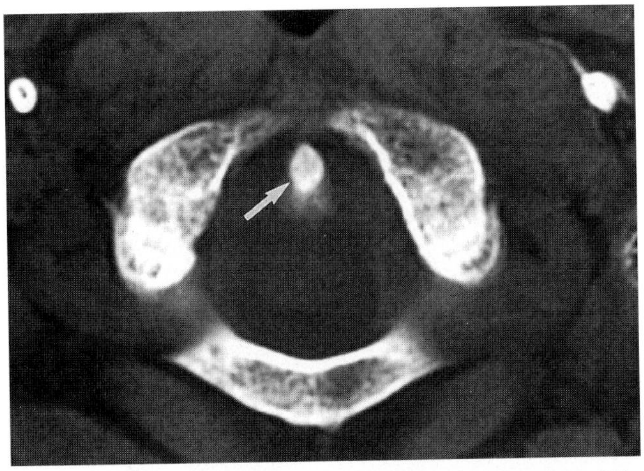

Figure 7G-57B: Axial CT image showing ossification at the base of the apical ligament (*arrow*) at the level of insertion into the odontoid apex.

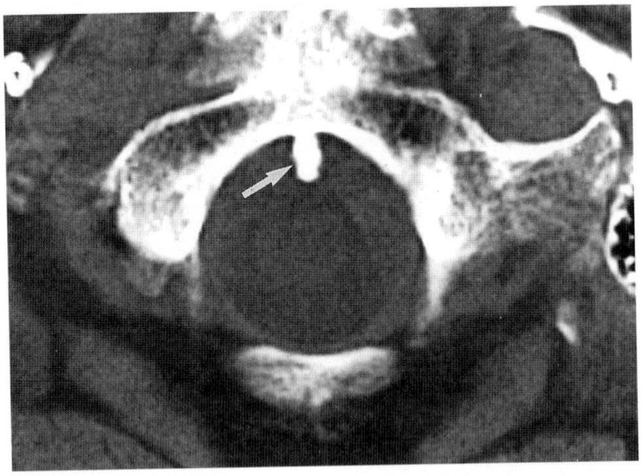

Figure 7G-57C: Axial CT image showing ossification at the distal end of the apical ligament (*arrow*) at the level of insertion into the clivus.

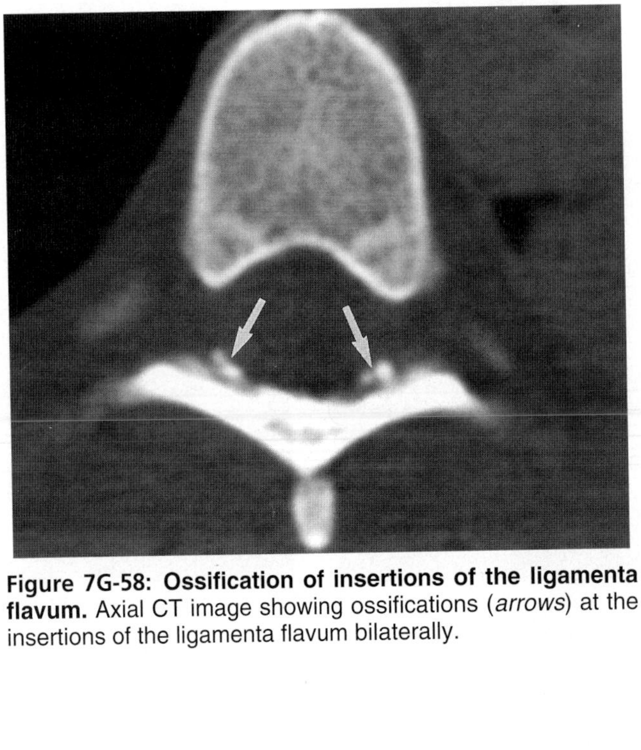

Figure 7G-58: Ossification of insertions of the ligamenta flavum. Axial CT image showing ossifications (*arrows*) at the insertions of the ligamenta flavum bilaterally.

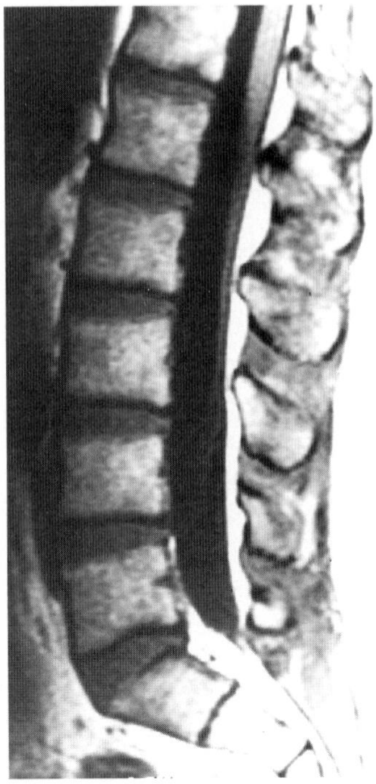

Figure 7G-59: Generally enlarged (patulous) central spinal canal and thecal sac. Unenhanced sagittal T1-weighted MR image showing an enlarged central spinal canal and a patulous lumbosacral thecal sac/ultraspinal canal.

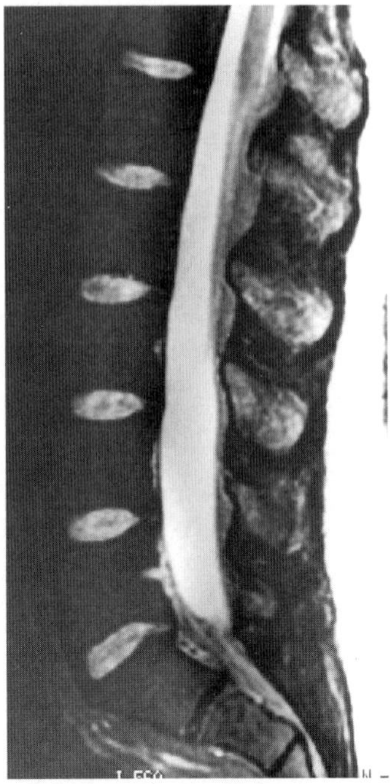

Figure 7G-60: Enlarged central spinal canal. Sagittal T1-weighted MR image with fat suppression in the same case as that in Figure 7G-59 again shows the patulous thecal sac.

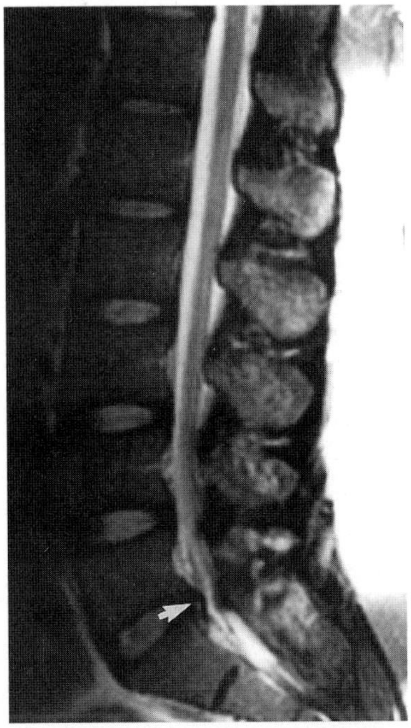

Figure 7G-61A: Developmental stenosis of the central spinal canal. Sagittal T2-weighted MR image showing caudally progressive central stenosis of the lumbar spinal canal. Also note the intervertebral disc protrusion at the L-5 to S-1 level (*arrow*).

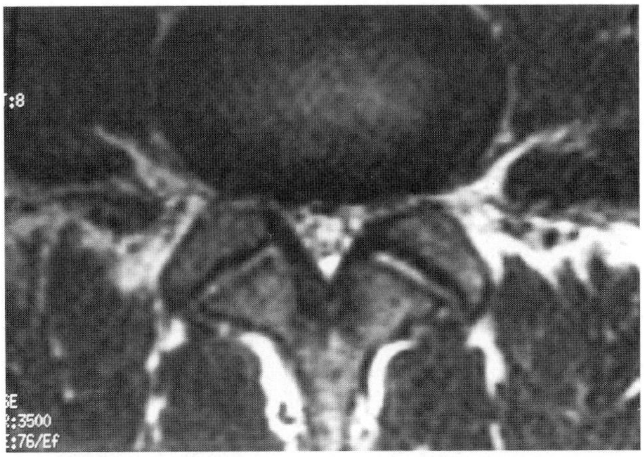

Figure 7G-61B: Axial T2-weighted MR image at the L-4 to L-5 level showing generalized central spinal canal stenosis.

CHAPTER 8

The Neck

THE CERVICAL MUSCLES AND TRIANGLES

1. The neck is divided into two large "triangles": anterior and posterior cervical triangles. The oblique division point between the two is the sternocleidomastoid muscle.
2. These larger triangles are further subdivided into a total of six smaller triangles. The *anterior cervical triangle* consists of the carotid, infrahyoid muscular, submental, and submandibular triangles. The *posterior cervical triangle* consists of the occipital and subclavian triangles. All of these so-called triangles are paired, with the exception of the single midline submental and infrahyoid muscular triangles.
3. These triangular divisions and subdivisions are primarily of clinical importance.

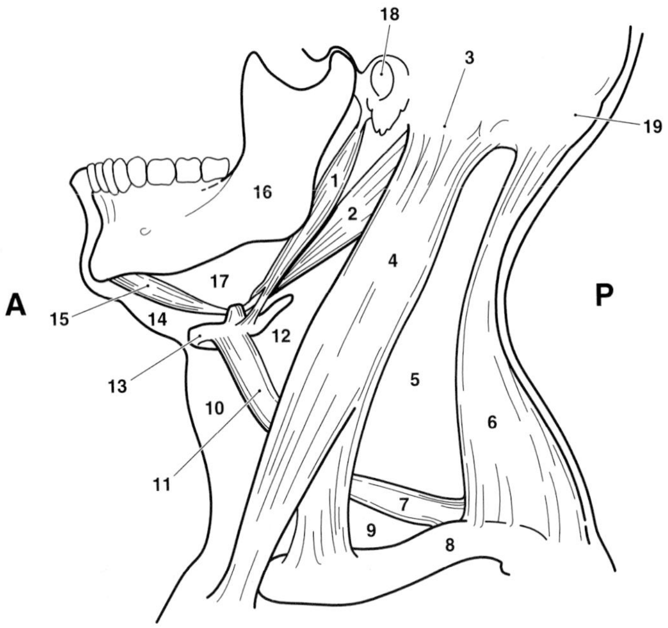

Figure 8-1: Lateral schematic of the triangles of the neck on the left side. *A*, anterior; *P*, posterior.
1 Stylohyoid muscle/ligament
2 Posterior belly of digastric muscle
3 Mastoid process of temporal bone
4 Sternocleidomastoid muscle
5 Occipital triangle
6 Trapezius muscle
7 Inferior belly of omohyoid muscle
8 Clavicle
9 Subclavian triangle
10 Infrahyoid muscular triangle
11 Superior belly of omohyoid muscle
12 Carotid triangle
13 Hyoid bone
14 Submental triangle
15 Anterior belly of digastric muscle
16 Mandible
17 Submandibular triangle
18 External auditory canal in temporal bone
19 Occiput

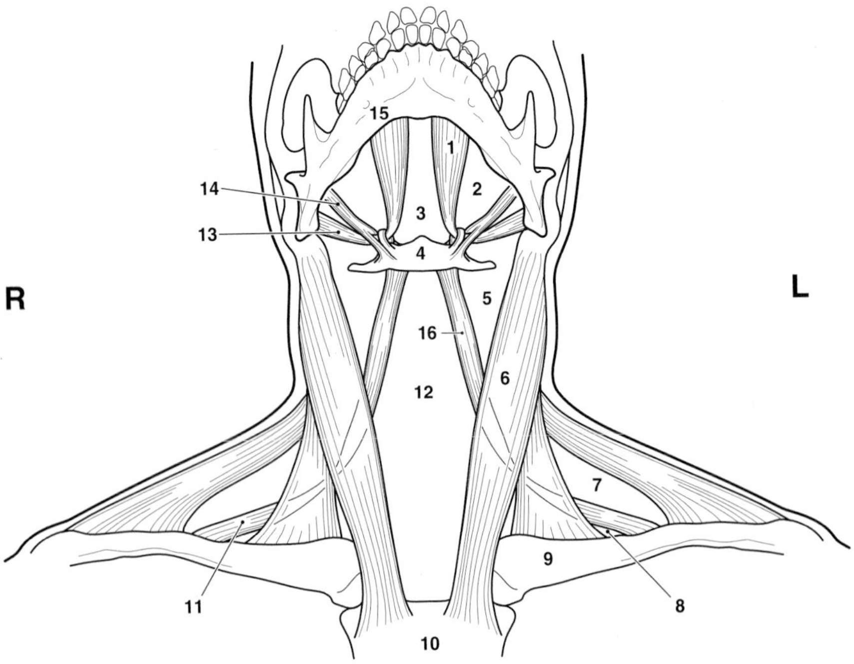

Figure 8-2: Frontal schematic of the triangles of the neck with the chin elevated. *R*, right; *L*, left.
1 Anterior belly of digastric muscle
2 Submandibular triangle
3 Submental triangle
4 Hyoid bone
5 Carotid triangle
6 Sternocleidomastoid muscle
7 Occipital triangle
8 Subclavian triangle
9 Clavicle
10 Sternum (manubrium)
11 Inferior belly of omohyoid muscle
12 (Infrahyoid) muscular triangle
13 Posterior belly of digastric muscle
14 Stylohyoid muscle/ligament
15 Mandible
16 Superior belly of omohyoid muscle

HEAD AND NECK MUSCLE INNERVATION AND FUNCTION

1. The motor innervation to the head and neck muscles is derived mainly from six cranial nerves: the mandibular division of the trigeminal nerve (CN-V3), facial nerve (CN-VII), glossopharyngeal nerve (CN-IX), vagus nerve (CN-X), spinal accessory nerve (CN-XI), and hypoglossal nerve (CN-XII). The functions of these muscles include facial expression, mastication, and deglutition.
2. All infrahyoid muscles, with the exception of the thyrohyoid, are supplied by the ansa cervicalis. The ansa cervicalis proper is formed by the junction of the inferior root of the ansa cervicalis, in turn composed of branches from the second and third cervical spinal nerves (C-2, C-3, and occasionally C-1 and C-4), and the "superior root." The superior root of the ansa cervicalis is composed of neural fibers destined for muscle innervation, originating from the hypoglossal nerve (CN-XII).

TABLE 8-1: The Origins, Insertions, and Innervation of Major and Minor Muscles of the Head and Neck Region

Muscle	Origin	Insertion	Motor innervation
A. Major muscles of the head and neck region:			
Sternocleidomastoid	Sternum and medial third of clavicle	Mastoid process of temporal bone and superior nuchal line	Spinal accessory nerve (CN-XI)
Digastric (anterior belly)	Lower border of mandible near symphysis	Into an intermediate tendon, where it is united with the posterior belly	Mylohyoid branch of the mandibular division of the trigeminal nerve (CN-V3)
Digastric (posterior belly)	Digastric notch of temporal bone	Into an intermediate tendon, where it is united with the anterior belly	Facial nerve (CN-VII)
Stylohyoid	Styloid process of temporal bone	Hyoid bone (lesser cornu)	Facial nerve (CN-VII)
Mylohyoid	Entire length of mylohyoid line of mandible	Midline fibrous raphe extending from mandibular symphysis to hyoid bone	Mylohyoid branch of the mandibular division of the trigeminal nerve (CN-V3)
Hyoglossus	Body and greater horn of hyoid bone	Posterior half of side of tongue	Hypoglossal nerve (CN-XII)
Omohyoid (superior belly)	Body and greater horn of hyoid bone	United with inferior belly by a tendon deep to the sternocleidomastoid muscle	Branches of the ansa cervicalis (C-2 to C-3 spinal nerves)
Omohyoid (inferior belly)	Upper border of scapula	United with the superior belly by a tendon deep to sternocleidomastoid muscle	Branches of the ansa cervicalis (C-2 to C-3 spinal nerves)
Sternohyoid	Manubrium of sternum medial third of clavicle	Lower border of hyoid bone	Branches of the ansa cervicalis (C-2 to C-3 spinal nerves)
Sternothyroid	Posterior aspect of manubrium and first costal cartilage	Oblique line on lateral surface of thyroid cartilage	Branches of the ansa cervicalis (C-2 to C-3 spinal nerves)

continued

TABLE 8-1 *(continued)*

Muscle	Origin	Insertion	Motor innervation
Thyrohyoid	Lateral surface of thyroid cartilage	Lower border of greater horn of hyoid bone	Hypoglossal nerve (CN-XII)
Trapezius (upper and middle fibers)	Medial portion of superior nuchal line, external occipital protuberance, ligamentum nuchae and the spine of C-7	Upper fibers: lateral third of clavicle Middle fibers: acromion and spine of scapula	Spinal accessory nerve (CN-XI)
Temporalis	Temporal fossa, temporal fascia	Ramus and coronoid process of mandible	Trigeminal nerve (CN-V3)
Masseter	Zygomatic arch	Ramus and coronoid process of mandible	Trigeminal nerve (CN-V3)
Pterygoid (lateral)	Infratemporal surface of greater wing of sphenoid bone, lateral pterygoid plate	Neck of mandible, articular capsule, and disc of temporomandibular joint	Trigeminal nerve (CN-V3)
Pterygoid (medial)	Medial pterygoid plate, palatine bone, maxillary tuberosity, pyramidal process	Mandibular ramus and angle	Trigeminal nerve (CN-V3)
B. Muscles of the soft plate:			
Tensor veli palatini	Medial pterygoid process, auditory (eustachian) tube	Palatine bone	Trigeminal nerve (CN-V3)
Musculus uvulae	Palatine aponeurosis	Palatine aponeurosis	Spinal accessory nerve (CN-XI)
Palatoglossus	Palatine aponeurosis	Palatine aponeurosis	
Palatopharyngeus	Palatine aponeurosis	Palatine aponeurosis	
Tensor tympani	Auditory (eustachian) tube	Handle of malleus	Trigeminal nerve (CN-VII)
Stapedius	Bony pyramidal eminence of inner ear	Neck of Stapes	Facial nerve (CN-VII)
Buccinator	Alveolar process of maxillary bone	Alveolar process of mandible, pterygomandibular raphe	Facial nerve (CN-VII)
Frontalis (anterior scalp)	Frontal superficial scalp fascia, superior periocular muscles	Epicranial aponeurosis	Facial nerve (CN-VII)
Occipital (posterior scalp)	Occipital bone, temporal bone (mastoid)	Epicranial aponeurosis	Facial nerve (CN-VII)
Temporalis (lateral scalp)	Zygomatic arch	Epicranial aponeurosis	Facial nerve (CN-VII)
C. Muscles of facial expression:			
Orbicularis oculi	Periorbital subcutaneous fascia	Periorbital subcutaneous fascia	Facial nerve (CN-VII)
Perioral muscles	Periorbital subcutaneous fascia	Periorbital subcutaneous fascia	Facial nerve (CN-VII)
Platysma	Fascia and skin over the upper part of pectoralis major and deltoid muscles	Lower border of mandible, muscles of lower lip, skin and subcutaneous tissues of lower face	Facial nerve (CN-VII)
Stylopharyngeus	Styloid process	Pharyngeal constrictor muscles, glossoepiglotic fold mucosa, thyroid cartilage	Glossopharyngeal nerve (CN-IX)

TABLE 8-1 *(continued)*

Muscle	Origin	Insertion	Motor innervation
D. Pharyngeal constrictors:			
Superior (pterygopharyngeal, buccopharyngeal, mylopharyngeal, glossopharyngeal)	Varied according to specific muscle	Median pharyngeal raphe	Vagal nerve component of pharyngeal plexus (CN-X)
Middle (chondropharyngeal and ceratopharyngeal)	Lesser and greater cornu of hyoid bone, stylohyoid ligament	Median pharyngeal raphe	Vagal nerve component of pharyngeal plexus (CN-X)
Inferior (cricopharyngeal and thyropharyngeal)	Cricoid cartilage, inferior thyroid cornu, thyroid cartilage	Median pharyngeal raphe	Vagal nerve component of pharyngeal plexus (CN-X)
E. Intrinsic laryngeal musculature:			
Cricothyroid	Cricoid cartilage	Thyroid cartilage	External laryngeal nerve (CN-X)
Posterior cricoarytenoid, lateral cricoarytenoid, transverse arytenoid, oblique arytenoid, thyroarytenoid, vocalis	Varied according to specific muscle	Varied according to specific muscle	Recurrent laryngeal nerve (CN-X)
F. Tongue musculature:			
Intrinsic tongue musculature (superior and inferior longitudinal [transverse and vertical])	Within tongue itself	Within tongue itself	Hypoglossal nerve (CN-XII)
Extrinsic tongue musculature (genioglossus, hyoglossus, chondroglossus, styloglossus, paletoglossus)	Varied according to specific muscle Palatine aponeurosis	Varied according to muscle Fascia of tongue	Hypoglossal nerve (CN-XII) Spinal accessory nerve component of pharyngeal plexus (CN-IX)
G. Suboccipital muscles:			
Rectus capitis posterior major	Spinous process of axis (C-2)	Posterior aspect of occipital bone	C-1 spinal nerve
Rectus capitus posterior minor	Tubercle and posterior arch of atlas (C-1)	Posterior aspect of occipital bone	C-1 spinal nerve
Obliquus capitis superior	Transverse process of atlas (C-1)	Posterior aspect of occipital bone	C-1 spinal nerve
Obliquus capitis inferior	Spinous process and lamina of axis (C-2)	Transverse process of atlas (C-1)	C-1 spinal nerve
H. Lateral perivertebral musculature: Scalenus anterior	Transverse process of C-3 to C-6	First rib	C-4 to C-6 spinal nerves
Scalenus medius	Transverse process C-1 and C-2, Posterior tubercles of transverse processes C-3 to C-7	First rib	C-3 to C-8 spinal nerves
Scalenus posterior	Posterior tubercles of transverse processes of C-4 to C-6	Second rib	C-6 to C-8 spinal nerves

TABLE 8-2: Cranial Nerves with Specific Head and Neck Muscle Innervation and Muscle Function

Cranial nerve number	Cranial nerve name	Muscles innervated	Muscle function
V	Trigeminal nerve, mandibular division (CN-V3)	Temporalis, masseter, medial and lateral pterygoids, mylohyoid, anterior belly of digastric	Mastication opens mouth, retracts chin
		Tensor veli palatini	Tenses palate, opens eustachian tube
		Tensor tympani	Acoustic dampening
VII	Facial nerve	Muscles of facial expression	Facial expression, buccinator prevents fluid from pooling in vestibule of mouth, orbicularis oculi closes eye and wink, perioral muscles close lips, smile, etc.
		Platysma	Function obscure, stretches skin of neck
		Frontalis (anterior scalp)	Frown and elevates eyebrows
		Posterior belly of digastric	Opens mouth, retracts chin
		Stapedius	Acoustic dampening
		Stylohyoid	Function obscure, elevates hyoid bone
IX	Glossopharyngeal nerve	Stylopharyngeus	Elevates laryngopharynx
		Muscles of soft palate, excluding tensor veli palatinus	Flap valve that can block oropharynx or nasopharynx
X	Vagus nerve	Pharyngeal constrictors: superior, middle, inferior	Aids swallowing
		Cricothyroid, endolaryngeal muscles	Aids speech, prevents aspiration
XI	Spinal accessory nerve	Sternocleidomastoid	Head movement
		Trapezius	Scapular rotation
XII	Hypoglossal nerve: superior root of ansa cervicalis	Intrinsic tongue muscles	Changes tongue shape
		Extrinsic muscles: genioglossus, hyoglossus, styloglossus;	Changes tongue position
		Geniohyoid, thyrohyoid muscles	Laryngeal depression

THE CERVICAL LYMPHATIC SYSTEM

1. The lymphatic system of the cervical region is complex and has many variations.
2. The cervical lymphatic system can be grouped as follows: the occipital nodes, postauricular nodes, parotid nodes (preauricular and intraglandular), submandibular nodes, facial nodes, submental nodes, sublingual nodes, retropharyngeal nodes, anterior cervical nodes (prelaryngeal, pretracheal, peritracheal), and lateral cervical nodes (superficial, deep [spinal accessory, transverse cervical, internal jugular chains]).
3. The lymphatic drainage of the head and neck can generally be divided into the deep (carotid or internal jugular chain) and the superficial groups (all others).
4. The normal lymphatic drainage is from the superficial to the deep layers of the neck and from the superior to the inferior levels.
5. The terminal lymphatic drainage is into the lymphatic duct on the right side and into the thoracic duct on the left side. Via these ducts, lymph eventually drains into the venous system at the level of the internal jugular or subclavian veins.

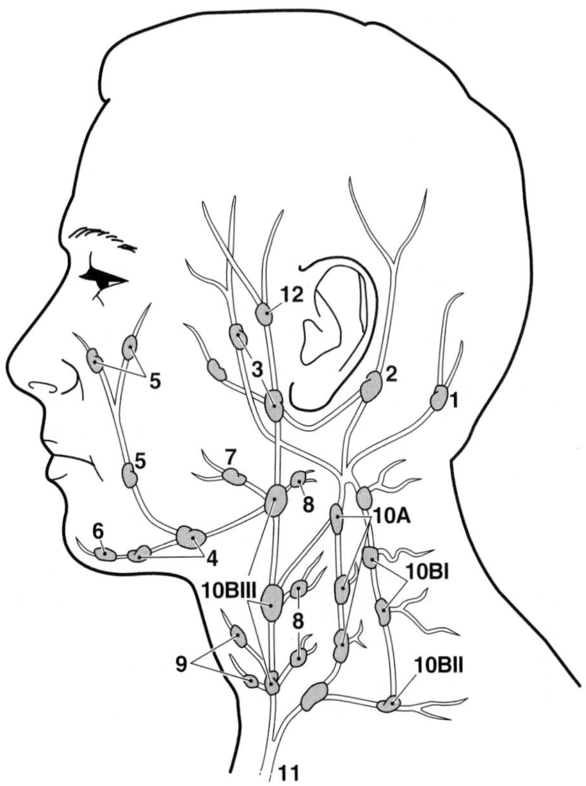

Figure 8-3: Lateral schematic of craniocervical lymphatic system on the left side.

1 Occipital nodes
2 Postauricular nodes
3 Intraglandular parotid nodes
4 Submandibular nodes
5 Facial nodes
6 Submental node(s)
7 Sublingual node(s)
8 Retropharyngeal node(s)
9 Anterior cervical nodes (prelaryngeal, pretracheal, peritracheal)
10 Lateral cervical nodes
 A. Superficial lateral cervical nodes
 B. Deep lateral cervical nodes
  I. Spinal accessory chain
  II. Transverse cervical chain
  III. Internal jugular chain
11 Thoracic duct (left side); lymphatic duct (right side)
12 Preauricular node(s) (part of parotid node system)

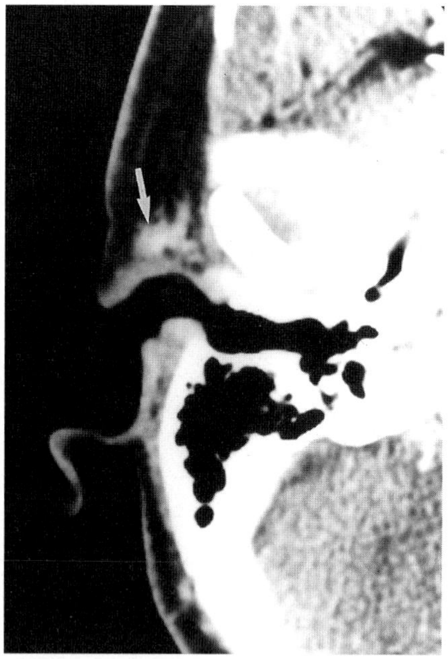

Figure 8-4A: Cervical lymph nodes. Axial CT image showing a preauricular (parotid group) lymph node (*arrow*) on the right side.

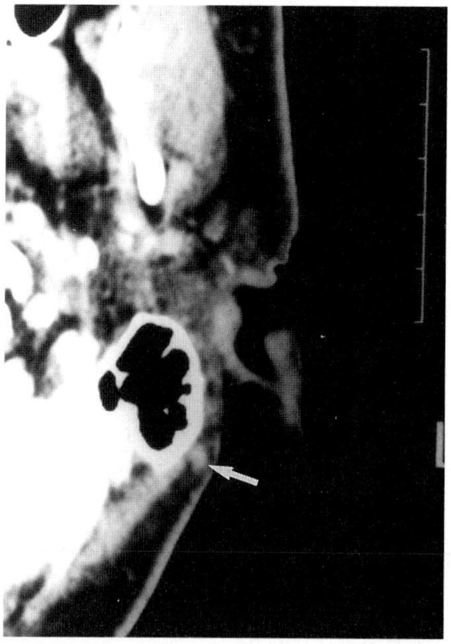

Figure 8-4B: Axial CT image showing a posterior auricular lymph node (*arrow*) on the left side.

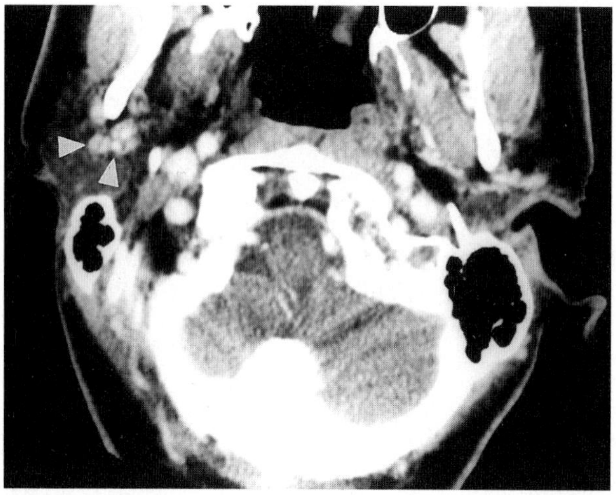

Figure 8-4C: Enhanced axial CT image showing several right intraglandular parotid lymph nodes (*arrowheads*).

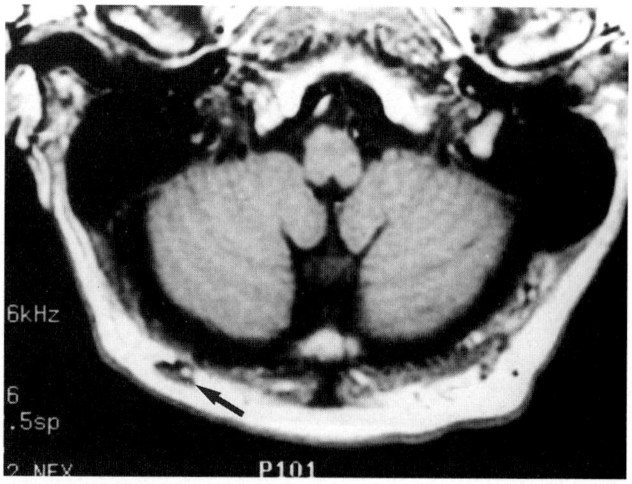

Figure 8-4D: Axial T1-weighted MR image showing an occipital lymph node (*arrow*) on the right side.

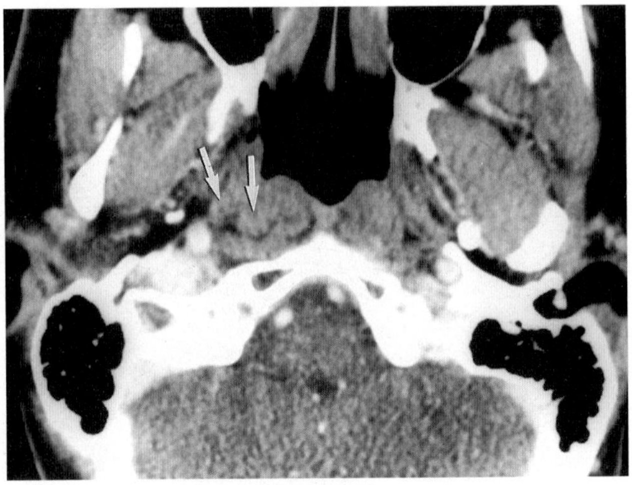

Figure 8-4E: Axial CT image showing two retropharyngeal lymph nodes (*arrows*) on the right side.

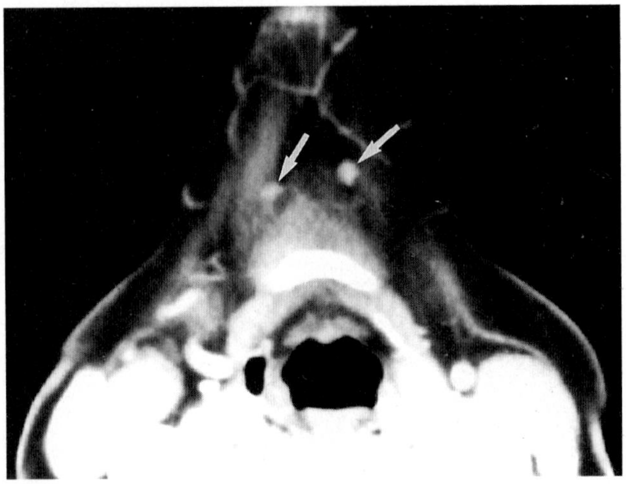

Figure 8-4F: Enhanced axial CT image showing two submental lymph nodes (*arrows*).

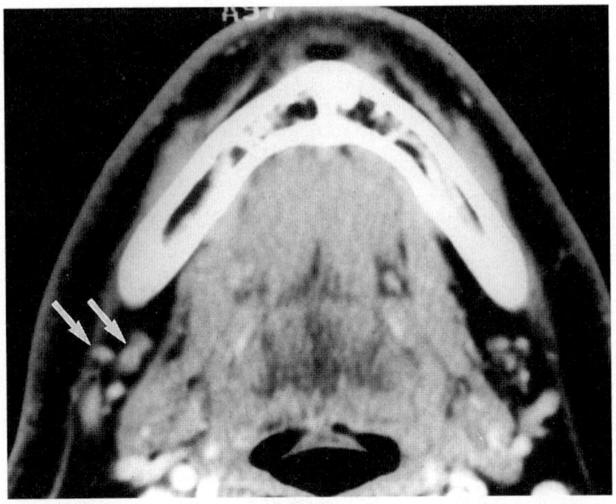

Figure 8-4G: Enhanced axial CT image showing several submandibular lymph nodes (*arrows*) on the left side.

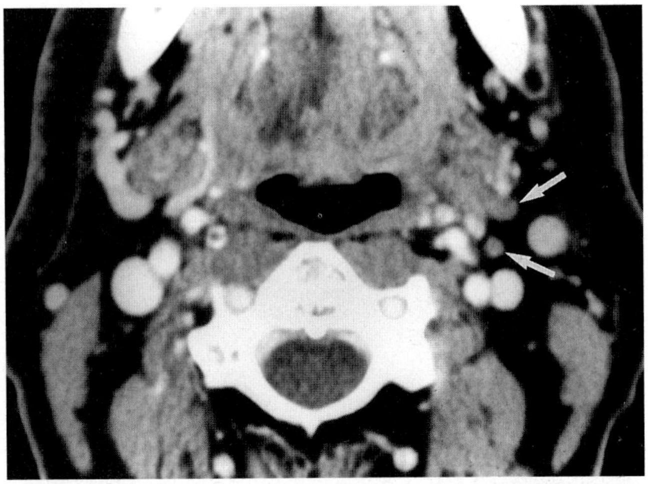

Figure 8-4H: Enhanced axial CT image showing several submandibular lymph nodes (*arrows*) on the right side.

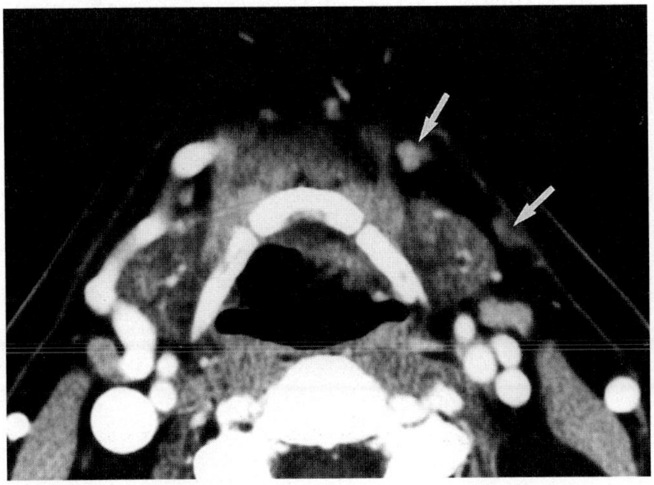

Figure 8-4I: Enhanced axial CT image showing several anterior cervical lymph nodes (*arrows*) superficially.

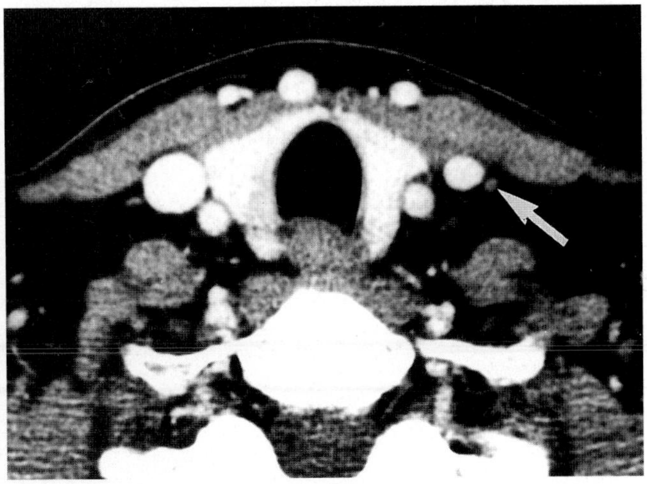

Figure 8-4J: Enhanced axial CT scan showing an anterior (peritracheal) cervical lymph node (*arrow*).

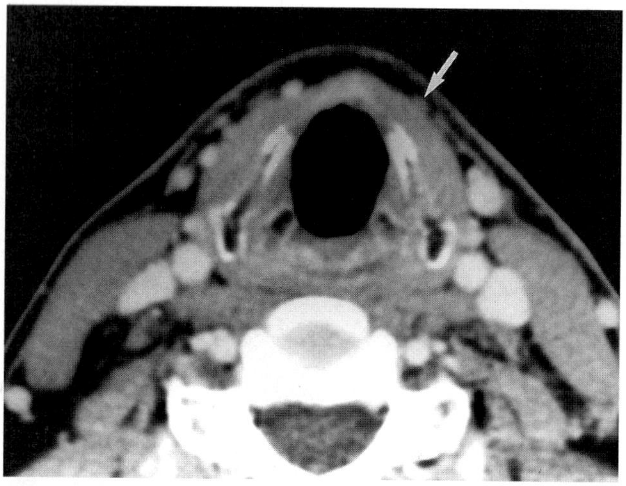

Figure 8-4K: Enhanced axial CT image showing a prelaryngeal anterior cervical lymph node (*arrow*) on the left side.

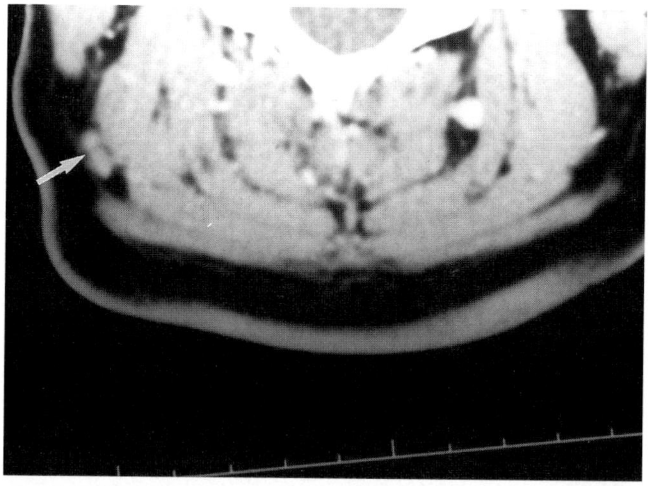

Figure 8-4L: Enhanced axial CT image showing two spinal accessory lymph nodes (*arrow*) on the right side (deep lateral cervical mode subgroup).

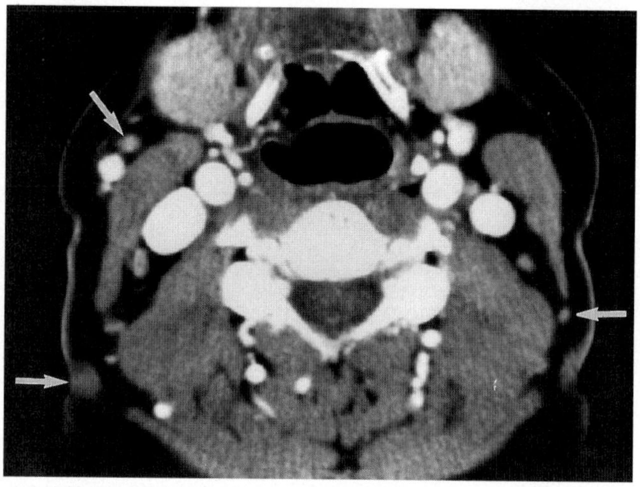

Figure 8-4M: Enhanced axial CT image showing several superficial lateral cervical lymph node(s) (*arrows*).

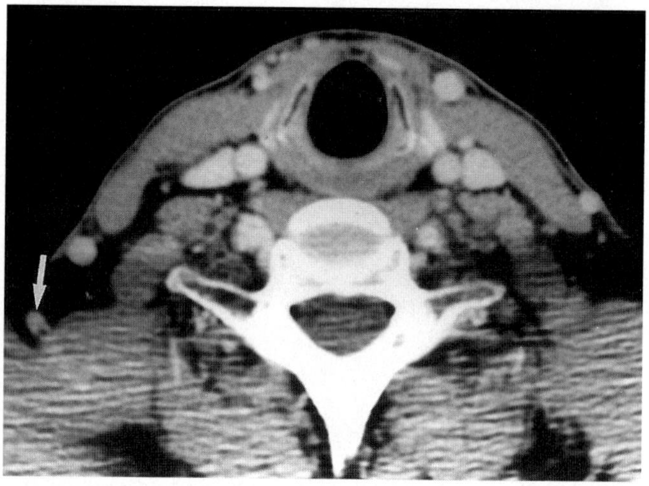

Figure 8-4N: Enhanced axial CT image showing a transverse cervical lymph node (*arrow*) on the right side (deep lateral cervical node group, transverse cervical chain).

THE UPPER AERODIGESTIVE TRACT

Overview

1. The upper aerodigestive tract consists of several linked structures, including the oral cavity, nasal passageways, nasopharynx, oropharynx, hypopharynx, larynx, trachea, and esophagus.
2. The margins and contents of these subdivisions are
   a. *The oral cavity:* Extends from the oral orifice anteriorly to palatoglossal arches (the anterior pillars of the fauces) posteriorly. The oral vestibule is located external to the teeth, while the oral cavity proper is found internal to the teeth. The palatal portion of the tongue is found within the oral cavity, and the salivary glands empty into it.
   b. *The nasal passageways:* Extends from the nares anteriorly to the posterior nasal apertures (choanae). The nasal passageways contain the nasal turbinates and receive drainage from the nasolacrimal and paranasal sinus ducts/foramina.
   c. *The nasopharynx:* Extends from the choanae to the pharyngeal isthmus (the aperture between the posterior aspect of the terminal margin of the soft palate and the posterior wall of the pharynx). The pharyngeal adenoids and the tubal tonsils are found in the nasopharynx. The eustachian tube on each side opens into the nasopharynx in the area of the tubal tonsils.
   d. *The oropharynx:* Extends from the palatoglossal arches to the laryngeal inlet. The pharyngeal portion of the tongue and lingual and palatine tonsils are found in the oropharynx.
   e. *The hypopharynx (laryngopharynx)*: Extends from the laryngeal inlet posterior to the larynx to the orifice of the esophagus.
   f. *The larynx:* Extends from the laryngeal inlet through the cricoid cartilage at its junction with the trachea. The laryngeal inlet (aditus) is bordered by the epiglottis anteriorly and superiorly, the mucosa over the arytenoid cartilages posteriorly and inferiorly, and by the aryepiglottic folds laterally. It contains the laryngeal cartilages, laryngeal musculature, the vestibular and vocal folds, the vestibule, and the laryngeal ventricles and saccules.
   g. *The trachea:* Extends inferiorly from the lower border of the cricoid cartilage to the tracheal bifurcation into the mainstem bronchi.
   h. *The esophagus:* Extends inferiorly from its orifice beneath the hypopharynx to the stomach.

THE PHARYNX

1. The pharynx consists of three connected parts: the nasopharynx, the oropharynx, and the hypopharynx (laryngopharynx).
2. The pharynx links the oral cavity with the larynx and the nasopharynx and oral passageway with the esophagus.
3. The pharynx is basically an internally mucosal-lined, fibromuscular tube. The intrinsic muscles of the pharynx include
   a. The superior pharyngeal constrictor (a combination of the pterygopharyngeal, buccopharyngeal, mylopharyngeal, glossopharyngeal muscles).
   b. The middle pharyngeal constrictor (a combination of the chondropharyngeal and ceratopharyngeal muscles).
   c. The inferior pharyngeal constrictor (a combination of the thyropharyngeal and cricopharyngeal muscles).
4. Other pharyngeal muscles include
   a. The palatopharyngeus muscle extending from the hard palate to the palatine aponeuroses.
   b. The salpingopharyngeus muscle extending from the submucosal cartilage of the eustachian tube to merge with the palatopharyngeus muscle.
   c. The stylopharyngeus muscle extending from the base of the styloid process to merge with the constrictor muscles and insert into the thyroid cartilage.

d. Passavant's muscle encircles the pharynx at the level of the palate. This muscle may in fact be a part of the superior pharyngeal constrictor.

5. The blood supply to the pharynx is derived from many sources including the ascending pharyngeal artery, the inferior thyroidal artery, ascending palatine and tonsillar branches of the facial artery, pharyngeal and greater palatine branches of the maxillary artery, the artery of the vidian (pterygoid) canal, and the lingual artery on each side. Venous drainage of the pharynx is primarily into the pharyngeal venous plexus which in turn drains into the internal jugular vein, the brachiocephalic vein, the facial vein, and the pterygoid venous plexus on each side.
6. The majority of the innervation of the pharynx is from the tonsillar and pharyngeal branches of the glossopharyngeal nerve (CN-IX). The anterior nasopharynx and soft palate are supplied by branches of the maxillary nerve (CN-V2). The lower aspect of the pharynx is supplied by the superior laryngeal branch of the vagus nerve (CN-X).

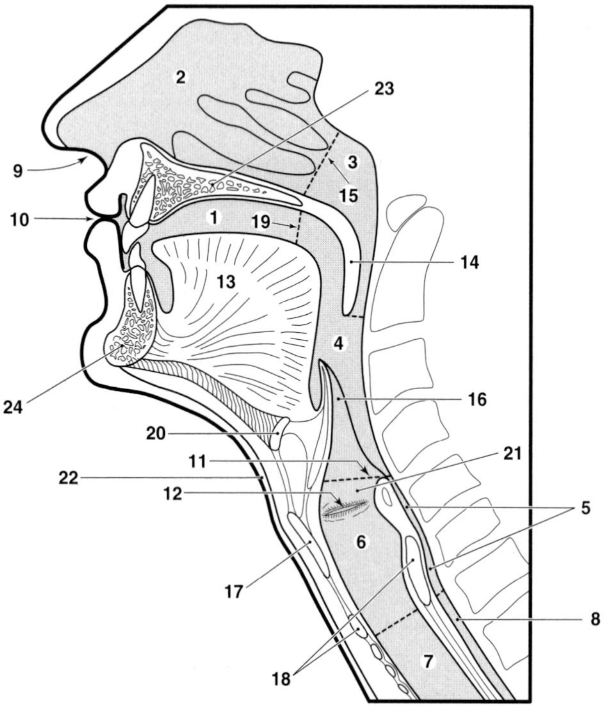

Figure 8-5: Sagittal schematic showing the divisions of the upper aerodigestive tract.
1 Oral cavity
2 Nasal passageways
3 Nasopharynx
4 Oropharynx
5 Hypopharynx (laryngopharynx)
6 Larynx
7 Trachea
8 Esophagus
9 Nasal orifices
10 Oral orifice
11 Laryngeal inlet
12 Vocal fold, laryngeal ventricle, and vestibular fold
13 Tongue
14 Soft palate and uvula
15 Choanae
16 Epiglottis
17 Thyroid cartilage
18 Cricoid cartilage
19 Palatoglossal arches (division between the oral cavity and the oropharynx)
20 Hyoid bone
21 Vestibule
22 Median thyrohyoid ligament
23 Hard palate
24 Anterior aspect of mandible

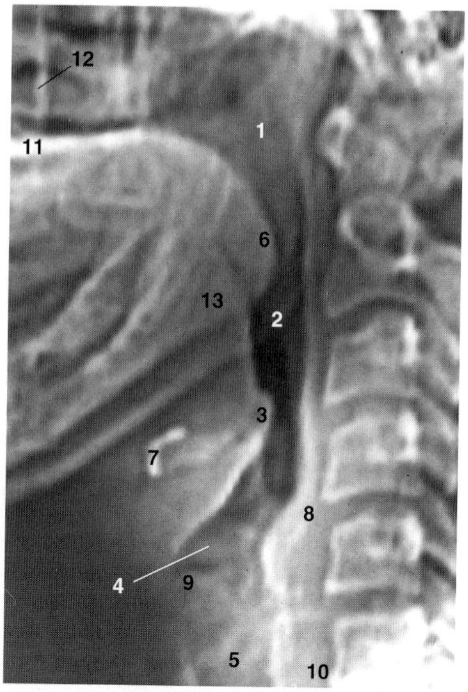

Figure 8-6A: The upper aerodigestive tract. Digital radiograph in the lateral projection showing the upper aerodigestive tract anatomy.

1 Nasopharynx
2 Oropharynx
3 Epiglottis
4 Laryngeal ventricle
5 Trachea
6 Soft palate and uvula
7 Hyoid bone
8 Hypopharynx (potential air-space)
9 Vocal cords
10 Esophagus
11 Hard palate
12 Nasal passageways
13 Root of tongue

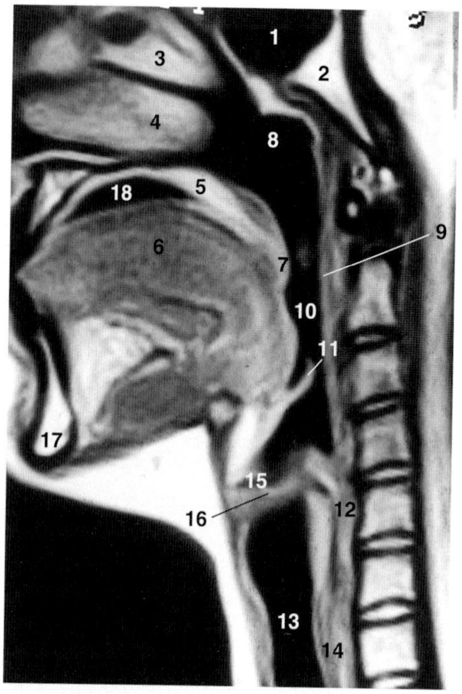

Figure 8-6B: Midline sagittal T1-weighted MR image showing the upper aerodigestive tract anatomy.

1 Sphenoid sinus
2 Clivus
3 Middle nasal turbinate
4 Inferior nasal turbinate
5 Hard palate
6 Tongue
7 Soft palate and uvula
8 Nasopharynx
9 Posterior wall of pharynx
10 Oropharynx
11 Epiglottis
12 Hypopharynx
13 Trachea
14 Esophagus
15 Laryngeal ventricle
16 True vocal cord
17 Anterior aspect of mandible
18 Oral cavity

THE SUPRAHYOID NECK

1. The suprahyoid neck encompasses the tissues between the skull base and the hyoid bone.
2. The suprahyoid neck is divided by the deep cervical fascia into three compartments: medial, lateral, and posterior.
3. Each compartment in the suprahyoid neck can be subdivided into a number of spaces. The *medial* compartment contains the pharyngeal mucosal space. The *lateral* compartment contains the parapharyngeal space, masticator, parotid, and carotid spaces. The *posterior* compartment contains the retropharyngeal, danger, and prevertebral spaces.

TABLE 8-3: Spaces and Contents of the Suprahyoid Neck

Space	Contents
Pharyngeal mucosal space	Pharyngeal tonsils Adenoids Superior pharyngeal constrictor muscle Middle pharyngeal constrictor muscle Salpingopharyngeus muscle Levator palatini muscle Torus tubarius Pharyngobasilar fascia Minor salivary glands
Parapharyngeal space	Fat Ascending pharyngeal artery Internal maxillary artery Pterygoid venous plexus Branches of mandibular division of trigeminal nerve (CN-V3)
Masticator space	Lateral pterygoid muscle Medial pterygoid muscle Masseter muscle Temporalis muscle Branches of the mandibular division of the trigeminal nerve (CN-V3: e.g., inferior alveolar nerve, masticator nerve) Ramus and posterior body of mandible Inferior alveolar artery Inferior alveolar vein
Parotid space	Parotid gland Facial nerve (CN-VIII) Parotid (intraglandular) lymph nodes External carotid artery Retromandibular vein
Carotid space	Internal carotid artery Internal jugular vein Vagus nerve (CN-X) Glossopharyngeal nerve (CN-IX) Spinal accessory nerve (CN-XI) Hypoglossal nerve (CN-XII) Sympathetic neural plexus (paraspinal) Lymph nodes

TABLE 8-3: *(continued)*

Space	Contents
Retropharyngeal space[a]	Fat Lymph nodes
Danger space[a]	Fat
Prevertebral space	Longus colli muscles Longissimus capitis muscles Rectus capitis muscles Vertebral arteries Vertebral veins Scalene muscles Brachial plexus Phrenic nerve (C-3 to C-5) Upper cervical vertebrae Upper cervical intervertebral discs Paraspinal muscles (anterior) Spinal cord and exiting upper cervical nerves

[a] These two spaces cannot be clearly differentiated on imaging and may be considered together for practical purposes.

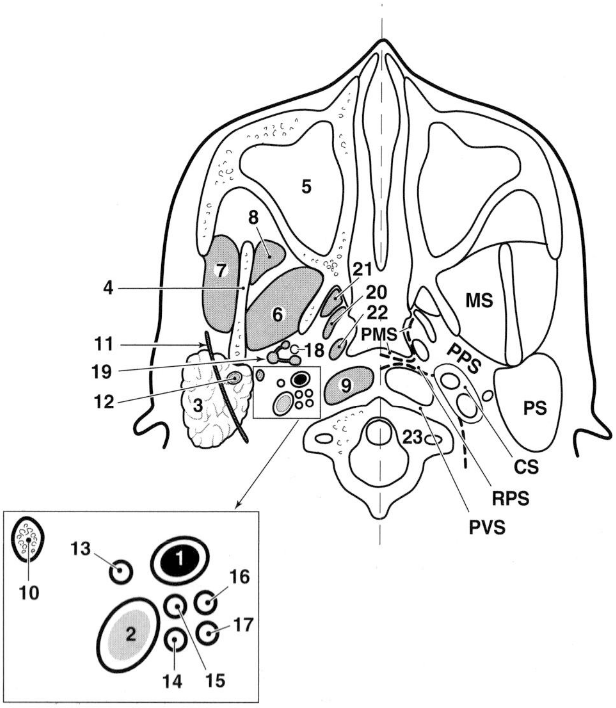

Figure 8-7A: Axial schematic of the anterior suprahyoid neck at the level of the mid-nasopharynx. *MS,* masticator space; *PS,* parotid space; *CS,* carotid space; *PVS,* prevertebral space; *RPS,* retropharyngeal space; *PPS,* parapharyngeal space; *PMS,* pharyngeal mucosal space.

1 Internal carotid artery
2 Internal jugular vein
3 Parotid gland
4 Ramus of mandible
5 Maxillary sinus
6 Lateral pterygoid muscle
7 Masseter muscle
8 Temporalis muscle
9 Longus colli muscle
10 Styloid process
11 Facial nerve (CN-VII) within and traversing the parotid gland
12 Retromandibular vein
13 Glossopharyngeal nerve (CN-IX)
14 Spinal accessory nerve (CN-XI)
15 Vagus nerve (CN-X)
16 Hypoglossal nerve (CN-XII)
17 Sympathetic neural plexus
18 Lingual nerve (branch of CN-V3)
19 Pterygoid venous plexus
20 Tensor palatini muscle
21 Medial pterygoid muscle
22 Levator palatini muscle
23 Atlas (C-1)

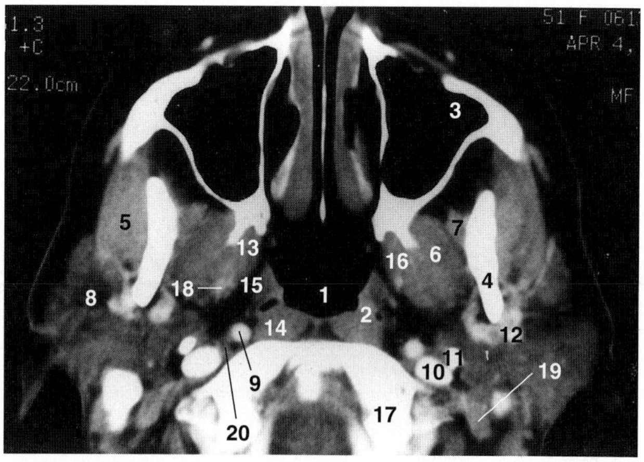

Figure 8-7B: Anatomy of the suprahyoid neck. Enhanced axial CT at the level of the mid-nasopharynx showing the normal anatomy.

1 Nasopharynx
2 Lateral parapharyngeal recess (fossa of Rosenmüller)
3 Maxillary sinus
4 Ramus of mandible
5 Masseter muscle
6 Lateral pterygoid muscle
7 Temporalis muscle
8 Parotid gland
9 Internal carotid artery
10 Internal jugular vein
11 Styloid process
12 Retromandibular vein
13 Medial pterygoid muscle
14 Longus colli muscle
15 Levator palatini muscle
16 Tensor palatini muscle
17 Atlas (C-1)
18 Pterygoid venous plexus
19 Upper extent of vertebral venous plexus
20 Region of traversing CNs IX–XII and upper cervical sympathetic neural plexus (carotid space)

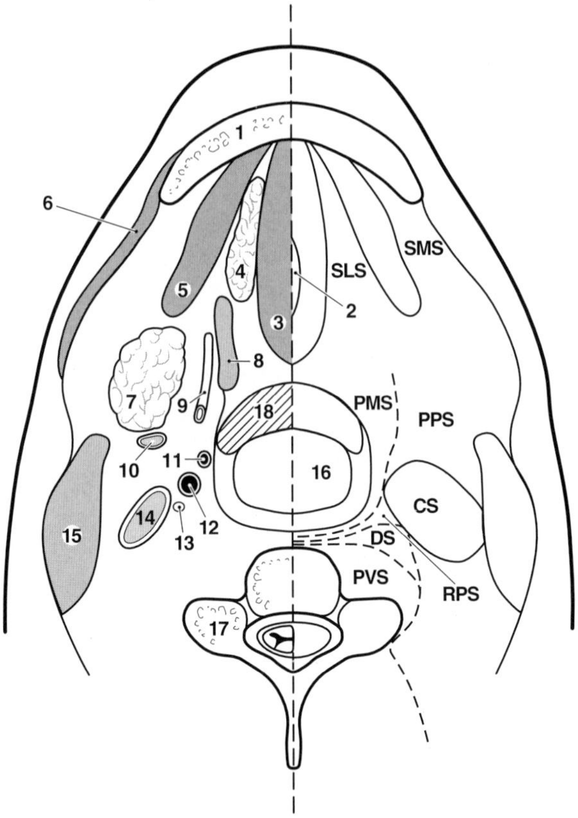

Figure 8-8A: Axial schematic at the level of the base of the oral cavity. *PMS,* pharyngeal mucosal space; *PPS,* parapharyngeal space; *SMS,* submandibular space; *SLS,* sublingual space; *RPS,* retropharyngeal space; *CS,* carotid space; *PVS,* prevertebral space; *DS,* danger space.

1 Mandible
2 Lingual septum
3 Genioglossus muscle
4 Sublingual gland
5 Mylohyoid muscle
6 Platysma muscle
7 Submandibular gland
8 Hypoglossal muscle
9 Hypoglossal nerve
10 Facial vein
11 External carotid artery
12 Internal carotid artery
13 Vagus nerve
14 Internal jugular vein
15 Sternocleidomastoid muscle
16 Oropharynx
17 Cervical vertebra
18 Lingual tonsil

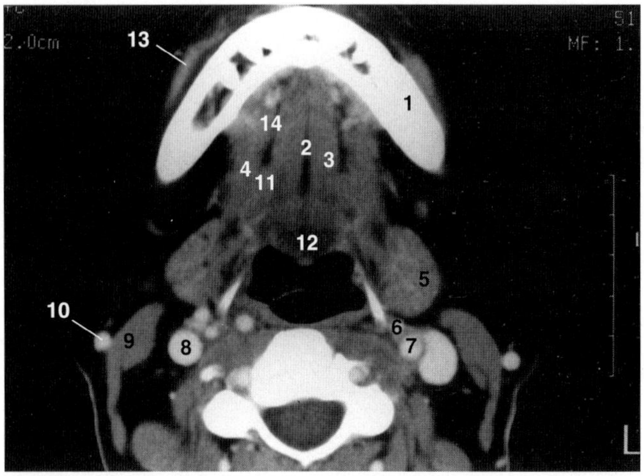

Figure 8-8B: Anatomy of the suprahyoid neck. Enhanced axial CT at the level of the base of oral cavity showing normal anatomy.

1 Mandible
2 Median longitudinal lingual septum
3 Genioglossus muscle
4 Mylohyoid muscle
5 Submandibular gland
6 External carotid artery
7 Internal carotid artery
8 Internal jugular vein
9 Sternocleidomastoid muscle
10 External jugular vein
11 Hypoglossal muscle
12 Lingual tonsil
13 Platysma muscle
14 Sublingual gland (inseparable from surrounding muscle)

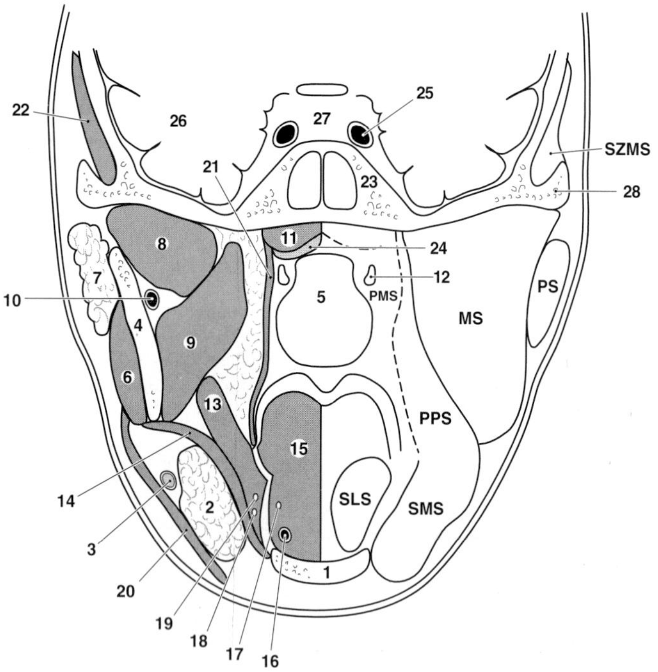

Figure 8-9: Coronal schematic of the deep facial anatomy. *MS,* masticator space; *PMS,* pharyngeal mucosal space; *PPS,* parapharyngeal space; *PS,* parotid space; *SLS,* sublingual space; *SMS,* submandibular space; *SZMS,* suprazygomatic masticator space.

1 Hyoid bone (corpus)
2 Submandibular gland
3 Facial vein
4 Ramus of mandible
5 Oropharynx
6 Masseter muscle
7 Parotid gland
8 Lateral pterygoid muscle
9 Medial pterygoid muscle
10 Internal maxillary artery
11 Prevertebral muscle (e.g., longus colli muscle)
12 Cartilaginous eustachian tube
13 Styloglossus muscle
14 Mylohyoid muscle
15 Intrinsic tongue muscles
16 Lingual artery
17 Glossopharyngeal nerve (CN-IX)
18 Hypoglossal nerve (CN-XII)
19 Lingual nerve (branch of mandibular [third] division of the trigeminal nerve: CN-V3)
20 Platysma muscle
21 Superior pharyngeal constrictor (combination of pterygopharyngeal, buccopharyngeal, mylopharyngeal, glossopharyngeal muscles)
22 Temporalis muscle
23 Sphenoid bone
24 Adenoids
25 Internal carotid artery (cavernous segment)
26 Temporal lobe
27 Sella turcica
28 Base of (temporal process of) zygomatic arch

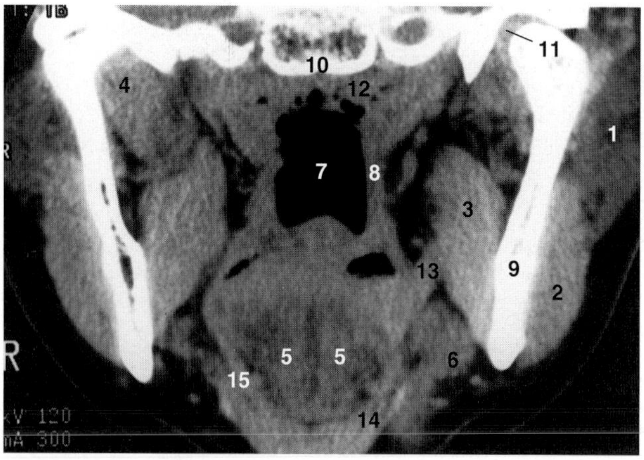

Figure 8-10: Coronal facial anatomy. Coronal CT image showing the normal deep structures of the face.

1 Parotid gland
2 Masseter muscle
3 Medial pterygoid muscle
4 Lateral pterygoid muscle
5 Intrinsic muscles of the tongue
6 Submandibular gland
7 Nasopharynx
8 Superior pharyngeal constrictor
9 Mandible
10 Body of sphenoid bone
11 Temporomandibular joint
12 Longus colli muscle
13 Styloglossus muscle
14 Geniohyoid muscle
15 Mylohyoid muscle

THE TONGUE

1. The tongue is an organ of taste, deglutition, and speech.
2. The tongue is highly muscular and is attached by its muscles to the hyoid bone, mandible, styloid processes, soft palate, and pharyngeal wall.
3. The tongue is divided sagittally by a midline (median) fibrous lingual septum into right and left halves. The (medial longitudinal lingual) fibrous septum attaches the tongue to the hyoid bone. Each half of the tongue has intrinsic tongue muscles, i.e., those wholly within the tongue proper; and extrinsic tongue muscles, i.e., those that extend outside of the confines of the tongue.
4. The extrinsic muscles of the tongue include the genioglossus, hyoglossus, styloglossus, chondroglossus, and palatoglossus muscles. All extrinsic tongue muscles are innervated by the hypoglossal nerve (CN-XII), with the exception of palatoglossus, which is supplied by the vagal (CN-X) component of the pharyngeal neural plexus.
5. The intrinsic muscles of the tongue include superior longitudinal, inferior longitudinal, transverse, and vertical muscles. The fiber groups are difficult to distinguish because their fibers intercalate. All intrinsic tongue muscles are innervated by the hypohypoglossal nerve (CN-XII).
6. The superior surface (dorsum) of the tongue is divided by the posteriorly directed "V"-shaped sulcus terminalis into an oral (anterior) part of the tongue and a pharyngeal (posterior) part of the tongue. The foramen cecum is located at the apex of the sulcus terminalis. The superior surface of the oral tongue is divided at the midline by the longitudinal median sulcus.
7. The mucosa of the oral tongue is papillated by several varieties of papillae, including filiform, fungiform, vallate (circumvallate), and foliate papillae. These papillae are mucous membrane modifications that effectively expand the surface area of the tongue, thereby effectively increasing tongue contact with oral contents.
8. The inferior surface of the tongue reflects onto the floor of the mouth and gums via the midline frenulum linguae and the paired paramedian plicae fimbriata.
9. The pharyngeal tongue is devoid of papillae. Submucosal lymphoid nodules that are embedded in the submucosa of the median pharyngeal tongue are collectively known as the (unpaired) lingual tonsil.
10. The taste buds are microscopic epithelial structures that harbor chemosensory cells; they are scattered over the superior surface of the tongue, sides of the tongue, epiglottis, and lingual aspect of the soft palate.
11. The lingual sensory nerves include (a) the lingual branch of the mandibular nerve (CN-V3: general sensation to mucosa of oral part of tongue, floor of mouth, and lingual gingivae); (b) the chorda tympani branch of the facial nerve (CN-VII: gustatory [taste] sensation); (c) the lingual branch of the glossopharyngeal nerve (CN-IX: general and gustatory sensation); and the superior laryngeal nerve (branch of the vagus nerve [CN-X]: general and gustatory sensation).
12. Stated a different way, gustatory (taste) nerve fibers originate from neurons in the geniculate ganglion of the facial nerve (CN-VII) and the inferior ganglia of the glossopharyngeal (CN-IX) and vagus (CN-X) nerves. The central axons of the gustatory pathway constitute the tractus solitarius, synapsing with the rostral aspect of the nucleus solitarius (solitary nucleus).

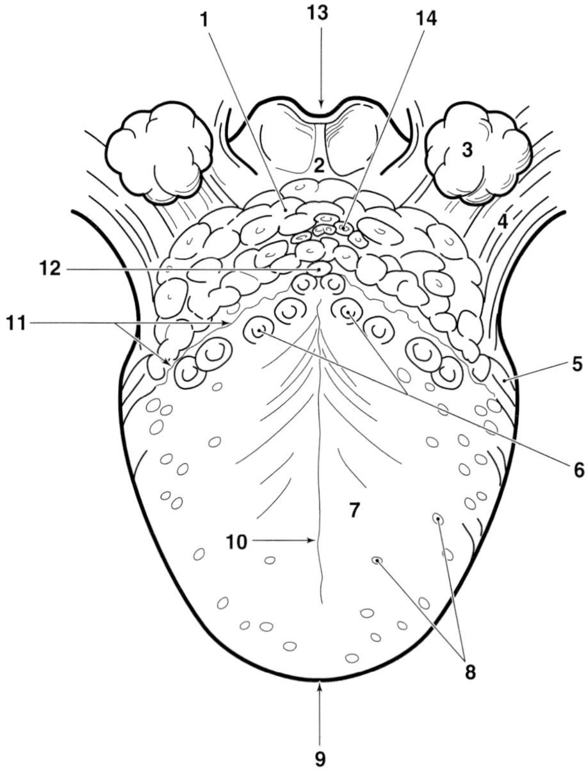

Figure 8-11: Anterosuperior schematic of the superior surface of the tongue.
1 Pharyngeal part of tongue
2 Median glossoepiglottic fold
3 Palatine tonsil
4 Palatoglossal arch
5 Foliate papillae
6 (Circum)vallate papillae
7 Oral part of tongue
8 Fungiform papillae
9 Apex of tongue
10 Longitudinal median sulcus
11 Sulcus terminalis
12 Foramen cecum
13 Epiglottis
14 Lingual tonsil

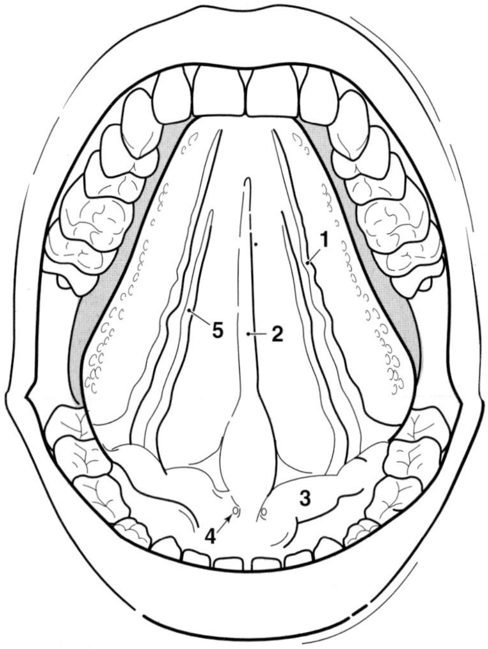

Figure 8-12: Frontal schematic of the floor of the mouth with the mouth open and the tongue elevated to show the undersurface of the tongue.
1 Plica fimbriata
2 Frenulum linguae
3 Sublingual fold
4 Orifice of submandibular duct on sublingual papilla
5 Deep lingual vein (beneath mucosa)

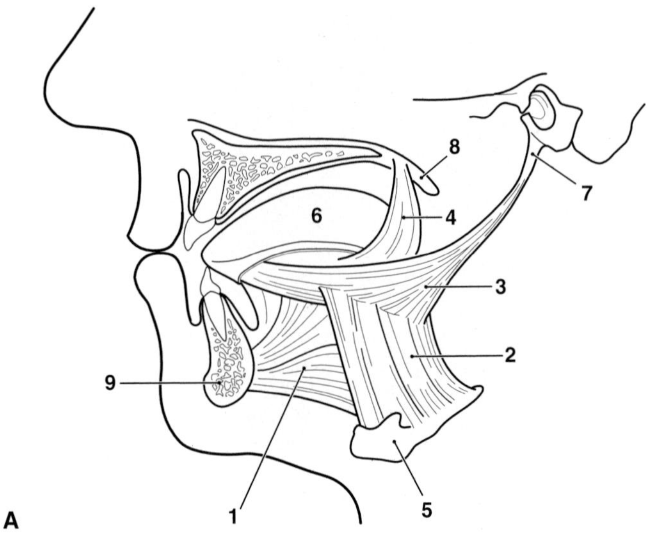

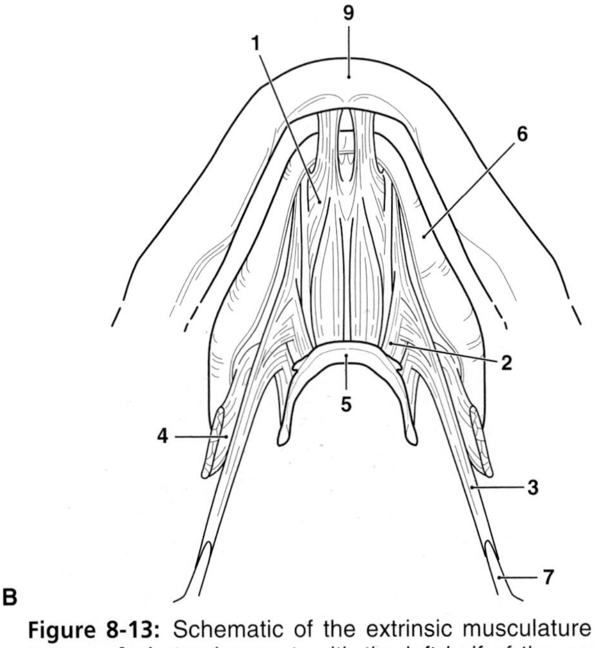

Figure 8-13: Schematic of the extrinsic musculature of the tongue. **A:** Lateral aspect, with the left half of the mandible, maxilla, and face removed. **B:** Inferior aspect, with many of the overlying tissues removed.

1 Genioglossus muscle
2 Hyoglossus muscle
3 Styloglossus muscle
4 Palatoglossus muscle
5 Hyoid bone
6 Tongue
7 Styloid process
8 Soft palate
9 Anterior aspect of mandible

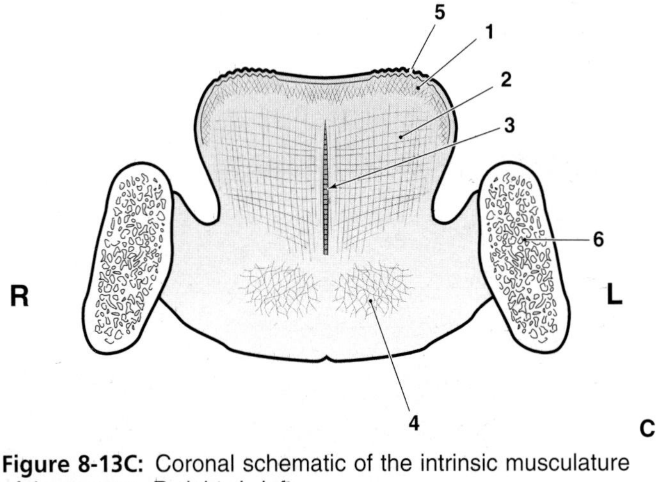

Figure 8-13C: Coronal schematic of the intrinsic musculature of the tongue. *R,* right; *L,* left.

1 Superior longitudinal lingual muscle
2 Vertical and transverse lingual muscles
3 Median longitudinal lingual septum
4 Inferior longitudinal lingual muscle
5 Mucosal surface of tongue
6 Mandible

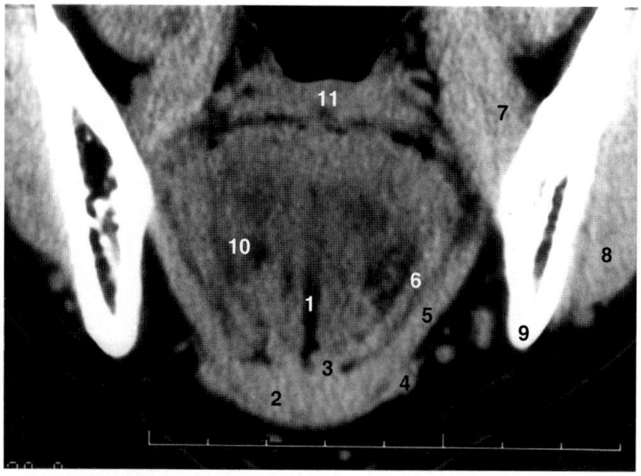

Figure 8-14A: Anatomy of the tongue. Coronal CT image showing the structure of the tongue and the surrounding tissues.

1 Median longitudinal lingual septum
2 Geniohyoid muscle
3 Genioglossus muscle
4 Anterior belly of digastric muscle
5 Mylohyoid muscle
6 Hyoglossus muscle
7 Medial pterygoid muscle
8 Masseter muscle
9 Mandible
10 Intrinsic tongue muscles
11 Lingual tonsil

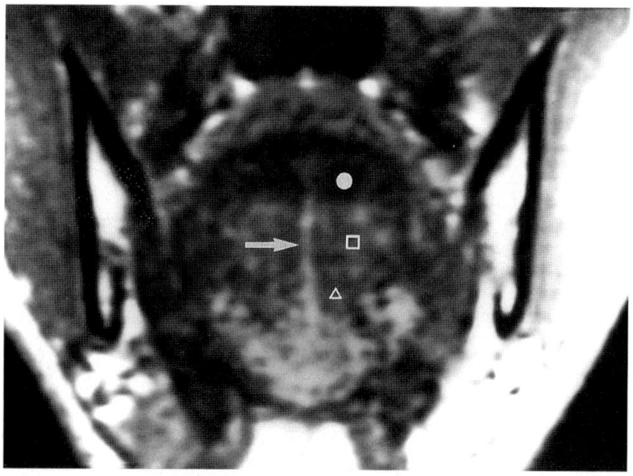

Figure 8-14B: The intrinsic muscles of the tongue. Coronal T1-weighted MR image showing the superior longitudinal muscles (*dot*), the vertical and horizontal muscles (*box*), the inferior longitudinal muscles (*triangle*), and the median longitudinal lingual septum (*arrow*).

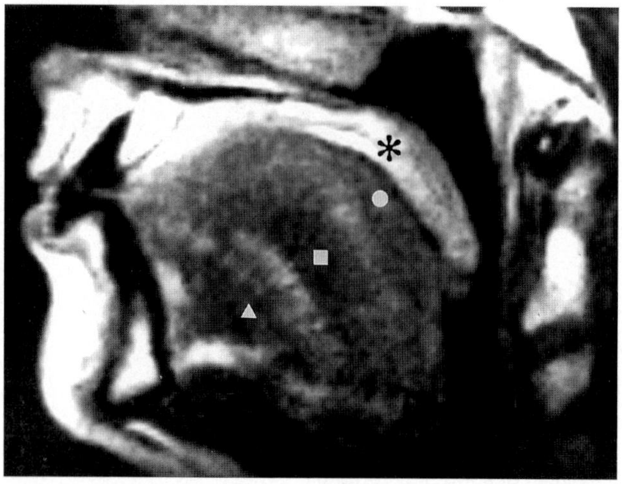

Figure 8-14C: The tongue. Parasagittal T1-weighted MR image in a child demonstrates little lingual fat separating the superior longitudinal muscles (*dot*), the vertical and horizontal muscles (*square*), and the inferior longitudinal muscle (*triangle*). Also noted is fat in the soft palate (*asterisk*).

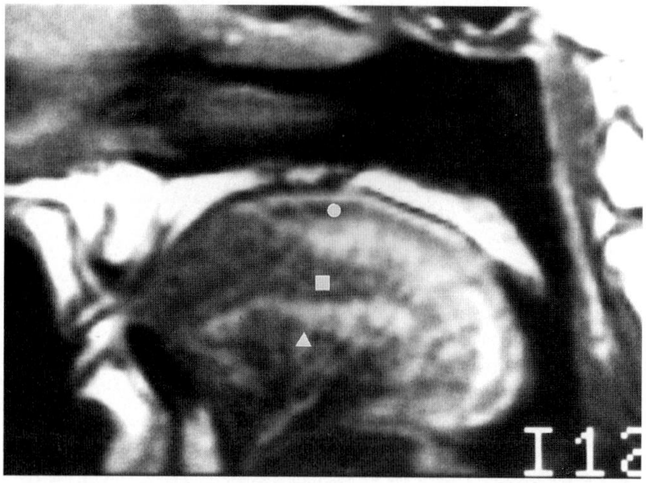

Figure 8-14D: Parasagittal T1-weighted MR image in an elderly adult showing an increase in the amount of lingual fat and a reduction of muscle mass with aging, separating the superior longitudinal muscle (*dot*), the vertical and horizontal muscles (*square*), and the inferior longitudinal muscle (*triangle*).

THE SALIVARY GLANDS

Paired Major Salivary Glands

1. The paired parotid glands are located anterior and inferior to the ear and superficial to the masseter muscle. The parotid (Stenson's) duct is about 5 cm long. It courses anteriorly and turns medially at the anterior border of the masseter muscle and then pierces the buccinator to open into the oral cavity opposite the second upper molar crown. An accessory part of the parotid gland, when present, may drain directly into the parotid duct. The parotid glands consist almost entirely of serous glandular tissue.
2. The paired submandibular glands are located inferior to the base of the tongue in the posterior-lateral part of the floor of the mouth. The submandibular (Wharton's) duct is about 5 cm in length and runs anteriorly to open in the floor of the mouth on the summit of the sublingual papilla lateral to the frenulum of the tongue. The submandibular glands are mixed seromucous in type.
3. The paired sublingual glands lie beneath the oral mucosa, anterosuperior to the submandibular glands. Each gland has 8 to 20 excretory ducts; of the smaller independent sublingual ducts, most open separately on the summit of the sublingual fold whereas a minority drain directly into the submandibular duct. From the anterior part of the gland, small rami sometimes join to form a major anterior sublingual duct opening into the oral cavity together with or near the orifice of the submandibular duct. The sublingual glands are primarily mucous glands.

Minor Salivary Glands

1. Small groups of minor salivary glands are often found scattered beneath the mucosa of the oral cavity. They include the labial, buccal, palatoglossal, palatal, and anterior and posterior lingual glands.
2. The minor salivary glands are serous, mucous, or mixed type.
3. Generally speaking, the minor salivary glands empty independently directly into the oral cavity via their own independent minor excretory ducts.

Innervation of the Salivary Glands

1. The secretomotor innervation of the parotid gland is from the glossopharyngeal nerve (CN-IX) via the otic ganglion.
2. The secretomotor innervation of the submandibular and sublingual glands is from the facial nerve (CN-VII) via the submandibular ganglion.
3. The secretomotor innervation of the minor salivary glands is from the trigeminal nerve (CN-V) via the pterygopalatine ganglion.

Functions of the Salivary Glands

The functions of the salivary glands and their secretions include lubrication, moistening, providing an aqueous solvent for taste, supplying a fluid seal for suckling, enzyme secretion (e.g., salivary amylase), and antimicrobial agent secretion (e.g., IgA, lysozyme, and lactoferrin).

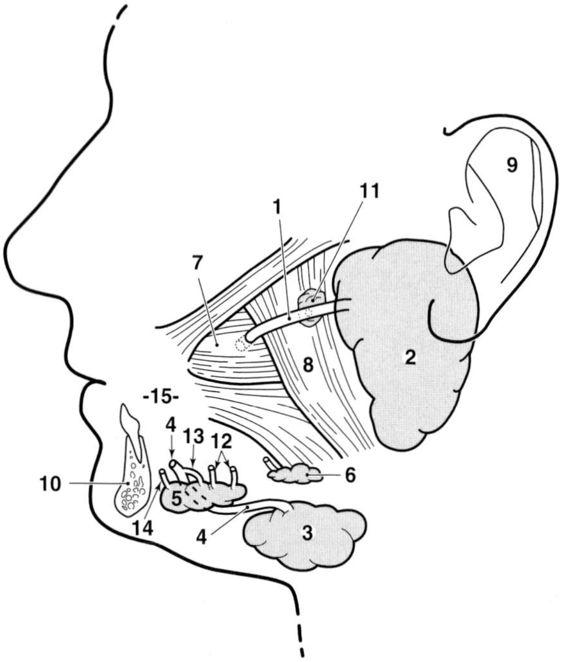

Figure 8-15: Lateral schematic of the salivary glands and ducts on the left side. The superficial tissues and mandible have been removed.

1 Parotid (Stenson's) duct piercing buccinator muscle to drain into the oral cavity
2 Parotid gland
3 Submandibular gland
4 Submandibular (Wharton's) duct draining into the floor of the oral cavity
5 Sublingual gland
6 Minor salivary gland and duct draining directly into the oral cavity
7 Buccinator muscle
8 Masseter muscle
9 Pinna of the ear
10 Anterior aspect of mandible (cut surface: left side removed)
11 Accessory part of the parotid gland and duct draining directly into the parotid duct
12 Posterior sublingual ducts independently draining directly into the floor of the oral cavity
13 Sublingual duct draining into submandibular duct
14 Anterior sublingual duct(s) draining independently into floor of the oral cavity

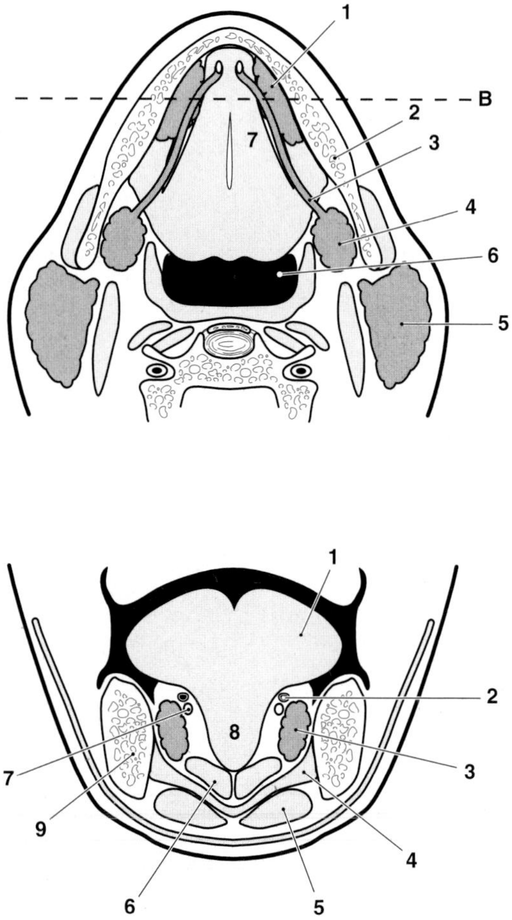

Figure 8-16A: Schematics showing the relationship of the sublingual glands to the surrounding tissues. *B,* plane of coronal section.

Top: Axial schematic.

1 Sublingual gland
2 Ramus of mandible
3 Wharton's duct
4 Submandibular gland
5 Parotid gland
6 Oropharynx
7 Genioglossus muscle

Bottom: Coronal schematic.

1 Intrinsic tongue muscles
2 Wharton's duct
3 Sublingual gland
4 Mylohyoid muscle
5 Anterior belly of digastric muscle
6 Geniohyoid muscle
7 Lingual nerve
8 Genioglossus muscle
9 Ramus of mandible

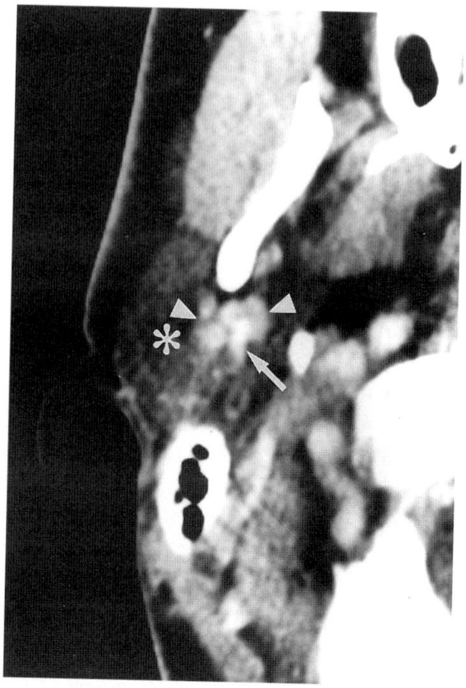

Figure 8-16B: The parotid gland. Enhanced axial CT image showing the parotid gland (*asterisk*), the retromandibular vein (*arrow*) and several normal parotid lymph nodes (*arrowheads*).

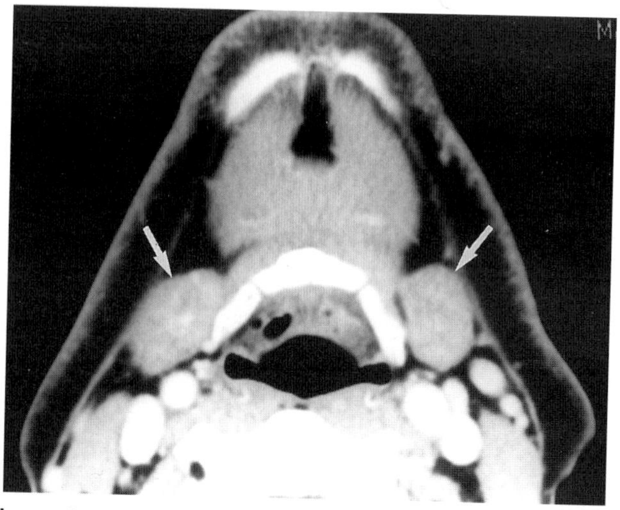

Figure 8-16C: The submandibular glands. Enhanced axial CT image showing the two submandibular glands (*arrows*).

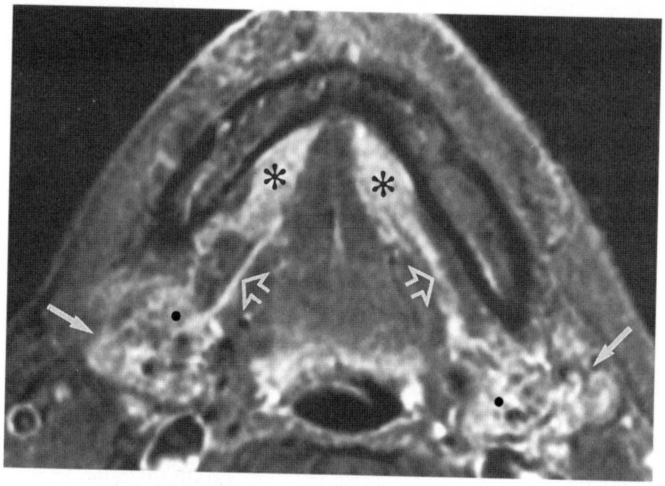

Figure 8-16D: Sublingual salivary glands. Axial intravenous gadolinium–enhanced T1-weighted fat-suppressed MR image showing the sublingual glands (*asterisks*), the submandibular glands (*dots*), the lower pole of the parotid glands (*solid arrows*), and Wharton's (submandibular) ducts (*open arrows*).

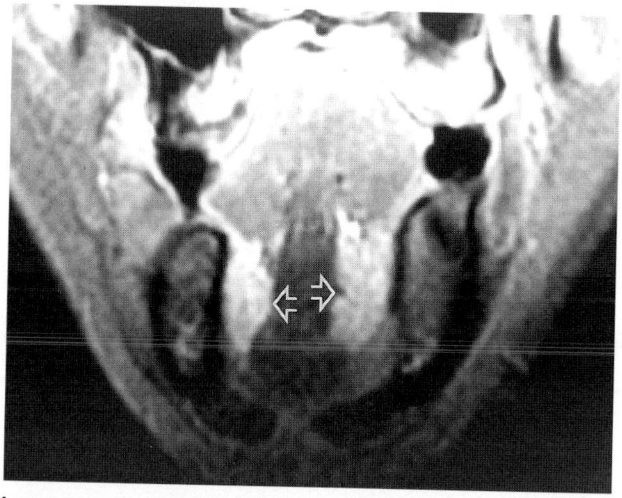

Figure 8-16E: Coronal intravenous gadolinium–enhanced T1-weighted fat-suppressed MR image showing the sublingual glands (*arrows*).

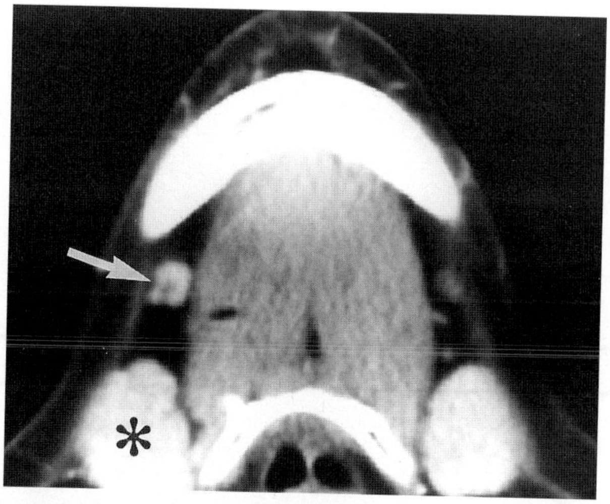

Figure 8-16F: Minor salivary gland. Axial CT image showing a minor salivary gland (*arrow*) anterior to the submandibular gland (*asterisk*) on the right side.

THE TONSILS

1. Waldeyer's ring is an annulus of lymphoid tissue associated with the oral and pharyngeal mucosa that surrounds the upper aerodigestive tract. It consists of seven designated tonsils, including the singular lingual tonsil, and the paired palatine, tubal, and nasopharyngeal tonsils (adenoids), as well as small unnamed collections of lymphoid tissue in the intertonsillar regions.
2. The lingual tonsil is a collection of lymphoid nodules embedded in the submucosa of the pharyngeal part of the superior surface of the tongue in the midline.
3. The paired palatine tonsils are masses of lymphoid tissue located in the oropharynx within the tonsillar recesses, situated between the palatopharyngeal and palatoglossal folds.
4. The paired nasopharyngeal tonsils (adenoids) are masses of lymphoid tissue located in the roof of the nasopharynx.
5. The paired tubal tonsils are collections of lymphoid tissue located at the junction between the eustachian (pharyngotympanic/auditory) tube and the nasopharynx.
6. The functions of the tonsils include (a) selecting clones of B and T cells that respond specifically to microorganisms on the pharyngeal surface, (b) acting as a site for the proliferation of selected B and T cell clones, and (c) producing IgA and IgG for local secretion.

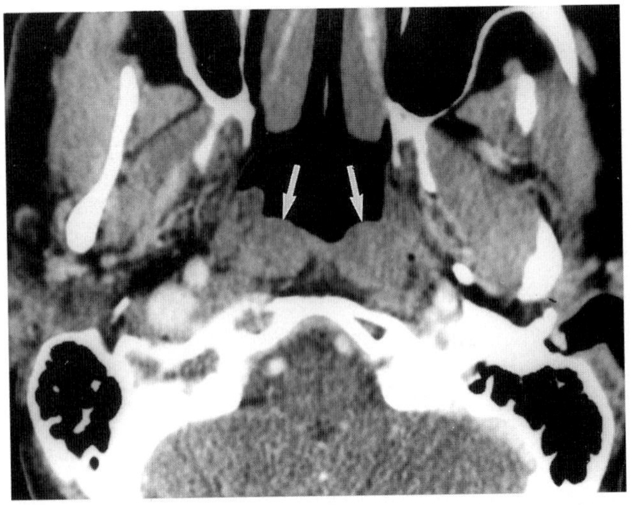

Figure 8-17A: The adenoids (nasopharyngeal tonsil[s]). Axial CT showing the paired adenoids (*arrows*).

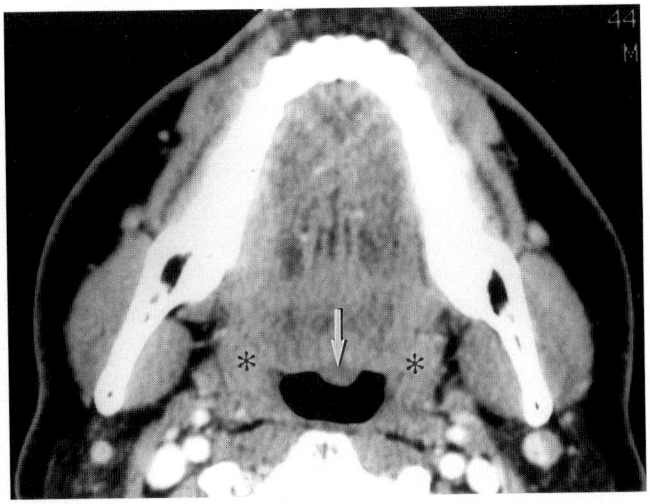

Figure 8-17B: The lingual and palatine tonsils. Axial CT image showing the lingual tonsil (*arrow*) and the palatine tonsils (*asterisks*).

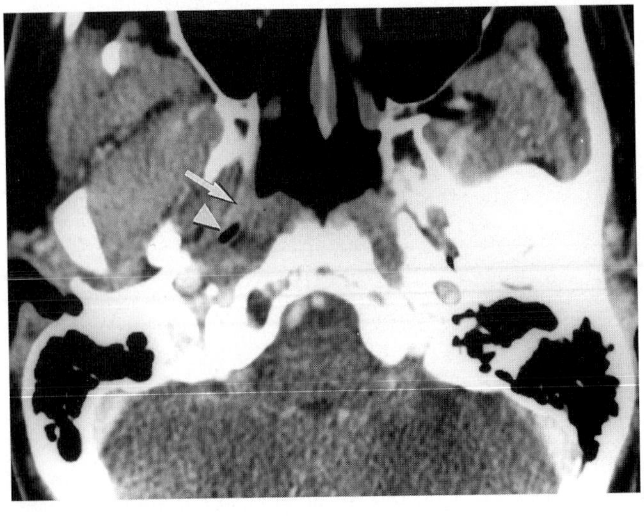

Figure 8-17C: The tubal tonsils. Axial CT showing the area of the tubal tonsil (*arrow,* relatively hyperdense tissue) at the origin of the eustachian tube on the right side. Note the air (*arrowhead*) within the proximal eustachian tube.

THE HYOID BONE

1. The U-shaped hyoid bone is composed of five parts: an unpaired body (ċorpus), paired lesser cornua, and paired greater cornua.
2. The muscles and ligaments attaching to the body of the hyoid bone include: anteriorly, the geniohyoid hyoglossus, mylohyoid, sternohyoid, and omohyoid muscles; superiorly, the genioglossus muscles, the hyoepiglottic ligament, and the thyrohyoid membrane; and inferiorly, the sternohyoid and omohyoid muscles, together with the thyrohyoid (occasionally) and the levator glandulae thyroideae (when present) muscles.
3. The paired greater cornua of the hyoid bone are initially united to the body by cartilage (*greater cornucorpal junction* [Jinkins]); later in life the greater cornua may fuse to the body. The muscles attaching to the greater cornua include the hyoglossus, the stylo- and thyrohyoid, and the middle pharyngeal constrictor group of muscles.
4. The paired lesser cornua of the hyoid bone are small conical bony structures located at the junctions of the body and greater cornua. They are connected to the hyoid body by fibrous tissue (*lesser cornucorpal junction* [Jinkins]); there may be a synovial joint between the lesser and greater cornua on each side (*intercornual joints* [Jinkins]). Fusion across these junctions or joints may occur later in life. The stylohyoid ligament on each side extends from the tip of the styloid process of the temporal bone to the lesser cornua of the hyoid bone on each side.

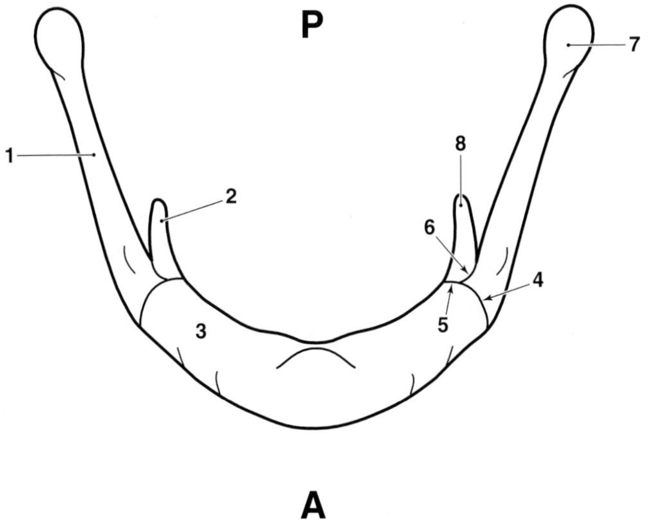

Figure 8-18: Frontal schematic of the hyoid bone. *A*, anterior; *P*, posterior.
1 Greater horn (cornu)
2 Lesser horn (cornu)
3 Body (corpus)
4 Greater cornu–corpal junction
5 Lesser cornu–corpal junction
6 Intercornual junction or joint (greater/lesser cornual junction or joint)
7 Apex of greater horn
8 Apex of lesser horn

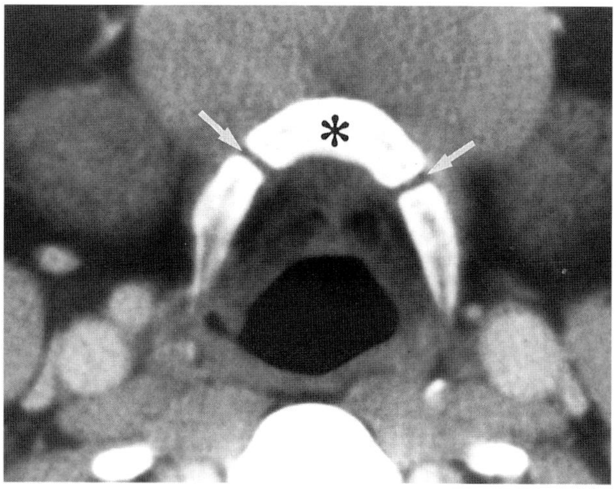

Figure 8-19A: The hyoid bone. Axial CT image showing the body (corpus) of the hyoid bone (*asterisk*) and the articulations (*arrows*) of the greater cornua with the hyoid body (i.e., greater cornu–corpal junctions).

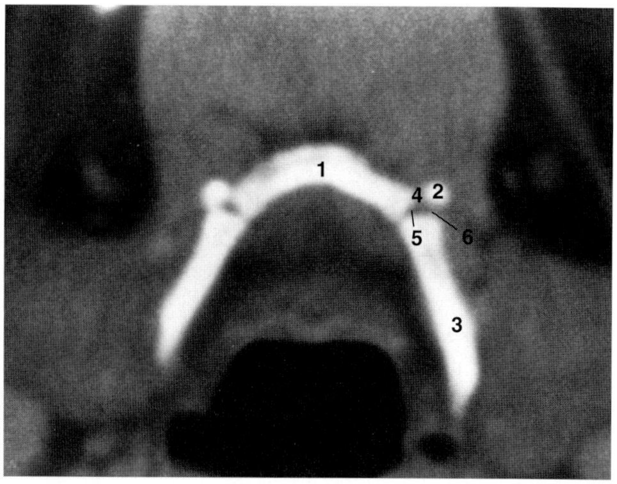

Figure 8-19B: Axial CT image showing the general structure of the hyoid bone.
1 Body (corpus) of hyoid bone
2 Lesser cornu (horn)of hyoid bone on left side
3 Greater cornu (horn) of hyoid bone on left side
4 Lesser cornu–corpal junction
5 Greater cornu–corpal junction
6 Intercornual joint or junction

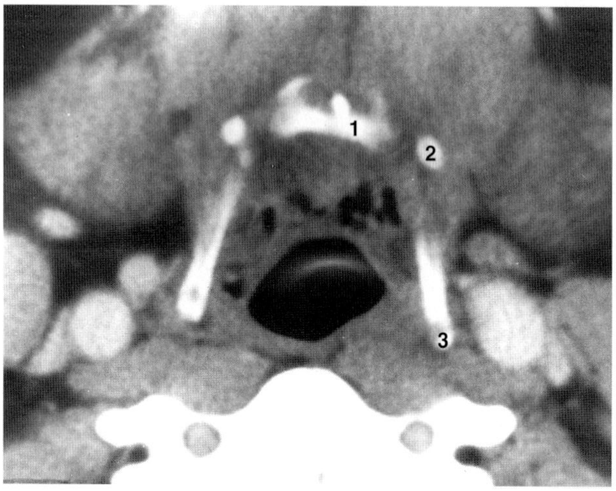

Figure 8-19C: Axial CT image showing the cornua of the hyoid bone.
1 Body (corpus) of hyoid bone
2 Apex of lesser horn (cornu) of hyoid bone on the left side
3 Apex of greater horn (cornu) of hyoid bone on the left side

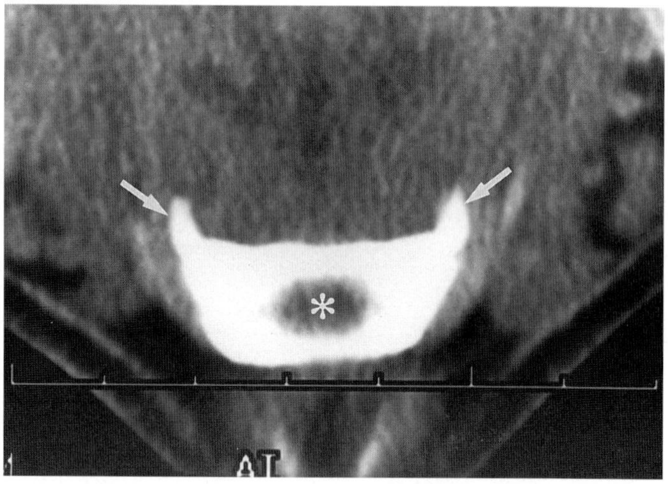

Figure 8-19D: Coronal CT image showing the body (*asterisk*) and lesser horns (*arrows,* cornua) of the hyoid bone.

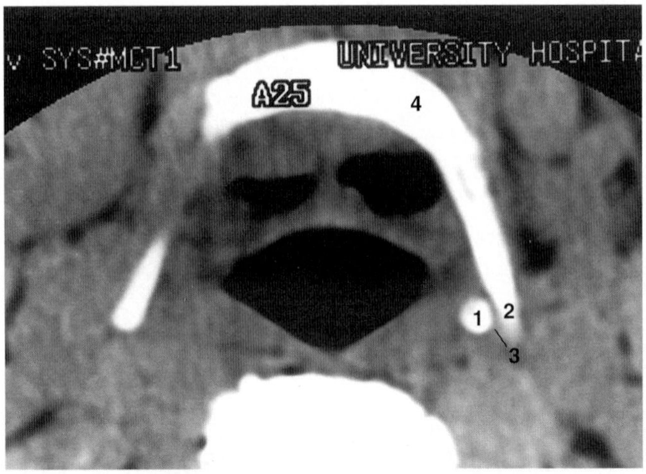

Figure 8-20: Ossified thyrohyoid ligament (superior cornu of thyroid cartilage). Axial noncontrast-enhanced CT image showing ossification of the superior aspect of the thyrohyoid ligament at its attachment (articulation) with the apex of the greater horn of the hyoid bone on the left side.

1 Ossified thyrohyoid ligament
2 Apex of greater horn of hyoid bone
3 Thyrohyoid articulation/junction
4 Body of hyoid bone

THE INFRAHYOID NECK

Overview

1. The infrahyoid neck encompasses the tissues between the hyoid bone and clavicles. It is divided into several spaces that are delineated in part by the superficial and deep cervical fascia.
2. The spaces of the infrahyoid neck include the superficial space, carotid space, visceral space, danger space, retropharyngeal space, prevertebral space, posterior cervical space, and anterior cervical space.

TABLE 8-4: Contents and Spaces of the Infrahyoid Neck

Space	Contents
Superficial space	Platysma muscles Sternocleidomastoid muscles Lymph nodes Inferior omohyoid muscles External jugular veins Trapezius muscles
Carotid space	Common carotid artery Internal jugular vein Vagus nerve (CN-X) Sympathetic chain Deep cervical lymph nodes
Visceral space	Pharynx Larynx Thyroid gland Parathyroid glands Trachea Esophagus Recurrent laryngeal nerves (branch of CN-X) Lymph nodes Strap muscles
Danger space	Fat
Retropharyngeal space	Fat
Prevertebral space	Prevertebral muscles Scalene muscles Brachial plexus nerve roots Phrenic nerves (C-3 to C-5) Vertebral arteries and veins
Posterior cervical space	Fat Spinal accessory nerve (CN-XI) Lymph nodes
Anterior cervical space	Fat

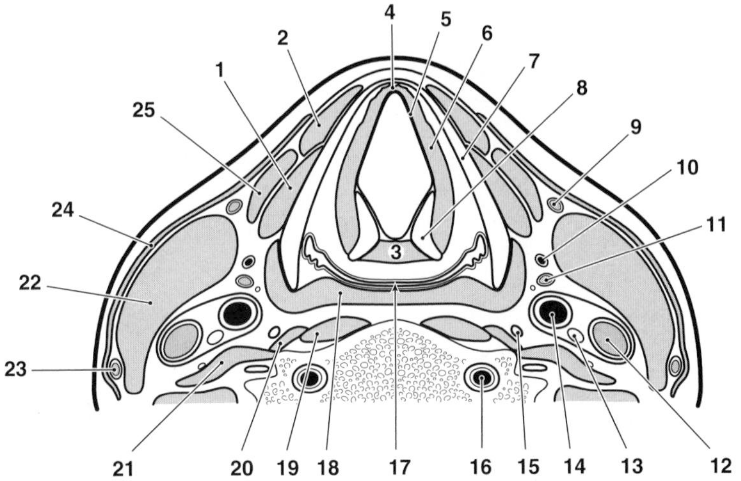

Figure 8-21A: Axial cross-section schematic through the ventral region of the neck at the level of the vocal folds (cords).

1 Thyrohyoid muscle
2 Sternohyoid muscle
3 Transverse arytenoid muscle
4 Anterior commissure
5 Vocal fold (cord)
6 Vocalis (medial thyroarytenoid) muscle
7 Thyroid cartilage (lamina)
8 Arytenoid cartilage
9 Anterior jugular vein
10 Superior thyroid artery
11 Superior thyroid vein
12 Internal jugular vein
13 Vagus nerve
14 Common carotid artery
15 Sympathetic trunk
16 Vertebral artery
17 Pharynx
18 Cricopharyngeus muscle
19 Longus colli muscle
20 Longissimus capitis muscle
21 Scalenius anterior muscle
22 Sternocleidomastoid muscle
23 External jugular vein
24 Platysma muscle
25 Omohyoid muscle

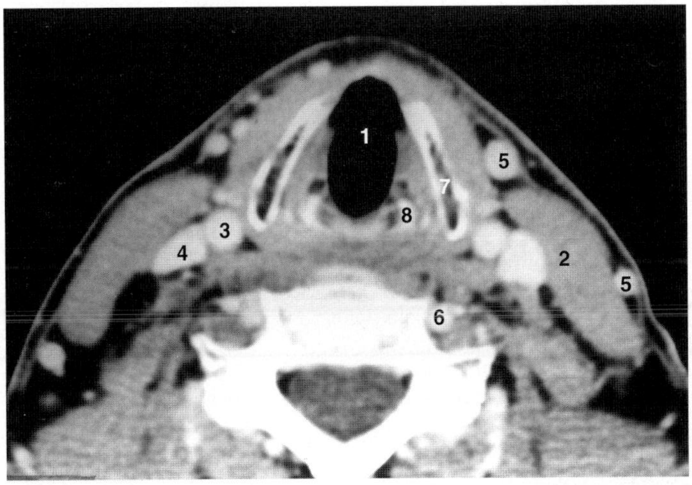

Figure 8-21B: Anatomy of the infrahyoid neck. Enhanced axial CT of the infrahyoid neck showing the normal anatomy.

1 Larynx
2 Sternocleidomastoid muscle
3 Common carotid artery
4 Internal jugular vein
5 External jugular vein(s)
6 Vertebral artery
7 Inferior thyroid cartilage
8 Arytenoid cartilage

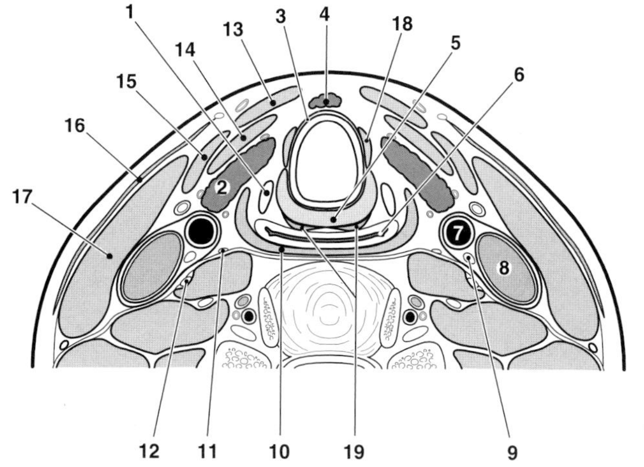

Figure 8-22: Axial schematic through the ventral region of the neck at the level of the cricoid cartilage.

1 Inferior cornu of thyroid cartilage
2 Right lobe of thyroid gland
3 Cricothyroid ligament (membrane)
4 Pyramidal lobe of thyroid gland
5 Lamina of cricoid cartilage
6 Laryngeal part of pharynx
7 Common carotid artery
8 Internal jugular vein
9 Vagus nerve
10 Cricopharyngeus muscle
11 Sympathetic trunk
12 Phrenic nerve
13 Sternohyoid muscle
14 Thyrohyoid muscle
15 Omohyoid muscle
16 Platysma muscle
17 Sternocleidomastoid muscle
18 Cricothyroid muscle
19 Posterior cricoarytenoid muscle

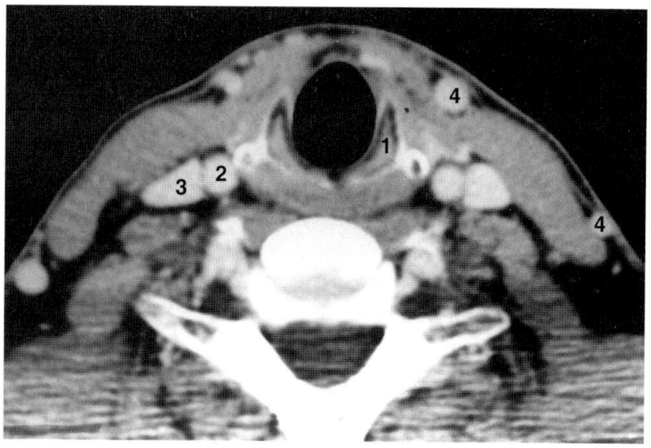

Figure 8-23: The infrahyoid neck at the level of the cricoid cartilage.

1 Cricoid cartilage
2 Common carotid artery
3 Internal jugular vein
4 Branches of external jugular vein

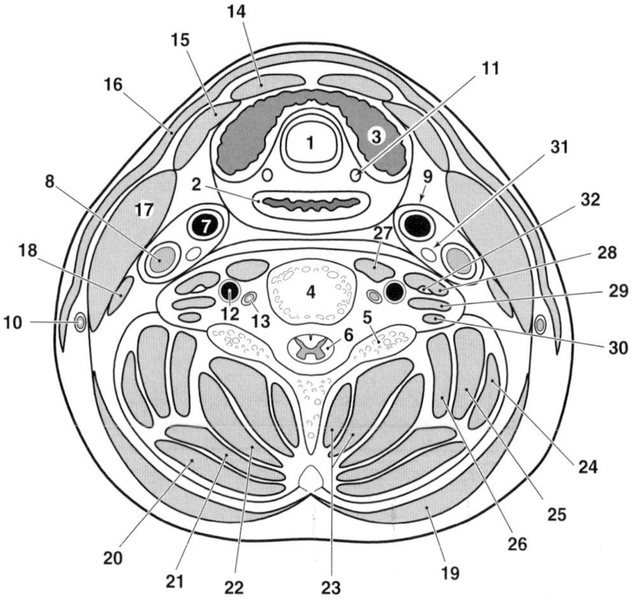

Figure 8-24: Axial schematic of the anatomy of the mid-infrahyoid neck at the level of the thyroid gland.

1 Trachea
2 Esophagus
3 Thyroid gland
4 Vertebral body
5 Posterior bony vertebral arch
6 Spinal cord
7 Common carotid artery
8 Internal jugular vein
9 Carotid sheath
10 External jugular vein
11 Recurrent laryngeal nerve
12 Vertebral artery
13 Vertebral vein
14 Sternohyoid muscle
15 Sternothyroid muscle
16 Platysma muscle
17 Sternocleidomastoid muscle
18 Omohyoid muscle
19 Trapezius muscle
20 Splenius muscle
21 Semispinalis cervicis muscle
22 Semispinalis capitis muscle
23 Multifidus muscles (greater and lesser)
24 Levator scapulae muscle
25 Longissimus capitis muscle
26 Longissimus cervicis muscle
27 Longus colli muscle
28 Anterior scalene muscle
29 Middle scalene muscle
30 Posterior scalene muscle
31 Vagus nerve (CN-X)
32 Phrenic nerve (contributions from C3 to C5 spinal nerves)

THE LARYNX

Anatomy

1. The larynx is an air passage, a sphincter, and an organ of phonation.
2. The upper extent of the larynx borders on the hypopharynx; the lower extent of the larynx borders on the upper trachea.
3. There are 11 laryngeal cartilages: single epiglottic, thyroid, and cricoid cartilages; and paired arytenoid, cuneiform, corniculate, and triticeal cartilages. Some authors do not include the epiglottic cartilage as a part of the larynx.
4. The cricoid cartilage forms a complete ring around the laryngeal airway. It is attached by synovial joints to the apices of the inferior cornua of the thyroid cartilage (*cricothyroid/joints* [Jinkins]) and the two arytenoid cartilages (*cricoarytenoid joints* [Jinkins]); it is attached inferiorly to the trachea. Cricothyroid and cricotracheal ligaments contribute to this craniocaudal linkage.
5. The thyroid cartilage consists of two laminae that are fused anteriorly along the inferior two thirds of their height; the unfused remainder is the thyroid notch (incisure). Paired horns (cornua) protrude from the upper and lower posterior borders posteriorly, the superior and inferior thyroid cartilage cornua. The superior cornua terminate in the thyrohyoid ligament that in turn attach or articulate (when ossified) with the apices of the greater cornua of the hyoid bone on each side; the inferior thyroid cartilage cornua end in paired facet joints that articulate on each side with the cricoid cartilage (cricothyroid joints). The other ligaments inserting into the thyroid cartilage include the unpaired thyroepiglottic and anterior (medial) cricothyroid ligaments, and the paired vestibular and vocal ligaments. The muscles inserting into the thyroid cartilage include the vocal, thyroarytenoid, thyroepiglottic, palatopharyngeus, stylopharyngeus, and salpingopharyngeus muscles.
6. The arytenoid cartilage is somewhat pyramidal in form with a base, apex, and two processes. The connections of this cartilage are complex and include, according to surface or process of attachment: apex, the articulation with the corniculate cartilage (arytenocorniculate joint); base, the articulation with the cricoid cartilage (cricoarytenoid joint); vocal process, the vestibular ligament and vocalis/cricoarytenoid muscles; posterior surface, the transverse arytenoid muscle; muscular process, the posterior cricoarytenoid and lateral cricoarytenoid muscles.
7. The paired corniculate cartilages articulate with the apices of the arytenoid cartilages (arytenocorniculate joint); they occasionally are fused with the arytenoid cartilages.
8. The paired cuneiform cartilages lie within each of the aryepiglottic folds, anterior and superior to the corniculate cartilages.
9. The epiglottic cartilage is connected to the thyroid cartilage by the thyroepiglottic ligament and to the arytenoid cartilages by the aryepiglottic folds. The epiglottis is also attached to the hyoid bone by the hyoepiglottic ligament. The upper surface of the epiglottis is reflected onto the tongue and pharyngeal walls by a single median, and paired lateral, glossoepiglottic folds. The bilateral depressions on either side of the median glossoepiglottic fold are the valleculae.
10. The triticeal cartilages are paired nodular structures within the free posterior edge of the thyrohyoid membrane; they are located approximately midway between the apex of the superior cornua of the thyroid cartilage and the apices of the greater cornua of the hyoid bone on each side.
11. The laryngeal airway has several distinguishing features including the paired aryepiglottic folds, mucosal ridges extending between the lateral margins of the epiglottis and the apexes of the arytenoid cartilages on each side; the laryngeal vestibule, the airspace extending between the laryngeal inlet and the vestibular folds or "false vocal cords"; the laryngeal sinus (ventricle), a slit between the vestibular folds and vocal folds or cords; and the laryngeal saccule, a pouch extending anteriorly from the laryngeal ventricle between the vestibular fold and the thyroid cartilage.
12. The arterial blood supply to the larynx is primarily supplied by two paired arteries: the superior and the inferior laryngeal arteries. The superior laryngeal artery originates

from the superior thyroidal artery, itself a branch of the external carotid artery. The inferior laryngeal artery arises from the inferior thyroidal artery, itself a branch of the thyrocervical trunk. The cricothyroid artery, originating from the superior thyroidal artery, may also provide arterial supply to the larynx. The venous drainage from the larynx is primarily via the superior and inferior laryngeal veins, which in turn drain into the superior and inferior thyroidal veins, respectively.

13. The innervation of the larynx is from the superior laryngeal nerve and the recurrent laryngeal nerve, both branches of the vagus nerve (CN-X), and from unnamed sympathetic nerves. The superior laryngeal nerve gives rise to the internal laryngeal nerve, consisting of sensory and autonomic components supplying the laryngeal mucosa from the epiglottis to the vocal folds; and the external laryngeal nerve, supplying motor fibers to the cricothyroid muscle. The recurrent laryngeal nerve supplies all of the intrinsic laryngeal muscles with the exception of the cricothyroid muscle and also innervates the mucosa of the larynx below the vocal folds.

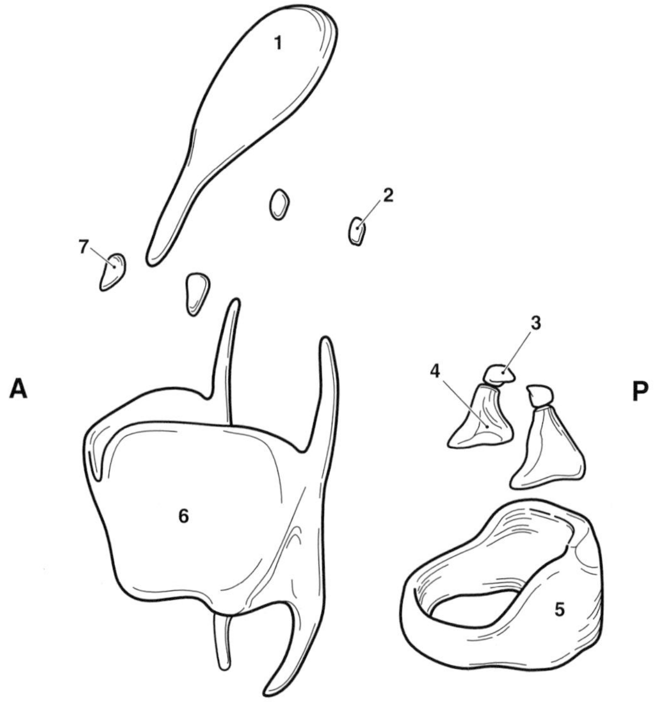

Figure 8-25: Exploded oblique schematic showing different cartilages of the larynx. *A,* anterior; *P,* posterior.
1 Epiglottis
2 Triticeal cartilage
3 Corniculate cartilage
4 Arytenoid cartilage
5 Cricoid cartilage
6 Thyroid cartilage
7 Cuneiform cartilage

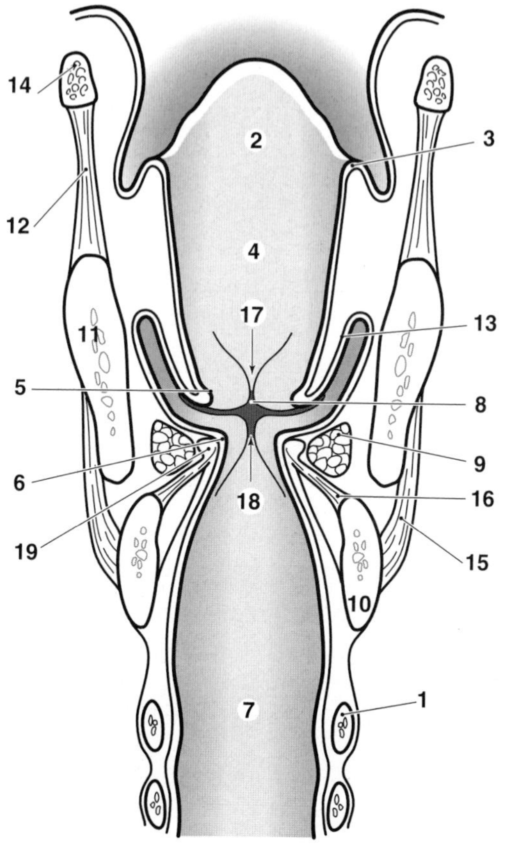

Figure 8-26: Coronal schematic through the larynx and the cranial end of the trachea from the posterior aspect. The posterior portion of the larynx and trachea have been removed.
1 Tracheal cartilage
2 Epiglottis
3 Aryepiglottic fold
4 Vestibule
5 Vestibular fold (false vocal cord)
6 Vocal fold
7 Trachea
8 Laryngeal ventricle (sinus)
9 Medial thyroarytenoid (vocalis) muscle
10 Cricoid cartilage
11 Thyroid cartilage
12 Thyrohyoid ligament (membrane)
13 Saccule of laryngeal ventricle
14 Greater cornu of hyoid bone
15 Cricothyroid muscle
16 Cricovocal membrane
17 Rima vestibuli (between the vestibular folds)
18 Rima glottidis (between the vocal folds)
19 Vocal ligament

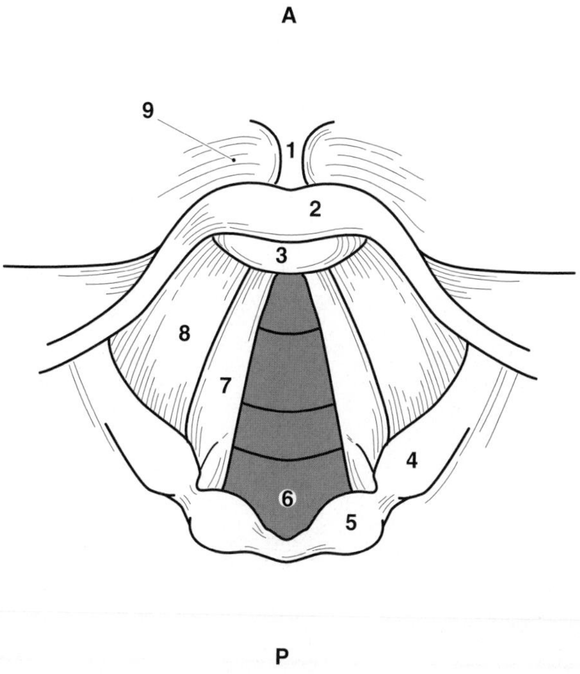

Figure 8-27: Superior schematic showing the interior of the larynx as viewed through laryngoscope. *A,* anterior; *P,* posterior.
1 Median glossoepiglottic fold
2 Epiglottis
3 Tubercle of epiglottis
4 Aryepiglottic fold
5 Arytenoid cartilage
6 Trachea seen through rima glottidis
7 Vocal fold
8 Vestibular fold
9 Vallecula

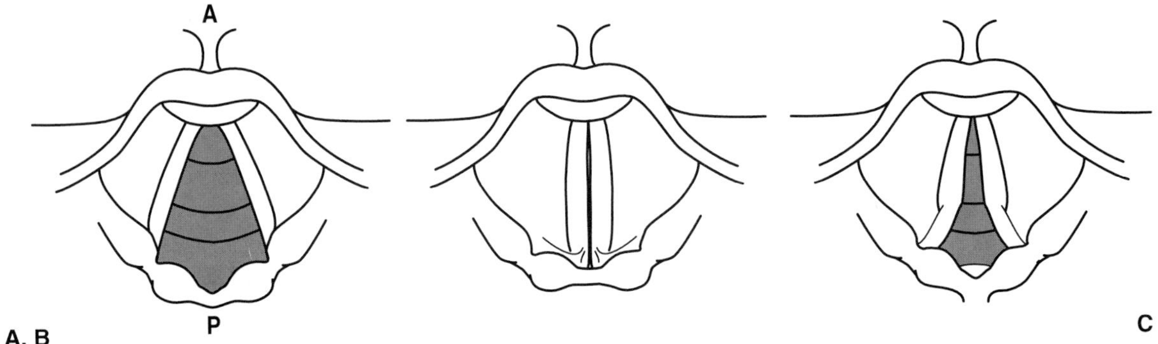

Figure 8-28: Schematics showing the rima glottidis during rest and various maneuvers. **A:** During quiet respiration. **B:** During speech. **C:** During whispering. *A,* anterior; *P,* posterior.

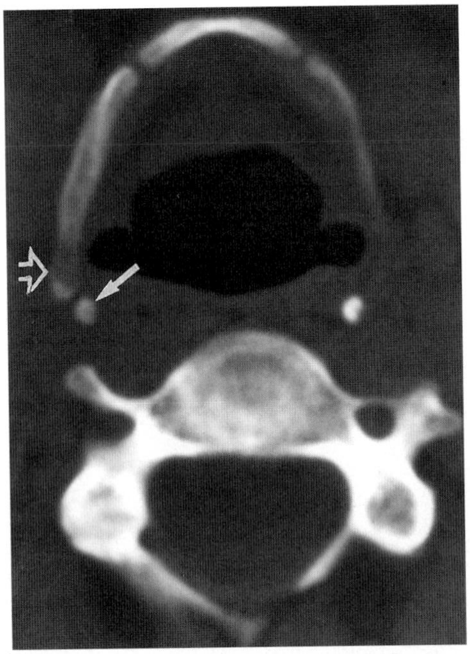

Figure 8-29A: CT of laryngeal anatomy from superior to inferior thyrohyoid ligament. Axial CT image showing calcification/ossification of the upper thyrohyoid ligament (*solid arrow*) at the junction of the thyrohyoid ligament with the apex of greater cornu of the hyoid bone (*open arrow*).

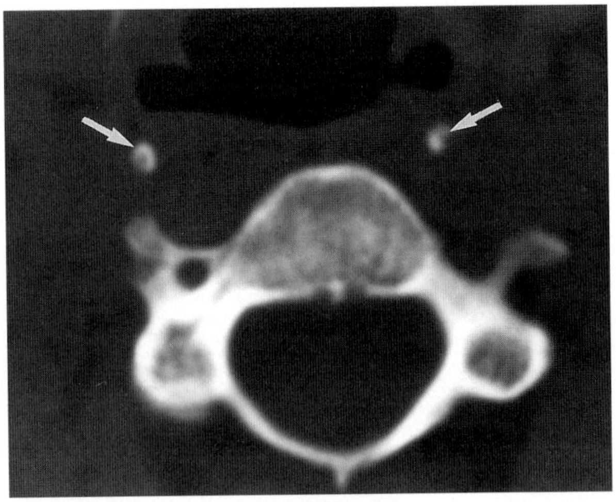

Figure 8-29B: Triticeal cartilage. Axial CT image showing calcifications within the triticeal cartilages (*arrows*) lying within the upper thyrohyoid ligaments bilaterally.

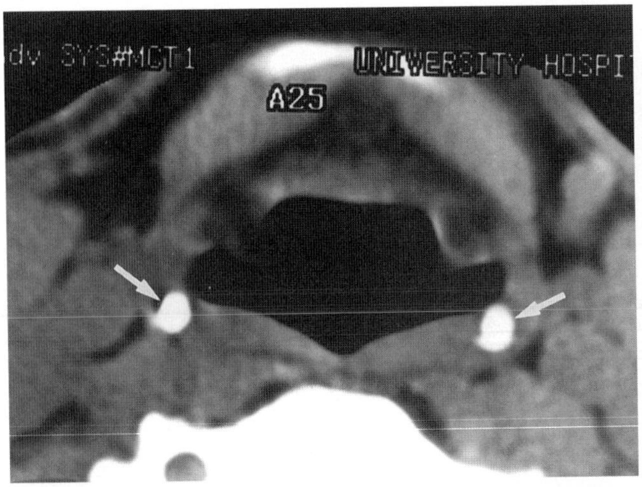

Figure 8-29C: Superior cornua of the thyroid cartilage. Axial CT image showing the superior cornua of the thyroid cartilage (*arrows*).

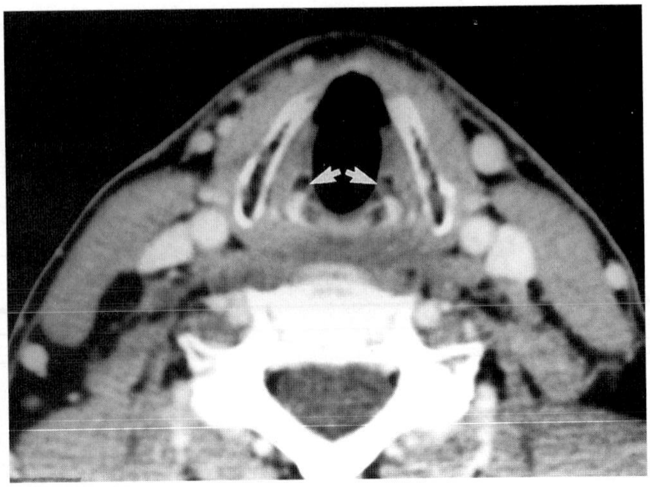

Figure 8-29D: Corniculate cartilages. Axial CT image showing the corniculate cartilages (*arrows*) arising from the arytenoid cartilages.

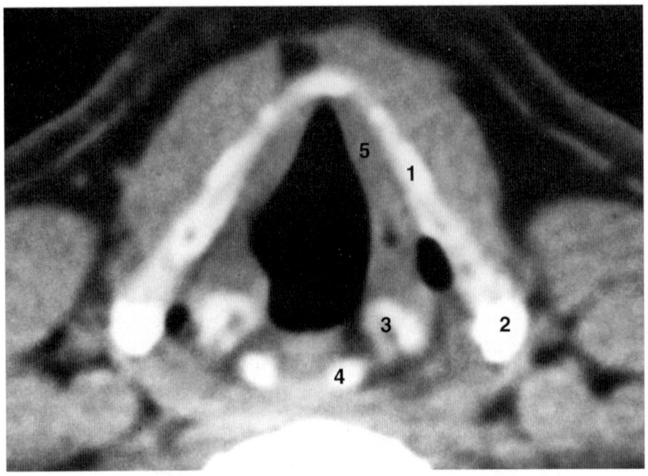

Figure 8-30A: Laryngeal anatomy. Axial CT image showing the laryngeal anatomy:
1 Lamina of thyroid cartilage
2 Superior cornu of thyroid cartilage
3 Arytenoid cartilage
4 Cricoid cartilage
5 True vocal cord

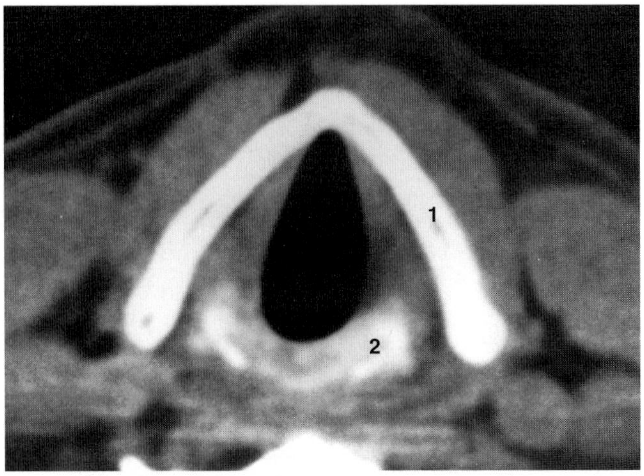

Figure 8-30B: Axial CT image showing the laryngeal anatomy.
1 Lamina of thyroid cartilage
2 Cricoid cartilage

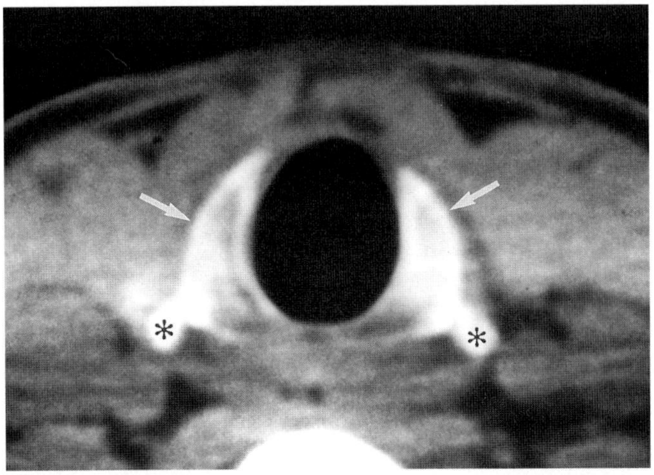

Figure 8-30C: Axial CT image showing the cricoid cartilage (*arrows*) and inferior cornua of the thyroid cartilage (*asterisks*).

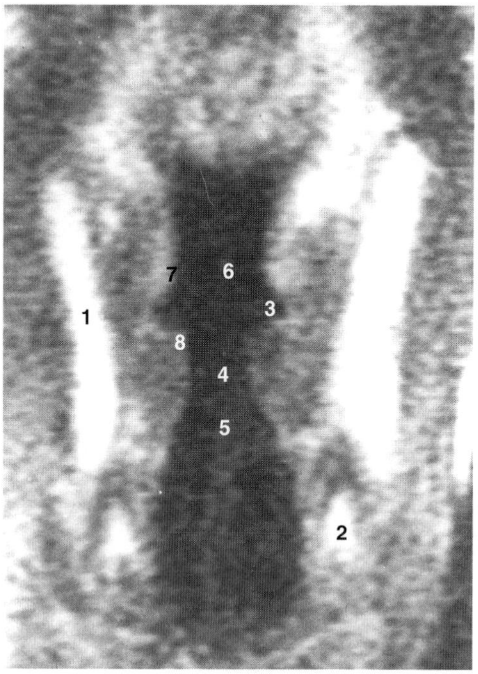

Figure 8-31A: MR of laryngeal anatomy. Coronal T1-weighted MR image showing laryngeal anatomy.
1 Thyroid cartilage lamina
2 Cricoid cartilage
3 Laryngeal vestibule
4 Glottis
5 Subglottis
6 Supraglottis
7 False vocal cord
8 True vocal cord

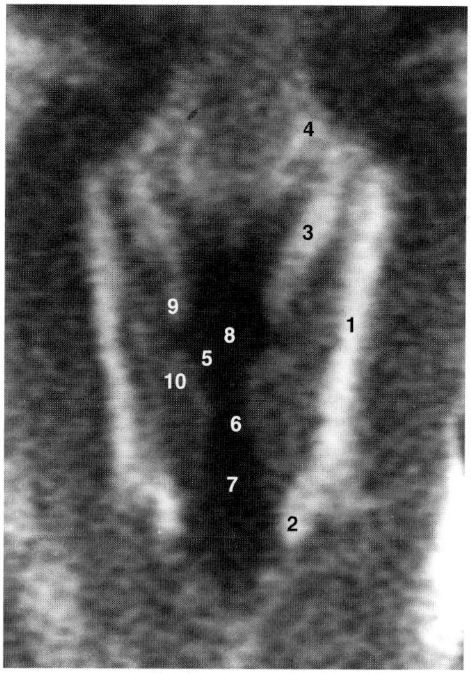

Figure 8-31B: Coronal T1-weighted MR image showing laryngeal anatomy.
1 Thyroid cartilage lamina
2 Cricoid cartilage
3 Arytenoid cartilage
4 Corniculate cartilage
5 Laryngeal ventricle
6 Glottis
7 Subglottis
8 Supraglottis
9 False vocal cord
10 True vocal cord

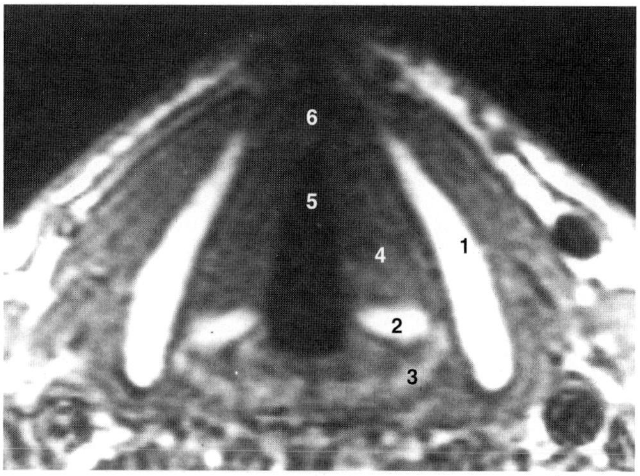

Figure 8-31C: Axial T1-weighted MR image showing some of the laryngeal cartilages.
1 Lamina of thyroid cartilage
2 Arytenoid cartilage
3 Cricoid cartilage
4 True vocal cord
5 Rima glottidis
6 Anterior commissure

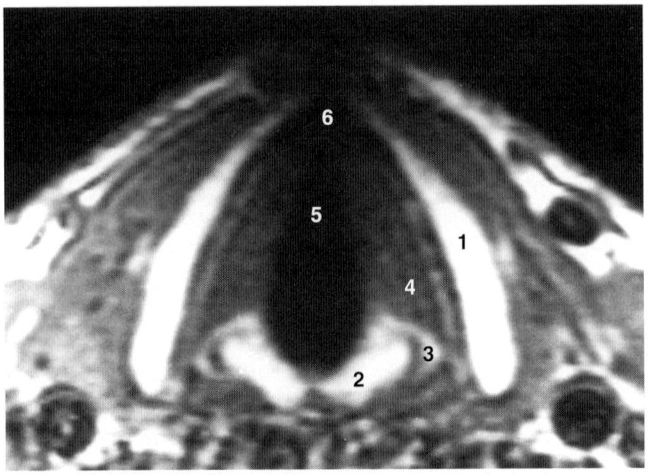

Figure 8-31D: Axial T1-weighted MR image showing some of the laryngeal cartilages.
1 Lamina of thyroid cartilage
2 Cricoid cartilage
3 Arytenoid cartilage
4 True vocal cord
5 Rima glottidis
6 Anterior commissure

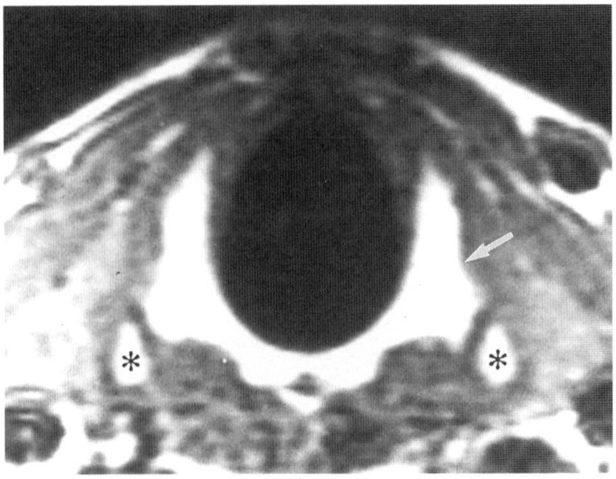

Figure 8-31E: Axial T1-weighted MR image showing the cricoid cartilage (*arrow*) and the inferior cornua of the thyroid cartilage (*asterisks*).

Laryngeal Ligaments and Membranes

The Laryngeal Membranes

The larynx has four membranes including the thyrohyoid (single), the cricovocal (single), and the quadrangular (paired).

1. The thyrohyoid membrane extends from the upper inner surface of the body and greater horns of the hyoid bone to the upper border of the thyroid cartilage. A single midline thickening of the ligament is termed the median thyrohyoid ligament. The paired thickenings of the lateral posterior margins are termed the lateral thyrohyoid ligaments; these connect the superior horns of the thyroid cartilage to the posterior tips of the greater horns of the thyroid bone; they may contain the triticeal cartilages (see below).
2. The cricovocal membrane extends from the inner anterior surface of the thyroid cartilage near the midline and from the vocal processes of the arytenoid cartilage to the upper border of the arch of the cricoid cartilage. The free margins of the cricovocal membrane are thickened to form the vocal ligaments (vocal cords) (see below).
3. The quadrangular membranes are paired structures extending from the lateral margin of the epiglottis on each side to the respective left and right arytenoid cartilages. The upper posterior border forms the aryepiglottic fold; the lower border (vestibular ligament) forms the vestibular fold. The cuneiform cartilages lie within the aryepiglottic folds.

The Laryngeal Ligaments

The larynx has 12 ligaments, including the cricotracheal (single), the lateral thyrohyoid (paired), the median thyrohyoid (single), the vestibular (paired), the vocal (paired), the hypoepiglottic (paired), the posterior cricoarytenoid (single), and the thyroepiglottic (single).

1. The anterior (median) cricothyroid ligament extends in the midline anteriorly between the lower border of the thyroid cartilage to the upper border of the cricoid cartilage. Some include this ligament as a part of the cricovocal membrane.
2. The paired lateral thyrohyoid ligament extends on both sides from the apex of the greater horns (cornua) of the hyoid bone to the superior horns of the thyroid cartilages; they may contain the triticeal cartilages.
3. The single median thyrohyoid ligament extends in the midline from the body of the hyoid bone to the upper anterior border of the thyroid cartilage.
4. The paired vestibular ligaments form the vestibular fold (false vocal cord) on each side at the lower borders of the quadrangular membranes.
5. The paired vocal ligaments (vocal cords) are the thickened free edges of the cricovocal membrane. It forms the anterior three-fifths of the vocal fold; the posterior two fifths of the vocal fold is composed of the vocal process of the arytenoid cartilage.
6. The paired hypoepiglottic ligaments extend from the middle portion of the epiglottis on each side to the lateral aspects of the body of the hyoid bone.
7. The paired posterior cricoarytenoid ligaments extend from the posterior base of the arytenoid cartilage to the upper-lateral posterior free margin of the cricoid cartilage lamina on each side.
8. The single, thyroepiglottic ligament extends from the base of the epiglottis anteriorly to the upper inner surface of the thyroid cartilage.
9. The single, circumferential cricotracheal ligament extends from the lower border of the cricoid cartilage to the first cartilaginous ring of the trachea.

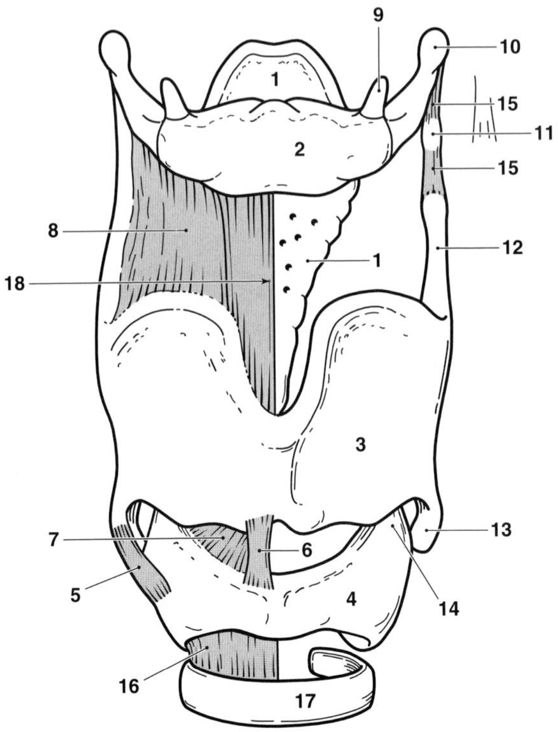

Figure 8-32: Frontal schematic of the cartilages, ligaments, capsules, and membranes of the larynx: membranes removed on left side.

1 Epiglottis
2 Body of hyoid bone
3 Lamina of thyroid cartilage
4 Cricoid cartilage
5 Capsule of cricothyroid joint
6 Anterior (median) cricothyroid ligament
7 Cricovocal membrane
8 Thyrohyoid membrane
9 Lesser horn (cornu) of hyoid bone (insertion of stylohyoid ligament/muscle)
10 Apex of greater horn (cornu) of hyoid bone
11 Triticeal cartilage
12 Superior horn (cornu) of thyroid cartilage
13 Inferior horn (cornu) of thyroid cartilage
14 Superior horn (cornu) of cricoid cartilage
15 Lateral thyrohyoid ligament
16 Cricotracheal ligament
17 First tracheal cartilage ring
18 Median thyrohyoid ligament

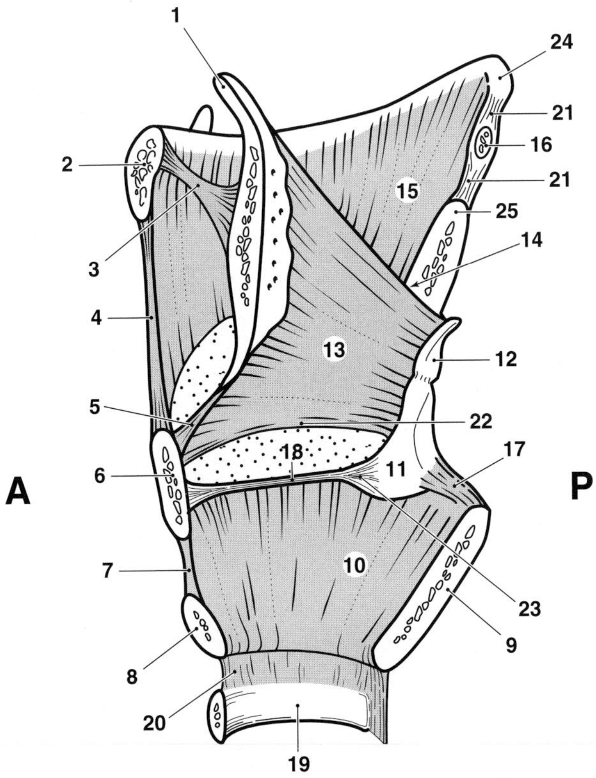

Figure 8-33: Sagittal midline schematic of the cartilages, ligaments, and membranes of the larynx: left half of larynx removed. *A*, anterior; *P*, posterior.

1 Epiglottis
2 Body of hyoid bone
3 Hyoepiglottic ligament
4 Median thyrohyoid ligament
5 Thyroepiglottic ligament
6 Thyroid cartilage
7 Anterior (median) cricothyroid ligament
8 Arch of cricoid cartilage
9 Lamina of cricoid cartilage
10 Cricovocal membrane
11 Arytenoid cartilage
12 Corniculate cartilage
13 Quadrangular membrane
14 Aryepiglottic fold
15 Thyrohyoid membrane
16 Triticeal cartilage in lateral thyrohyoid ligament
17 Posterior cricoarytenoid ligament
18 Vocal ligament (vocal cord: anterior three-fifths of vocal fold)
19 First tracheal cartilage ring
20 Cricotracheal ligament
21 Lateral thyrohyoid ligament
22 Vestibular ligament (vestibular fold)
23 Vocal process of arytenoid cartilage (posterior 2/5 of vocal fold)
24 Apex of greater horn (cornu) of hyoid bone
25 Superior horn (cornu) of thyroid cartilage

The Laryngeal Musculature

1. The muscles of the larynx may be divided into extrinsic and intrinsic muscle groups.
2. The extrinsic muscles of the larynx, 14 in total, join the larynx to regional structures and move the larynx vertically during swallowing and phonation. The paired extrinsic muscles include the thyrohyoid, sternothyroid, thyropharyngeal, cricopharyngeal (part of the inferior pharyngeal constrictor), and stylo-, palato-, and salpingopharyngeal muscles.
3. The intrinsic muscles of the larynx, numbering 17 in total, include the cricothyroid, posterior and lateral cricoarytenoid, transverse and oblique interarytenoid, aryepiglotticus, thyroarytenoid and its subcomponents (lateral thyroarytenoid muscle and medial thyroarytenoid muscle [vocalis muscle]), and thyroepiglottic muscles. With the exception of the transverse arytenoid, each of these muscles is paired.
4. The actions of the intrinsic laryngeal musculature may be divided into three types: (a) muscles that vary the rima glottidis (the glottis, or fissure between the mucosa covering the vocal folds and arytenoid cartilages): the posterior and lateral cricoarytenoid, oblique and transverse interarytenoid muscles; (b) muscles that regulate tension on the vocal ligaments: the cricothyroid, posterior cricoarytenoid, and thyroarytenoid (with its vocalis subcomponents) muscles; and (c) muscles that vary the laryngeal inlet: the oblique interarytenoid, aryepiglotticus, and thyroepiglotticus muscles.

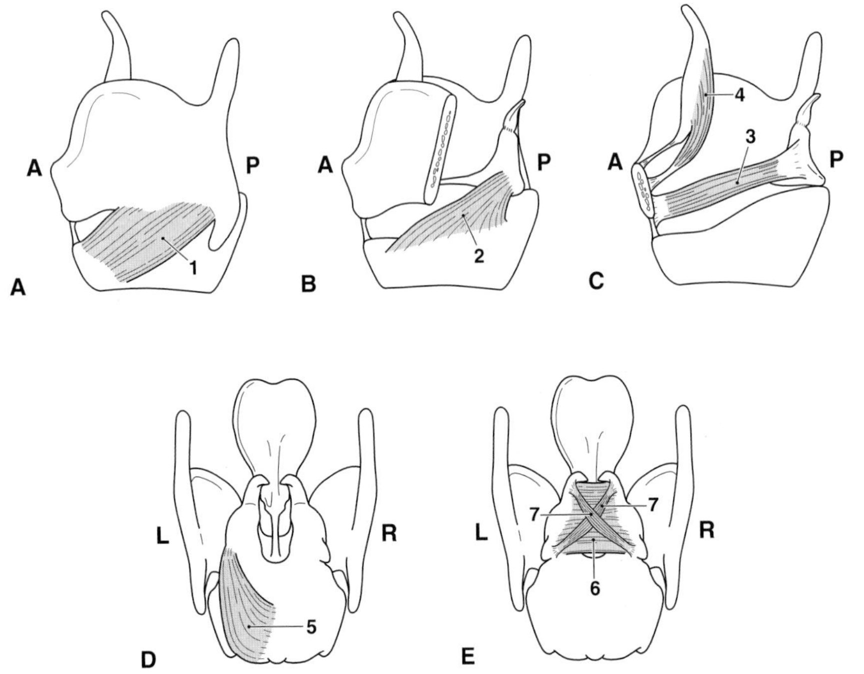

Figure 8-34: Schematics of the intrinsic muscles of the larynx. **A:** Cricothyroid muscle (*1*, lateral aspect). **B:** Lateral cricoarytenoid muscle (*2*, medial aspect—half of thyroid cartilage on left removed). **C:** Medial thyroarytenoid (vocalis muscle) *(3)* and thyroepiglottic *(4)* muscle (medial aspect—half of thyroid cartilage on left removed). **D:** Posterior cricoarytenoid muscle (*5*, posterior aspect). **E:** Interarytenoid muscle (*6*, transverse and *7*, oblique fibers—posterior aspect). *A*, anterior; *P*, posterior; *L*, left; *R*, right.

THE THYROID GLAND

1. The thyroid gland is located in the anterior neck, typically lying at a level between the fifth cervical to the first thoracic vertebrae.
2. The thyroid gland is composed of paired lateral lobes connected by a narrow isthmus in the midline; the location of the isthmus varies somewhat, but it usually connects the lower portions of the gland.
3. The apex of each lobe extends upward to the level of the thyroid cartilage; the base of each lobe extends downward to the level of the fourth or fifth tracheal cartilage.
4. Posteromedially each lobe of the thyroid gland is attached to the cricoid cartilage by a lateral thyroid ligament; laterally it is bordered by the sternothyroid muscle; anteriorly it is bordered by parts of the sternohyoid, the superior belly of the omohyoid, and the anterior border of the sternocleidomastoid muscles; medially it is bordered by the larynx and trachea; superiorly it is bordered by the inferior pharyngeal constrictor and the cricothyroid muscles; and posterolaterally it is bordered by the carotid sheath and the parathyroid glands.
5. A pyramidal lobe of the thyroid gland is frequently present; this lobe is conical in shape and extends upward from either the isthmus or directly from one of the lateral thyroid lobes toward the hyoid bone; a fibromuscular band, the levator of the thyroid gland, occasionally extends from the body of the hyoid bone to the pyramidal lobe or the thyroid isthmus.
6. The arterial supply to the thyroid gland is from the superior and inferior thyroid arteries. The superior thyroid artery originates from the external carotid artery; the inferior thyroid artery arises directly from the thyrocervical trunk, itself a branch of the subclavian artery. Occasionally a supplemental thyroid artery, called the arteria thyroidea ima, arises from the brachiocephalic trunk or aortic arch to directly supply the thyroid gland.
7. The innervation of the thyroid gland is sympathetic and is derived primarily from the middle cervical sympathetic ganglion; the superior and inferior cervical sympathetic ganglia may also contribute to this innervation. These nerves serve vasomotor function and possibly stimulate the follicular cells to produce or secrete thyroid hormones.
8. Basically, hypophyseal (pituitary gland) thyroid-stimulating hormone stimulates follicular cells of the thyroid gland to synthesize thyroglobulin and to eventually release the thyroid hormones T_3 (triiodothyronine) and T_4 (thyroxine) into the bloodstream.
9. The parafollicular cells of the thyroid gland store a form of calcitonin or thyrocalcitonin. Thyrocalcitonin release into the bloodstream is controlled by the serum calcium concentration: high blood calcium levels result in thyrocalcitonin secretion; low blood thyrocalcitonin levels cause thyrocalcitonin secretion inhibition. There is a reciprocal relationship between the secretion of thyrocalcitonin and parathyroid hormone (see below).

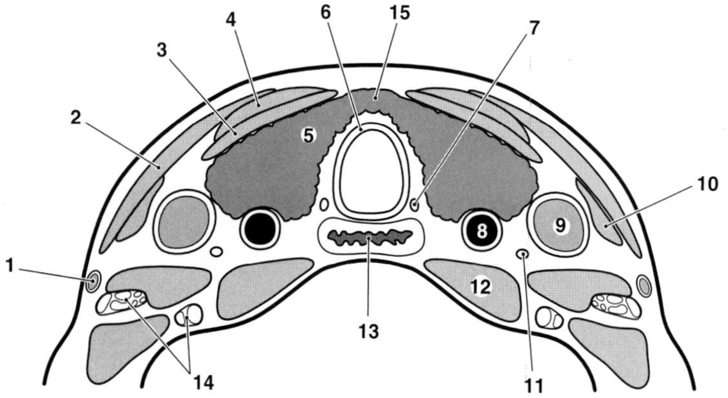

Figure 8-35: Axial schematic of the ventral region of the neck at the level of the thyroid gland.
1 External jugular vein
2 Sternocleidomastoid muscle
3 Sternothyroid muscle
4 Sternohyoid muscle
5 Right lobe of thyroid gland
6 Trachea
7 Recurrent laryngeal nerve
8 Common carotid artery
9 Internal jugular vein
10 Omohyoid muscle
11 Vagus nerve
12 Longus colli muscle
13 Esophagus
14 Roots of the brachial plexus
15 Isthmus of thyroid gland

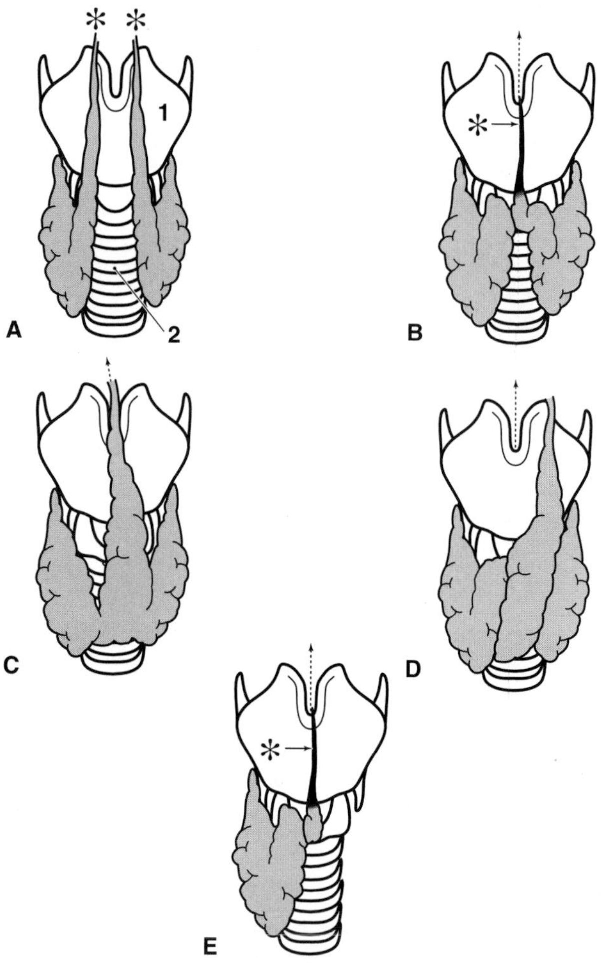

Figure 8-36: Frontal schematics showing the various final forms of the mature thyroid gland. **A:** No agenetic isthmus. *Asterisks*, extension of fibromuscular bands, the levator(s) of the thyroid, to body of hyoid bone. **B:** Normal isthmus—fibrous band (*asterisk*) extending from the thyroid isthmus superiorly to body of hyoid bone (*dashed arrow*). **C:** Midline pyramidal lobe. *Dashed arrow*, levator of the thyroid. **D:** Off-midline pyramidal lobe with levator of thyroid extending to body of hyoid bone (*dashed arrow*). **E:** Hemiagenesis of the thyroid gland. *Asterisk*, fibrous band to body of hyoid bone (*dashed arrow*).
1 Thyroid cartilage
2 Trachea

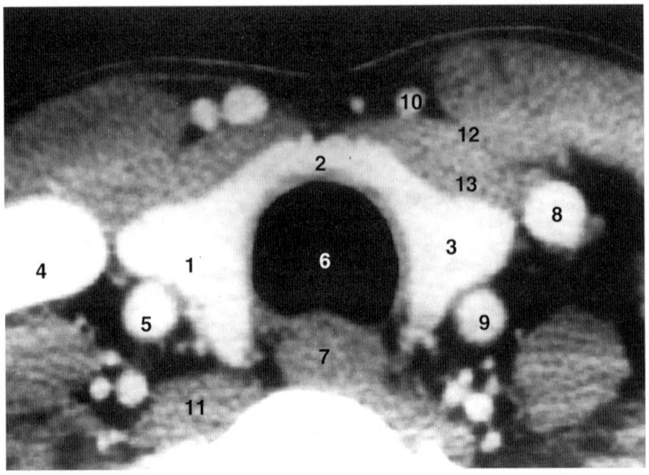

Figure 8-37A: CT of the thyroid gland. Axial enhanced CT image showing the normal anatomy of the thyroid gland.
1 Right lobe of the thyroid gland
2 Isthmus of the thyroid gland
3 Left lobe of the thyroid gland
4 Right jugular vein
5 Right common carotid artery
6 Trachea
7 Esophagus
8 Left jugular vein
9 Left common carotid artery
10 Anterior jugular vein
11 Longus colli muscle
12 Sternohyoid muscle
13 Sternohyoid muscle

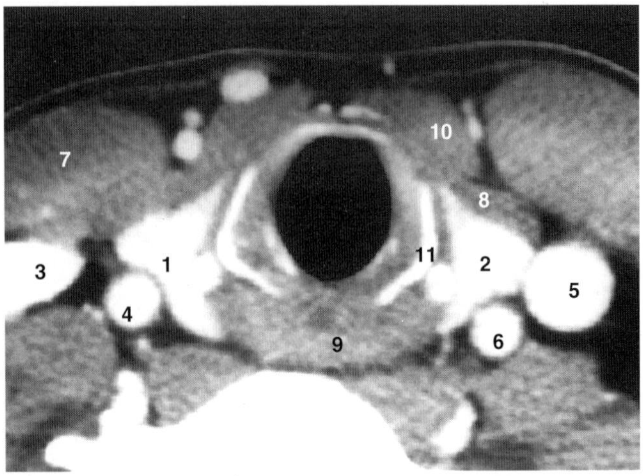

Figure 8-37B: Axial magnified enhanced CT image acquired at a higher level than that of Figure 8-37A showing the normal anatomy of the thyroid gland. Note the absence of the thyroid isthmus at this level.
1 Right lobe of thyroid gland
2 Left lobe of thyroid gland
3 Right jugular vein
4 Right common carotid artery
5 Left jugular vein
6 Left common carotid artery
7 Sternocleidomastoid muscle
8 Sternohyoid muscle
9 Esophagus
10 Sternohyoid muscle
11 Tracheal cartilage

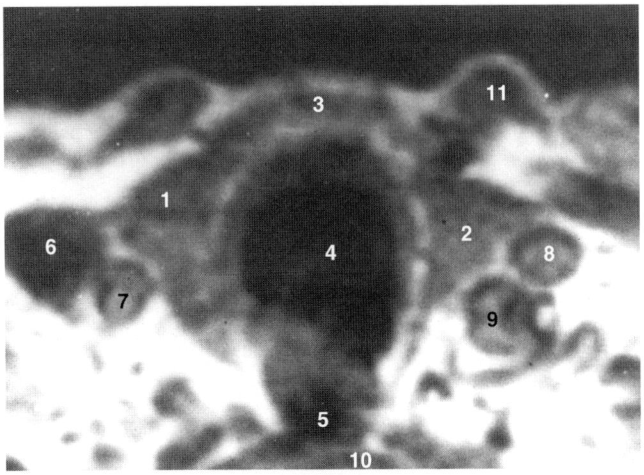

Figure 8-38: MR of the thyroid gland. Axial T1-weighted MR image showing the thyroid gland and surrounding structures.
1 Right lobe of thyroid gland
2 Left of thyroid gland
3 Isthmus of thyroid gland
4 Trachea
5 Esophagus
6 Right internal jugular vein
7 Right common carotid artery
8 Left internal jugular vein
9 Left common carotid artery
10 Cervical vertebral body
11 Sternocleidomastoid muscle

THE PARATHYROID GLANDS

1. The parathyroid glands are ovoid structures typically individually located between the thyroid gland proper and its capsule.
2. The parathyroid glands usually number four in total, i.e., two superior and two inferior.
3. The left and right superior parathyroid glands are usually found midway along the posterior surface of the thyroid gland.
4. The left and right inferior parathyroid glands vary more widely in their location, including: within the thyroid facial sheath near the inferior poles of the thyroid gland; immediately outside the thyroid facial sheath above the inferior thyroid artery; or within the substance of the inferior poles of the thyroid gland.
5. Although the foregoing is the idealized anatomic configuration, in practice the total number of parathyroid glands varies; they may number only three in total (i.e., aplasia of one or more parathyroid glands), or many (i.e., greater than four), being scattered within the connective tissue surrounding the thyroid gland near the typical sites (supernumerary parathyroid glands).
6. The parathyroid glands receive their vascular supply from the inferior thyroid arteries and/or from anastomoses between the inferior and superior thyroid arteries.
7. The innervation of the parathyroid glands is sympathetic; the relevant nerves are vasomotor in function.
8. Parathyroid hormone secretion is stimulated by variations in blood calcium levels: low blood calcium results in parathyroid hormone secretion; high blood calcium results in parathyroid hormone release inhibition.

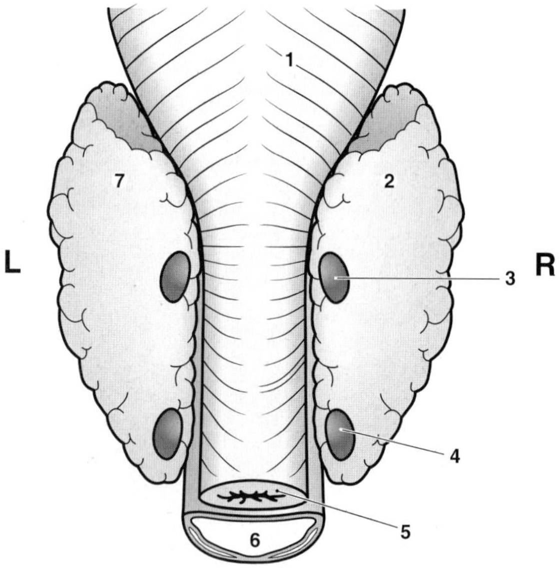

Figure 8-39: Posterior schematic of the thyroid and parathyroid glands. *L*, left; *R*, right.
1 Pharynx
2 Left lobe of thyroid gland
3 Superior parathyroid gland on the right side
4 Inferior parathyroid gland on the right side
5 Esophagus
6 Trachea
7 Right lobe of thyroid gland

NECK VARIANTS

Vascular (Arterial, Venous, Lymphatic) Variants
- Lateral asymmetry in size in the paired neck veins/arteries
- Minor variations in location and size of cervical lymph nodes (one or more sites on one or both sides)
- Vascular/lymphatic aplasia, hypoplasia on one or both sides

Ligamentous Variants
- Ligamentous calcification/ossification (i.e., stylohyoid ligament[s], thyrohyoid ligament[s])

Degree of Calcification/Ossification of the Laryngeal Cartilage Variants
- Noncalcified laryngeal cartilages (e.g., triticeal cartilages)
- Calcified laryngeal cartilages (e.g., triticeal cartilages)

Glandular Variants
- Accessory salivary gland(s) (e.g., parotid)
- Minor salivary gland(s) presence (e.g., labial, buccal palatoglossal, palatal, lingual [anterior and posterior]) (one or more sites on one or both sides)
- Lateral asymmetry in size of the paired salivary glands
- Variations in size and pattern of salivary gland ducts (one or more sites on one or both sides)
- Asymmetry of the lobes of the thyroid gland
- Pyramidal lobe of the thyroid gland (presence, absence, lateralization, hyperplasia)
- Aplasia/hypoplasia of thyroid gland isthmus
- Aplasia/hypoplasia of lobe of thyroid gland
- Ectopic thyroid tissue (along path of embryonic migration of thyroid tissue)
- Thyroglossal duct cyst
- Reactive tonsillar hypertrophy (one or more sites on one or both sides)
- Aplasia of one or more parathyroid glands
- Supernumerary parathyroid glands
- Duplication of parathyroid gland

Head and Neck Muscle Variants
- Muscle hemihypertrophy (one or more muscles)
- Muscle hemiatrophy (one or more muscles)

Tongue Variants
- Variations in the size, number, and type of lingual papillae

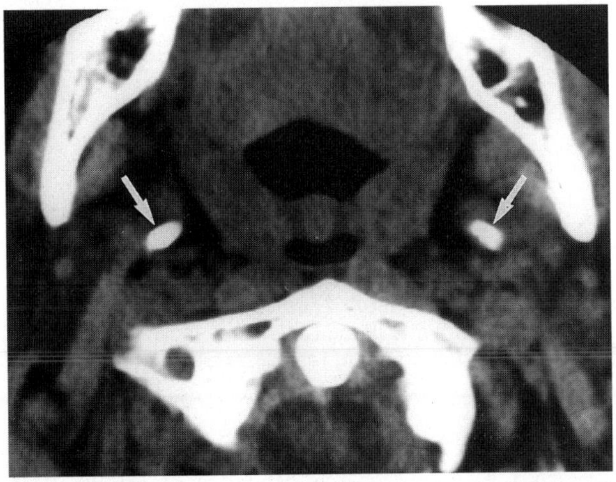

Figure 8-40A: Calcified/ossified stylohyoid ligaments. Axial CT image showing calcification of the stylohyoid ligaments bilaterally (*arrows*).

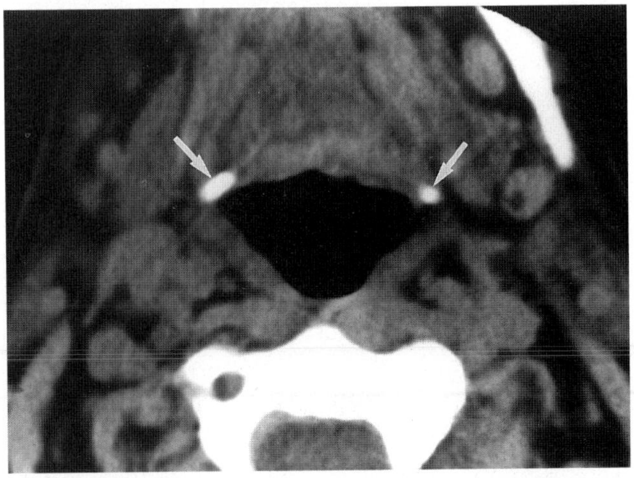

Figure 8-40B: Magnified axial CT image at a lower level than that of Figure 8-40A showing calcification of stylohyoid ligaments bilaterally (*arrows*).

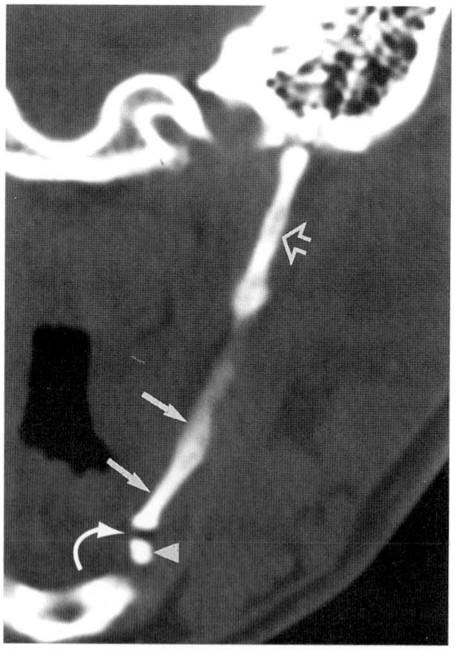

Figure 8-41A: Ossification of the stylohyoid ligament. Coronal CT image showing ossification of the left stylohyoid ligament (*solid arrows*) joining the styloid process (*open arrow*) superiorly and the apex of the lesser cornu (horn) of the hyoid bone (*arrowhead*) inferiorly. Also note the body of the hyoid bone (*asterisk*), and the nonossified junction (*curved arrow*) of the apex of the lesser cornu and the ossified stylohyoid ligament.

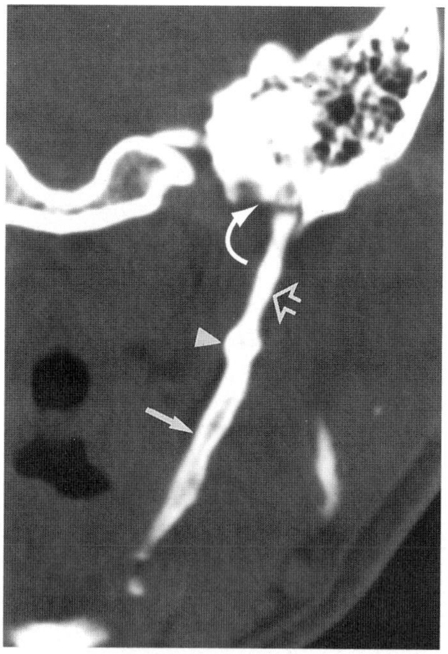

Figure 8-41B: Coronal CT image again showing the ossified stylohyoid ligament (*solid arrow*) joining the styloid process (*open arrow*). The bulbous junction (*arrowhead*) between the styloid process and the ossified stylohyoid ligament is also noted, as is the nonossified junction (*curved arrow*) between the styloid and mastoid processes of the temporal bone.

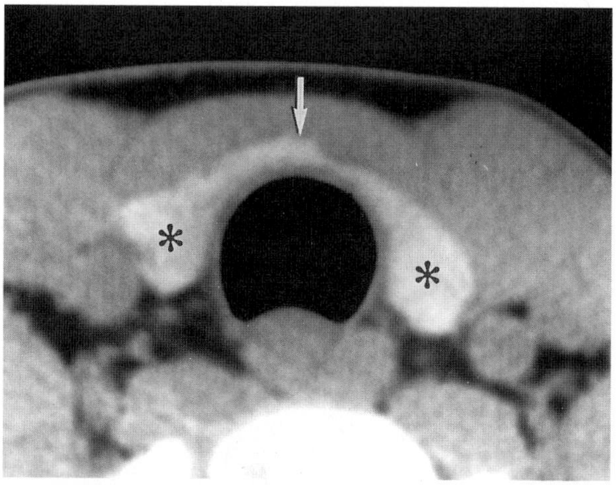

Figure 8-42A: Pyramidal lobe of thyroid gland. Contrast-enhanced axial CT image showing the right and left lobes (*asterisks*) and isthmus (*arrow*) of the thyroid gland.

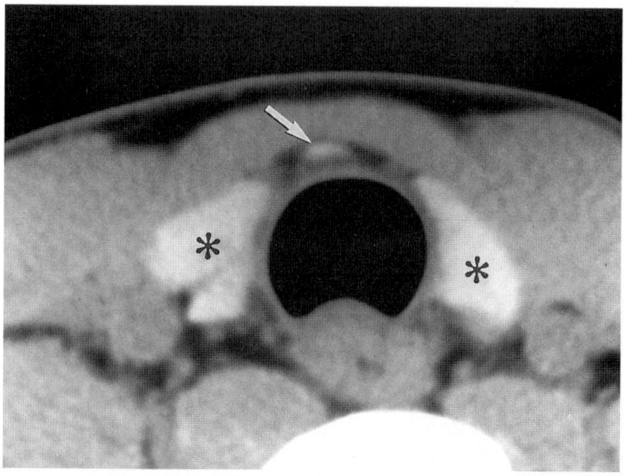

Figure 8-42B: Contrast-enhanced axial CT image acquired at a higher level than that of Figure 8-42A showing the right and left lobes of the thyroid gland (*asterisks*) as well as the pyramidal lobe of the thyroid gland (*arrow*) extending superficially.

APPENDIX 1: Cervicothoracic Segmental Innervation of Muscles Not Intimately Related to the Spine

Muscle	Spinal nerve(s)
Sternocleidomastoid	C1C2C3C4
Trapezius	C3C4
Levator scapulae	C3C4C5
Diaphragm	C3C4C5
Rhomboids	C4**C5**C6
Supraspinatus	**C5**C6
Infraspinatus	**C5**C6
Teres minor	C5C6
Deltoid	**C5**C6
Biceps	C5C6
Brachialis	C5C6
Brachioradialis	C5**C6**
Subscapularis	C5C6
Extensor carpi radialis (longus and brevis)	C5**C6**
Serratus anterior	C5C6C7
Teres major	C5C6C7
Pectoralis major	C5C6C7C8T1
Coracobrachialis	C6**C7**
Supinator	C6C7
Pronator teres	C6C7
Flexor carpi radialis	C6C7
Pectoralis minor	C6C7C8
Latissimus dorsi	C6**C7**C8
Triceps	C6**C7**C8
Extensor carpi ulnaris	**C7**C8
Extensor digitorum	**C7**C8
Extensor digiti quinti	**C7**C8
Abductor policis longus	**C7**C8
Extensor policis longus and brevis	**C7**C8
Extensor indicis	**C7**C8
Flexor digitorum profundus (all digits)	C7**C8**
Flexor pollicis longus	C7**C8**
Palmaris longus	C7**C8**T1
Flexor digitorum superficialis	C7**C8**T1
Pronator quadratus	C7**C8**T1
Flexor carpi ulnaris	C7**C8**T1
Abductor pollicis brevis	C8**T1**
Flexor pollicis brevis (superficial and deep)	C8**T1**
Opponens pollicis	C8**T1**
Lumbricals (I–IV)	C8**T1**
Hypothenar muscles	C8**T1**
Palmar and dorsal interossei	C8**T1**
Adductor pollicis	C8**T1**

C1–8, T1, specific segmental spinal nerve innervation.
Boldface type indicates predominant innervation

APPENDIX 2: Lumbosacral Innervation of Muscles Not Intimately Related to the Spine

Muscle	Spinal nerve(s)
Iliacus	**L1L2**L3
Obturator externus	**L2L3**L4
Adductor longus, brevis, magnus	**L2L3**L4
Gracilis	**L2L3**L4
Rectus femoris: vastus, lateralis, intermedius, medialis	L2**L3L4**
Pectineus	**L2L3**L4
Sartorius	**L2L3**L4
Tibialis posterior	L4L5
Tibialis anterior	**L4**L5
Adductor magnus	L4L5S1
Plantaris	L4L5S1
Popliteus	L4L5S1
Peroneus tertius	L4**L5**S1
Gluteus medius and minimus	**L4L5**S1
Tensor fasciae latae	**L4L5**S1
Peroneus longus and brevis	L5S1
Extensor digitorum longus	**L5**S1
Extensor hallucis longus	**L5**S1
Extensor digitorum brevis	L5S1
Semitendinosus	L5**S1**S2
Biceps femoris	L5**S1**S2
Semimembranosus	L5**S1**S2
Flexor digitorum longus	L5**S1S2**
Flexor hallucis longus	L5**S1S2**
Gluteus maximus	**L5S1**S2
Gastrocnemius	S1S2
Soleus	S1S2
Small foot muscles	S1S2

L1–S2, specific segmental spinal nerve innervation.
Boldface type indicates predominant innervation.

Bibliography

CHAPTER 1: EMBRYOLOGY

General References

DeMyer W. *Neuroanatomy*. Media, PA: Harwal Publishing, 1988:34–35, 352–387.
Moore K. *The developing human*. Philadelphia: WB Saunders, 1988:214, 385–409, 433–439.
Moore KL, Persaud TVN. *The developing human*. Philadelphia: WB Saunders, 1993:186–225, 405–408, 423–430, 433–439.
Sadler TW. *Langman's medical embryology*. Baltimore: Williams & Wilkins, 1990:140–145, 207–210, 297–337, 352–387.

Notochord and Neural Tube Formation

Barkovich JA. Brain development: normal and abnormal. In: Atlas SW, ed. *Magnetic resonance imaging of the brain and spine*. New York: Raven Press, 1991:129–138.
Burt AM. *Textbook of neuroanatomy*. Philadelphia: WB Saunders, 1993:3–24.
Hansen PE, Ballesteros MC, Soila K, Garcia L, Howard JM. MR imaging of the developing human brain. *Radiographs* 1993; 13:21–36.
Osborn AG, ed. *Diagnostic neuroradiology*. St. Louis: Mosby, 1994:3–10.
Pansky B, Allen DJ. *Review of neuroscience*. New York: Macmillan, 1988:4–31.
van der Knaap MS, Valk J. Classification of congenital abnormalities of the CNS. *AJNR* 1988; 9:315–326.
Volpe JJ. Normal and abnormal human brain development. *Clin Perinatol* 1977; 4:3–30.
Wolpert SM, Barnes PD, eds. *MRI in pediatric neuroradiology*. St. Louis: Mosby, 1992:331–344.

Formation of the Brain Vesicles and Regional Adult Derivatives

Romero-Sierra C. *Neuroanatomy: a conceptual approach*. New York: Churchill Livingstone, 1986:15–20.

Development of the Cerebral Commissures

Wonsiewicz MJ, Finn S, eds. *Neuroradiology: a study guide*. New York: McGraw-Hill, 1998:309–322.

Development of the Calvaria (Skull)

Jacobson RI. Abnormalities of the skull in children. *Neurol Clin* 1985; 3:117–145.
Kaplan SB, Kemp SS, Oh KS. Radiographic manifestation of congenital anomalies of the skull. *Radiol Clin North Am* 1991; 29:195–218.

Normal Development of the Aortic Left-sided Arch

Haughton VM, Rosenbaum AE. The normal anomalous aortic arch and brachycephalic arteries. In: Newton TH, Potts DG, eds. *Angiography*. Radiology of the skull and brain, vol 2, book 4. Great Neck, NY: MediBooks, 1974:1145–1163.
Padget DH. The development of the cranial arteries in the human embryo. *Contrib Embryol* 1948; 32:205.

Embryologic Anatomy of Common (Typical) Aortic Arch and Cephalic Artery Anomalies

Kaplan HA, Ford DH. *The brain vascular system*. New York: American Elsevier Publishing, 1966:27–40.
Padget DH. The cranial venous system in man in reference to development, adult configuration, and relation to the arteries. *Am J Anat* 1956; 98:307–356.
Padget DH. The development of the cranial venous system in man, from the viewpoint of comparative anatomy. *Contrib Embryol* 1957; 36:79–140.
Stein RL, Rosenbaum AE. Normal deep cerebral venous system. In: Newton TH, Potts DG, eds. *Angiography*. Radiology of the skull and brain, vol 2, book 4. Great Neck, NY: MediBooks, 1974:1904–1998.
Stephens RB, Stilwell DL. *Arteries and veins of the human brain*. Springfield, Ill.: Charles C Thomas, 1969.

Normal Development of the Anterior Cerebral Artery

Lin JP, Kricheff II. The anterior cerebral artery complex. In: Newton TH, Potts DG, eds. *Angiography*. Radiology of the skull and brain, vol 2, book 4. Great Neck, NY: MediBooks, 1974:1391–1409, 1441.

Normal Development of the Middle Cerebral Artery

Ring BA. The middle cerebral artery. In: Newton TH, Potts DG, eds. *Angiography*. Radiology of the skull and brain, vol 2, book 4. Great Neck, NY: MediBooks, 1974:1442–1470.

Normal Development of the Posterior Cerebral Artery

Hoyt WF, Newton TH, Margolis MT. The posterior cerebral artery. In: Newton TH, Potts DG, eds. *Angiography*. Radiology of the skull and brain, vol 2, book 4. Great Neck, NY: MediBooks, 1974:1540–1560.

Normal Development of the External Carotid Artery

Salamon G, Faure J, Raybaud C, Grisoli F. The external carotid artery. In: Newton TH, Potts DG, eds. *Angiography*. Radiology of the skull and brain, vol 2, book 4. Great Neck, NY: Medibooks, 1974:1246–1274.

Normal Development of the Cranial Vertebrobasilar Vascular System

Congdon ED. Transformation of the aortic-arch system during the development of the human embryo. *Contrib Embryol* 1922; 14:47–110.

Evans HM. The development of the vascular system. In: Kiebel F, Mall FP, eds. *Manual of human embryology*. Philadelphia: JB Lippincott, 1912.

Gillilan LA. Anatomy and embryology of the arterial system of the brain stem and cerebellum. In: Vinken PJ, Bruyn GW, eds. *Handbook of clinical neurology*, vol. 11. Amsterdam: North Holland Publishing, 1972.

Kier EL. Development of cerebral vessels. In: Newton TH, Potts DG, eds. *Angiography*. Radiology of the skull and brain, vol 2, book 4. Great Neck, NY: Medibooks, 1974:1089–1130.

Sabin FR. Origin and development of the primitive vessels of the chick and the pig. *Contrib Embryol* 1917; 6:61–124.

Intermediate and Late Cerebral Venous Development

Huang UP, Wolf BS. Veins of the white matter of the cerebral hemispheres (the medullary veins): diagnostic importance in carotid angiography. *Am J Roentgenol* 1964; 92:739–755.

Kaplan HA, Ford DH. *The brain vascular system*. New York: American Elsevier Publishing, 1966:27–40.

Development of the Spinal Column

Naidich TP, Raybaud C. Embryogenesis of the spine and spinal cord. *Riv Neuroradiol* 1992; 5:101–112.

Development of the Hypophysis

Kollias SS, Ball WS, Prenger EC. Review of the embryologic development of the pituitary gland and report of a case of hypophyseal duplication detected by MRI. *Neuroradiology* 1995; 37:3–12.

Overview of the Embryologic Development of the Neck

Patten BM. The normal development of the facial region. In: Pruzansky S, ed. *Congenital anomalies of the face and associated structures*. Springfield, Ill.: Charles C Thomas, 1961:11.

Remmick H. *Embryology of the face and oral cavity*. Rutherford, N.J.: Fairleigh Dickinson University Press, 1970.

Shepard TH. Development of the thyroid gland. In: Gardner LI, ed. *Endocrine and genetic diseases of childhood and adolescence*. Philadelphia: WB Saunders, 1975:2.

Sperber GH, ed. *Craniofacial embryology*, 2nd ed. Chicago: Year Book Medical Publishers, 1976.

Sulik KK, Schoenwolf GC. Highlights of craniofacial morphogenesis in mammalian embryos, as revealed by scanning electron microscopy. *Scanning Electron Microsc* 1985; 4:1735–1752.

CHAPTER 2: CRANIUM

General References

Berkovitz BKB, Moxham BJ, Brown MW. *A textbook of head and neck anatomy*. Chicago: Year Book Medical Publishers, 1988:25–50, 103–111, 514, 534–535.

Burt AM. *Textbook of neuroanatomy*. Philadelphia: WB Saunders, 1993:162–166, 172–179, 335–336, 357–360, 403–430, 433–435.
Carpenter M. *Core text of neuroanatomy*. Baltimore: Williams & Wilkins, 1978:35–40, 41–42, 181–248, 203–205, 236–238, 258–262.
Morris P. *Practical neuroangiography*. Baltimore: Williams & Wilkins, 1997:94–95, 117–277.
Osborn AG. *Introduction to cerebral angiography*. Hagerstown, MD: Harper and Row, 1980:33–59, 78–96, 109–120, 142–154, 185–237, 239–293, 295–325, 406–418.
Osborn A. *Handbook of neuroradiology*. St. Louis: Mosby–Year Book, 1991:30–55.
Pansky B, Allen DJ, Budd GC. *Review of neuroscience*. New York: Macmillan, 1988:80, 133–136, 209, 570.
Romero-Sierra C. *Neuroanatomy: a conceptual approach*. New York: Churchill Livingstone, 1986:35, 89–108, 135–145, 147–165, 261–275, 309–334, 345.
Williams PL. *Gray's anatomy*. New York: Churchill Livingstone, 1995.

The Sutures, Synchondroses, and Fontanelles of the Calvarium

Gooding CA. Cranial sutures and fontanelles. In: Newton TH, Potts DG, eds. *Radiology of the skull and brain: the skull*. Great Neck, NY: MediBooks, 1974:216–237.
Madeline LA, Elster AD. Postnatal development of the central skull base: normal variants. *Radiology* 1995; 196:757–764.
Meschan I. Roentgenology of the skull. In: *Roentgen signs in diagnostic imaging*. Philadelphia: WB Saunders, 1985:219–234.
Okamoto K, Ito J, Tokiguhi S, Furusawa T. High-resolution CT findings in the development of the sphenooccipital synchondrosis. *AJNR* 1996; 17:117–120.
Som PM, Bergeron RT. Embryology. In: Som PM, Bergenon RT, eds. *Head and neck imaging*. St. Louis: Mosby, 1991:881–895.
Williams PL. Cranial synchondroses. In: *Gray's anatomy*. New York: Churchill Livingstone, 1995:490.

Foramina of the Skull and the Structures Transmitted

Ginsberg LE, Pruett SW, Chen MY, Elster AD. Skull-base foramina of the middle cranial fossa: reassessment of normal variation with high-resolution CT. *AJNR* 1994; 15:283–291.
Sondheimer FK. Basal foramina and canals. In: Newton TH, Potts DG, eds. *Radiology of the skull and brain: the skull*. Great Neck, NY: MediBooks, 1986:287–347.

The Clivus

Kim H, Him D, Chung I, Lee W, Kim K. Topographical relationship of the facial and vestibulocochlear nerves in the subarachnoid space and internal auditory canal. *Am J Neuroradiol* 1998; 19:1155–1161.
Newton TH, Potts DG. Skull base. In: *Radiology of the skull and brain: the skull*. Great Neck, NY: MediBooks, 1974:348–356.

The Petrous Portion of the Temporal Bone

Grossman RI, Yousem DM. *Neuroradiology: the requisites*. St. Louis: Mosby, 1994:335–356.

Cerebral Hemisphere Variants

LeMay M, Culebras A. Human brain: morphological differences in the hemispheres demonstrable by carotid arteriography. *N Engl J Med* 1972; 287:168–170.
LeMay M, Geschwind N. Hemispheric differences in the brains of great apes. *Brain Behav Evol* 1975; 11:48–52.
LeMay M, Kido DK. Asymmetries of the cerebral hemispheres on computed tomograms. *J Comput Assist Tomogr* 1978; 2:471–476.
McGlone J. Sex difference in human brain asymmetry: a critical survey. *Behav Brain Sci* 1980; 3:215–263.

The Diencephalon

Alvin B. Diencephalon. In: *Textbook of neuroanatomy*. Philadelphia: WB Saunders, 1993:137–139, 150–155.
DeMyer W. Diencephalon. In: *Neuroanatomy*. Media, PA: Harwal Publishing, 1988:251–272.
Potts DG. Diencephalon. In: Newton T, Potts DG, eds. *Angiography*. Radiology of the skull and brain, vol 2, book 4. Great Neck, NY: MediBooks, 1974:2942–2946.

Connections of Limbic System

DeMyer W. Connections of the olfactory and limbic lobes. In: *Neuroanatomy*. New York: John Wiley and Sons, 1988:284–288.
Duvernoy HM. *The human hippocampus: an atlas of applied anatomy*. Munich: JF Berman Verley, 1988.
Mark LP, Daniels DL, Naidich TP, Borne JA. Limbic system anatomy: an overview. *AJNR* 1993; 14:349–352.

The Cerebellar Blood Supply

Willard FH. *Medical neuroanatomy: a problem-oriented manual with annotated atlas.* Philadelphia: JB Lippincott, 1993:99–114.

Peripheral Segments of the Cranial Nerves

Grant JCB. *Atlas of anatomy.* Baltimore: Williams & Wilkins, 1962:653–662.
Hollinshead WH. *Textbook of anatomy.* New York: Harper & Row, 1967:829–831.
Kretschmann HJ, Weinrich W. *Cranial neuroimaging and clinical neuroanatomy: MRI and CT.* New York: Thieme, 1992:299–302.
Leblanc A. Anatomy and imaging of the cranial nerves: a neuroanatomic method of investigation using MR and CT. New York: Springer-Verlag, 1992:1–259.
Liebman M. *Neuroanatomy made easy and understandable.* Baltimore: University Park Press, 1979:43–52.
Miller NR. *Clinical neuroophthalmology.* Baltimore: Williams & Wilkins, 1982:41–78.

Sympathetic and Parasympathetic Neural Supply to the Head and Neck

Beausang-Linder M, Bill A. Cerebral circulation in acute arterial hypertension: protective effects of sympathetic nervous activity. *Acta Physiol Scand* 1981; 111:193–199.
Edvinsson L, Owman C, Sjoberg N-O. Autonomic nerves, mast cells and amine receptors in human brain vessels: histochemical and pharmacologic study. *Brain Res* 1976; 115:377–393.
MacKenzie ET, Strandgaard D, Graham DI, Jones JV, Harper AM, Ferrer JK. Effects of acutely induced hypertension in cats on pial arteriolar caliber, local cerebral blood flow and the blood–brain barrier. *Circ Res* 1976; 39:33–41.
Netter FH, Brass A, Dingle RV. Autonomic nervous system. In: *Nervous system.* (*The Ciba collection of medical illustrations*, vol. 1; part 2: *Anatomy and physiology.*) West Caldwell, N.J.: Ciba Pharmaceutical, 1983:73–78.
Pansky B, Allen DJ, Budd GC. Autonomic nervous system. In: *Review of neuroscience.* New York: McGraw-Hill, 1988:226–237.

The Association (Arcuate) Fibers

Curnes JT, Burger PC, Djang WT, Boyko OB. MR imaging of compact white matter pathways. *AJNR* 1988; 9:1061–1068.

Cerebral Commissural Fibers

Hayman LA, Jinkins JR, Kirkpatrick JB. Cerebral commissures. In: Hayman LA, Hinck VC, eds. *Clinical brain imaging: normal structure and functional anatomy.* St. Louis: Mosby–Year Book, 1992:154–166.

Circumventricular Organs

Jinkins JR, Xiong L, Reiter RJ. The midline pineal "eye": MR and CT characteristics of the pineal gland with and without benign cyst formation. *J Pineal Res* 1995; 19:64–71.
Niewenhuys R, Voogd J, Vanhuizen C. *The human central nervous system: a synopsis and atlas.* Berlin: Springer-Verlag, 1988:309–323.
Scott DE, Krobisch-Dudley G. Ultrastructural analysis of the mammalian median eminence. In: Knigge KM, Scott DE, Kobayashi H, Ishii S, eds. *Brain-endocrine interaction II.* Basel: Karger, 1975:29–39.
Summy-Long JY, Keil LC, Severes WB. Identification of vasopressin in the subfornical organ region: effects of dehydration. *Brain Res* 1978; 140:241–250.
Weindel A, Sofroniew MV. Relation of neuropeptides to mammalian circumventricular organs. In: *Neurosecretion and brain peptides.* New York: Raven Press, 1981:303–320. (Martin JB, Reichlin S, Bick KL, eds. *Advances in biochemical psychopharmacology*, vol. 28.).

Overview of the Anatomy of the Meninges

Amundsen P, Newton TH. Subarachnoid cisterns. In: Newton TH, Potts DG, eds. *Radiology of the skull and brain: cisterns and ventricles,* vol. 4. Great Neck, NY: MediBooks, 1978:3588–3711.
Wilson M. *The anatomic foundation of neuroradiology of the brain.* Boston: Little, Brown, 1972.
Yasargil MG, Kasdaglis K, Jain KK, Weber HP. Anatomical observations of the subarachnoid cisterns of the brain during surgery. *J Neurosurg* 1976; 44:298–302.

Anatomy of the Dural Folds/Reflections

Parent A. Meninges and cerebrospinal fluid. In: Parent A, ed. *Carpenter's human neuroanatomy.* Baltimore: Williams & Wilkins, 1996:3–23.
Williams PL. Fluid compartments and fluid balance in the central nervous system. In: *Gray's anatomy.* New York: Churchill Livingstone, 1995:1202–1223.

Anatomy of the Cerebrospinal Fluid Pathways

Bell WO. Cerebrospinal fluid reabsorption: a critical appraisal. *Pediatr Neurosurg* 1995; 23:42–53.
Greitz D, Franck A, Nordell B. On the pulsatile nature of intracranial and spinal CSF-circulation demonstrated by MR imaging. *Acta Radiol* 1993; 34:1–8.

Maillot C. Anatomy of meninges and physiology of cerebro-spinal fluid. *Riv Neuroradiol* 1995; 5[Suppl 2]:59–62.
McComb JG. Recent research into the nature of CSF formation and absorption. *J Neurosurg* 1983; 59:369–383.

Anatomy of the Arachnoid Granulations

Upton ML, Weller RO. The morphology of cerebrospinal fluid drainage pathways in human arachnoid granulations. *J Neurosurg* 1985; 63:867–875.

Anatomy of the Perivascular or Virchow-Robin Spaces

Adachi M, Hosoya T, Haku T, Yamaguchi K. Dilated Virchow-Robin spaces: MRI pathological study. *Neuroradiology* 1998; 40:27–31.
Hutchings M, Weller RO. Anatomical relationships of the pia mater to the cerebral blood vessels in man. *J Neurosurg* 1986; 65:316–325.
Kaplan GP, Hartman BK, Creveling CR. Localization of cathecolo-methyltransferase in the leptomeninges, choroid plexus and ciliary epithelium: implications for the separation of central and peripheral cathecols. *Brain Res* 1981; 204:353–360.
Leurer DJ, Weller RO. Barrier functions of the leptomeninges: a study of normal meninges and meningiomas in tissue culture. *Neuropathol Appl Neurobiol* 1991; 11:391–405.
Weller RO. Anatomy and pathology of the subpial space. *Riv Neuroradiol* 1994; 7:15–21.
Zhang ET, Inman CBE, Weller RO. Interrelations of the pia mater and the perivascular (Virchow-Robin) spaces in the human cerebrum. *J Anat* 1990; 170:111–123.

The Left Aortic Arch

Haughton VM, Rosenbaum AE. The normal and anomalous aortic arch and brachiocephalic arteries. In: Newton TH, Potts DG, eds. *Angiography.* Radiology of the skull and brain, vol 2, book 4. Great Neck, NY: MediBooks, 1974:1145–1163.

Normal Variations and Anomalies of the Left Aortic Arch

Takahashi M. Angiographic anatomy of arterial system. In: *Atlas of carotid angiography.* Tokyo: Igaku-Shoin Medical Publishers, 1977:17–57.

The External Carotid Artery

Day A. Arterial distribution and variants. In: Wood JH, ed. *Cerebral blood flow.* New York: MacGraw-Hill, 1987:19–35.
Lasjaunias P. *Craniofacial and upper cervical arteries: functional, clinical, and angiographic aspects.* Baltimore: Williams & Wilkins, 1981.
Lasjaunias P, Berenstein A. *Surgical neuroangiography: functional anatomy of craniofacial arteries.* Berlin: Springer-Verlag, 1987.
Ramsey RG. External carotid artery. In: *Neuroradiology with computed tomography.* Philadelphia: WB Saunders, 1981:199–200.
Salamon G, Faure J, Raybaud C, Grisoli F. The external carotid artery. In: Newton TH, Potts DG, eds. *Angiography.* Radiology of the skull and brain, vol 2, book 4. Great Neck, NY: MediBooks, 1974:1246–1274.
Taveras JM, Wood EH. External carotid angiography. In: *Diagnostic neuroradiology.* Baltimore: William & Wilkins, 1977:971–972.

The Internal Carotid Artery

Dilenge D, Heon MM. The internal carotid artery. In: Newton TH, Potts DG, eds. *Angiography.* Radiology of the skull and brain, vol 2, book 4. Great Neck, New York: MediBooks, 1974:1145–1163.
Takahashi M. Angiographic anatomy of arterial system. In: *Atlas of carotid angiography.* Tokoyo: Igaku-Shoin Medical Publishers, 1977:17–57.
Taveras JM, Wood EH. Carotid angiography. In: *Diagnostic neuroradiology.* Baltimore: William & Wilkins, 1977:576–620.

The Anterior Cerebral Artery

Perlmutter D, Rhoton AL. Microsurgical anatomy of the anterior cerebral–anterior communicating–recurrent artery complex. *J Neurosurg* 1976; 45:259–272.
Perlmutter D, Rhoton AL. Microsurgical anatomy of the distal anterior cerebral artery. *J Neurosurg* 1978; 49:204–228.
Taveras JM, Wood EH, Carotid angiography. In: *Diagnostic neuroradiology.* Baltimore: William & Wilkins, 1977:576–620.

The Middle Cerebral Artery

Gibo H, Carver CC, Rhoton AL, et al. Microsurgical anatomy of the middle cerebral artery. *J Neurosurg* 1981; 54:151–169.

Ring BA, Michaty P, Moscow N, Salamon G. The middle cerebral artery. In: Newton TH, Potts DG. *Angiography.* Radiology of the skull and brain, vol 2, book 4. Great Neck, NY: MediBooks, 1974:1420–1525.

Taveras JM, Wood EH. Carotid angiography. In: *Diagnostic neuroradiology.* Baltimore: William & Wilkins, 1977:576–620.

Umansky F, Juarez SM, Dujovny M, et al. Microsurgical anatomy of the proximal segments of the middle cerebral artery. *J Neurosurg* 1984; 61:458–467.

Variants of the Internal Carotid Artery

Anderson RA, Sondheimer FK. Rare carotid-vertebrobasilar anastomoses with note on the differentiation between proatlantal and hypoglossal arteries. *Neuroradiology* 1976; 11:113–118.

Beresini DC, Hieshima GB, Mehringer CM, et al. Bilateral absence of the internal carotid artery with sellar enlargement due to anomalous vascularity. *Surg Neurol* 1980; 16:9–12.

Fantini GA, Reilly LM, Stoney RJ. Persistent hypoglossal artery: diagnostic and therapeutic considerations concerning carotid thromboendarterectomy. *J Vasc Surg* 1994; 20:995–999.

Guinto FC, Garrabrant EC, Radcliffe WB. Radiology of the persistent stapedial artery. *Radiology* 1979; 105:365–369.

Karasawa J, Kikuchi R, Furuse S, et al. Bilateral persistent carotid-basilar anastomoses. *Am J Roentgenol* 1976; 127:1053–1056.

Midkiff RB, Boykin MW, McFarland DR, et al. Agenesis of the internal carotid artery with intercavernous anastomosis. *Am J Neuroradiol* 1995; 16:1356–1359.

Reynolds AF, Stovring J, Turner PT. Persistent otic artery. *Surg Neurol* 1980; 13:115–117.

Siqueira M, Piske R, Ono M, et al. Cerebellar arteries originating from the internal carotid artery. *Am J Neuroradiol* 1993; 14:1229–1235.

Staples G. Transsellar intracavernous intercarotid collateral artery associated with agenesis of the internal carotid artery. *J Neurosurg* 1979; 50:393–394.

Suzuki S, Nobechi T, Itoh I, et al. Persistent proatlantal intersegmental artery and occipital artery originating from the interior carotid artery. *Neuroradiology* 1979; 17:105–109.

Teal JS, Rumbaugh CL, Segall HD, et al. Anomalous branches of the internal carotid artery. *Radiology* 1973; 106:567–573.

Tomsick TA, Lukin RR, Chambers AA. Persistent trigeminal artery: unusual associated findings. *Neuroradiology* 1979; 17:253–257.

Variants of the Middle Cerebral Artery

Komiyama M, Nakajima H, Nishikawa M, Yasui T. Middle cerebral artery variations: duplicated and accessory arteries. *AJNR* 1998; 19:45–49.

Teal JS, Rumbaugh CL, Bergeron RT, Segall HD, Anomalies of the middle cerebral artery: accessory artery, duplication, and early bifurcation. *AJR* 1973; 118:567–575.

The Cranial Vertebrobasilar Arterial System

Caruso G, Vinventelli F, Guidicelli G, et al. Perforating branches of the basilar bifurcation. *J Neurosurg* 1990; 73:259–265.

Hardy DG, Peace DA, Rhoton AL. Microsurgical anatomy of the superior cerebellar artery. *Neurosurgery* 1980; 6:10–28.

Mani RL, Newton TH, Glickman MG. The superior cerebellar artery: an anatomic–roentgenographic correlation. *Radiology* 1968; 91:1102–1108.

The Posterior Cerebral Artery

Margolis MT, Newton TH, Hoyt WF. Gross and roentgenologic anatomy of the posterior-cerebral artery. In: Newton TH, Potts DG, eds. *Angiography.* Radiology of the skull and brain, vol 2, book 4. Great Neck, NY: MediBooks, 1974:1551–1576.

Zeal AA, Rhoton AL. Microsurgical anatomy of the posterior cerebral artery. *J Neurosurg* 1978; 48:534–559.

The Choroidal Point

Huber P. Branches of the vertebral artery. In: *Cerebral angiography.* Stuttgart: Georg Thieme Verlag, 1982:141–150.

Margolis MT, Newton TH. The posterior inferior cerebellar artery. In: Newton TH, Potts DG, eds. *Angiography.* Radiology of the skull and brain, vol 2, book 4. Great Neck, NY: MediBooks, 1974:1710–1774.

Variants of the Vertebrobasilar System

Haughton VM, Rosenbaum AE, Pearce J. Internal carotid artery origins of the inferior cerebellar arteries. *AJR* 1978; 130:1191–1192.

Hoffman HB, Margolis MT, Newton TH. The superior cerebellar artery. In: Newton TH, Potts DG, eds. *Angiography.* Radiology of the skull and brain, vol 2, book 4. Great Neck, NY: MediBooks, 1974:1809–1848.

Ito J, Takeda N, Suzuki Y, Takeuchi S, Osugi S, Yoshida Y. Anomalous origin of the anterior inferior cerebellar arteries from the internal carotid artery. *Neuroradiology* 1980; 19:105–109.

Kretschman HJ, Weinrich W. *Cranial neuroimaging and clinical anatomy.* New York: Thieme Medical Publishers, 1992.

Lie TA. Congenital anomalies of the carotid arteries: variations in cerebrovascular anatomy. In: Fox JL, ed. *Intracranial aneurysms*. New York: Springer-Verlag, 1983:432–489.
Margolis MT, Newton TH. The posterior inferior cerebellar artery. In: Newton TH, Potts DG, eds. *Angiography*. Radiology of the skull and brain, vol 2, book 4. Great Neck, NY: MediBooks, 1974:1710–1774.
Naidich TP, Kricheff II, George AE, Lin JP. The normal anterior inferior cerebellar artery. *Radiology* 1976; 119:355–373.
Padget DH. The development of the cranial arteries in the human embryo. *Contrib Embryol* 1948; 32:207–261.
Saeki N, Rhoton AL. Microsurgical anatomy of the upper basilar artery and the posterior circle of Willis. *J Neurosurg* 1977; 46:563–578.
Scotti G. Anterior inferior cerebellar artery originating from the cavernous portion of the internal carotid artery. *Radiology* 1975; 116:93–94.
Takahashi M. The anterior inferior cerebellar artery. In: Newton TH, Potts DG, eds. *Angiography*. Radiology of the skull and brain, vol 2, book 4. Great Neck, NY: MediBooks, 1974:1796–1808.
Taveras JM, Wood EH. In: *Diagnostic neuroradiology*, 2nd ed. Baltimore: Williams & Wilkins, 1977.
Teal JS, Rumbaugh CL, Segall HD, Bergeron RT. Anomalous branches of the internal carotid artery. *Radiology* 1973; 106:567–573.
Torche M, Mahmood A, Araujo R, et al. Microsurgical anatomy of the lower basilar artery. *Neurol Res* 1992; 14:259–262.

Arterial Territories of the Cerebrum, Cerebellum, and Brain Stem

Amarenco P, Rosengart A, DeWitt LD, Pessin MS, Caplan LR. Anterior inferior cerebellar artery territory infarcts: mechanisms and clinical features. *Arch Neurol* 1993; 50:154–161.
Berkovitz BKB, Moxham B, Brown MW. *The vasculature of the cerebral nervous system. A textbook of head and neck anatomy*. Chicago: Year Book Medical Publishers, 1988:575–584.
Bonafe A, Maneife C, Scotto B, Pradere MY, Rascol A. Role of computed tomography in vertebrobasilar ischemia. *Neuroradiology* 1985; 27:484–493.
Hinshaw DB, Thompson JR, Hasso AN, Casselman ES. Infarctions of the brainstem and cerebellum: a correlation of computed tomography and angiography. *Radiology* 1980; 137:105–112.
Kase CS, White JL, Joslyn JN, Williams JP, Mohr JP. Cerebellar infarction in the superior cerebellar artery distribution. *Neurology* 1985; 35:705–711.
Savoiardo M, Bracchi M, Passerini A, Visciani A. The vascular territories in the cerebellum and brainstem: CT and MR study. *AJNR* 1987; 8:199–209.
Takahashi M. Angiographic anatomy of arterial system. In: *Atlas of carotid angiography*. Tokoyo: Igaku-Shoin Medical Publishers, 1977:17–33.
Taveras JM, Wood EH. Carotid angiography. In: *Diagnostic neuroradiology*. Baltimore: Williams & Wilkins, 1997:576–620.
Wicks L. *Atlas of radiologic anatomy*. Philadelphia: Lea & Febiger, 1994:575–584.

The Circle of Willis

Krabbe-Hartkamp MJ, van der Grond J, de Leeuw F-E, et al. Circle of Willis: morphologic variation on three-dimensional time-of-flight MR angiograms. *Radiology* 1998; 207:103–111.
Taveras JM, Wood EH. Carotid angiography. In: *Diagnostic neuroradiology*. Baltimore: William & Wilkins, 1977:576–620.
Wollschlaeger G, Wollschlaeger PB. The circle of Willis. In: Newton TH, Potts DG, eds. *Angiography*. Radiology of the skull and brain, vol 2, book 4. Great Neck, NY: MediBooks, 1974:1171–1201.

Anastomoses Between the Intracranial Vessels

Anderson RA, Sondheimer FK. Rare carotid-vertebrobasilar anastomoses with note on the differentiation between proatlantal and hypoglossal arteries. *Neuroradiology* 1976; 11:113–118.
Guinto FC, Garrabrant EC, Radcliffe WB. Radiology of the persistent stapedial artery. *Radiology* 1972; 105:365–369.
Hoyt W, Newton TH, Morgolis T. The posterior cerebral artery. In: Newton TH, Potts DG, eds. *Angiography*. Radiology of the skull and brain, vol 2, book 4. Great Neck, NY: MediBooks, 1974:1540–1550.
Karasawa J, Kikuchi R, Furuse S, et al. Bilateral persistent carotid-basilar anastomoses. *Am J Roentgenol* 1976; 127:1053–1056.
Kolbinger R, Heindel W, Pawlik G, et al. Right proatlantal artery type 1, right internal artery occlusion, and left internal carotid stenosis: case report and review of the literature. *J Neurol Sci* 1993; 117:232–239.
Lui CC, Liu YH, Wai YY, et al. Persistence of both proatlantal arteries with absence of vertebral arteries. *Neuroradiology* 1987; 29:304–305.
Runge VM. Normal arterial anatomy. In: *Review of neuroradiology*. Philadelphia: WB Saunders, 1996:8–19.
Siqueira M, Piske R, Ono M, et al. Cerebellar arteries originating from the internal carotid artery. *Am J Neuroradiol* 1993; 14:1229–1235.
Suzuki S, Nobechi T, Itoh I, et al. Persistent proatlantal intersegmental artery and occipital artery originating from the interior carotid artery. *Neuroradiology* 1979; 17:105–109.
Takahashi M. Angiographic anatomy of arterial system. In: *Atlas of carotid angiography*. Tokoyo: Igaku-Shoin Medical Publishers, 1977:17–57.
Takahashi M. Stenotic and occlusive diseases. In: *Atlas of carotid angiography*. Tokoyo: Igaku-Shoin Medical Publishers, 1977:351–352.
Taveras JM, Wood EH. Carotid angiography. In: *Diagnostic neuroradiology*, 2nd ed. Baltimore: William & Wilkins, 1977:576–620.
Tomsick TA, Lukin RR, Chambers AA. Persistent trigeminal artery: unusual associated findings. *Neuroradiology* 1979; 17:253–257.

Overview of the Cerebral Veins

Andrews BT, Dujovny M, Mirchandani HG, et al. Microsurgical anatomy of the venous drainage into the superior sagittal sinus. *Neurosurgery* 1989; 24:514–520.
DiChiro G. Angiographic patterns of cerebral convexity veins and superficial dural sinuses. *Am J Roentgenol* 1962; 87:306–321.
Oka K, Rhoton AL, Barry M, et al. Microsurgical anatomy of the superficial veins of the cerebrum. *Neurosurgery* 1985; 17:711–748.
Ono M, Rhoton AL, Peace D, et al. Microsurgical anatomy of the deep venous system of the brain. *Neurosurgery* 1984; 15:621–657.
Takahashi M. Angiographic anatomy of venous system. In: *Atlas of carotid angiography*. New York: Igaku-Shoin Medical Publishers, 1977:58–86.
Taveras JM, Wood EH. Cerebral veins. In: *Diagnostic neuroradiology*. Baltimore: Williams & Wilkins, 1977:620–634.

The Veins of the Posterior Fossa

Matsushima T, Rhoton AL, De Oliveira E, et al. Microsurgical anatomy of the veins of the posterior fossa. *J Neurosurg* 1983; 59:63–105.

The Cranial Emissary Veins

Andrews BT, Dujovny M, Mirchandani HG, et al. Microsurgical anatomy of the venous drainage into the superior sagittal sinus. *Neurosurgery* 1989; 24:514–520.
DiChiro G. Angiographic patterns of cerebral convexity veins and superficial dural sinuses. *Am J Roentgenol* 1962; 87:306–321.
Huang YP, Wolf BS. Veins of posterior fossa: superior or galenic draining group. *Am J Roentgenol* 1965; 95:808–821.
Huang YP, Wolf BS. Precentral cerebellar vein in angiography. *Acta Radiol (Diagn)* 1966; 5:250–262.
Huang YP, Wolf BS. The vein of the lateral recess of the fourth ventricle and its tributaries: roentgen appearance and anatomic relationships. *Am J Roentgenol* 1967; 101:1–21.
Huang YP, Wolf BS, Antin SP, et al. The veins of the posterior fossa: anterior or petrosal draining group. *Am J Roentgenol* 1968; 104:36–56.
Matushima T, Rhoton AL, De Oliveira E, et al. Microsurgical anatomy of the veins of the posterior fossa. *J Neurosurg* 1983; 59:63–105.
Oka K, Rhoton AL, Barry M, et al. Microsurgical anatomy of the superficial veins of the cerebrum. *Neurosurgery* 1985; 17:711–748.
Ono M, Rhoton AL, Peace D, et al. Microsurgical anatomy of the deep venous system of the brain. *Neurosurgery* 1984; 15:621–657.
Wolf BS, Huang YP. The subependymal veins of the lateral ventricles. *Am J Roentgenol* 1964; 91:406–426.
Wolf BS, Huang YP, Newman CM. Superficial sylvian venous drainage system. *Am J Roentgenol* 1963; 89:398–410.

CHAPTER 3: THE SELLA TURCICA, PITUITARY GLAND, AND CAVERNOUS VENOUS SINUSES

General Reference

Williams PL. *Gray's anatomy*. New York: Churchill Livingstone, 1995.

The Sella Turcica Bony Anatomy

Berkovitz BKB, Moxham BJ, Brown MW. The sphenoidal air cells. In: *A textbook of head and neck anatomy*. London: Year Book Medical Publishers, 1988:251–252.
Taveras JM, Morello F. Sella turcica. In: Taveras JM, Morello F. *Normal neuroradiology: an atlas of the skull, sinuses and facial bones*. Chicago: Year Book Medical Publishers, 1979:25.

Anatomy of the Pituitary Gland

Brooks BS, El Gammal T, Allison JD, Hoffman WH. Frequency and variations of the posterior pituitary bright signal on MR images. *AJNR* 1989; 10:943–948.
Elster AD. Modern imaging of the pituitary. *Radiology* 1993; 187:1–14.
Elster AD, Chen MYM, Williams DW, Key LL. Pituitary gland: MR imaging of physiologic hypertrophy in adolescence. *Radiology* 1990; 174:681–685.
Fujisawa L, Asato R, Kawata M, et al. Hyperintense signal of the posterior pituitary on T1-weighted MR images: an experimental study. *J Comput Assist Tomogr* 1989; 13:371–377.
Swartz JD, Russell KB, Basile BA, O'Donnell PC, Popky GL. High-resolution computed tomography appearance of the intrasellar contents in women of childbearing age. *Radiology* 1983; 147:115–117.
Wiener SN, Rzeszotarski MS, Droege RT, Pearistein AE, Shafron M. Measurements of pituitary gland height with MR Imaging. *AJNR* 1985; 6:717–722.

Wolpert SM, Molitch ME, Goldman JA, Wood JB. Size, shape, and appearance of the normal female pituitary gland. *AJR* 1984; 143:377–381.

Variations of the Pituitary Infundibulum

Ahmadi H, Larsson EM, Jinkins JR. Normal pituitary gland: coronal MR imaging of infundibular tilt. *Radiology* 1990; 177:389–392.
Burt AM. Magnocellular and parvocellular neurosecretory systems. In: *Textbook of neuroradiology*. Philadelphia: WB Saunders, 1993:390–392.
Nieuwenhuys R, Voogd J, van Huijzen C. Olfactory and limbic systems. In: *The human central nervous system: a synopsis and atlas*, 3rd ed. Berlin: Springer-Verlag, 1988:297–302.
Spickler EM, Hirsch WL, Hayman LA. Neurosecretory regions. In: Hayman LA, Hinck VC, eds. *Clinical brain imaging: normal structure and functional anatomy*. St. Louis: Mosby–Year Book, 1992:417–426.

Anatomy of the Cavernous Venous Sinuses

Daniels DL, Pech P, Mark L, Pojunas K, Williams AL, Haugton VM. Magnetic resonance imaging of the cavernous sinus. *AJNR* 1985; 6:187–192.
Eister AD. Modern imaging of pituitary. *Radiology* 1993; 187:1–14.
Grossman RI, Yousem DM. Sella and central skull base. In: *Neuroradiology: the requisites*. St. Louis: Mosby, 1994:305–333.
Melloni JL, Dox I, Melloni HP, Melloni BJ. In: *Review of human anatomy*. Philadelphia: JB Lippincott, 1988:210–211.

CHAPTER 4: THE ORBIT

General Reference

Williams PL. *Gray's anatomy*. New York: Churchill Livingstone, 1995.

Overview of the Anatomy of the Bony Orbit

Burt AM. *Textbook of neuroanatomy*. Philadelphia: WB Saunders, 1993:407–416.
Taveras JM, Morello F. Orbital cavity. In: Taveras JM, Morello F, eds. *Normal neuroradiology: an atlas of the skull, sinuses and facial bones*. Chicago: Year Book Medical Publishers, 1979:25–27.

Overview of the Anatomy of the Globe and Optic Nerve/Sheath Complex

Brown MR. The eye. In: Berkovitz BKB, Moxham BJ. *A textbook of head and neck anatomy*. London: Year Book Medical Publishers, 1988:200–209.
Brown MR. The eyelids. In: Berkovitz BKB, Moxham BJ. *A textbook of head and neck anatomy*. London: Year Book Medical Publishers, 1988:200–213.
Goss CM. *Anatomy of the human body*. Philadelphia: Lea & Febiger. 1975:1059–1062.

The Optic Pathway

DeMyer W. *Neuroanatomy*. Media, PA: Harwal Publishing, 1988:207–235.

The Visual Pathway

Brown MW. Visual areas. In: Berkovitz BKB, Moxham BJ, eds. *A textbook of head and neck anatomy*. London: Year Book Medical Publishers, 1988:550–552.

The Extraocular Muscles of the Orbit

Hall-Craggs ECB. *Anatomy as a basis for clinical medicine*. Munich: Urban Schwarzenberg, 1985:523.
Harnsberger HR. Anatomy of the orbit. In: *Handbook of head and neck imaging*. St. Louis: Mosby–Year Book, 1990:309–315.

Anatomy of the Lacrimal Apparatus

Berkovitz BKB, Moxham BJ, Brown MW. *A textbook of head and neck anatomy*. London: Year Book Medical Publishers, 1988:213–214.
Lloyd GAS. *Radiology of the orbit*. Philadelphia: WB Saunders, 1975:189–195.
Tortora GJ. Accessory structures of the eye. In: *Principles of human anatomy*. New York: HarperCollins, 1995:550–551.

Arterial Supply and Venous Drainage of the Orbit

Doyon DL, Aron-Rosa DS, Ramée A. Orbital veins and cavernous sinus. In: Newton TH, Potts DG, eds. *Angiography.* Radiology of the skull and brain, vol. 2, book 4. Great Neck, NY: MediBooks, 1974:2220–2254.

CHAPTER 5: FACIAL STRUCTURES

General Reference

Williams PL. *Gray's anatomy.* New York: Churchill Livingstone, 1995.

Overview of Facial Bone Anatomy

Goss CM. The skull. In: Goss CM, ed. *Anatomy of the human body by Henry Gray.* Philadelphia: Lea & Febiger, 1975:133–152.

Hollinshead WH. Skull, face and jaws. In: Hollinshead WH, ed. *Textbook of anatomy.* New York: Harper & Row, 1967:791–852.

Taveras JM, Morello F, eds. *Normal neuroradiology: an atlas of the skull, sinuses and facial bones.* Chicago: Year Book Medical Publishers, 1979:23–25.

Anatomy of the Mandible

Agur AMR, Lee MJ. Mandible. *Grant's atlas of anatomy*, 9th ed. Baltimore: Williams & Wilkins, 1991:500–501.

Overview of the Temporomandibular Joint

Berkovitz BKB, Moxham BJ, Brown MW. The capsule and ligaments of the temporomandibular joint. In: *A textbook of head and neck anatomy.* London: Year Book Medical Publishers, 1988:173–174.

Katzberg RW, Westesson PL. Temporomandibular joint imaging. In: Som PM, Bergeron RT, eds. *Head and neck imaging.* St. Louis: Mosby–Year Book, 1991:249–353.

CHAPTER 6: PARANASAL SINUSES AND NASAL PASSAGEWAYS

General References

Calhoun KH, Waggenspack GA, Simpson BC, Hokanson JA, Bailey BJ. CT evaluation of the paranasal sinuses in symptomatic and asymptomatic populations. *Otolaryngol Head Neck Surg* 1991; 104:480–483.

Earwaker J. Anatomic variations in sinonasal CT. *Radiographics* 1993; 13:381–415.

Williams PL. *Gray's anatomy.* New York: Churchill-Livingstone, 1995.

Zinreich SJ, Mattox DE, Kennedy DW, Chisholm HL, Diffley DM, Rosebaum AE. Concha bullosa: CT evaluation. *J Comput Assist Tomogr* 1988; 12:778–784.

Anatomy of the Nasal Passageways

Taveras JM, Morello F. Nasal cavity. In: Taveras JM, Morello F. *Normal neuroradiology: an atlas of the skull, sinuses and facial bones.* Chicago: Year Book Medical Publishers, 1979:23–24.

CHAPTER 7: THE SPINE

General References

Romero-Sierra C. *Neuroanatomy: a conceptual approach.* New York: Churchill Livingstone, 1986:87–88, 169–183, 369–371.

Williams PL. *Gray's anatomy.* New York: Churchill Livingstone, 1995.

Gray Matter Nuclei and Columns of the Spinal Cord

Burt AM. Grey matter. In: *Textbook of neuroanatomy.* Philadelphia: WB Saunders, 1993:126–131.

Ascending and Descending Tracts of the Spinal Cord

DeMeyer W. Ascending pathways of the spinal white matter. In: *Neuroanatomy.* New York: John Wiley & Sons, 1988:112–118, 120–123.

Arterial Supply to the Spinal Cord and Spinal Column

Burt AM. Spinal cord vasculature. In: *Textbook of neuroanatomy.* Philadelphia: WB Saunders, 1993:177–178.

Crock HV, Yoshizawa H. *The blood supply of the vertebral column and spinal cord in man.* New York: Springer-Verlag, 1977.
DeMyer W. Neuroanatomy. In: *The national medical series for independent study.* Media, Penn.: Harwal Publishing, 1988:336–338.
Ratcliffe JF. The arterial anatomy of the adult human lumbar vertebral body: a microarteriographic study. *J Anat* 1980;131:57–59.
Taveras JM, Morello F, eds. *Normal neuroradiology: an atlas of the skull, sinuses and facial bones.* Chicago: Year Book Medical Publishers, 1979:608–611.

The Venous Drainage of the Spine

Hanley EN, Howard BH, Brigham CD, et al. Lumbar epidural varix as a cause of radiculopathy. *Spine* 1994; 19:2122–2126.

The Coccygeal Neural Plexus

Tortora GJ. The spinal cord and the spinal nerves. In: *Principles of human anatomy.* New York: HarperCollins, 1995:454–479.

Spinal Innervation

Inman VT, Saunders JB. The clinico-anatomical aspects of the lumbosacral region. *Radiology* 1942;38:669–678.
Jinkins JR. The pathoanatomic basis of somatic, autonomic and neurogenic syndromes originating in the lumbosacral spine. *Riv Neuroradiol* 1995; 8[Suppl 1]:35–51.
Kellgren JH. The anatomical source of back pain. *Rheumatol Rehabil* 1977;16:3–12.
Kellgren JH. On the distribution of pain arising from deep somatic structures with charts of segmental pain areas. *Clin Sci* 1938–42;4:35–46.

The Autonomic Nervous System

Parent A. *Carpenter's human neuroanatomy.* Baltimore: Williams & Wilkins, 1996:397–399.

The Intrinsic Muscles of the Spine

Tortora GJ. *Principles of human anatomy.* New York: HarperCollins, 1995:258, 279–280.
Williams PL, ed. *Gray's anatomy.* New York: Churchill Livingstone, 1995:809–813, 831–838.

Superficial Muscles of the Back and Trunk Attaching to the Extremities

Tortora GJ. *Principles of human anatomy.* New York: HarperCollins, 1995:258, 279–280.

CHAPTER 8: THE NECK

General References

Brown MW. *Head and neck anatomy.* London: Year Book Medical Publishers, 1988:291–294, 310–318, 332–346.
Williams PL. Gray's anatomy. New York: Churchill-Livingstone, 1995.

The Cervical Muscles and Triangles

Harnsberger HR. *Handbook of head and neck imaging.* St. Louis: Mosby, 1995:152.

The Anatomy of the Hyoid Bone

Agur AMR, Lee MJ. Hyoid bone. In: Agur AMR, Lee MJ, eds. *Grant's atlas of anatomy.* Baltimore: Williams & Wilkins, 1991:563.

Figure Credits

CHAPTER 1: EMBRYOLOGY

Figs. 1-1A, 1-2, 1-5A, 1-6, 1-11, 1-13, 1-14, 1-35, 1-40, 1-41, 1-42, 1-43, 1-44, 1-45, 1-46, 1-47, 1-48, and 1-50 modified from Sadler TW. *Langman's medical embryology*. Baltimore: Williams & Wilkins, 1990:63–64, 141, 142, 298, 299, 306, 307, 311, 312, 315–316, 317, 318, 323–324, 353, 354, 354, 375, 372, 401.

Figs. 1-1B–D, 1-5B, 1-5C, 1-33, 1-34, 1-36, 1-37, 1-38, and 1-49 modified from Moore K. *The developing human*. Philadelphia: WB Saunders, 1988:213–214, 386, 405, 410, 423–430, 435, 436.

Fig. 1-4 modified from McLaurin R. *Pediatric neurosurgery: surgery of the developing nervous system*. Philadelphia: WB Saunders, 1989:11–13.

Figs. 1-7 and 1-10 modified from Romero-Sierra C. *Neuroanatomy: a conceptual approach*. New York: Churchill Livingstone, 1986:16, 17.

Figs. 1-8 and 1-9 modified from Moore KL, Persaud TVN. *The developing human: clinically oriented embryology*. Philadelphia: WB Saunders, 1998:465–477.

Fig. 1-12 modified from Pansky B, Allen DJ. *Review of neuroscience*. New York: Macmillan, 1988:31.

Fig. 1-15 modified from Som PM, Bergeron RT. Embryology. In: Som PM, Bergeron RT, eds. *Head and neck imaging*. St. Louis: Mosby–Year Book, 1991:881–883; and Smoker WRK. Craniovertebral junction: normal anatomy, craniometry, and congenital anomalies. *Radiographics* 1994;14:255–277.

Figs. 1-21 and 1-28 modified from Padget DH. The development of the cranial arteries in the human embryo. *Contrib Embryol* 1948;32:205.

Fig. 1-22 modified from Lin JP, Kricheff II. The anterior cerebral artery complex. In: Newton TH, Potts DG (eds.) *Angiography*. Radiology of the skull and brain, vol. 2, book 2. Great Neck, NY: Medibooks, 1974:1391–1409.

Fig. 1-23 modified from Ring BA. The middle cerebral artery. In: Newton TH, Potts DG (eds.) *Angiography*. Radiology of the skull and brain, vol. 2, book 2. Great Neck, NY: Medibooks, 1974:1442–1470.

Fig. 1-25 modified from Hoyt WF, Newton TH, Margolis MT. The posterior cerebral artery. In: Newton TH, Potts DG (eds). *Angiography*. Radiology of the skull and brain, vol. 2, book 2. Great Neck, NY: Medibooks, 1974:1540–1560.

Fig. 1-26 modified from Padget DH. The development of the cranial venous system in man, from the viewpoint of comparative anatomy. *Contrib Embryol* 1957;36:79–140; Padget DH. The cranial venous system in man in reference to development, adult configuration, and relation to the arteries. *Am J Anat* 1956;98:307–356; Salamon G, Faure J, Raybaud C, Grisoli F. The external carotid artery. In: Newton TH, Potts DG (eds). *Angiography*. Radiology of the skull and brain, vol. 2, book 2. Great Neck, NY: Medibooks, 1974:1246–1274.

Fig. 1-30 modified from Naidich TP, Raybaud C. Embryogenesis of the spine and spinal cord. *Riv Neuroradiol* 1992;5:101–112.

Fig. 1-31 modified from Barnes PD. Wolpert SM, Barnes PD, eds. *Pediatric neuroradiology*. St. Louis: Mosby, 1992:333.

Fig. 1-32B modified from Lemire RJ, Loesser JD, Leech RW, et al. *Normal and abnormal development of the human nervous system*. New York: Harper & Row, 1976.

Fig. 1-39 modified from Scuderi AJ, Harnsberger HR, Boyer RS. Pneumotization of the paranasal sinus: normal features of importance to the accurate interpretation of CT scans and MR images. *AJR* 1993;160:1101–1104.

CHAPTER 2A: THE SKULL

Figs. 2A-4 and 2A-7 modified from Hall-Craggs ECB. In: *Anatomy as a basis for clinical medicine*. Munich: Urban Schwarzenberg, 1985:482, 483.

Fig. 2A-8 modified from Smoker WRK. Craniovertebral junction: normal anatomy, craniometry, and congenital anomalies. *Radiographics* 1994;14:255–277.

CHAPTER 2B: SKULL BASE

Fig. 2B-1 modified from Romero-Sierra C. *Neuroanatomy: a conceptual approach*. New York: Churchill Livingstone, 1986:36.

Fig. 2B-3 modified from DiChiro G, Fisher RL, Nelson KB. The jugular foramen. *J Neurosurg* 1964;21:447–460.
Figs. 2B-9 and 2B-10 modified from Agur AMR. In:*Grant's atlas of anatomy*. Baltimore: Williams & Wilkins, 1991:536.
Figs. 2B-11 and 2B-12 modified from Williams PL. *Gray's anatomy*. New York: Churchill Livingstone, 1995:1375, 1376.
Fig. 2B-13 modified from Harnsberger HR. Normal anatomy of the inner ear. In: *Handbook of head and neck imaging*. St. Louis: Mosby–Year Book, 1995.
Fig. 2B-14 modified from Bergeron RT. The temporal bone. In: Som P, Bergeron RT, eds. *Head and neck imaging*. St. Louis: Mosby–Year Book, 1991:941.
Fig. 2B-15 modified from Tortora GJ. *Principles of human anatomy*. New York: HarperCollins Publishers, 1995:568.
Fig. 2B-19 modified from Sherman JL. The craniocervical junction. In: Rao KCVG, Williams JP, Lee BCP, Sherman JL, eds. *MRI and CT of the spine*. Baltimore: Williams & Wilkins, 1994:74.

CHAPTER 2C: CEREBRAL HEMISPHERES

Fig. 2C-1 modified from Pansky B, Allen DJ. *Review of neuroscience*. New York: Macmillan, 1988:91.
Fig. 2C-2A modified from Carpenter MB. *Core text of neuroanatomy*. Baltimore: Williams & Wilkins, 1978:17.
Fig. 2C-2C modified from Taveras JM, Morello F. *Normal neuroradiology and atlas of the skull, sinus and facial bones*. Chicago: Year Book Medical Publishers, 1979:276, 277.
Fig. 2C-2H modified from Burt AM. *Textbook of neuroanatomy*. Philadelphia: WB Saunders, 1993:159.
Fig. 2C-2I modified from DeMyer W. In: *Neuroanatomy*. Media, PA: Harwal Publishing, 1988:279. (Three-dimensional MR images courtesy of J. Lancaster.)
Fig. 2C-3A modified from Williams PL. *Gray's anatomy*. New York: Churchill Livingstone, 1995:1114.
Fig. 2C-4 modified from Pansky B, Allen DJ, Budd GC. *Review of neuroscience*. New York: Macmillan, 1988:209.
Fig. 2C-5 modified from Penfield W, Rasmussen T. *The cerebral cortex of man*. New York: Hafner Publishing, 1968:44–57.

CHAPTER 2D: DIENCEPHALON

Figs. 2D-1 and 2D-3 modified from Williams PL. *Gray's anatomy*. New York: Churchill Livingstone, 1995:1085, 1095.
Fig. 2D-2 modified from Berkovitz BKB, Moxham BJ, eds. *A textbook of head and neck anatomy*. London: Year Book Medical Publishers, 1988:531.
Fig. 2D-4 modified from Parent A. Hypothalamus. *Carpenter's human neuroanatomy*. Baltimore: Williams & Wilkins, 1996:727.

CHAPTER 2E: BASAL GANGLIA

Fig. 2E-1 modified from Pansky B, Allen DJ, Budd GC. *Review of neuroscience*. New York: Macmillan, 1980:187.
Figs. 2E-2 and 2E-4A modified from Romero-Sierra C. The cerebral hemispheres. In: *Neuroanatomy: a conceptual approach*. New York: Churchill Livingstone, 1986:127–146.

CHAPTER 2F: LIMBIC SYSTEM AND HIPPOCAMPUS

Fig. 2F-1A modified from Pansky B, Allen DJ, Budd GC. *Review of neuroscience*. New York: Macmillan, 1988:264–265.
Fig. 2F-1B modified from Hayman LA, Bronen RA, Charletta DA. Adult cerebrum. In: Hayman LA, Hinck VC, eds. *Clinical brain imaging*. St. Louis: Mosby, 1992:121.
Fig. 2F-2 modified from Carpenter MB. *Neuroanatomy*. Baltimore: Williams & Wilkins, 1985:275.
Fig. 2F-3 modified from Romero-Sierra C. *Neuroanatomy: a conceptual approach*. New York: Churchill Livingstone, 1986:134.
Fig. 2F-5 modified from Williams PL. *Gray's anatomy*. New York: Churchill Livingstone, 1995:1126.
Fig. 2F-6 modified from DeMyer W. *Neuroanatomy*. Media, PA: Harwal Publishing, 1988:287.

CHAPTER 2G: CEREBELLUM

Fig. 2G-1 modified from Taveras JM, Morello F. *Normal neuroanatomy*. Chicago: Year Book Medical Publishers, 1979:287.
Fig. 2G-3 modified from Press GA, Courchesne E. Cerebellar hemispheres and vermis. In: Hayman LA, Hinck VC, eds. *Clinical brain imaging: normal structure and functional anatomy*. St. Louis: Mosby, 1992:283.

Figs. 2G-4 and 2G-5 modified from Pansky B, Allen DJ, Budd GC. *Review of neuroscience*. New York: Macmillan, 1988:241.
Fig. 2G-6 modified from Williams PL. *Gray's anatomy*. New York: Churchill Livingstone, 1995:1032.
Figs. 2G-7 and 2G-9 modified from Burt AM. *Textbook of neuroanatomy*. Philadelphia: WB Saunders, 1993:350, 360.
Figs. 2G-8, 2G-10, and 2G-11 modified from Berkovitz BKB, Moxham BJ, eds. *A textbook of head and neck anatomy*. London: Year Book Medical Publishers, 1988:515, 519, 522.

CHAPTER 2H: BRAIN STEM

Figs. 2H-1, 2H-2, and 2H-4 modified from DeMyer W. *Neuroanatomy*. New York: Harwal Publishing, 1988:132, 134, 170.
Figs. 2H-3A and 2H-3B modified from Romero-Sierra C. *Neuroanatomy: a conceptual approach*. New York: Churchill Livingstone, 1986:100, 103.
Figs. 2H-3C and 2H-6H modified from Williams PL. *Gray's anatomy*. New York: Churchill Livingstone, 1995:1017, 1193.
Fig. 2H-5 modified from Berkovitz BKB, Moxham BJ, eds. *A textbook of head and neck anatomy*. London: Year Book Medical Publishers, 1988:490.
Figs. 2H-6A–G modified from Martin JH. *Neuroanatomy: text and atlas*. New York: Elsevier, 1989:145, 179, 196, 198, 202.

CHAPTER 2I: PERIPHERAL SEGMENTS OF THE CRANIAL NERVES

Figs. 2I-1 and 2I-2 modified from Parent A. Olfactory system. *Carpenter's human neuroanatomy*. Baltimore: Williams & Wilkins, 1996:749.
Fig. 2I-3 modified from Pansky B, Allen DJ, Budd GC. Visual (retinogeniculostriate) pathways. *Review of neuroscience*. New York: McGraw-Hill, 1988:321.
Figs. 2I-4, 2I-5, 2I-6A, 2I-6C, 2I-7, 2I-8, 2I-9, 2I-10, and 2I-12 modified from Grant JCB. *Grant's atlas of anatomy*. Baltimore: Williams & Wilkins, 1962:653–657, 659, 662.
Fig. 2I-11 modified from Romero-Sierra C. Brain stem. In: Agur AMR (ed.) *Neuroanatomy: a conceptual approach*. New York: Churchill Livingstone, 1986:93.
Fig. 2I-19 modified from Williams PL. Nervous system. In: *Gray's anatomy*. New York: Churchill Livingstone, 1995:1235.

CHAPTER 2J: COMMISSURES AND ASSOCIATION AND PROJECTION SYSTEMS OF THE CEREBRUM

Figs. 2J-1, 2J-8, and 2J-9 modified from DeMyer W. *Neuroanatomy*. Media, PA: Harwal Publishing, 1988:295, 298, 299.
Fig. 2J-2 modified from Romero-Sierra C. Projection fibers. *Neuroanatomy: a conceptual approach*. New York: Churchill Livingstone, 1986:149.
Fig. 2J-3 modified from Parent A. Forebrain. *Carpenter's human neuroanatomy*. Baltimore: Williams & Wilkins, 1996:684.
Fig. 2J-4 modified from Williams PL. Internal capsule. In: *Gray's anatomy*. New York: Churchill Livingstone, 1995:1093.
Fig. 2J-6 modified from Carpenter MB. Circumvetricular organs. *Core text of neuroanatomy*. Baltimore: Williams & Wilkins, 1985:18.
Fig. 2J-7 modified from Pandya DN, Seltzer B. The topography of commissural fibers. In: Lepore F, Ptito M, Jasper HH, eds. *Two hemispheres—one brain: functions of the corpus callosum*. New York: Alan R. Liss, 1986:47–73.

CHAPTER 2K: CEREBRAL VENTRICULAR SYSTEM, CHOROID PLEXI, AND ARACHNOID GRANULATIONS

Fig. 2K-1 modified from Romero-Sierra C. *Neuroanatomy: a conceptual approach*. New York: Churchill Livingstone, 1986:17.
Fig. 2K-9 modified from Carpenter MB. *Core text of neuroanatomy*. Baltimore: Williams & Wilkins, 1985:18–19.
Fig. 2K-7 modified from Williams PL. Arachnoid granulations and villi. *Gray's anatomy*. New York: Churchill Livingstone, 1995:1214–1215.
Figs. 2K-15 and 2K-16 modified from Nieuwenhuys R, Voogd J, Van Huijzen C. *The human central nervous system: a synopsis and atlas*. Berlin: Springer-Verlag, 1988:55.

CHAPTER 2L: MENINGES AND SUBARACHNOID PATHWAYS

Figs. 2L-1 and 2L-5 modified from Nieuwenhuys R, Voogd J, Van Huijzen C. Vessels and meninges. *The human central nervous system*. Berlin: Springer-Verlag, 1978:54, 56.
Fig. 2L-6 modified from Warwick R, Williams PL. *Gray's anatomy*. Philadelphia: WB Saunders, 1973:991.
Fig. 2L-21 modified from Williams PL. *Gray's anatomy*. New York: Churchill Livingstone, 1995:1216;and Weller RO. Anatomy and pathology of the subpial space. *Riv Neuroradiol* 1994;7:15–21.

CHAPTER 2N: SUBCLAVIAN ARTERIES

Fig. 2N-1 modified from Morris P. Aortic arch. *Practical neuroangiography*. Baltimore: Williams & Wilkins, 1997:99–101.

CHAPTER 2P: EXTERNAL CAROTID ARTERY

Fig. 2P-1 modified from Takahashi M. Angiographic anatomy of arterial system. In: *Atlas of carotid angiography*. Tokyo: Igaku-Shoin, 1977:17–57.

CHAPTER 2Q: INTERNAL CAROTID ARTERY

Figs. 2Q-5, 2Q-9, 2Q-13, 2Q-14, 2Q-21, and 2Q-34 modified from Taveras MJ, Morello F. *Normal neuroradiology and atlas of the skull, sinuses and facial bones*. Chicago: Year Book Medical Publishers, 1979:407, 412, 416, 418, 425.
Fig. 2Q-7 modified from Osborn AG. *Introduction to cerebral angiography*. Hagerstown, MD: Harper & Row, 1980:251.
Fig. 2Q-8 modified from Osborn AG. In: *Diagnostic neuroradiology*. St. Louis: Mosby, 1994:137.
Figs. 2Q-22 and 2Q-28 modified from Krayenbuhl HA, Yasargil MG. *Cerebral angiography*. London: Butterworth Scientific Publication, 1968:40.
Fig. 2Q-23 modified from Kombos T, Meisel HJ, Janz C, Brock M. Paraplegia due to rupture of an anterior communicating artery aneurysm: consequence of a rare anatomic variant of the A2 segment. *Interventional Neuroradiol* 1996;2:53–57.

CHAPTER 2R: VERTEBROBASILAR ARTERIAL SYSTEM

Figs. 2R-1A and 2R-1B modified from Morris P. The extradural vertebral arteries. *Practical neuroangiography*. Baltimore: Williams & Wilkins, 1997:209.
Fig. 2R-3A modified from Wood JH. *Cerebral blood flow*. New York: McGraw-Hill, 1987:30.
Fig. 2R-3B modified from Osborn AG. *An introduction to cerebral angiography*. Baltimore: Harper and Row, 1980:382.
Fig. 2R-5 modified from Kretschmann HJ, Weinrich W. *Cranial neuroimaging and clinical neuroanatomy*. Stuttgart: Thieme Medical Publishers, 1992:195; and Morris P. The posterior cerebral artery. In: *Practical neuroangiography*. Baltimore: Williams & Wilkins, 1997:193–202.
Fig. 2R-7 modified from Ross P, du Boulay GH. *An atlas of normal vertebral angiograms*. Boston: Butterworth, 1976:25.

CHAPTER 2S: ARTERIAL VASCULAR TERRITORIES OF THE CEREBRUM, BRAIN STEM, AND CEREBELLUM

Fig. 2S-1 modified from Berman SA, Hayman LA, Hinck VC. Cerebrovascular territories. In: Hayman LA, Hinck VC, eds. *Clinical brain imaging: normal structure and functional anatomy*. St. Louis: Mosby, 1992:402–416, and Meder JF, Chiras J, Roland J, Guinet P, Bracard S, Bargy F. Venous territories of the brain. *J Neuroradiol* 1994:21:118–133.
Fig. 2S-2 modified from Savoiardo M, Bracchi M, Passerini A, Visciani A. The vascular territories in the cerebellum and brainstem: CT and MR study. *AJNR* 1987;8:199–209.
Fig. 2S-3 modified from Carpenter MB. Arterial supply of the medulla and pons. *Core text of neuroanatomy*. Baltimore: Williams & Wilkins, 1985:408.

CHAPTER 2T: ANASTOMOTIC PATTERNS

Fig. 2T-1 modified from Burt AM. The cerebral arterial circle of Willis. *Textbook of neuroanatomy*. Philadelphia: WB Saunders, 1993:179.
Fig. 2T-3 modified from Taveras JM, Wood EH. *Diagnostic neuroradiology*. Baltimore: Williams & Wilkins, 1976:972.

Fig. 2T-6 modified from Lasjaunias P. The occipital artery. *Neuroradiology* 1978;15:31–37.
Fig. 2T-8 courtesy of Corr P, Hoffman M. Positional transient ischemic attacks due to a persistent primitive hypoglossal artery. *Intern Med Imag Regist* 1995;2:85–86.
Fig. 2T-10 modified from Kirkwood JR. *Essentials of neuroimaging*. New York: Churchill-Livingstone, 1990:14.

CHAPTER 2U: VENOUS DRAINAGE OF THE CRANIUM

Figs. 2U-1 and 2U-2 modified from Morris P. *Practical neuroangiography*. Baltimore: Williams & Wilkins, 1997:237.
Fig. 2U-3 modified from Melloni L, Dox I, Melloni HP, Melloni BJ. *Review of human anatomy*. Philadelphia: JB Lippincott, 1988:221.
Fig. 2U-6 modified from Osborn AG. *Introduction to cerebral angiography*. Hagerstown, MD: Harper & Row, 1980:394.
Fig. 2U-7 modified from Ross P, du Boulay GH. *An atlas of normal vertebral angiograms*. Boston: Butterworth, 1976:27.
Fig. 2U-9 modified from Meder JF, Chiras J, Roland J, Guinet P, Bracard S, Bargy F. Venous territories of the brain. *J Neuroradiol* 1994;21:118–133.
Fig. 2U-10 modified from Gray H. In: Goss CM, ed. *Anatomy of the human body*. Philadelphia: Lea & Febiger, 1966.
Fig. 2U-11 modified from Kretschmann HJ, Weinrich W. In: *Cranial neuroimaging and clinical neuroanatomy*. Stuttgart: Thieme Medical Publishers, 1992:215.
Figs. 2U-30 and 2U-31 modified from Kadir S. *Atlas of normal and variant angiographic anatomy*. Philadelphia: WB Saunders, 1991:486.
Fig. 2U-34 modified from Taveras JM, Morello F. *Normal neuroradiology and atlas of the skull, sinuses and facial bones*. Chicago: Year Book Medical Publishers, 1979:435.

CHAPTER 2W: CENTRAL NERVOUS SYSTEM BARRIERS AND INTERFACES

Fig. 2W-1 modified from Nieuwenhuys R, Voogd J, van Huijzen C. Vessels and meninges. In: *The human central nervous system*. Berlin: Springer-Verlag, 1978:54.
Fig. 2W-2 modified from Burt AM. *Textbook of neuroanatomy*. Philadelphia: WB Saunders, 1993:46.
Fig. 2W-6 modified from Parent A. Blood–brain barrier, the blood–CSF barrier, and the brain–CSF interface that separate the brain and CSF from the cerebral vascular compartment. In: *Carpenter's human neuroanatomy*. Baltimore: Williams & Wilkins, 1996:20–21.

CHAPTER 3: THE SELLA TURCICA, PITUITARY GLAND, AND CAVERNOUS VENOUS SINUSES

Fig. 3-1 modified from Woodruff WW. Sella. *Fundamentals of neuroimaging*. Philadelphia: WB Saunders, 1993:5.
Fig. 3-2 modified from Agur AMR. Interior base of the skull. In: Agur AMR, ed. *Grant's atlas of anatomy*. Baltimore: Williams & Wilkins, 1991:476–477.
Fig. 3-6 modified from Elster AD. Modern imaging of the pituitary. *Radiology* 1993;187:1–14.
Fig. 3-12 modified from Ahmadi H, Larsson EM, Jinkins JR. Normal pituitary gland: coronal MR imaging of infundibular tilt. *Radiology* 1990;177:389–392.
Fig. 3-13 modified from Williams PL. Vessels of the hypophysis. *Gray's anatomy*. New York: Churchill Livingstone, 1995:1887–1888.
Fig. 3-14 modified from Osborn AG. Cranial nerves minus VIII: anatomy, pathology, and imaging considerations. In: *Core curriculum course in neuroradiology*. ASNR Annual Meeting, Nashville, May 1–2, 1994.

CHAPTER 4: THE ORBIT

Fig. 4-1A modified from Woodruf WW. *Fundamentals of neuroimaging*. Philadelphia: WB Saunders, 1993:290.
Fig. 4-8 modified from Mafee MF. The eye. In: Som PM, Bergeron RT, eds. *Head and neck imaging*. St. Louis: Mosby–Year Book, 1991:695–702.
Fig. 4-9 modified from Williams PL. Peripheral visual apparatus. *Gray's anatomy*. New York: Churchill Livingstone, 1995:1322–1367.
Fig. 4-12 modified from Brown MW. Visual areas. In: Berkovitz BKB, Moxham BJ, eds. *A textbook of head and neck anatomy*. London: Year Book Medical Publishers, 1988:551.
Fig. 4-13 modified from Hall-Craggs ECB. *Anatomy as a basis for clinical medicine*. Munich: Urban Schwarzenberg, 1985:523.
Fig. 4-14 modified from Harnsberger HR. *Handbook of head and neck imaging*. St. Louis: Mosby–Year Book, 1995:318–319.
Fig. 4-15 modified from Berkovitz BKB, Moxham BJ, eds. *A textbook of head and neck anatomy*. London: Year Book Medical Publishers, 1988:208.

Fig. 4-16 modified from Brown MW. Visual areas. In: Berkovitz BKB, Moxham BJ, eds. *A textbook of head and neck anatomy*. London: Year Book Medical Publishers, 1988:218.

Fig. 18A modified from Russell EJ, Czervionke L, Huckman M, Daniels D, McLachlan D. CT of the inferomedial orbit and the lacrimal drainage apparatus: normal and pathologic anatomy. *AJNR* 1985;6:759–766.

Fig. 4-19 modified from Taveras JM, Wood EH. *Diagnostic neuroradiology*. Baltimore: Williams & Wilkins, 1976:581–584.

Fig. 4-20 modified from Doyon DL, Aron-Rosa D, Ramée A. Orbital veins and cavernous sinus. In: Newton TH, Potts DG, eds. *Radiology of the skull and brain*. Great Neck, N.Y.: Medibooks, 1974:2221; and Melloni L, Dox I, Melloni HP, Melloni BJ. *Illustrated review of human anatomy*. Philadelphia: JB Lippincott, 1988:215.

Fig. 4-29 modified from Hayreh SS. The ophthalmic artery. In: Newton TH, Potts DG, eds. *Radiology of the skull and brain*. Great Neck, NY: MediBooks, 1974:1333–1350.

CHAPTER 5: FACIAL STRUCTURES

Fig. 5-3 modified from Hall-Craggs ECB. *Anatomy as a basis for clinical medicine*. Munich: Urban Schwarzenberg, 1985:483.

Fig. 5-6 modified from Agur AMR. The head. In: Agur AMR, ed. *Grant's atlas of anatomy*, 9th ed. Baltimore: Williams & Wilkins, 1991:454.

Fig. 5-7 modified from Taveras JM, Morello F. *Normal neuroradiology and atlas of the skull, sinuses and facial bones*. Chicago: Year Book Medical Publishers, 1979:43.

Figs. 5-9, 5-10, 5-18, and 5-25 modified from Williams PL. Mandible. *Gray's anatomy*. New York: Churchill-Livingstone, 1995:576–578, 576–578, 562–563, 1700–1704.

Fig. 5-13 modified from Nance EP, Powers TA. Imaging of temporomandibular joint. *Radiol Clin North Am* 1990;28:1019–1031.

Fig. 5-14 modified from Blaschke DD, Solberg WK, Sanders B. Arthrography of the temporomandibular joint: review of current status. *J Am Dent Assoc* 1980;100:388–395.

Fig. 5-15 modified from Brown MW. The innervation and vasculature of the temporomandibular joint. In: Berkovitz BKB, Moxham BJ, eds. *Textbook of head and neck anatomy*. London: Year Book Medical Publishers, 1988:173.

Figs. 5-16A and 5-16B courtesy of RF Ribeiro, MD, Goias, Brazil, RH Tallents, MD, Rochester, NY, and RW Katzberg, MD, Sacramento, CA.

CHAPTER 6: PARANASAL SINUSES AND NASAL PASSAGEWAYS

Fig. 6-1 modified from Hall-Crags ECB. *Anatomy as a basis for clinical medicine*. Munich: Urban Schwarzenberg, 1985:521.

Fig. 6-10 modified from Som PM, Brandwein M. The sinonasal cavities: anatomy, physiology, and plain film normal anatomy. In: Som PM, Bergeron RT, eds. *Head and neck imaging*. St Louis: Mosby, 1996:57.

CHAPTER 7A: SPINAL COLUMN

Fig. 7A-1 modified from Hollinshead WH, Rosse C. In: *Textbook of anatomy*. Hagerstown: Harper & Row, 1985:288.

Fig. 7A-2 modified from Gerlock A. *The cervical spine in trauma*. Philadelphia: WB Saunders, 1978:288.

Figs. 7A-11, 7A-15, and 7A-19 modified from Woodruff WW. *Fundamentals of neuroimaging*. Philadelphia: WB Saunders, 1993:430, 431, 433.

Figs. 7A-22, 7A-23, 7A-34, and 7A-35 modified from Grant JCB. In: Agur AMR, ed. *Grant's atlas of anatomy*. Baltimore: Williams & Wilkins, 1962:272, 366, 373, 374.

Fig. 7A-24 modified from Goss CM. In: *Gray's anatomy of the human body*. Philadelphia: Lea & Febiger, 1975:113–118.

Fig. 7A-26 modified from Prassopoulos PK, Faflia CP, Voloudaki AE, Gourtsoyiannis NC. Sacroiliac joints: anatomical variants on CT. *J Comput Assist Tomogr* 1999;23:323–327.

Fig. 7A-32 modified from Rogg JM, Kemp SS. CT anatomy of the spine. In: Latchwaw RE, ed. *MR and CT imaging of the head, neck, and spine*. St. Louis: Mosby—Year Book, 1991:1071–1088.

Figs. 7A-37 and 7A-38 modified from Brasch JC. In: *Cunningham's manual of practical anatomy*. London: Oxford University Press, 1958:258–295.

Fig. 7A-39A modified from Taveras JM, Morello F. *Normal neuroradiology*. Chicago: Year Book Medical Publishers, 1979:53.

Figs. 7A-39B and 7A-39E modified from Tao KCVG. Anatomy. In: Rao KCVC, Williams JP, Lee BCP, Sherman LD, eds. *MRI and CT of the spine*. Baltimore: Williams & Wilkins, 1994:45–56.

Fig. 7A-43 modified from Singer KP, Breidahl PD. Accessory ossification centers at the thoracolumbar junction. *Surg Radiol Anat* 1990;12:53–58.

Fig. 7A-44 modified from Williams PL. Skeletal system. In: *Gray's anatomy*. New York: Churchill Livingstone, 1995:533.

CHAPTER 7B: SPINAL CORD

Figs. 7B-2A, 7B-8A, and 7B-9 modified from Romero-Sierra C. Spinal cord and its coverings. *Neuroanatomy: a conceptual approach*. New York: Churchill Livingstone, 1986:86, 87.

Figs. 7B-3 and 7B-4 modified from Burt AM. Spinal cord. *Textbook of neuroanatomy*. Philadelphia: WB Saunders, 1995:125, 128.

Figs. 7B-5, 7B-6A, and 7B-7 modified from DeMyer W. *Neuroanatomy*. Media, PA: Harwal Publishing, 1988:114, 116, 117.

Fig 7B-6B and 7B-8B modified from Parent A. *Carpenter's human anatomy*. Baltimore: Williams & Wilkins, 1996:375, 385.

CHAPTER 7C: SPINAL VASCULATURE

Figs. 7C-1, 7C-2, 7C-10, 7C-13, 7C-15, and 7C-16 modified from Taveras JM, Morello F. *Normal neuroradiology and atlas of the skull, sinuses and facial bones*. Chicago: Year Book Medical Publishers, 1979:608–611.

Fig. 7C-3 modified from Romero-Sierra C. *Neuroanatomy: a conceptual approach*. New York: Churchill Livingstone, 1986:370.

Fig. 7C-11 modified from DeMyer W. *Neuroanatomy*. Media, PA: Harwal Publishing, 1988:338.

Fig. 7C-14 modified from Williams PL. Veins of the vertebral column. *Gray's anatomy*. New York: Churchill Livingstone, 1995:1594–1595.

Fig. 7C-25 modified from Jinkins JR. Magnetic resonance imaging of benign nerve root enhancement in the unoperated and postoperative lumbosacral spine. *Neuroimaging Clin North Am* 1993;3:537.

Fig. 7C-26 modified from Lane JI, Koeller KK, Atkinson JLD. Enhanced lumbar nerve roots in the spine without prior surgery: radiculitis or radicular veins? *AJNR* 1994;15:1317–1325.

Fig. 7C-27 modified from Garfin SR, Rydevik B, Lind B, Massie J. Spinal nerve compression. *Spine* 1995;20:1801–1820.

CHAPTER 7D: ANATOMY OF THE SPINAL NERVE ROOTS, SPINAL NERVES, AND SPINAL NERVE PLEXI

Fig. 7D-1 modified from Haymaker W, Woodhall B. Peripheral nerve injuries. In: *Principles of diagnosis*. Philadelphia: WB Saunders, 1953:32.

Figs. 7D-10, 7D-11, 7D-13, and 7D-14A modified from Williams PL. *Gray's anatomy*. New York: Churchill Livingstone, 1995:1264, 1267, 1283.

Figs. 7D-12, 7D-18, and 7D-25 modified from Parent A. *Carpenter's human neuroanatomy*. Baltimore: Williams & Wilkins, 1996:284, 295, 398.

Fig. 7D-14B modified from Netter FH. *Nervous system*. New York: CIBA Collection of Medical Illustrations, 1968:55.

Figs. 7D-15, 7D-16, 7D-17 modified from DeMyer W. The development and innervation of somites. *Neuroanatomy*. Media, PA: Harwal Publishing, 1988:46–48, 62–64, 69.

Fig. 7D-19 modified from Romero-Sierra C. *Neuroanatomy: a conceptual approach*. New York: Churchill Livingstone, 1986:169–183.

Fig. 7D-20 modified from Jinkins JR, Whittemore AR, Bradley WG. The anatomic basis of vertebrogenic pain and the autonomic syndrome associated with lumbar disk extrusion. *AJNR* 1989;10:219–231.

Fig. 7D-21 modified from Jinkins JR. The pathoanatomic basis of somatic and autonomic syndromes originating in the lumbosacral spine. *Neuroimaging Clin North Am* 1993;3:444, 446, 452.

Fig. 7D-22 modified from Jinkins JR. The pathoanatomic basis of somatic, autonomic and neurogenic syndromes originating in the lumbosacral spine. *Riv Neuroadiol* 1995;8[Suppl 1]:35–51.

Figs. 7D-23 and 7D-24 modified from Burt AM. In: *Textbook of neuroanatomy*. Philadelphia: WB Saunders, 1993:370, 371.

CHAPTER 7E: SPINAL MENINGES

Fig. 7E-1 modified from Taveras JM, Morello F. *Normal neuroradiology*. Chicago: Year Book Medical Publishers, 1979:572.

CHAPTER 7F: PARASPINAL MUSCLES

Fig. 7F-1 modified from Smoker WRK, Harnsberger HR. Differential diagnosis of head and neck lesions based on their space of origin. II. The infrahyoid portion of the neck. *AJR* 1991;157:155–159.

Figs. 7F-3 and 7F-5 modified from Agur AMR, Lee MJ. *Grant's atlas of anatomy*. Baltimore: Williams & Wilkins, 1991:239.

CHAPTER 7G: VARIANTS OF THE SPINAL COLUMN

Fig. 7G-30 modified from Singer KP, Breidhahl PD. Accessory ossification centres at the thoracolumbar junction. *Surg Radiol Anat* 1990;12:53–58.

CHAPTER 8: THE NECK

Figs. 8-1 and 8-2 modified from Som PM, Curtin HD. In: *Head and neck imaging*. St. Louis: Mosby, 1996:503.
Fig. 8-3 modified from Jinkins JR. Computed tomography of the cranio-cervical lymphatic system: anatomical and functional considerations. *Neuroradiology* 1987;29:317–326.
Figs. 8-5, 8-11, 8-12, 8-15, 8-18, 8-21A, 8-22, 8-25, 8-26, 8-35, and 8-39 modified from Williams PL. In: *Gray's anatomy*. New York: Churchill Livingstone, 1995:582, 1271, 1639, 1640, 1643, 1690, 1721, 1726, 1896.
Figs. 8-7A and 8-8A modified from Harnsberger HR. Introduction to the suprahyoid neck. *Handbook of head and neck imaging*. St. Louis: Mosby, 1995, :10, 123.
Fig. 8-9 modified from Hardin CW, Harnsberger HR, Osborn AG, et al. CT in the evaluation of the normal and diseased oral cavity and oropharynx. *Semin Ultrasound CT MR* 1986;7:131–153.
Figs. 8-13A, 8-13B, 8-26, 8-27, 8-28, 8-33, and 8-34 modified from Berkovitz BKB, Moxham BJ, eds. *A textbook of head and neck anatomy*. London: Year Book Medical Publishers, 1988: 282, 291–294, 333, 335, 336.
Fig. 8-16A modified from Sumi M, Izumi M, Yonetsu K, Nakamura T. Sublingual gland: MR features of normal and diseased states. *AJR* 1999;172:717–722.
Fig. 8-24A modified from Smoker WRK, Harnsberger HR. Differential diagnosis of head and neck lesions based on their space of origin: the infrahyoid portion of the neck. *AJR* 1991;157:155–159.
Fig. 8-36 modified from Zodvinshis DP, Benson MT, Som PM, Smoker WRK. Embryology and congenital cystic lesions. In: Som PM, Curtin HD. *Head and neck imaging*. St. Louis: Mosby, 1996:760.

Subject Index

Note: Page numbers in *italics* indicate figures; page numbers followed by t indicate tables.

N

T

W

Y

Z